Health Promotion Strategies Through the Life Span

Eighth Edition

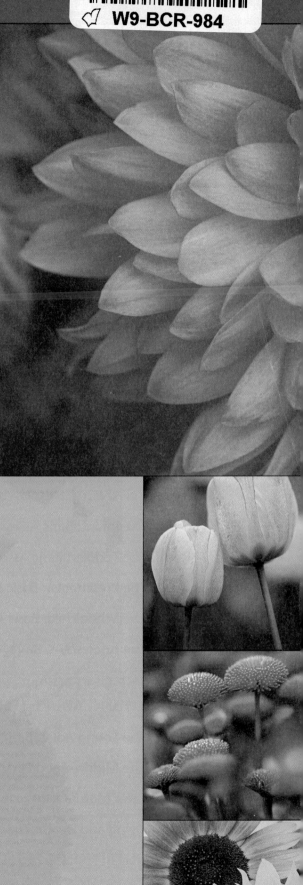

Health Promotion Strategies Through the Life Span (8th Edition)

Health Promotion Strategies Through the Life Span

Eighth Edition

➤ **RUTH BECKMANN MURRAY, EDD, MSN, N-NAP, FAAN**

Psychiatric/Mental Health Nursing Educator and Clinical Nurse Specialist
Professor Emerita
School of Nursing
Saint Louis University
St. Louis, Missouri

➤ **JUDITH PROCTOR ZENTNER, MA, BS, FNP-BC**

Hickory Hill Furniture Corporation Health Clinic
Director of Health Care, Retired
Valdese, North Carolina

➤ **RICHARD YAKIMO, PHD, PMHCNS-BC, N-NAP**

Assistant Professor
School of Nursing
Southern Illinois University Edwardsville
Edwardsville, Illinois

PEARSON
Prentice Hall

Upper Saddle River, NJ 07458

Library of Congress Cataloging-in-Publication Data

Murray, Ruth Beckmann.
  Health promotion strategies through the life span / Ruth Beckmann Murray, Judith Proctor
Zentner, Richard Yakimo.—8th ed.
      p. ; cm
  Includes bibliographical references and index.
  ISBN-13: 978-0-13-513866-3
  ISBN-10: 0-13-513866-3

  1. Nursing assessment. 2. Health promotion. 3. Life cycle, Human. 4. Developmental
psychology. I. Zentner, Judith Proctor. II. Yakimo, Richard. III. Title.
  [DNLM: 1. Nursing Assessment—Nurses' Instruction. 2. Health Promotion—Nurses'
Instruction. 3. Human Development—Nurses' Instruction. WY 100.4 M983h 2009]
  RT48.M8 2009
  613—dc22

                                                        2008020982

Publisher: Julie Levin Alexander
Assistant to Publisher: Regina Bruno
Editor-in-Chief: Maura Connor
Assistant to the Editor-in-Chief: Marion Gottlieb
Executive Acquisitions Editor: Pamela Lappies
Assistant to the Executive Acquisitions Editor: Sarah Wrocklage
Development Editor: Barbara Price
Media Product Manager: John J. Jordan
Director of Marketing: Karen Allman
Senior Marketing Manager: Francisco del Castillo
Marketing Specialist: Michael Sirinides
Managing Editor, Production: Patrick Walsh

Production Editor: Emily Bush, S4Carlisle Publishing Services
Production Liaison: Anne Garcia
Media Project Manager: Stephen Hartner
Manufacturing Manager: Ilene Sanford
Senior Design Coordinator: Christopher Weigand
Interior Design: Wanda España
Cover Design: Wanda España
Cover Illustration: Courtesy Corbis and Getty Images
Composition: S4Carlisle Publishing Services
Printer/Binder: Quebecor World Color/Versailles
Cover Printer: Phoenix Color Corp./Hagerstown

Notice:
Care has been taken to confirm the accuracy of information presented in this book. The authors, editors, and the publisher, however, cannot accept any responsibility for errors or omissions or for consequences from application of the information in this book and make no warranty, express or implied, with respect to its contents.

    The authors and publisher have exerted every effort to ensure that drug selections and dosages set forth in this text are in accord with current recommendations and practice at time of publication. However, in view of ongoing research, changes in government regulations, and the constant flow of information relating to drug therapy and reactions, the reader is urged to check the package inserts of all drugs for any change in indications or dosage and for added warnings and precautions. This is particularly important when the recommended agent is a new and/or infrequently employed drug.

Pearson Prentice Hall is a trademark of Pearson Education, Inc.
Pearson is a registered trademark of Pearson plc
Prentice Hall is a registered trademark of Pearson Education, Inc.

Pearson Education Ltd., London
Pearson Education Singapore, Pte. Ltd
Pearson Education Canada, Inc., Toronto
Pearson Education—Japan
Pearson Education Australia PTY, Limited

Pearson Education North Asia, Ltd., Hong Kong
Pearson Educación de Mexico, S.A. de C.V.
Pearson Education Malaysia, Pte. Ltd.
Pearson Education Upper Saddle River, New Jersey

10 9 8 7 6 5 4 3 2 1
ISBN-13: 978-0-13-513866-3
ISBN: 0-13-513866-3

Dedication

"This book is dedicated to

Our students—for their inspiration

Our friends—for their assistance

Our families—for their patience

Our clients/patients—for their trust in us"

Ruth Beckmann Murray, EdD, MSN, N-NAP, FAAN

Dr. Murray received her basic nursing education from Deaconess Hospital School of Nursing, St. Louis, Missouri, and graduated with a baccalaureate degree from Lindenwood College in St. Charles, Missouri. She graduated from Washington University School of Nursing in St. Louis with a major in psychiatric/mental health nursing, and in 1983 earned a doctorate degree in education from Southern Illinois University Edwardsville. During her professional career she was a school nurse at Lindenwood College, staff nurse on medical-surgical and psychiatric hospital units, and supervisor of obstetrics-gynecology. For 42 of her 48 years as an active professional, nursing education was her primary role. She retired as professor emerita from Saint Louis University School of Nursing in St. Louis, Missouri.

As an educator, she was active in the community in the role of mental health counselor and educator and as consultant to agency staff and schools of nursing locally and nationally. She conducted evaluation research and was a member of agency committees and boards of directors. In addition to being senior author of the first text on health promotion and development through the life span, she was senior author of several other books, authored many articles, and contributed chapters to a number of books. She received numerous awards for her contributions as educator, consultant, author, and for community service. She is a fellow in the American Academy of Nursing, member of Sigma Theta Tau International, Delta Lambda Chapter, the American and Missouri Nurses Association, other nursing organizations, and Distinguished Practitioner in the National Academies of Practice-Nursing.

As professor emerita, she has not really retired, but is "retreading." She is active on committees, as a board member of several community agencies, and with her church. She continues to do telephone crisis counseling, a professional activity for more than three decades. Free time is spent with people, her garden, botanical photography, and continuing to learn.

Judith Proctor Zentner, MA, BS, FNP-BC

Judith Zentner received her basic nursing education from Deaconess Hospital School of Nursing, St. Louis, Missouri. She received a bachelor of science degree with majors in English and history from Anderson University, Anderson, Indiana. She received a master of arts degree with a concentration in English/education from Ball State University, Muncie, Indiana. Her nurse practitioner education was obtained from the University of North Carolina branch program in Asheville.

The last 25 years have been devoted to starting and directing a health program in industry with a primary care focus for employees and their families. Also, the last 25 years have been devoted to funding clinics and shelter for the homeless in Kenya, East Africa.

During the 44 years as a nurse and the 28 years as a nurse practitioner, Judith has used her background skills in English to teach both English and nursing in a college setting. She has held various positions in the emergency room, medical-surgical units, visiting nurse association, private duty cases, hospital occupational health, and in an HMO.

In addition to being the co-author of the first text on health promotion and development through the life span, Judith has written six articles and has spoken to various college nursing students and professional organizations. She is a member of several professional organizations and was honored with being selected for Who's Who in American Nursing.

Going forward, Judith plans to continue with the Africa projects, substitute for nurse practitioners when needed, as well as have more time to spend with the children and grandchildren who live in other states.

Richard Yakimo, PhD, PMHCNS-BC, N-NAP

Dr. Yakimo received his bachelor's, master's, and doctoral nursing degrees from Saint Louis University in St. Louis, Missouri. He also completed a postdoctoral fellowship in psychiatric epidemiology at Washington University in St. Louis. He is certified as a clinical specialist in adult psychiatric-mental health nursing and is especially interested in the mental health of older adults, trauma clients, and the psychosocial care of the physically ill.

Dr. Yakimo is currently an assistant professor at Southern Illinois University Edwardsville School of Nursing, where he teaches psychiatric nursing and epidemiology and also serves as a consultant in evidence-based practice and research to a local hospital. His research interests focus on the quality of care and the analysis of outcomes within nursing practice. Dr. Yakimo is a member of the American Nurses Association, the International Society of Psychiatric-Mental Health Nurses, and Sigma Theta Tau, International, Honor Society of Nursing. He was recently elected as a Distinguished Practitioner in the National Academies of Practice.

Preface

To provide holistic health promotion and preventive care, we believe the nurse and other health care providers must consider all dimensions of development and the total health of the person and family. The physical, mental, emotional, sociocultural, and spiritual needs and characteristics are interrelated. Your emphasis must be on comprehensive assessment of the whole person and on health promotion and appropriate interventions and strategies, rather than on patchwork remedies or fragmented understanding. This has been an emphasis in each of our previous editions. We are gratified to see the emphasis of nursing and health care dramatically following our projection. Now in the eighth edition, we have retained and updated the most important of these concepts.

Organization

This text introduces you to the highly complex, normal person and the family during the entire life span—from birth to death. For this edition, all chapters have been reorganized to present the most essential information. A new chapter has been added, Chapter 2, Health Promotion: Concepts and Theories, which focuses on health promotion trends, models, and strategies.

Chapters 1, 2, and 3 present theories, models, and principles that apply to practice in any setting, across age groups. In Chapters 4, 5, 6, 7, and 8, you will explore the influences on the developing person—environmental, sociocultural, family, religion, and the prenatal stage. We realize the prenatal stage could be called the first developmental stage. However, Chapter 8, which includes content on prenatal development, is placed with other chapters that discuss influences on the person or family because prenatal development significantly influences all the life eras, even into the older years. Chapters 9 through 16 present each life stage from infancy through later maturity. Chapter 17 presents dying and death as the last developmental stage.

Each chapter on developmental eras is presented in a consistent format:

1. Family development, relationships, and developmental tasks.
2. Physiologic concepts, including physical characteristics, special considerations in physical assessment, nutrition, exercise, rest and sleep, play or leisure, and health promotion.
3. Psychosocial concepts, including cognitive, emotional, social, moral, and spiritual development, individual developmental tasks, and health promotion.
4. Health care and nursing applications, including common health problems and special concerns.

Abstracts for evidence-based practice and case situations further highlight significant findings for the individual and family throughout the life span. We believe that the integrated holistic approach of this text provides the most comprehensive review possible of each developmental stage and, in a sense, a critical pathway paradigm for health and health promotion.

We do not cover diseases, their treatment, or specific assessment techniques in detail. These are covered in many clinical texts that can be used in conjunction with this text. Before you can understand the ill person and the family, you must understand the well person in the usual family, cultural, and community settings. Only then can your assessment be thorough and your interventions individualized and culturally competent. Only then will you be prepared to give the community-focused care that is now emphasized.

Nurses have always had to cope with death. The focused study of the phases of dying, how to assist the person and family in making decisions related to death, and specific care measures will enhance your ability to foster a naturalness about this last event in life.

Using This Text

As you use this book, keep in mind that although each person is unique, the uniqueness occurs in the predictable patterns discussed in this text. Your knowledge of normal mental and physical health and influences on development and health at each life stage can help you detect deviations from the norm and implement the intervention measures appropriate to the person's or family's development. In this text, intervention focuses on measures that foster and maintain health within the family unit and cultural context and major points of care for common health problems.

Before reading any chapters you should orient yourself by, (1) reading the table of contents, (2) looking at the list of objectives that precede each chapter, (3) noting key terms listed at the beginning of the chapter, (4) glancing at chapter headings and subheadings, and (5) noting the key terms in bold type and their italicized definitions that appear throughout each chapter. Orient yourself to the Companion Website in order to integrate the additional information with the content in the text. Critical thinking questions have been added to stimulate integration, discussion, and application of the content.

This text has been used successfully at the beginning of course work and for all levels and disciplines of health care students in the clinical practicum. Graduate-level students in programs for advanced practices such as clinical nurse specialists and nurse practitioners, and students enrolled in a doctorate for nursing practice program will benefit from the review of the holistic perspective, regardless of specialty focus. Wherever you encounter this text, we invite you to be an active participant as you read. Our ideas are presented with conviction and directness. We want you to integrate and adapt our ideas into your specific circumstances. Each of you will have to apply this information to your setting—be it hospital, clinic, home, community agencies, or populations in the community—to promote health and prevent illness among people of diverse backgrounds.

Special Features

This book presents many boxes, tables, charts, and other features designed to facilitate learning. Becoming familiar with them will allow you to obtain the maximum benefit from your textbook.

Interventions for Health Promotion. Strategies for promoting health are woven into the narrative of this book, but primary interventions are called out in this new feature to make them more visible.

Healthy People 2010. Goals for the health of individuals and families are included in boxes highlighting the U.S. Department of Health and Human Services Initiative to set objectives for health.

Practice Point. These statements support the well-being and ethical and cultural competency of the nurse or health care provider, with key concepts and tips for practice.

Client Education. These boxes provide tips and instructions to relay to clients about issues involving family life, health practices, and other aspects of healthy living.

Case Situations. These studies provide examples of real-life situations involving concepts and topics related to the chapter.

Abstract for Evidence-Based Practice. Incorporating research into practice is essential to good practice. This helpful feature provides a clear example of how to read and assess a study.

Nursing Diagnoses. NANDA nursing diagnoses related to specified topics appear in these boxes.

Chapter-Opening Features. Each chapter begins with **Objectives** to alert students to content they will be expected to know and a list of **Key Terms.**

End-of-Chapter Features. Every chapter concludes with a **Summary** of key concepts, **Chapter Review Questions,** and **References.**

Companion Website

www.prenhall.com/murray

The Companion Website is an extension of this book, and we believe that it is important for you to explore it before using your text so that you will understand how to access chapter-related material. The Me-diaLink icons along the outside edges of some pages indicate that material related to the topic being discussed can be found on the Companion Website. Each chapter provides the following categories.

- **Objectives**—These are the same as those found at the start of the chapter.
- **Key Terms**—The list of terms from the start of the chapter is presented here.
- **Tools**—Tables, charts, figures, boxes, and other useful material related to the chapter appear in this section.
- **Challenge Your Knowledge**—These essay-style questions require you to apply information from the chapter.
- **Learning Activities**—For these exercises, you are asked to consider how chapter-related material and personal experiences support the chapter objectives.
- **Additional References** or **Additional Information**—These categories appear when relevant to a chapter to provide more information.
- **Critical Thinking Questions**—These essay-style questions ask you to consider various aspects of health promotion in relation to your own experiences and to the information from the chapter.
- **MediaLink Applications**—These exercises require you to access a specific Website to gather information and apply it.
- **MediaLinks**—Online resources for further study of chapter content are provided in this section.

Instructor Resources

The Instructor Resource Center is an online store for classroom resources. It can be accessed through the Pearson Education online catalog at www.prenhall.com. On it, instructors will find valuable tools for class preparation, teaching, and assessment.

- **Online Instructor's Resource Manual**—The chapter-specific tools in this manual equip instructors with Concepts for Lecture, Classroom Activities, Clinical Activities, and lecture slides.
- **PowerPoint Lecture Slides**—Chapter-specific PowerPoint slides provide customizable teaching aids.
- **TestGen Testbank**—Questions in varied formats are available for assessment. Rationales for the answers are provided, along with cognitive level and other descriptors.

Acknowledgments

This eighth edition, as all prior editions, is the result of considerable effort, collaboration, and assistance on the part of many people. Ruth and Judith are especially pleased to have a new senior author join the team; Richard Yakimo brings a freshness and special talents to the project. We are grateful to the new contributors, as well as to the prior contributors, for continuing with this edition.

Several people deserve special recognition. This edition would not have been initiated without the patient guidance and continuing assistance of Pamela Lappies, executive acquisition editor. It could not have been completed without the skill, patient assistance, mentoring, and conscientious, cheerful, and kind approach of Barbara Price, development editor. Barbara, Patrick Walsh, and the staff in the production department at Prentice Hall gave considerable time and talent to shepherd this project to completion. However, all of this professional competence would have been for naught without the continuing skillful efforts, cheerful countenance, rapid work, and commitment of Patti Gray Baygents, administrative assistant to Ruth. Her talents exceeded that of typing the electronic copy of the manuscript.

Equally important to Ruth, Judith, and Richard has been the support and encouragement of family, friends, and colleagues. Ruth was inspired by the encouragement of Charles Edwin Murray to complete this project, even as he was in a trajectory through the final developmental stage that we discuss. Ruth has realized during content preparation how her parents, Viola and Ferdinand Beckmann, but especially her mother, lived the principles of nurturing, guidance, and generativity discussed in the text.

Judith reminded Ruth of how we have moved from young-young adults into late middle age, and that her children have moved from toddlerhood to young adulthood. We have experienced a great deal of the life span development as well as inclusion of comprehensive health promotion in nursing practice.

Richard, with an educational range from psychology, through a doctorate in nursing, and a post-doctoral research fellowship, brings a unique developmental and health promotion perspective and practice. He utilizes the holistic approach presented in this text as he educates and intervenes to promote health.

Richard gratefully acknowledges the incisive and sensitive mentoring of Ruth Murray, who has overseen his development from baccalaureate to advanced practice nurse, and to nurse researcher and educator. He also recognizes the support of his parents, Mike and Dunya Yakimo, who highly valued education and would have been proud to see the publication of this book.

Our efforts have focused on what students and practitioners need to know to give holistic care in a fragmented health care system. We extend wishes to future nurses and other health care providers for a rewarding and productive career.

Ruth Beckmann Murray
Judith Proctor Zentner
Richard Yakimo

Contributors

The authors wish to thank the people below for their excellent contributions to this edition.

Sylvia Pye Adams, MSN, PMHCNS-BC
Chief Nurse Executive
St. Louis Psychiatric Rehabilitation Center,
    Missouri Department of Mental Health
St. Louis, MO

Frances D. Atkins, PhD, PMHCNS-BC
Psychiatric/Mental Health Nurse
Private Practice and Healthy Living Institute
Higginsville, MO

Mildred Heyes Boland, MSN, RN
Nursing Educator and Coordinator of Wellness
    Program, Retired
Tempe, AZ

Kathy Borcherding, PhD, MSN, RN
Assistant Professor
College of Nursing
University of Missouri at St. Louis
St. Louis, MO

Gina Bufe, PhD, MSN(R), PMHCNS-BC
Director of Nursing for Education, Quality, and
    Research
NewYork-Presbyterian
University Hospital of Columbia and Cornell
New York, NY

Jill Zentner Burns, RD, BS
Registered Dietitian, Home Office
Greenville, SC

Father Peter J. Klink, S.J.
President
Red Cloud Indian School
Holy Rosary Mission
Pine Ridge, SD

Carole Piles, PhD, RN
Nursing Educator and Administrator, Retired
Fenton, MO

Norma Nolan Pinnell, RN, MSN
Nursing Educator in Medical-Surgical Nursing,
    Retired
Godfrey, IL

Caroline Samiezadi-Yazd, MSN, PNP, RN
Researcher in Transcultural Nursing,
    Self-Employed
Littleton, CO

Rita Sander, PhD, MSN, RN
Assistant Professor
Southern Illinois University Edwardsville,
    School of Nursing
Edwardsville, IL

Sharon Stecher, MSN, PMHCNS-BC
Private Practice, Psychiatric/Mental Health
    Nursing
St. Louis, MO

Carol Stubblefield, PhD, MSN, RN
Nursing Educator, Medical-Surgical and
    Psychiatric/Mental Health Nursing and
    Interdisciplinary Health Care
Professor Emerita
Barnes-Jewish Hospital College of Nursing
St. Louis, MO

Pamela Talley, MSN, CNS-BC, CSAC II
Private Practice, Psychiatric/Mental Health
    Nursing
Therapeutic Solutions
St. Louis, MO

Nina Kelsey Westhus, PhD, RN
Associate Professor
School of Nursing, Saint Louis University
St. Louis, MO

Recognition of Contributors to the Prior Editions

Joyce Dees Brockhaus, RN, PhD
Robert H. Brockhaus, PhD
Elaine Cox, RN, MSN
Ellen Duvall, RN, MSN, MA, Ed
Dorothy Fox, RN, PhD
Mary Ellen Grohar-Murray, RN, MSN, PhD
Joanne Jenkins
Joan Haugh, RN, BSN, MSW
M. Marilyn Huelskoetter, RN, MSN
Ruth Launius Jenkins, RN, MSN, PhD
Beverly Leonard, RN, MSN, PhD
Barbara Levy, RN, BSN
Mary Ann Lough, RN, MSN, PhD
Virginia Luetje, RN, MSN
K. Michele McConville, RN, MSN
Peggy M. McDowell, RN, CFNP, CPNP
Patricia Meili, RN, MSN, PhD
Sister Juliann Murphy, CCVI, RN, MSNE
Marilyn Smith, RD
Eleanor Sullivan, RN, MSN, PhD

Contributors to Supplements

Angeline Bushy, PhD, RN, FAAN
University of Central Florida–Daytona Beach Regional Campus
Daytona Beach, FL

Barbara M. Carranti, RN, MS, CNS
Le Moyne College
Syracuse, NY

Donna Jeanne Pugh, RN, MSN/ED
University of Florida
Jacksonville, FL

Thank You!

Our sincere thanks and appreciation goes out to the instructors and clinicians who gave so generously of their time and expertise by reviewing the chapters of this book.

Glenda Avery
Troy University
Phoenix City, AL

Connie Booth
Des Moines Area Community College
Boone, IA

Angeline Bushy
University of Central Florida
Daytona Beach, FL

Debra L. Carter
The University of Virginia's College at Wise
Wise, VA

Barbara Cheuvront
Regis University
Denver, CO

Karen Clark
Indiana University East
Richmond, IN

Pamela N. Clarke
University of Wyoming
Laramie, WY

Kim Clevenger
Morehead State University
Morehead, KY

Nancy J. Cooley
University of Maine at Augusta
Augusta, ME

Alayne Fitzpatrick
Mercy College
Dobbs Ferry, NY

Patricia E. Freed
Saint Louis University
St. Louis, MO

Brenda L. Hosley
Eastern Kentucky University
Richmond, KY

Hendrika Maltby
University of Vermont
Burlington, VT

Barbara Maxwell
SUNY Ulster
Stone Ridge, NY

Jeanne Morrison
Kaplan University

Martha J. Morrow
Shenandoah University
Winchester, VA

Stephanie A. Navarro-Silvera
Montclair State University
Montclair, NJ

Judith Pratt
Weber State University
Ogden, UT

Cindy Rieger
Oklahoma Baptist University
Shawnee, OK

Linda L. Robertson
La Roche College
Pittsburgh, PA

Anne Schappe
Webster University
St. Louis, MO

George F. Shuster
University of New Mexico
Albuquerque, NM

Kim White
Southern Illinois University Edwardsville
Edwardsville, IL

Bobbie Sue Whitworth
Kaplan University
IL

Karen Zapko
Kent State University
Salem, OH

Contents

CHAPTER 7   Spiritual and Religious Influences   181

Primary Contributor: Judith Proctor Zentner

Other Contributors: Ruth Beckmann Murray

Sylvia Adams

Pamela Talley

Frances Atkins

Carole Piles

CHAPTER 8   Prenatal and Other Developmental Influences   212

Primary Contributor: Ruth Beckmann Murray

Other Contributors: Judith Proctor Zentner

Sharon Stecher

Richard Yakimo

UNIT III   THE DEVELOPING PERSON AND FAMILY UNIT: INFANCY THROUGH ADOLESCENCE   247

CHAPTER 9   The Infant: Basic Assessment and Health Promotion   248

Primary Contributors: Ruth Beckmann Murray

Nina Kelsey Westhus

Other Contributors: Judith Proctor Zentner

Richard Yakimo

Jill Zentner Burns

CHAPTER 10 The Toddler: Basic Assessment and Health Promotion 298

Primary Contributors: Ruth Beckmann Murray

Nina Kelsey Westhus

Other Contributors: Judith Proctor Zentner

Richard Yakimo

Carole Piles

Consultant: Jill Zentner Burns

CHAPTER 13   The Adolescent: Basic Assessment and Health Promotion 435

Primary Contributors: Ruth Beckmann Murray

Nina Kelsey Westhus

Other Contributors: Judith Proctor Zentner

Norma Nolan Pinnell

Richard Yakimo

Carole Piles

Gina Bufe

Consultant: Jill Zentner Burns

UNIT IV   THE DEVELOPING PERSON AND FAMILY UNIT: YOUNG ADULT THROUGH DEATH 489

CHAPTER 14   The Young Adult: Basic Assessment and Health Promotion 490

Primary Contributors: Rita Acosta Sander

Ruth Beckmann Murray

Other Contributors: Judith Proctor Zentner

Norma Nolan Pinnell

Richard Yakimo

Carole Piles

Consultant: Jill Zentner Burns

CHAPTER 15   The Middle-Aged Person: Basic Assessment and Health Promotion   556

Primary Contributors: Ruth Beckmann Murray

Richard Yakimo

Other Contributor: Judith Proctor Zentner

Consultant: Jill Zentner Burns

CHAPTER 16   Later Maturity: Basic Assessment and Health Promotion   609

Primary Contributors: Ruth Beckmann Murray

Richard Yakimo

Other Contributors: Judith Proctor Zentner

Mildred Boland

Consultant: Jill Zentner Burns

CHAPTER 17   Dying and Death: The Last Developmental Stage 688

Primary Contributors: Richard Yakimo

Ruth Beckmann Murray

Other Contributor: Judith Proctor Zentner

UNIT I

Concepts and Theories Basic to Human Development

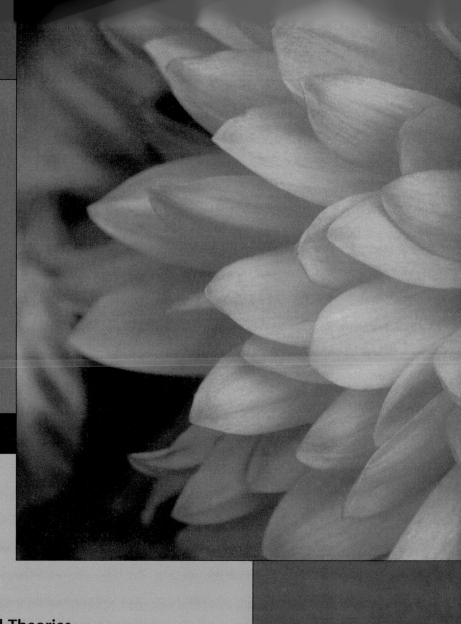

CHAPTERS

CHAPTER 1

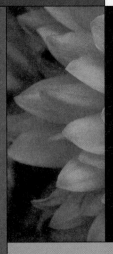

Biological, Ecological-Social, Psychological, and Moral Dimensions of the Person: Overview of Theories

OBJECTIVES

Study of this chapter will enable you to:

1. Identify major theoretical perspectives for understanding the developing person.

2. Describe some physiologic theories about aspects of the developing person.

3. Discuss systems theories and ecological systems as they apply to the developing person.

4. Identify major psychological developmental theorists, according to their views about the developing person.

5. Compare major concepts of behavioral, psychoanalytic and neo-analytic, existential-humanistic, and cognitive theories.

6. Describe major concepts of moral development as proposed in the theories by Kohlberg and Gilligan.

7. Apply concepts from theories of development during care of the client.

MediaLink **www.prenhall.com/murray**

Go to the Companion Website for interactive resources that accompany this chapter.

Glossary
Review Questions
Challenge Your Knowledge
Learning Activities

Critical Thinking
Tools
Media Link Applications
Media Links

Progression of Study of Human Development

Human development has been described for millennia. Confucius, in ancient China, described five stages and the main tasks for the person. Shakespeare, in *As You Like It*, wrote of life stages from infancy to old age and characteristics of each. You have read the works of poets and playwrights who have described human development and dynamics of family life.

The science of **psychology**, *the study of human behavior*, led people to better understand themselves by learning about child behavior. Gradually the child was seen as a distinct person different from the adult. Study of the child became more systematic and research-based. Theories about human behavior were developed. Until the 20th century, study of child development and advice in child care was not based on the scientific method but on observation and folklore.

As the 20th century progressed and societal and life span changes occurred, study was expanded to include the adolescent and different stages of adulthood, including young and middle adulthood. As people lived longer, the elderly became a focus, and several stages of older adulthood have been described.

The life span is studied physically, emotionally, cognitively, spiritually, and socially. Dying is seen as the last developmental phase, the final attempt to come to terms with self, others, and life in general. Learning more about self and others, including how people respond to surrounding influences to meet basic needs, helps people become better able to meet individual potential and health care needs.

Theories that explain the developing person and behavior use either a physical-biological, ecologic-sociocultural, psychological, or moral-spiritual basis. How theories are developed and applied is influenced by the historical time in which they are developed, just as development is influenced by the historical time. Major theories applicable to the developing person and family unit and to health promotion are summarized in this chapter. Keep in mind that *no theory explains all aspects of the person. The whole person is best understood when several theories are combined to explain the person's total development.* The theories have been developed by one or several methods for studying people. Use the theories described in this chapter in assessment, goal setting, and interventions for health promotion.

Physical-Biological Theories

Basic to the person is anatomic and physiologic structure and function. Various areas of the brain control functions and influence development and behavior. The concept that behavior is an expression of neural activity is central to the philosophy of modern neuroscience. The **mind** *represents a range of brain functions*—simple to complex, including physical, sensory, cognitive, and affective functions. The **brain** *controls behavior—how we perceive, think, feel, behave, act, and interact*. The two halves of the brain are mutually involved in all high levels of psychological functioning. **Consciousness** is a *dynamic result of brain activity, neither identical with, nor reducible to, the neural events of which it is composed.*

Consciousness is *an active integral part of the cerebral process; it exerts control over the biophysical and chemical activities at subordinate levels* (2, 37).

The huge quantity and vast range of sensory information that is transmitted to the cerebral cortex and the way in which the brain sorts, classifies, organizes, and interprets sensory information; handles input and output; considers expectations, past experiences, and other sources of information; and sends messages throughout the body are complex and not fully understood. In many ways the human brain may be like those of other animals, but it differs in its capacity to think, make judgments, remember, use symbols, store maps of the body and the world, and create.

Research on the physiologic basis for behavior has gained sophistication with advancing technology that studies the complexity of the brain and nervous system, endocrine and immune functions, and physiologic responses in a variety of situations. These findings affect current beliefs about health, normality, and development. In the following discussion, theories related to genetic, biochemical, neurophysiologic, immunologic, maturational, and other factors are covered briefly. For further study, refer to references listed at the end of the chapter (2, 37). Refer to Chapters 8 through 16, which present physiologic factors that affect the person. ∞

GENETIC FACTORS

Genetics is the *study of individual genes and their functions, the effects of heredity, and the combined impact of genes on disorders or specific characteristics.* Understanding of the role of genetic factors has been derived historically from studies focusing on pedigree descriptions and incidence of abnormalities in generations of families. Recent data come from direct visual examination of chromosomes, biochemical analyses of genetic material and enzymatic processes, and study of genes and DNA through the Human Genome Project (23). An understanding of genetic concepts is essential in order to effectively educate the client about health promotion and development.

Traditionally, genetics has focused on the **Mendelian Law of Inheritance**, *which states that a dominant gene for a trait or characteristic in at least one parent will cause, on the average, 50% of the children to inherit the trait. If both parents have the dominant gene, 75% of their children will inherit the trait.* When the trait is attributed to a **recessive gene**, *the offspring does not manifest it unless the gene was received from both parents.* If the gene was received from only one parent, the offspring is not affected but will probably pass on the gene to the next generation child (the grandchild). If the parents are **heterozygous** for a recessive gene (*both received the same gene type from only one of their parents*), 25% of the children probably will be affected. If the parents are **homozygous** for the recessive gene (*the same gene type was received from both of their parents*), all the children probably will inherit the trait or characteristic (2, 37, 60, 71). The Mendelian law explains the occurrence of many physical traits, such as eye color and height, and may explain certain physiologic characteristics or behavioral tendencies.

To isolate environmental factors from genetic effects, researchers have used several methodologic designs, such as the family resemblance method, the twin study method, and a combination of the two. The **family resemblance method** *looks for similarity between a person with a disorder and his or her relatives.* The **twin study method** *relies on differences* between two groups: **monozygotic twins** *(from a single ovum and therefore identical)* and **dizygotic twins** *(from two ova fertilized by two sperm and therefore not identical, i.e., fraternal twins).* Monozygotic twins have been found to resemble each other more in mood level and lability than dizygotic twins. Research is also being done on identical and fraternal twins reared apart to determine the physiologic versus environmental influences (8, 57, 60).

Definitions and Concepts

Basic genetic concepts that promote understanding of the developing person can be found in several references (8, 37, 39, 60, 71). The following are some important definitions:

1. **Deoxyribonucleic acid (DNA)**–*Chemical inside the cell nucleus that is the molecular basis of heredity,* constructed of double helix with parallel strands of both pairs held together by hydrogen bonds.
2. **Chromosome**–*Threadlike package of genes and DNA in the cell nucleus; contains instructions to make all the proteins a living being needs.* Humans have 46 chromosomes (23 pairs—44 autosomes and two sex chromosomes).
3. **Genome**–*All the DNA and full set of chromosomes with all the genes they contain, which make up the genetic material of an organism.* Each human genome contains about 30,000 genes.
4. **Gene**–*Basic functional and physical unit for transmission of hereditary instructions.*
   a. Each gene is a separate section of the chromosome, and each contains instructions for a specific protein, made up of strings of blocks of amino acids.
   b. Four chemicals, adenine (A), thiamine (B), guanine (G), and cytosine (C), are found in various combinations.
   c. Each molecule of DNA is made up of two strands of these chemicals, twisted into a double helix or what looks like a twisted ladder. Each rung is made up of a pair of these chemicals, A-T, T-A, G-C, and C-G. These pairs are arranged in triplets. Each triplet is a genetic code for a specific amino acid.
   d. A gene is a series of triplets corresponding to the string of 20 amino acids that make up a protein and do the work of the cells. Genes are dominant or recessive, and interact directly or indirectly with many other genes.
   e. Some genes are "regulator" genes; they direct other genes to guide growth and development and account for genetic differences between humans and animals. In each cell, some genes are expressed while others remain dormant.

The genetic code is immense, accounting for the uniqueness of each person. Conception brings together genetic instructions from both parents for every characteristic. A **gamete** or *reproductive cell* produces a new individual when it combines with a gamete from the opposite sex. Each person can produce about 8 million chromosomally different ova or sperm. Upon conception, a **zygote**, the *single cell formed by fusing of sperm and ovum,* begins development

of the person. **Genotype** is the *person's entire genetic inheritance or potential but is not shown outwardly.* Every behavioral tendency is affected by many genes, including additive or dominant-recessive patterns. **Phenotype** is the *person's observable appearance and behavior, the result of genetic and environmental influences.*

Gene interaction patterns occur in several ways (8, 37, 39, 60, 71):

1. **Additive genes**–A *trait reflects fairly equal distribution of all involved genes,* for example, skin color, height, and hair texture or curliness. Additive traits depend on contributions of whichever genes a child inherits (half from each parent). Each additive gene affects the phenotype.
2. **Nonadditive genes**–The *phenotype shows influence of one gene more than another gene,* which results in the following patterns:
   a. Dominant-recessive patterns
      (1) **Dominant**–The *phenotype reveals influence of a dominant gene,* for example, brown rather than blue eyes. **Incomplete dominance** may occur; the *phenotype is influenced primarily, but not exclusively, by the dominant gene.* A dominant gene, for example, height, *may not completely be shown in the phenotype* due to nongenetic factors, such as nutritional status.
      (2) **Recessive**–The *phenotype does not reveal that the person carries the gene.* For example, brown-eyed parents may have the gene for blue eyes, and their child may have blue eyes.
   b. **Sex or X-linked pattern**–*Genes located on the X chromosome affect the offspring.*
      (1) Females have two X chromosomes; males have one X and one Y chromosome.
      (2) In females, a normal dominant gene on the X chromosome from the father generally overrides a defective gene on the X chromosome from the mother.
      (3) Sex-linked recessive traits are carried on one of the X chromosomes of an unaffected mother. She is a carrier; she does not have the disease but can pass it on to her children.
      (4) Whatever recessive gene is inherited on the male Y chromosome cannot be counterbalanced by the female X chromosome. Thus, recessive genes will be expressed. Traits on the X chromosome can be passed from mother to son, not father to son. Thus, males have more X-linked disorders, for example, red-green color-blindness.
3. **Parental "imprinting" or "tagging" of genes**–*Certain genes may behave differently, depending on whether they came from the mother or father.* For example, genes for height, insulin production, and some forms of mental retardation affect the child in different or opposite ways, depending on which parent the gene came from.
4. **Mutation**–*A change in the normal DNA pattern of a particular gene is caused by environmental factors, including **teratogens** (agents that produce adverse effects),* such as radiation or toxic chemicals. Most mutations are lethal; however, sometimes the person with a mutation may live, thrive, and reproduce. Inherited mutations account for a small number of disorders.

Relatively few people are born with abnormal chromosomes, with characteristics apparent in the phenotype, but *everyone* carries abnormal genes that could produce serious diseases or disabilities in the next generation. Some chromosome abnormalities are inherited; others result from adverse effects or accidents in prenatal development and are not inherited. An additive abnormal gene could give rise to **multifactorial disorders**, in which *effect of the gene is expressed only if specific other genes are also present in the genotype and influenced by environment as well*. A related concept is **multifactorial effects**, meaning that *genetic traits are influenced by many factors, including environment*. Thus, without genes, no traits or behavior would exist. Without environment, no gene could be expressed (8, 39).

Polygenic inheritance, the *combination or interaction of many genes acting together to produce a behavioral characteristic*, is believed to be a factor if certain characteristics or behavioral defects occur. Environmental effects contribute to the person's development of genetic potential from the moment of conception (60, 63). For example, three factors determine cholesterol levels: presence of a single gene, polygenetic inheritance, and environment. One gene plays a key role in determining serum cholesterol levels and subsequent risk for coronary artery disease. This gene causes blood cholesterol levels of 300 mg/dL and results in heart attacks for males between 30 and 39 years of age and for females in their 60s. Polygenetic inheritance determines blood cholesterol levels (120 to 300 mg/dL). Some people have a higher level of high-density lipoproteins (the good ones) and a lower level of low-density lipoproteins (the bad ones). The low-density lipoproteins carry most of the cholesterol in the bloodstream; the high-density lipoproteins carry cholesterol to the liver for metabolism or removal from the body (37). Environmental factors that increase risk of high cholesterol include cigarette smoking, inactivity, stress, and diet (60).

Two principles explain how differences in heredity may exert influence on development. The **Principle of Differential Susceptibility** suggests that *individual differences in heredity exist that make people susceptible to the influence of certain environments. Given different experiences, a person with certain hereditary potential could develop in different ways*. The **Principle of Differential Exposure** suggests that *inherited characteristics cause differing reactions from people, which in turn affect or shape the personality of the individual*. For example, body build, facial structure, and presence or absence of overall physical attractiveness result primarily from inheritance. People perceive, judge the actions of, and react more favorably to physically attractive children than to less attractive children. Over time, reactions of others contribute to formation of the self-concept, positive or negative feelings about self, and a sense of competency or incompetency that may affect behavior toward others or general performance. Excessive negative reaction from others may predispose to abnormal behavior and even mental illness if the stress is great enough (60).

Genomics is *the study of the functions and interactions of all the genes in the genome, including interaction of genes with each other and of genes with the environment, and the relationships among genes, environment, health, and disease*. The completion of the Human Genome Project (HGP), an international effort, made possible the study of genomics. The HGP involved the mapping and sequencing of all human genes and analysis of interactions and relationships (22, 23). Thus, the **genomic era** has begun. *Research will continue*.

Diseases appear to "run in families." *Inherited genes are only one of the explanations*. For example, families pass on traits (or behaviors) besides genes, such as portion sizes at mealtime and eating habits. A family may carry the gene for cleft palate, but if the family regularly eats food high in folic acid, the chance that a child is born with cleft palate is reduced (*multifactorial or polygenic inheritance*).

Interconnections between genes and genotype and between external environmental factors and the person's genomic pattern and penetrance (intensity of effect) are discussed by Chui and Dover (13) and Nadeau (58). Childhood chronic diseases and conditions with a genetic basis are summarized by Kenner, Gallo, and Bryant (42). The **Stress-Diathesis Model** *explains that numerous genes each create a biological bias toward certain behaviors but do not guarantee those behaviors. Genes produce changes at biological but not behavioral levels*. However, the *biological changes increase the probability of abnormal behavior or disease*, due to combinations of genetic influences with sufficient environmental input (13).

Information about genomics and genetics can be obtained from the following sources.

1. Centers for Disease Control and Prevention: National Office of Public Health Genomics *http://www.cdc.gov.genomics/*
2. GenEd Net (American Society of Human Genetics and Genetics Society of America) *http://www.genednet.org*
3. International Society of Nurses in Genetics *http://www.isong.org*
4. National Health Service (United Kingdom), National Genetics Education and Development Centre *http://www.geneticseducation.ngs/uk/*
5. National Human Genome Research Institute *http://www.genome.gov/*

Health Care and Nursing Applications

Assessment and intervention related to genomics must consider various factors (39):

1. **Preawareness Phase**–*Person lacks knowledge about a genetic disease risk factor.*
2. **Nonsymptomatic Phase**–*Person is aware of genetic risk but has no symptoms.* The phase may extend years to decades until disease onset, or may extend for the person's lifetime, because genetic risk does not result in disease expression. Interventions focus on increased monitoring and education to prevent or delay onset through changes in health behaviors.

If a person or family is considered high risk for a certain condition, based on family history, or if a screening test is positive, expanded definitive testing is preferred while the person is in the pre- or nonsymptomatic phase. Education, screening, and referral are then based on test results and risk profile in order to provide specialized follow-up and genetic counseling (22, 23, 82).

In your health care practice, genetic counseling will be needed by clients in relation to the specific disease, personal or family history, and individual questions. A summary of terms related to genomics and their definitions are presented by Jenkins, Grady, and Collins (39). The successful completion of the HGP in April 2003 marked the beginning of the genomic era in health care. The sequenced map of 3 billion DNA base pairs in the human genome reveals the biological pathways involved in physical and mental illnesses. As a result, better methods of diagnosis, treatment, and prevention can be evolved, and genetic counseling can be more effective (63). The process of genetic counseling is described in detail by Pestka. Internet resources for constructing a family pedigree are also presented (63). Keep abreast as knowledge continues to be generated about application of genomics to care of clients (42, 63). Technology will continue to be developed for genomic care. Current genomic technologies are summarized by Loescher and Merkle (50).

If you engage in genetic education or counseling, be aware of social, ethical, and legal implications of genomic health care. Clients are concerned about social stigma associated with psychiatric and some physical disorders, which may affect employment, insurance benefits, or accessibility to care. However, genomics could be used to place psychiatric disorders on an equal level with medical diseases in relation to funding for care and public acceptance. Ethical and legal concerns relate to the extent to which clients and families are given information and review of the informed consent process. Privacy laws prohibit a provider from discussing confidential patient information with family members without the client's consent (63, 82).

Just as genomics gives new options, so it also raises cultural, ethnic, racial, and family dilemmas. If there is a genetic predisposition to a disease, the person has an advanced warning and may take precautions to avoid disease development. The person may think about the implication of passing along the genetic legacy to children. Or the person may become preoccupied about the possibility of a genetic-linked disease and change the life patterns un-

necessarily (82). As a result of biotechnology, another industry, **bioinformatics**, *a field that focuses on the storage and retrieval of biological information from a database in a biologically meaningful way, is developing.* The new research and computerized information is important; it is equally essential to remember that genetics alone cannot explain human behavior (25, 29, 63, 81).

In **evaluation**, realize that much remains unknown about the manner and extent to which early individual differences result in later personality differences, and the extent to which early transactions between parents and child either enhance or obscure genetic characteristics. Intellect, emotions, societal factors, values, and learned life patterns are crucial to consider in development and health promotion of the person and family. Research is being done to determine response to and effectiveness of educating about genetic disease risk factors. Refer to the Abstract for Evidence-Based Practice.

BIOCHEMICAL FACTORS

Research on the relationship between biochemical factors and behavior involves the study of neurochemistry and hormones. The chemical processes and endocrine system are complex in structure and function. For more information, refer to a physiology textbook. A brief overview related to developmental processes and health promotion practice is presented.

Neurochemistry is implicated in behavioral development. **Neurotransmitters**, *chemicals involved in transfer or modulation of nerve impulses from one cell to another, are related to mood.* Acetylcholine, norepinephrine, dopamine, serotonin, and gamma-aminobutyric acid (GABA) are important neurotransmitters in the brain and are involved in such emotional states as arousal, fear, rage, pleasure, motivation, exhilaration, sleep, and wakefulness. Brain opioids and peptides aid in control of pain and maintain a happy or euphoric mood (2, 37). Such behavior, in turn, affects re-

INTERVENTIONS FOR HEALTH PROMOTION

Practice applications related to genetics include:

1. Obtain a genetic history as part of assessment; include family, ethnic, racial, and cultural variables.
2. Explain diagnostic tests related to genetic-based disease and the meaning of positive and negative results.
3. Provide emotional support to persons with genetic disorders and to their families.
4. Offer genetic screening and testing to those who do not request it.
5. Teach that the person may not want, and has a right not to have, genetic testing.
6. Address ethical issues related to expansion of genetic information, such as reproductive issues, individual rights, confidentiality, and treatment issues.
7. Learn about gene therapy, gene transfer, rationale, and constraints.
8. Educate that genetic tests can tell if the client carries the disease but do not predict eventual diagnoses.
9. Teach that environmental or other events may have to occur with positive genetic findings before a disease, such as cancer or depression, is manifested. Genes are only one explanation.
10. Teach that negative genetic findings (not having a gene for a disease) do not mean that the disease will not occur for other reasons.
11. Counsel the client who expresses feelings of guilt about having the gene.
12. Advocate for the client with genetic predisposition to disease in relation to employment and health insurance coverage.
13. Apply data from the Human Genome Project (HGP); work with the interdisciplinary team.

Abstract for Evidence-Based Practice

Psychological Adaptation to Genetic Information Scale (PAGIS)

Read, C., Perry, D., & Duffy, M. (2005). Design and psychometric evaluation of the Psychological Adaptation to Genetic Information Scale. *Journal of Nursing Scholarship, 37*(3), 203–208.

KEYWORDS

research, instruments, factor analysis, genetics.

Purpose ➤ To design and evaluate the Psychological Adaptation to Genetic Information Scale (PAGIS), an instrument to measure the person's response to learning about having a disease-related gene.

Conceptual Framework ➤ Skirton's grounded theory of the client's view of genetic counseling proposed variables related to positive psychological adaptation to a genetic condition. The Roy Adaptation Model addressed self-concept, self-esteem, and emotional concerns of daily life.

Sample/Setting ➤ Participants affected by genetic diseases were recruited via the Internet. The survey Website was visited by 452 people. The final sample of 323 respondents (70% return rate) was composed primarily of White females, median age of 36 to 45 years, who lived in North America, Europe, Oceania, Asia, and South America. Most (*n*=264; 82%) had attended college. Self-rated health for 137 (42%) of the participants, who had information about the disease, was 3 points on a scale of 1 (excellent) to 5 (poor). Genetic transmission of disease to a child occurred in 143 (44%) of the sample; rating of their child's health was 2.7, using the same point scale.

Method ➤ A preliminary 75-item PAGIS questionnaire included 15 items for each of five proposed constructs: nonintrusiveness, support, self-worth, certainty, and self-efficacy. Focus group discussion led to revision and reduction to 50 items, with 10 items per construct. A panel of four professional experts evaluated the items for content validity and reliability, as well as readability (10th-grade level). Participants who were recruited electronically followed university-approved protocol, were given directions for completion of the study, and could exit at any point.

Findings ➤ Psychometric evaluation of the 50-item PAGIS used by the respondents revealed an internal consistency reliability estimate of .93. Further statistical analysis resulted in a 26-item, five-factor PAGIS scale, with the original five constructs developed as subscales.

Implications ➤ A reliable, valid instrument is needed to measure the multidimensional phenomenon of psychological adaptation to personal genetic disease information. Subsequent research is needed. The five subscales may be useful in designing education, support, and counseling interventions for clients.

actions of others to the child, and the child's moods may affect childrearing behavior.

Hormonal factors, based on changes in the endocrine system, may contribute to certain behaviors. Steroid hormones are increased during stress behavior, which in turn may interfere with normal developmental processes physically and cognitively (2, 60). Excess steroid hormone intake (prescribed for illness or to build muscles and strength in athletes) causes mental as well as physical problems. The changing hormone production (estrogen, progesterone, and estradiol) that occurs during the menstrual cycle phases contributes to elevation or decline in neurotransmitter production. In turn, emotional status and mood are affected in the female after puberty (37, 60).

The pineal gland secretes the hormone melatonin, a metabolite of serotonin. It is produced during darkness and appears to keep the mind synchronized with environmental light and the outside world. An imbalance may be linked to inducing sleep disorders and melancholia (37).

Thyroid hormones are necessary for normal metabolism and function. Gland dysfunction may cause hypothyroidism or autoimmune thyroiditis, which results in thyroid atrophy, causing signs, symptoms, and behavior that match the criteria for depression: fatigue, constipation, vague aches and pains, feeling cold, poor memory, anxiety, and low mood. Eventually, the person may manifest confusion, cognitive impairment, and psychosis. Hyperthyroidism or excessive hormone production may manifest as anxiety, irritability, restlessness, euphoria, or mild manic disorder (2, 37, 60).

Biochemical differences exist between persons and can be identified. What is not clear is whether the biochemical changes precede—and thus contribute to—abnormal behavior or result from changes that occur interpersonally or socially as a result of the person's abnormal behavior. The person in acute or short-term stress or crisis may have an abnormal level of a neurotransmitter as a result of normal feelings precipitated by and related to the event; yet, that person is not determined to be, and does not become, mentally ill (2, 60).

Incorporate biochemical knowledge and research in health promotion and the nursing process. Refer to physiology textbooks for more information. Stress management techniques can be taught to help the client prevent or manage biochemical responses. Medications may also be necessary to maintain health and prevent or treat illness.

NEUROPHYSIOLOGIC FACTORS

The central and peripheral nervous systems are complex in structure and function. Neurologic structures generally have a prime time for development. If this development is interfered with, the child may not develop to the fullest potential. However, the brain continues to develop as neurons are added for decades. Brain structure is malleable, and use of a skill or talent expands competence. Neurophysiologic factors mediate all physiologic processes and behavior via the nervous system.

Some specific motor and speech functions and various sensations in different body parts can be traced to specific brain areas. Neurophysiologic factors in behavior and personality development are not fully understood. **Localization of brain function** *means that certain areas of the brain are more concerned with one kind of function than another.* It does not imply that a specific function is mediated by only one brain region. Specific brain function requires the integrated action of neurons located in many different brain regions (37). Understanding general neurologic functions is necessary for determining developmental progress of the child and adolescent and the general health status of the person, which in turn may direct health promotion measures.

Brain regions and some of their specialized functions are described in references (2, 37, 71, 77). In the *cerebral cortical lobes,* the frontal lobe regulates planning, movement, concentration, anxiety, guilt, aggression, and mental fatigue. The parietal lobe is responsible for somatic sensation. The temporal lobe regulates hearing, memory, learning, and emotion. The occipital lobe is responsible for vision. There are also major association cortices. The prefrontal cortex regulates highest brain or executive functions. The limbic cortex regulates memory, emotion, and motivation of behavior. The parietal-temporal-occipital cortex is responsible for higher sensory function and language. The premotor association cortex regulates planning of action and initiation of movement; damage to the area affects execution of movement. The parietal-temporal-occipital association cortex links information from the senses that is necessary for perception. Damage causes deficit in body image and spatial relations and impaired ability to speak, recognize familiar objects or persons, or identify objects by touch. Dysfunction in any of these areas affects normal developmental progress and interferes with health.

Linkage of the hypothalamus, limbic system, and cerebral cortex maintains homeostasis directly by regulating the endocrine and autonomic nervous systems and indirectly by regulating emotions and drives, including sexual preference, and any pleasure, by acting through the external environment. The hypothalamus is involved in a number of functions. It integrates cardiovascular and respiratory functions and motor and endocrine responses; mediates stress response; suppresses emotional responses and behavior; and controls weight, appetite, and sleep-wake cycles. The forebrain delays responses to external events, which allows for planning, and is crucial to conscious experiences of emotion (2, 51).

The *limbic system* is the seat of emotion and is involved in affective and cognitive function and motivation, feelings, and behavioral homeostasis. The limbic structures are involved in comparison of external stimuli with internal states and in learning, memory, and motivation. The limbic system is especially prone to pathology because neurotransmitter effects are rapid (2, 8, 37).

Motivated behavior can be regulated by factors other than tissue needs, including learned habits and subjective pleasurable feelings. The ***central reward system (CRS)***, *located within the limbic system, is responsible for the pleasure response.* It is not fully known how the CRS mediates and registers reward or reinforcement. The reward cascade begins in the hypothalamus and affects the opioid peptide, methionine enkephalin, which is released in the substantia nigra, where enkephalin inhibits release of gamma-aminobutyric acid (GABA). GABA is inhibited; dopamine supply is increased and acts to give a feeling of reward, pleasure, or elation (2, 37).

Teach parents that children apparently are born with a predisposition to be outgoing or quiet, or there may be a chemical predisposition to seeking danger or high risk. Yet neurophysiology does not supply all the answers. A supportive environment may cause further development of certain neurophysiologic rudiments and promote further development of the neurophysiologic processes that are manifested; thus environment helps to produce a well-adjusted child. A hostile home environment, especially in early life, contributes to the opposite result (8).

IMMUNOLOGIC FACTORS

The *immune system* functions to protect the body against disease; it recognizes and distinguishes foreign substances, such as bacteria, toxins, and cancer, from the body's own tissue. There are two major types of attack cells. The B cells, manufactured by bone marrow, create antibodies to destroy specific invading bacteria and viruses. Antibodies remain in the body so that some diseases occur only once. The T cells are manufactured by the thymus gland and produce substances to destroy any infected cells. The B and T cells strengthen other aspects of the immune system. The natural killer (NK) cells and white blood cells are other components of the immune system (37). Immune suppression and stimulation are both necessary at different times to maintain health. At times the system responds excessively and destroys normal tissues.

The immune system and brain communicate directly and indirectly through a complex array of hormones and neurotransmitters. Pituitary hormones affect the immune system. The sympathetic nervous system affects lymph nodes and the spleen. Stress may predispose the person to illness through effects on the immune system that either decrease or alter immune functions (2, 77). Excess stress affects the immune system adversely, causing a variety of physical illnesses (e.g., musculoskeletal disease, cancer, asthma, thyroid and heart disease, colitis) with concomitant emotional effects (2, 37).

Educate clients about **psychoneuroimmunology,** the *connections between stress in the environment and physical and emotional health.* Certain mechanisms produce greater physical health when there is emotional well-being. The stress of rapid or unexpected change can negatively affect health (2). Research on immune function has applications to immunizations, as well as to cancer, HIV/AIDS, and a variety of other disorders.

MATURATIONAL FACTORS

The **maturational view** *emphasizes the emergence of patterns of development of organic systems, physical structures, and motor capabilities under the influence of genetic and maturational forces.* Because of an inherent predisposition of the neurologic, hormonal, and skeletal-muscular systems to develop spontaneously, *physiologic and motor development occurs in an inevitable and sequential pattern in children throughout the world.* The growth of the nervous system is critical in this maturation, *unless the normal process is inhibited by severe environmental, physiologic, or emotional deprivation.*

Gender differences may be inherent for some characteristics. For example, women generally have a greater response to the intuitive part of the brain, whereas men have a greater response to the spatial part of the brain. Yet many characteristics are the result of sociocultural influences; women from certain cultures may demonstrate characteristics common to men in some cultures (57, 71). Gender differences are described in Chapters 9 through 16. ∞

Foster development of maturational factors as you work with clients. Chapters 9 through 16 ∞ present more information for assessment and intervention.

BIOLOGICAL RHYTHMS

Biorhythms are *self-sustaining, repetitive, rhythmic patterns established in plants, animals, people, and seasonal-environmental events.* These daily or monthly biological cycles affect a number of physical functions, such as blood cell production, levels of blood glucose and hormones, body temperature, heartbeat, blood pressure, renal and gastrointestinal function, sleep, and muscular strength and coordination (2, 37, 60, 71). Mental skills and emotional changes are also apparently affected.

Biological rhythm is unique to the individual and may be recorded through (a) interview, (b) a detailed diary recording quantitative information about body processes and subjective experiences, and (c) **autorhythmometry**, *in which the person records and rates physiologic processes and mood* (8, 60, 71). Biological rhythms are discussed in Chapter 14. ∞ Refer to physiologic textbooks for more information.

BIOLOGICAL DEFICIENCIES

Biological stressors, such as certain kinds of foods; lack of food, fluids, and electrolytes, or malnutrition; and lack of sleep may change behavior and the course of development and negatively affect health (58). These factors are discussed further in other chapters.

Ecological-Social Concepts and Theories

ECOLOGICAL CONCEPTS

Ecology is a *science that studies the community and the total setting in which life and behavior occur. A basic ecological principle is that the continuity and survival of a person depends on a deliberate balance of factors influencing the interactions between the family or person and the environment.* System factors are discussed in the following paragraphs.

Family Social System, *a unit dependent on the resources and groups in the community to survive and continue its own development and to nurture development of offspring.* Climate, terrain, and natural resources affect family lifestyle and development and behavior of family members. The neighborhood may adversely affect development, especially if the person is reared in a family that lives in a deteriorating neighborhood or in an area with poor schools, inadequate housing, and a high crime rate. Excessively crowded housing may create stresses within the family that contribute to sleep deprivation, bickering, incest, or other types of abuse that affect developmental progress in all spheres of the person. Job loss because of a changing community and job market and the resultant financial problems may affect health care practices and nutrition and, in turn, physical growth and emotional security. See Chapter 6 ∞ for more information on family development.

Urbanization, *creation of large population centers, fosters many opportunities and services but also contributes to rapid social changes, social stressors, discrimination, unemployment, poor housing, inadequate diet and health care, poverty, and feelings* of **anomie** (*not being part of society and negative self-image*). These all contribute to stress, developmental difficulties, and health problems in various ways. The person in poverty or poor health; the young, elderly, or immature person; and the person or family without an adequate support system are especially affected by such stressors (8).

Sociologic variables, *including family socioeconomic level and position in the community, and the prestige related to birth, race, age, cultural ties, and power roles,* affect development, behavior, and adaptation of the person and family. Certain behaviors may be expected from a person because of age, gender, race, religion, or occupation. The individual may experience role conflicts and developmental problems when there are discrepancies between norms and values and these demands (8).

Cultures *vary in their definitions of normal and abnormal behavior;* cross-cultural comparisons of developmental norms are difficult. Theorists in each culture describe their research findings about normal child or adult characteristics or behavior based on norms of their culture and their cultural bias. For example, cognitive impairment in elderly adults is rare in cultures that revere their elderly or where people do not live to an advanced age. What might be associated with homosexuality in our culture, such as men embracing, is considered normal male heterosexual behavior in the Arab world.

Some authorities believe that non-Caucasian racial groups must be evaluated by psychological criteria different from those used for Caucasians. They cite adaptive personality traits that members of ethnic groups have adopted to survive in American society (8).

Geographic moves *may create many adjustments for the person as he or she attempts to meet norms of the new community.* Developmental and behavioral problems may occur among those who migrate (8). Persons who move often as children may never form "chumships" or close relationships later in adulthood; however, the mobile family and individual do learn coping skills that help them adjust to unfamiliar or stressful situations.

Some professionals and some laypeople think abnormal behavior results from individual failure. In this view an individual's psychological problems are the result of some personal circumstances, such as deficient achievement of developmental tasks, immaturity, character defect, or maladjustment. An alternative view is to see the individual's problems as stemming from social system causes. The broad economic, political, cultural, and social patterns of the nation, and particular subcultures, can be viewed as system determinants of individual developmental responses. Then the community is the place to begin making changes if individual dysfunction is to be decreased (8, 14, 60, 71). Chapters 4 through 7 ∞ discuss environmental, cultural, family, and religious/spiritual variables, and Chapters 9 through 16 present the interrelationship of these variables on the person. ∞ See **Figure 1-1**■, which depicts social systems and their interactions.

SOCIAL SYSTEMS PERSPECTIVE: GENERAL SYSTEMS THEORY APPLIED TO BEHAVIOR

First proposed by von Bertalanffy (79, 80), **General Systems Theory** *presents a comprehensive, holistic, and interdisciplinary study of any aspect of life. Nothing is determined by a single cause or explained by a single factor.* Nothing can be studied as a lone entity. This theory proposes that the family, individual, various social groups and organizations, health care agencies, and cultures are systems.

A **system** is an *assemblage, group, unit, or organism of interrelated, interacting, interdependent parts. Persons or objects are united by some form or order into a recognizable unit and are in equilibrium* (2, 8, 9, 51, 59, 71).

Synergy exists, meaning that *the whole is greater than the sum of its parts or units.* Within a system, **subsystems,** *smaller units within the whole, exist,* such as spouses and children in the family, or the mental health clinic within the larger health care center. **Suprasystems** *refer to the large environment, community, or an organization or agency on a global, national, or state level.* All systems need energy and activity to maintain self. Input of energy allows **differentiation**, *the tendency for the system to advance or mature to a higher level of complexity and organization.*

The elements or components that are common to all systems are listed in **Table 1-1.** A given entity is not a system unless these characteristics are present (2, 9, 43, 49, 51, 79, 80).

People satisfy their needs within social systems. The **social system** is a *group of people joined cooperatively to achieve common goals, using an organized set of practices to regulate behavior* (9, 43). The person occupies various positions and has defined roles in the social system. The person's development is shaped by the system; in turn, people create and change social systems (2, 43, 51). Social systems include the family, churches, economic systems, politicolegal and educational institutions, and health care agencies. See **Figure 1-1** for a summary.

All living organisms (i.e., every person) comprise an open system. Change occurs constantly within and between the system and other systems. An **open system** is *characterized by the ability to exchange energy, matter, and information with the environment to*

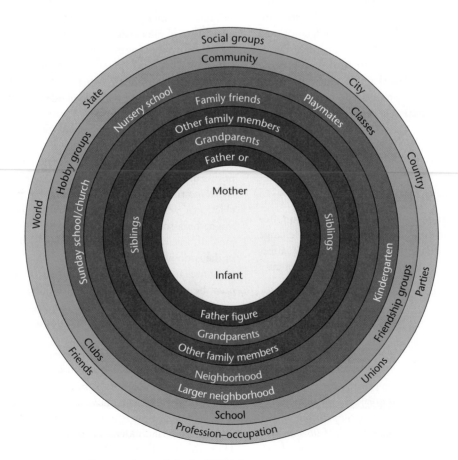

FIGURE ■ **1-1** Social systems and interactions of the individual.

TABLE 1-1

Elements and Characteristics of a System

Element	Definition/Example
Parts	Definition: *The system's components that are interdependent units. None can operate without the other. Change in one part affects the entire unit.* Example: The person as a whole system is composed of physical, emotional, mental, spiritual, cultural, and social aspects. Physically, he or she is composed of the body systems—neurologic, cardiovascular, and so on. The health agency is one part of the health care system, and it, in turn, is composed of parts: physical plant, employees, clients, departments that give services.
Attributes	Definition: *Characteristics of the parts.* Example: Temperament, roles, education, age, or health of the person or family members.
Information/ communication	Definition: *Sending of messages and feedback, the exchange of energy.* Example: A system has input and output with the environment; information exchange varies with the system but is essential to achieve goals.
Feedback	Definition: *Internal and external responses to behavior (output), dynamic, self-regulating.* Example: Monitoring and reporting allows the system to readjust or change if needed.
Equilibrium	Definition: *Steady state or state of balance that is maintained through adaptive, dynamic, self-regulating processes, and information input, transformation, output, and feedback.* Example: Complex hormonal processes maintain blood glucose levels. Predictable behaviors of the administrator of an agency improve employee performance.
Boundary	Definition: *A barrier or area of demarcation that limits or keeps a system distinct from its environment and within which information is exchanged.* Example: The skin of the person, home of the family, or walls of the health agency are boundaries. Boundary is not always rigid. Relatives outside the home are part of the family. Boundary may be an imaginary line, such as the feeling that comes from belonging to a certain racial or ethnic group.
Organization	Definition: *The formal or informal arrangement of parts to form a whole entity so that the organism or institution has a working order that results in established hierarchy.* Example: The person is organized into a physical structure, basic needs, cognitive stages, and achievement of developmental tasks. Hierarchy in the family or health agency provides organization that is based on power (*ability to control others*) and responsibility. Specialization of medical and nursing practice is a way of organizing care. Organization in an institution or family is maintained by norms, roles, and customs that each member must follow.
Goals	Definition: *Purposes of or reasons for the system to exist, either short- or long-term.* Example: Goals include survival, development, and socialization of the individual or the family.
Environment	Definition: *The social and physical world outside the system, boundaries, or the community in which the system exists.* Example: The person's or family's environment may be a tribal enclave, farm, small town, or an urban neighborhood. Environment of a health care system may be the city in which the agency is located or may extend to other states and countries.
Evolutionary processes	Definition: *Changes in the system and the environment, proceeding from simple to complex.* Example: The person undergoes physical, psychological, and social changes throughout the life span. All systems continually change in some way.

evolve into higher levels of heterogeneity, organization, order, and development (2, 49). Physically, there is a *hierarchy of components,* such as cells and organ systems. Emotionally, there are levels of needs and feelings. Cognitively, a person has memories, knowledge, and cognitive strategies. Socially, the person is in a relative rank in a hierarchy of prestige roles, such as boss, worker, adult, or child. Although internal stimuli, such as those governed by the

nervous and endocrine systems, are at work, outer stimuli also affect the person. The *boundaries or environment,* such as one's skin, the limits set by others, social status, home, and community, influence the person's *needs* and *goal achievement.* To remain healthy, the person must be able to *communicate* and must have *feedback.* The condition of the skin tells about temperature control; an emotional reaction signifies a sense of security, a job well done, or a failure; a pain signifies malfunction or injury. In turn, the person influences the external world through his or her developmental behavior. A constant *exchange of energy and information* must exist with the surrounding specified environment if the system is to be open, useful, and creative. If this *information or energy exchange does not occur, the system becomes a* **closed system:** ineffective, disorganized, and diseased. Death may result.

Linkage *occurs when two systems exchange energy across their boundaries* (10). Industry, the church, or the health agency, for example, draws energy from its linkage to the family. In return, industry may contribute to employee benefits, community or societal mental health campaigns, or societal improvements. The church maintains its role as prime defender of family stability. The health agency sets standards of health care and refines policies and procedures based on feedback from consumers, employees, and accrediting bodies.

Other terms explain social systems. **Equifinality** *means that the system endpoint, goal, or influence is unpredictable. The end is not determined by the beginning action.* **Entropy** refers to *the tendency of a system to go from a state of order to disorder.* **Negentropy** refers to positive movement, the tendency of a system to go from a state of disorder to order (9, 60). These terms are applicable to the individual or family system, as well as the political, educational, social service, or health care systems.

Each person and family you care for is a system interacting with other systems in the community. Development and function are greatly affected by the interdependence and interrelationships of each component part and by all other surrounding systems.

ECOLOGIC SYSTEMS THEORY

Bronfenbrenner formulated **Ecologic Systems Theory** to describe *how the person's development is influenced by a broad range of situations and from interactive and overlapping contextual levels. The levels of these systems are still applicable and are described as follows* (10, 11):

1. **Microsystem.** *Face-to-face physical and social situations that directly affect the person,* such as family, schoolroom, workplace, church, peers, and health services.
2. **Mesosystem.** *Connections and relationships among the person's microsystems.*
3. **Exosystem.** *Settings or situations that indirectly influence the person,* such as the extended family, friends, neighbors, spouse's workplace, mass media, legal services, various levels of government, and community agencies and organizations.
4. **Macrosystem.** *Sociocultural values, beliefs, and policies that provide a framework for organizing individuals' lives and indirectly affect the person* through the exosystem, mesosystem, and microsystem.
5. **Chronosystem.** *Effect of time and timing of events and the extent of change upon development,* caused by the event, or remaining stability in the person's world. Events include changing place of residence or family structure, loss of extended family members, employment variables such as the working mother, or larger events such as war, terrorism, disasters, economic cycles, and waves of migration.

A person's development is influenced by these systems. The person also shapes personal development and influences other systems through appearance, personality traits, use of talents and skills, or disabilities (10, 11).

You will be working within a system (health care) and with systems (clients, families, groups, communities). You also are an individual system. Use holistic assessment and consider system factors in interventions.

Evaluation criteria can be generated from the elements of a system presented in **Table 1-1.** Evaluation must include feedback from all parts of the system.

Behavioral Theories

OVERVIEW

Behaviorists *adhere to stimulus-response conditioning theories.* This scientific approach to the study of the person generalizes results from animal experiments to people. The **neo-behaviorists,** *contemporary behavioral theorists, obtain data by observing the human's behavioral response to stimuli.* The person is considered in terms of component parts. *The focus is on specific units of behavior or parts of behavioral patterns that are objectively observed or measured by various instruments and analyzed from the perspective of physiologic associations.*

VIEW OF THE PERSON

Behavioral theorists view the living organism as a self-maintaining mechanism. The person has sensory input and, in turn, acts to reduce a need or meet a goal. There is a natural tendency and drive to satisfaction. The person is seen as a reactive organism responding overtly and quantitatively to past conditioning and present situations. The person is regarded as a product of learning (60, 71).

The *focus is on physiologic processes and identifiable aspects of the person; subjective, unobservable aspects of the human are not studied.* Physiologic concepts explain feelings and human behavior. There are no biases except for past conditioning. The person or the client engages in *activity or behavior* called **learning.** Rest or cessation of behavior follows **reinforcement** or *reward* for learning.

Behaviorists believe emotions arise from body changes, are learned through **classical conditioning,** or arise in the present situation based on past learning that is associated with the present event. For example, a person likes men with beards because he or she learned this response during childhood as a result of associating beards with a kindly, bearded grandfather. Behaviorists propose that maladaptive behaviors are also reinforced and learned.

VIEW OF EDUCATION AND THERAPY

Goals of education and treatment are to (a) control the person's behavior; (b) help the person become more efficient and realistic, as defined by others in the environment; (c) move toward a goal set by external standards; and (d) create learning by forming bonds, connections, or associations. Responses that are appropriate are rewarded and therefore are stamped in to form habits (12, 38, 61). A treatment approach is to identify factors in the environment or in prior learning that must be modified to change the problem behavior.

The teacher, health care provider, or therapist is at the center of and in control of the educational or treatment process and functions as a reinforcer to help the student or client achieve behavioral objectives. For example, in education about child rearing or health care or in changing parenting or health behavior, the external situation is set up to elicit the desired response. Organized sequential steps are created so that the person achieves a goal and receives a reward. Insight is not considered as a variable in behavior. Inefficient behavior is removed from the person by **shaping**, *setting up the situation so that the person acts in a desired way, and then rewarding the desired behavior.* Rewards are arranged to continue behavior. If education or treatment is individualized, the emphasis is on the preconceived end product rather than on the process (12, 61).

Evaluation of application of behavioral theory includes several considerations. An *ethical issue with this approach is that the person may feel he or she is being manipulated, that something is being done to rather than with the person, or that something is being done for the person rather than allowing the person to do for self.* Further, who defines which behavior is maladaptive—the client or health care provider? What the therapist considers maladaptive, such as hypervigilance, may be adaptive for the client's life situation. To change that behavior would make the client more vulnerable to harm. Also, the approach may seem too superficial or simplistic. The person may develop different symptoms to express the underlying problem or pathology. The person may resist behavioral change. Or the person may not return for treatment after the initial visit because he or she felt misunderstood. Further, behavioral change may not last when the program of learning ends, when life situations change, or when prior situations reassert themselves.

BEHAVIORAL THEORISTS
Skinner: Operant Conditioning Theory

B.F. Skinner is well known for his Operant Conditioning Theory. According to Skinner, **behavior** is an *overt response that is externally caused and is controlled primarily by its consequences.* The environmental stimuli determine how a person alters behavior and responds to people or objects in the environment. Feelings or emotions are not the cause of behavior; they result from the behavior (38, 72, 75). **See Figure 1-2▢,** Development as viewed by learning theorists. **Table 1-2** lists key terms and definitions, with examples (38, 72–75).

Learning is a *change in the form or probability of response as a result of conditioning.* **Operant conditioning** is the *learning process whereby a response (operant) is shaped and is made more probable or frequent by reinforcement.* **Transfer** is an *increased probability of response in the future.* **Operant responses** are a set of acts that *operate on the environment and generate consequences.* The *important stimulus is the one immediately following the response,* not the one preceding it (72, 74).

According to Operant Conditioning Theory, certain kinds of events are reinforcers; when such an event or operant follows a response, similar responses are more likely to occur. The reinforcing events can be identified, and responses can be planned. The stimulus sets the occasion in which the response is likely to occur, in spite of infrequent or intermittent reinforcement. Behavior may continue as the result of more than one reinforcer. Certain behaviors that have a genetic basis are more likely to respond to reinforcers. When there is no reinforcement, the behavior is extinguished or no longer occurs (38, 72–75).

Operant Conditioning occurs in most everyday activities, according to Skinner. People constantly cause others to modify their behavior by reinforcing certain behavior and ignoring other behavior. During development, people learn to balance, walk, talk, play games, and handle instruments and tools because they are reinforced after performing a set of motions, thereby increasing

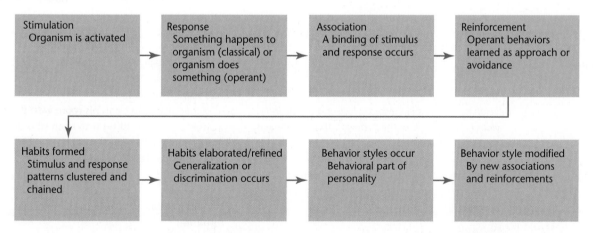

FIGURE ▢ **1-2** Development as viewed by learning theorists. Stimuli from inside or outside the organism are reinforced on a particular schedule that determines response force and strength. Habits develop. The response processes of generalization and discrimination elaborate these habits and modify them. Effective habits are equated with effective development. New habits are learned when new stimuli, associations, and reinforcers are encountered.

TABLE 1-2

Selected Terminology Pertaining to Application of Behavioral Theory

Term	Definition	Example
Respondent conditioning	Pairing a neutral stimulus with a nonneutral stimulus until the person learns to respond to the neutral stimulus as to the nonneutral stimulus	Baby learns to "love" a sibling (nonneutral stimulus) because the sibling shakes a rattle and offers other toys (neutral stimulus) while cooing, touching, and smiling at baby.
Operant conditioning	Rewarding or punishing a response until the person learns to repeat or avoid that response in anticipation of positive or negative consequences	Preschooler returns toys to the toy box at the end of the day because he remembers the consequences: Doing so is followed by 10 minutes of time with the parent; failure to do so results in sitting alone in his room for 5 minutes.
Positive reinforcement	Rewarding desired behavior to maintain or strengthen behavior	Parent buys a desired item for the child who earns an A in a course.
Negative reinforcement	Removing an aversive stimulus in response to behavior, which maintains behavior that is not desired or appropriate	Parent allows the child to skip household tasks if he complains when asked to do them, yet the child receives an allowance weekly.
Extinction	Suppressing behavior by removing reinforcers that are maintaining the behavior	Parent does not give the child who complains about doing household tasks the allowance at the end of the week and explains why.
Punishment	Suppressing an undesirable behavior by using an aversive stimulus in response to the person's behavior	Parent spanks the child for running into the street.
Time-out	Suppressing maladaptive behavior by removing the subject to a neutral environment, void of reinforcements, when the behavior is manifested	Parent makes the 4-year-old child sit facing a corner for 5 minutes after hitting a sibling.
Generalization	Transferring a conditioned response from the conditional stimulus to another stimulus	Child who is bitten by a dog fears all animals.
Systematic desensitization	Pairing an anxiety-causing stimulus with an induced state of relaxation to extinguish fearful behavior	Parent remains with the child who has been bitten by a dog when the child is in the vicinity of animals, gradually helps the child to relax, and eventually to pet a very friendly dog.
Discrimination	Responding only to a specific stimulus	Toddler learns via punishing encounters with mother that playing in water in the bathtub is acceptable and playing in the water in the toilet is not.
Escape behavior	Initiating a response to escape an unpleasant or aversive stimulus	Adolescent brings the parents a gift when returning late from a weekend with a friend.
Avoidance learning	Arranging responses to avoid exposure to an aversive stimulus	Adolescent verbally refuses the offer and walks away from the person offering a marijuana joint after a bad experience with it.
Chaining	Developing complex behavior by focusing on the individual components of the behavior; this is done in a backward fashion	Schoolchild learns to clean his room with the parent instructing and assisting with each step of the task and then verbally repeating in reverse order the steps after the task is finished.
Shaping	Reinforcing successive approximations or small units of a desired response until that behavior is gradually achieved	Parent teaches the child to clean his room by praising him for doing every step of the process—vacuuming the rug, dusting each piece of furniture.
Fading	Removing gradually the reinforcement given to the person	Parent gives less and less verbal approval to the schoolchild for doing assigned household tasks.

TABLE 1-2

Selected Terminology Pertaining to Application of Behavioral Theory—continued

Term	Definition	Example
Satiation	*Providing excessive amount of reinforcer, which causes loss of effectiveness*	Chocolate candy is reward for behavior. Child is given extra candy and loses desire for candy and for behavior change.
Token	*Object that serves as general reinforcer; may be exchanged for other reinforcers*	Client earns tokens for helpful behavior, and exchanges 10 tokens for trip to science museum.
Contingency	*Systematic use or management of rewards to obtain desired behavior; reward is contingent on behavior or performance*	Condition a desired response or suppress maladaptive response by drawing up contract indicating rewards and punishments contingent on or related to responses in the contract.

the repetition of these motions. Health, social, and ethical behaviors are imitated and learned as people are reinforced to continue them; in turn, they reinforce others for the same behaviors. Operant reinforcement improves the efficiency of behavior, whether the behavior is appropriate or inappropriate. *Any attention, even if negative, reinforces response to a stimuli* (72, 75).

Some present-day relaxation methods used by health care providers are based on behavioral conditioning. The client is trained to respond to a therapist's direction by relaxing a muscle group; music is then played while the therapist gives directions for relaxing. Later the person is able to respond automatically by relaxing when music plays. Conditioning is also used in childbirth preparation classes.

Positive reinforcement occurs when the *presence of a stimulus strengthens a response.* A positive reinforcer is food, water, a smile, or a pleasant, friendly interchange with another person. A person waves to someone because of the reinforcement, not because of the stimulus of the other person's hand waving. The person selects a motion because it was reinforced. In this process, reinforcement must be immediate. The person wants attention and will change behavior in the desired direction to receive approval (72–75). Ignoring inappropriate behavior may cause continual inappropriate behavior in order for the person to get attention. Skinner emphasized positive reinforcement. He rejected use of negative reinforcement, punishment, or aversive control, contending that this merely produces escape or avoidance behavior (72, 75).

A **reinforcement schedule** is a *pattern of rewarding behavior at fixed time intervals, with a fixed number of responses between reinforcements.* Reinforcement strengthens a general tendency to make the response, or a class of responses, in the future (72).

Application of Skinner's theory for client care and teaching is threefold:

1. **Behavior modification** *is the theory applied to clinical and classroom problems.*
2. **Programmed learning** *is the theory applied to courses of study.*
3. **Biofeedback** *is the theory applied to correction of physiologic problems.*

INTERVENTIONS FOR HEALTH PROMOTION

Behavior modification involves the following steps after the initial analysis:

1. Target behavior to be changed is identified.
2. Tentative duration time and place of treatment are specified.
3. **Shaping**, *breaking complex behavior into small steps and reinforcing each small step of behavior that is closer to the final desired behavior, is used to gradually modify behavior.*
4. The desired behavior is reinforced consistently and continuously each time it occurs.
5. When the desired response has been maintained, an **intermittent schedule of reinforcement**, *whereupon reward is contingent on increasing demonstrations of the desired behavior, is used.*
6. When the behavior is learned, occasional reinforcement will maintain the desired behavior.
7. Behavior that has been maintained by an intermittent schedule of reinforcement or partial reinforcement is highly resistant to extinction.
8. Interventions by designated professionals are specified.

TABLE 1-3

Factors to Be Analyzed by Therapist Before Beginning a Behavior Modification Program

1. Maladaptive behavior, or the behavior to be decreased
2. Target or desired observable outcome
3. Current repertoire of behaviors, which is starting point to get to desired behaviors
4. Environmental factors supporting present behavior
5. Specific steps to lead client from current to desired behaviors
6. Consequences considered as rewards and punishments by the client that can be manipulated to alter the client's behavior, for example:
   - Material rewards (money, food, trinkets)
   - Surrogate rewards (tokens, stars, points on a chart)
   - Social rewards (approval or joining in group activities)
   - Behavioral rewards (opportunity to do special activities)
   - Avoidance of punishment

Presentation of each new program step or behavioral unit is contingent on meeting the requirements of the preceding one. Behavior therapy deals with one specific problem at a time, rather than with a combination of all the perceived behavioral problems.

Behavior modification is the *deliberate application of Learning Theory and conditioning, thereby structuring different social environments to teach alternative behaviors and to help the person gain control over behavior and environment.* **Table 1-3** gives basic information (72, 75).

Operant conditioning is used in many situations, including to:

1. Replace undesirable behaviors of children with or without developmental disabilities.
2. Reduce abnormal or self-destructive behavior.
3. Reduce specific maladaptive behaviors such as stuttering, tics, poor hygiene, and messy eating habits.
4. Control physical symptoms through biofeedback.
5. Teach social skills training through rehearsal of appropriate social behaviors.
6. Use role-playing, modeling, feedback, and social reinforcers to change communication patterns.
7. Train parents, teachers, probation officers, and health care workers for their roles.

For example, the child learns to talk not only through imitation of others but because of parental approval and verbal responses that serve as rewards or reinforcement. To teach a client who is mute to talk, you would first give a reward, possibly food or drink, every time there was the slightest movement of lips. Later, the reward would be given only for an utterance. Eventually, reward would be given only for sounds or words, then for phrases, and then for meaningful sentences. The aim of behavioral therapy is maximum benefit for the client and society, but behavioral therapy is primarily reliant on the therapist's judgment and goals for the client.

Psychological Theories

The following theories contribute to understanding developmental levels, effects of internal stimuli, unconscious processes, social relationships, and environmental factors. Concepts from these theories are useful in teaching parents about child rearing, in understanding the developing person through the life span, to educate about health promotion practices, and to understand, assess, and treat the client.

OVERVIEW

Psychoanalytic and neo-analytic theorists *study the person more comprehensively and as a social being, using experimentation, objective observation, and self-report methods. These theorists seek information about changes within the developing person, observe interpersonal relationships, and analyze the impact of social units, norms, and laws on the person. Information from unconscious processes, early development, and the past is used to understand present behavior and goal direction. These theorists give us a perspective of developmental stages, influences on behavior, and methods of dealing with developmental and behavioral problems* (38, 61). Such information can also be relevant in using a developmental approach to client education about health practices.

VIEW OF THE PERSON

Reality is external and interpersonal—what people agree on. The person is a reactive social organism with a developmental past on which to build and a level of readiness that influences or contributes to learning and behavior. The person has maturational and social needs that affect development, learning, and behavior; he or she seeks social role satisfaction and reacts to social values and symbolic processes. The person internalizes societal rules to gain approval, can understand cause-and-effect relationships and complex abstract issues, is capable of insight and emotions, and initiates action and makes choices. The goal of behavior is seen as reduction of symbolic or internal needs or tension (61).

VIEW OF EDUCATION AND THERAPY

Development, learning, and behavior are influenced strongly by the person's developmental level, personal history, cognitive processes and intellect, and intrapsychic processes. The goal of developmental guidance and education or therapy is to help the person become an adaptive, effective social being, aware of and responsive to social reality and patterns. The person has to learn and follow socially prescribed values, customs, and norms to fit into society (38, 61).

As the health care provider, teacher, or therapist, you are a social role model who directs the client. Emphasis is on the person, even in the younger years, understanding the inner self and overt behavior. Increased insight promotes development and maturation. If the person is not ready to learn or change behavior, the parent, teacher, or health care provider acts as an external motivator or facilitator of readiness to change. Rewards are given through approval, affiliation, and various verbal and nonverbal methods. Learning and behavioral change also are self-reinforcing to the person.

Evaluation of application of psychological theory is achieved through gaining feedback from the person, observing and measuring levels of anxiety, interpersonal relationships, or developmental processes. The person's perceptions, feelings, or internal responses and overt behavior present evaluative information, and may lay the base for development and use of research instruments.

PSYCHOANALYTIC AND NEO-ANALYTIC THEORISTS AND THEORIES

Psychoanalytic Theory was developed by Sigmund Freud, and he wrote prolifically about his theory. A number of neo-analytic theorists, such as Erik Erikson, Harry S. Sullivan, and Carl Jung, reinterpreted Freud's theory. **Neo-analysts** *follow Freud's theory in general but have modified some of the original propositions. They maintain the medical model and share the view of intrapsychic determinism as the basis for external behavior. Some take into account the social and cultural contexts in which the person lives.* **The psychodynamic perspective** *refers to*:

1. *Inner psychic and unconscious processes of the person—drives, needs, motivations, feelings, and conflicts.*
2. *Past developmental experiences in causation of behavior and for achieving present developmental tasks and maturity.*
3. *Thoughts and feelings that are not directly observable, but inferred from the individual's overt behavior.*
   (31, 38, 60)

Theories of Freud (26–29), Harry S. Sullivan (38, 76), Erik Erikson (20, 21), and Carl Jung (38, 40, 41) are described briefly. Erikson is referred to in Chapters 9 through 16. ∞ Freud, Sullivan, and Erikson are known as **Stage Theorists** *because they emphasize that the person develops in sequential stages.*

Freud: Psychoanalytic Theory

Sigmund Freud, a Viennese neurologist, developed Psychoanalytic Theory, the first psychological theory to include an explanation of abnormal behavior. Little was known about biological factors; thus he used the medical model of emphasizing pathology and symptoms.

Freud's study of personality laid the foundation for many diverse psychological theories. Many theorists either built on his

work directly or generated other theoretical and therapy approaches. For more information about these theorists, refer to several references (1, 2, 8, 38, 52, 60, 61, 71). Freud's *theory of personality* seems complicated, because it *incorporates many interlocking factors.* Some of his theory is discussed here and referred to in the chapters on childhood. Refer to **Table 1-4** for a summary of Freud's theory (34–38).

Freud proposed five stages of psychosexual development and contended that personality was formed by age 5 (29). See **Table 1-5** for a summary of each stage (28, 29). These stages are described in relation to the developmental era in Chapters 9 through 13. ∞

Commonly used ego adaptive (defense) mechanisms are summarized in **Table 1-6**. They are described throughout the text in relation to the developmental era during which they arise (26, 27, 29).

Anxiety is the *response of tension or dread to perceived or anticipated danger or stress and is the primary motivation for behavior.* There are two types of anxiety-provoking situations. Anxiety may be caused by excessive stimulation that the person cannot handle. Anxiety may also arise from intrapsychic or unconscious conflicts, unacceptable wishes, unknown or anticipated events, superego inhibitions and taboos, and threatened loss of self-image (26). Anxiety at the mild level is probably always present in the awake state but can escalate to panic levels. **Table 1-7** describes the four levels of anxiety and manifestations of each level that were first conceptualized by Hildegard Peplau (62), building on Freud's theory. If anxiety cannot be managed by direct action or coping strategies, the ego initiates unconscious defenses by warding off awareness of the conflict to keep the material unconscious, to lessen discomfort, and to maintain the self-image. Because everyone experiences psychological danger, the use of defense mechanisms clearly is not a special characteristic of maladaptive behavior. Positive mechanisms can also be learned (83). Such mechanisms are used by all people, either singly or in combination, at one time or another, and are considered adaptive (26, 27, 29, 62).

Psychoanalytic Theory has been criticized for many reasons. See an objective critique by Graves (35). In contrast, Greenberg and Fisher (36) reviewed scientific studies done worldwide to check the validity of Freud's ideas and found that Freud's model of personality development and behavior is supported by other studies. His theory continues to influence thought and research, especially in Western cultures, in relation to development and therapy of the ill person (38, 60, 61, 71). Feminist scholars have begun to reassess Freud's theory, in relation to current culture, and recognize the value of some of his ideas and their applicability to understanding men, women, boys, and girls (8).

Freud described the complexities of mental life, which are applicable to client assessment and intervention. *Utilize his insights through the following* (1): (a) much of what we do is motivated by the unconscious or what is outside of conscious awareness; (b) dreams have psychological meaning; (c) infants are active, thinking individuals who have sensual and painful experiences; (d) listening to a client can help the person and therapist gain insights; (e) psychoanalysis (therapy) and biology should be brought together for greater understanding of the person; (f) counseling, recollection, and reflection in the presence of an empathic professional can treat or cure diagnosable diseases.

TABLE 1-4

Summary of Freud's Theory of Personality

Psychic determination	All behavior determined by prior thoughts and mental processes
Psychic structures of the personality	**Id**—*Unorganized reservoir of psychic energy;* furnishes energy for ego and superego, *biological drives, and impulses necessary for survival*
	Operates on **pleasure principle** *(seeking of immediate gratification and avoidance of discomfort)*
	Discharges **tension** *(increased energy)* through reflex physiologic activity and **primary process thinking** *(image formation, drive-oriented behavior, free expression of feelings and impulses, dream-like state, unconscious)*
	Ego—*Establishes relations with environment through conscious perception, feeling, action*
	Controls impulses from id and demands of superego
	Operates on **reality principle** *(external conditions considered and immediate gratification delayed for future gains that can be realistically achieved)*
	Controls access of ideas to conscious
	Appraises environment and reality
	Uses various mechanisms to help person feel emotionally safe
	Guides person to acceptable behavior
	Assists with **secondary process thinking** *(realistic delayed or substitute gratification; realistic thoughts; conscious processes; cognitive strategies)*
	Superego—*Represents internalized moral code based on perceived social rules and norms; restrains expression of instinctual drives; prevents disruption of society*
	Made up of two systems:
	Ego ideal—*Perfection to which person aspires; corresponds to what parents taught was good*
	Conscience—*Responsible for guilt feelings; corresponds to those things parents taught were bad*
Conscious-unconscious continuum	**Conscious**—*All aspects of mental life currently in awareness or easily remembered*
	Preconscious—*Aspects of mental life remembered with help; not currently in awareness*
	Unconscious—*Thoughts, feelings, actions, experiences, dreams not remembered; difficult to bring to awareness; not recognized*
	Existence inferred from effects on behavior
Instincts (drives)	*Inborn psychological or physiologic source of energy*
	Kinds of instincts: self-preservation, preservation of species, life, death
Libido (sexuality or psychic energy)	*Energy arising from hidden drives or impulses involved in conflict*
	Desire for pleasure, sexual gratification, preservation of species
	Not limited to biology or genital areas; includes capacity for loving another
Anxiety	*Response to presence of unconscious conflict, tension, or dread; perceived or anticipated danger; and stress—primary motivation for behavior*
	Basic source is the unconscious; related to loss of self-image
	Kinds of anxiety: (1) neurotic—id-ego conflict; (2) realistic—in response to real dangers in world; (3) moral anxiety—id-superego conflict
	Managed by direct action, coping strategies, or unconscious defense mechanisms
Primary process thinking	*Thought processes based in the id and unconscious; drive-oriented, unable to distinguish between reality and nonreality, primitive, illogical, labile, and without synthesis; process carried out through pictorial, images or dreams*
Secondary process thinking	*Realistic, conscious thought processes based in the ego and occurring in normal waking life;* association of ideas subject to reality conditions and conform to ethical and moral laws; process based on use of words
Cathexis	*Energy responsible for behavior*

TABLE 1-5

Freud's Stages of Psychosexual Development

Stage (years)	Major Body Zone	Activities	Extension to Others
Oral (0–1½)	Mouth (major source of gratification and exploration)	Security—primary need Pleasure from eating and sucking Major conflict—weaning Incorporation (suck, consume, chew, bite, receive)	Sense of *we*—no differentiation or extension Sense of *I* and *other*—minimum differentiation and total incorporation Beginning of ego development at 4–5 months
Anal (1½–3)	Bowel (anus) and bladder source of sensual satisfaction, self-control, and conflict (mouth continues in importance)	Expulsion and retention (differentiation, expelling, controlling, pushing away) (Incorporation still is used) Major conflict—toilet training	Sense of *I* and *other*—separation from *other* and increasing sense of *I* Beginning control over impulses
Phallic (4–6)	Genital region—penis, clitoris (mouth, bowel, and bladder sphincters continue in importance)	Masturbation Fantasy Play activities Experimentation with peers Questioning of adults about sexual topics Major conflict—Oedipus complex, which resolves when child identifies with parent of same sex (Mastery, incorporation, expulsion, and retention continue)	Sense of *I* and *other*—fear of castration in boy Sense of *I* and *other*—strengthened with identification process with parents Sense of *other*—extends to other adults
Latency (6–puberty)	No special body focus	Diffuse activity and relationships (Mastery, incorporation, expulsion, and retention continue)	Sense of *I* and *other*—extends out of nuclear family and includes peers of same sex
Genital (puberty and thereafter)	Penis, vagina (mouth, anus, clitoris)	Develop skills needed to cope with the environment Full sexual maturity and function (Mastery, incorporation, expulsion, and retention continue) Addition of new assets with each stage for gratification Realistic sexual expression Creativity and pleasure in love and work	Sense of *I* and *other*—extends to other adults and peers of opposite sex

Sullivan: Interpersonal Theory of Psychiatry

Harry Stack Sullivan (38, 76), a neo-analyst, formulated the **Interpersonal Theory of Psychiatry**. *This theory was the first to focus on relationships between and among people*, in contrast to Freud's emphasis on the intrapsychic and sexual phenomena and Erikson's focus on biological, emotional, and sociocultural aspects. *Experiences in major life events are the result of either positive or negative interpersonal relationships. Personality development is largely the result of the mother-child relationship, childhood experiences, and interpersonal encounters; however, development continues into adult-*hood. There are two basic needs: **satisfaction** (*biological needs*) and **security** (*emotional and social needs*). Biological and interpersonal needs are interrelated. How biological needs are met in the interpersonal situation determines sense of satisfaction and security and provides avoidance of anxiety.

Sullivan implied that the need to avoid anxiety and the need to gratify basic needs are the primary motivations for behavior. His **concept of anxiety** states that *anxiety has its origin in the prolonged dependency of infancy, urgency of biological and emotional needs, and how the mothering person meets those needs. Anxiety is the result of*

TABLE 1-6

Ego Adaptive or Defense Mechanisms

Mechanism	Definitions/Example
Compartmentalization	*Separation of two incompatible aspects of the psyche from each other to maintain psychological comfort,* behavioral manifestations show the inconsistency. **Example:** The person who attends church regularly and is overtly religious conducts a business that includes handling stolen goods.
Compensation	*Overachievement in one area to offset deficiencies, real or imagined, or to overcome failure or frustration in another area.* **Example:** The student who makes poor grades devotes much time and energy to succeed in music or sports.
Condensation	*Reacting to a single idea with all of the emotions associated with a group of ideas;* expressing a complex group of ideas with a single word or phrase. **Example:** The person says the word *crazy* for many types of mental illness and for feelings of fear and shame or *awesome* for joy and surprise.
Conversion	*Unconscious conflicts are disguised and expressed symbolically by physical symptoms* involving portions of the body, especially the five senses and motor areas. Symptoms are frequently not related to innervation by sensory or motor nerves. **Example:** The person who is under great pressure on the job awakes at 6 A.M. and is unable to walk but is unconcerned about the symptoms.
Denial	*Failure to recognize an unacceptable impulse or undesirable but obvious thought, fact, behavior, conflict, or situation, or its consequences or implications.* **Example:** The alcoholic person believes that he or she has no problem with drinking even though family and work colleagues observe the classic signs.
Displacement	*Release or redirection of feelings and impulses on a safe object or person as a substitute for that which aroused the feeling.* **Example:** The person punches a punching bag after an argument with the boss.
Dissociation	*Repression or splitting off from awareness of a portion of a personality or of consciousness;* however, repressed material continues to affect behavior (compartmentalization). **Example:** A client discusses a conflict-laden subject and goes into a trance.
Emotional isolation	*Repression of the emotional component of a situation, although the person is able to remember the thought, memory, or event;* dealing with problems as interesting events that can be rationally explained but have no feelings attached. **Example:** The person talks about the spouse's death and details of the accident that caused it with an apathetic expression and without crying or signs of grieving.
Identification	*Unconscious modeling of another person so that basic values, attitudes, and behavior are similar to those of a significant person or group, but overt behavior is manifested in an individual manner.* (Imitation is not considered a defense mechanism per se, but imitation usually precedes identification. Imitation is consciously copying another's values, attitudes, movements, etc.) **Example:** The adolescent over time manifests the assertive behavior and states ideas similar to those that she admires in one of her instructors, although she is unaware that her behavior is similar.
Projection	*Attributing one's unacceptable or anxiety-provoking feelings, thoughts, impulses, wishes, or characteristics to another person.* **Example:** The person declares that the supervisor is lazy and prejudiced; colleagues note that this person often needs help at work and frequently makes derogatory remarks about others.
Rationalization	*Justification of behavior or offering a socially acceptable, intellectual, and apparently logical explanation for an act or decision actually caused by unconscious or verbalized impulses.* Behavior in response to unrecognized motives precedes reasons for it. **Example:** A student fails a course but maintains that the course was not important and that the grade can be made up in another course.
Reaction formation	*Unacceptable impulses repressed, denied, and reacted to by opposite overt behavior.* **Example:** A married woman who is unconsciously disturbed by feeling sexually attracted to one of her husband's friends treats him rudely and keeps him at a safe distance.

TABLE 1-6

Ego Adaptive or Defense Mechanisms—continued

Mechanism	Definitions/Example
Regression	*Adopting behavior characteristic of a previous developmental level;* the ego returns to an immature but more gratifying state of development in thought, feeling, or behavior. **Example:** The person takes a nap, curled in a fetal position, on arriving home after a stressful day at work.
Repression	*Automatic, involuntary exclusion of a painful or conflicting feeling, thought, impulse, experience, or memory from awareness.* The thought or memory of the event is not consciously perceived. **Example:** The mother seems unaware of the date or events surrounding her child's death and shows no emotions when the death is discussed.
Sublimation	*Substitution of a socially acceptable behavior for an unacceptable sexual or aggressive drive or impulse.* **Example:** The adolescent is forbidden by her parents to have a date until she graduates from high school. She gives much time and energy to editorial work and writing for the school paper. The editor of the school paper and the faculty advisor are males.
Suppression	*Intentional exclusion of material from consciousness.* **Example:** The husband carries the bills in his pocket for a week before remembering to mail in the payments.
Symbolization	*One object or act unconsciously represents a complex group of objects and acts.* External objects or acts stand for internal or repressed desires, ideas, attitudes, or feelings. The symbol may not overtly appear to be related to the repressed ideas or feelings. **Example:** The husband sends his wife a bouquet of roses, which ordinarily represents love and beauty. But roses have thorns, and his beautiful wife is hard to live with. He consciously focuses on her beauty.
Undoing	*An act, communication, or thought that cancels the significance or partially negates a previous one;* treating an experience as if it had never occurred. **Example:** The husband purchases a gift for his wife after a quarrel the previous evening.

uncomfortable interpersonal relationships, is the chief disruptive force in interpersonal relationships, is contagious through empathic feelings, and can be relieved by being in a secure interpersonal relationship. Relief of anxiety fosters a sense of "good-me" (76).

An important principle for the study and care of people is the **One-Genus Postulate**, which states *we are all more simply human than otherwise, hence more similar than different in basic needs, development, and the meaning of our behavior* (76). This is basic to how nurses perceive clients although cultural differences are acknowledged.

Sullivan's developmental stages and concepts are described in relation to each developmental era. These concepts are pertinent to understanding and care of the developing person and family unit (38, 76).

Erikson: Epigenetic Theory of Personality Development

Erik Erikson (20, 21), a neo-analytic theorist, formulated the **Epigenetic Theory** *based on the principle of the unfolding embryo: Anything that grows has a ground plan and each part has its time of special ascendancy until all parts have arisen to form a functional whole.* A result of mastering the developmental tasks of each stage is a **virtue**, *a feeling of competence or direction.*

Erikson's psychosexual theory enlarges on Psychoanalytic Theory. It is not limited to historical era, specific culture, or personality types. It encompasses development through the life span, is universal to all people, and acknowledges that society, heredity, and childhood experiences all influence the person's development (20, 21). See **Figure 1-3** for Erikson's eight stages of development of the person. The developmental task or crisis for each stage and related virtue are depicted (16, 20, 21).

The *following are basic principles of Erikson's theory, based on cross-cultural studies* (16, 20, 21, 38):

1. There is a step-by-step (stage-by-stage) unfolding of emotional and social development during encounters with the environment. Each stage lays the groundwork for the next stage.
2. Each phase has a specific developmental task to achieve or solve. These tasks describe the order and sequence of human development and the conditions necessary to accomplish them, but actual accomplishment is done at an individual pace, tempo, and intensity.
3. Each psychosexual stage of development is a developmental crisis because there is a radical change in the person's perspective, a shift in energy, and an increased emotional vulnerability. How the person copes with the task and crisis depends on previous developmental strengths and weaknesses.

TABLE 1-7

Levels and Manifestations of Anxiety

Level	Type	Effect
Mild	Physiologic	Tension of needs motivates behavior
		Adaptive to variety of internal and external stimuli
	Cognitive	Attentive, alert, perceptive to variety of stimuli, effective problem solving
	Emotional	No intense feelings, self-concept not threatened
		Use of ego adaptive mechanisms minimal, flexible
		Behavior appropriate to situation
Moderate	Physiologic	Some symptoms may be present
		Accelerated rate of speech; change in pitch of voice
	Cognitive	Perceptual field narrows; responds to directions; repetitive questioning
		Tangible problems solved fairly effectively, at least with direction and support
	Emotional	Selective inattention—focus is on stimuli that do not add to anxiety
		Impatient, irritable, forgetful, demanding, crying, angry
		Uses any adaptive mechanism (e.g., rationalization, denial, displacement) to protect from feelings and meaning of behavior
		(Physiologic, cognitive, and emotional changes of alarm and resistance stages of stress response. Individual functions in normal pattern but may not feel as healthy physically or emotionally as usual; illness may result if feeling persists.)
Severe	Physiologic	Alarm stage changes intensify, and stage of resistance may progress to stage of exhaustion stress response
	Cognitive	Perceptual field narrows; stimuli distorted, focus is on scattered details
		Selective inattention prevails
		Learning and problem solving ineffective
		Clarification or restatement needed repeatedly
		Misinterprets statements
		Unable to follow directions or remember main points
		Unable to plan or make decisions; needs assistance with details
		Disorganized; unable to see connection between events
		Consciousness and lucidity reduced
	Emotional	Self-concept threatened; sense of helplessness or impending doom; mood changes
		Behavior erratic, inappropriate, regressive, inefficient; may be aware of inappropriate behavior but unable to improve
		Many ego defense mechanisms used; dissociation and amnesia may be used
		Disorientation, confusion, suspicion, hallucinations, and delusions may be present
		(Psychoses or physical illness or injury may result.)
Panic	Physiologic	Severe symptoms of exhaustion stage may be ignored
	Cognitive	Sensory ability and attention reduced so that only object of anxiety noticed
		May fail to notice specific object of concern or disastrous event but will be preoccupied with trivial detail
	Emotional	Self-concept overwhelmed; feeling of personality disintegration
		Ego defense mechanism used, often inappropriately and uncontrollably
		Behavior focused on finding relief; may scream, cry, pray, thrash limbs, run, hit others, hurt self
		Often easily distracted; cannot attend or concentrate
		No learning, problem solving, decision making, or realistic judgments
		May become immobilized, assume fetal position, become mute, or be unresponsive to directions
		Needs protection
		(Psychoses may occur.)

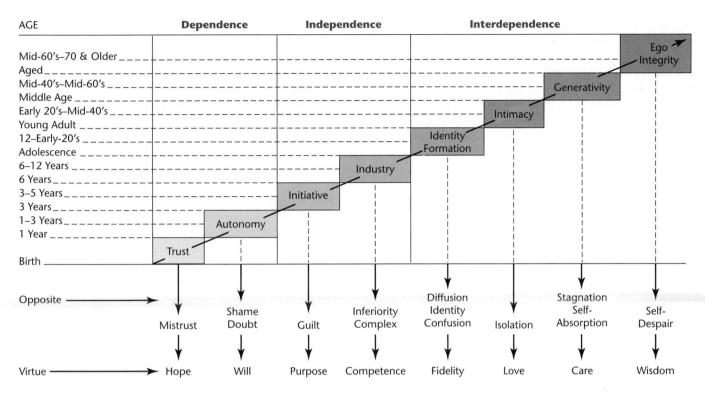

FIGURE ■ 1-3 Erikson's eight stages of the person.

4. The potential inherent in each person evolves if given adequate chance to survive and grow. Anything that distorts the environment essential for development interferes with evolution of the person. Society attempts to safeguard and encourage the proper rate and sequence of the unfolding of human potential so that humanity is maintained.

5. Each developmental task is redeveloped, reworked, and redefined in subsequent stages. Potential for further development always exists.

6. Internal organization is central to development. Maturity increases as the tasks of each era are accomplished, at least in part, in proper order.

Utilize Erikson's theory as described in relation to each developmental era. His theory is pertinent to assessing and understanding the developing person and in implementing nursing and health care.

Jung's Theory

Carl Jung, another neo-analytic theorist, proposed the following assumptions about personality structure (19, 38, 44, 45, 61):

1. **Ego** or **consciousness** includes *awareness of self and the external world.*

2. **Persona** *is the image presented to the outer world, depending on the person's role.*

3. **Shadow** consists of *traits and feelings that cannot be admitted to the self; it is the opposite of ego or self-image.*

4. **Anima** and **animus** in the personality *refer to the characteristics traditionally considered feminine and masculine. Each person has both characteristics or is androgynous or bisexual with the feminine, nurturing, feeling side and the masculine, logical, assertive side.* Socialization forces the person to overemphasize gender characteristics so that the opposite aspect of the person is not usually fully developed.

5. **Personal unconscious** *is unique, contains all the repressed tendencies and feelings that build over the lifetime, and includes the shadow and some of the anima or animus.*

6. **Self** *is the most important force, the unconscious centeredness, wholeness, and meaning. There is an inner urge to balance and reconcile the opposing aspects of personality.*

7. **Individuation** *involves finding the unique way, achieving a measure of psychic balance while separating self from social conformity to goals and values.*

8. There are *two basic personality types or tendencies:*
   a. **Introvert** *refers to being inner-reflective; caught up in one's inner state, fears, hopes, and feelings.* The introvert hesitates in relationships, is more secure in his or her inner world, and takes pleasure in activities that can be done alone.
   b. **Extrovert** *refers to direct and confident initiation of interactions with others.* The extrovert moves outward toward the world and prefers and seeks activities with people.

The early childhood years are not emphasized in this developmental theory. The first period, until age 35 or 40, is a time of outward expansion. After age 40, the person undergoes a transformation and looks for meaning in personal activities. With increasing age, there is increasing reflection. The late 30s and early 40s are important in life transition; this is a time when energy from youthful interests is channeled to cultural and spiritual pursuits (41). Jung's theory is referred to again in the chapters on adulthood. This theory is gaining wider acceptance in understanding of the developing adult. Use concepts of his theory in assessment, counseling, and interdisciplinary conferences.

Existential and Humanistic Theories

OVERVIEW

Existential and humanistic psychologies acknowledge the dynamic aspect of the person but emphasize the impact of environment to a greater degree.

Existentialism has its roots in philosophy, theology, literature, and psychology and *studies the person's uniqueness and existence in a hostile or indifferent world and within the context of history. Existentialism emphasizes freedom of choice, responsibility, satisfaction of ideals, the burden of freedom, discovery of inner self, and consequences of action. Themes addressed include suffering, death, despair, meaninglessness, nothingness, isolation, anxiety, hope, self-transcendence, and finding spiritual meaning.* The transcendence of inevitable suffering, anxiety, and alienation is emphasized (24, 25, 38, 78).

Humanism *emphasizes self-actualization, satisfaction of needs, the individual as a rule unto self, the pleasure of freedom, and realization of innate goodness and creativity. Humanism shares the following assumptions with existentialism* (12, 38, 78): (a) uniqueness of the person, (b) potential of the person, and (c) necessity of listening to or studying the person's perceptions.

Both existentialists and humanists seek to answer the following questions (12, 31, 69, 70, 78):

1. What are the possibilities of the person?
2. From these possibilities, what is an optimum state for the person?
3. Under what conditions is individuality and developmental potential of the person most likely to be reached?

Because all behavior is considered a function of the person's perceptions, *data for study of the person are subjective and come from self-reports, including* (a) feelings at the moment about self and the experience, (b) meaning of the experience, and (c) personal values, needs, attitudes, beliefs, behavioral norms, and expectations. Perception is synonymous with reality and meaning. The person has many components—physical, physiologic, cognitive, emotional, spiritual, cultural, social, and familial—and cannot be adequately understood if studied by individual components. The person is also affected by many variables, both objective and subjective. All behavior is pertinent to and a product of perceptions.

VIEW OF THE PERSON

The person is viewed as a significant, complex, unique whole individual in dynamic interaction with the environment, in the process of becoming, and more than the sum of the parts. The person is constantly changing, expanding perceptual processes, learning, and gaining insights. The person is never quite the same as he or she was even an hour or day earlier, which affects education and counseling practices in health care. The goals of the creative being are feeling adequate and reaching the potential, regardless of age or stage of life. Basic needs are the maintenance and enhancement of the self-concept and a sense of adequacy and self-actualization (12, 53, 54, 69, 78).

Various factors affect perception, including (a) the sensory organs and central nervous system of the person, (b) time for observation, (c) opportunities available to experience events, (d) the external environment, (e) interpersonal relationships, and (f) self-concept (12, 54, 69, 70). What is most important to the person is conscious experience, what is happening to the self at a given time. The person is aware of social values and norms but lives out those values and norms in a way that has been uniquely and personally defined (54).

Self-concept is learned as a consequence of meaningful interactions with others and the world, has a high degree of stability at its core, and changes only with time and opportunity to try new perceptions of self. This person is open to all experiences, develops trust in self, and feels a sense of oneness with other people, depending on the nature of previous contacts.

VIEW OF EDUCATION AND THERAPY

Characteristics of the learner or client are described as follows (69, 70):

1. Is unique, has dignity and worth.
2. Brings a cluster of understandings, skills, values, and attitudes that have personal meaning.
3. Presents total self as sum of reactions to previous experiences and cultural and family background.
4. Wants to learn that which has personal meaning; learns from experience.
5. Wants to be fully involved; learning involves all dimensions of the person.
6. Believes finding the self is more important than facts.

Education and therapy are (a) growth-oriented rather than controlling, (b) rooted in perceptual meaning rather than facts, (c) concerned with people rather than things, (d) focused on the immediate rather than the historical view of people, and (e) hopeful rather than despairing. The goals of education and therapy are the same goals as those of the client: to achieve full functioning and ongoing development, meet individual potential, and continue

---

Practice Point

The health care provider, teacher, or therapist is also a unique, whole person with a self-concept that directly affects the philosophy and style of teaching or counseling. In those roles, consider yourself as central, but be *learner- or client-centered.*

INTERVENTIONS FOR HEALTH PROMOTION

Use the following existential approaches in your health care role:

1. Present the personality as a caring presence.
2. Act as a permissive facilitator.
3. Provide a warm, accepting, supportive environment that is as free from threat and obstacles as possible.

4. Provide an enriched environment and a variety of ways for the person to perceive new experiences and to learn.
5. Demonstrate that all people are perceived and related to in an empathic, cooperative, forward-looking, trustworthy, and responsible approach.
6. Reject the traditional, pessimistic, or mechanical view of people.

movement toward self-actualization. Education and therapy should be presented as a process, not a condition or institution; through the process the person achieves effective behavior. The basic tenets of freedom and responsibility are essential focal points in this approach (12, 61, 69, 70, 78).

Evaluation of this intervention approach includes the client's statements of increased self-esteem and positive self-concept, problem solving to achieve goals, and achievement of optimal functioning. The client validates your use of a supportive therapeutic relationship characterized by warmth, nonpossessive caring, and fostering the person's worth and dignity.

EXISTENTIAL AND HUMANISTIC THEORISTS AND THEORIES

Theorists in this group include the humanist Abraham Maslow (Theory of Motivation and Hierarchy of Needs [52–55]) and the humanist-existentialist Carl Rogers (Theory on Self-concept and Client-centered Therapy [44, 69, 70]). Humanism is the basis for the views of Hildegard Peplau (62). Maslow and Rogers are discussed in this chapter. Peplau's Interpersonal Theory of Nursing and therapeutic relationship concepts are discussed in Chapter 2. ∞

Maslow: Theory of Motivation and Hierarchy of Needs

Abraham Maslow's theory *is based on the study of normal people and mental health, in contrast to other developmental and personality theories.* One of his most important concepts is **self-actualization**, the *tendency to develop one's potential and become a better person* and the need to achieve the sense of self-acceptance and direction implicit in self-actualization. Thus, people are not static but are always in the process of becoming different and more mature (52–55). In self-actualizing people, the unconscious is creative, loving, and positive.

The needs that motivate self-actualization can be represented in a hierarchy of relative order and predominance. The basic needs are listed in **Table 1-8**. Although *Maslow ranked these basic human needs from lowest to highest, they do not necessarily occur in a fixed order.* The physiologic and safety needs (deficiency needs), however, are dominant and must be met before higher needs can be se-

cured. Personal growth needs are those for love and belonging, self-esteem and recognition, and self-actualization. The highest needs of self-actualization, knowledge, and aesthetic expression may never be as fully gratified as those at lower levels. Individual growth and self-fulfillment are a continuing, lifelong process of becoming (53, 55).

To motivate the person toward self-actualization and health, there must be freedom to speak, to pursue creative potential, and to inquire; an atmosphere of justice, honesty, fairness, and order; and environmental stimulation and challenge. Many have trouble moving toward self-actualization because of the environment in which they live. For example, socialization practices may hinder females in fully using their intellectual abilities. Males may be inhibited from expressing emotions of tenderness, love, or need for others by cultural norms. Deprivation of growth needs results in feelings of despair and depression and a sense that life is meaningless (52–55).

Utilize this theory in all client care. Basic needs are always considered in client care, whether teaching health promotion strategies or caring for the ill or injured person, including family members.

Evaluate care pertinent to the needs and progress of recovery or maintenance of health manifested by the client. Some needs may be more urgent or dominant than others.

Carl Rogers: Theory on Self-Concept and Client-Centered Therapy

Carl Rogers' Theory on Self-Concept *presents a humanistic-existentialist perspective on personality and a focus on self-concept. Self-actualization is a key concept in his theory.* Rogers assumed that the person sees self as the center of a continually changing world and responds to the world as it is perceived. The ability to achieve self-understanding, self-actualization, and acceptance by others is based on experience and interaction with other people. The person who felt wanted and highly valued as a child is likely to have a positive self-image, be thought well of by others, and have the capacity to achieve self-actualization. Optimal adjustment results in what Rogers called the *fully functioning person who demonstrates the following behaviors:* (a) accepts self, (b) avoids a personality facade, (c) is genuine and honest, (d) is increasingly self-directive and autonomous, (e) is open to new experiences, (f) avoids being driven

TABLE 1-8

Maslow's Theory of Hierarchy of Needs

Needs*	Characteristics
Physiologic (most basic)	Requirements for oxygen, water, food, temperature control, elimination, shelter, exercise, sleep, sensory stimulation, and sexual activity met
	Needs cease to exist as means of determining behavior when satisfied, reemerging only if blocked or frustrated
Safety	Able to secure shelter
	Sense of security, dependency, consistency, stability
	Maintenance of predictable environment, structure, order, fairness, limits
	Protection from immediate or future danger to physical well-being
	Freedom from fear, anxiety, chaos, and certain amount of routine
Love and belonging	Sense of affection, love, and acceptance from others
	Sense of companionship and affiliation with others
	Identification with significant others
	Recognition and approval from others
	Group interaction
	Not synonymous with sexual needs, but sexual needs may be motivated by this need
Esteem from others	Awareness of own individuality, uniqueness
	Feelings of self-respect and worth and respect from others
	Sense of confidence, independence, dignity
	Sense of competence, achievement, success, prestige, status
	Recognition from others for accomplishments
Self-actualization (highest level)	Acceptance of self and others
	Empathetic with others
	Self-fulfillment
	Ongoing emotional and spiritual development
	Desire to attain standards of excellence and individual potential
	Use of talents, being productive and creative
	Experiencing fully, vividly, without self-consciousness
	Having peak experiences
Aesthetic	Desire for beauty, harmony, order, attractive surroundings
	Interest in art, music, literature, dance, creative forms
Knowledge and understanding	Desire to understand, systematize, organize, analyze, look for relations and meanings
	Curiosity; desire to know as much as possible
	Attraction to the unknown or mysterious

*Needs are listed in ascending order. Physiologic needs are most basic and self-actualization is highest level of needs. Adapted from references 52 and 53.

by other people's expectations or the cultural norms, and (g) has a low level of anxiety (38, 61, 69–71).

Each person is basically rational, socialized, and constructive. Behavior is goal directed and motivated by needs. Unlike the intrapsychic and interpersonal theorists, Rogers stated that current needs are the only ones the person endeavors to satisfy (70).

Utilize Rogers' technique of client-centered therapy to bring about behavioral change. Convey complete acceptance, respect, and empathy for the client. Avoid interpretations and advice. Providing this high degree of acceptance helps the person to meet health needs. Perceptions and behavior change. The person may then continue the self-actualizing process. Chapter 2 ∞ discusses use of Rogers's technique as it can be applied to the nurse-client relationship.

Cognitive Theories

Cognitive Theory *deals with the person as an information processor and problem solver. The cognitive perspective is concerned with internal processes but emphasizes how people acquire, interpret, and use information to solve life's problems and to remain normal or healthy.* It emphasizes conscious processes, present thoughts, and problem-solving strategies. Relationships among emotions, motivations, and cognitive processes are studied.

BANDURA: SOCIAL LEARNING THEORY

Albert Bandura's **Social Learning Theory** states that *learning occurs without reinforcement, conditioning, or trial-and-error behavior* *because people can think and anticipate consequences of behavior and act accordingly. This theory emphasizes* (3–7):

1. Cognitive processes, modeling, environmental influences, and the person's self-directed capacity to influence development, learning, and behavior.
2. Importance of vicarious, symbolic, and self-regulatory processes in psychological functioning.
3. Capacity of the person to use symbols, represent events, analyze conscious experience, communicate with others at any distance in time and space, and plan, create, imagine, and engage in foresightful action.

The person does not simply react to external forces; he or she selects, organizes, and transforms impinging stimuli and thus exercises some influence over personal behavior. **Bandura's Model of Causation** *involves the interaction of three components: (a) the person with unique characteristics, perceptions, beliefs, feelings, attitudes, values, and goals, which are affected by cognitive and biological events; (b) the external environment, physical setting, and various stimuli; and (c) behavior choices. Each component affects the others* (5–7).

The person may be motivated by ideas or fantasies of future consequences or by personal goal-setting behavior. If the person wants to accomplish a certain goal and there are distractions from the task, the person visualizes how he or she will feel when the goal is attained. People respond evaluatively to their own behavior and tend to persist until the behavior or performance meets the goal (3, 6, 7).

Bandura proposes that learning occurs through **modeling**, *imitation of another's behavior. Four interacting mental processes must be present for modeling to occur* (3, 4):

1. **Attention:** *The learner must perceive the model.*
2. **Memory:** *The learner must encode the information obtained from observing the model in a form that can be used at a later time.*
3. **Motor control:** *The learner must be able to use this coded information to guide his or her own actions.*
4. **Motivation:** *The learner must have some reason or inducement to perform the modeled actions.*

These processes are involved in behavior that depends on information gained from the environment. Learning is achieved primarily through interactions with other people. Social rewards such as praise and acceptance help motivate and reinforce such learning, as well as simple observation of other people. People learn and modify their cognitive constructs throughout life as they interact with others. The person acts on the environment (and the environment on the person) in a continuous lifelong process (3, 4, 6, 7).

According to Bandura's theory, the client can learn about achieving normal development and health through modeling. Imitation is one of the most effective forms of learning. Teach parents that babies learn to speak by imitating the sounds of their parents, and older children learn a number of behaviors by watching their teachers, parents, or peers. People learn how to be normal. Maladaptive behavior arises from modeling when the child imitates ineffective behavior in parents or others. Teach that research also shows the power of watching television on people's behavior and that for some people the model of aggressive behavior will cause later unhealthy or acting-out behavior (3). This research is discussed further in Chapter 12. ∞

Bandura identified self-efficacy as a mediator in behavior. **Self-efficacy** is a *judgment about one's ability to organize and execute action and to accomplish a certain level of performance in a situation.* Self-efficacy is based on mastered experiences, vicarious experiences or observation of other people doing the behavior, verbal persuasion from another to adjust behavior, and physiologic states or internal cues that are evidence of the capability or deficit. Bandura also described the importance of health care professionals and parents giving information, rather than just fear-producing statements, to motivate change (6, 7).

Utilize Bandura's research, which combines aspects of behavioral and psychodynamic theories and is pertinent to understanding certain aspects of the developing person. His theory is pertinent to nursing and health care, especially the educational role in promoting health (3–7, 38, 61).

PIAGET: COGNITIVE DEVELOPMENT THEORY

Jean Piaget's (64–67) **Theory of Cognitive Development** *is concerned with the child's thinking at particular periods of life and with differences among well children of a specific age.* A great amount of empirical data was used in developing the theory. Development is not just **maturation,** an *unfolding of the innate growth process,* or **learning,** an *accumulation of experiences.* Rather, development is an active process resulting from **equilibration**, an *internal force that is set in motion to organize thinking when the child's belief system develops sufficiently to contain self-contradictions.*

Four factors interact within the person to stimulate mental development (66):

1. Maturation of the nervous and endocrine systems, which provides physical capabilities.
2. Experience involving action, with a consequent discovery of properties of objects.
3. Social interaction with opportunity to observe a wide variety of behaviors and gain direct instruction and to receive feedback about individual performance.
4. An internal self-regulation mechanism that responds to environmental stimuli.

Intelligence is an adaptive process by which the person modifies and structures the environment to fit personal needs and also modifies self in response to environmental demands. By interaction with the environment, the person constructs reality by assimilation, accommodation, and adaptation. **Assimilation** is *taking new content and experiences into the mind or cognitive structure.* **Accommodation** is the *revising, realigning, and readjusting of cognitive structure to take into account the new content.* **Adaptation** is the *change that results from the first two processes.* The innate, inborn processes of the person are the essential force to start the process of equilibration or cognitive growth. Cognitive development proceeds from motor activity to interaction with the wider social world and, finally, to abstract ideas. Development is seen as solidly rooted in what already exists, and it displays a continuity with the past. Adaptations do not develop in isolation; all form a coherent pattern so that the totality of biological life is adapted to its environment (64–67, 81).

The thinking process is explained by schematic mental structures or mental pictures formed in response to stimuli. A **schema** is a *cognitive structure, a complex concept encompassing both motor behavior and internalized thought processes.* A schema involves paying attention and the mental picture that is formed as a result of the sensory process. Thinking eventually involves using unique combinations of mental pictures, forming concepts, internalizing use of language or subvocal speech, drawing implications, and making judgments. When these internal actions become integrated into a coherent, logical system, they are considered logical operations and, in turn, structure future learning. *Learning is determined by* (a) what is observed, (b) whether new information is fit into old schemata accurately or in a distorted way, and (c) how much increase in competence results from the encounter or experience (64–67).

Piaget, a stage theorist, divided human development into four periods: sensorimotor, preoperational, concrete operations, and formal operations. Table 1-9 summarizes the periods and stages. In each stage, the person demonstrates interpretation and use of the environment through certain behavior patterns. He or she incorporates and restructures the previous stage and refines the ability to perceive and understand. Suggested ages for each stage are indicated, but innate intellectual ability and environmental factors cause variation (64, 65–67, 81). These periods are discussed with development of the infant, toddler, preschooler, schoolchild, adolescent, and adult.

Use information about these stages to determine the client's mental development. Develop educational approaches and activities that correspond to the client's cognitive developmental level.

NEO-PIAGETIAN THEORY: INFORMATION PROCESSING

The **Neo-Piagetian approach** *does not propose stages of cognitive development but, like Piaget, sees people as active thinkers about their world. People learn by becoming efficient at processing information.* These theorists *study mental processes underlying intelligent behavior; perception, attention, memory, and problem solving; and how people acquire, transform, and use sensory information through active manipulation of symbols or mental images.* They look at the mind as a computer. Practice enables learning, since there is a limit to what a person can keep in mind. *With practice, an idea or skill becomes automatic, which frees the person to learn additional information and do more complex problem solving.* These theorists believe learning does not occur in demarcated stages but is more gradual and continuous. However, Information-Processing Theory neglects study of creativity, motivation, and social interaction as they relate to cognitive development (8, 60, 71).

According to this theory, information is taken from the environment, through the senses, and held in memory: the first memory storage. If the person pays attention, the information is transferred to the short-term memory storage. The short-term memory can hold only about seven pieces of information at a time, so the information is either forgotten or processed to the long-term memory storage. To save information at this third level, organizing and hearing it is necessary. Retrieval may be difficult. As the child grows older, information is processed more efficiently and comprehensively. The child develops **metacognition**, *an awareness of how to think and learn, and an understanding of self as a learner.* Thus, a knowledge base is developed through the life span. However, knowledge is specialized, depending on the information and skills accumulated (8, 60, 71).

Acknowledge that what you taught the person earlier about health behaviors or practices that foster development of the child may be forgotten. Review and demonstrate what has been taught; and have the client repeat the directions or the demonstration.

VYGOTSKY: SOCIOCULTURAL THEORY

Russian psychologist Lev Vygotsky was a prominent proponent of the culture's contextual perspective, particularly as it applies to children's cognitive development. In contrast with Bronfenbrenner, who described contextual systems as centered around the individual person, Vygotsky's central focus was the social, cultural, and historical environment and time of the child. To understand cognitive development, he maintained, one must look to the social processes from which a child's thinking is derived. The culture provides the practices, the tools, and the information or knowledge (8, 60).

Vygotsky's Sociocultural Theory, like Piaget's theory, *emphasizes children's active engagement with their environment. Cognitive growth is a collaborative* process. *Children learn through social interaction. Shared activities help children to internalize their society's ways of thinking and behaving and to make those ways their own* (83). Adults and children learn from each other, and children learn from their peers (9). In contrast, Piaget described the solo mind taking in and interpreting information about the world.

According to Vygotsky, adults (or more advanced peers) must help direct and organize a child's learning before the child can master and internalize it. This guidance is most effective in helping children cross the **zone of proximal (nearby) development (ZPD),** *the gap between what they are already able to do and what they are not quite ready to accomplish by themselves.* With the right kind of guidance, however, they can perform the task successfully. In the course of the collaboration, parents, teachers, peers, or others engage in **scaffolding,** *temporarily supporting the child to do the task and, when the child is ready, shifting responsibility for directing and monitoring learning* to the child (8, 60). For example, when an adult teaches a child to float, the adult first supports the child in the water and then lets go gradually as the child's body relaxes into a horizontal position. When the child seems ready, the adult withdraws all but one finger and finally lets the child float free. The process of apprenticeship in thinking or guided participation begins with teaching the child and extends into adulthood.

When you are in your educator role, the client (novice) develops competencies in knowledge, behavior, or any skill from interactions with you, the more skilled person or mentor. In guided participation neither the client (student) nor you (teacher) is passive; each learns from the other in words and activities. As you

TABLE 1-9

Summary of Piaget's Theory of Cognitive Development

Period	Age	Characteristics
Sensorimotor Period		
Stage 1: Use of reflexes	0–1 month	Behavior innate, reflexive, specific, predictable to specific stimuli
		Example: sucking, grasping, eye movements, startle (Moro reflex)
Stage 2: First acquired adaptations and primary circular reactions	1–4 months	Initiates, prolongs, and repeats behavior not previously occurring
		Acquires response to stimulus that creates another stimulus and response
		Modifies innate reflexes to more purposeful behavior, repeated if satisfying
		Learns feel of own body as physiologic stabilization occurs
		Example: looks at object, reaches for it, and continues to repeat until vision, reaching, and mouthing are coordinated
Stage 3: Secondary circular reactions	4–8 months	Learns from unintentional behavior
		Motor skills and vision further coordinated as infant learns to prolong or repeat interesting act
		Interest in environment around self
		Explores world from sitting position
		Assimilates new objects into old behavior pattern
		Behavior increasingly intentional
		Example: looks for object that disappears from sight, continues to drop object from different locations, which adult continues to pick up
Stage 4: Coordination of secondary schema acquisition of instrumental behavior, active search for vanished objects	8–12 months	Uses familiar behavior patterns in new situation to accomplish goal
		Differentiates objects, including mother from stranger (stranger anxiety)
		Retains memory of object hidden from view
		Combines actions to obtain desired, hidden object; explores object
		Imitates others when behavior finished
		Develops individual habits
		Cognitive development enhanced by increasing motor and language skills
Stage 5: Tertiary circular reactions and discovery of new means by active experimentation	12–18 months	Invents new behavior not previously performed
		Uses fewer previous behaviors
		Repeats action without random movements
		Explores variations that occur when same act accomplished
		Varies action deliberately as repeats behavior
		Uses trial-and-error behavior to discover solution to problem
		Differentiates self from object and object from action performed by self; increasing exploration of how objects function
		Invents new means to solve problems and variation in behavior essential to later symbolic behavior and concept formation
Stage 6: Internal representation of action in external world	18–24 months	Pictures events to self; follows through mentally to some degree
		Imitates when model out of sight
		Forms mental picture of external body, of body in same space with another object, and of space in limited way
		Uses deliberate trial and error in solving problems
Preoperational Period		
	2–7 years	Internalizes schemata of more and more of the environment, rules, and relationships
		Forms memories to greater extent
		Uses fantasy or imitation of others in behavior and play
		Intermingles fantasy and reality
		Uses words to represent objects and events more accurately; symbolic behavior increases

continued

TABLE 1-9

Summary of Piaget's Theory of Cognitive Development—continued

Period	Age	Characteristics
		Egocentric (self-centered in thought)—focuses on single aspect of object and neglects other attributes because of lack of experience and reference systems, which results in false logic
		Follows rules in egocentric way; rules external to self
		Is static and irreversible in thinking; cannot transform from one state to another (e.g., ice to water)
		Develops story or idea while forgetting original idea so that final statements disconnected, disorganized; answer not connected to original idea in monologue
		Tries logical thinking; at times sounds logical but lacks perspective so that false logic and inconsistent, unorganized thinking result
		Is magical, global, primitive in reasoning
		Begins to connect past to present events, not necessarily accurate
		Links events by sequence rather than causality
		Deals with information by recall; begins to categorize
		Is **anthropomorphic** (attributes human characteristics to animals and objects)
		Unable to integrate events separated by time, past to present
		Lacks reversibility in thinking
		Unable to anticipate how situation looks from another viewpoint
Preconceptual stage	2–4 years	Forms images or preconcepts on basis of thinking just described
		Lacks ability to define property or to denote hierarchy or relationships of objects
		Constructs concepts in global way
		Unable to use time, space, equivalence, and class inclusion in concept formation
Intuitive stage	4–7 years	Forms concepts increasingly; some limitations
		Defines one property at a time
		Has difficulty stating definition but knows how to use object
		Uses transductive logic (from general to specific) rather than deductive or inductive logic
		Begins to classify in ascending or descending order; labels
		Begins to do seriation; reverses processes and ordinality
		Begins to note cause-effect relationships
Concrete Operations Period		
	7–11 years (or beyond)	Organizes and stabilizes thinking; more rational
		See interrelationships increasingly
		Does mental operations using tangible, visible references
		Able to **decenter** (sees other perspectives; associates or combines events; understands reversibility [e.g., add-subtract, ice–water transformation])
		Recognizes number, length, volume, area, weight is the same even when perception of object changes
		Develops conversation as experience is gained with physical properties of objects

TABLE 1-9

Summary of Piaget's Theory of Cognitive Development—continued

Period	Age	Characteristics
Formal Operations Period		
	12 years and beyond	Manifests adultlike thinking
		Not limited by own perception or concrete references for ideas
		Combines various ideas into concepts
		Coordinates two or more reference systems
		Develops morality or restraint and cooperation in behavior
		Uses rules to structure interactions in socially acceptable way
		Uses probability concept
		Works from definition or concept only to solve problem
		Solves problem mentally and considers alternatives before acting
		Considers number of variables at one time
		Links variables to formulate hypotheses
		Begins to reason deductively and inductively instead of solving problem by action
		Relates concepts or constructs not readily evident in external world
		Formulates advanced concepts of proportions, space, destiny, momentum
		Increases intellectual ability to include art, science, humanities, religion, philosophy
		Is increasingly less egocentric

teach about parenting and healthy behaviors, incorporate an understanding of the client's cultural context. Foster relationships or scaffolding with supportive others who can be a role model or teach the client. Close the gaps (ZPD) between what is known and what needs to be learned through questions, teaching materials, and activities. Be accepting that the client may learn more from others than from you.

Moral Development Theories

KOHLBERG'S THEORY OF MORAL DEVELOPMENT

Kohlberg's Theory of Moral Development *is related to cognitive and emotional development and to societal values and norms and is divided into stages* (45–48). Moral reasoning focuses on 10 universal values: punishment, property, affection, authority, law, life, liberty, distribution of justice, truth, and sexual behavior. A conflict between two or more of these values necessitates a moral choice and justification by the individual, requiring systematic problem solving and other cognitive capabilities (45–48, 68).

Kohlberg theorized that a person's moral reasoning process and behavior develop through stages over varying lengths of time. *Each* **moral stage** *is based or dependent on the* **reason** *for behavior and shows an organized system of thought. The person's thinking and behavior is consistent with the level of moral judgment. The person is considered in a specific stage when the same level of reason for action*

is given at least half the time. More advanced logical thinking is needed for each successive moral stage. One criterion of moral maturity, the ability to decide autonomously what is right and caring, is lacking in the Preconventional and Conventional Levels because the person is following the commands of authority figures. If the person is at Piaget's Stage of Concrete Operations, the person is limited to the Preconventional or Conventional Levels of moral reasoning. Even the person in the Stage of Formal Operations may not be beyond the Conventional Level of moral maturity. Kohlberg found that 50% of late adolescents and adults are capable of formal operations thinking, but only 10% of these adults demonstrated the Postconventional Level of behavior. Thus the person moves through stages, but few people progress through all six stages. However, certain types of educational experiences can stimulate development of moral reasoning (48). **Table 1-10** shows the three levels and six stages (45–48).

Kohlberg added a seventh stage of moral reasoning shortly before his death. This stage moves beyond considerations of justice and has more in common with self-transcendence and faith explained in religious and Eastern philosophies. He asked: Why be moral? He believed the answer was to achieve a cosmic perspective, a sense of unity with the cosmos, nature, or God. This perspective enables the person to see moral issues from a universal whole, seeing that everything is connected. All actions of a person affect everyone else and everything else, and consequences rebound on the doer. The person experiences a oneness with the ultimate conditions of life and being (60, 68, 71). Moral development is discussed in relation to each developmental era in Chapters 9 through 16. ∞

TABLE 1-10

Kohlberg's Theory of Moral Development

Level	Stage
Preconventional Person is responsive to cultural rule of labels of good and bad, right or wrong. Externally established rules determine right or wrong actions. Person reasons in terms of punishment, reward, or exchange of favors.	I. *Punishment and Obedient Orientation* Fear of punishment, not respect for authority, is the reason for decisions, behavior, and conformity. *Good* and *bad* are defined in terms of physical consequences to the self from parental, adult, or authority figures. The person defers to superior power or prestige of the person who dictates rules ("I'll do something because you tell me and to avoid getting punished"). Average age: toddler to 7 years
Egocentric focus	II. *Instrumental Relativist Orientation* Conformity is based on egocentricity and narcissistic needs. The person's decisions and behavior are usually based on what provides satisfaction out of concern for self. Something is done to get something in return. Occasionally the person does something to please another for pragmatic reasons. There is no feeling of justice, loyalty, or gratitude. These concepts are expressed physically ("I'll do something if I get something for it or because it pleases you"). Average age: preschooler through school age
Conventional Person is concerned with maintaining expectations and rules of the family, group, nation, or society. A sense of guilt has developed and affects behavior. The person values conformity, loyalty, and active maintenance of social order and control. Conformity means good behavior or what pleases or helps another and is approved.	III. *Interpersonal Concordance Orientation* A. Decisions and behavior are based on concerns about others' reactions; the person wants others' approval or a reward. The person has moved from egocentricity to consideration of others as a basis for behavior. Behavior is judged by the person's intentions ("I'll do something because it will please you or because it is expected"). B. An empathic response, based on understanding of how another person feels, is a determinant for decisions and behavior ("I'll do something because I know how it feels to be without; I can put myself in your shoes"). Average age: school age through adulthood
Societal focus	IV. *Law-and-Order Orientation* The person wants established rules from authorities, and the reason for decisions and behavior is that social and sexual rules and traditions demand the response. The person obeys the law just because it is the law or out of respect for authority and underlying morality of the law. The law takes precedence over personal wishes, good intentions, and conformity to group stereotypes ("I'll do something because it's the law and my duty"). Average age: adolescence and adulthood

TABLE 1-10

Kohlberg's Theory of Moral Development—continued

Level	Stage
Postconventional The person lives autonomously and defines moral values and principles that are from personal identification with group values. He or she lives according to principles that are universally agreed on and that the person considers appropriate for life.	V. *Social Contract Legalistic Orientation* The social rules are not the sole basis for decisions and behavior because the person believes a higher moral principle applies, such as equality, justice, or due process. The person defines right actions in terms of general individual rights and standards that have been agreed on by the whole society but is aware of relativistic nature of values and opinions. The person believes laws can be changed as people's needs change. The person uses freedom of choice in living up to higher principles but believes the way to make changes is through the system. Outside the legal realm, free agreement and contracts are the binding elements of obligation ("I'll do something because it is morally and legally right, even if it isn't popular with the group"). Average age: middle-age or older adults
Universal focus	VI. *Universal Ethical Principle Orientation* Decisions and behavior are based on internalized rules, on conscience rather than on social laws, and on self-chosen ethical and abstract principles that are universal, comprehensive, and consistent. The rules are not concrete moral rules but instead encompass the Golden Rule, justice, reciprocity, equality of human rights, and respect for the dignity of human beings as individual persons. Human life is inviolable. The person believes there is a higher order than social order, has a clear concept of civil disobedience, and will use self as an example to right a wrong. The person accepts injustice, pain, and death as an integral part of existence but works to minimize injustice and pain for others ("I'll do something because it is morally, ethically, and spiritually right, even if it is illegal and I get punished and even if no one else participates in the act"). Average age: middle-age or older adult (Few people maintain this stage. Examples of this stage are seen in times of crisis or extreme situations.)

Data from references 45–48.

Development of moral judgment is stimulated whenever the person (45):

1. Can work through inadequate modes of thinking.
2. Has opportunity for group discussion of values and can participate in a group decision making about moral issues.
3. Has opportunity to assume responsibility for the consequences of behavior.

Kohlberg's theory has application to nursing, education, and family counseling. Studies show that moral development continues as he described through adulthood (15). The client's willingness or ability to stop unhealthy behavior and change life patterns to foster health may be influenced by the client's moral stage of development and associated behaviors. Continued avoidance of your educational suggestions or continued practices that negatively affect the self or others may be associated with a Preconventional Level of development. The person may need more overt positive attention in order to try new behaviors, if he or she feels those efforts will result in your overt approval.

GILLIGAN'S THEORY OF MORAL DEVELOPMENT

Gilligan's research on moral development has focused on women in contrast to Kohlberg's research focus on men. Gilligan found that moral development proceeds through three levels and two transitions, with each level representing a more complex understanding of the relationship of self and others and each transition resulting in a crucial reevaluation of the conflict between selfishness and responsibility. Women define the moral problem in the context of human relationships, exercising care and avoiding hurt. In Gilligan's studies, women's moral judgment proceeded from initial concern with survival, to a focus on goodness, to a principled understanding of others' need for care. **Table 1-11** summarizes

TABLE 1-11

Gilligan's Theory of Moral Development

Level	Characteristics
Orientation of Individual Survival	*Concentrates on what is practical and best for self;* selfish; dependent on others.
Transition 1: From Selfishness to Responsibility	Realizes connection to others; thinks of responsible choice in terms of another as well as self.
Goodness as Self-Sacrifice	*Sacrifices personal wishes and needs to fulfill others' wants* and to have others think well of her; feels responsible for others' actions; holds others responsible for her choices; dependent position; indirect efforts to control others often turn into manipulation through use of guilt; aware of connectedness with others.
Transition 2: From Goodness to Truth	*Makes decisions on personal intentions and consequences of actions rather than on how she thinks others will react;* takes into account needs of self and others; wants to be good to others but also honest by being responsible to self; increased social participation; assumes more responsibilities.
Morality of Nonviolence	*Establishes moral equality between self and others; assumes responsibility for choice in moral dilemmas;* follows injunction to hurt no one, including self, in all situations; conflict between selfishness and selflessness; judgment based on view of consequences and intentions instead of appearance in the eyes of others.

Data from references 32–34.

the three levels and two transitions of moral development proposed by Gilligan (32, 33).

In your practice with individual clients and in the broader health care system, the concepts by Kohlberg and by Gilligan can be incorporated to address concerns and advocacy for individual care and for eliminating inequality or disparity in health care services.

Focus on justice and issues of inequality and oppression related to populations, and the value of reciprocal rights and equal respect for individuals. The care focus proposed by Gilligan is concerned with issues of abandonment and values the ideals of attention and response to need (32, 33). Cooper describes how Gilligan's value of caring makes it pertinent to nursing (18). As you combine both perspectives in your client care, help clients incorporate them into their moral development. More research in all age groups, men and women, and all races and ethnic groups is needed to better understand moral development.

Health Care and Nursing Applications

Theory application to assessment and understanding the developing person, and to intervention and health promotion has been incorporated throughout the chapter in relation to each theory.

Table 1-12 summarizes how the theories discussed in this chapter can be applied in nursing and health care practice. Applications will be discussed in chapters throughout the book in relation to the developing person and the family, understanding influences on the person and family unit, and fostering healthy behaviors.

Evaluations of intervention statements have been interwoven throughout the chapter. Other evaluation criteria can be developed from theory descriptions and described applications.

TABLE 1-12

Health Promotion Implications of Selected Theories

Theorist/Theory	Practice Implications
Biological Theory	1. In assessment, planning, intervention, and evaluation, relate information previously presented about genetic inheritance and biochemical, neurophysiologic, immunologic, maturational, and other biological factors.
	2. In assessment, consider multifactorial effects and polygenic inheritance.
	3. Relate other physiologic theory to presented content to promote health, foster developmental processes, and assist clients during nursing and health care.
Ecological and Social Systems Theory	1. Consider self as an individual system as well as part of other systems.
	2. Consider client (individual, family, group, or community) as part of a system in implementing nursing process and health care.
	3. Assess client in totality and the relationships and interactions between parts: physiologic, psychological, spiritual, and sociocultural. Dysfunction in one part affects all parts.
	4. Consider client as a system that has definite range for absorption, processing, and retention of stimuli. Avoid overstimulation or deprivation of stimuli. Assess needs and intervene accordingly.
	5. Help client determine resources and supportive systems that will maintain or return function and wellness.
Skinner's Operant Conditioning Theory	1. Assess, intervene, teach, and evaluate, using the guidelines previously described for Behavioral Theory application.
	2. Follow the general procedure for behavior modification:
	a. Plan what behavior is to be established; plan what is to be taught and at what specific time. Objectives are specific. Follow the teaching or treatment plan explicitly.
	b. Determine available reinforcers. Feedback from physical sensations, excelling over others, or the teacher's affection—all may reinforce. The only way to determine whether a consequence is rewarding is to observe its effect on the behavior associated with it.
	c. Identify the responses that can be made by the person.
	d. Plan how reinforcements can be efficiently scheduled so the behavior will be repeated. Reinforcements must immediately and intermittently follow the desired behavior.
	e. Evaluate evidence of behavior change.
Freud's Psychoanalytic Theory	1. Gain insight into own behavior to add to personal maturity and understanding of others.
	2. Use constructs of id, ego, superego, conscious–unconscious continuum, manifestations of anxiety and defense mechanisms, and psychosexual development in assessment and intervention.
	3. Consider all behavior as meaningful; overt behavior may hide inner need or conflict.
	4. Use knowledge of psychosexual development to teach parents about norms and meaning of child's behavior.
Sullivan's Interpersonal Theory	1. Use the One-Genus Postulate for nursing practice with clients from all settings and backgrounds.
	2. Assess developmental stage and task; teach family about basic needs during development and need for nurturing parent and others.
	3. Promote positive experiences for client so that anxiety is reduced and positive self-concept can develop.
Erikson's Epigenetic Theory	1. Assess and gain insight into own stage of development.
	2. Use knowledge of eight stages and psychosexual tasks in assessment and intervention with clients and teaching parents about child development.
	3. Help clients and staff realize that emotional development is lifelong process and that society influences health and behavior.
Jung's Theory	1. Assess personality tendencies.
	2. Promote self-acceptance, including masculine and feminine characteristics.
	3. Assist person in finding unique self; balance spirituality.
	4. Promote reflection, finding meaning of life.

continued

TABLE 1-12

Health Promotion Implications of Selected Theories—continued

Theorist/Theory	Practice Implications
Existential Theory	1. Realize each person is in charge of own destiny; each person is primary agent of change and is responsible for own future. Destiny is not in hands of others. 2. Consider basic conflicts that are outgrowths of confrontation with existence—death, freedom, helplessness, loss, isolation, aloneness, anxiety, and meaninglessness—and promote reflection about these life issues. 3. Be a facilitator who understands and accepts the person as being and becoming. Main themes of therapy are self-awareness, self-determination, search for meaning, and relatedness. 4. Assist person in learning how to confront self, how behavior is viewed by others, how others feel about own behavior, and how behavior contributes to opinions about self. 5. Assist person to learn how to change; give support to reduce anxiety, low self-esteem, and loneliness. 6. Help person move to self-actualization and achieve maximum potential.
Maslow's Theory of Motivation and Hierarchy of Needs	1. Assess with a focus on hierarchy of needs. Planning and intervention must consider need hierarchy and priorities in care. 2. Care for person as a unified whole, not divided into components of needs. 3. Meet higher-level needs simultaneously with some lower-level needs. 4. Use concepts of needs and motivation in teaching and therapy. By meeting needs of client on one level, you can help client mature and feel motivated to meet growth needs.
Carl Rogers's Theory on Self-concept and Client-centered Therapy	1. Assess own self-concept and self-actualization needs prior to teaching and counseling clients. 2. Assess client's self-concept; promote positive experiences and contribute to development of positive self-concept. 3. Assume as much as possible the client's frame of reference to perceive world as he or she does. 4. Be accepting, warm, genuine, and empathic to help client discover self and mature.
Bandura's Social Learning Theory	1. Consider your appearance and behavior as a model for client. 2. Determine who significant adults were in the person's life and who role models were. 3. Demonstrate desired self-care behavior during intervention and teaching. 4. Utilize recovered person visiting an ill client as model for rehabilitation and a normal life, e.g., person with mastectomy, colostomy, amputation, alcoholism. 5. Demonstrate nurturing approaches or discipline methods to child client so that parents can learn effective childrearing methods. 6. Implement nurse-client relationship as a behavioral model of trust and interpersonal relations for the client.
Piaget's Theory of Cognitive Development	1. Teach parents about process of child's cognitive development and the implications for education, purchase of toys, interactions, and guidance. 2. Assess cognitive stage of client as basis for planning content and presentation in teaching sessions. 3. Assess cognitive development to determine language and abstraction level to use in interventions or teaching with client. 4. Use knowledge of cognitive development in play therapy.
Kohlberg's Theory of Moral Development/Gilligan's Theory of Moral Development	1. Assess own level of moral development. 2. Assess client's level of moral development when working with children, adolescents, or adults. 3. Use your modeling, clarification, explanation, and validation to contribute to client's moral development.

Summary

1. Various theories describe aspects of the developing person; no theory describes all dimensions (physiologic, emotional, cognitive, cultural, social, moral, spiritual) of development.
2. Biological theories include study of genetics, biochemistry, neurophysiology, immunology, maturational factors, biological rhythms, and biological deficiencies.
3. Ecological and social theories include study of family, urbanization, sociologic and cultural variables, geographic environments, and systems perspectives, such as the person, family, school, community, and organization.
4. Psychological theories include behavioral, psychoanalytic, and neo-analytic theories.
5. Behavioral theories include study of behavior that is learned or modified through various kinds of conditioning or learning and shows a measurable outcome.
6. Psychoanalytic and neo-analytic theories include study of the intrapsychic processes, psychological stage, and interpersonal development of the person, and their effects on behavior of the person and family unit.
7. Existential and humanistic theories include study of the needs, perceptions, self-concept, and dynamic aspects of the person, and development within the self in relation to the environment or society.
8. Cognitive theories include study of the stages of the person's cognitive development, the person as an information processor and problem solver, and effects of modeling, imitation, or environment on behavior.
9. Moral development theories study how the person learns to incorporate societal and philosophic norms into behavior and the relationship of moral development to cognitive, emotional, and social behavior.
10. The theories presented in this chapter form the basis for effective approaches in nursing, health care, and therapy or other interventions designed to promote health.
11. During client care, you may apply several of these theories and related concepts to any one client or family unit.

Review Questions

1. A student nurse is researching theories on causation of a particular disease process and is reviewing several twin studies. Many of these studies conclude that there is a familial tendency toward this particular disease. These conclusions support which category of theory of human behavior?
   1. Physical-biological
   2. Ecological-sociocultural
   3. Behavioral
   4. Moral
2. A 50-year-old woman is concerned about a persistent "blue" mood and lack of interest in previously enjoyed activities. The nurse may anticipate which measure to evaluate the biochemical cause of this client's condition?
   1. A referral to a psychologist
   2. Evaluation of hormone levels
   3. A social work evaluation
   4. A recommendation to take a vacation
3. The nurse is working with the employees of a community service agency, which due to loss of a major financial grant has been forced to cut several positions. The remaining employees have expressed to the nurse that they are unable to get answers to their questions and concerns about the future of the agency. There is an atmosphere of chaos within the agency. According to General Systems Theory, this can best be described as:
   1. A closed system
   2. Negentropy
   3. Entropy
   4. Linkage
4. The school nurse is working with a parent of a child who has displayed significant behavioral and emotional issues since starting school. The parent is concerned that because the child was adopted as a toddler, the lack of maternal bond in early childhood is the cause of his problems. Which developmental theorist would support the parent's concern?
   1. Sullivan
   2. Freud
   3. Erikson
   4. Kohlberg

References

1. Adler, J. (2006, March 27). Freud in our midst. *Newsweek*, 43–49.
2. Antai-Otong, D. (2003). *Psychiatric nursing: Biological & behavioral concepts.* London: Thomson-Delmar Learning.
3. Bandura, A. (1986). *Social foundations of thought and action: A social cognitive theory.* Englewood Cliffs, NJ: Prentice-Hall.
4. Bandura, A. (1989). Social cognitive theory. In R. Vasta (Ed.), *Annals of child development: Six theories of child development: Revised formulations and current issues* (pp. 1–60). Greenwich, CT: JAI Press.
5. Bandura, A. (1991). Social cognitive theory of moral thought and action. In W. Kurtines & J. Gerwitz (Eds.), *Handbook of moral behavior and development* (pp. 45–103). Hillsdale, NJ: Lawrence Erlbaum.
6. Bandura, A. (1991). Social cognitive theory of self-regulation. *Organizational Behavior and Human Decision Processes, 50,* 248–287.
7. Bandura, A., Barbaranelli, C., Caprara, G.V., & Pastorelli, C. (2001). Self-efficacy beliefs as shapers of children's aspirations and career trajectories. *Child Development, 72*(1), 187–206.
8. Berger, K. (2005). *The developing person through the lifespan* (6th ed.). New York: Worth Publishers.
9. Berrien, K. (1968). *General and social systems.* New Brunswick, NJ: Rutgers University Press.
10. Bronfenbrenner, U. (1989). Ecological systems theory. In R. Vasta (Ed.), *Annals of child development: Vol. 6. Six theories of child development: Revised formulations and current issues.* Greenwich, CT: JAI Press.
11. Bronfenbrenner, U., & Morris, P. A. (1998). The ecology of developmental processes. In W. Damon (Series Ed.) & R. Lerner (Vol. Ed.), *Handbook of child psychology: Vol. 1. Theoretical models of human development* (13th ed., pp. 993–1028). New York: Wiley.
12. Carter, S. (1978). The nurse educator: Humanist or behaviorist? *Nursing Outlook, 26*(9), 554–557.
13. Chui, D., & Dover, G. (2001). Sickle cell disease: No longer a single gene disorder. *Current Opinion in Pediatrics, 13,* 23–37.
14. Clark, M. (2008). *Community health nursing: Advocacy for population health* (5th ed.). Upper Saddle River, NJ: Pearson/Prentice Hall.
15. Colby, A., Kohlberg, L., Gibbs, J., & Lieberman, M. (1983). A longitudinal study of moral behavior. *Monographs of the Society of Research in Child Development, 48*(1–2), 1–124.
16. Coles, R. (Ed.). (2000). *The Erik Erikson reader.* New York: W. W. Norton.
17. Contingency management. (2006). *Harvard Mental Health Letter, 22*(8), 6–7.
18. Cooper, M. (1989). Gilligan's different voice: A perspective for nursing. *Journal of Professional Nursing, 5*(1), 10–16.
19. DeLaszio, V. (1990). *The basic writings of C.G. Jung.* Princeton, NJ: Princeton University Press.
20. Erikson, E. (1963). *Childhood and society* (2nd ed.). New York: W. W. Norton.
21. Erikson, E. H. (1992). *The life cycle completed.* New York: Norton.
22. Feetham, S., Thomson, E., & Hinshaw, A. S. (2005). Nursing leadership in genomics for health and society. *Journal of Nursing Scholarship, 37*(2), 102–110.
23. Feetham, S. I., & Williams, J. K. (Eds.). (2004). *Nursing and genetics in the 21st century—Leadership for global health.* Geneva, Switzerland: International Council of Nurses.
24. Frankl, V. (2000). *Man's search for ultimate meaning.* New York: Basic Books.
25. Frankl, V. (1988). *The will to meaning.* New York: Meridian.
26. Freud, S. (1936). *The problem of anxiety.* New York: W. W. Norton.
27. Freud, S. (1937). *The ego and the mechanisms of defense.* London: Hogarth Press.
28. Freud, S. (1947/1989). *Ego and the id.* New York: W. W. Norton.
29. Freud, S. (1969). *An outline of psycho-analysis.* New York: W. W. Norton.
30. Friedman, W. J., Robinson, A. B. and Friedman, B. L. (1987). Sex differences in moral judgments: A test of Gilligan's theory. *Psychology of Women Quarterly, 7*(1), 87.
31. Fromm, E. (1963/2000). *The art of loving.* New York: Harper & Row.
32. Gilligan, C. (1982). *In a different voice: Psychological theory and women's development.* Cambridge, MA: Harvard University Press.
33. Gilligan, C., & Attanucci, D. (1988). Two moral orientations: Gender differences and similarities. *Merrill-Palmer Quarterly, 34*(3), 332–333.
34. Gilligan, C., Murphy, J. M., & Tappan, M. B. (1990). Moral development beyond adolescence. In C. N. Alexander & E. J. Langer (Eds.), *Higher stages of human development* (pp. 208–228). New York: Oxford University Press.
35. Graves, J. (1973). Psychoanalytic theory. A critique. *Perspectives in Psychiatric Care, 11*(3), 114–120.
36. Greenberg, R., & Fisher, S. (1978). Testing Dr. Freud. *Human Behavior, 7*(9), 28–33.
37. Guyton, A., & Hall, J. E. (2006). *Textbook of medical physiology* (11th ed.). Philadelphia: Elsevier.
38. Hall, C., Lindzey, G., & Campbell, J. (1998). *Theories of personality* (4th ed.). New York: John Wiley & Sons.
39. Jenkins, J., Grady, P., & Collins, F. (2005). Nurses and the genomic revolution. *Journal of Nursing Scholarship, 37*(2), 98–101.
40. Jung, C. G. (1969). *The structure and dynamics of the psyche.* Princeton. NJ: Princeton University Press.
41. Jung, C. (1971). Psychological types. In G. Adler, Fordham, M. and Read, H. (Eds.), *Collected works of Carl G. Jung* (Vol. 6). Princeton, NJ: Princeton University Press.
42. Kenner, C., Gallo, A., & Bryant, K. (2005). Promoting children's health through understanding of genetics and genomics. *Journal of Nursing Scholarship, 37*(4), 308–314.
43. Killeen, M., & King, I. (2007). Viewpoint: Use of King's conceptual system, nursing informatics, and nursing classification systems for global communication. *International Journal of Nursing Terminologies and Classifications, 18*(2), 51–58.
44. Kirschenbaum, H., & Henderson, V. (Eds.). (1989). *A Carl Rogers reader.* Boston: Houghton Mifflin.
45. Kohlberg, L. (Ed.). (1973). *Collected papers on moral development and moral education.* Cambridge, MA: Moral Educational Research Foundation.
46. Kohlberg, L. (1976). Moral stages and moralization: The cognitive developmental approach. In T. Lickona (Ed.), *Moral development and behavior.* New York: Holt, Rinehart, & Winston.
47. Kohlberg, L. (1977). *Recent research in moral development.* New York: Holt, Rinehart, & Winston.
48. Kohlberg, L. (1978). The cognitive-developmental approach to moral education. In P. Scharf (Ed.), *Readings in moral education* (pp. 36–51). Minneapolis: Winston Press.
49. Lilly, L., & Guanci, R. (1995). Applying systems theory. *American Journal of Nursing, 95*(11), 14–15.
50. Loescher, L., & Merkle, C. (2005). The interface of genomic technologies and nursing. *Journal of Nursing Scholarship, 37*(2), 111–119.
51. Loomis, C.P. (1960). *Social systems.* New York: D. Van Nostrand.
52. Maslow, A. (1968). *Towards a psychology of being* (2nd ed.). New York: Harper & Row.
53. Maslow, A. (1970). *Motivation and personality* (2nd ed.). New York: Harper & Row.
54. Maslow, A. (1971). *The farther reaches of human nature.* New York: Viking Press.
55. Maslow, A. (1982). *The journals of Abraham Maslow* (R. J. Lowry, Ed.). Lexington, MA: Lewis.
56. Metheny, N. (2000). *Fluid and electrolyte balance: Nursing considerations* (4th ed.). Philadelphia: Lippincott.
57. Mohr, W. (2003). Discarding ideology: The nature/nurture endgame. *Perspectives in Psychiatric Care, 39*(3), 113–121.
58. Nadeau, J. H. (2005). Listening to genetic background noise. *New England Journal of Medicine, 352*(15), 1598–1599.

59. Neuman, B. (1988). The Betty Neuman health-care systems model: A total person approach to patient problems. In J. P. Riehl & C. Roy (Eds.), *Conceptual models for nursing practice* (3rd ed.). New York: Appleton-Century-Crofts.

60. Papalia, D., Olds, S., & Feldman, R. (2004). *Human development* (9th ed.). Boston: McGraw Hill.

61. Patterson, C., & Watkins, C. E. (1996). *Theories of psychotherapy* (5th ed.). New York: Harper Collins.

62. Peplau, H. (1952/1991, reissued). *Interpersonal relations in nursing: A conceptual frame of reference for psychodynamic nursing.* New York: Springer.

63. Pestka, E. (2006). Genetic counseling for mental health disorders. *Journal of American Psychiatric Nurses Association, 11*(6), 338–343.

64. Piaget, J. (1963). *The origins of intelligence in children.* New York: W. W. Norton.

65. Piaget, J. (1974). *Understanding causality.* New York: W. W. Norton.

66. Piaget, J., & Inhelder, B. (1969). *The psychology of the child.* New York: Basic Books.

67. Piaget, J., & Inhelder, B. (1975). *The origin of the idea of chance in children.* New York: W. W. Norton.

68. Rest, J. (1988). The legacy of Lawrence Kohlberg. *Counseling and Values, 32*(3), 156–162.

69. Rogers, C. (1961). *On becoming a person.* Boston: Houghton-Mifflin.

70. Rogers, C. (1980). *Way of being.* Boston: Houghton Mifflin.

71. Santrock, J. (2004). *Life span development* (9th ed.). Boston: McGraw Hill.

72. Skinner, B. F. (1969). *Contingencies of reinforcement: A theoretical analysis.* New York: Alfred A. Knopf.

73. Skinner, B. F. (1971). *Beyond freedom and dignity.* New York: Appleton-Century-Crofts.

74. Skinner, B. F. (1985). Cognitive science and behaviorism. *British Journal of Psychology, 76,* 291–301.

75. Skinner, B. F. (1987). *Upon further reflection.* Englewood Cliffs, NJ: Prentice-Hall.

76. Sullivan, H. S. (1953). *The interpersonal theory of psychiatry.* New York: W. W. Norton.

77. Swift, R. (2005). Symptoms, circuits, and stress. *Clinical Psychiatry News, 37*(10), 4.

78. Urban, H. (1991). Humanist, phenomenological, and existential approaches. In M. Hersen, A. Kadzin, & A. Bellak (Eds.), *The clinical psychology handbook* (2nd ed., pp. 200–219). New York: Pergamon Press.

79. von Bertalanffy, L. (1968). *General systems theory.* New York: George Braziller.

80. von Bertalanffy, L. (1972). The history and status of general systems theory. In G. Klir (Ed.), *Trends in general systems theory.* New York: Wiley.

81. Wadsworth, B. (2004). *Piaget's theory of cognitive and affective development* (5th ed.). Boston: Pearson.

82. Williams, J., Skirton, H., & Masny, A. (2006). Ethics, policy, and educational issues in genetic testing. *Journal of Nursing Scholarship, 38*(2), 119–125.

83. Zook, R. (1998). Learning to use positive defense mechanisms. *American Journal of Nursing, 98*(3), 16B–16H.

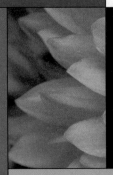

Health Promotion: Concepts and Theories

OBJECTIVES

Study of this chapter will enable you to:

1. Relate information about health care issues and national and international initiatives to advance health services.

2. Differentiate primary, secondary, and tertiary levels of prevention, and apply them to health promotion/disease prevention with the client at various developmental stages.

3. Examine barriers to health care service delivery that affect people at any developmental level and from any sociocultural group or population in the United States.

4. Relate the focus on improving quality of care to the issue of health care disparities.

5. Relate major concepts of stress and crisis theories to development, and utilize the theories in health promotion and disease prevention.

6. Contrast complementary and alternative therapies used by various populations to promote health or prevent or treat illness.

MediaLink www.prenhall.com/murray

Go to the Companion Website for interactive resources that accompany this chapter.

Glossary	Critical Thinking
Review Questions	Tools
Challenge Your Knowledge	Media Link Applications
Learning Activities	Media Links

Overview: Health Promotion and Disease Prevention

Health promotion and disease prevention—old concepts—have been inadequately applied and are currently being widely publicized. Headlines in the popular press reiterate the theme: "A Culture of Health" (1), "Searching for Hidden Heart Risks" (54), and "Five Top Child Killers" (3). This chapter introduces responses to health care, barriers to and disparities in health care services, models and theories that relate to health promotion, and some trends in providing improved health care.

THE NATIONAL RESPONSE

The alarming increase in preventable diseases and strategies to promote health for all populations in the United States are being addressed by the *Healthy People 2010* Initiative (91), the American Nurses Association (28), Sigma Theta Tau, International (22), and the American Academy of Nursing (46). Examples of objectives from *Healthy People 2010* are presented in Units III and IV (see the index for page numbers). ∞ The nursing professional organizations, along with those of other health care disciplines, generally agree that improving quality of care requires short-term and long-term action. The National Alliance on Mental Illness (NAMI) has addressed quality and inequities of mental health care for the mentally ill and mentally retarded (27), the cost of mental illnesses, the disability and premature death that results from mental illness (just as with physical illness) (62), and the human and economic benefits of treatment (62). *All involved organizations agree with the American Academy of Nursing, which has proposed* (46):

1. Public education.
2. Research for direct practice.
3. Change in accessibility of delivery systems.
4. Improved databases and clinical information systems.
5. Altered incentives for health promotion practices.

On a national level, *Healthy People 2010* presents 28 specific areas for health improvement, 467 objectives, and ways to achieve and evaluate progress to the goals for health promotion and disease prevention (91). Further, the Institute of Medicine (IOM), in its 2005 report, addressed the need for strategies to improve health care for all populations (44). Obtain information about this comprehensive report from the IOM Website, www.iom.edu.

One IOM report, *To Err Is Human: Building a Safer Health System*, documents serious and pervasive problems in health care. Over 98,000 hospitalized patients die each year as a result of errors in their care—more than die annually from auto accidents, breast cancer, and AIDS. In addition, unnecessary suffering and disability result from medical errors. An estimated 7,000 medication errors occur annually, in and out of hospitals—more events than workplace injuries. Some errors are caused by dependence on technology rather than by poor personal judgment. Nurses are expected to practice astute assessment, use relevant rationale and theory, apply scientific principles, be assertive in communication and persistent in advocacy, and practice commitment to quality care interventions (88).

The second IOM report, *Crossing the Quality Chasm: A New System for the 21st Century*, highlights other defects in the U.S. health care system. Changes have been identified for the next decade that emphasize safe, effective, timely, equitable, efficient, and evidence-based nursing and health care (88).

The potential for diseases being brought to the United States from countries around the world has increased with more transportation of people and goods (17, 22, 45, 53). Thus, *global health initiatives, as well as national and local strategies, are needed to ensure disease prevention and consequent health for all populations* (44).

GLOBAL HEALTH RESPONSE

The World Health Organization (WHO) emphasizes a broad approach to disease prevention and treatment and health promotion, and more can be found at the Website, www.who.int. To focus efforts on education of individuals, or even family units, is not acceptable in some countries. Further, there is poor or no accessibility to health care services in some places. Rather, according to WHO, there must be organizational and governmental changes, legislation and policy development, and community development (64). Infectious diseases, such as tuberculosis, HIV/AIDS, severe acute respiratory syndrome (SARS), monkeypox, West Nile virus, Hantavirus pulmonary syndrome, and other diseases transmitted through animal and insect vectors, cross international borders (45).

The United States has responded to such threats at various times with more extensive screening of immigrants, immunizations for people at risk, embargo on imports of certain animals, quarantine, and travel advisories (17, 45). These measures prevent spread; they do not prevent occurrence.

The broad approach recommended by WHO for globalization of health can also be approached by comparing health care practices and outcomes in different countries to foster use of best practices, improve health management, influence governmental policy, and foster communication between health care professionals and workers (46). A comparative study of health care delivery systems in Korea and Thailand is an example (53).

Global health issues, including the challenges of overcoming disease, unhealthy environmental conditions for populations, socioeconomic disparities, difficult work environments for nurses, educational needs, and practice issues, were studied by Sigma Theta Tau, International in worldwide conferences. Both common and unique themes were identified in various world regions (22). The urgency of working on these issues is apparent. For more information, access the Website www.nursingsociety.org.

Because of widespread international travel and transportation of products, there is increasing emphasis on a global health agenda. *Strategies to achieve better health care for more people, preferably all people, throughout the world include to* (65):

1. Empower people through information, education, and decision-making opportunities, including use of communication networks such as the World Wide Web.
2. Strengthen local primary health care systems and services.
3. Improve education for health care professionals.
4. Apply science and technology to critical health problems.

MediaLink | World Health Organization

MediaLink | Nursing Society

5. Use new approaches to old problems (e.g., violence, environmental pollution).
6. Provide culturally appropriate assistance to less developed countries.
7. Establish a process to examine world challenges to health.

Definitions

Health is an evolving concept, defined differently by various cultures and each individual, family, community, and nation. Health is more than the absence of illness. Health *is a state of well-being in which the person uses adaptive responses physically, mentally, emotionally, spiritually, and socially, in response to external and internal stimuli or stressors, to maintain relative stability and comfort and to achieve personal objectives.* Health emphasizes *strength, resilience, resources, and capabilities* rather than focusing on pathology. However, **morbidity** *(prevalence of disease)* and **mortality** *(death)* are most commonly used to measure health (65).

Pender, Murdaugh, and Parsons *differentiate health promotion and disease prevention* as follows (65):

1. **Health promotion** is *behavior motivated by the person's desire to increase well-being and health potential.* It is not disease specific.
2. **Disease prevention** is *behavior motivated by a desire to avoid disease, detect it early,* or *maintain functioning within the constraints of illness or disability.*

Both are essential at each developmental stage. The terms are often used interchangeably, which is incorrect. Health promotion and disease prevention have been defined *traditionally* in terms of three levels: primary, secondary, and tertiary (8, 13, 15, 18, 23, 52, 65).

Primary prevention *refers to activities that prevent or decrease the probability of occurrence of an injury, physical or mental illness, or health-threatening situation in an individual or family, or an event or illness in the population, by combating harmful forces that operate in the individual or the community and by strengthening the capacity of people to withstand these forces.* Examples of primary prevention are wellness or health promotion measures, including immunizations, health education and safety programs, nutrition education and healthy diet to prevent disease, environment policies and efforts toward clean air and sanitation (garbage removal and chlorinated water), smoking cessation, exercise, and parenting classes. In an epidemiologic focus, all primary prevention activities have the goal to reduce risky behaviors and occurrence of disease, injury or harm, and negative aftereffects (5). Treatment and follow-up care given to the ill person can in turn foster primary prevention of other events or illness.

Secondary prevention *refers to screening and early diagnosis and prompt treatment of the existing health problem, disease, or harmful situation, thereby shortening duration and severity of consequences, preventing disability or complications, and enabling the person to return to maximum potential health or normal function as quickly as possible. Secondary prevention, in an epidemiologic focus, refers also to identification of asymptomatic individuals before the onset of disease and occurrence of symptoms* (5). *Early detection occurs in the window of time just before symptoms are apparent, which fosters early treat-*

ment and delays onset of more serious symptoms. An example would be HIV screening, which can delay the consequences of AIDS through early treatment, or early detection of asymptomatic breast cancer (5).

Tertiary prevention *refers to restoring the person to optimum function or maintenance of life skills through long-term treatment and rehabilitation and within the constraints of an irreversible problem, thereby preventing progression of sequelae, complications, or deterioration. Tertiary prevention, in an epidemiologic focus, may include prompt treatment, proper follow-up, rehabilitation, and client education* (5). An example would be care of the person with diabetes; the goal is to improve survival and quality of life (5).

These three levels of prevention are interrelated and may lack clear boundaries. Brownson, Baker, and Novick address all prevention issues, from primary risk reduction to secondary screening to prevention of disability from existing chronic diseases, within a cohesive, seamless framework that indicates the overlap between the levels (13). The Case Situation presents an example. These levels of prevention will be addressed in Chapters 9 through 16 ∞, relevant to the specific developmental level.

Your practice will include any one or all of these levels of prevention as you work with individuals, families, the community, or the overall environment or society. Educate the public and clients to engage in primary prevention.

Unhealthy lifestyles and environmental conditions are responsible for a major percentage of morbidity and mortality. These are compounded by the **health care disparities,** *the inequality of services that exist* related to cultural factors, unavailability of care facilities, and financial factors, which must be overcome if there is to be true health promotion or any level of disease prevention (56). According to one Website (www.covertheuninsured.org), 45 million Americans, including 8 million children, have *no* health insurance.

Barriers to and Disparities in Health Care Services

Demographic, cultural, and health care system and related barriers are summarized in **Table 2-1** and discussed in depth by Huff and Kline (42). Refer to Unit II ∞ for more information about influences on the person and family unit that may contribute to or diminish these barriers. Information presented about the developing person and family unit in Chapters 9 through 16 ∞ is also relevant for understanding barriers that exist and how they can be overcome.

Health disparities are *differences in incidence, prevalence, mortality, and burden of disease and other adverse conditions that exist among specific population groups* (31). Barriers or obstacles to obtaining needed health promotion and disease prevention services in the United States are being addressed by the U.S. Department of Health and Human Services (DHHS), Health Resources and Services Administration (HRSA). Efforts and policy making are directed to research, screening or assessment, education, and expanding access to health care for a variety of vulnerable populations, including people in ethnic/racial groups, immigrants, homeless people, and medically underserved rural and urban communities (90). A number of clini-

Case Situation

Levels of Prevention

A clinic located in a metropolitan neighborhood of newly arrived immigrants and new citizens gives multiple and integrated services. The pregnant woman brings her family. She receives prenatal care; her 6-month-old infant is given a well-baby checkup and immunizations (primary prevention). The toddler has a beginning respiratory infection and is given medication (secondary prevention). The mother is taught about measures to care for the toddler at home. The maternal grandmother accompanies the family. She is given a thorough physical examination, including vision, hearing, and bone density index (primary prevention). She is referred to an optometrist for eyeglasses (secondary prevention). Safety measures are explained to her (primary prevention). She demonstrates the progress in rehabilitation following surgery for a fractured hip (tertiary prevention) and is reminded to continue taking prescribed medication and the calcium and vitamin D tablets (secondary prevention).

This clinic is special to this community. The staff are bilingual with competence in Spanish. Translators for other languages come on assigned days, and residents in the area are advised to come on the day that medical specialists and specific language translators are present. Professional staff and volunteers work closely together; the clinic day always extends past the posted time schedule. This clinic works to reduce health care disparities.

Contributed by Ruth Murray, EdD, MSN, N-NAP, FAAN

TABLE 2-1

Barriers to Health Promotion and Disease Prevention

Demographic Barrier	Cultural Barriers	Health Care System Barrier
Age	Perception of age by cultural group	Access to care for infants, women, elders, or other groups
Gender	Value on men and women in family, economic class, or cultural group	Insurance or other financial resources
Ethnicity	Worldview/perceptions of life	Lack of understanding by providers of cultural perceptions
Primary language spoken	Time orientation	Orientation to preventive health services, timed appointments
Religion	Religious beliefs and practices	Perceptions of need for health care services, beliefs about healing and acceptable healing methods
Education and literacy level	Primary language spoken	Ignorance and/or distrust of Western medical practices and procedures
Occupation, income, and health insurance benefits	Social customs, values, and norms, economic resources	Cultural insensitivity to needs of individuals, competence of providers to individualize care and secure resources
Area of residence	Traditional health beliefs and practices of geographic areas	Western versus folk health beliefs and practices
Transportation	Access of services, preferences for certain kinds of services	Poor doctor-patient communications; flexible availability of service
Time and/or generation in the United States	Communication patterns and customs	Lack of bilingual and bicultural staff

Adapted from Huff, R., & Kline, M. (1999). Health promotion in the context of culture. In R. Huff & M. Kline (Eds.), *Promoting health in multicultural populations: A handbook for practitioners* (p. 16). Thousand Oaks, CA: Sage.

MediaLink   HRSA

cal areas are addressed, including need for immunizations and services for people with diabetes, cardiovascular disease, cancer, asthma, HIV/AIDS, mental illness, and substance abuse (90). Maternal/child health services and causes of infant mortality are addressed (90). Health problems and services in the workplace are also being explored (90). A full report is available at the HRSA Website. Refer to **Table 2-1** and selected references for more information about disparity concerns related to primary care, insurance coverage, hospital characteristics, and cultural and communication barriers (9–11, 22, 24, 25, 40, 44, 45, 90, 93).

The National Alliance on Mental Illness (NAMI) is also addressing the significant barriers to mental health care experienced by African American, Asian American and Pacific Islander, American Indian, and Latino/Hispanic populations. NAMI is developing national partnerships and strategies to overcome the crisis. For more information, refer to the Website www.nami.org.

There is also increasing emphasis on improving quality of health care within the existing services in the United States. To achieve quality, there must be (11):

1. Improved access to care for all people.
2. Appropriate and acceptable treatment plans that incorporate multidisciplinary knowledge.
3. A workforce of sufficient numbers and qualifications.
4. Agreement on indicators for health care quality.
5. Responsible practices and follow-through on the part of patients.

The graduate-prepared, advanced practice nurse can be a key person in this endeavor (8). More research is needed related to evidence-based practice in order to achieve higher quality of care.

Because disparities or inequity in health care services are increasing problems in the United States, considerable research and publication has been directed to learning more about the problem and ways to make the necessary care available for all people. Without essential health services, the person and family unit cannot develop their capabilities or meet their developmental tasks. For example, one issue is how to conduct research to obtain meaningful information. Selected references discuss the use of several research methods (9, 10, 25, 33, 58, 64, 70, 74, 88, 90, 93). Selected references report vulnerable groups that have been studied, such as rural Mexican American women (57), African American populations (2, 39, 85, 90), Native American Indians (89), and Chinese Americans (56). Issues of availability of services and the number of qualified nurses in the workplace are being addressed (10, 70). Cost factors have to be considered in relation to quality care. One study of infants revealed the cost of hospitalizing premature infants, the need to improve prenatal care to women at high risk for delivering preterm or low-birth-weight infants, and the need to improve outcomes for those infants (20). Obtain more information from a variety of professional journals, and the websites presented in this chapter and on the Companion Website.

The Canadian system of health care is increasingly examined by health care professionals in the United States as one way to reduce U.S. health care disparities. Canada's system has advantages in relation to improved health level of the population, amount of money spent per person, and expected longevity. More information is available at their Website, www.organicconsumers.org.

Health Promotion Theories and Models

Research has contributed to development of theories and models about health promotion behavior. Such knowledge can be applied to overcome barriers to or disparities in health care as well as to prevent illness. These theories and models explain the dynamics behind behavior related to maintaining health or the secondary or tertiary levels of prevention. Assessment, intervention, and evaluation of outcomes will in turn be more effective for people in different developmental levels and from different backgrounds (65). Health beliefs, perceptions, and behaviors are complex; theoretical knowledge fosters understanding and effective action.

Frankish, Lovato, and Shannon describe theories and models for health behavior, health promotion, and illness prevention that have been developed in the past 40 to 50 years (31). *The theories can be categorized as follows* (31):

1. Behavioral and social learning
2. Cognitive and decision making (e.g., Health Belief Model), coping
3. Motivation and emotional arousal, such as learned helplessness
4. Communication methods
5. Interpersonal relationships (e.g., social support, nurse or health care provider–client relationship)

BEHAVIORAL AND SOCIAL LEARNING THEORIES

Refer to Chapter 1 ∞ for explanation of these theories. **Using Behavioral Theory,** the toddler and preschooler may learn health behaviors because of *parental conditioning processes,* for example, hygiene and self-care practices. The schoolchild may imitate parents, family members, or peers. **Social Learning Theory** may apply to the health habits of the adolescent or adult in relation to (a) **imitational learning** (*doing what others do*), (b) **behavioral capacity** (*having the cognitive abilities and skills to learn and perform desired behaviors*), or (c) **efficacy** (*believing the behavior will have the desired consequences*) (6).

HEALTH BELIEF MODEL

This model describes interrelated and multiple variables that motivate people to learn and engage in health-seeking behavior. *The model is composed of several major constructs* (31, 65, 72, 73):

1. Perceived personal susceptibility
2. Perceived severity of the condition
3. Perceived benefits of a particular action against the threat
4. Perceived barriers or obstacles to taking such action

The person is motivated when a health issue seems relevant and is sufficiently severe to threaten comfort, health, or longevity. "Minor" symptoms motivate some people; other people have to be severely ill or unable to work before they perceive themselves as vulnerable. See **Table 2-1** for a summary of demographic, cultural, and health care system barriers that apply to preventive measures (42).

Perceived benefits of action depend upon the personal and family system, past experiences, cognitive level, or other variables (see Chapter 1). ∞ Chapters 9 through 16 ∞ also describe developmental influences on perceptions. For behavioral change to occur, the person must believe that a change will be beneficial, that the benefits will outweigh the costs or demands, and that the person is competent to accomplish the change.

Abstract for Evidence-Based Practice

Health Belief Model

Al-Ali, N., & Haddad, L. (2004). The effect of the Health Belief Model in explaining exercise participation among Jordanian myocardial infarction patients. *Journal of Transcultural Nursing, 15*(2), 114–121.

KEYWORDS

health belief, exercise, myocardial infarction.

Purpose ➤ To describe the effect of the Health Belief Model in explaining participation in an exercise program by Jordanian patients who had a myocardial infarction.

Conceptual Framework ➤ The concepts of the Health Belief Model guided the research design.

Sample/Setting ➤ A convenience sample of 98 patients in cardiology clinics who had been discharged from four government hospitals in the northern part of Jordan were recruited during a 2-month period. Patients had experienced their first myocardial infarction (MI), were alert and oriented, and were able to ambulate. Exclusion criteria were presence of dysrhythmias, neuromuscular disorder, psychiatric problems, and chronic renal failure. The participants were male, middle-aged (*M*=50 years), and Moslem (90%); 92% were married. Over half (57%) had at least a high school education.

Method ➤ The Health Belief Questionnaire, a self-report instrument combined with a structured interview of 20 to 25 minutes, was utilized for data collection after each patient gave written consent for participation.

Findings ➤ Forty percent of the participants reported receiving no physician recommendation for exercise. Patients reported a range of exercise frequency from 0 to 30 times in the month prior to data collection. Only 3% of the patients ranked exercise as the most important factor in preventing or treating myocardial infarction. Most (80%) of the patients reported they contacted their physician immediately when chest pain was experienced. Most (61%) ranked heart disease as second in concern to cancer.

Implications ➤ Participants may not have perceived exercise as beneficial, especially if they had regularly exercised and still developed the MI. The absence of mass media health education messages about exercise benefits may contribute to this perception. Further, Moslems in the Arab Jordanian culture strongly believe in reliance on God's will and absolute dependence on the beneficence of Higher Power. Thus, many Jordanians may not think about prevention. Differences in roles for men and women would also affect participation in exercise and reducing certain risk factors. Research is needed to develop a culturally sensitive instrument that takes into consideration the cultural variation and specific needs of MI patients.

HEALTH PROMOTION MODEL

Pender developed this model in the early 1980s, proposing a framework for integrating nursing and behavioral science perspectives to factors influencing health behaviors (65). This model offered a guide to explore the complex biopsychosocial processes that motivate people to engage in behaviors that enhance health. The model was revised in the 1990s and incorporated constructs from Social Learning Theory (see Chapter 1) ∞ and Expectancy Value Theory (65). According to **Expectancy Value Theory,** a *person pursues a goal or engages and persists in an action* (65):

1. To the extent it has value and a change is desired.
2. To the degree it is likely to achieve positive results.
3. Whether or not it is perceived as possible to achieve.

The *variables and their interrelationships are described briefly* (65):

1. **Individual characteristics and experiences:** *Each person is unique in personal characteristics and life experiences,* which in turn may be highly relevant or not at all relevant to a specific health behavior.
2. **Prior related behavior:** *The past is a predictor for repeating the same or similar behavior.* Every incident of behavior is accompanied by emotions, which also affect future behavior. If a behavior has been pleasurable, it is more likely to be repeated and become a habit.

3. **Personal factors:** These either can or cannot be changed:
   a. **Biological factors** *include age, body mass index, pubertal or menopausal status, aerobic capacity, agility, and strength.*
   b. **Psychological factors** *include self-esteem, self-motivation, and perceived health status.*
   c. **Sociocultural factors** *include race or ethnicity, education, and socioeconomic status.*
4. **Behavior-specific cognitions (thoughts) and affect (emotions):** *These affect motivation to change* and must be considered in planning interventions.
5. **Perceived benefits of action:** *Change is pursued if it increases comfort or leads to decreased symptoms.*
6. **Perceived barriers to action:** *Expense, inconvenience, time factors, loss of satisfaction, and discomfort are barriers.* Refer also to **Table 2-1.**
7. **Perceived self-efficacy:** *The person perceives self as able to organize and carry out a course of action,* to accomplish a goal.
8. **Activity-related affect:** *The subjective feeling that accompanies the behaviors and the overall event* ("the high") may be the main reason for change in some people.

9. **Interpersonal influences:** *Beliefs and attitudes of others,* such as family, peers, or health care providers, have a powerful influence on behavior. Examples of interpersonal influences include:
   a. Norms or expectations of others.
   b. Social and emotional support from others.
   c. Observing and imitating others' behavior.

10. **Situational influences:** *Environmental constraints, company regulations, or stressful events* may foster movement to or away from behavioral change.

11. **Commitment to a plan of action:** The *emotional and cognitive set propels the person* to be organized, pursue strategies, and continue the behavior. However, "good intentions" must be reinforced by some kind of reward.

12. **Immediate competing demands and preferences:** *Situations arise and needs change, which necessitate alternative behaviors that in turn can change plans or the course of action.* A competing demand may be another person's expectations for help on a project or negative attitudes. A competing preference may be a high-caloric dessert rather than fruit.

13. **Health-promoting behavior:** *The outcome is that a healthy lifestyle integrates the variables described* and fosters a quality of life at all stages of development.

COPING THEORY

The ability to stay healthy is reflective of **coping abilities,** the *person's constantly changing cognitive and behavioral efforts to manage specific external or internal demands* (31, 49–51). These abilities are dependent on a number of variables, such as developmental level, personal and social resources, and family and environmental support (49–51). Whether or not the person tries to cope with a situation or tries health behaviors depends on whether the demands are considered manageable, are too stressful, or carry an actual or perceived threat of harm (50, 51). *Coping abilities are also influenced by* (50, 51):

1. Ability for self-control.
2. Willingness to accept responsibility for behavior.
3. Desire to avoid or distance self or to confront the situation.
4. Capacity for problem solving.
5. Ability to view the situation or practice from a positive perspective.

Health promotion includes regular physical examinations and screening. This sounds easy to handle; the health care professionals make appointments for diagnostic tests. It's not so easy and straightforward for the single parent with three young children who is balancing many demands or for the elderly adult who is frail and has few resources to help plan action or get to the various sites for screening. In either situation, the best coping action may be to avoid the screenings.

The patient's ability to cope with all the activities necessary to continue a treatment plan, such as chemotherapy and radiation for advanced cancer, involves multiple variables. The treatment plan may be the answer from the physician's viewpoint. It may be overwhelming for the patient and family. They may consider stopping treatment so there is some comfort, some quality of life, some enjoyment of favorite activities, or energy to maintain close friendships—even if it means a shorter life span. Be an advocate for clients to foster their coping.

MOTIVATION AND EMOTIONAL AROUSAL THEORY

Emotional arousal refers to *feelings that affect behavior during health and illness* (31). A health behavior such as exercise serves as a **motivator** for personal appearance and positive self-esteem in the adolescent and to improve stamina and self-confidence in the older adult. The person who faces an apparently insurmountable task may behave in a manner consistent with feelings of **helplessness** (*inability to handle events*), depression, or sense of failure. The young adult who has not been very active physically may "give up" at the prospect of a long rehabilitation period after suffering paralysis of both legs due to an auto accident (**learned helplessness**) (31).

COMMUNICATION THEORY

Use communication approaches that are based on therapeutic techniques and that are relevant to the person's developmental level. Consider also the family and cultural norms of the client as you interview, assess, and intervene. The person or family will then be more likely to act on education or engage in behaviors to promote health or prevent illness (24, 58, 86). See **Table 2-2** for effective communication methods and their rationale (43, 67, 71) and **Table 2-3** for guidelines for an effective interview (43, 66, 67, 71). **Table 2-4,** Barriers to Effective Communication, describes actions that can contribute to client avoidance of your assessment or health education (43, 67, 71). Shattell and Hogan (86) present guidelines to facilitate and **evaluate** communication.

You may find the *following communication guidelines helpful* in **evaluating** *your communication methods:*

1. Examine the purpose of your communications.
2. Consider the total physical and human setting.
3. Plan the communication to clarify ideas, present information, and provide or seek consultation.
4. Analyze the methods used and their effectiveness.
5. Identify hidden meanings as well as the basic content of the message you conveyed.
6. Support the communication delivered through actions.
7. Follow up communication to determine if the purpose was accomplished.

Evaluation can also be based on *analyzing your communication methods or having someone observe you,* utilizing content presented in **Tables 2-2, 2-3,** and **2-4.**

THERAPEUTIC RELATIONSHIP THEORY

The therapeutic relationship is key to health promotion, disease prevention, and treatment, and to your work with people in any developmental stage. The **therapeutic or helping relationship** or **alliance,** or **therapeutic nurse-client relationship,** is a *purposeful interaction over time between an authority in health care and a person, family, or group with health care needs, with the focus on needs*

TABLE 2-2

Effective Communication Methods and Their Rationale

Communication Method	Rationale
Be accepting in nonverbal and verbal behavior (does not mean agreement with person's words or behavior).	All behavior is motivated and purposeful. Promotes climate in which person feels safe and respected. Indicates that you are following the person's trend of thought and encourages further talking while you remain nonjudgmental.
Use thoughtful silence at intervals, while continuing to look at and focus on person.	Indicates accessibility. Encourages person to talk and set own pace. Gives both you and client time to organize thoughts. Aids consideration of alternative courses of action, provides opportunity for explanation of feelings, gives time for contemplation. Conserves energy and promotes relaxation.
Use "I" and "we" in proper context; call person by name and title, as preferred.	Strengthens identity of person in relation to others.
State open-ended, general, leading statements or questions: "Tell me about it." "What are you feeling?"	Encourages person to take the initiative in introducing topics and to think through problems. May gain pertinent information that you would not think to ask about because client has freedom to pursue feelings and ideas important to him or her.
Ask related or peripheral questions when indicated: "And what else happened?" "You have four children. What are their ages?"	Explores or clarifies pertinent topic. Adds to database. Encourages person to work through larger or related issues and to engage in problem solving. Explores subject in depth without appearing to pry. Helps person see implications, relationships, or consequences. Helps keep communication flowing and person talking.
Encourage description of feelings: "Tell me what you feel."	Helps person identify, face, and resolve own feelings. Validates your observation. Deepens your empathy and insight.
Place described events in time sequence: "What happened then?" "What did you do after that?" "And then what?"	Clarifies how event occurred or explains relationships associated with given event. Places event in context or manageable perspective. Helps identify recurrent patterns or difficulties or significant cause-effect relationships.
State your observations about the person: "You appear . . ." "I sense that you . . ." "I notice that you . . ."	Acknowledges client's feelings, needs, behavior, or efforts at a task. Offers content to which person can respond. Encourages comparisons or mutual understanding of client's behavior. Validates your impressions. Helps person notice own behavior and its effects; encourages self-awareness. Reinforces behavior. Adds to person's self-esteem.
State the implied, what client has hinted, or a feeling that you sense may be a consequence of an event.	Expresses acceptability of feeling or idea. Clarifies information. Conveys your attention, interest, and empathy. May be used as subtle form of suggestion for action.
Paraphrase; translate into your own words the feelings, questions, ideas, key words of other person: "I hear you saying . . ." "You feel . . ."	Indicates careful listening and focus on client. Encourages further talking. Validates and summarizes what you think client has said. Conveys empathy and understanding. Indicates that person's words, ideas, feelings, opinions, or decisions are important. Promotes integration of feelings with content being discussed.
Restate or repeat main idea expressed by client.	Conveys interest and careful listening or desire to clarify a vague point. Helps to reformulate certain statements or to emphasize key words to help client recognize less obvious meanings or associations.
Clarify: "Could you explain that further?" "Explain that to me again."	Indicates interest and desire to understand. Helps the person become clearer to himself or herself. Encourages exploration of subject in depth or of meaning behind what is being said.

continued

TABLE 2-2

Effective Communication Methods and Their Rationale—continued

Communication Method	Rationale
Make reflective statement, integrating feelings and content.	Indicates active listening and empathy. Synthesizes your perceptions and provides feedback to client. Shares your perception of congruity between person's statements and other behavior. Provides client with new ways of considering ideas, behavior, or a situation. Identifies and encourages understanding of latent meanings.
Suggest collaboration and a cooperative relationship.	Offers to do activities with, not for or to, person. Encourages person to participate in identifying and appraising problems. Involves person as active partner in care. Tells person you are available and interested. Provides reassurance.
Offer information; self-disclose by sharing own thoughts and feelings briefly, if appropriate.	Makes facts available whenever client needs or asks for them. Builds trust; orients; enables decision making. Reduces client's anxiety, frustration, or other distressing feelings that hinder comfort, recovery, or realistic action. Helps client focus on deeper concerns.
Encourage evaluation of situation.	Helps client appraise quality of his or her experience and consider people and events in relation to own and others' experience and values. Assists person in determining how others affect him or her, and personal effect on others. Promotes understanding of own situation and avoidance of uncritically adopting opinions, values, or behavior of others.
Encourage formulation of plan of action.	Conveys that person is expected to be active participant in own care. Helps person consider alternative courses of action. Helps person plan how to handle future problems.
Voice doubt; present own perceptions or facts; suggest alternative line of reasoning: "What gives you that impression?" "Isn't that unusual?" "I find that hard to believe." Respond to underlying feeling.	Promotes realistic thinking. Helps person consider that others do not perceive events as he or she does nor do they draw the same conclusions. May reinforce doubts person already has about an idea or course of action. Avoids argument. May help to gradually reduce delusion. Conveys acceptance that delusion is the client's reality; acknowledges the communication.
Seek consensual validation of words; give definition or meaning when indicated.	Ensures that words being used mean the same to both you and client. Clarifies ideas for you and client as client defines meaning for self. Avoids misunderstanding. May help to reduce self-centered thinking.
Summarize; condense what speaker said, using speaker's own words.	Synthesizes and emphasizes important points of dialogue. Helps both you and client leave session with same ideas in mind. Emphasizes progress made toward self-awareness, problem solving, and personal development. Provides sense of closure.

Source: References 43, 67, 71.

of the clients, being empathic, and using knowledge. The therapeutic relationship/alliance must be differentiated from mere association. Social contact with another individual, verbal or nonverbal, may exercise some influence on one of the participants and needs may be met. But inconsistency, nonpredictability, or partial fulfillment of expectations often results. Develop a therapeutic relationship in order to be effective.

Phases of the therapeutic relationship/alliance were first researched and formulated by a nurse, Hildegard Peplau (66–68). The phases are (1) orientation, establishment, or initial phase; (2) identification phase; (3) working or exploitation phase; and (4) termination or resolution phase. *Certain behaviors and feelings, for both the nurse/helper and client/patient, are typical of these phases.* **Table 2-5** summarizes phases of the helping relationship. *Because*

TABLE 2-3

Guidelines for an Effective Interview

Method	Rationale
1. **Wear clothing that conveys the image of a professional and is appropriate for the situation.**	1. Consider expectations the interviewee may have of you. In some cases he or she will respond more readily to your casual dress; at other times the person may need your professional dress as part of the image to help him or her talk confidentially.
2. **Avoid preconceived ideas, prejudices, or biases.** Avoid imposing personal values on others.	2. Acceptance of client promotes feelings of self-respect and security and promotes more accurate assessment.
3. **Control the external environment** as much as possible. Try to minimize external distractions or noise, regulate ventilation and lighting, and arrange the setting.	3. Minimize discomfort, external distractions, and sense of distance. Comfort factors show respect to client and promote expression of feelings.
4. **Arrange comfortable positions** for yourself and the client.	4. Full attention can be given to the interview.
5. **Establish rapport.** Create a warm, accepting climate and a feeling of security and confidentiality.	5. The person feels free to talk about what is important to him or her.
6. **Use a vocabulary on the level of awareness or understanding of the person.** Avoid professional jargon or abstract words. **Be precise in what you say.**	6. Convey respect for and respond to the interviewee's level of understanding or health condition. Convey that you want client to understand the meaning of what you say and that you consider the client as part of the health care team.
7. **Begin by stating and validating with the client the purpose of the interview.** Either you or the interviewee may introduce the theme. You may start the session by briefly expressing friendly interest in the everyday affairs of the person, but avoid continuing trivial conversation. Maintain the proposed structure.	7. The client realizes the importance of the interview, that he or she is taken seriously and will be listened to. Client does not confuse interview with social event.
8. **Say as little as possible to keep the interview moving.** Ask questions that are well-timed, open-ended, and pertinent to the situation. **Avoid overwhelming the client with questions asked too rapidly.**	8. This pattern allows the person to place his or her own style, organization, and personality on the answers and on the interview. Getting unanticipated data can be useful in assessment. Questions that bombard the person produce unreliable information. Open-ended sentences usually keep the person talking at his or her own pace. Careful timing of your messages, verbal and nonverbal, allows time for the interviewee to understand and respond and increases accuracy and meaning of response.
9. **Avoid asking questions in ways that elicit socially acceptable answers.**	9. The interviewee often responds to questions with what he or she thinks the interviewer wants to hear, either to be well thought of, to gain status, or to show that he or she knows what other people do and what is considered socially acceptable.
10. **Ask questions beginning with "What . . . ?" "Who . . . ?" "Where . . .?" and "When . . . ?" to gain factual information. Avoid "How . . . ?" and "Why. . . ?"**	10. Words connoting moral judgments are not conducive to a feeling of neutrality, acceptance, or freedom of expression. The "How" question may be difficult for the person to answer because it asks, "In what manner . . . ?" or "For what reason . . . ?" and the individual may lack sufficient knowledge to answer. The "Why" question asks for insights that the person should not be expected to give.

continued

TABLE 2-3

Guidelines for an Effective Interview—continued

Method	Rationale
11. **Be gentle and tactful when asking about home life or personal matters.** If a subject meets resistance, change the topic; when the anxiety is reduced, return to the matter for further discussion. Be alert to what the person omits or avoids, "forgets" to mention, or deliberately refuses to discuss.	11. What you consider common or usual information may be considered very private by some. Matters about which it would be tactless to inquire directly can often be arrived at indirectly by peripheral questions. Remember, what the person does not say is as important as what is said.
12. **Be an attentive listener.** Show interest by nodding, responding with "I see," etc. Remain silent and **control your responses when another's comments evoke a personal meaning and thus trigger an emotional response in you.** While the person is talking, **seek answers to the following:** What does this experience mean? Why is this content being told at this time? What is the meaning of the choice of words, the repetition of key words, the inflection of voice, the hesitant or aggressive expression of words, the topic chosen? **Listen for feelings, needs, and goals. Listen for what is not discussed. Do not answer too fast or ask a question too soon.** If necessary, learn if the words mean the same to you as to the interviewee. Explore each clue as you let the person tell his or her story.	12. Careful listening conveys respect, promotes self-esteem and a sense of security and safety, and aids assessment. Listening is an important intervention and evaluation tool.
13. **Carefully observe nonverbal messages for signs of anxiety, frustration, anger, loneliness, or guilt.** Look for feelings of pressure hidden by the person's attempts to be calm. Encourage the free expression of feelings, for feelings often bring facts with them. Focus on emotionally charged topics when the person is able to share deep feelings.	13. Nonverbal behavior is often the key to the message and is usually not under the client's voluntary control or in his or her awareness. Nonverbal behavior often conveys more directly the client's feelings. Ventilation of feeling is the key resolution of many emotional difficulties and opens the door to new data as well as increased understanding and insight in the client.
14. **Encourage spontaneity.** Provide movement in the interview by **picking up verbal leads, clues, bits of seemingly unrelated information, and nonverbal signals** from the client. If the person asks you a personal question, redirect it to him or her; it may be the topic he or she unconsciously (or even consciously) wishes to speak about.	14. Movement of the interview gives you understanding about the person, his or her behavior, needs, health, illness, and relationships. Only occasionally will it be pertinent for you to answer personal questions. Sometimes brief self-disclosure will help the interviewee feel comfortable and elicit additional data. Be sure to disclose such information for the benefit of the client, not yourself.
15. **Indicate when the interview is terminated,** and terminate it graciously if the interviewee does not do so first. **Make a transition in interviewing or use a natural stopping point** if the problem has been resolved, if the information has been obtained or given, or if the person changes the topic. You may say, "There is one more question I'd like to ask," or "Just two more points I want to clarify," or "Before I leave, do you have any other questions, comments, or ideas to share?"	15. The client feels more secure with structure. Avoid social conversation or a feeling in the client that you lack skill. Skillful and distinct termination prevents you from feeling manipulated by the client's prolonging of the interview.

TABLE 2-3

Guidelines for an Effective Interview—continued

Method	Rationale
16. **Keep data obtained in the interview confidential, and share this information only with the appropriate and necessary health team members,** leaving out personal assumptions. If you are sharing an opinion or interpretation, state it as such, rather than have it appear to be what the other person said or did. The person should be told what information will be shared and with whom and the reason for sharing.	16. Show respect for the individual. Confidentiality is the client's right and your responsibility, as well as a professional and legal mandate.
17. **Evaluate the interview. Were the purposes accomplished?**	17. Evaluate yourself in each situation. Recognize that not everyone can successfully interview everyone. Others may see you differently from the way you see yourself. Validation with someone who is a skilled interviewer is helpful.

Source: References 43, 67, 71.

TABLE 2-4

Barriers to Effective Communication

1. **Conveying your feelings of anxiety, anger, judgment, blame, ambivalence, condescension, placating approach, denial, isolation, lack of control, or lack of physical or emotional health.**
2. **The appearance of being too busy, of not having time or desire to listen, of not giving sufficient time for an answer, or of not really wanting to hear.**
3. **Not paying attention to what is being said verbally and nonverbally; rehearsing** what you plan to say as the other is talking; **filtering** (listening selectively); **trying to second-guess the other person; daydreaming while the other talks.**
4. **Using the wrong vocabulary**—vocabulary that is abstract or intangible, or full of jargon, slang, or implied status; talking too much; or using unnecessarily long sentences or words out of context.
5. **Failing to understand the reason for the person's reluctance to make a message clear.**
6. **Making inappropriate use of facts, twisting facts, introducing unrelated information, offering premature interpretation, or saying something important when the person is upset or not feeling well and thus unable to hear what is really said.**
7. **Making glib statements, offering false reassurance** by saying, "Everything is OK."
8. **Using clichés, stereotyped responses, trite expressions, and empty or patronizing verbalisms** stated without thought, such as "It's always worse at night," "I know," "You'll be OK," or "Who is to say?"
9. **Expressing unnecessary approval.** Stating that something the person does or feels is particularly good implies that the opposite is bad.
10. **Expressing undue disapproval.** Denouncing another's behavior or ideas implies that you have the right to pass judgment and that he or she must please you.
11. **Giving advice; stating personal experiences, opinions, or value judgments; giving pep talks; telling another what should be done.**
12. **Requiring explanations, demanding proof, challenging or asking "Why . . .?"** when the person cannot provide a reason for thoughts, feelings, and behavior for events.
13. **Belittling the person's feelings** (equating intense and overwhelming feelings expressed by the client with those felt by everyone or yourself). This implies that such feelings are not valid; that he or she is bad; or that the discomfort is mild, temporary, and unimportant.

TABLE 2-5

Phases of the Helping Relationship

Orientation Phase (Problem-defining phase)

Nurse Behaviors

- Initiates interaction:
  - Introduces self
  - Listens to client's/family's perception of problem, expectations, and needs
  - Establishes rapport with client
  - Demonstrates acceptance
  - Explains own role to person/family
- Establishes contract (verbal or written):
  - Explains nature of relationship
  - Schedules time, duration, and plan of treatment
  - Discusses issues of confidentiality
  - Gathers information from person or family
- Collaborates with client to analyze situation and establish goals:
  - Validates whether care plan matches client's impression of problem
  - Acts as a resource to person and/or family
  - Refers person and/or family to services within the agency or elsewhere
  - Continues assessment, promotes security
- Demonstrates therapeutic emotional response:
  - Demonstrates empathy, remains objective
  - Demonstrates unconditional positive regard
  - Demonstrates trustworthiness to client
  - Examines own thoughts, feelings, expectations, and actions

- Demonstrates ability to control countertransference behavior
- Reduces anxiety/tension in the relationship through use of communication and relationship principles
- Provides experiences for client to release anxiety and tension feelings
- Assists client to focus on goals, coping with problems, and treatment

Patient/Client Behaviors

- Describes perceived need(s) or may be unable to identify need for assistance
- Seeks assistance; clarifies problems
- Demonstrates trust in the nurse; responds to teaching

Mutual Behaviors

- Define existing problems and perceptions
- Clarify facts; express feelings
- Make decisions about assistance needed
- Develop goals and care plan
- Validate that implementation of a care plan meets expectations; collaborate with goals
- Continue interventions as indicated

Working Phase

Nurse Behaviors

- Continues assessment:
  - Encourages client to express feelings and thoughts
  - Listens carefully; client does more talking than nurse
  - Evaluates problems and goals and redefines as necessary
  - Helps client overcome resistance to change
  - Assists client as necessary with tasks and meeting goals
  - Intervenes, using communication principles
  - Confronts incongruities in client's verbal and nonverbal behavior and life patterns in a way that does not threaten client
  - Clarifies possible solutions, resources, options with client
  - Educates and supports client's behavior in a way that client can accept and use the information to change behavior, gain new self-view
- Promotes client's development: emotional, interpersonal, and behavioral:
  - Assists client in developing healthy methods to reduce anxiety and relate to others

- Provides opportunities for client to become more independent and interdependent
- Facilitates behavioral change in person/family
- Discusses strengths and positive factors in person/family
- Supports, instills optimism, conveys hope, and reinforces positive directions in client's behavior
- Teaches client as needs emerge, pertinent to life situation and illness:
  - Teaches problem-solving skills
  - Teaches about illness/treatment regimen
  - Accepts that client may not follow nurse's suggestions/teaching
- Discusses approaching discharge and rehabilitation plans:
  - Initiates discharge and rehabilitation plans and specific measures
  - Teaches family about their role in rehabilitation and recovery of patient
  - Accepts that family may not consider or follow nurse's suggestions or teaching

TABLE 2-5

Phases of the Helping Relationship—continued

- Demonstrates therapeutic emotional response:
  - Demonstrates deeper empathy
  - Continues to convey attitudes of acceptance, concern, and positive attitude
  - Controls countertransference feelings

Patient/Client Behaviors

- Maintains relationship with nurse; may imitate
- Describes feelings of trust in nurse
- Fluctuates between dependency and independency
- Demonstrates increasing ability to establish own goals:
  - Demonstrates increasing assertiveness and self-reliance in self-care and goal attainment
  - Insists on doing tasks in his or her own way
  - Demonstrates attention-seeking and self-centered behavior at times
- Participates increasingly in decision making about own welfare, treatment, rehabilitation, and postdischarge plans
- Utilizes services and resources offered by the nurse and health team that meet his or her needs:
  - Makes demands on nurse and other health care members
  - Pursues helpful resources
  - Carries out assignments between sessions

- Demonstrates increasingly more open and effective communication skills
  - Describes willingness to accept help while recognizing own strengths, abilities, and limits
  - Describes sense of hope and self-confidence about own potential: increasing self-esteem
- Demonstrates increasingly the signs of physical and emotional health or a higher level of functioning
  - Demonstrates increasing skills in interpersonal relationships and problem solving
  - Describes feelings of wellness and readiness for approaching discharge, explores deeper feelings

Mutual Behaviors

- Examine together the relationship and its meaning
- Collaborate as partners in meeting health care goals
- Utilize multidisciplinary team members in various facets of intervention and rehabilitation plans
- Formulate discharge and rehabilitation plans/goals

Termination Phase

Nurse Behaviors

- Continues to demonstrate empathy, support, and caring for the client
- Sustains relationship as long as client demonstrates need
- Plans for discharge and termination of relationship with client
- Teaches measures to help person prevent further illness and maintain self-care
- Promotes interaction between person and family
- Discusses community resources or networks that could be utilized by person/family

Patient/Client Behaviors

- Demonstrates fewer or diminished symptoms
- Demonstrates defensive maneuvers that are meant to delay discharge and termination:
  - Does not keep interview appointments
  - Is sarcastic or hostile to nurse or others
  - Demonstrates temporary dependency
  - Describes lack of confidence in ability to manage postdischarge; receptive to support
  - Does not come to final appointment
- Demonstrates or describes that needs have been met and goals accomplished:
  - Demonstrates improved social functioning
  - Demonstrates being independent of helping person

- Explores feelings about impending separation and discharge
- Indicates verbally and/or behaviorally that he or she is ready for discharge:
  - Demonstrates more adaptive mechanisms of behavior
  - Describes increased self-esteem, self-confidence, and significance to others
  - Describes hope for the future
  - Demonstrates or describes ability to live independently
  - Maintains behavioral and communication changes

Mutual Behaviors

- Discuss what was accomplished in treatment, goals set and accomplished
- Examine uncertainty about client's ability to manage after discharge
- Plan together how the client will continue to interact and manage life's patterns and stresses
- Utilize community resources as necessary
- Resolve mourning process that is part of separation and termination with long-term relationship
- Demonstrate more mature behavior as result of relationship
- Terminate relationship

Generated by Ruth Murray, EdD, MSN, N-NAP, FAAN, adapted from reference 68.

TABLE 2-6

Characteristics of a Helping Relationship

Respectful: Feeling and communicating an attitude of seeing the client as a unique human being, filled with dignity, worth, and strengths, regardless of outward appearance or behavior; being willing to *work* at communicating with and understanding the client because he or she is in need of emotional care

Genuine: Communicating spontaneously, yet tactfully, what is felt and thought, with proper timing and without disturbing the client, rather than using professional jargon, façade, or rigid counselor or nurse role behaviors

Attentive: Conveying active listening to verbal and nonverbal messages and an attitude of working with the person

Accepting: Conveying that the person does not have to put on a façade and that the person's statements will not shock you; enabling the client to change at his or her own pace; acknowledging personal and client's feelings aroused in the encounter; "being for" the client in a nonsentimental, caring way

Positive: Showing warmth, caring, respect, and agape love; being able to reinforce the client for what he or she does well

Strong: Maintaining a separate identity from the client; withstanding the testing

Secure: Permitting the client to remain separate and unique; respecting his or her needs and your own; feeling safe as the client moves emotionally close; feeling no need to exploit the other person

Knowledgeable: Having an expertise based on study, experience, and supervision

Sensitive: Being perceptive to feelings; avoiding threatening behavior; responding to cultural values, customs, norms as they affect behavior; using knowledge that is pertinent to the client's situation; being kind and gentle

Empathic: Looking at the world from the client's viewpoint; being open to the client's values, feelings, beliefs, and verbal statements; stating your understanding of his or her verbal or nonverbal expressions of feelings and experiences

Nonjudgmental: Refraining from evaluating the client moralistically, or telling the client what to do

Congruent: Being natural, relaxed, honest, trustworthy, and dependable; demonstrating consistency in behavior

Unambiguous: Avoiding contradictory messages

Creative: Viewing the client as a person in the process of becoming, not being bound by the past, and viewing yourself in the process of becoming or maturing

Adapted from reference 71.

of the nature of mutual participation in a therapeutic relationship, mutual behaviors are also noted (7, 29, 30, 66–68). Descriptions of behaviors of these phases have been modified over time. These *modifications are also incorporated* into this table. You will use these behaviors.

Incorporate into your behavior, during assessment and intervention, information from **Table 2-6,** which summarizes how to use the humanistic approach with a client (71). These characteristics were first combined into a total approach by Carl Rogers. They are considered basic to a professional therapeutic relationship or alliance, and to any counseling or educational role (71). Your use of therapeutic communication and a client-centered approach will move you through the relationship with a family or individual.

The behaviors presented in **Tables 2-5 and 2-6** can be used to **evaluate** progress and the effectiveness of your approach in the therapeutic relationship.

Stress and Crisis Theories

Stressors and crises are a part of development throughout the life span and do affect health. An understanding of stress and crisis theories is essential for health promotion assessment and interventions.

Two theories describe how a person responds to stressors, both routine and severe, and to overwhelming events. The **Theory of Stress and General Adaptation Syndrome,** as formulated by Selye, *describes the physiologic adaptive response to stress, the everyday*

wear and tear on the person (78–84). However, continued studies show that the stress response has emotional, cognitive, and sometimes social effects as well.

Crisis Theory *was formulated to explain how people respond psychologically and behaviorally when they cannot cope adequately with stressors.* Crises or overwhelming events have physical and psychological effects. The theories together explain a range of adaptive responses, for stress response always occurs in crisis to some extent, although not every stressful event is a crisis (4, 15, 40).

THEORY OF STRESS RESPONSE AND GENERAL ADAPTATION SYNDROME

Stress *is a physical and emotional state always present in the person, influenced by various environmental, psychological, and social factors. It is uniquely perceived by the person and intensified in response when environmental change or threat occurs internally or externally and the person must respond.* The manifestations of stress are both overt and covert, purposeful, and *initially* protective, maintaining equilibrium, productivity, and satisfaction to the extent possible (78–84).

The person's survival depends on constant mediation between environmental demands and adaptive capacities. Various self-regulatory physical and emotional mechanisms are in constant operation, adjusting the body to a changing number and nature of internal and external stressors, or factors causing intensification of the stress state. **Stressors** *(stress agents) encompass a number of types of stimuli* (18, 21, 49, 60, 61, 78–84):

1. **Physical:** excessive or intense cold or heat, sound, light, motion, gravity, or electrical current.
2. **Chemical:** alkalines, acids, drugs, toxic substances, hormones, gases, or food and water pollutants.
3. **Microbiologic:** viruses, bacteria, molds, parasites, or other infectious organisms.
4. **Physiologic:** disease processes, surgery, immobilization, mechanical trauma, fever, organ hypo- and hyperfunction, or pain.
5. **Psychological:** anticipated marriage or death, imagined events, intense emotional involvement, anxiety or other unpleasant feelings, distortions of body image, threats to self-concept, others' expectations of behavior, rejection by or separation from loved ones, role changes, memory of negative past experiences, or actual or perceived failures.
6. **Developmental:** genetic endowment, prematurity, immaturity, maturational impairment, or the aging process.
7. **Sociocultural:** sociocultural background and pressures, unharmonious interpersonal relationships, demands of our technologic society, social mobility, changing social mores, job pressures, economic worries, childrearing practices, redefinition of sex roles, or minority status.
8. **Environmental:** unemployment, air and water pollution, overcrowding disasters, war, or crime.

Eustress is the *stress that comes with successful adaptation and is beneficial or promotes emotional development and self-actualization.* It is *positive stress,* an optimum orientation to life's challenges coupled with the person's ability to regulate life and maintain optimum levels of stress for a growth-promoting lifestyle (84). A moderate amount of stress, when regulatory mechanisms act within limits and few symptoms are observable, is constructive. **Daily hassles** *are the repeated and chronic strains of everyday life.* Daily hassles have a negative effect on both somatic health and psychological status (18, 21). **Distress** is *negative, noxious, unpleasant, damaging stress* that results when adaptive capacity is decreased or exhausted (18, 21, 83).

What is considered a stressor by one person may be considered normal or pleasurable by another. The amount of stress in the immediate environment cannot be determined by examining only the stressor or source of stress. *Certain principles, however, apply to most people* (14, 19, 21, 60, 78–84):

1. **The primary response to a stressor is behavioral.** When an event or situation is perceived as threatening, the person reacts to meet the threat. Physiologic impact is secondary.
2. **The impact is cumulative.** Most stressors in the environment occur at levels below that which would cause immediate physical or emotional damage.
3. **Circumstances alter the impact or harm done by a stressor.** The social and emotional context and the attitude and previous experiences of the person are as important as the nature of the stimuli.
4. **People are remarkably adaptable.** Each person has evolved a plasticity and a normal range of response or a unique pattern of defense. What may at first be considered uncomfortable or intolerable may eventually be perceived as normal. The immediate impact of a stressor is apparently different from long-term or indirect consequences.
5. **Various psychological or social factors can ease or exaggerate the effects of a stressor.** If a stressor is predictable, it will not be as harmful as an unpredictable one. If the person feels in control of the situation or can relate positively or directly to the stressor, the effects are less negative. For example, the person in a noisy environment suffers less startle reaction if sudden noises come regularly and are anticipated.
6. **Conditioning is an important protection.** The person whose heart, lungs, and skeletal muscles are conditioned by exercise can withstand cardiovascular and respiratory effects of the Alarm Stage better than someone who leads a sedentary life.

Responses to stress throughout life are both local and general. The **Local Adaptation Syndrome,** *typified by the inflammatory response,* is the *method used to wall off and control effects of physical stressors locally.* When the stressor cannot be handled locally, the *whole body responds to protect itself and ensure survival in the best way possible through the* **General Adaptation Syndrome.** The *general body response augments body functions that protect the organism and suppresses those functions nonessential to life.* The General Adaptation Syndrome is *characterized by the Alarm and Resistance Stages. When body resistance is not maintained, the Exhaustion Stage occurs* (78–84). **Figure 2-1** ◼ depicts the hypothalamic-pituitary-adrenal and autonomic nervous system. **Figure 2-2** ◼ depicts the physiologic responses in acute stress.

General Adaptation Syndrome

The **Alarm Stage** is an *instantaneous, short-term, life-preserving, and total sympathetic nervous system response* when the person consciously or unconsciously perceives a stressor and feels helpless, insecure, or biologically uncomfortable. This stage is typified by a *fight-or-flight* reaction (69, 75). Perception of the stressor—the alarm reaction—stimulates the anterior pituitary to increase production of adrenocorticotropic hormone (ACTH). The adrenal cortex is stimulated by ACTH to increase production of glucocorticoids, primarily hydrocortisone or cortisol, and mineralocorticoids, primarily aldosterone. Catecholamine release triggers increased sympathetic nervous system activity, which stimulates production of epinephrine and norepinephrine by the adrenal medulla and release at the adrenergic nerve endings. The alarm reaction also stimulates the posterior pituitary to release increased antidiuretic hormone (37, 38, 48, 78–84). *Generally the person is prepared to act, is more alert, and is able to adapt.* See **Figures 2-1 and 2-2** for a summary. Physiologically, the responses that occur during the Alarm Stage when the sympathetic nervous system is stimulated are summarized in **Figure 2-3** ◼ (78–84).

To complicate assessment, there are times when *parts of the parasympathetic division of the autonomic nervous system are inadvertently stimulated during a stressful state because of the proximity of sympathetic and parasympathetic nerve fibers.* With intensification of stress, *opposite behaviors are then observed.* Normal parasympathetic body functions are diminished, which can cause cardiopulmonary collapse, and even sudden death (37, 38, 48, 84).

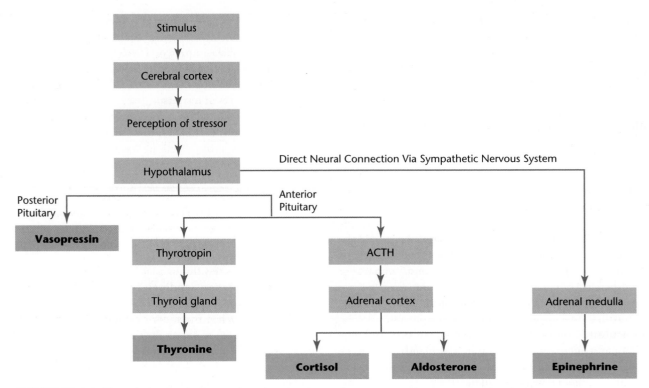

FIGURE ☐ **2-1** Hypothalamic-pituitary-adrenal and autonomic nervous system response to stress.

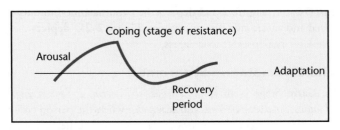

FIGURE ☐ **2-2** Reaction pattern in acute stress.

Lazarus identified three psychological stages that occur during the Alarm Stage: *threat, warning, and impact.* Stimuli are perceived as a *threat* cognitively, emotionally, and perhaps also physically. This serves as a *warning* to respond to the meaning, recall of past memories, anxiety, fear, anger, guilt, or shame. *Impact* of the warning brings forth physical or physiologic responses (49–51).

The **Allostatic Load Model** *further explains the Alarm Stage and effects of stress on body* **homeostasis** *or* **equilibrium.** The model integrates the body's response to cortisol secretion and subsequent pathology and *integrates other factors that combine to affect the person on a biochemical and cellular level.* These factors include the person's past learning, interpretation of event, perception of threat, genetic influence, developmental stages, gender, social history, and context (60, 61, 78).

The **Stage of Resistance** is the *body's way of adapting, through an adrenocortical response, to the disequilibrium caused by the stressors of life.* Increased use of body resources, tissue anabolism, antibody production, hormonal secretion, and changes in blood sugar levels and blood volume sustain the body's fight for preservation

(37, 38, 78, 84). Lazarus described coping with resistance to stress as more complicated than a physical response to stimuli. Personal and environmental factors influenced appraisal or perception of the stressor, the use of biopsychosocial resources for coping or adaptation, and the ability to act to maintain health or wellness and avoid maladaptation, such as illness, social dysfunction, or emotional dysfunction (48–51). Refer to **Figure 2-4**☐ for a summary of the Stage of Resistance and signs of emotional, intellectual, and physiologic distress.

The tissue tranquilizers that are released help us adapt to stimuli, and the enzymes and blood cells release attack pathogens. Moderate anxiety is felt; habitual ego defenses are unconsciously used. *Responses eventually return to normal when stressors diminish or when the person has found adaptive mechanisms* that meet emotional needs and physical demands (38, 48, 78–84).

If biological, psychological, or social stresses, alone or in combination, occur over a long period without adequate relief, the **resistance stage** is maintained for a time. *With continued stressors, the person becomes distressed and manifests objective and subjective emotional, intellectual, and physiologic responses,* as shown in **Figure 2-4**☐ **and Figure 2-5**☐, which depicts the reaction pattern in chronic stress (10, 14, 18, 21, 48, 78–84). Although responses to stressful situations vary, anxiety is a common one (see **Chapter 1, Table 1-6**). ∞ Protective factors *modify, ameliorate, or alter the person's response to stressors and to a potentially maladaptive outcome.* They include such factors as positive temperament, intelligence, ability to relate well to others, participation in achievements, success in school or the job, family support, friends, and a safe environment (21, 48, 60).

The **Stage of Exhaustion** occurs when the *person is unable to continue to adapt to internal and external environmental demands.*

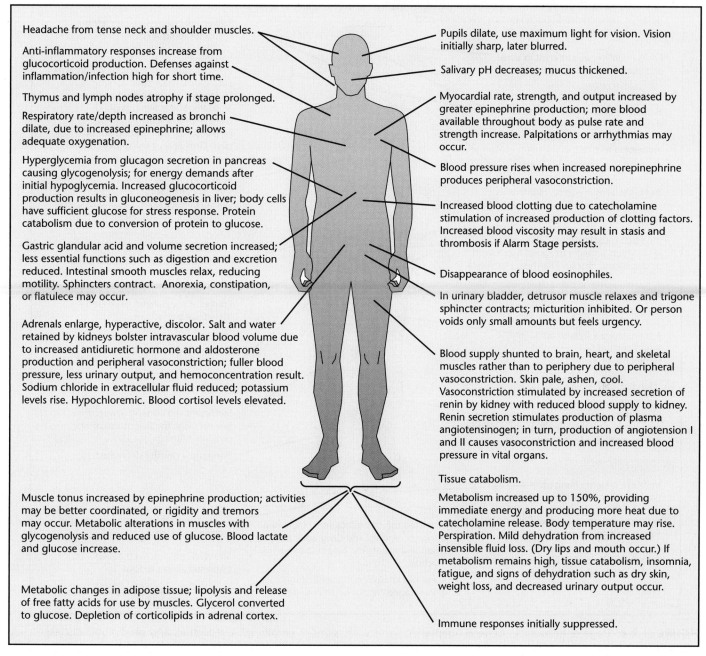

Headache from tense neck and shoulder muscles.

Anti-inflammatory responses increase from glucocorticoid production. Defenses against inflammation/infection high for short time.

Thymus and lymph nodes atrophy if stage prolonged.

Respiratory rate/depth increased as bronchi dilate, due to increased epinephrine; allows adequate oxygenation.

Hyperglycemia from glucagon secretion in pancreas causing glycogenolysis; for energy demands after initial hypoglycemia. Increased glucocorticoid production results in gluconeogenesis in liver; body cells have sufficient glucose for stress response. Protein catabolism due to conversion of protein to glucose.

Gastric glandular acid and volume secretion increased; less essential functions such as digestion and excretion reduced. Intestinal smooth muscles relax, reducing motility. Sphincters contract. Anorexia, constipation, or flatulece may occur.

Adrenals enlarge, hyperactive, discolor. Salt and water retained by kidneys bolster intravascular blood volume due to increased antidiuretic hormone and aldosterone production and peripheral vasoconstriction; fuller blood pressure, less urinary output, and hemoconcentration result. Sodium chloride in extracellular fluid reduced; potassium levels rise. Hypochloremic. Blood cortisol levels elevated.

Muscle tonus increased by epinephrine production; activities may be better coordinated, or rigidity and tremors may occur. Metabolic alterations in muscles with glycogenolysis and reduced use of glucose. Blood lactate and glucose increase.

Metabolic changes in adipose tissue; lipolysis and release of free fatty acids for use by muscles. Glycerol converted to glucose. Depletion of corticolipids in adrenal cortex.

Pupils dilate, use maximum light for vision. Vision initially sharp, later blurred.

Salivary pH decreases; mucus thickened.

Myocardial rate, strength, and output increased by greater epinephrine production; more blood available throughout body as pulse rate and strength increase. Palpitations or arrhythmias may occur.

Blood pressure rises when increased norepinephrine produces peripheral vasoconstriction.

Increased blood clotting due to catecholamine stimulation of increased production of clotting factors. Increased blood viscosity may result in stasis and thrombosis if Alarm Stage persists.

Disappearance of blood eosinophiles.

In urinary bladder, detrusor muscle relaxes and trigone sphincter contracts; micturition inhibited. Or person voids only small amounts but feels urgency.

Blood supply shunted to brain, heart, and skeletal muscles rather than to periphery due to peripheral vasoconstriction. Skin pale, ashen, cool. Vasoconstriction stimulated by increased secretion of renin by kidney with reduced blood supply to kidney. Renin secretion stimulates production of plasma angiotensinogen; in turn, production of angiotension I and II causes vasoconstriction and increased blood pressure in vital organs.

Tissue catabolism.

Metabolism increased up to 150%, providing immediate energy and producing more heat due to catecholamine release. Body temperature may rise. Perspiration. Mild dehydration from increased insensible fluid loss. (Dry lips and mouth occur.) If metabolism remains high, tissue catabolism, insomnia, fatigue, and signs of dehydration such as dry skin, weight loss, and decreased urinary output occur.

Immune responses initially suppressed.

FIGURE ■ 2-3 Alarm Stage, General Adaptation Syndrome: physiologic responses to sympathetic nervous system stimulation.

Disease or death results because the body can no longer compensate for or correct homeostatic imbalances, as shown in **Figure 2-5** (10, 37, 61, 78–84).

The **mind-body relationship**, the *effect of emotional responses to stress on body function and the emotional reactions to body conditions*, has been established through research and experience. Emotional factors are important in the precipitation or exacerbation of nearly every organic disease and may increase susceptibility to disease. Stress and emotional distress, including depression, influence function of the immune system via central nervous system and endocrine mediation. Apparently, adrenocortical steroid hormones are immunosuppressive. Recurring or chronic emotional stress has a cumulative physiologic effect and eventually may produce chronic illness or disease (37, 38, 48, 61, 77, 80–84). The **Glucocorticoid Cascade Hypothesis** formulated by Sapolsky, Krey, and McEwen (75) *discussed how genetic predisposition or exposure to stressful events at a young age disturb the hypothalamic-pituitary-adrenal (HPA) axis.* High serum cortisol levels and consequent cumulative effect on brain tissue result. *Eventually the whole body responds* to damage to cells in the hippocampus and hypothalamus, *which contributes to long-term physical and psychological effects* (32, 60, 61).

When physical or organic symptoms or disease result from feeling states, the process is called **psychosomatic** *or* **psychophysiologic**. *The opposite process, feeling states of depression or worry in response to physical states, is called* **somatopsychic**.

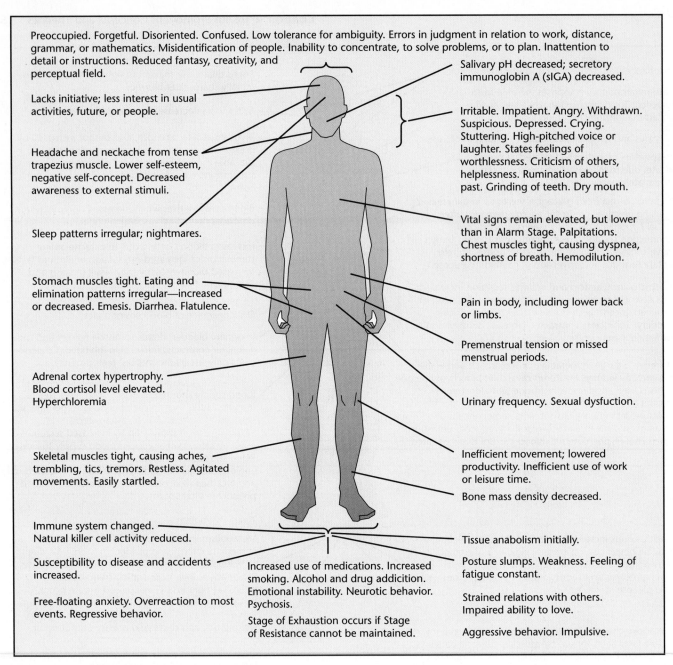

Preoccupied. Forgetful. Disoriented. Confused. Low tolerance for ambiguity. Errors in judgment in relation to work, distance, grammar, or mathematics. Misidentification of people. Inability to concentrate, to solve problems, or to plan. Inattention to detail or instructions. Reduced fantasy, creativity, and perceptual field.

Lacks initiative; less interest in usual activities, future, or people.

Headache and neckache from tense trapezius muscle. Lower self-esteem, negative self-concept. Decreased awareness to external stimuli.

Sleep patterns irregular; nightmares.

Stomach muscles tight. Eating and elimination patterns irregular—increased or decreased. Emesis. Diarrhea. Flatulence.

Adrenal cortex hypertrophy. Blood cortisol level elevated. Hyperchloremia

Skeletal muscles tight, causing aches, trembling, tics, tremors. Restless. Agitated movements. Easily startled.

Immune system changed. Natural killer cell activity reduced.

Susceptibility to disease and accidents increased.

Free-floating anxiety. Overreaction to most events. Regressive behavior.

Salivary pH decreased; secretory immunoglobin A (sIGA) decreased.

Irritable. Impatient. Angry. Withdrawn. Suspicious. Depressed. Crying. Stuttering. High-pitched voice or laughter. States feelings of worthlessness. Criticism of others, helplessness. Rumination about past. Grinding of teeth. Dry mouth.

Vital signs remain elevated, but lower than in Alarm Stage. Palpitations. Chest muscles tight, causing dyspnea, shortness of breath. Hemodilution.

Pain in body, including lower back or limbs.

Premenstrual tension or missed menstrual periods.

Urinary frequency. Sexual dysfuction.

Inefficient movement; lowered productivity. Inefficient use of work or leisure time.

Bone mass density decreased.

Tissue anabolism initially.

Posture slumps. Weakness. Feeling of fatigue constant.

Strained relations with others. Impaired ability to love.

Aggressive behavior. Impulsive.

Increased use of medications. Increased smoking. Alcohol and drug addiction. Emotional instability. Neurotic behavior. Psychosis.

Stage of Exhaustion occurs if Stage of Resistance cannot be maintained.

FIGURE ▪ 2-4 Stage of Resistance, General Adaptation Syndrome: signs of emotional, intellectual, and physiologic distress.

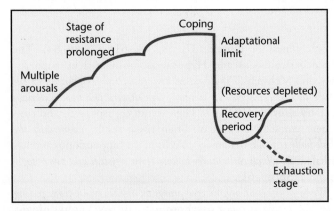

FIGURE ▪ 2-5 Reaction pattern in chronic stress.

Source: Adapted from reference 82.

The field of **psychoneuroimmunology** *focuses on the links between the mind, or mental processes, physiologic brain, and immune system.* This is a newer perspective of the mind-body relationship in psychophysiologic causation of illness. Research shows that the immune system responds to the mind. In turn, other body systems are affected—positively or negatively.

Use of **positive adaptive mechanisms,** such as compensation, identification, and sublimation (described in Table 1-6) ∞, and positive coping behaviors (described in Client Education: Positive Coping Strategies), as well as visualization, imagery, and positive thinking all promote a healthy response in the immune and other body systems. All of these also help to handle stressors (92). Other stress management strategies are presented later.

Client Education

Positive Coping Strategies

Affiliation:	Seek help and support from others.
Altruism:	Dedicate self to meet the needs of others.
Anticipation:	Prepare by thinking of future problems, realistic solutions, and consequences.
Assertiveness:	Express one's feelings and thoughts directly.
Humor:	Recognize the amusing aspects of a situation; maintain the ability to laugh.
Self-observation:	Reflect on one's thoughts, feelings, motivations, and behavior, and respond appropriately to self-evaluation.

Health Care and Nursing Applications

Health care providers are concerned with helping people cope with the Alarm Stage, maintain the Resistance Stage, and foster a return to normal function. In turn, the Exhaustion Stage is prevented or reversed. Identify potential stressors that the person might encounter (14, 41, 63, 69). Teach the client how to recognize signs of the stress response. Then teach the client how to activate the relaxation response. One method is to use PBR3: pause, breathe, relax, reflect, and rewrite. It is important for the client to change the mental self-talk when encountering stress, to rewrite the story he or she is telling self. The story—positive or negative—that is repeated to self mentally sets the stage for future responses to and coping with stress (35). Determine how to alter the stressors or best support the person's adaptive mechanisms and resources physically, emotionally, and socially, because the person will respond as a whole entity to the stressors. The relationship of stress to life crises or changes must be considered whenever you are doing health promotion measures or intervening with the ill person. **Evaluate** the effectiveness of stress management methods. Refer to **Table 2-7** for criteria for evaluation related to stress management interventions.

Websites of selected complementary and alternative therapies, including methods that can be utilized to prevent or reduce stress response, are presented later in **Table 2-10**. These methods are effective for health promotion and can be modified as necessary to the capacity of the person in different developmental stages.

CRISIS THEORY
Definitions and Characteristics

Crisis is any *temporary situation that threatens the person's self-concept, necessitates reorganization of psychological structure and behavior, causes a sudden alteration in the person's expectation of self, and cannot be handled with the person's usual coping mechanisms* (4, 15, 40). Crises always involve change and loss. Either the changes or losses that occur result in the person's inability to cope, or as a result of the crisis, the person is no longer the same. He or she will have to change behavior to remain adaptive and functional; in the process, loss will be felt. Crisis resolution means that something is lost even while something else is gained (4, 40). Both emotional and physical health is threatened.

During crisis, the person's ordinary behavior is no longer successful—emotionally, intellectually, socially, or physically (4, 40). The person may refer to a crisis as a "tough time" or speak of the lack of coping ability by saying, "I'm at the end of my rope. I can't manage anymore." The usual coping skills or adaptive mechanisms do not work in the situation; old habits and daily patterns are disturbed. Thus, the person feels motivated to try new behavior to cope with the new situation. Although behavior during crisis is inadequate or inappropriate to the present situation and may be different from normal, *it should not be considered pathologic.* For example, rage or bitterness or prolonged crying by a usually jovial person may be an emotional release that paves the way for problem solving.

INTERVENTIONS FOR HEALTH PROMOTION

Practice application for the Theory of Stress Response and Adaptation includes the following:

1. Assess physical, emotional, and cognitive manifestations of stress response.
2. Assess level of anxiety.
3. Determine stage of adaptation.
4. Teach stress management methods.
5. Counsel as necessary.
6. Intervene as necessary to prevent exhaustion stage.
7. Evaluate results of intervention.

TABLE 2-7

Criteria for Evaluation of Intervention Related to Stress Management

1. Client identifies stressors, stressful relationships, and lifestyle that interferes with personal functioning and interpersonal relationships.
2. Client identifies physical (psychosomatic) manifestations of stress.
3. Client describes feelings related to anxiety state and accepts assistance in coping with anxiety as necessary.
4. Client describes and uses at least one strategy to reduce frequency of stress response.
5. Client describes and demonstrates at least one strategy to avoid a stressor.
6. Client describes at least one situation whereby a stressful situation is perceived as challenging or positive rather than distressful.
7. Client practices at least one method of relaxation.
8. Client describes and practices one positive health habit and one other method to prevent disease and promote health.
9. Client describes positive characteristics about self and lifestyle.
10. Client demonstrates improved interpersonal relationships; changed behavior is validated by significant others.
11. Client sets priorities and goals appropriate to developmental stage and life situation that do not predispose to excessive stress.

The crisis may also reactivate old, unresolved crises or conflicts, which can impose an additional burden to be handled at the present time. *The crisis is a turning point;* it operates as a second chance for resolving earlier crises or for correcting faulty problem solving. If all goes well, a state of equilibrium or behavior that is more mature than the previous status results. On the other hand, because of the stress involved and the felt threat to the equilibrium, the person is also more vulnerable to regression and emotional or physical illness. The outcome—either increased, the same level of, or decreased maturity, or illness—depends on how the person handles the situation and on the help others give. Encountering and resolving a crisis is a normal process that each person or family faces many times during a lifetime (4, 15, 40).

Not all persons facing the same hazardous event will be in a state of crisis, but *some events or situations are viewed as a crisis by all persons,* of any age, in that some behavioral adjustment must be made by anyone facing that situation. (4, 40, 41, 69). *Crises also vary in degree;* a situation may be perceived as major, moderate, or minimal in the discomfort caused and amount of behavioral change demanded. A person may view minimal crises as stressful life situations, but the objective observer would see that the individual is ineffective in coping.

Crisis differs from transition. **Transition** refers to a *passage or movement from one state or place to another that occurs over time, involving changes that can be managed* (76).

Types of Crises and Influencing Factors

Crises are divided into two major categories: (a) developmental, maturational, or normative; and (b) situational, accidental, or catastrophic (4, 40). **Developmental crises** *occur during transition points, those periods that every person and family typically experience in the process of biopsychosocial maturation.* These are times in development when new relationships are formed and old relationships take on new aspects. There are new expectations of the person. Certain emotional tasks must be accomplished to move on to the next phase of development. The onset of the developmental or maturational crisis is gradual because it occurs as the person moves from one stage of development to another. *The crisis resolves* when the individual succeeds in new age-level behaviors; disruption does not last for the entire developmental phase.

There are *three main reasons why someone may be unable to make healthy role changes necessary to prevent a developmental or maturational crisis* (40):

1. The person may be unable to picture self in a new role. Roles are learned, and adequate role models may not exist.
2. The person may be unable to make role changes because of a lack of intrapersonal resources, lack of communication skills, or lack of past opportunities to learn how to cope with crises.
3. Others in the social system may refuse to let the person assume a different role. For example, when the adolescent tries to move from childhood to the adult role, the parent may persist in keeping him or her in the child role.

Several factors help the person adjust to a new life era, including (a) desire for a change, or boredom with the present, (b) goals and future plans, (c) accomplishments in the present era, (d) past success in coping with turning points, (e) group support in meeting turning points, and (f) examples of how peers have coped with similar situations.

The more clear-cut the cultural definitions, the less frightening is the future situation, because the person has models of behavior and can prepare in advance for change.

A **situational crisis** *is an external event or situation, not necessarily a part of normal living, often sudden, unexpected, and unfortunate, that looms larger than the person's immediate resources or ability to cope. This demands a change in behavior* (12, 32, 40). Life goals are threatened; tension and anxiety are evoked; unresolved problems and crises from the past are reawakened. The amount of time taken for healthy or unhealthy adaptation to occur usually ranges from 1 to 6 weeks, although resolution may take longer. A situational crisis may occur at the same time as a developmental crisis.

Situational crises include:

1. Natural disasters, such as hurricane, tornado, earthquake, and flood.
2. Separation, divorce, or incapacitation or death of a loved one.
3. Loss of job, money, or valued possessions; or a job change.

4. Illness, hospitalization, or institutionalization.
5. Additions to the family, such as an unwanted pregnancy, or a return of a prisoner of war.
6. Adoption of a child, or remarriage resulting in a stepparent and stepsiblings.
7. Power struggle on the job, or a sudden change in role responsibilities.
8. Forced geographic relocation.
9. Rape, suicide, homicide, imprisonment, or being taken as a hostage.

Crisis events for the family include the developmental and situational crises previously discussed. Family crises are also classified as follows (4, 40):

1. **Dismemberment.** *Medical emergencies;* loss of family member through death, divorce, separation, marriage, or geographic move.
2. **Accession.** *Addition of family member* through birth, adoption, marriage, or foster placement, or older relative moving into the home.
3. **Demoralization.** *Loss of morale* in the family unit through delinquency or crime, legal problems, economic problems, job loss, child or spouse abuse, certain illnesses such as AIDS, or events that cause alienation from the community or carry a social stigma, such as imprisonment.
4. **A combination of the above.**

Various factors influence how prone a group or community is to crisis (34):

1. Personal strengths, characteristics, and level of need satisfaction of its members.
2. Social and economic stability of family units or groups versus social and economic inequities among ethnic, racial, or socioeconomic groups.
3. Adherence to versus rebellion against social norms by families and groups.
4. Adequacy of community resources to meet social, economic, health, welfare, and recreational needs of individuals and families.
5. Geographic, environmental, and climatic resources and characteristics that surround the group or community.

The community is also affected by natural disasters; by disasters resulting from advances in our civilization, such as chemical or radiation spills and electrical blackouts; and by disasters for which humans are responsible, such as shootings in a schoolyard or workplace, fire, and war. *Reactions of a community to any of these disasters will be influenced by* (a) the extent of preparedness, (b) leadership and organization, (c) availability of outside help, (d) communication channels, (e) ability of families to remain together, and (f) availability of emergency services, shelter, and health care (32, 38, 47, 55).

Phases of Crisis and Responses

All crises require a sudden and then a later restructuring of biopsychosocial integration before normal function can be restored. The *phases are* (a) shock, followed closely by general realization of the crisis; (b) defensive retreat; (c) acknowledgment and mourning; and, finally, (d) adaptation or resolution (26).

Table 2-8 presents the feelings and behaviors that may be experienced by the person during the phases of crisis. These behaviors are normal when a crisis is encountered; be aware of that fact in your assessment (4, 26, 40, 55). Grief and mourning processes are discussed further in Chapter 17. ∞

Table 2-9 summarizes influences on the reactions and coping ability how the person, family, or community will react to and cope with crisis and, thereby, the crisis outcome (4, 15, 26, 40, 68).

The family unit undergoes essentially the same phases of crisis and manifests similar reactions as the designated client, although the intensity and timing may be different for each person. Furthermore, members of the family in crisis interact with each other, compounding the crisis reaction and creating more intense or complex behavioral responses. Roles are disorganized; expectations of self, other family members, and outsiders change; and individual needs intensify.

Communities in crisis have characteristics in common with individuals and groups in crisis. The most immediate social consequence of a disaster is disruption of normal social patterns and services; the community is socially paralyzed. Furthermore, one disaster, such as a chemical spill, may contribute to another disaster, such as an explosion or fire.

Response to external emergencies is often quicker than the response to internal stresses or crises. Some survivors remain reality-oriented, calm, and able to develop and implement a plan of action. These people often are those with advanced training. These people may experience the crisis phases later and need intervention at that time. Other survivors may suffer long-term effects previously discussed.

Health Care and Nursing Applications

You will be caring for people in crisis every day, for example, a hospitalized patient with illness or injury; a student, employee, or family member with a developmental crisis; or a resident in an elder apartment complex with chronic illness who has just suffered the death of a spouse. Your knowledge of crisis and the stress responses associated with crisis will be useful in both your professional and personal life.

Comprehensive information on assessing crisis responses to various types of disasters and interventions with individuals, families, groups, and communities is available in the text by Langan and James. Developmental and cultural considerations are included (47).

Evaluate effectiveness of your **interventions. See Table 2-9** for factors influencing the outcome of crisis. These factors are relevant to evaluation criteria. Review your communication approach, as previously discussed, and the client's demonstration of progression through the phases of crisis, ability to use stress management techniques, and utilization of community resources and other support systems. Short-term crisis therapy can achieve great results, but you may not have ongoing contact to see the client's change. It may be 6 to 12 months before crisis resolution occurs. Realize the assistance you give makes a difference in recovery. Use information from this chapter to foster your effectiveness.

TABLE 2-8

Individual Reactions in the Crisis Phases

Phase and Duration	Feelings	Cognitive Manifestations	Physical Symptoms	Interpersonal/ Social Behavior
Initial Impact; Shock (duration of 1 to 24–48 hours)	Anxiety. Helplessness. Chaos. Overwhelmed. Hopeless. Incomplete. Detached. Despair. Depersonalized. Panic. Self-concept threatened. Self-esteem low. Anguish may be expressed by silent, audible, or uncontrollable crying.	Altered sensorium. Disorganized thinking. Unable to plan, reason logically, or understand situation. Impaired judgment. Preoccupation with image or hallucination of last object/person.	Somatic distress. May suffer physical illness or injury and ignore symptoms. Shortness of breath. Choking. Sighing. Hyperventilation. Weakness. Fatigue. Tremors. Anorexia. Lump in throat or abdomen. Respiratory or other infection may develop.	Disorganized behavior. Habitual or automatic behaviors used unsuccessfully. Withdrawn. Docile. Hyperactive. May appear overtly as if nothing happened or may be unable to carry out routine behavior. Lacks initiative for daily tasks. May need assistance meeting basic needs. Very suggestible, even if contrary to values or well-being.
	Developmental Crisis Response more gradual. Feelings less intense. May feel anxiety, frustration, lack of confidence, discouragement, imperfection, unfamiliarity with self, loss of self-control as realizes new responsibilities. Cannot move emotionally into next stage or change life perception.			*Developmental Crisis* May try to do more than is biologically or emotionally realistic. Unable to achieve behavior appropriate to role or to change inappropriate behavior in relationships.
Defensive Retreat (duration of hours to weeks)*	May feel tense and inadequate, but usually feels as if nothing is wrong because of use of repression and defense mechanisms. Apathetic or euphoric. Feelings displaced onto other objects.	Tries habitual coping mechanisms unsuccessfully. States nothing is wrong. May try to redefine problem unrealistically. Fantasizes about what could be done, how well past problems handled. Avoids thinking about event. May be disoriented. Maintains rigid thinking. States same ideas over and over. May be unable to devise alternative courses of action or predict effects of behavior. Denies through rationalization cause for situation.	Denies symptoms including presence of physical illness.	Tries habitual behaviors and defense mechanisms unsuccessfully. May seek support of others indirectly. Usually withdraws from others. Superficial response. May avoid reality with overactivity. Resistant to change suggested by others. Unwilling to initiate new behavior. Ineffective, disorganized behavior. May be unable to maintain daily activities, work performance, or social roles. Denies through demands, complaints, or projections of inadequacy.

TABLE 2-8

Individual Reactions in the Crisis Phases

Phase and Duration	Feelings	Cognitive Manifestations	Physical Symptoms	Interpersonal/ Social Behavior
		Developmental Crisis Denies that physical, emotional, or role changes are occurring or that different behavior is expected; behavior reflects earlier developmental stage; developmental tasks not worked out or met.		
Acknowledgment of Reality (duration varies)	Tension and anxiety rise. Loneliness. Irritable. Depressed. Agitated. Apathetic. Self-hate. Low self-esteem. Grief—mourning occurs. Gradually self-satisfaction increased. Self-concept becomes more positive. Gains self-confidence in ability to cope.	Becomes aware of facts about change, loss, event. Asks questions about situation. Slowly redefines situation. Attempts problem solving. May be disorganized in thinking. Trial-and-error approach to problems. Gradually perceives alternatives. Makes appropriate plans. Gives up undesirable goals. Validates personal experiences and feelings. Coping skills improved.	Symptoms may reappear or intensify. New symptoms may occur. May somatize feelings. Gradually regains physical health.	Exhibits mourning behaviors. Gradually demonstrates appropriate behaviors and resumes roles. Uses suggestions. Tries new approaches. Greater maturity demonstrated.
Resolution Adaptation, Change (duration of mourning and crisis work may be 6–12 months)	Painful feelings integrated into self-concept and sense of maturity. New sense of worth. Firm identity. Gradual increase in self-satisfaction about mastery of situation. Gradual lowering of anxiety. Does not feel bitter, guilty, or ashamed.	Perceives crisis situation in positive way. Integrates crisis event into self. Problem solving successful. Discusses feelings about event. Organizes thinking and planning. Redefines priorities. Does not blame self or others. Remembers comfortably and realistically pleasures and disappointments of last relationship.	Functions at optimum level.	Discovers new resources. Uses support systems and resources appropriately. Resumes status and roles. Strengthens relations with others. Adaptive in relationships. Lifestyle may be changed. Initiates measures to prevent similar crisis if at all possible.

*(Note: Temporary retreat emotionally, mentally, and socially is adaptive and protective from perceived stress and loss and overwhelming anxiety. Allows time to gradually realize what has happened; avoids debilitating effects of high anxiety or panic. Initially person fluctuates between the phases of Defensive Retreat and Acknowledgment of Reality.)

TABLE 2-9

Factors Influencing the Outcome of Crisis

1. **Perception of the event.** If the event (or the implications or consequences of it) threatens the self-concept; conflicts with the value system, self-expectations, or wishes for the future; contributes to a sense of shame or guilt; or is demoralizing or damaging to self, family, or personal objects, the situation is defined as hazardous. The perception of the event is reality for the person or family, regardless of how others might define reality. How the event is perceived depends in large measure on past experience.
2. **Degree of perceived dependency on a lost object.** This is also crucial; the greater the dependency, the more difficult the resolution of loss.
3. **Physical and emotional status.** This includes level of health, amount of energy present, age, genetic endowment, and biological rhythms of the person or family, or the general well-being of the community. Working through crisis takes considerable energy.
4. **Coping techniques or mechanisms and level of personal maturity.** If adaptive capacities are already strained, or if the stress is overwhelming, the person will cling to old habits or existing defenses, and behavior will very likely be inappropriate to the task at hand. The person or family who has met developmental tasks all along and who perceives self as able to cope will adapt more easily in any crisis. The group or community that has mechanisms, policies, or procedures defined and in operation to cope with the unexpected event or disaster can better meet the crisis.
5. **Previous experiences with similar situations.** The person, family, or group needs to learn to cope with stress, change, and loss. If past crises were handled by distorting reality or by withdrawing, when similar crises arise, burdens of the prior failure will be added to the problem of coping with the new situation. Unresolved crises are cumulative in effect. The most recent crisis revives the denial, depression, anger, or maladaptation that was left unsettled from past crises. If the person, family, or group successfully deals with crises, self-confidence and self-esteem will thereby be increased, and future crises will be handled more effectively.
6. **Realistic aspects of the current situation.** These include personal, material, or economic losses; the extent to which group ties or community services are interrupted; and changes in living pattern or family life necessitated by the loss.
7. **Cultural influences.** How the person is trained and socialized in the home to solve problems and meet crisis situations; the use of religious, cultural, or legal ceremonies or rituals to handle separation or loss and facilitate mourning; expectations of how the social group will support the person or family during crisis; and the method established by the community to provide help—all influence present behavior.
8. **Availability and response of family and close friends, community groups, or other helping resources, including professional persons.** The less available the environmental or emotional support systems are to decrease stress or buttress the coping response, the more hazardous the event will be. The family system, by its influence on development of self-concept and maturity, can increase or decrease the person's vulnerability to crisis.

INTERVENTIONS FOR HEALTH PROMOTION

Use of the following crisis intervention principles will foster crisis resolution and return to optimum function for the person or family unit:

1. Assess anxiety level, feelings, and perceptions of client.
2. Assess presence of emotional and physical symptoms.
3. Determine whether person is suicidal or homicidal.
4. Explore support system and usual coping patterns.
5. Clarify crisis event, including its onset and impact.
6. Provide comfort measures for client.
7. Help client work through feelings about situation.
8. Develop plan with client to resolve crisis; develop alternative options to achieve goal.
9. Reinforce strengths and healthy adaptive patterns.
10. Involve client in decisions and working on specific tasks.
11. Help person establish necessary social relationship; assist person in seeking and accepting help.
12. Collaborate with client to determine effectiveness of interventions.
13. Refer as necessary for additional services.
14. Maintain follow-up care as necessary.

Complementary and Alternative Therapies

Millions of Americans and people throughout the world use **complementary or alternative medicine/therapies (CAM or CAT)**, *nontraditional or nonmedical approaches that are considered holistic or integrative to promote health or prevent and treat illness and treat even severe and complex disease.* These therapies are **alternative,** *not part of conventional medical practice,* such as American Indian or Asian practices, or they **complement** (*supplement*) *conventional therapies taught in Western medical schools.*

Today's health care consumer may combine a variety of healing methods. Selected references present information. Gladstar and Hirsch (34) and Gutmanis (36) describe the uses of many herbs and medicinal plants. Gutmanis (36) describes herbal medicines based on interviews with Hawaiians. Assessment, diagnosis, and treatments are included for children, and a section is presented on special illnesses of women. Refer to references (24, 59, 65, 87) and the following Websites:

1. American Holistic Nurses Association, www.ahna.org
2. American Psychological Association, www.apa.org
3. Department of Health and Human Services, www.dhhs.gov
4. *Healthy People 2010*, www.healthypeople.gov
5. National Center for Complementary and Alternative Medicine, www.nccam.nih.gov
6. National Institute of Mental Health, www.nimh.gov
7. Office of Disease Prevention and Health Promotion, www.dhhs.gov

Refer also to **Table 2-10,** Websites for Stress Management and Complementary/Alternative Therapies, for more detailed information about types of therapies.

TABLE 2-10

Websites for Stress Management and Complementary/Alternative Therapies

Therapy	Website
I. Mind-Body Interventions	
Potential for mind to influence body and symptoms	
• Biofeedback	Association for Applied Biopsychology and Biofeedback http://www.aapb.org/
• Progressive Relaxation	A Guide to Psychology and Its Practice: Progressive Relaxation http://www.guidetopsychology.com
• Yoga	Yoga Journal http://www.yogajournal.com
• Imagery	Academy for Guided Imagery http://www.academyforguidedimagery.com
• Meditation	Worldwide Online Meditation Center http://www.meditationcenter.com
• Vedic Medicine/Ayurveda	Maharishi Ayurveda http://www.mapi.com
• Visualization	Success Consciousness: Creative Visualization http://www.successconsciousness.com/
• Hypnosis	American Association for Professional Hypnotherapists http://www.aaph.org
II. Biological-Based Interventions	
Focus of therapy is the neurologic or musculoskeletal system	
• Acupuncture	Acupuncture.com: Gateway to Chinese Medicine, Health, and Wellness http://www.acupuncture.com/
• Acupressure	Acupressure Institute http://www.acupressure.com/
• Shiatsu	Shiatsu Information Page http://homepage.ntlworld.com/
• Craniosacral Therapy	Craniosacral Therapy Association of North America http://www.craniosacraltherapy.org/
• Magnet Therapy	WholeHealthMD.com: Magnet Therapy http://www.wholehealthmd.com/
• Eye Movement Desensitization Reprocessing (EMDR)	EMDR Institute http://www.emdr.com
III. Botanical Interventions	
Use of pharmacologic principles with plant/herbal preparations	
• Herbal medicine	Herb Research Foundation http://www.herbs.org
IV. Manipulations: Body-Based Interventions	
Use of manipulation and/or musculoskeletal body movement	
• Tai Chi	What Is Tai Chi? http://www.chebucto.ns.ca/
• Massage	American Massage Therapy Association http://www.amtamassage.org
• Chiropractic	Foundation for Chiropractic Education and Research http://www.fcer.org
• Osteopathy	American Academy of Osteopathy http://www.academyofosteopathy.org/

continued

TABLE 2-10

Websites for Stress Management and Complementary/Alternative Therapies—continued

Therapy	Website
V. Biophilia Therapy	
Use of natural environment to enhance psychotherapy	
• Horticultural Therapy	American Horticultural Therapy Association http://www.ahta.org/
• Wilderness Therapy	Wilderness Therapy and Treatment http://www.wilderness-therapy.org/
VI. Positive Thinking	
Use of cognitive strategies to reduce stress or enhance coping	
• Positive Thinking	Mayo Clinic—Positive Thinking: A Skill for Stress Relief http://www.mayoclinic.com/health/
• Time Management	Mind Tools: Time Management Skills http://www.mindtools.com/
VII. Spiritual Interventions	
Use of spiritual/religious beliefs to enhance healing	
• Christianity	
• Catholic	CharisCenter: National Service Committee of the Catholic Charismatic Renewal http://www.nsc-chariscenter.org/
	St. Louis Catholic Charismatic Center http://www.stlcharismatic.org
• Protestant	Christian Healing Ministries http://www.christianhealingmin.org/
	Stephen Ministries http://www.stephenministries.org/
• Orthodox	Greek Orthodox Archdiocese of America http://www.goarch.org/
• Judaism	National Center for Jewish Healing http://www.ncjh.org/
• Islam	Islamic Traditional Healing Methods http://www.crescentlife.com/
• Hindu	Sanskrit Mantras and Spiritual Power http://www.sanskritmantra.com/
• Buddhist	The Art of Healing: A Tibetan Buddhist Perspective http://www.dharma-haven.org/
VIII. Energy Field Interventions	
Diverse group of energies based on two types of therapies	
Biofield Therapies	
Based on the existence of life energy, chi, prana, ki, or spiritual forces	
• Healing/Therapeutic Touch	Welcome to Healing Touch http://www.healingtouch.net/
• Reiki (Japanese)	International Center for Reiki Training http://www.reiki.org
• Mana (Hawaiian)	Kahuna Concepts http://www.active-stream.com/
• Prana (Asian)	Pranic Healing http://www.pranichealing.com/
• Chi (Chinese)	Qi Journal http://qi-journal.com/
• Light (Christian)	Christian Healing Ministries http://www.christianhealingmin.org/
Bioelectromagnetic Therapies	
Use of magnetism or electricity	
• Magnets	WholeHealthMD.com: Magnet Therapy http://www.wholehealthmd.com/
• Electromagnetic radiation	Electromagnetic Therapy http://alternative-medicine-and-health.com/therapy/
IX. Sensory Therapies	
Classification of therapies that focus on the five senses	The Well-Arts Institute http://www.well-arts.org
• Aromatherapy	National Association for Holistic Aromatherapy http://www.naha.org/
• Art Therapy	American Art Therapy Association http://www.arttherapy.org/
• Color Therapy	About.com: Chromotherapy http://healing.about.com/
• Dance Therapy	American Dance Therapy Association http://www.adta.org/
• Laughter/Humor Therapy	American Association for Therapeutic Humor http://www.aath.org
• Music Therapy	American Music Therapy Association http://www.musictherapy.org/

TABLE 2-10

Websites for Stress Management and Complementary/Alternative Therapies—continued

Therapy	Website
X. Pet Therapy	
	Therapy Dogs http://www.therapydogs.com
Use of human/animal bond to foster physical, emotional, and social health/well-being	North American Riding for the Handicapped Association http://www.narha.org
	Delta Society http://www.deltasociety.org
XI. Homeopathy	
Based on the theory that disease can be cured by giving small doses of drugs which in healthy persons and in large doses would cause like disease	Homeopathic Educational Services http://www.homeopathic.org

INTERVENTIONS FOR HEALTH PROMOTION

Health care providers have the following responsibilities when clients use complementary or alternative therapies:

1. Be familiar with purpose, use, effectiveness, and potential risks of the therapies.
2. Assess the client's knowledge about and use of these therapies, singly or in combination.
3. Give additional information as needed, based on available data, about adverse effects and contraindications, to assist the client in decision making.
4. Explain that botanical preparations and some dietary supplements have no governmental regulated guarantees of safety or effectiveness.

5. Suggest the client keep a daily diary or journal on each therapy used and extent of changes in the symptoms.
6. Review the journal with the client to determine cause and effect of symptoms and explore possible lifestyle changes.
7. Encourage the client not to substitute these therapies for necessary conventional treatment and to report any therapies being used.
8. Assist the client to gain access to and understanding of current research information on the therapy.
9. Encourage the client to determine if the therapist is qualified.

Improving Health Care Practice and Advocacy

CURRENT TRENDS

Assessment, intervention, and evaluation strategies have been integrated throughout the chapter. Sources of information to keep abreast of practice trends will assist you in maintaining your own health and in your role as advocate for the client and family unit at any stage of development. Client health promotion, education, and advocacy also depend on remaining abreast of trends. For example, you are likely to engage in telehealth practice.

Telehealth practice, *electronically transmitted clinician consultation, and treatment descriptions,* has improved access to care for people in rural or underserved areas but is also increasingly used in health promotion education, illness prevention, and prevention of unnecessary hospitalizations. Telehealth can also reduce the number of home care visits because the computer monitoring that is possible through audiovisual transmission over phone lines enables the client and care provider to see and

Practice Point

Use modern technology to continue your own professional education for practice, to collaborate with members of the disciplinary team, and to educate the client. The client may share information with you gained from his or her use of technology or media and demand changes in your practice as a result. Collaborate with and learn from your clients.

hear each other. The client controls the video monitor, which prevents intrusion into privacy. The American Nurses Association was instrumental in obtaining Medicare reimbursement for telehealth services in specific rural areas.

You can use modern technology to continue learning about cultural and CAM care as well as contribute to improved specialized care. Further, you will participate in **multidisciplinary care;** *all members of the team work together for optimum client care and advocacy.*

Health protection involves risk reduction behaviors and changing threatening environmental and social conditions. Screening and immunizations continue to be important, but changing personal health behaviors of people before the clinical disease develops is essential. *Frequency and specific facets of the periodic health examination should be tailored to the unique health risks, age, and sex of the individual client.* Counseling and education that help the person, family, or group assume greater responsibility for health may be of more value than screenings every year. Further, health promotion and protection must focus on the community as well.

Health promotion and disease prevention must also focus on the community. *Strengths of a community-based approach compared with individual approaches include the following* (24, 65):

1. The power of intervention is greater, owing to the opportunity for diffusion and change of social norms.
2. Public awareness of health-promoting behaviors and barriers to such behaviors is increased, providing a basis for informed social actions.
3. Programs are geared to the "real world" in which people live.
4. Programs can be delivered to larger groups than services targeted to individuals in circumscribed clinical settings.
5. Costs are generally lower for community programs than for one-on-one clinical services.
6. An environment of social support can be developed for risk-lowering and health-enhancing behaviors.

Community health protection strategies must be carefully planned and well coordinated. *The following guidelines are useful for community health programming* (13, 24, 65, 87):

1. Involve as many small groups, organizations, interorganizational networks, community-wide structures, and respected community leaders as possible.
2. Obtain official endorsement of your program from governmental agencies (mayor's office, city council, governor's office,

local and state health departments), local school districts, and churches in the community.
3. Focus on intensive community action with a trained and well-organized health service structure and the media as backup.
4. Plan so that adequate time is allowed for each program phase and the overall time frame is manageable.
5. Develop and maintain a sense of community ownership and control of the program; enlist community volunteers as change agents.
6. Incorporate strategies to promote both maintaining healthful lifestyles and acquiring new habits.
7. Attend to ethnic and sociocultural aspects of the community in designing the program and tailoring health promotion strategies to subpopulations. Monitor and evaluate the success of the program and provide feedback to participating populations concerning progress in reaching program goals.

SITES FOR HEALTH PROMOTION AND WELLNESS PROGRAMS

Traditionally the main health concerns for employees in the workplace were safety and accident prevention. A yearly physical examination was also included in many industries.

Today *industries, health care settings, and other work settings have programs for their employees that generally include emphasis in four areas:* stress reduction, exercise, smoking cessation, and nutritional and weight guidance, particularly for obesity and sodium and cholesterol dietary reduction. *Employee Assistance Programs (EAPs)* are established to provide counseling services to employees related to work-related problems and family crises or "stresses." EAPs also work with the chemically dependent employee to reduce alcohol or drug intake and remain a safe, dependable worker. Day care for workers with young children is offered to reduce the worker's stress related to child care. The workplace may make available a fully equipped exercise room, gymnasium, handball court, and whirlpool bath. For example, a rough running track has been measured around a furniture factory in rural North Carolina. In some cities, the employer uses existing exercise facilities in various clubs or organizations, such as the local chapter of the American Heart Association, for screening or teaching programs.

Health promotion sites are also established on university campuses and in retirement centers, day care centers, stores, housing projects, neighborhood community centers, schools, churches, laundry facilities, or senior nutrition sites. Such sites are more acceptable to many cultural populations for health screening, well-child checkups, immunizations, or counseling than is the hospital or traditional outpatient setting. Innovative city and county public health agencies have for years used nontraditional settings for health promotion and illness prevention. The master's prepared clinical nurse specialist and nurse practitioner frequently work in nontraditional sites, engage in entrepreneurial opportunities, or combine practice, research, and academic roles.

Health care services must be given in nontraditional sites to reach people who are homeless, refugees, or migrant workers. The following Case Situation is an example.

Case Situation

A Nontraditional Approach to Health Promotion

Community agencies can combine health and social services. For example, one author (RM) has volunteered for over 20 years with a private community agency that provides a combination and variety of programs and services not offered in the surrounding metropolitan community. The walk-in *day treatment program* is for people who are homeless and chronically mentally ill and/or substance abusing. Each client is given a membership card to foster a sense of inclusion. Basic needs can be met at the facility in addition to *private and group counseling* and *educational programs.* A continental breakfast and lunch are served every day. Personal care and hygiene supplies, clothing, showers, and laundry facilities are available. The agency is a safe place during the daytime for a wide mix of people; there is a *women's night shelter program* for mentally ill homeless women who have access to the same provisions and services as the daytime clients. Clients have access to a telephone, if needed, and can obtain employment through the *employment program.* Employment skills may first be learned in the *restaurant program;* McMurphy's Grill is part of the agency. The *employment program presents classes for homeless veterans* who have no illness, chronically ill veterans, and other homeless clients. Computer classes are incorporated into all employment readiness classes. The agency address can be used as a personal address until the *housing program* secures affordable housing, such as an apartment or a single room in a hotel or group home. Some individuals are referred to the *transitional residential program,* whereby clients have housing for up to a year and access to the agency's other programs. Individuals can enroll in the *Adult Basic Education/General Equivalency Diploma (ABE/GED) program* to obtain a basic or high school equivalency diploma, or they may enroll in the *living skills classes program* to gain more information about tenant living, budgeting, nutrition, or child care/parenting. The *health clinic* is available daily for clients who need care for minor injury or illness, immunizations, or health education. A *child care drop-in center* is available for preschool children of single parents who are attending classes during the daytime hours and need babysitting services. Chronically ill homeless individuals who meet criteria for more independent living are enrolled in the *Assertive Community Treatment (ACT) program,* whereby they are given housing placement in a renovated hotel or one of several apartment buildings. Clients receive case management, medical and psychiatric treatment, and medication monitoring with holistic follow-up care for a year, during which they can enroll in any of the other programs or receive other services as appropriate.

The local *College of Chiropractic Medicine* gives health services to clients at the agency. *Legal Aid of Eastern Missouri* is also at the site to assist clients in obtaining entitlements, such as Social Security or disability benefits or pensions, and to give other paralegal services. Individuals who have successfully completed the programs they needed and are employed and independently housed are invited to participate in the *Alumni Club Program,* where they can meet each evening for social activities, educational sessions, and monthly case management follow-up.

This agency provides health promotion and all levels of prevention—physically, emotionally, cognitively, and socially—through its many programs and services. Throughout the agency and in each program, the spirituality dimension is addressed, based on the needs of the individual client.

Contributed by Ruth Murray, EdD, MSN, N-NAP, FAAN

Summary

1. Health promotion and disease prevention are a concern for the clients for whom you care; for local, national, and international populations; and for you as an individual.
2. You will encounter disparities in available services and quality of care issues; be involved as a professional to reduce these disparities.
3. Goals of the *Healthy People 2010* Initiative include to increase quality of life and the number of healthy years for individuals and to eliminate health care disparities in the United States.
4. Concepts from relevant health promotion models and theories and communication and therapeutic relationship theories will be applicable in every setting, with all clients, in combination with any other theoretical approach.
5. Each client for whom you care will be experiencing stress response and will likely be in a developmental and/or situational crisis. Assessment and intervention must include application of General Adaptation Syndrome and Crisis Theories. Utilize stress management and crisis intervention strategies.
6. Stay abreast of practice trends and the literature related to complementary and alternative therapies, and the extent to which they enhance or interfere with optimum health.
7. Continue to build on the information base presented in this chapter as you care for, educate, or counsel clients and collaborate with other professionals in a variety of settings.

Study Questions

1. A local hospital has offered a reduction in insurance premiums for employees who enroll in an on-site fitness program. This strategy supports the *Healthy People 2010* Initiative by:
   1. Addressing access to health care
   2. Enhancing screening opportunities
   3. Reducing health care costs
   4. Encouraging healthy lifestyles
2. An education session offered at a local middle school for parents of preteen girls regarding the human papilloma virus (HPV) vaccine is an example of what type of activity on the part of the nurse?
   1. Tertiary prevention
   2. Secondary prevention
   3. Primary prevention
   4. Screening
3. Holding frequent hypertension and diabetes screening programs on Native American reservations is an important health promotion initiative for the nurse to engage in because:

   1. These conditions have a high prevalence in the Native American population.
   2. These conditions are difficult to treat.
   3. Dietary issues may influence response to treatment in this population.
   4. Lack of access may prevent Native Americans from seeking treatment.
4. The nurse is working with a client who expresses a desire to begin taking an herbal preparation for the treatment of depression. In order to effectively teach the client, the nurse should first:
   1. Determine why the client is interested in this particular preparation and what the client knows about its use.
   2. Tell the client that herbal remedies are generally harmless and there will likely be no ill effects.
   3. Report this desire to the client's primary care provider for further evaluation.
   4. Tell the client that herbal remedies are never recommended for treatment of depression.

References

1. A culture of health. (2005, October 3). *Newsweek*, 67.
2. Adderley-Kelly, B., & Green, P. (2005). Strategies for successful conduct of research with low-income African-American populations. *Nursing Outlook, 53*(3), 149–152.
3. Addis, J. (2005, Autumn). Top five child killers. *World Vision News, 8*(4), 4.
4. Aguilera, D.C. (1998). *Crisis intervention: Theory and methodology* (8th ed.). St. Louis, MO: Mosby.
5. Aschengrau, A., & Seage, G., III. (2007). *Essentials of epidemiology in public health* (2nd ed.). Boston: Jones and Bartlett.
6. Bandura, A. (1991). Social cognitive theory of self-regulation. *Organizational Behavior and Human Decision Processes, 50*, 248–287.
7. Bedi, R. P., et al. (2005). Critical incidents in the formation of the therapeutic alliance from the client's perspective. *Psychotherapy: Theory, Research, Practice, Training, 42*(31), 311–323.
8. Berger, K. (2005). *The developing person through the life span* (6th ed.). New York: Worth.
9. Berkowitz, B., & McCubbin, M. (2005). Advancement of health disparities research: A conceptual approach. *Nursing Outlook, 53*, 153–159.
10. Brewer, C. (2005). Health services research and the nursing workforce: Access and utilization issues. *Nursing Outlook, 53*(12), 281–290.
11. Brogten, D., Youngbluf, J., Kutcher, J., & Bobo, C. (2004). Quality and the nursing workforce: APNs, patient outcomes, and health care costs. *Nursing Outlook, 52*(1), 45–52.
12. Brown, G., & Harris, T. (Eds.). (1989). *Life events and illness* (pp. 49–93). New York: Guilford Press.
13. Brownson, R., Baker, E., & Novick, L. (1999). *Community-based prevention: Programs that work.* Gaithersburg, MD: Aspen.
14. Bryne, D. G. (1984). Personal assessment of life event stress and future onset of psychological symptoms. *British Journal of Medical Psychology, 57*, 241–248.
15. Caplan, G. (1964). *Principles of preventive psychiatry.* New York: Basic Books.
16. Carlson, E., & Chamberlain, R. (2003). Social capital, health, and health disparities. *Journal of Nursing Scholarship, 35*, 325–331.
17. Cava, M., Fay, K., Beanlands, H., McCay, E., & Wignall, R. (2005). Risk perception and compliance with quarantine during the SARS outbreak. *Journal of Nursing Scholarship, 37*(4), 343–347.
18. Clark, M. J. (2008). *Community health nursing: Advocacy for population health* (5th ed.). Upper Saddle River, NJ: Pearson Education.
19. Clements, K., & Turpia, G. (2000). Life event exposure, physiological reactivity, and psychological strain. *Journal of Behavioral Medicine, 23*(1), 73–94.
20. Cuevas, K., Silver, D., Brooter, D., Youngblut, J., & Bobo, C. (2005). The cost of prematurity: Hospital charges at birth and frequency of rehospitalizations and acute care visits over the first year of life. *American Journal of Nursing, 105*(7), 56–64.
21. DeLongis, A., Folkman, S., & Lazarus, R. (1988). The impact of daily stress on health and mood: Psychological and social resources as mediators. *Journal of Personality and Social Psychology, 54*, 486–495.
22. Dickenson-Hazard, N. (2004). Global health issues and challenges. *Journal of Nursing Scholarship, 36*(1), 6–10.
23. Dunn, H. L. (1961). *High-level wellness.* Washington, DC: Mount Vernon Publishing.
24. Edelman, C., & Mandel, C. (2005). *Health promotion throughout the lifespan* (6th ed.). St. Louis, MO: Mosby.
25. Esparat, M., Feng, D., Owen, D., & Green, A. (2005). Transformation for health: A framework for health disparities research. *Nursing Outlook, 53*(3), 113–120.
26. Fink, S. (1967). Crisis and motivation: A theoretical model. *Archives of Physical Medicine and Rehabilitation, 48*(11), 592–597.
27. Fisher, K. (2004). Health disparities and mental retardation. *Journal of Nursing Scholarship, 36*(1), 48–53.
28. Foley, S. (2004). To die for. *American Journal of Nursing, 104*(1), 20.
29. Forchuk, C., & Brown, B. (1989). Establishing a nurse client relationship. *Journal of Psychosocial Nursing, 27*(2), 30–34.
30. Forchuk, C. (1991). Peplau's theory: Concepts and their relationships. *Nursing Science Quarterly, 4*(2), 54–59.
31. Frankish, C. J., Lovato, C., & Shannon, W. (1999). Models, theories, and principles of health promotion with multicultural populations. In R. Huff & M. Kline (Eds.), *Promoting health in multicultural populations* (pp. 41–72). Thousand Oaks, CA: Sage.
32. Gast, R., & Lubin, B. (Eds.). (1989). *Psychological aspects of disasters.* New York: John Wiley & Sons.
33. Gesler, W., Haynes, M., Arcury, T., Skelly, A., Nash, S., & Soward, A. (2004). Use of mapping technology in health intervention research. *Nursing Outlook, 52*, 145–146.
34. Gladstar, R., & Hirsch, P. (Ed.). (2000). *Planting the future: Saving our medicinal herbs.* Rochester, VT: Healing Arts Press.

35. Graner, B. (2007). Break the cycle of stress with PRB3. *American Nurse Today, 2*(5), 56–57.

36. Gutmanis, J. (2005). *Hawaiian herbal medicine Kahuma la'au lapa'au.* Waipahu, HI: Island Heritage Publishers.

37. Guyton, A., & Hall, J. E. (2006). *Textbook of medical physiology* (11th ed.). Philadelphia: Elsevier.

38. Henry, J. P. (1992). Biological basis of the stress response. *Integrative Physiological and Behavioral Science, 27*(1), 66–83.

39. Hines-Martin, V. (2002). African American consumers: What should we know to meet their mental health needs? *Journal of the American Psychiatric Association, 8*(6), 189–193.

40. Hoff, L.A. (2001). *People in crisis: Clinical and public health perspective* (5th ed.). San Francisco: Jossey Bass.

41. Holmes, T., & Rahe, R. (1967). The Social Readjustment Rating Scale. *Journal of Psychosomatic Research, 11*(8), 213–217.

42. Huff, R., & Kline, M. (1999). Health promotion in the context of culture. *Promoting health in multicultural populations: A handbook for practitioners* (pp. 3–22). Thousand Oaks, CA: Sage.

43. Hutchins, D., & Cole, C. (1992). *Helping relationships and strategies* (2nd ed.). Belmont, CA: Brooks/Cole.

44. Institute of Medicine. (2006). *Improving the quality of health care for mental and substance abuse conditions: Quality chasm series.* Washington, DC: National Academy Press.

45. Katz, J., & Hirsch, A. (2003). When global health is local health. *American Journal of Nursing, 103*(12), 75–79.

46. Lamb, G., Jennings, B., Mitchell, P., & Lang, N. (2004). Quality agenda: Priorities for action. Recommendations of the American Academy of Nursing Conference on Health Care Quality. *Nursing Outlook, 52*(1), 60–65.

47. Langan, J., & James, D. (2005). *Preparing nurses for disaster management.* Upper Saddle River, NJ: Pearson Prentice Hall.

48. Lavallo, W. (1997). *Stress and health. Biological and psychological interactions.* Thousand Oaks, CA: Sage.

49. Lazarus, R. (1966). *Psychological stress and the coping process.* New York: McGraw-Hill.

50. Lazarus, R. (1999). *Stress and emotion: A new synthesis.* New York: Springer.

51. Lazarus, R., & Folkman, S. (1984). *Stress, appraisal, and coping.* New York: Springer.

52. Leavell, H., & Clark, E.G. (1963). *Prevention medicine for the doctor in his community: An epidemiologic approach.* New York: McGraw-Hill.

53. Lee, C. Y., Phanchareanworakul, K., Cho, W. J., Suwonnaroop, N., Storey, M., Sanaeha, C., et al. (2003). A comparative study of the health care delivery system of Korea and Thailand. *Nursing Outlook, 51*, 115–119.

54. Libby, P., & Skerrett, P. (2005, October 3). Health for life: Searching for hidden health risks. *Newsweek,* 73–74.

55. Lindemann, E. (1944). Symptomology and management of acute grief. *American Journal of Psychiatry, 101*, 141–148.

56. Luo, M. (2005). Chinese-American mental health outreach in New Jersey. *NAMI Advocate, 3*(2), 24–25.

57. Mann, A., Hoke, M., & Williams, J. (2005). Lessons learned. Research with rural Mexican-American women. *Nursing Outlook, 53*, 141–146.

58. Manning, M., & Lee, G. L. (2001, Summer). Working with parent's cultural and linguistic considerations. *Kappa Delta Pi Record,* 160–164.

59. Massage therapy offers multiple benefits. (2007). *Mount Sinai School of Medicine: Focus on Healthy Aging, 10*(2), 6–7.

60. McEwen, B. (1998). Protective and damaging effects of stress mediators. *New England Journal of Medicine, 338*(3), 171–179.

61. McEwen, B., & Stellar, E. (1993). Stress and the individual: Mechanisms leading to disease. *Archives of Internal Medicine, 153*, 2093–2101.

62. NAMI releases new factsheets on the uninsured and the costs of mental illnesses. (2007, Summer). *NAMI Advocate, 6*, 9–11.

63. Napholz, L. (2002). Stress-reduction psychoeducational interventions for Black working women. *Nursing Clinics of North America, 37*, 263–272.

64. Olshansky, E., Sacco, D., Bruxler, B., Dodge, P., Hughes, E., Ondeck, M., et al. (2005). Participatory action research to understand and reduce health disparities. *Nursing Outlook, 53*, 121–126.

65. Pender, N., Murdaugh, C., & Parsons, M. (2006). *Health promotion in nursing practice* (5th ed.). Upper Saddle River, NJ: Pearson Prentice Hall.

66. Peplau, H. (1952/1991). *Interpersonal relations in nursing.* New York: G.P. Putnam's Sons.

67. Peplau, H. (1969). *Basic principles of patient counseling* (2nd ed.). Philadelphia: Smith, Kline, and French.

68. Peplau, H. (1997). Peplau's theory of interpersonal relations. *Nursing Science Quarterly, 10*(4), 162–167.

69. Rahe, R., & Arthur, R. (1968). Life change patterns surrounding illness perception. *Journal of Psychosomatic Research, 11*(3), 341–345.

70. Ricketts, T., & Goldsmith, L. (2005). Access in health services research: The battle of frameworks. *Nursing Outlook, 53*, 274–280.

71. Rogers, C. (1951). *Client centered therapy.* Boston: Houghton.

72. Rosenstock, I.M. (1974). Historical origins of the health belief model. *Health Education Monographs, 2*, 328–343.

73. Rosenstock, I. M., Strecher, V., & Becker, M. (1988). Social learning theory and the health belief model. *Health Education Quarterly, 15*, 175–183.

74. Ruff, C., Alexander, I., & McKie, C. (2005). The use of focus group methodology in health disparities research. *Nursing Outlook, 53*, 134–140.

75. Sapolsky, R., Krey, I., & McEwen, B. (1986). The neuroendocrinology of stress and aging: The glucocorticoid cascade hypothesis. *Endocrinology Review, 7*, 284–301.

76. Schumacher, K., & Meleis, A. (1994). Transitions: A general concept in nursing. *IMAGE: Journal of Nursing Scholarship, 26*(2), 119–127.

77. Seeman, T., & McEwen, B. (1996). Impact of social environment characteristics on neuroendocrine regulation. *Psychosomatic Medicine, 58*(5), 459–471.

78. Selye, H. (1965). Stress syndrome. *American Journal of Nursing, 65*(3), 97–99.

79. Selye, H. (1974). *Stress without distress.* Philadelphia: J.B. Lippincott.

80. Selye, H. (1975, October). Implications of stress concepts. *New York State Journal of Medicine,* 2139–2145.

81. Selye, H. (1976, July 3). Forty years of stress research: Principal remaining problems and misconceptions. *Canadian Medical Association Journal, 115*, 53–56.

82. Selye, H. (1976). *The stress of life* (rev.). New York: McGraw-Hill.

83. Selye, H. (1979). Stress and the reduction of distress. *Primary Cardiology, 5*(8), 22–30.

84. Selye, H. (1980). The stress concept today. In I. C. Kutash & L. B. Schlesinger (Eds.), *Handbook on stress and anxiety* (pp. 127–144). New York: Jossey-Bass.

85. Shambley-Ebron, D., & Boyle, J. (2004). New paradigms for transcultural nursing: Framework for studying African-American women. *Journal of Transcultural Nursing, 15*(1), 11–17.

86. Shattell, M., & Hogan, B. (2005). Facilitating communication: How to truly understand what patients mean. *Journal of Psychosocial Nursing, 43*(10), 29–32.

87. Snyder, M., & Lindquist, R. (2002). *Complementary alternative therapies in nursing* (4th ed.). New York: Springer.

88. Stevens, K., & Staley, J. (2006). The *Quality Chasm Reports,* evidence-based practice, and nursing: Response to improve health care. *Nursing Outlook, 54*(2), 94–101.

89. Struthers, R., Lauderdale, J., Nichols, L., Tom-Orme, L., & Strickland, C. (2005). Respecting tribal traditions in research and publications: Voices of five Native American nurse scholars. *Journal of Transcultural Nursing, 16*, 193–201.

90. Sullivan-Bolyai, S., Bova, C., & Harper, D. (2005). Developing and refining interventions in persons with health disparities: The use of qualitative description. *Nursing Outlook, 53*, 127–133.

91. U.S. Department of Health and Human Services. (2000). *Healthy People 2010: With understanding and improving health and objectives for improving health* (2nd ed.). 2 Vols. Washington, DC: U.S. Government Printing Office.

92. Zook, R. (1998). Learning to use positive defense mechanisms. *American Journal of Nursing, 98*(3), 16B–16H.

93. Zust, B., & Moline, K. (2003). Identifying underserved ethnic populations within a community: The first step in eliminating health care disparities among racial and ethnic minorities. *Journal of Transcultural Nursing, 14*(1), 66–74.

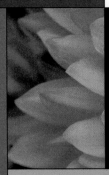

CHAPTER 3

Growth and Development: Concepts and Principles

KEY TERMS

OBJECTIVES

Study of this chapter will enable you to:

1. Define growth, development, and related terms.

2. Describe general beliefs about and principles of development and human behavior.

3. Define principles of human growth and development.

4. Relate information in this chapter to yourself as a developing person.

5. Apply information from this chapter when assessing or caring for the person or family unit through the life span.

6. Teach the person and family about beliefs and principles described in this chapter, when relevant to the client situation.

MediaLink www.prenhall.com/murray

Go to the Companion Website for interactive resources that accompany this chapter.

Glossary	Critical Thinking
Review Questions	Tools
Challenge Your Knowledge	Media Link Applications
Learning Activities	Media Links

Study of the person and family unit throughout the life span centers around certain beliefs about and principles of growth and development. Growth and development are usually thought of as a forward movement, a kind of adding on, such as increase in height and weight or the self-actualizing personality. However, reversal, decay, deterioration, and death also occur. *Three kinds of reversals occur:* (a) loss of some part, such as occurs with **catabolism** (*changing of living tissue into wastes or destructive metabolism*), (b) purposefully changing behavior when it is no longer useful, and (c) death (8, 11).

Growth and development are generally characterized by the following (2, 19):

1. Direction, goal, or end state
2. Identifiable stage or era
3. Forward progression, so that once a stage is worked through, the person does not return to the same position
4. Increasing specialization
5. Causal forces that are either genetic or environmental
6. Potentialities and capabilities for various behaviors and achievements

Dimensions of Time

Use theory about time dimensions, descriptions about behavior, and principles of growth and development in assessment and health promotion interventions. This knowledge is applicable to all age eras.

Lifetime or *chronologic age* is frequently used as an index of maturation and development but is only a rough indicator of the person's position on any one of the numerous physical or psychological dimensions. Furthermore, the society is a reference point for understanding the behavior; what is appropriate for a 14-year-old in one society is not appropriate in a different society.

Historical time refers to a *series of economic, political, and social events that directly shape the life course of the person and long-term processes*, such as industrialization and urbanization, that create the sociocultural context and changing definitions of the phases of the life cycle (2, 3, 17, 19). *A group of people born at a certain calendar or historical time* (**cohort**) has, as a group, a particular background and demographic composition. Most of the people of a specific age or generation will have similar experiences, behavior and life patterns, work and leisure patterns, value systems, consumer behavior, and ideas about life generally (2, 16). Refer to the Abstract for Evidence-Based Practice for information related to time perception.

Social time, *social expectations of behavior for each age era*, is not necessarily synchronous with biological age as prescribed by each society. Societies divide life into socially relevant or normative units. Age grading occurs. Duties, rights, and rewards are differential for each age group. In societies in which division of labor is simple and social change is slow, family, work, religious, and political roles for each age are set. A modern, complex, rapidly changing society, which has overlapping systems of age status, has some tasks and roles that are tied to chronologic age and some that are less defined. In every society there is a time to do what is the norm or expected: to be a child and dependent, to be educated to whatever level is needed, to go to work, to have a family, to retire. The members of the society have a general consensus about these age expectations and norms, although perceptions may vary somewhat by age, sex, or social class. Thus there is some pressure to conform. If the person engages in the tasks earlier or later than others in the society, he or she may be considered deviant. Patterns of timing can play an important role with respect to self-concept and self-esteem, depending on the person's level of awareness about his or her fit to social age norms and the rigidity in the culture (1–4). To be too far ahead or behind in one's developmental stage may involve negative consequences. Many of the major markers in the life cycle are ordered and sequential and are social rather than biological, and their time is socially regulated (2, 17).

This book is organized along chronologic lines, with the life cycle divided into different periods rather than having content organized around a topical approach. The person's life is divided into the following chronologic stages: the **prenatal period** (*from the moment of conception to birth*), **infancy** (*birth to 1 year*), **toddlerhood** (*1 to 3 years*), **preschool** (*3 to 6 years*), **school years** (*6 to 12 years*), **adolescence** (*12 to 20 or 25 years*), **young adulthood** (*20 or 25 to 45 or 50 years*), **middle age** (*45 or 50 to 65 or 70 years*), and **older adulthood** (*65 or 70 years and older*). *The divisions are somewhat arbitrary because it is difficult to assign definite ages; individual lives are not marked off so precisely.* In discussion of stage theories, such as those of Freud, Erikson, and Piaget, we use their age ranges, and the same reservations apply to them. Neugarten and Neugarten (16) state that we are becoming an **age-irrelevant society;** *age designations for adult life eras are difficult to assign* in the United States. There is the 14-year-old mother, the 35-year-old grandmother, and the father of young children who is 65 or 85 (12). The university graduate student may be age 84. *People are often at one level in one area of development and at another level in another area.*

Ideal **norms**, *standards* or *expectancies*, for different behaviors vary among different groups of people (1). The entire life cycle is speeded up for people who are poor. They tend to finish education earlier than middle- or upper-class people, take their first jobs sooner, marry younger, have children earlier, reach their career peak earlier, and become grandparents earlier. These differences are related to financial needs (1, 2). People from more affluent backgrounds can pursue their educations for a longer time, use young adulthood to explore options, and delay becoming financially independent and beginning a family.

General Descriptions About Behavior

The study of development is not merely a search for facts about people at certain ages. The study involves finding *patterns* or *general principles that apply to most people most of the time.* **The following statements are drawn from previously described theories and are relevant to your understanding of the developing person and client.**

All persons are similar and have the same basic needs, but they are also unique in following and expressing their own developmental patterns. The **One-Genus Postulate** states that *people are more similar than different simply because they are all Homo sapiens* (20).

Abstract for Evidence-Based Practice

Effect of Age on Time Perception

Wettman, M., & Lehnhoff, S. (2005). Age effects in perception of time. *Psychological Reports, 97,* 927–935.

KEYWORD

time perception

Purpose ➤ Determine whether time perception differs from the teen to older adult years, and whether older people report perception of time passing faster than do youth.

Conceptual Framework ➤ Time is perceived in three dimensions. Time perspective is the concept of past, present, and future. Time estimation is the ability to accurately estimate clock time. Time awareness is the subjective impression of time movement being rapid or slow. Time perception changes with age.

Sample/Setting ➤ A total of 499 participants, 196 men and 303 women, ages 14 to 94 years who lived at home were included in the sample. Participants from Germany and Australia were surveyed. Participants reported at least 9 years of education and no disorders.

Method ➤ Each participant completed two Likert-type scales designed to assess subjective time perception and the person's experience with time dimensions. Data were analyzed using Pearson correlation.

Findings ➤ There were small to moderate correlations between age and perception of time passing. Subjective sense of speed of time passage increased as the person ages. Participants 20 to 50 years of age reported more sense of time pressure than participants of other ages.

Implications ➤ Age *per se* may not influence the perception of time passage. Sociocultural influences may be a major influence in perceptions about time. People who live in a less industrialized society may perceive time dimensions differently. More research is needed.

The person is a unified but open system composed of body, mind, feelings, and spirit, which are continually influenced by the environment. The person, in turn, influences the environment. Change in one part produces change in all parts of the system (6, 7, 17, 18, 21).

Stability and change are constant in any system, including the individual. The person and family unit evidence **stability,** *maintaining some characteristics.* **Changes,** *demonstrating differences in various aspects of the self,* also occur throughout life. Both earlier and later life experiences contribute to stability and the capacity for change (18).

The person's life process evolves irreversibly; the person cannot totally return to something he or she was developmentally in the past (13, 17, 19). Nevertheless, the past influences the person to some degree whether or not he or she is aware of the influence. The past sets the direction for present and future patterns of behavior (13, 18, 20).

The person responds as a total organism at any given moment to events, persons, or objects in terms of personal perception, needs, and expectations (13, 18).

Relative influences of biology and culture, both essential, shift over the life span. Visual acuity diminishes in old age. Social relationships become more important as the child enters into the preschool period (13).

Each person is a social being who has the capacity to communicate and react to other people and the environment. Thus the person can function in the social system and its various institutions, such as family, school, and church (13).

The person cannot understand the self without understanding others, and he or she cannot understand others without understanding the self. Understanding the past and the parents helps to understand the self, as developmental patterns of the parents are repeated in the child (20).

Culture and society determine guidelines for normal progression of development and behavior patterns. What is normal in one group may be considered undesirable in another. Or, the child may show abnormally slow development in one area and unusually accelerated development or a mature quality in another. Yet despite these differences, the child may be perceived generally by others as a normal person (5, 15).

Nature and nurture are both basic to development. **Nature** *means people grow and develop in an orderly way based on genetic and physiologic foundations.* There is a basic genetic blueprint or pattern for physical growth progression and sequence, for language development, and for gradual physical decline in strength. However, **nurture** *(environmental experiences)* is a powerful influence and may suppress or enhance genetic capacity for expression of certain talents, cognitive abilities, language or physical achievements, or social skills. Environment is biological (nutrition, health care, or exposure to extreme conditions) or social (caring people, education, community resources, or media) (12, 18, 20).

Throughout life the person strives to reach optimum physical and emotional potential, barring great interferences. An inner drive or motivation propels him or her onward to meet the various developmental tasks. The person tries all types of adaptive behavior when interferences occur. He or she may regress to work through unsolved problems from the past. Once a need is met or a goal is accomplished, the person is free to move on to new arenas of behavior (10, 14, 17).

Principles of Growth and Development

DEFINITIONS

Certain words are basic to understanding the person and are used often. They are defined as follows for the purpose of this book.

Growth refers to *increase in body size or changes in structure, function, and complexity of body cell content and metabolic and biochemical processes.* Growth changes occur through incremental or replacement growth. **Incremental growth** refers to *maintaining an excess in growth over normal daily losses from catabolism, seen in urine, feces, perspiration, and oxidation in the lungs.* Incremental growth is observed as increases in weight or height. **Replacement growth** refers to *normal refills of essential body components* necessary for survival (8). For example, once a red blood cell (erythrocyte) has entered the cardiovascular system, it circulates an average of 120 days before disintegrating, when another red blood cell takes its place (11). Growth occurs through **hypertrophy,** *increase in the size of cellular structures*, and **hyperplasia,** *an increase in the number of cells* (8, 11). Growth during the fetal and infancy periods is achieved primarily through hyperplasia, which is gradually replaced by hypertrophic growth. Each body organ has its own optimum period of growth. Body tissues are most sensitive to permanent damage during periods of the most rapid hyperplastic growth.

Development is the *patterned, orderly, lifelong changes in structure, thought, feelings, or behavior that evolve as a result of maturation of physical and mental capacity, experiences, and learning and results in a new level of maturity and integration* (5, 6, 17. 18). Development permits the person to adapt to the environment by either controlling the environment or controlling responses to the environment. **Developmental processes** *involve interplay among the physiologic characteristics and the environmental forces, culture, and psychological mechanisms that mediate between them.* **Psychological processes** *include the person's perception of self, others, and the environment, and the behaviors acquired in coping with needs and the environment.* Development combines growth, maturation, and learning and involves organizing and maintaining behavior (5, 6, 17, 18).

A **developmental task** is a *growth responsibility that arises at a certain time in the course of development, successful achievement of which leads to satisfaction and success with later tasks.* Failure leads to unhappiness, disapproval by society, and difficulty with later developmental tasks and functions (9).

Biological age is the *level of physical growth and development related to physical health and capacity of vital organs* (17). It refers to *how the body functions over time.* **Psychological age** *is the adaptive capacity of the person compared with other people of a similar age* (18). It involves the person's *perception of aging processes.* **Social age** *refers to society's roles and expectations of the person at a specific age or stage.* As described earlier, social age relates to historical and social time (1). **Chronologic age** is the *time since birth.* It is not always identical to the other ages.

Learning is the *process of gaining specific knowledge or skills and acquiring habits and attitudes as a result of experience, training, and*

behavioral changes. **Maturation** refers to the *emergence of genetic potential for changes in form, structure, complexity, integration, organization, and function, physically and mentally* (17). *Maturation is the unfolding of a natural sequence of physical changes and behavior patterns, including readiness to master new activities* (17). Maturation and learning are interrelated. No learning occurs unless the person is mature enough to be able to understand and change his or her behavior (6, 17, 18).

GENERAL PRINCIPLES OF DEVELOPMENT

The following statements apply to the overall development of the person. Principles are italicized.

Childhood is the foundation period of life. Attitudes, habits, patterns of behavior and thinking, personality traits, and health status are established during the early years (2, 6, 17, 18). Early patterns of behavior may persist throughout life.

Development is lifelong; follows a definable, predictable, and sequential pattern; and occurs continually through adulthood. All persons progress through similar stages, but the age for achievement varies because of the inherent maturational capacity interacting with the physical and social environment. The different areas of growth and development—physical, mental, emotional, social, and spiritual—are interrelated, proceed together, and affect each other; yet these areas mature at their own pace. The stages of development overlap, and the transition from one stage to another is gradual (1, 3, 6, 10, 17, 18, 20).

Growth and development evidence both **continuity** (*cumulative change*) *and* **discontinuity** (*distinct stages, abrupt occurrence, or even regression*). The first action or word of a child may seem to be a sudden or discontinuous event; yet it is the result of weeks or months of practice (continuity). Puberty or aging manifestations may seem abrupt in onset but are the result of a gradual process occurring over several years (1, 18).

Growth is accompanied by behavior change. Development is multidirectional (1). As the child matures, he or she retains earlier ways of behaving, but there will be a developmental revision of habits. Some dimensions gain an expanded focus; others become less prominent at certain life periods. For example, the high-activity infant becomes a high-activity toddler or adult, but the object of the activity changes from diffuse interests to concentrated play to work. Behavior changes also occur because of others' reactions and expectations, which change as the person matures physically. Peers are important to the child through adolescence; the young adult focuses on an intimate relationship or several close friends.

Human behavior has purpose. It is goal directed and involves both gain and loss. Some abilities are diminished or lost (e.g., skipping typical of a 4-year-old) while new goals are met and abilities developed (e.g., greater strength and coordination of the late teen years). Therefore, the behavior is commonly preceded by imagining the desired result. The person visualizes the future and tries to bring it about. Behavior is directed to meeting needs and goals (14, 17, 20).

Critical periods in human development **occur** *when specific organs and other aspects of a person's physical and psychosocial growth undergo marked rapid change and the capacity to adapt to stressors is underdeveloped. During critical periods when tremendous demands* are placed on the person, the susceptibility to adverse environmental factors increases. See Chapters 4 and 8 ∞ for a description of teratogens. For example, implantation of the ovum is a critical period, and at certain times during pregnancy certain substances are more likely to damage fetal structures (8, 11). The form of the brain is established by the 12th week of gestation. *Critical periods of brain growth are* (8):

1. From the third to ninth weeks of gestation.
2. During brain growth spurt from 12 to 20 weeks of gestation.
3. During the time of rapid neuronal additions from 30 to 40 weeks of gestation.
4. During the first 18 to 24 months after birth.

Exposure of the nervous system to a teratogen during these time frames affects specific brain regions that are growing the most rapidly at that time. During adolescence the rapid physical growth may negatively affect social relationships or feelings about self. Middle or old age may be another critical period (8, 11, 19, 22).

If appropriate stimuli and resources are not available at the critical time or when the person is ready to receive and use particular stimuli for the development of a specific psychomotor skill, the skill may be more difficult to learn later in the developmental sequence. Learning of any psychomotor skill, however, is also influenced by sociocultural factors.

Mastering developmental tasks of one period is the basis for mastering the next developmental era, physically and emotionally. Certain periods exist when the task can be best accomplished, and the task should be mastered then. Each phase of development has characteristic traits and a period of equilibrium when the person adjusts more easily to environmental demands, and a period of disequilibrium when he or she experiences difficulty in adjustment (4–6, 9, 10, 15, 17, 18, 22).

Progressive differentiation of the self from the environment results from increasing self-knowledge and autonomy. The young child first separates as an object apart from mother, gradually becoming less dependent on the parents. Into adulthood, increased cognitive development enables more control over behavior. The ability to be autonomous and interdependent is reworked throughout life (10, 15, 17, 22).

Development involves changing allocation of resources—time, energy, talent, social skills, or money—for growth, improvement, maintenance, recovery, or dealing with loss. From birth through adolescence, resources are allocated for growth. In old age, more energy may be directed to coping with loss (1–4, 19).

Development is multidimensional. The developing person simultaneously acquires competencies in four major areas:

1. **Physical competency** includes *various motor and neurologic capacities* to attain mobility and manipulation and to care for self physically.
2. **Cognitive competency** includes *learning how to perceive, think, solve problems, and communicate thoughts and feelings* that, in turn, affect emotional and social skills.
3. **Emotional competency** includes *developing an awareness and acceptance of self as a separate person, responding to other people and factors in the environment because others have been respon-*

sive to him or her, coping with inner and outer stresses, and becoming increasingly responsible for personal behavior.

4. **Social competency** includes *learning how to affiliate securely with the family first and then with various people in various situations.*

These four competencies constantly influence one another. Lack of care or stimulation in any one area inhibits development of the other three areas. Repetition and practice are essential to learning. Rewarded behavior is usually repeated. The person optimally uses personal assets, inner resources, competencies, and abilities to keep energy expenditures at a minimum while focusing toward the achievement of a goal (10, 13, 14, 17).

Readiness and motivation are essential for learning to occur. Hunger, fatigue, illness, pain, and the lack of emotional feedback or opportunity to explore inhibit readiness and lower motivation (14, 15).

Development is contextual (1). *Many factors contribute to the formation of permanent characteristics and traits, including:*

1. The child's genetic inheritance.
2. Undetermined prenatal environmental factors.
3. Family and society when he or she is an infant and young child.
4. Nutrition and the physical and emotional environment.
5. Degree of intellectual stimulation in the environment.

Development is modifiable; the person demonstrates plasticity. Use of skills stimulates neuronal development and dendritic branching, and related abilities are improved. Not using certain skills or abilities causes neuronal loss (dendritic pruning) and consequent decrease or loss of function (1–4, 17, 19).

PRINCIPLES OF GROWTH

Several principles of growth are emphasized in the following pages, but the primary determinant of normal growth is the development of the central nervous system, which in turn governs or influences other body systems. Refer to Chapters 9 through 16 ∞ for information related to developmental eras.

The **Principle of Readiness** states that the *child's ability to perform a physical task depends not only on maturation of neurologic structures in the brain but also on maturation of the muscular and skeletal systems* (11, 17, 22). Until a state of physiologic readiness is reached, the child cannot perform a function, such as toilet training.

The **Principle of Differentiation** means that *development proceeds from (a) simple to complex, (b) homogeneous to heterogeneous, and (c) general to specific* (8, 11, 22). For example, movement from *simple to complex* is seen in mitotic changes in fetal cell structures as they undergo cell division immediately after ovum fertilization by a sperm. **Figure 3-1 □ depicts** how the brain structures differentiate and become more complex and specific in function. All human embryos are anatomically female for the first 6 weeks of life; only through the action of testosterone does the male embryo develop between the 6th and 12th weeks of life. Androgens or steroids administered prenatally can masculinize a genetic female brain (8, 11, 22). *Differentiation from general to simple motor skill*

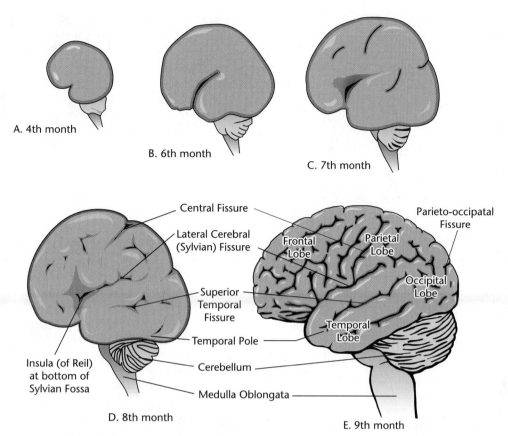

A. 4th month

B. 6th month

C. 7th month

Central Fissure

Lateral Cerebral
(Sylvian) Fissure

Parieto-occipatal
Fissure

Frontal
Lobe

Parietal
Lobe

Occipital
Lobe

Superior
Temporal
Fissure

Temporal Pole

Temporal
Lobe

Insula (of Reil)
at bottom of
Sylvian Fossa

Cerebellum

Medulla Oblongata

D. 8th month

E. 9th month

FIGURE ▢ 3-1 Principle of Differentiation: simple to complex and general to specific. Lateral views of the fetal brain at various stages of development.

is seen after birth as the baby first waves his or her arms and then later learns to control finger movements. The general body configurations of male and female at birth are much more similar than during late adolescence, thus indicating *movement from homogeneity to heterogeneity*. The mass of cells in the embryo is at first homogeneous, but the limbs of the 5-week-old embryo show considerable differentiation as the elbow and wrist regions become identifiable and finger ridge indentations outline the progressive protrusion of future fingers from the former paddle-shaped arm bud (8, 11). *General to specific* development is observed in motor responses, which are diffuse and undifferentiated at birth and become more specific and controlled later. The baby first moves the whole body in response to a stimuli; later he or she reacts with a specific body part (15, 22). The behavior of the child becomes more specific to the person or situation with increasing age.

The **Cephalocaudal, Proximodistal,** and **Bilateral Principles** all indicate that *major physical and motor changes invariably proceed in three bipolar directions.* **Cephalocaudal** (*head to tail*) means that the *upper end of the organism develops with greater rapidity than and before the lower end of the organism.* Increases in neuromuscular size and maturation of function begin in the head and proceed to hands and feet. For example, a comparison of pictures of a 5-week-old embryo during a period of several days clearly shows the extensive head growth, caused mainly by development of the brain, accompanied by further elongation of the body structure from

head to tail. Further, auditory, visual, and other sensory mechanisms in the head develop sooner than motor systems of the upper body. At the same time, the arm buds, first appearing paddle shaped, continue to change in shape and size more rapidly than do the lower limbs. After birth the infant will be able to hold the head erect before being able to sit or walk (6, 8, 11, 15, 17, 18, 22). **Proximodistal** (*near to far*) means that *growth progresses from the central axis of the body toward the periphery or extremities.* **Bilateral** (*side to side*) means that the *capacity for growth and development of structures is symmetric* (8, 15, 17, 22). Growth that occurs on one side of the body occurs simultaneously on the other. **Figure 3-2▢** depicts cephalocaudal and proximodistal directions of growth.

The **Principle of Asynchronous Growth** focuses on *developmental shifts at successive periods in development.* A comparison of pictures of persons of different ages indicates that the young child is not a "small adult." The proportional size of the head to the chest and of the torso to the limbs of younger and older persons is vastly different. Length of limbs in comparison to torso length is smaller in the infant than in the schoolchild and greater in the older adult than in the adolescent because of the biological changes of aging. **Figure 3-3▢** depicts asynchronous growth from prenatal to adulthood eras. **Figure 3-4▢** depicts asynchronous growth through how parts of the body increase length at different rates. As individuals develop from infancy through adulthood, one of the most noticeable physical changes is that the head becomes smaller in relation

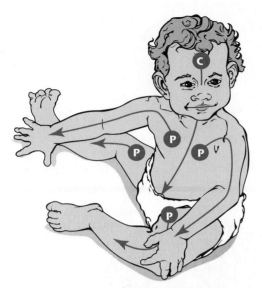

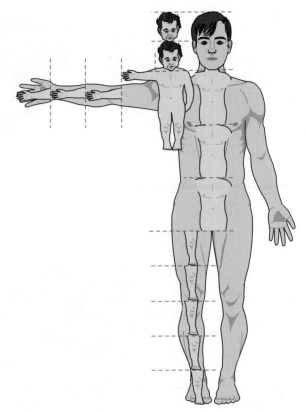

FIGURE ☐ **3-2** Cephalocaudal and proximodistal directions of growth. Cephalocaudal sequence of growth is from head (brain) to trunk to feet. Proximodistal sequence of growth is from the center of the body to the extremities.

to the rest of the body. The fractions listed refer to head size as a proportion of total body length at different ages (17).

The **Principle of Discontinuity of Growth Rate** refers to the *different rate of growth changes at different periods during the life span.* The *whole* body does not grow as a total unit simultaneously. Instead, various structures and organs of the body grow and develop at different rates, reaching their maximum at different times throughout the life cycle. For instance, in its rudimentary form the heart and circulatory system begin to function during the third week of embryonic life, continue to mature slowly compared with the rest of the body, and after the age of 25 years remain fairly constant in size. Before birth the head is the fastest growing body part.

FIGURE ☐ **3-4** Principle of Asynchronous Growth. General portions of the body increase their length at different rates.

The brain grows and develops according to a different pattern; this vital organ grows very rapidly during fetal life and infancy, reaching 80% of its maximum size at the age of 2 years. Full growth is seen at approximately 6 years of age (8, 11, 22). Body growth is rapid in infancy and adolescence and relatively slow during the school years. **Figures 3-1 through 3-4** demonstrate this principle.

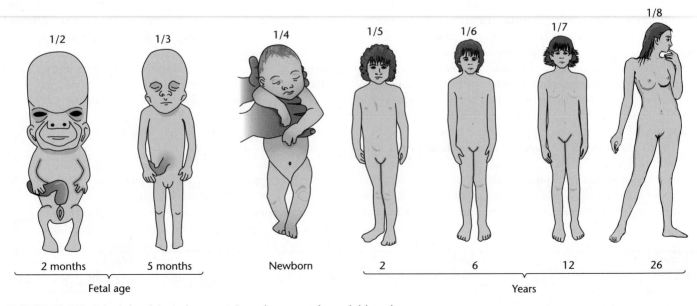

FIGURE ☐ **3-3** Principle of Asynchronous Growth: prenatal to adulthood.

INTERVENTIONS FOR HEALTH PROMOTION

1. You will apply the beliefs about people and principles of growth and development as you care for people throughout the life span.
2. The information in this chapter is also applicable to people from various cultural backgrounds and in any health care agency or in the community.

3. Knowledge of the beliefs and principles will help you evaluate progression of development as well as effectiveness of interventions.

Summary

1. The developing person changes at varying chronologic periods and is affected by historical and social time.
2. General descriptions about the person as a developing organism promote understanding for assessment and intervention.
3. Principles of growth are relevant to assessment of the person through the life span.
4. All body systems normally continue to work in unity through the life span. Some physiologic changes remain fairly stable (e.g., blood oxygen concentration); other changes (e.g., body temperature, pulse) depend on age, organ size, or maturity.
5. Age-related changes occur at varying chronologic periods.
6. Some developmental eras (prenatal, young childhood) are considered critical periods; the organism is extremely vulnerable to negative forces.

7. Structural deterioration usually precedes functional decline. Some organs and systems deteriorate more rapidly than others. In late life, the capacity for adaptation changes and finally death results.
8. The study of growth and development processes must focus on the complete continuum of the life cycle—from conception through death.
9. Seek a comprehensive understanding in order to assess the complexity of these processes and how these principles are activated throughout the life span.

Review Questions

1. A group of college freshmen is discussing marriage and parenthood. When sharing that many of their parents married and started families right out of high school, but do not consider this acceptable for their children, the students are discussing the concept of:
   1. Chronologic age
   2. Historical time
   3. Social time
   4. Age-irrelevant societies
2. By measuring height, weight, and head circumference during a well-child visit, the nurse is measuring which type of growth?
   1. Development
   2. Psychological
   3. Replacement
   4. Incremental
3. A woman enrolled in a childbirth preparation class asks the nurse if it is safe to take over-the-counter medications during the last trimester of pregnancy. The nurse should base the response to this inquiry on the fact that:

    1. A critical period of brain development occurs in the third trimester.
    2. Neurologic development is completed by the end of the first trimester.
    3. It is never safe to take medications while pregnant, regardless of stage of the pregnancy.
    4. All over-the-counter medications are teratogenic.
4. A parent is concerned that a 3-year-old is not yet toilet trained. The nurse can explain toilet training in this age group by applying the Principle of Readiness. In using this principle the nurse would explain to the parent that:
    1. Development occurs from the simplest task to the more complex.
    2. Development begins with the head and progresses downward.
    3. Development is not synchronous, and children are not "small adults."
    4. This task depends on nervous system maturity as well as the child's musculoskeletal maturity.

References

1. Baltes, P. B. (1987). Theoretical perspectives of life-span development psychology: On the dynamics between growth and decline. *Developmental Psychology, 23*(5), 611–626.

2. Baltes, P. B. (2003). On the incomplete architecture of human ontogeny: Selection, optimization, and compensation as foundations of developmental theory. In U.M. Staudinger & U. Lindenberger (Eds.), *Understanding human development: Dialogues with life-span psychology* (pp. 17–43). Dordrecht, Netherlands: Kluwer.

3. Baltes, P. B., Lindenberger, U., & Staudinger, U.M. (1998). Life-span theory in developmental psychology. In R.M. Lerner (Ed.), *Handbook of child psychology: Vol. 1. Theoretical models of human development* (pp. 1029–1143). New York: Wiley.

4. Baltes, P. B., Reese, H.W., & Lipsitt, I. (1980). Life-span developmental psychology. *Annual Review of Psychology, 31*, 65–110.

5. Bee, H. (1998). *Lifespan development* (2nd ed.). New York: Longman.

6. Berger, K. (2005). *The developing person through the life span* (6th ed.). New York: Worth.

7. Berrien, K. (1968). *General and social systems.* New Brunswick, NJ: University Press.

8. Cunningham, F., MacDonald, P., & Gant, N. (2005). *Williams obstetrics* (22nd ed.). Norwalk, CT: Appleton & Lange.

9. Duvall, E., & Miller, B. (1984). *Marriage and family development* (6th ed.). New York: Harper & Row.

10. Erikson, E. (1963). *Childhood and society* (2nd ed.). New York: W.W. Norton.

11. Guyton, A., & Hall, J.E. (2006). *Textbook of medical physiology* (11th ed.). Philadelphia: Elsevier.

12. Karaim, R. (2006, February). Mr. Johnson's new family. *AARP Bulletin*, 39.

13. King, I. (1981). *Theory for nursing: Systems, concepts, and process.* New York: Delmar.

14. Maslow, A. (1970). *Motivation and personality* (2nd ed.). New York: Harper & Row.

15. Mussen, P., et al. (1990). *Child development and personality* (7th ed.). New York: Harper & Row.

16. Neugarten, B. L., & Neugarten, D. (1989, May). The changing meaning of age. *Psychology Today*, 44–51.

17. Papalia, D., Olds, S., & Feldman, R. (2004). *Human development* (9th ed.). Boston: McGraw-Hill.

18. Santrock, J. (2004). *Life-span development* (9th ed.). Boston: McGraw-Hill.

19. Staudinger, U. M., & Bluch, S. (2001). A view of midlife development from life-span theory. In M.E. Lachman (Ed.), *Handbook of midlife development* (pp. 3–39). New York: Wiley.

20. Sullivan, H. S. (1953). *Interpersonal theory of psychiatry.* New York: W.W. Norton.

21. von Bertalanffy, L. (1968). *General systems theory.* New York: George Braziller.

22. Wong, D. (2003). *Whaley and Wong's nursing care of infants and children* (7th ed.). St. Louis, MO: C.V. Mosby.

UNIT II

Influences on the Developing Person and Family Unit

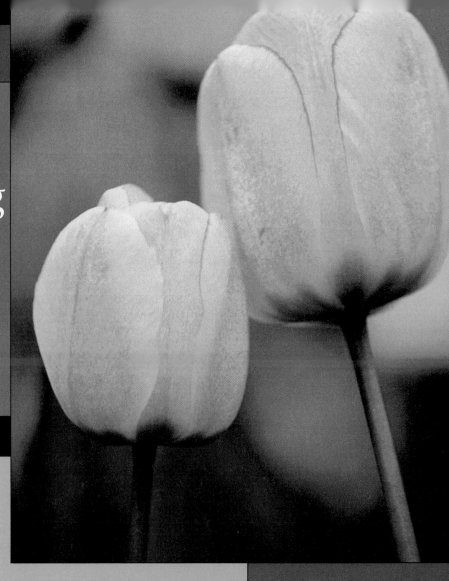

CHAPTERS

CHAPTER 4

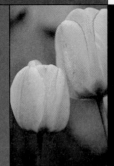

Environmental Influences

KEY TERMS

OBJECTIVES

Study of this chapter will enable you to:

1. Examine the scope of environmental pollution and the interrelationship of various pollutants with each other and their effects on people.

2. Observe sources of pollution in your community and identify resulting hazards to human health.

3. Assess health hazards encountered in the home and the workplace, their effects, and intervention measures.

4. Discuss and practice ways that you can prevent or reduce various types of environmental pollution.

5. Examine your professional responsibility in assessing for and intervening in illness caused by environmental pollutants.

6. Discuss the importance of disaster planning and management, including bioterrorism.

MediaLink www.prenhall.com/murray

Go to the Companion Website for interactive resources that accompany this chapter.

Glossary	Critical Thinking
Review Questions	Tools
Challenge Your Knowledge	Media Link Applications
Learning Activities	Media Links

Ecology *refers to the relationships between organisms and their environment.* The ecological perspective of a specific discipline provides a focus for looking at people's transactions with some portion of their physical or psychosocial surroundings. In the ecological models that provide a framework for health promotion, the term **environment** *usually refers to the space outside of the individual—the physical environment* (76). Human health is determined through the interaction of genetics and the environment. The purpose of this chapter is to focus on aspects of people's physical environment in relationship to promoting health and to supporting positive health behavior. **Figure 4-1**☐ depicts a summary of human interrelationships with the environment.

Health care in the past was concerned primarily with the client's immediate environment in the hospital or home. Today, *health care extends to include assessment and intervention directed toward promoting a healthy environment for individuals and families, well or ill, and for the community.* Chapter 2 ∞ refers to the global community and international health problems, some induced by the environment. Environmental illness occurs when one is exposed to a noxious agent in the environment that is absorbed through inhalation, ingestion, skin contact, or sensory overstimulation. Whether an individual becomes ill depends on susceptibility, the toxic agent itself, and the intensity and duration of exposure (92). As discussed in Chapter 2, the presence of health hazards in the environment affects health promotion efforts and all the levels of prevention.

Understanding the sources and negative effects of specific environmental health problems enables you to function both as an individual and a health care professional who promotes health. The concept of environment should be included in each step of the nursing process.

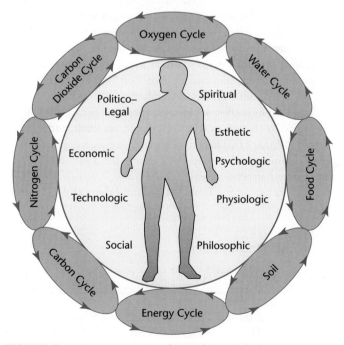

FIGURE ☐ **4-1** Human interrelationships with the environment.

Historical Perspective

In their quest to conquer nature, early people discovered fire and the wheel. These discoveries played major roles in early civilization and in the later industrialization of the world. Fire was essential to survival, but with its advent, natural or man-made sparks and pollutants were sent into the atmosphere—the beginning of environmental pollution. With the Industrial Revolution came the technologic advances that gave people increased power and comforts. Progress, however, can make us both comfortable and sick (15, 36, 96).

As cities grew, population growth and changing agricultural and industrial practices resulted in changes in the climate and environment. Megacities, factory farms, and jet planes have opened even more new avenues for environmental change. Over 30 new diseases have appeared since the mid-1970s, some as the result of climatic conditions and some as the result of human intervention. A global effect of climatic conditions on the environment is not uncommon. As an example, an unusually warm winter in the Southwest caused by an ocean disturbance led to an explosion of the rodent population and the hantavirus that they carry, causing a SARS-like syndrome in young adults. Clearing forests to increase cropland and suburban development can also increase the number of disease-carrying rodents, with global health implications (15, 96).

Antipollution legislation in the United States can be traced back to the early 1900s, but most legislative moves were poorly funded and had little effect on growing pollution problems. However, Rachel Carson's revelations about the hazards of chemicals in *Silent Spring* resulted in an increased interest in the environment in the 1960s. The United States became the world's environmental leader. The Environmental Protection Agency (EPA) was established in 1970. Legislation passed during that period included the National Environmental Policy Act (1969), the Clean Air and Solid Waste Disposal Act (1965), and the Clean Water Act (1972). However, corporate America turned back these gains in what journalist Bill Moyers has called Washington's mercenary culture (43, 57, 59, 80, 96). This is in contrast with the movement of the European Union to "go green" with the development of laws to curb toxic pollution and waste from manufacturing (50). However, all is not lost. At the state and local level, there is considerable movement toward combating global warming, decreasing pollution, and promoting the use of renewable energy sources (57, 59, 65, 85, 96). Although the U.S. federal government refused to participate in the 2005 **Kyoto Protocol**, *an international agreement to curb heat-trapping emissions caused by burning fossil fuels,* 203 mayors of major U.S. cities have signed a climate protection agreement to reduce global warming pollution in cities throughout the nation (13, 54).

The environment is a vital part of our existence. Human skill in manipulating the environment has produced tremendous benefits; but none has been without a price, the high price of global warming and pollution. Global warming (71, 72) is increasingly being accepted as a real risk to population lifeways, health, and future quality of life worldwide, as attested to by response to efforts and leadership by former Vice President Al Gore, environmentalists, and various researchers and political leaders. For example, the film *An Inconvenient Truth* has been widely circulated, viewed, and discussed. Refer to the Website, www.participate.net. Environmental pollution is a complex problem requiring multiple solutions. As both climactic changes and people can influence the environment, so can one form of environmental pollution influence another form. To illustrate, when a person inhales harmful particles from the soil that have become airborne, soil pollution becomes air pollution; and soil or surface pollution becomes water or food pollution if the harmful particles are swept into the water, consumed first by fish, and then consumed by people. Human health and development may be adversely affected by air, water, soil, food, noise, and surface pollution and by occupational hazards. The CLEAN Energy Act of 2007 passed by Congress would invest money in clean, renewable energy and energy efficiency—a step to reducing global warming and pollution.

Air Pollution

You will assess and care for patients in a variety of settings who have diseases caused or aggravated by outdoor and indoor air pollution. The sources of these air pollutants vary, and their effect on humans differs according to duration and extent of exposure to the pollutant. Air pollution is most harmful to the very young, the very old, and persons with respiratory and cardiac disease. It is critical to promote health by educating the public, participating in policy and legislation development with advocacy groups, and individually making lifestyle changes, if necessary, related to reduction of air pollution (36, 79, 92).

PROBLEMS OF OUTDOOR AIR POLLUTION

Air pollution is not a new problem; people have known for centuries that air can carry poisons. Natural processes, such as forest and prairie fires, volcanic eruptions, and wind erosion, contaminate the air. Air pollution and water pollution act interchangeably; together they present a global problem. Given enough time, the oceans can cleanse the atmosphere through the processes of precipitation, oxidation, and absorption; but if the amount of pollution exceeds the ocean's capacity to neutralize the waste, harmful materials are dispersed into the atmosphere. We realize the effects of breathing contaminated air. The primary sources of air pollution are due to excessive use of fossil fuels that contribute to an increase in greenhouse gases, depletion of the upper atmosphere ozone layer and the presence of photochemical ozone at ground level, industrial chemical releases, and the presence of acid deposition (6, 24, 28).

Increase in Greenhouse Gases

Some **greenhouse gases**—*water vapor, carbon dioxide, methane, nitrous oxide, and ozone—occur naturally in the atmosphere whereas others, such as fluorocarbons, result from human activity.* They allow sunlight to freely enter the atmosphere and absorb heat, maintaining the temperature of the earth at a constant level and creating a natural greenhouse effect. Human activity, however, has increased the levels of carbon dioxide, methane, and nitrous oxide, which intensifies the heat-trapping capability of the earth's atmosphere and

heightens the greenhouse effect. In addition, the gases become part of a feedback loop that triggers the development of water vapor. Heating the atmosphere allows it to take up and retain more moisture, exacerbating the greenhouse effect (6, 24, 28).

Fossil fuels *are formed from the fossilized remains of prehistoric plants and animals that drew carbon from the atmosphere. When we burn fossil fuels, we release carbon that has been out of the atmosphere for eons* (24). It combines with oxygen to form carbon dioxide. Our reliance on fossil fuels—coal, oil, and natural gas—to run cars and trucks, heat homes and businesses, and power factories is responsible for about 98% of carbon dioxide emissions, 24% of methane emissions, and 18% of nitrous oxide emissions in the United States (32). In 2002, 23 billion tons of carbon dioxide were released into the atmosphere—41% from burning coal, 39% from oil, and 20% from natural gas (24). During this process, methane and nitrous oxide are also emitted. At present, fossil fuels provide 66% of the world's electrical power and 95% of its total energy demands (28). Large sport utility vehicles, with their low gas mileage, are exacerbating the greenhouse effect because of the tonnage of carbon dioxide produced. As an example, a Hummer emits 24,100 pounds of carbon dioxide per year whereas a Honda Accord emits 10,300 pounds (8).

Soil and trees act as natural sinks or reservoirs to uptake chemical elements such as carbon. **Deforestation**, *cutting large forests of old tree growth to increase cropland or suburban development*, leads to an increase in atmospheric carbon dioxide. In addition, if trees or other wood products are burned, carbon that has been out of the atmosphere for years is released into the air to bond with oxygen and form carbon dioxide (24, 32).

In addition to the emissions that result from fossil fuel consumption, methane and nitrous oxide are by-products of other processes. **Methane (swamp gas) emissions** *are an outcome of the decomposition of organic waste in landfills, of rice cultivation in flooded areas, and of raising livestock as they emit methane during digestion.* **Nitrous oxide emissions** *result from the use of nitrogen-based fertilizers and from waste disposal in sewage treatment plants.* Methane and nitrous oxide occur in lower concentrations in the atmosphere than carbon dioxide, but their heat-absorbing capacity is 60 to 270 times greater, respectively (24).

The greenhouse effect may lead to increased global warming accompanied by changes in weather, climate, sea levels, and land use patterns (57, 71, 72). There may be positive effects associated with global warming, such as decreased energy use and increased economic growth in certain areas (22). However, it is projected to negatively affect health. See **Table 4-1**, Health Effects of Air Pollution (24, 28, 32, 92).

Changing Ozone Levels

Ozone *is a gas that occurs in the upper atmosphere and at ground level.* It can be good or bad for health depending on its location in the atmosphere. A thin layer of ozone surrounds the earth and blocks much of the sun's ultraviolet radiation from reaching the earth's surface. This ozone layer is endangered by the continued use of ozone-depleting substances found in coolants, pesticides, solvents, foaming agents, fire extinguishers, and aerosol propellants. These substances are broken down by strong ultraviolet light

TABLE 4-1

Health Effects of Air Pollution

Pollutant	Symptoms	Diseases
Greenhouse gases	Related to increased environmental heat and effects on human physiology	Diseases caused by insects, pests due to increased warmth Heat strokes, heat-related deaths Myocardial infarction Respiratory diseases, bronchitis, asthma
Ozone	Sunburn Compromised immune functions	Cataracts Nonmelanoma skin cancer Malignant melanoma Immune system diseases
Photochemical ozone (urban smog)	Respiratory difficulty in healthy people, children, outdoor workers, people exercising outdoors Cardiac and respiratory symptoms increase in ill people	Bronchitis, emphysema, asthma Scarring of lung tissue Cardiac diseases All respiratory and cardiac diseases increase in severity
Acid deposition (acid rain)	Cardiac and respiratory symptoms increase, especially in ill people	Cardiac diseases Respiratory diseases Death
Asbestos	Respiratory difficulty, depending on number of fibers inhaled	Asbestosis, depending on length of exposure Lung cancer, risk increased in smokers Mesothelioma Respiratory diseases
Biological contaminants	Allergic reactions on skin Respiratory difficulty, especially children and elderly	Specific allergies, e.g., mold, dog and cat hair and saliva, dust, mites, cockroaches, pollen Asthma
Carbon monoxide	*Low concentration: Fatigue, Flulike symptoms, headaches* in healthy person; chest pain if heart disease present Nausea, vomiting *Moderate concentration:* Respiratory difficulty due to tissue ischemia Impaired vision, dizziness, poor coordination More severe headache Confusion; symptoms relieved if go outdoors immediately when suspected	Acute myocardial injury Permanent cognitive impairment Death from high concentrations or prolonged exposure
Formaldehyde	Watery eyes Burning sensation in eyes and throat Nausea Respiratory difficulty, wheezing, coughing Skin rash, allergic reactions	Asthma attacks from high concentrations Lung cancer
Lead	Physical and mental developmental delays Shortened attention span Behavioral/conduct disorders Mental retardation, lower IQ levels depend on exposure	Damage to red blood cells Kidney disease Nervous system damage Convulsions, coma, death from high blood lead levels
Nitrogen oxide	Irritation to eyes, nose, throat, and respiratory tract mucosa	Respiratory infections, especially young children Low levels: Bronchial reaction in asthmatics; decreased lung capacity in chronic obstructive pulmonary disease High levels, continued exposure: Bronchitis

continued

TABLE 4-1

Health Effects of Air Pollution—continued

Pollutant	Symptoms	Diseases
Pesticides	Headache	Chronic exposure: Liver and kidney disease
	Dizziness, weakness	Damage to endocrine and central nervous system
	Nausea	
Volatile organic compounds	Immediate: Eye, nose, throat irritation	Short-term contact: Skin allergic reactions
	Short-term contact: Headache, nausea, visual disorders, dizziness, uncoordination	Long-term contact: Liver, kidney, and central nervous system damage
	Long-term contact: Memory impairment	
Radon	No immediate symptoms	Lung cancer 2 to 5 years after exposure
	Respiratory difficulty with prolonged contact	
Secondhand smoke	Irritation of eyes, nose, and throat	Ear infections in children
	Respiratory difficulty	Asthma attacks
		Bronchitis
		Pneumonia
		Lung cancer

releasing chlorine and bromine molecules into the stratosphere that then destroy the good ozone. **Table 4-1** presents problems that will result from depletion of the ozone layer (28, 33, 92).

Conversely, **photochemical ozone** *at ground level is a harmful pollutant and the major ingredient of urban smog.* It is created by chemical reactions between nitrogen oxides and volatile organic compounds in the presence of sunlight. Emissions from industrial facilities and electric utilities, motor vehicle exhaust, gasoline vapors, and chemical solvents are some of its major sources. Breathing ozone may trigger numerous health problems (See **Table 4-1**) (16, 28, 87, 92).

The EPA developed the **Air Quality Index (AQI)** *to replace the Pollutant Standards Index (PSI) as a means of reporting how clean or polluted the air is and what associated health effects might be of concern* (4). The levels of five major air pollutants regulated by the Clean Air Act—ground level ozone, particle pollution, carbon monoxide, sulfur dioxide, and nitrogen dioxide—are calculated to determine air quality. The **AQI** is *a scale that runs from 0 to 500. The higher the AQI value the greater the level of air pollution and the greater the health risk.* An AQI value of 50 represents good air quality. An AQI value of 100 represents the national air quality standard set by the EPA to protect public health. AQI values above 100 are considered to be unhealthy, at first for certain sensitive groups of people, such as those with lung or heart disease, and then for everyone as AQI values get higher. For ease of use, *the EPA has assigned a specific color to each AQI category—green or yellow means safe air, orange means air is unhealthy for sensitive groups, and red means that conditions are unhealthy for everyone* (4). The EPA is considering revising these standards, however, a recent study conducted by the EPA and the Centers for Disease Control and Prevention (CDC) found evidence that even low levels of ozone exposure are dangerous. *Even at the EPA's current acceptable level of*

ozone, the study found a statistically significant increased risk of premature death (16, 23).

Educate people with cardiac or respiratory disease to follow directions in their community to remain indoors, related to AQI values, in order to prevent adverse effects. Advocate for control of air pollution.

Acid Deposition

Although we generally speak of acid rain, **acid deposition** is the more precise term. **Wet deposition** *refers to acidic rain, fog, and snow that affect plants and animals.* **Dry deposition** *refers to acidic gases and particles in the atmosphere.* Dry deposition is blown onto buildings, cars, and trees. Rain washes the acidic particles from these objects, increasing the acidity of the falling rain itself. Sulfur dioxide and nitrogen oxide are the primary causes of acid deposition and enter the atmosphere from power plants powered by fossil fuels, from iron and copper smelters, and from automobile exhaust. Although acid rain looks, feels, and tastes just like clean rain, it has numerous negative effects. It can damage forests, soil, fish, and human health. The gases cause it to interact in the atmosphere to form fine sulfate and nitrate particles that can be inhaled. Studies have shown a relationship between elevated levels of these particles and increased illness and death from heart and lung disorders. (See **Table 4-1**.) At present, the only solution is to decrease sulfur dioxide and nitrogen oxide emissions into the atmosphere (1, 21, 98).

PROBLEMS OF INDOOR AIR POLLUTION

Indoor air quality is of concern in homes, schools, and workplaces because we spend 90% of our time indoors. Indoor air pollutants include asbestos, biological pollutants, carbon monoxide, formaldehyde, volatile organic compounds, lead, nitrogen dioxide, pesticides, radon, respirable particles, and secondhand and third-hand smoke. The levels of some of these pollutants are much higher indoors than outdoors (41, 79, 83, 92).

Educate clients about indoor air pollution. Health effects can range from minor irritation to life-threatening illness.

Asbestos

Until the 1970s, **asbestos**, *a mineral fiber, was added to a variety of products to strengthen them, provide heat insulation, or increase fire resistance*. Unless they are labeled otherwise, most products made today do not contain asbestos. See **Table 4-1** for effects from breathing high levels of asbestos fibers. The risk of developing asbestosis is correlated with length of exposure. We are all exposed to small amounts of asbestos in our daily lives. Repeated inhalation of the fibers, however, may result in an accumulation in the lungs and increase the risk of disease (5, 77, 83).

Educate the client that if there is asbestos in the home, the best thing to do is to leave it alone unless there is a danger that fibers are being released and inhaled. If removal is necessary, a professional trained in asbestos removal should be contacted.

Biological Pollutants

Biological contaminants include *bacteria, molds, mildew, viruses, animal dander and cat saliva, house dust, mites, cockroaches, and pollen*. Mold, dust mites, pet dander, pollen, and pest droppings or body parts can trigger allergic reactions and some types of asthma. Certain infectious illnesses are transmitted through air containing these contaminants, and some diseases are associated with exposure to toxins in heating and cooling systems and in humidifiers. Children, elderly people, and people with breathing problems, allergies, and lung diseases are particularly susceptible. See **Table 4-1** for health effects (79, 83, 86).

Educate the client that general good housekeeping, maintenance of heating and air conditioning equipment, adequate ventilation, pest management, and moisture control are key to minimizing the risk. Dampness serves as a breeding ground for some of these pollutants; a relative humidity of 30% to 50% should be maintained in the home.

Carbon Monoxide

Carbon monoxide (CO) *is an odorless, colorless, and toxic gas that binds with hemoglobin, reducing the number of binding sites for oxy-gen, which inhibits oxygen uptake, causing various symptoms.* Sources of the gas are unvented heaters, leaking chimneys and furnaces, gas water heaters, wood stoves and fireplaces, generators and other gasoline-powered equipment, and automobile exhaust from attached garages. See **Table 4-1** for the range of symptoms: insidious to severe, and even death. Symptoms relate to CO concentration (79, 83).

Educate clients and the public about CO pollution and effects. Prevention involves ensuring that any combustion equipment is in good condition. Every home should have at least one carbon monoxide detector and the batteries must be checked regularly.

Formaldehyde

Formaldehyde, *a colorless, pungent-smelling gas, is widely used in the manufacture of building materials and household products.* Formaldehyde emissions generally decrease as products age. It may be present in substantial concentrations indoors and outdoors. In homes, the most significant source is likely to be pressed wood products, including furniture, cabinets, and paneling. Formaldehyde release is accelerated by heat and may be affected by humidity level. Health effects are listed in **Table 4-1** (81).

Lead

Lead is a *highly toxic metal* that was used for years in products found around the home, such as paint, water pipes, and gasoline. Today, the most common sources of lead exposure are deteriorating lead-based paint, lead-contaminated dust, vehicles that use leaded gasoline, and residential soil (79, 84).

An estimated 38 million housing units in the United States have been identified as containing lead-based paint at levels that are a serious health hazard, according to the EPA. A bipartisan bill introduced in 2006 would provide federal funding for lead removal in residences that house low-income people, women of childbearing age, and young children. The federal government has a goal to eliminate by the year 2010 toxic blood levels in children under 6 years of age (61).

Airborne lead enters the body when an individual breathes or swallows lead particles or dust. Fetuses, infants, and children are most vulnerable because lead is more readily absorbed into growing bodies. Their tissues are more sensitive to its damaging effects, and children are more likely to get lead dust or particles on their hands and then put their fingers into their mouths. Although lead poisoning is seen most frequently in children from

---

INTERVENTIONS FOR HEALTH PROMOTION

*Educate clients and the public about the following measures that reduce exposure to **formaldehyde** (81):*

1. Use exterior-grade pressed wood products whenever possible as they emit lower concentrations of the gas.
2. Avoid the use of formaldehyde-emitting products.

3. Use air conditioners and dehumidifiers to maintain moderate temperature and humidity levels.
4. Provide adequate ventilation, particularly after bringing any new source of formaldehyde into the home.

INTERVENTIONS FOR HEALTH PROMOTION

*Educate clients and the public that **prevention of lead exposure** involves the following measures* (79, 83):

1. Keep the environment as free of lead as possible by keeping surfaces clean and dust-free.
2. Take care not to bring lead dust into the home from another location.
3. Leave lead-based paint undisturbed if it is in good condition.
4. Seek professional help if removal of lead-based paint is necessary.
5. Keep children away from chipping paint; keep them from eating dirt or chewing on windowsills.
6. Make sure children wash their hands when they come inside and before meals.
7. Maintain good nutrition; the child who gets enough iron and calcium will absorb less lead.
8. Participate in screening for lead exposure, which is readily available.

---

inner cities due to the preponderance of older housing, no economic or racial subgroup of children is exempt from lead toxicity. Children who display a behavior called **pica,** *the habit of eating nonfood substances,* are at increased risk for lead exposure. Effects of lead exposure on fetuses and young children are presented in **Table 4-1** (79, 83).

Educate families about prevention and early screening. Be an active community advocate to overcome hazards from environmental lead. Further, educate about the importance of follow-up diagnostic testing for children with elevated screening blood lead levels. This is often neglected, especially for poor, urban children, and can lead to other health problems (46).

Nitrogen Oxide

Nitrogen oxide (NO) *is a colorless, odorless, nonflammable gas* used as an anesthetic and in aerosols. Other sources include kerosene heaters, unvented gas stoves and heaters, and tobacco smoke. Nitrogen oxide effects are listed in **Table 4-1** (77, 83). The average level of nitrogen oxide in homes without combustion appliances is about half that of outdoors. In homes with combustion appliances, indoor levels often exceed outdoor levels. As with carbon monoxide, ensuring that any combustion equipment is in good condition will reduce exposure (77, 83).

Pesticides

Pesticides *are toxic semivolatile organic compounds used to kill or control pests,* such as bacteria, fungi, insects, and rodents. Studies suggest that 75% of U.S. households used at least one pesticide product indoors during the last year, that 80% of pesticide exposure occurs indoors, and that measurable levels of up to a dozen pesticides have been found in the air in homes (37, 51, 79, 83). In these studies, the pesticide levels that were found could not be explained by recent pesticide use in the home alone. Other potential sources included contaminated soil that floated or was tracked in, especially in rural and agricultural areas, stored pesticide containers, and household surfaces that collected and later released pesticides. Health effects are listed in **Table 4-1.** At present, it is not

known what pesticide concentrations are necessary to produce these effects (37, 79, 83).

Teach clients and the public the steps to minimize exposure (37, 51, 79, 83):

1. Choose a pest control company carefully, which is likely to be safer than self-administration.
2. Follow the manufacturer's directions for pesticide use in the home or outdoors.
3. Provide adequate ventilation during and after use indoors; stay out of the building for the recommended time duration.
4. Dispose of unwanted pesticides safely; follow directions on the label.
5. Keep exposure to moth repellents to a minimum.
6. Consider the use of organic or biopesticides and integrated pest management for both indoors and outdoors.

Biopesticides, *or biological pesticides, are derived from natural materials* such as animals, plants, bacteria, and certain minerals. For example, canola oil and baking soda are biopesticides. They are less harmful than conventional pesticides, are targeted at specific pests rather than having a more global effect, are effective in small quantities, and decompose quickly, thus avoiding pollution problems. Integrated pest management relies on the use of "good" bugs (such as ladybugs) to kill "bad" bugs in conjunction with minimal pesticide use (79, 83).

Volatile Organic Compounds

Volatile organic compounds *are emitted as gases from certain solids or liquids.* They may be given off by household products such as cleaning supplies, drain openers, paints and paint removers, pesticides, building materials and furnishings, office equipment such as copiers and printers, craft materials such as glues and adhesives, permanent markers, and photographic solutions. Concentrations of these compounds are much higher indoors than outdoors. These fumes may have short- and long-term health effects, especially if used in a confined space with inadequate ventilation. See **Table 4-1** for health effects (57, 82, 83). The extent and nature of the health effects are related to many factors, including level of exposure and length of time exposed (82, 83).

Educate clients and the public about steps to reduce exposure:

1. Provide adequate ventilation.
2. Discard unneeded chemicals per toxic waste guidelines; gases may leak from closed containers.
3. Minimize exposure to methylene chloride, benzene, and perchloroethylene as they are carcinogenic.

Radon

Radon *is an invisible, odorless, radioactive gas produced by the natural decay of uranium in soil and rocks that moves up through the ground.* It is harmlessly dispersed in outdoor air. If it enters homes through cracks or holes in the foundation or walls or gaps around pipes and becomes trapped inside, it can be harmful at elevated levels. Because it is odorless, people tend to minimize its risk but *it is the most serious health threat of the common indoor pollutants.* See **Table 4-1** for a summary of health effects (12, 79, 83). It decays into radioactive particles that can enter the lungs, leading to the risk of damage to lung tissue. It is a major cause of lung cancer. The EPA estimates that radon is responsible for up to 21,000 deaths from lung cancer each year. About 2,900 of these deaths occur among nonsmokers. Although the risk of lung cancer due to radon exposure is much higher in smokers, it is a major cause of lung cancer among nonsmokers. The risk of radon exposure is based on how much radon is in the home, the amount of time spent in the home, and whether or not the person is a smoker or has smoked. There is no evidence that it increases the risk of other respiratory diseases, and children are not believed to be at greater risk than adults (12, 79, 83).

Any home may have a radon problem, and it is estimated that 1 out of every 15 homes in the United States has an elevated radon level. Other sources of radon include well water and building materials. One can breathe in radon released into the air when well water contaminated with radon is used for showering. In addition, ingesting well water contaminated with radon to some extent increases the risk of developing stomach cancer. Building materials rarely cause radon problems by themselves (12, 79, 83).

Teach preventive measures, such as sealing cracks and other sources of radon. A do-it-yourself kit can be used to test the home for radon, or a qualified tester can be hired. If an elevated radon level is present, a radon reduction system can be installed.

Respirable Particles

Respirable particles, *such as dust, soot, and ash,* may be inhaled into the lungs. Sources include fireplaces, wood stoves, and kerosene heaters. Particle levels in homes without these sources are the same as, or lower than, outdoor levels. Respirable particles may cause eye, nose, and throat irritation; respiratory infections and bronchitis; and lung cancer (83).

Teach home measures to reduce exposure. Adequate ventilation and venting of combustible sources, inspection, cleaning and changing filters, and repair of heating and air conditioning systems are essential measures.

Secondhand Smoke and Thirdhand Smoke

Secondhand smoke *refers to inhalation of smoke that people who smoke cigarettes or cigars exhale into the air.* Smoking, radon, and secondhand smoke are the leading causes of lung cancer. Secondhand smoke is the cause of approximately 3,000 lung cancer deaths a year—about 1,000 of these are people who never smoked. *It is especially harmful to children's health because they are still developing physically and have higher respiratory rates than do adults.*

Thirdhand smoke *refers to the effects on the fetus when the pregnant woman is around people who smoke, although they may not be smoking at that time* (3).

The Surgeon General's report "The Health Consequences of Involuntary Exposure to Tobacco Smoke" states that even brief exposure to secondhand smoke, which contains more than 50 cancer-causing chemicals, can cause immediate harm to nonsmokers (89). See **Table 4-1** for more information about the effects of secondhand smoke (30, 79, 83, 89). Fetal exposure to thirdhand smoke may contribute to the child demonstrating aggressive and defiant behaviors, which may progress to attention deficit/hyperactivity disorder and conduct disorder (3).

Teach families that *the best way to alleviate the effects of secondhand smoke is to not allow smoking in the home or car.* Support family members who make this decision in the face of general family oppositions.

Indoor Environmental Quality

Indoor air quality *refers to the quality of the air in an office environment.* In the 1970s, virtually airtight buildings were constructed in order to conserve fossil fuels. In some of these buildings, office workers began to complain of a variety of similar symptoms, including headache, fatigue, itching or burning eyes, skin irritation, nasal congestion, dry or irritated throats, and nausea. Workers often consider the workplace the cause of the symptoms if they are alleviated when they leave the office. It is believed that the symptoms are often related to ventilation system deficiency, overcrowding, release of gas from materials in the office and from mechanical equipment, tobacco smoke, microbiological contamination, and outside air pollutants. These buildings have been referred to as "sick buildings," giving rise to the "sick building syndrome" (41).

The National Institute for Occupational Safety and Health (NIOSH) uses the term **indoor environmental quality (IEQ)** *to describe the problems occurring in buildings throughout the nation.* This term encompasses not only the quality of the air but other factors, such as comfort, noise, lighting, ergonomic stressors, and job-related psychosocial factors (41).

Hospitals are associated with specific forms of indoor air pollution. Fumes from disinfectants, such as glutaraldehyde, a sterilizing agent for instruments; surgical smoke or laser plume from tissue being cut, vaporized, or coagulated; and waste gases from anesthetic agents affect health care workers and patients. A small amount of glutaraldehyde fumes can cause respiratory and dermatologic problems. Surgical smoke or laser plume can cause respiratory symptoms, burning and watery eyes, nausea, and viral contamination and regrowth. Individuals who work in the recovery room are likely to feel fatigue from breathing the patients' exhaled anesthesia gases (78, 92).

Educate clients and the public that all forms of indoor air pollution are physically irritating, and some may present a potential hazard to long-term health, either by direct damage to the respiratory tract mucous membranes or through the indirect effects of continuously breathing contaminated air. Support the professional organizations and legislators as they work to foster a healthy environment (36).

Water Pollution

Although water is our most valuable natural resource, we disregard its value by polluting rivers, lakes, and oceans. About 1 billion people in the world lack access to clean drinking water; more than 40% of the world's population in 80 countries regularly experience serious water shortages (6). **Water is considered polluted** *when it is unfit for its intended use.* Man-made water pollution has two major origins: point sources and nonpoint sources. **Point sources** *are those that discharge pollutants directly into a body of water, such as from an oil spill.* **Nonpoint sources** *pollute water indirectly through environmental changes, such as runoff soil from surface-polluted areas or from a fertilized field.* Although point sources can be regulated, nonpoint sources account for most contamination and are much more difficult to control (47).

WATER PURIFICATION PROCESS

The natural water purification process involves bacterial action in the presence of oxygen to decompose organic matter. If too much waste is dumped into a given body of water, oxygen is used up and the natural cleansing process is slowed or halted. In addition, many types of aquatic organisms cannot survive when the oxygen level is too low (43). Higher levels of life are also affected. See **Figure 4-2** for various forms of life affected by pollution (47).

SOURCES OF WATER POLLUTION

The major sources of water pollution can be classified as municipal, industrial, and agricultural. **Municipal water pollution** *consists of wastewater from homes and commercial establishments.* **Industrial pollutants** *vary based on the industry or mining operation involved.* **Agricultural pollutants** *include many organic and inorganic compounds from commercial livestock and poultry farming, including* animal waste, pesticides, commercial fertilizers, and sediment from cropland erosion (47).

One source of pollution is the result of sewage, grass clippings, and fertilizers containing nutrients, such as nitrates and phosphates, which stimulate the growth of some aquatic plants and algae. This growth clogs waterways, uses up oxygen as it decomposes and interferes with the water purification process, and blocks light to deeper water, affecting fish respiration and the growth of certain aquatic organisms. Pollution also results from silt entering the water when it rains, filling the water body with sediment and organic matter that reduces water depth and interferes with oxygen use (47).

Pesticide runoff has the potential to contaminate the water supply. A recent U.S. Geological Survey found pesticides in 97% of

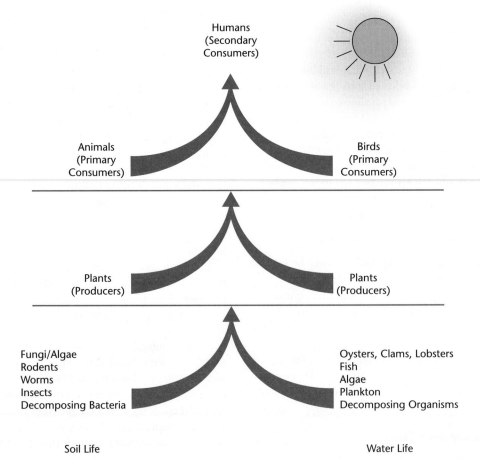

FIGURE ■ 4-2 Various forms of life affected by pollution.

streams in agricultural and urban areas. Pesticides were found in 50% of the groundwater in those same areas. At present levels, pesticides are not considered harmful to humans but may contribute to health problems with prolonged contact (69).

Pathogens associated with foodborne illness, such as *Escherichia coli* O157:H7, *Giardia lamblia*, and *Cryptosporidium*, may also pollute water, resulting in illnesses ranging from typhoid and dysentery to minor respiratory and skin diseases. Pathogens enter waterways through untreated sewage, storm drains, runoff from septic tanks, and farms and boats that dump sewage. Metropolitan sewer services in the United States must place the EPA Required Overflow Sign where there is possible sewage overflow exposure to water, whether or not related to storm water overflow. The sign warns people not to play, swim, or fish in the area, in order to prevent illness. Other pollutants include petroleum from oil spills, radioactive materials from nuclear power plants and industry, and heat that increases water temperature resulting in the deaths of aquatic organisms (47). Chemical contamination, for example, mercury contamination of water, is of increasing concern because of the effect on aquatic life and eventually on animals and people who eat fish and other aquatic life.

Drinking water in the United States is considered to be some of the world's cleanest water, with 9 out of 10 sources meeting federal standards. However, many inhabitants of small towns obtain their drinking water from municipal sources that can become polluted under certain conditions, such as when a heavy rain overtaxes the sewage system. They live under the constant threat of a "boil order." In rural areas, inhabitants may rely on well water that is not subject to testing. Even in large cities, tap water can become tainted due to aging pipes that break, leach contaminants into water, and breed bacteria. Old-fashioned treatment facilities may not be up to today's standards. *Let tap water run for 60 seconds before using it because the lead content of water sitting in a pipe may be higher. Avoid drinking hot tap water as heat pulls more lead from pipes* (11, 38, 79).

Because more and more people drink bottled water, teach them that bottled water must meet federal and state safety standards but standards are not always enforced. They should look for the International Bottled Water Association (IBWA) logo. Bottled water may be safe, but the opened container that sits for days at room temperature is an ideal breeding ground for bacteria. Bottles should be washed in a dishwasher before being refilled (11, 38, 79).

One of the most frightening results of water pollution is the threat to the oceans. The global practice of dumping sewage and trash in violation of the Ocean Dumping Act (1977) may permanently pollute the oceans. Results from failure to enforce the Ocean Dumping Act are apparent. Some beaches have been closed because of the health hazard, and litter clutters some shorelines. In addition to the danger to humans, the pollution endangers aquatic life.

PROBLEMS IN WATER PURIFICATION

Water pollution stems from our using natural resources in greater and greater amounts because of increased industrialization and population growth, increasing the need for sewage disposal.

Drinking water and the ability to use water for recreational purposes are affected; more important is the effect on the sustainability of water quality and aquatic life in various bodies of water.

Educate that water shortage and pollution is a global problem with health and economic implications. Misuse of water has far-reaching consequences that threaten people all over the world. Take personal responsibility for stopping needless pollution of water by exercising careful personal use of and disposal of agents that can destroy the water. Support legislation to prevent undue dumping of wastes into lakes, rivers, and streams. Educate that pregnant women and children should limit fish and shellfish intake unless the aquatic source is known to be relatively free of chemicals.

Soil Pollution

Soil pollution *refers to contamination of soil by various substances or agents.* It can result in a loss of land to cultivation or development, but even more important, it can affect people's health (37). *Sources of pollution may include* (37):

1. Air pollutants previously described that fall to earth as particles or are dissolved in rain.
2. Discharge of industrial wastes including radioactive substances.
3. Increased agricultural and home garden use of fertilizers containing fungicides, herbicides, and pesticides.
4. Discharge of toxic materials from sewage plants or animal waste deposits.
5. Heavy metals, including arsenic, cadmium, lead, mercury, and cyanide.
6. Landfills containing chemicals or contaminated wastes from homes, health care agencies, and industries.

Soil pollutants may be drawn up through plant roots or otherwise ingested. See **Box 4-1** for the effects of pesticide soil pollutants.

Teach that prevention involves careful handling of all products and their containers and following disposal recommendations printed on the label. Keep abreast of information from the EPA, environmental advocacy groups such as the state Public Interest Research Group, and state and national conservation agencies.

Food Pollution

We expect to have a wide array of food available year-round. This expectation carries with it the potential for health risks from additives, pesticides, hormones, antibiotics, arsenic, and other toxins such as mercury and dioxin from food grown in the United States and imported from other countries. In addition, bacterial contamination from food handlers or from international food suppliers may result in foodborne illness.

ADDITIVES

There are two types of food additives: direct and indirect. **Direct food additives** *are those added to food for a specific purpose,* such as salt, herbs, sugar, and spices that have been added to food for centuries to preserve it and improve flavor. **Indirect food additives** *are agents that become part of food in trace amounts due to packaging, storing, or handling.* Today, additives are used to maintain

BOX 4-1 Effects of Pesticide Soil Pollutants

Source	Where Found	Effects
Pesticide manufacturing plants	Farms	May be undiagnosed
Exposure by inhalation of dust or spray, direct skin contact, ingestion of contaminated food and water, contact with contaminated equipment	Industry	Toxic effects vary, but most remain in soil long periods, causing water, soil, and food pollution, and disease
	Homes	Cholinesterase inhibition
	Gardens	Central nervous system depression or stimulation:
	Federal, state, and local agencies	Forgetfulness
	Storage bags	Attention impairment
	Spray equipment	Short attention span
	Surface water contamination by dust or spray	Anxiety
	Rain washes into streams and lakes, affecting food supply	Depression
		Nervousness
		Hyperirritability
		Insomnia
		Skin rashes and diseases
		Eye disease
		Respiratory disease
		Digestive disorders
		Reproductive problems
		Birth defects
		Cancer
		Leukemia
		Destruction of insects, bees, and birds reduces cross-pollination essential in food chain
		Water pollution from spray, dust, or rain affects food chain
		Destruction of earthworms and rodents interferes with food cycle for animals and people
		Farmers, workers in pesticide-manufacturing plants, agricultural workers, commercial pest-control operators are at high risk

freshness, prevent spoilage, and improve nutritional value, taste, texture, and appearance. All additives are regulated by federal authorities and international organizations to ensure that foods are safe to eat and accurately labeled (22, 26). Teach parents and the public that, despite regulation, there are health risks associated with some color additives, nitrites, and sulfites. Share the following information.

A **color additive** *is a dye or pigment added to impart color.* Additives are used in food to offset color loss, correct natural variations in color, enhance color, or provide color to colorless and "fun" food. Without color additives, cola would not be brown and margarine would not be yellow. Since the 1970s, there has been some concern that color additives cause hyperactivity in children. Some children with attention deficit/hyperactivity disorder

(ADHD) and confirmed food allergy have shown behavioral improvement with dietary modification that removes color additives from their diet. *There is evidence that a small number of people are sensitive to tartrazine (FD&C Yellow No. 5). Yellow No. 5 must be shown on the ingredients list to allow the few who are sensitive to avoid it* (25, 29).

Functional foods are *foods to which components that appear to enhance health or prevent disease have been added, such as vitamins, minerals, herbs, or manufactured chemicals.* Herbs or excess iron added to foods may cause health problems, especially since these additions are poorly regulated (20).

Nitrite, *a salt or ester of nitrous acid,* is used to preserve food and to flavor and fix color in meat, poultry, and fish products. Nitrite can react with certain amines (derivatives of ammonia) to produce nitrosamines, many of which are known to cause cancer. In order to use nitrites, *food manufacturers must show that nitrosamines will not form in hazardous amounts.* In addition, *antioxidants may be added to the food product to inhibit the formation of nitrosamines* (25, 29).

Sulfite, *a salt or ester of sulfurous acid,* is used to preserve food. Sensitive individuals—asthma sufferers or anyone with airway hypersensitivity—can react if sulfites are ingested in unexpectedly large amounts. Sulfite ingestion can lead to difficulty breathing, asthmatic attacks, rashes, and abdominal upset. There are regulations in place to reduce the likelihood that sulfite-sensitive individuals will unknowingly consume sulfited foods. *Raw fruits and vegetables made available in restaurants, on salad bars, and in grocery store produce sections may no longer be treated with sulfites.* Sulfites added to food must be stated on the label (25, 29, 94).

PESTICIDES

Pesticides *are a group of chemicals used to control insects, weeds, fungi, diseases, or other pests on crops, the landscape, or animals. The most commonly used pesticides are insecticides, fungicides, and herbicides.* They are used to increase crop yield, extend growing seasons, and maintain product quality. If used improperly, however, *pesticides can pose health risks.* To protect the consumer from harmful levels of pesticides, the EPA sets a **tolerance** *or limit on how much pesticide residue can remain on food.* In setting tolerance levels, an additional margin of safety is added to protect infants, children, and other sensitive people. Various agencies, including the Food and Drug Administration (FDA) and the United States Department of Agriculture (USDA), monitor imported food, food transmitted interstate, packing sheds, wholesale markets, chain store distribution centers, retail markets, and ports of entry. Samples are analyzed for the presence of more than 200 pesticides. If **illegal residue**, *pesticide residue that exceeds the legal limit or is not licensed for use on that crop,* is found, it is tracked to the source; distribution of the item is halted and sanctions are imposed. Records reveal that about 1% of samples tested contain illegal residues. State and federal residue monitoring programs show that imported produce violates tolerance limits more frequently, but the violation rates are still low. The presence of an illegal residue does not necessarily equate to a health risk (14, 37, 68, 100). Teach the client that although tolerance levels serve to protect the consumer, we can easily consume small amounts of more than 30 pesticides a day (68). Pesticide risk can be minimized by selecting produce that is free of cuts or insect holes, washing it in water (not soap that is not intended for ingestion), and eating a wide variety of foods. Buying food produced by organic farmers and choosing an organic diet can limit further exposure. An EPA study found that after 5 days on an organic diet, specific markers for commonly used pesticides in the urine of 23 children decreased to undetectable levels (20, 29, 37, 68, 100).

HORMONES

Growth hormones may be added to animal feed. Studies show that synthetic growth hormones may be carcinogenic and exposure to them may be linked to the precocious onset of puberty in girls.

The USDA bans the use of such hormones in all poultry (organic or not), but when it comes to hogs, beef cattle, or dairy cattle, only organic products are legally bound not to use them (99, 100).

Educate about hormones and organically grown foods. The public can reduce ingestion by changing consumer patterns.

ANTIBIOTICS AND ARSENIC

Farmers' widespread use of antibiotics to speed animal growth and to deal with health issues that arise when animals are in overcrowded and unsanitary pens has helped spawn antibiotic-resistant bacteria. In turn, human resistance to the same family of antibiotics has increased when they are later administered therapeutically (100). Chickens, hogs, beef cattle, and dairy cattle may eat feeds that contain drugs designed to promote growth and kill microbes. An FDA-approved antibiotic, roxarsone, also contains arsenic. FDA tests show samples from chickens that have received roxarsone test well below the tolerance limit set for arsenic. However, independent testing by Consumer Reports found that, according to EPA standards, the amount present could cause neurologic problems in a child who ate 2 oz of chicken liver a week or in an adult who ate 5.5 oz of chicken liver a week. In these tests, there is no way to tell if the arsenic in the chicken liver came from the drug or was taken up from the environment, but the lack of arsenic in organic chicken meat is suggestive of its source because *arsenic is not allowed in organic chicken feed* (27, 98, 100).

Educate the public about potential health risks, either antibiotic sensitivity or more severe illness, that may occur. Suggest purchase of meat that has been raised by organic farmers.

OTHER TOXINS

Another health issue is the extent to which animal feed is protected from **infectious prions**, *proteins believed to be the cause of mad cow disease.* Mammalian blood and meat scraps are allowed in cow feed. Chickens are not susceptible to mad cow disease, and meat from diseased cows is allowed in their feed. Cow remains can be fed to chickens and pigs, whose remains can then be fed back to cows. If blood and scraps harbor infectious prions or if contaminated nonruminant feed is accidentally mixed with ruminant feed, cattle could sicken and pass along the disease. *Some consumer groups are calling for a ban of all mammalian material from animal feed* (99, 100). Prior to agribusiness, animals on smaller farms were usually fed organic products, not mammalian material. Mad cow disease has been reported only recently.

Mercury, *a by-product of coal-burning power plants,* usually stays airborne, but some is emitted as a water-soluble compound formed when mercury reacts with chlorine. Precipitation washes this form of mercury into natural bodies of water where microorganisms take it up and convert it into toxic methylmercury. The mercury passes up the food chain into fish, reaching the highest levels in large predatory species like shark and swordfish, and from there into people, who unknowingly eat contaminated fish (2, 20, 39, 53, 79).

Educate the public and clients that high levels can cause learning problems or retardation in children and neurologic damage in developing fetuses.

INTERVENTIONS FOR HEALTH PROMOTION

Pregnant and lactating females, and females who may become pregnant, can reduce risk of methylmercury poisoning by (20):

1. Omitting shark, swordfish, king mackerel, or tilefish from the diet.
2. Limiting intake of other fish (excluding tuna) and shellfish to 12 oz per week.
3. Limiting intake of the same type of fish or shellfish to no more than one time weekly.
4. Eating no more than 6 oz of local fish weekly if the chemical safety of local waters is unknown, or checking with the local health department or EPA to determine whether local fish are safe to eat.

People are constantly exposed to *toxins such as* **dioxin** through ingestion of it at low levels as an environmental contaminant in food. As examples, dioxin can get into farmed salmon feed because the feed may contain oil and meal from fish caught in polluted waters, or it may be found in the clay used as a filler in some animal feeds. It is slowly removed from the body and may accumulate in fatty tissue. Highly exposed people may develop cancer, reproductive and developmental problems, or increased heart disease and diabetes. The effect of long-term, low-level exposure is not known (18, 100).

FOODBORNE ILLNESS

Foodborne illness *is caused by consuming contaminated foods or beverages.* The most commonly occurring infections are caused by the bacteria *Campylobacter, Salmonella,* and *E. coli* O157:H7, and a group of viruses called caliciviruses or Norwalk-like viruses (26). Share the following information with clients and the public. You may work with local food suppliers to prevent the following foodborne illnesses. Notify the local health department if necessary.

Campylobacter

Campylobacter is the most commonly identified bacterial cause of diarrhea in the world. These bacteria live in the intestines of healthy birds, and most raw poultry contains it. Eating undercooked chicken or other foods contaminated with juices from raw chicken is the most frequent source of infection (26).

Salmonella

Salmonella is an organism widespread in the intestines of birds, reptiles, and mammals. The chance of buying a chicken contaminated with *Salmonella* has increased rather than decreased in recent years. The government states that 16.3% of all chickens are contaminated. Symptoms include fever, diarrhea, and abdominal cramps. In persons with poor health or weakened immune systems, it can cause life-threatening infections (7, 26, 100).

E. coli O157:H7

E. coli O157:H7 is an organism found in cattle and other animals. Illness usually follows consumption of food such as hamburger or water contaminated with microscopic amounts of cow feces. Symptoms include severe, bloody diarrhea and abdominal cramps,

usually without much fever. In 3% to 5% of cases, severe complications, including hemolytic uremic syndrome, can occur (26).

Calicivirus or Norwalk-like virus

Calicivirus or Norwalk-like virus is an extremely common cause of illness that usually is associated with vomiting. It is believed to spread from one infected person to another through contact with food (26).

Other Organisms

Some foodborne diseases are caused by a microbe in the food producing a toxin. For example, botulism occurs when the bacterium *Clostridium botulinum* produces a powerful paralytic toxin (26). In addition, some common diseases are occasionally foodborne, including shigellosis, hepatitis A, and the parasitic diseases caused by *Giardia lamblia* and *Cryptosporidium* (26).

Raw foods of animal origin are the most likely to be contaminated. Foods that combine the products of many individual animals, such as bulk raw milk, pooled raw eggs, or ground beef, are particularly hazardous because a pathogen present in any one of the animals may contaminate the whole batch. Raw fruits and vegetables prepared under less than sanitary conditions are of concern. Washing can decrease but not eliminate contamination (26).

Prevention

Educate that the World Health Organization (WHO) and the CDC provide precautions for consumers to follow to protect themselves from foodborne illness. *Protective precautions include* (26):

1. Prepare foods in a sanitary manner.
2. Cook foods thoroughly.
3. Store foods at safe temperatures.
4. Separate foods to avoid cross-contamination.
5. Report suspected foodborne illness to the local health department.

Noise Pollution

Sensory stimulation such as sound plays a major role in human development. **Sound overload/noise pollution** *is defined as unwanted or offensive sounds that unreasonably intrude into our daily*

TABLE 4-2

Common Sound Pollutants and Their Decibel Reading

Sound	Decibels	Sound	Decibels
Rustle of leaves	10	Food blender in home	93
Watch ticking	20	Pneumatic hammer	95
Library whisper	30	Air compressor	95
Refrigerator humming	40	Power lawnmower	80–95
Normal conversation	60	Dirt bike	95
Electric shaver	60–86	Farm tractor	98
Dishwasher	60	Diesel truck	100
Car	60–90	Power drill	100
Office (busy)	70–85	Street sweeper	100
Vacuum cleaner	72–75	Chain saw	100–110
Minibike	76	Outboard motor	102
Garbage disposal, noisy restaurant	80	Jet flying at 1,000 ft	103
Shop tools	80–95	Ambulance siren	105
Loud street noise	80–100	Stereo headset	110
Alarm clock	80	Riveting gun	110
Washing machine	80	Jackhammer	115–130
Video arcade	80–105	Motorcycle	115
Subway	80–114	Live rock music	120
Screaming child	85	Gunshot	130–140
Snowmobile	85–120	Jet plane at takeoff	150
Heavy city traffic	90–95	Rocket engine	180

activity. The loudness of sound is measured in units called **decibels.** Most sources of noise pollution are associated with urban development; road, air, and rail transport; industrial noise; and neighborhood and recreational noise. See **Table 4-2** for a list of common sound pollutants and their decibel readings (5, 62, 63, 70). *Noise can affect human health and well-being in numerous ways, including* (55, 62, 63, 70):

1. Annoyance reaction; interference with communication.
2. Sleep disturbance.
3. Effects on performance and social behavior.
4. Hearing loss.

People experiencing high noise exposure report (55, 62, 63, 70):

1. Increased number of headaches.
2. Greater susceptibility to minor illness or accidents.
3. Increased reliance on sedatives and sleeping pills.
4. General fatigue.
5. Severe noise-induced hearing loss (NIHL).

There is evidence that regular exposure to noise levels at or above 80 decibels can cause deafness. Sounds less than 80 decibels are unlikely to cause hearing loss (55, 62, 63).

More than 30 million Americans are exposed to hazardous sound levels on a regular basis. Of the 28 million Americans who have some degree of hearing loss, about 33% can attribute it in part to noise. Individuals of any age can develop NIHL resulting from damage to the sensitive hair cells of the inner ear and the acoustic nerve. Hearing can be damaged by two kinds of noise: loud impulse noise such as an explosion, or loud continuous noise such as in a factory. The hearing loss may be temporary or permanent (62, 63, 70).

Teach, especially to youth and young adults, that NIHL is preventable. The Occupational Safety and Health Administration (OSHA) requires that hearing protectors be provided to workers who are exposed for 8 hours to a noise level of 85 decibels or higher. Understand the hazards of noise and teach others about them. Be aware of hazardous noise in the environment and, if possible, take action to decrease it. We all need to protect ourselves and our children from noise above 80 decibels.

Surface Pollution

Until the mid-1960s, U.S. residents were not concerned with problems of waste disposal or recycling. Raw materials were plentiful, and the open-dump method of disposal was convenient and economical. In the early 1970s, however, people became more concerned with the health problems created by open dumps. Today, the EPA's Office of Solid Waste (OSW) regulates waste disposal under the Resource Conservation and Recovery Act (RCRA). Waste is categorized as nonhazardous or hazardous. **Hazardous waste** *is waste that is potentially harmful or dangerous to human health or the environment.* Unfortunately, some nonhazardous waste is potentially harmful but does not meet the OSW definition of hazardous waste. The OSW aims to protect human health and the environment by ensuring responsible national management of hazardous and nonhazardous waste. Its goals are to conserve resources by reducing waste, preventing future waste disposal problems, and cleaning up areas where waste may have spilled, leaked, or been improperly disposed. Individual states adopt federal standards and operate their own industrial waste management programs. Unfortunately, these programs do not eliminate all improper waste disposal (95).

The total quantity of solid waste is large and increasing. The extent of the problem can be seen in the fact that Americans generate millions of tons of household waste a year. The EPA estimates that 1.6 million tons of this waste is **household hazardous waste (HHW)**, including paints, cleaners, oils, batteries, and pesticides that contain corrosive, toxic, ignitable, or reactive ingredients. The average home may accumulate as much as 100 pounds of HHW in storage areas (19, 92).

You have a role in public education. Improper disposal of hazardous household waste can endanger human health and the environment. Each citizen has a role in reducing surface pollution by reducing, reusing, and recycling materials to decrease the amount and toxicity of the generated waste. He or she should learn what constitutes HHW and take the time to dispose of the product properly. Older computers and printers also need to be disposed of properly. Improper disposal of HHW, such as pouring such material down the drain, on the ground, or into storm sewers, or putting it in the trash, can pollute the environment and pose a threat to human health. Many communities offer a collection facility or special collection days for the disposal of HHW.

Occupational Hazards

The amount of time adults spend at the workplace supports the need to recognize occupational hazards in health promotion efforts. The Occupational Safety and Health Act of 1970, the Coal Mine Health and Safety Act of 1969, and the Toxic Substances Control Act of 1976 are some of the laws passed by Congress that have been responsible for making occupational safety and health a public concern rather than a private matter. Through these laws the federal government works to prevent work-related accidents and disease, correct hazardous working conditions, and promote good health for employees. *OSHA's mission is to* (66):

1. Assure the safety and health of workers by setting and enforcing standards.
2. Provide training, outreach, and education; establishing partnerships.
3. Encourage continual improvement in workplace safety and health.

Almost all workers are under OSHA jurisdiction with the exception of miners, transportation workers, some public employees, and the self-employed. OSHA has forced industries to become more active in reducing workplace hazards, providing health services for employees, and offering additional services related to disease prevention and education of employees (66).

Educate employers and the public about the *Healthy People 2010* document, which presents two *specific goals for workplace health promotion:* (a) increase the proportion of work sites that offer a comprehensive employee health promotion program, and (b) increase the proportion of employees who participate in employer-sponsored health promotion activities (90). When you assess clients, determine whether they have programs at work that foster health and education. Be an advocate for such programs.

Environmental hazards in the workplace include physical, chemical, and biological threats. Workplace hazards may be common to many work sites where there is exposure to various forms of air pollution. The hazards may be site specific, such as exposure to certain industrial chemicals, to the risk of needle sticks, or to products containing latex. Workers in manufacturing, construction, health care services, and agriculture are at higher risk for work-related injuries, but most occupations involve some form of health hazard, sometimes in the form of emotional stress. Information on job-specific occupational hazards is readily available through numerous Websites.

Assess for specific workplace hazards in your health promotion efforts. Analyze the relationship between individual susceptibility to certain risks and risk exposure to be more thorough and careful in assessment. Advocate for enforcement of preventive measures for known hazards and for continued environmental research (56, 66). Support professional or societal organizations that advocate for occupational safety (36).

Health Promotion and Nursing Applications

GLOBAL RESPONSIBILITY

The environment, social institutions, population groups, professionals, and individual citizens are a complex set of interacting, interdependent systems. We need to recognize this complexity in efforts to cooperate with other countries to control pollution worldwide. Some of the suggestions presented in **Box 4-2**, Conservation Solutions, may have a global impact.

PROFESSIONAL RESPONSIBILITY

An ecological approach to health care involves recognizing the impact of the environment on people's health and health behavior. It requires understanding the multiple relationships between aspects of the physical environment and associated health problems in order to provide health-promoting environments. Nurses can work with their professional organizations to establish environmental task forces and to restructure the national or state organization, if necessary, to better address environmental issues, health care implications, and legislative development and advocacy (36).

As a health care professional, your primary responsibilities are to:

1. Detect environmental health risks through thorough assessment.
2. Collaborate with other professionals for intervention.

Abstract for Evidence-Based Practice

Environmental Nursing Diagnoses

Green, P.M., Polk, L.V., & Slade, D.S. (2003). Environmental nursing diagnoses: A proposal for further development of Taxonomy II. *International Journal of Nursing Terminology and Classifications, 14(1), 17–29.*

Purpose ➤ To propose further development of environmental diagnoses and to offer recommendations to expand the taxonomy to further encompass the environmental domain.

Sources ➤ Literature review in the disciplines of nursing, biology, public health, toxicology, sociology, and anthropology.

Data Synthesis ➤ Nurses need diagnostic labels to describe human responses to environmental health threats.

Practice Implications ➤ Proposed environmental nursing diagnoses include actual or risk for:

Poisoning

Pesticide contamination

Decreased reproductive capacity

Pollution

Solid waste contamination

Indoor pollution

Outdoor pollution

Community-wide infection

Workplace environmental exposure/contamination

Day care/school environmental exposure

Global spread of infection

Transboundary environmental exposure/contamination

Society violence

Conclusions ➤ New environmental diagnoses will help to describe nursing's contribution in understanding the effect of these factors on health as an international and community health priority.

3. Provide health teaching to individuals, families, and the public.
4. Advocate for policy development and legislation designed to protect and preserve the environment, and thereby health.

During assessment and intervention, consider the client's immediate environment while receiving health care, and the physical environment in which the person lives and works, if employed. Use the environmental nursing diagnoses reported in the Abstract for Evidence-Based Practice as a starting point to develop interventions. Also see the **Box, Nursing Diagnoses Related to Environmental Considerations** (60). The client's surroundings should constitute a milieu free of environmental hazards and conducive to recovery (34, 85).

Health teaching can increase community awareness, contribute to maintaining a healthy environment, and decrease the incidence of illness from pollutants or hazards. Educate the public about current issues influencing health and the environment.

Prevention of environmental damage can begin with informed consumer groups (77).

Be an advocate for environmental control through membership in professional organizations. There is power in numbers, and professional organizations can effectively lobby at local, state, and national levels for policies and legislation that support environmental safety (36). For example, the American Nurses Association (ANA) has advocated and lobbied for legislation for safe working conditions for nurses and for safe environments for patients. Refer to the *American Journal of Nursing* and *The American Nurse;* most issues inform about the ANA's achievements.

Personal Responsibility

Be aware of what individuals and industries are doing to the air, water, and land. *Conserve natural resources* to the best of your ability as much as possible, and learn about and try to reduce

Nursing Diagnoses Related to Environmental Considerations

- Latex **A**llergy Response
- Readiness for Enhanced **C**oping
- Ineffective Community **C**oping
- Ineffective **H**ealth Maintenance
- **H**ealth-Seeking Behaviors (Specify)
- Impaired **H**ome Maintenance

- Risk for **I**nfection
- Risk for **I**njury
- Deficit **K**nowledge
- Risk for **P**oisoning
- **P**owerlessness
- Risk for **T**rauma

Source: Reference 60.

BOX 4-2 Conservation Solutions

ENERGY SOLUTIONS

- Use **public transportation**; carpool; bike or walk rather than drive a car if feasible.
- Invest in **ample insulation**, weatherstripping, and caulking for home and workplace.
- **Use electricity and hot water efficiently**. Buy energy-saving household appliances.
- **Reduce demand for energy** by turning off lights, radio, and television when no one is using them; run dishwasher and washer and dryer only when they have full loads.
- **Make the most of oven heat**—bake foods in batches; turn oven off shortly before baking is finished and use remaining heat to complete the job.
- **Dry clothes outdoors** on a line.
- **Use clothes dryer efficiently**; separate loads into heavy- and lightweight items as lighter ones take less time.
- In **winter turn down thermostat** a few degrees, especially at night and when house is empty. In **summer** if using **air conditioning, turn thermostat up a few degrees**. Regularly service the furnace and air conditioner.
- **Close off** and do not heat or cool **unused rooms**; use insulating shades and curtains on cold winter nights and hot summer days.

FOOD SOLUTIONS

- **Eat foods lower on the food chain**—vegetables, fruits, and grains; decrease consumption of meat and animal products.
- **Read the labels on food**; buy foods that have not been heavily processed. Learn which additives are harmful.
- **Support laws that ban harmful pesticides**, drugs, and other chemicals used in food production. Support markets that offer contaminant-free food.
- **Avoid food from endangered environments**, such as rain forests.

WATER SOLUTIONS

- **Fix leaks** promptly.
- Install sink faucet aerators and **water-efficient showerheads**, which use two to five times less water with no noticeable decrease in performance.
- Take showers, not baths, to **reduce water consumption**.
- **Do not let water run** when it is not actually being used while showering, shaving, brushing teeth, or hand washing clothes.
- **Use ultra-low-flush or air-assisted toilets**, saving 60% to 90% water. Composting toilets use no water and recycle organic waste.

- **Buy phosphate-free, biodegradable soaps and detergents**; ask your supermarket to carry them if it does not.
- Do not run the tap until the water is cold to get a drink. Instead, **keep water in a refrigerator bottle**.
- **Economize water** when washing the car, sprinkling the lawn, and removing debris from surfaces; repair leaks.

TOXINS AND POLLUTANTS SOLUTIONS

- Read labels; **buy the least toxic products** available; find out the best disposal methods for toxic products. Use nonharmful substitutes.
- Avoid purchasing clothes that require dry cleaning, which uses toxic chlorinated solvents. **Dry clean only when necessary**.
- **Avoid contact with pesticides** by thoroughly scrubbing or peeling foodstuffs; if possible, maintain your own garden without use of pesticides.
- **Test your home for radon**, especially if you live on the East Coast or in Wisconsin, Minnesota, North Dakota, Colorado, or Wyoming.
- **Ask your service station to use CFC recovery equipment** when repairing auto air conditioners.
- **Use more energy-efficient cars**.
- **Keep your automobile in top working condition** with a regular tuneup; make sure antipollution controls are working properly.
- **Operate your vehicle properly**; do not idle or rev engine; drive at steady pace; obey speed limits.
- **Support legislative initiatives that encourage industry to modify manufacturing processes** to eliminate the production of hazardous wastes and to reuse and recycle wastes when possible.

WASTE REDUCTION AND RECYCLING SOLUTIONS

- **Buy products in bulk or with the least amount of packaging**. (A major contributor to acid rain is sulfur dioxide, one of the chemicals used to process virgin paper. In the very-low-oxygen environment of the trash dump, paper or plastic may take 40 or more years to degrade.)
- **Buy products that are recyclable**, repairable, reusable, and biodegradable; avoid disposables. (Every 3 months enough aluminum cans are thrown away to rebuild an entire commercial fleet.)
- **Separate your recyclable garbage** such as newspaper, glass, paper, aluminum, and organic waste if you have a garden. Send to the landfill what cannot be used. (Only 10% of garbage is recycled in the United States.)
- **Recycle newspapers** through paper drives. Each Sunday, thousands of trees are made into newspapers that are not recycled.

- **Use recycled products**. Landfills are rapidly being exhausted, and the cost of recycling must be recovered.
- **Buy recycled paper for all uses**. It takes 16,320 kilowatt-hours of electricity to produce 1 ton of paper from virgin wood pulp. It takes 64% fewer kilowatt-hours (5,919) to produce 1 ton of recycled paper from waste paper.
- **Recycle used oil** to be re-refined for lubricants.
- If you do not have a **recycle center**, ask your city council to **establish one**. Find local groups that can use your recyclables.
- Urge your area to use **Glasphalt** from recycled glass for parking areas and roadways.

HOUSEKEEPING SOLUTIONS

- **Use simple substances for cleaning**. An all-purpose cleaner, safe for all surfaces, is 1 gallon hot water, ¼ cup sudsy ammonia, ¼ cup vinegar, and 1 tablespoon baking soda. After use, wipe surface with water to rinse.
- **Keep drains open by using the following mix** once weekly: 1 cup baking soda, 1 cup salt, 1 cup cream of tartar. Pour ¼ cup of the mixture weekly into the drain; follow with a pot of boiling water. If drain is clogged, pour in ¼ cup baking soda followed by ½ cup vinegar. Close drain until fizzing stops. Then flush with boiling water.
- **Use low-phosphate or phosphate-free detergents** to wash clothes and dishes.
- **Use natural furniture and floor polish products**; such products use lemon oil or beeswax in a mineral oil base.
- **Use nontoxic products to control pests**. Control ants by sprinkling barriers of talcum power, chalk, bone meal, or boric acid across their trails. Control cockroaches by dusting lightly with borax. Control ticks and fleas on pets by applying an herbal rinse. Boil ¼ cup of fresh or dried rosemary in a quart of water: Steep herb 20 minutes, strain, and cool. Then sponge on pet. Air-dry.
- **Maintain air circulation and clean ventilation systems** and ducts to remove fungi, mold, pollen, toxic residues, sprays, and other contaminants. Avoid hair spray and cleaning sprays.
- **Manage household hazardous waste**; buy only what is needed; do not store with household products; give unused product to someone else who may be able

to use it rather than disposing of it. Do not pour oil, grease, or hazardous chemicals down the drain.

TREE-SAVER SOLUTIONS

- **Plant trees**; as trees grow, they remove carbon dioxide from the atmosphere through photosynthesis, slowing buildup of carbon dioxide. (Carbon dioxide causes over 50% of the greenhouse effect.)
- **Plant fast-growing poplar tree hybrids** that suck contamination from soil and groundwater through **phytoremediation**, *a process that stores or metabolizes chemicals and releases volatile compounds through leaves*.
- Join efforts to **save forests** from being cleared or burned. When forests are burned, carbon is released, adding to carbon dioxide buildup and global warming.

PRESERVATION OF LIFE AND ENVIRONMENT SOLUTIONS

- **Do not burn leaves** or garbage; instead, compost organic materials.
- **Do not buy endangered plants**, animals, or products made from overexploited species (furs, ivory, reptile skin, or tortoise shell).
- **Avoid buying wood from the tropical rain forests** unless it was propagated by sustainable tree farming methods.
- **Buy products from companies that do not pollute** or damage the environment.
- **Join, support, and volunteer your time to organizations working on environmental causes**.
- **Contact your elected representatives** through letters, telegrams, calls, or visits to communicate your concerns about conservation and environmental issues.
- **Contact environmental authorities** before using nonnative plants for decorative, conservation, or gardening purposes to avoid invasions that kill native plants and destroy habitats.
- **Advocate saving America's wetlands**, which help filter pollution out of waterways, protect communities from floods, and sustain fish and wildlife.
- **Use wind turbines to produce energy** for electric power, which avoids pollution and nuclear waste of conventional power plants.

environmental pollution in your own area. *Personal practices* to promote environmental control *include lifestyle changes, support for conservation, and advocacy*. Refer to the Case Situation, Fostering an Environmentally Safe Lifestyle, for practical suggestions.

Lifestyle change involves considering what type of car to drive, the extent to which you use public transportation, how to dispose

of household waste, buying habits, and other actions that may negatively affect the environment. For some people, lifestyle change may be difficult; others may already be living in an environmentally friendly way.

Support conservation by joining an organization such as the Sierra Club, National Wildlife Federation, Audubon Society, or

Case Situation

Fostering an Environmentally Safe Lifestyle

Matthew and Joan live with their 4-year-old daughter, Sarah, in an older condominium (condo) near a large metropolitan city in the eastern United States. Both are professionals in the business world and commute to their city work sites via the subway. Before they moved into their renovated condo, they investigated to be sure there was no remaining asbestos or lead-based paint in their home. They decided to have hardwood floors and cabinets, although expensive, to avoid formaldehyde concentrations to the extent possible in their home. They do monthly cleaning of air filters, keeping the furnace and air conditioner as clean as possible. They installed a radon detector in the basement and carbon monoxide detectors in the bedrooms when they installed smoke detectors. They are working to conserve electricity and water use in their home.

Joan and Matthew do not smoke. Few of their visitors smoke; they relate closely to those who do not smoke to avoid second- and thirdhand smoking effects. If visitors smoke, they are invited to smoke in the condo parking lot. Joan and Matthew work to keep Sarah away from secondhand smoke.

They purchase their food at a store that sells only organic foods. They believe the extra cost incurred is worth it, especially for Sarah's health. Their current challenge is to work with the condo association and tenants to better dispose of waste products such as leftover paint.

Sarah is in preschool during the day. Joan and Matthew investigated carefully several centers before enrolling Sarah in the home-based preschool. The woman who runs the preschool has six children come daily to her home day care. She has a similar philosophy about child care and has similar values. Additionally, her home is as environmentally safe as their own home. On weekends, Matthew, Joan, and Sarah spend time at a wooded area about 25 miles from their home; they enjoy the fresh air and exploring the outdoors.

Matthew and Joan admit it is difficult to consistently consider environmental influences on their family, especially in a large urban area. They tell their friends about their efforts and find that those with young children are receptive to their suggestions, especially about food purchases.

Contributed by Ruth Murray, EdD, MSN, N-NAP, FAAN

Nature Conservancy. These organizations study the environment; alert citizens about pollutants, hazardous wastes, and toxins in the environment; and support legislation related to a healthy environment.

Join citizens' crusades for a clean environment. The Coalition for the Environment in St. Louis is an example. Such organizations work closely with state and federal legislators to pass protective legislation, hold public hearings to initiate protective measures, and conduct educational meetings to inform citizens about problems,

preventive measures, and means of strengthening legislation. *Support municipal and health agencies in their attempts at pollution control and recycling.* Citizen support given to these types of organizations and to legislative efforts is important. In the process, it means contributing to the health of your family, community, nation, and clients.

Refer to suggestions presented in **Box 4-2,** Conservation Solutions. Some suggestions may be applicable to you. Some of the suggestions you may already practice. Refer to the Case Situation, Fostering an Environmentally Safe Lifestyle, for a summary of how a family can practice suggestions presented in this chapter.

Practice Point

It is past time for all of us to ask ourselves some basic questions:

1. How much energy and natural resources do we really need to maintain an acceptable standard of living in the United States?
2. Are we willing to pay more for resources that will not pollute the environment or food that is organically grown?
3. Will strictly controlled energy and water allocation be necessary because people refuse to abide by suggested limits?
4. What more can each of us do personally and professionally to maintain a health-promoting environment?

Bioterrorism: Threat to Environmental Health

This section contributed by Rita Acosta Sander, PhD, RN.

INTRODUCTION

We live in an ever-changing environment. People in many nations throughout the world have experienced both natural and man-made disasters. Either can cause much environmental devastation, injury, illness, and loss of life. In the past decade, more attention has focused on man-made disasters, often referred to as bioterrorism, as people in Israel, the Middle East, Africa, Europe, the United Kingdom, and Asia have experienced political terrorism and bioterrorism. People in the United States experienced this directly on September 11, 2001, when the World Trade Center in

New York City, the Pentagon in Washington, D.C., and an area of Pennsylvania were attacked. Media reports in the following weeks of anthrax spores in the mail added to the sense of vulnerability. Public awareness of disaster, war, terrorism, and bioterrorism is part of everyday language for most people throughout the world (44, 93). Such events affect the development and health of people of all ages; long-term effects have not been well established.

DEFINITIONS

Disasters are classified into two groups: natural and man-made. The World Health Organization defines a ***natural disaster*** as an *ecologic disruption or threat that exceeds the adjustment capacity of the affected community or populations* (52, 90). Natural disasters refer to earthquakes, volcanoes, hurricanes, floods, and fires. ***Man-made disasters*** refer to *war, pollution, nuclear explosions, fires, hazardous materials exposures, explosions, and transportation accidents* (91, 100). Information about types of and preparedness for natural disaster can be obtained through the local American Red Cross and Salvation Army, a governmental and a private agency, respectively. Both assist their counterpart agencies worldwide when a natural disaster occurs. The following section focuses on the global environmental health threats known collectively as bioterrorism and weapons of mass destruction (WMDs).

CHEMICAL, BIOLOGICAL, RADIOLOGICAL, NUCLEAR, AND EXPLOSIVE AGENTS

In the United States, **weapons of mass destruction** are now *categorized as chemical, biological, radiological, nuclear, and explosive (CBRNE) agents* (58, 88). One survey reported 79% of health care providers lacked competence in handling patients affected by CBRNE-related agents and had neither seen nor treated patients with such chemical exposure or infectious diseases (40).

Nurses must continue to add to their knowledge and capability to assess and respond to terrorist incidents involving weapons of mass destruction. As professionals, it is important to be involved in prevention efforts.

Chemical Agents

Chemical releases can be ***unintentional*** (*industrial accident*) or ***intentional*** (*a terrorist attack*). Military organizations developed hazardous chemicals for use in warfare. *Chemical terrorism involves hazardous materials* and is known as a ***HAZMAT event***. Hazardous materials can be disseminated through inhalation, skin absorption, or ingestion.

Examples of chemical agents include (17, 93):

1. Biotoxins, poisons that come from plants or animals (e.g., digitalis, nicotine, strychnine, and ricin).
2. Blister agents, mustard agents, and phosgene.
3. Blood agents, poisons absorbed into the blood (e.g., arsine, carbon monoxide, cyanide).
4. Caustic acids.
5. Choking/pulmonary agents such as ammonia, hydrogen chloride, and phosgene.
6. Incapacitating agents, fentanyls, opioids.
7. Long-acting super warfarins.
8. Metals, arsenic, mercury.
9. Nerve agents, sarin, V agents.
10. Organic solvents, benzene.
11. Riot control agents, mace.
12. Toxic alcohols, ethylene glycol.
13. Vomiting agents.

Refer to the Department of Health and Human Services (17) and Veenema (93) for more information.

Biological Agents

History documents that military leaders and armies have used infectious agents since 600 B.C. (73). Unfortunately, biowarfare agents have been used since World Wars I and II because of their invisibility and delayed effect. Biological weapons are more destructive than chemical weapons, such as nerve gas, and can be as devastating as nuclear weapons. For a biological attack to occur, a vulnerable target, a person or group with the capability to attack, and the intent by the person responsible to carry out such an attack must be in place (81).

The Centers for Disease Control and Prevention (CDC) classifies biological agents into three categories: A, B, and C (67). ***Category A agents*** *have the greatest potential for adverse impact with mass casualties and require public health preparedness efforts* (e.g., surveillance, laboratory diagnosis, and stockpiling of specific medications). Category A agents include disease organisms for smallpox, anthrax, plague, botulism, tularemia, Ebola hemorrhagic fever, and Lassa fever (67).

Category B agents *have the potential for large-scale dissemination with resultant illness.* These have lower illness and mortality potential and therefore would be expected to have lower medical and public health impact. Examples of category B agents include Q fever, brucellosis, ricin toxin, *Salmonella*, and *Shigella dysenteriae* (75).

Category C agents *are not believed to present a high bioterrorism risk but could emerge as future threats.* Examples of category C agents are yellow fever and multidrug-resistant tuberculosis (75).

Radiological/Nuclear Agents

Radiation consists of alpha, beta, and gamma particles. ***Alpha particles*** *are the least penetrating.* ***Beta particles*** *can penetrate skin.* ***Gamma particles*** *can easily pass through the human body and be absorbed by the tissues.* All radiation damage is caused by penetration into the body. Geiger counters can detect beta and gamma particles; a special counter is needed for alpha particles. Radiation/nuclear agents can be delivered intentionally or accidentally (42). To end World War II, a nuclear bomb was dropped intentionally on Hiroshima, Japan, on August 6, 1945. Another was dropped on Nagasaki, Japan, on August 9, 1945. Great injury, loss of life, and devastation resulted. The accidental explosion of a reactor at the Chernobyl nuclear power station in the then Soviet Union on April 26, 1986, spewed radiation around the globe; the heaviest contamination was in the Soviet Union and Northern Norway and Finland. The evacuation of more than 300,000 people from an exclusion zone surrounding the reactor was a traumatic crisis. Radioactive cesium-137 and strontium-90 continue to contaminate all animal life and the food chain in the humanless habitat.

Explosive Agents

The U.S. Federal Bureau of Investigation reported that bombings accounted for nearly 70% of all terrorist attacks in the United States and its territories between 1980 and 2001 (100). Several mechanisms of blast injuries cause injuries primarily to the lungs, ears, and gastrointestinal tract. *Brisance involves the movement of particles from more to less dense areas.* For example, liquid in the lungs moves into the gas area of the alveoli and causes pulmonary hemorrhage. *Implosion, compression and decompression of gaseous compartments with rupture,* can cause rupture of tympanic membranes. Finally, with pressure differentials, the blast wave drives fluids from their spaces, causing pulmonary hemorrhage; death may occur hours, or even days, after the explosion (48, 49).

DISASTER PLANNING AND RESPONSE

Disaster response consists of three phases: activation, implementation, and recovery (48, 49). The first element in the *activation phase* is a 2- to 4-day survey to assess the geographic extent of damage, number of people involved, extent of the local response, and establishment of communication and information facilities. Communication is the most significant problem in a disaster recovery effort.

The *implementation phase* is search and rescue. Initially, survivors among the local population, even those injured, pull together and quickly become involved in looking for survivors. Most lives are saved in the first day or two; sometimes the rescuers themselves can become victims (48, 49). When victims are found, they are **triaged** to *classify for treatment.* The goal is the "greatest good for the greatest number." Color-coded tagging systems are frequently used to identify those who have minor injuries, moderate injuries, or severe injuries. The black tag is reserved for persons who have died. Once the patients are triaged, they are taken to various collection points. The first is a clearing and staging area, a safe distance from the disaster. Patients receive basic medical interventions—intravenous lines, wound care, oxygen, pain medications, and splints. From there, they receive secondary assessment and further field treatment at a casualty collection point (48, 49).

The *recovery phase* consists of reassessing the scene for missed victims, withdrawing prehospital services, and debriefing those involved. Debriefing involves critical incident stress management. Health care workers assisting disaster victims often become stressed and depressed. Professionals within the Federal Emergency Management Agency (FEMA) and the Red Cross help the workers to vent and resolve their feelings (48, 49).

AGENCIES AND RESOURCES FOR DISASTER RESPONSE

In the event of a terrorist attack, natural disaster, or other large-scale emergency, the U.S. Department of Homeland Security (DHS) assumes primary responsibility for ensuring that emergency response professionals are prepared (16). In the 1970s, the Federal Emergency Management Agency (FEMA) developed the Incident Command System, a military-type command center that is set up at or near a disaster site. The senior official of the first responder team assumes the lead role, and actions follow a formal-ized chain of command. The Medical Command System, a branch of the Incident Command System, determines the hospitals to which the patients will be transported for definitive care and arranges for medically supported transport.

President Carter established FEMA in 1979. It includes the National Fire Administration, Civil Defense, and insurance programs. It has authority to request assistance from other federal agencies as needed, including the Department of Transportation, the U.S. Army Corps of Engineers, the Environmental Protection Agency (EPA), and the Department of Agriculture (USDA). FEMA does not respond to disasters on its own accord but only at the invitation of a governor. The Robert T. Stafford Disaster Relief and Emergency Assistance Act, PL 100-707, signed into law November 23, 1988, gave statutory authority for most federal disaster response activities pertaining to FEMA programs. In 1992, the American Red Cross joined resources with the 26 federal agencies under FEMA.

On March 1, 2003, FEMA became part of the U.S. Department of Homeland Security (DHS), including the Emergency Preparedness and Response Directorate. The National Response Plan (NRP) is based on the National Incident Management System (NIMS). Together the NRP and the NIMS provide a nationwide template for working together to prevent or respond to natural or man-made threats and incidents, regardless of cause, size, or complexity (18). Preparation and readiness for a bioterrorist event is based on the principles of disaster planning. *The Incident Command System remains the center for all operations:* (a) system integration (communications with outside agencies and hospital response), (b) logistics (plan supply management system), (c) security, (d) clinical care, (e) human resources, and (f) public relations (45).

The Joint Commission is a not-for-profit, private-sector entity in the United States that was founded in 1951 and is dedicated to improving the safety and quality of care provided to the public. The Joint Commission on Accreditation of Healthcare Organizations Standards, developed in January 2001, mandates the creation and testing of hospital disaster plans. The new plan emphasizes *four specific phases of disaster planning:* (a) mitigation, (b) preparedness, (c) response, and (d) recovery (31).

INDIVIDUAL DISASTER PREPAREDNESS

Each family, or individual if living alone, should have a plan for coping with natural or man-made disasters. Part of a plan is to predetermine where to seek shelter and safety for self, family, and pets (it should consider work, school, and home sites). The plan should include how to contact each other if separated. Families are increasingly providing cell phones with specific "help" numbers and give instructions to children as young as 4 or 5 years of age. Each person should always carry a list of diagnoses, medications taken, and emergency contact numbers. A tote bag or kit for the home, work site, and car is advisable with supplies for emergency or disaster. *Contents of the kit should include* (a) an identification bracelet; (b) 3 to 7 days supply of prescription medications or other medications used frequently; (c) a flashlight, portable radio, and batteries; (d) a pair of sunglasses, an extra pair of prescription eyeglasses, and hearing aids and batteries; (e) bottled water;

(f) games or activities for the children; (g) copies of important family documents and pictures; and (h) adhesive bandages, tissues, and essential hygiene products. Supplies such as medications must be rotated through for daily use. Supplies such as batteries must be updated as necessary when the kit is not used. Preparedness depends upon the age of the respective family members.

Health Promotion and Nursing Applications

Most communities have developed more extensive disaster plans for health care agencies, businesses, and other organizations. You may be involved in this process. Langan and James present practical and holistic information for disaster planning, intervention, and evaluation of services. Physical and emotional health and cultural considerations are presented relative to people throughout the life span (46). Refer also to Websites listed in the References and other sources of information in the community and workplace that will educate you for responses as a professional and citizen.

The International Nursing Coalition for Mass Casualty Education (INCMCE) recommends nurses to be prepared to respond to terrorism as well as to natural disasters (9, 10, 42, 50, 97). Organizations representing various health care disciplines and public health professionals also recommend preparation.

Summary

1. Health and development are adversely affected by air, water, soil, food, noise, and surface pollution and by occupational hazards.
2. Problems associated with air pollution include increased emission of greenhouse gases, changes in ozone levels, and acid deposition.
3. Sources of indoor air pollution include asbestos, biological pollutants, carbon monoxide, formaldehyde, lead, nitrogen oxide, pesticides, volatile organic compounds, radon, respirable particles, and secondhand and thirdhand smoke.
4. Sources of water pollution are sewage and pathogenic organisms, plant nutrients, chemicals, silt, radioactive material, oil spills, and heat from industrial processes.
5. Sources of soil pollution include air pollution, industrial and agricultural wastes, toxic products, sewage, and heavy metals.
6. Sources of food pollution include food additives, pesticides, antibiotics and hormones fed to animals that are produced for food, mercury, and contamination from pathogens during food processing or handling.
7. Noise pollution in the home and workplace produces numerous adverse health and safety effects, including noise-induced hearing loss and client discomfort in the health care setting.
8. Sources of surface pollution include improper disposal of hazardous and nonhazardous waste.
9. Health care professionals must be aware of various health hazards in the workplace, both for their clients and themselves.
10. Health care professionals have global, professional, and personal responsibilities for controlling pollution effects and preventing further hazards to health and development.
11. Health care professionals are responsible for promoting a safe physical environment for the client.
12. Health care professionals must engage in legislative advocacy, public education, and public policy changes to foster a healthy environment.
13. Terrorist incidents and bombings remain a significant threat in the United States and throughout the world.
14. Threats of bioterrorism extend worldwide; preparedness is essential.
15. Development of all people is negatively affected by these threats.
16. Education is essential to professionals and citizens about the threats and management of chemical, biological, radiological/nuclear, and explosive agents.
17. As a professional and citizen, work with agencies and resources in the community to foster disaster preparedness.

Study Questions

1. The nurse in a large manufacturing plant is case managing an employee who has developed asthma that is believed to be related to inhaled workplace irritants. The employee, who has worked in the plant for many years, asks why his problem has only recently developed. The nurse's response should be based on the fact that:
   1. There is no explanation for why illness related to toxic exposure does not occur immediately.
   2. The condition may have been present for sometime but the individual has been asymptomatic.
   3. The development of the illness may be the result of duration of exposure.
   4. The client likely did not report the condition when symptoms first occurred.
2. The nurse is participating in a community-wide disaster plan. The nurse has been assigned to coordinate the recovery phase of the disaster. Which of the following will be a goal of this phase?
   1. Establishment of communication
   2. Triage of victims

3. Secondary assessment
4. Stress management
3. A local hospital has instituted a new security policy requiring all visitors to sign in, produce identification, and have their personal bags searched by a security officer. Instituting these measures addresses which phase of disaster planning?
   1. Mitigation
   2. Preparedness
   3. Response
   4. Recovery

4. The nurse in a pediatric office noted that several children from the same household have been treated for repeated otitis media and upper respiratory infections over the last 3 years. During well-child visits, the nurse should question the parents regarding:
   1. Proper use of over-the-counter medications
   2. Sleeping arrangements in the household
   3. Smoking habits of care providers and relatives
   4. Allergy history of the parents

References

1. *Acid rain.* (n.d.). Retrieved February 28, 2006, from http://www.epa.gov/acidrain/index.html
2. Administration plan fails to protect public from toxic mercury in fish. (2004). *Environmental Defense Solutions, 35*(2), 8.
3. *ADHD linked to third-hand smoke exposure.* Retrieved July 16, 2007, from http://www.aphroditewomanshealth.com/news/20070527-163205_health_newsshtml
4. *Air quality index.* (n.d.). Retrieved February 27, 2006, from http://www.airnow.gov/index.html
5. *Asbestos in your home.* (n.d.). Retrieved March 7, 2006, from http://www.epa.gov/asbestos/pubs/ashome.html
6. Begley, S., & Murr, A. (2007, July 2–9). Which of these is not causing global warming today? *Newsweek,* 48–50.
7. Burros, M. (2006, March 8). More salmonella is reported in chickens. *The New York Times,* p. D4.
8. By the numbers. (2004, January–February). *Sierra, 89*(1), 13.
9. Center for Health, Columbia University School of Nursing. (2002). *Bioterrorism and emergency readiness: Competencies for all public health workers: Preview version III.* New York: Author. Retrieved March 13, 2006, from http://cpmcnet.columbia.edu/dept/nursing/institutescenters/chphsr/btcomps.pdf
10. Center for Health, Columbia University Mailman School of Public Health. (2004). *Emergency preparedness and response competencies for hospital workers.* New York: Author. Retrieved March 13, 2006, from http://www.mailman.hs.columbia.edu/CPHP/hospcomps.pdf [Context Link]
11. Chalupka, S. (2005). Tainted water on tap. *American Journal of Nursing, 105*(11), 40–52.
12. *Citizen's guide to radon.* (n.d.). Retrieved February 27, 2006, from http://www.epa.gov/radon/pubs.html
13. Clean your town. (2006, February 22). *Citizen Journal,* p.1.
14. *Consumers' guide to pesticides and food safety.* (1995). Retrieved March 9, 2006, from http://www.ific.org
15. Cowley, G. (2003, May 5). How progress makes us sick. *Newsweek,* 33–35.
16. Cut methane, save a life. (2006, March 7). *The New York Times,* p. D3.
17. Department of Health and Human Services: Centers for Disease Control and Prevention. (2006). *Chemical categories.* Retrieved March 24, 2006, from http://www.bt.cdc.gov/agent/agentlistchem-category.asp#biotoxins
18. Department of Homeland Security. (2004). *National response plan.* Washington, DC: U.S. Government Printing Office. Retrieved March 12, 2006, from http://www.dhs.gov/interweb/assetlibrary/NRP_FullText.pdf
19. *Dioxin research at the National Institute of Environmental Health Sciences.* (2001). Retrieved March 7, 2006, from http://www.niehs.nih.gov/oc/factsheets/doxin.html
20. Dudek, S. (2007). *Nutrition essentials for nursing practice* (8th ed.). Philadelphia: Lippincott Williams & Wilkins.
21. *Effects of acid rain: Human health.* (n.d.). Retrieved February 27, 2006, from http://www.epa.gov/acidrain/effects/health.html
22. Ehrlich, R. (2004). Heat exchange. *Natural History, 113*(3), 58–64.
23. Even approved amount of ozone is found harmful. (2006, February 28). *The New York Times,* p. D6.
24. Flannery, T. (2005). *The weather makers.* New York: Atlantic Monthly Press.
25. *Food ingredients and colors.* (2004, November). International Food Information Council and U.S. Food and Drug Administration. Retrieved March 9, 2006, from http://www.cfsan.fda.gov
26. *Foodborne illness.* (2005). Retrieved February 28, 2006, from http://www.cdc.gov/incidod/dbmd/diseaseinfo/foodborne_infectionsg.html
27. Foodservice giant says "no" to antibiotics in poultry. (2004, March–April). *Environmental Defense Solutions, 35*(2), 7.
28. *Fossil fuels.* (2001). Retrieved February 26, 2006, from http://www.eia.doc.gov.html
29. Foulke, J. E. (1998). *A fresh look at food preservatives* (revised). Retrieved March 9, 2006, from http://www.cfsan.fda.gov
30. Gaffney, K. F. (2001). Infant exposure to environmental tobacco smoke. *Journal of Nursing Scholarship, 33*(4), 343–347.
31. Gebbie, K. M. (2000). *Bioterrorism and emergency readiness: Competencies for all public health workers.* Retrieved March 13, 2006, from http://www.nursing.hs.columbia.edu/institutes-centers/chphsr/hospcomps.pdf
32. *Global warming.* (2000). Retrieved February 27, 2006, from http://www.yosemite.epa.gov/oar/globalwarming.nsf/content/Climate.html
33. *Good up high, bad nearby.* (2003). Retrieved February 26, 2006, from http://epa.gov/oar/oaqps/gooduphigh/ozone.html#2
34. Green movement gaining momentum in health care. (2005). *Clinical News, 9*(12), 1, 16.
35. Green, P. M., Polk, L. V., & Slade, D. S. (2003). Environmental nursing diagnoses: A proposal for further development of Taxonomy II. *International Journal of Nursing Terminologies and Classification, 14*(1), 19–29.
36. Hall, K., Afzal, B., & Sattler, B. (2007). Healing our hazards environment. *American Nurse Today, 2*(7), 38–39.
37. Hallenbeck, W. (1985). *Pesticides and human health.* New York: Springer-Verlag.
38. Hennen, L. (2006, April). Water wise. *Real Simple,* 147–152.
39. Hooked on fish? There might be some catches. (2003). *Harvard Health Letter, 28*(3), 4–5.
40. Hsu, C. E., Mas, F. S., Jacobson, H., Papenfuss, R., Nkhoma, E. T., & Zoretic, J. (2005). Assessing the readiness and training needs of non-urban physicians in public health emergency and response. *Disaster Management & Response: DMR, 3*(4),106–111.
41. Indoor environmental quality. (1997, June). *NIOSH Facts.* Retrieved February 28, 2006, from http://www.cdc.gov/niosh.html
42. International Nursing Coalition for Mass Casualty Education. (2003). *Competencies for entry-level nurses in response to mass casualty incidents (MCIs) resulting from chemical, biological, radiological, nuclear and explosive agents.* Nashville, TN: Author. Retrieved March 13, 2006, from http://www.incmce.org/competenciespage.html
43. Is the EPA listening on clean air? (2003). *MoPIRG, 17*(1), 1.
44. Kapur, G. B., Hutson, H. R., Davis, M. A., & Rice, P. L. (2005). The United States twenty-year experience with bombing incidents: Implications for terrorism preparedness and medical response. *Journal of Trauma-Injury Infection & Critical Care, 59*(6), 1436–1444.
45. Karwa, M., Currie, B., & Kvetan, V. (2005). Bioterrorism: Preparing for the impossible or the improbable. *Critical Care Medicine, 33*(1), Supplement: S75–S95.

46. Kemper, A. R., Cohn, L., Fant, K. E., et al. (2005). Follow-up testing among children with elevated screening blood lead levels. *Journal of the American Medical Association, 293,* 2232–2237.

47. Kranz, D., & Kifferstein, B. (n.d.). *Water pollution and society.* Retrieved February 28, 2006, from http://www.umich.edu/~265/society/waterpollution.html

48. Landesman, L. Y., Malilay, J., Bissell, R. A., Becker, S. M., Roberts, L., & Ascher, M. S. (2001a). Roles and responsibilities of public health in disaster preparedness and response. In L.F. Novick & G.P. Mays (Eds.), *Public health administration: Principles for population-based management.* Gaithersburg, MD: Aspen Publishers.

49. Landesman, L. Y., Malilay, J., Bissell, R. A., Becker, S. M., Roberts, L., & Ascher, M. S. (2001b). Roles and responsibilities of public health in disaster preparedness and response. In L.F. Novick & G.P. Mays (Eds.), *Public health issues in disaster preparedness: Focus on bioterrorism.* Gaithersburg, MD: Aspen Publishers.

50. Langan, J., & James, D. (2005). *Preparing nurses for disaster management.* Upper Saddle River, NJ: Pearson Prentice Hall.

51. Lanson, S., Kutcher, J., & Frey, R. (1997). Pesticide poisoning: An environmental emergency. *Journal of Emergency Nursing, 23*(6), 516–517.

52. Lechat, M. F. (1979). Disasters and public health. *Bulletin of the World Health Organization, 57*(1), 11–17.

53. Levine, S. (2004). Who'll stop the mercury rain? *U.S. News & World Report, 136*(11), 70–71.

54. Loewenberg, S. (2004, January–February). Old Europe's new ideas. *Sierra, 89*(1), 40–43.

55. Lusk, S. L. (2002). Preventing noise-induced hearing loss. *Nursing Clinics of North America, 37,* 257–262.

56. Lusk, S. L., & Raymond, D. M., III. (2002). Impacting health through the worksite. *Nursing Clinics of North America, 37,* 247–256.

57. Malakoff, D. (2003, December). Global warming. *Audubon,* 45–48.

58. Markenson, D., DiMaggio, C., & Redlener, I. (2005). Preparing health professions students for terrorism, disaster, and public health emergencies: Core competencies. *Academic Medicine, 80*(6), 517–526.

59. McManus, R. (2004, January–February). Out front in the air wars. *Sierra, 89*(1), 12.

60. NANDA International. (2007). *NANDA nursing diagnoses: Definitions & classification, 2007–2008.* Philadelphia: Author.

61. National Low Income Housing Coalition. (2006). *Senator introduces bill to expedite lead-based paint removal.* Retrieved March 7, 2006 from http://www.nlihc.org/mtm/mtm/10_16html

62. *Noise-induced hearing loss.* (n.d.). National Institute on Deafness and Other Communication Disorders. Retrieved March 7, 2006, from http.www.nidcd.nih.gov/health/hearing/noise.asp

63. *Noise pollution.* (n.d.) Retrieved February 28, 2006, from http://www.epa.nsw.gov.au/soe/97/ch1/15_html

64. Noji, E.K. (2001). Bioterrorism: A 'new' global environmental health threat. *Global Change & Human Health, 2*(1), 1–10.

65. North Carolina passes landmark clear air law, setting precedent for other states. (2002). *Environmental Defense Solutions, 33*(5), 2–3.

66. Occupational Safety and Health Administration. (n.d.). *OSHA's mission.* Retrieved February 28, 2006, from http://www.osha.gov/oshinfo/mission.html

67. Persell, D. J., Arangie, P., Young, C., Stokes, E. N., Payne, W. C., Skorga, P., & Gilbert-Palmer, D. (2001). Preparing for bioterrorism: Category A agents. *Nurse Practitioner, 26*(12), 12–15, 19–24, 27.

68. *Pesticides and food.* (2003). Retrieved March 7, 2006, from http.www.epa.gov/pesticides/food/viewtols.html

69. Pesticides in nearly all U.S. streams. (2006, March 4). *Arizona Daily Star,* p. A5.

70. Protecting your ears. (2002). In *Hearing loss: A guide to prevention and treatment* (pp. 38–40). Palm Coast, FL: Harvard Health.

71. Revkin, A. (2006). *The North Pole was here. Puzzles and perils at the top of the world.* New York: Houghton Mifflin.

72. Revkin, A. (2007, July–August). Global meltdown. *AARP Magazine,* 50–55.

73. Riedel, S. (2004). Biological warfare and bioterrorism: A historical review. *Baylor University Medical Center Proceedings, 17*(4), 400–406.

74. Rosenthal, L. (2006). Carbon monoxide poisoning. *American Journal of Nursing, 106*(3), 40–45.

75. Roth, L. D., Khan, A. S., Lillibridge, S. R., Ostroff, S. M., & Hughes, J. M. (2002). Public health assessment of potential biological terrorism agents. *Emerging Infectious Diseases, 8*(2), 225–230.

76. Sallis, J. F., & Owen, N. (2002). Ecological models of health behavior. In K. Glanz, B. K. Rimer, & F. M. Lewis (Eds.), *Health behavior and health education* (3rd ed., pp. 462–484). San Francisco: Jossey-Bass.

77. Salazar, M. K. (2001). Environmental health responding to the call. *Public Health Nursing, 17*(2), 73–74.

78. Sattler, B. (2002). Environmental health in the health care setting. *American Nurse,* 25–40.

79. Sattler, B., Afzal, B. M., Condon, M. E., Belka, E. K., & McKee, T. M. (2001). Environmentally healthy homes and communities. *American Nurse,* 25–40.

80. Schultheis, R. (2004). The forecast: Hazy skies to continue. *National Parks,* 26–29.

81. Siegrist, D. (1999). The threat of biological attack: Why concern now? *Emerging Infectious Diseases, 5*(4), 505–508.

82. Slater, D. (2002, May–June). What's under your sink? *Sierra, 88*(3), 32–33.

83. *Sources of indoor air pollution.* (n.d.). Retrieved March 7, 2006, from http://www.epa.gov/iaq.html

84. Spake, A. (2003). A market for wellness. *U.S. News and World Report, 135*(23), 76.

85. Trossman, S. (2004). Catching the environmental health wave. *American Journal of Nursing, 104*(3), 73–74.

86. The truth about mold. (2003). *Harvard Health Letter, 28*(3), 1–3.

87. Turner, K. (2003, December). Playing it cool—Global warming solutions. *Audubon,* 74–76.

88. U.S. Department of Defense, Office of Joint Chiefs of Staff. (2001). *Joint publication 1-02: Department of Defense dictionary of military and associated terms.* Washington, DC: United States Department of Defense (as amended through 31 August 2005). Retrieved March 26, 2006, from http://www.dtic.mil/doctrine/jel/new_pubs/jp1_02.pdf

89. U.S. Department of Health and Human Services. (2006). *New Surgeon General's report focuses on effects of secondhand smoke.* Retrieved July 9, 2006, from http://www.hhs.gov/news/press/2006pres/20060627.html

90. U.S. Department of Health and Human Services. (2000). *Healthy people 2010: Understanding and improving health, Vol. 2.* Washington, DC: U.S. Government Printing Office.

91. U.S. Department of Justice, Federal Bureau of Investigation. (2004). *Terrorism 1980–2001.* Retrieved March 13, 2006, from http://www.fbi.gov/publications/terror/terror2000_2001.htm

92. VanDongen, C. J. (1998). Environmental health risks. *American Journal of Nursing, 98*(9), 16B, 16D–E.

93. Veenema, T. G. (2003). *Disaster nursing and emergency preparedness for chemical, biological, and radiological terrorism and other hazards.* New York: Springer Publishing.

94. Warner, C. R., Diachenko, G. W., & Bailey, C. J. (2000, August–September). Sulfites: An important food safety issue. *Food Testing & Analysis.* Retrieved February 27, 2006, from http://vm.cfsan.fda.gov

95. *Wastes.* (2006). Retrieved March 7, 2006, from http://www.epa.gov/epaoswer/osw

96. We need to cool it. (2005, July 11). *Newsweek,* 48, 50.

97. Weiner, E., Irwin, M., Trangrangenstein, P., & Gordon, J. (2005). Emergency preparedness curriculum in nursing schools in the United States. *Nursing Education Perspectives, 26*(6), 334–339.

98. *What society can do about acid deposition.* (n.d.). Retrieved February 27, 2006, from http://www.epa.gov/airmarkets/acidrain/society/index.html

99. When it pays to buy organic. (2006, February). *Consumer Reports,* 12–17.

100. You are what you eat. (2005, January). *Consumer Reports,* 26–31.

101. Zibulewsky, J. (2001). Defining disaster: The emergency department perspective. *Baylor University Medical Center Proceedings, 14*(2), 144–149.

CHAPTER 5

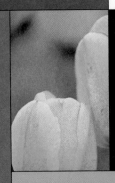

Sociocultural Influences

OBJECTIVES

Study of this chapter will enable you to:

1. Define culture and subculture and describe various types of cultures and subcultures and their general components.

2. Identify the dominant cultural and socioeconomic level values in the United States and discuss how they influence you as a health care worker, as well as the client and family.

3. Contrast traditional and current values with values of major diverse racial or ethnic groups in the United States.

4. Discuss the influences of culture and socioeconomic level on the health status of the person and group.

5. Assess a person from another culture and contrast his or her values with those described in this chapter.

6. Analyze how knowledge of cultural and socioeconomic level values and attitudes toward daily living practices, health, and illness can contribute to the effectiveness of health promotion.

7. Relate ways to give culturally competent care to a person with cultural values and a socioeconomic level different from your own.

8. Assess and care for a person or family from another culture and socioeconomic level and identify your own ethnocentric tendencies.

MediaLink www.prenhall.com/murray

Go to the Companion Website for interactive resources that accompany this chapter.

Glossary
Review Questions
Challenge Your Knowledge
Learning Activities

Critical Thinking
Tools
Media Link Applications
Media Links

Humans are unique; we are born into a culture. Culture includes all the components discussed in this chapter. Humans are heir to the accumulation of wisdom and folly of preceding generations, and, in turn, they teach others their beliefs, feelings, and practices. The client, family, and you are deeply affected by the culture learned during the early years, often more so than by cultural knowledge acquired later. Information from this chapter is designed to foster **culturally competent care** by *increasing knowledge of how the client's cultural background influences the life patterns, health practices, and expectations about health care services. In turn, your communication, interaction patterns, education, counseling, and service delivery with clients will be directed toward the unique background of the client and adapted in a way that is biopsychosocially satisfactory and effective for the client* (2, 17, 37, 95, 96).

Definitions

A number of definitions are presented to assist you in correctly using words that are relevant to cultures.

Culture *is the sum total of the learned ways of doing, feeling, and thinking, past and present, of a social group within a given period. These ways are transmitted from one generation to the next or to immigrants who become members of the society. Culture is a group's design for living, a shared set of socially transmitted assumptions about the nature of the physical and social world, goals in life, attitudes, roles, and values. Culture is a complex integrated system that includes knowledge, beliefs, skills, art, morals, laws, customs, norms, and any*

other acquired habits and capabilities of the human being. All provide a pattern for living together.

A **subculture** *is a group of persons within a larger culture who have an identity of their own but are related to the total culture in certain ways.* For example, Latinos or Spanish-speaking Americans, American Indians, and people of Asian, African, Middle Eastern, Asian Indian, or Polynesian descent practice their own cultures within the overall culture of the United States. In addition to ethnic and racial cultural groups, regional, socioeconomic, religious, and family subcultures also exist. See **Table 5-1** for definitions (2, 37, 62, 69, 107, 117).

Cultural Populations in the United States

An understanding of different types of cultures and their influence on development of behavior is essential to understanding yourself and the people for whom you care.

The United States has been called a melting pot, made up of people from diverse backgrounds. Various terms, including "people of color," are used to refer to this diversity. *A description of several racial and ethnic groups follows:*

1. African descent (Caribbean, Central American, South American), African American, Hispanic Black, or non-Hispanic Black.
2. Latino, Hispanic or Spanish, Mexican, Central American, or Caribbean descent; designation of specific country for people

TABLE 5-1

Types of Cultures or Subcultures

Racial:	Group of people or population with genetic and biological similarities in body structure and overall appearance. A less frequently used concept because differences among people of the same race may be greater than average differences among people of different races.
Biracial:	Group of people who have genetic heritage from two or more racial groups, such as combinations of African, Asian, and Caucasian, yet are distinguished from any one racial or ethnic group. Their values, language, or lifestyle patterns are influenced by each racial group or the dominant racial culture in which they live.
Ethnic:	Group of people or population who have a common national origin or country of birth and are distinguished from people of other nationalities or races. People who share an ancestral heritage, common physical traits as a result of heredity, and a common history or lineage, values, traditions, customs, language, and sometimes the same or similar religions. The words "ethnic" or "ethnicity" are sometimes used interchangeably with the words "race" or "racial."
Regional:	Group of people who live within a specific geographic area who demonstrate specific values or life patterns relevant to the location or environment, but also values and life patterns of the larger culture.
Socioeconomic:	Group of people who have similar financial position or wealth and the consequent social influence and position or status, values, language, political attitudes, cultural interests, lifestyle and consumption patterns, and opportunities for social mobility.
Religious:	Group of people who share a belief system that influences values, attitudes, behaviors, thinking about situations, and lifestyle patterns.
Neighborhood:	A community. A collective, functional, informal network of people within a specific residential area who share at least some values and lifestyle patterns. They demonstrate concern for each other and the residential area, and utilize services and resources of nearby institutions, agencies, organizations, and businesses.
Family:	Distinct unit or group of people who usually share lineage and who share commitment to each other. The unit shares common values and life patterns, including sexuality, and also manifest characteristics of the dominant culture in which they live.

who are American citizens, such as Mexican American, or Puerto Rican; or designation of country of birth, such as Belize.

3. American Indian or designation of Indian nation, such as Nez Perce or Navajo, Eskimo (or name of tribe), and Aleut. There are over 500 American Indian nations or tribes in the United States.

4. Asian Pacific Islander or Oceania descent, Asian American, Polynesian, or designations of specific people who have origins in a specific Asian country and are American citizens, such as Chinese American.

African Americans represent about 13% of the U.S. population; over half live in the southern states. People from a number of African countries, especially in West Africa, were brought as slaves to the United States from the 16th to the 19th centuries. Although people from other countries—the English, Germans, and Scotch-Irish—came as paupers and indentured servants, they were able to work to regain freedom. In contrast, slavery became a social institution when Virginia proclaimed slavery as legal in 1667; only Pennsylvania of the original 13 colonies protested the system of slavery. For some, the African American experience is entrenched in these roots and influences the person's and the population's worldview, attitudes and beliefs, and family structure, which has been matrifocal, or female-centered. In turn, interactions of African Americans with persons from other cultural groups may be affected. However, there are wide differences among the individuals in this population, related to educational, occupational, and socioeconomic background, as well as geographic region (2, 112). Today, a number of people of African heritage have immigrated voluntarily to the United States from African countries, the West Indies, the Dominican Republic, Haiti, Jamaica, and other Caribbean Islands (112).

The *Asian, Asian American, and Pacific Islander population is diverse,* composed of more than 51 cultures in the United States. Asians include Japanese, Chinese, Filipinos, Koreans, Vietnamese, Asian Indians, Thais, Hmong, Malaysians, Indonesians, Pakistanis, Cambodians, Laotians, and those from Singapore, Taiwan, and Hong Kong. Pacific Islanders include Polynesians (Hawaiians, Maoris, Tahitians, and Samoans), Micronesians (such as the indigenous people of Guam), and Melanesians (such as people from Fiji, Tonga, the Cook Islands, and the Marquesas Islands) (2, 37, 48).

Hispanic, *referring to persons from Spain or persons of Spanish origin, is often a term reserved for Latinos or Spanish or Latin Americans who have mixed ancestry,* without identifying country of origin. Most of those who are called Latino or Hispanic speak Spanish or Portuguese. *Among the Latino or Hispanic population, however, there are wide differences in genetic background, culture, tradition, lifestyle, and health behavior, depending on place of origin, ancestry, and current socioeconomic status. The person who is designated Latino or Hispanic may have an olive or dark complexion and may have come from Spain, Mexico, Puerto Rico, Cuba, The Dominican Republic, or any Central American or South American country.* For statistical purposes, specific birthplace should be recorded (37). For a general discussion of culture in this text, the term *Latino* or *Spanish-speaking* will be used (115).

Caucasians represent people from every European country, countries in the United Kingdom, and countries in the Middle East. People may refer to themselves in relation to country or region of origin as well as to their American citizenry, such as Iranian, Middle Easterner, Arabian American, Irish American, or Italian American. In the United States, there are many European Caucasian ethnic cultures, for example, German, Italian, Polish, Slavic (representing a number of Slovakian countries), Scandinavian (Danish, Norwegian, Icelandic, Finnish, or Swedish), Swiss, French, Dutch, and Russian. There are also ethnic subcultures from the United Kingdom: English, Irish, Welsh, and Scot. There are over 100 different ethnic groups in the United States (115).

The population in Hawaii, our 50th state, is composed of (a) native Hawaiians; (b) people born in Hawaii whose ancestors were the mainland Caucasians who arrived in the late 1800s or during the 1900s and established a home or business; (c) people of Polynesian descent from islands such as Tonga, Fiji, Tahiti, Samoa, Aotearoa, and Marquesas; and (d) people from Asian countries such as the Philippine Islands, Japan, or China. The population is diverse in ancestry, color, and lifestyles. There is no "majority" and no "minority." The U.S. Department of Commerce, Bureau of the Census, estimated in 2002 that by 2050 about half of the total American population will be non-White, eliminating the meaning of *minority* (37).

The markers of racial or ethnic identity include every conceivable hue of color. Sometimes values, socialization behaviors, language, ideology, or attitude are more of a marker than pigmentation. *Differences exist within each cultural group, just as differences exist between cultural groups.* In fact, dark-skinned East Indians, Pakistanis, and Bangladeshis, despite their dark pigmentation, are of the Caucasian race (37).

An increasing number of people claim to be **biracial** and therefore **bicultural,** *crossing two racial and cultural groups in lifestyles and values, and usually in appearance* (22, 37). Courtney (22) describes the challenges and hurts that he has encountered because he is biracial. He states that being biracial has frequently meant denying half of his identity; which half depended on whether he was with White Americans or African Americans. Tiger Woods, a professional golfer, is an example of a new generation of multiracial individuals who believe ethnic diversity and ambiguity confer both individuality and a sense of shared values. Some biracial people don't identify themselves with any race.

Regional culture *refers to the local, regional, or sectional variant of the national culture*—for example, rural or urban, or Yankee, Southern, or Midwestern. Regional culture is influenced and defined by geography, climate, natural resources, trade, and economics; variations may be shown in values, beliefs, housing, food, occupational skills, and language. One type of regional culture is **urban,** *which is defined by the U.S. Bureau of Census as a population within a specific area of 1,000 people per square mile and 500 people per square mile in the surrounding periphery* (115). **Urban areas** *include a population of at least 50,000 people;* an **urban cluster** *refers to populations between 2,500 and 50,000 people* (18). *At an international level, urban or city refers to a settlement of 20,000 or more people* (18). Another type is rural, which is a term that is difficult to define, partially because it prompts different images for different people. **Rural** *is defined by the U.S. Bureau of Census as an area or town with less than 500 people per square mile, a territory located outside the urban cluster* (115). Another definition for **rural** *is an area larger than 400 square miles with a population density of* *less than 30 people per square mile* (18). *Areas more sparsely popu-lated, for example, 6 persons per square mile, are designated as* **frontier** (115). Numerical values defining rural areas vary from one governmental agency to another. Population density, popula-tion size, and distance from health care facilities are criteria frequently used in defining rural areas. Rural is a matter of perspec-tive; to some people it means "smaller than here."

Rural dwellers use the same adaptive strategies and products as urban dwellers, and value systems may be similar. Yet, rural dwellers are more likely to live traditional values. Differences within and between rural populations may depend more on the geography, climate, and history of the area than on socioeconomic status, race, ethnicity, or religion. *Yet several characteristics are com-mon in rural areas in the United States and Canada* (8, 32, 44, 55, 72, 101, 106, 119):

1. Limited accessibility to at least some necessary resources to promote health and, sometimes, geographic isolation from people.
2. Assumption that what is done locally is the norm (e.g., "We've always done it this way") in spite of rules and regulations on a state or national level.
3. Lack of anonymity, because everyone knows, directly or indi-rectly, everyone else for miles around, and sometimes, the family history for generations.
4. A sense of independence or autonomy (e.g., a desire to be one's own boss and to be left alone).

These characteristics may have a negative impact on care of the ru-ral person, even though isolation, independence, and lack of anonymity are seen as positive attributes. However, the Internet potentially can bridge disparities in health care access for geo-graphically dispersed areas. Emerging technologies could be useful in preventing, assessing, and treating illness.

Cattle ranchers, migrant workers, coal miners, loggers, people who live in Appalachia, American Indians who live on reserva-tions, the Amish, and grain farmers each bring to mind life in ru-ral America. Ancestry, residence, age, income, and occupation all contribute to different values, customs, and definitions of health among rural people.

Socioeconomic level *is a cultural grouping of persons who have a consciousness of cohesion.* Socioeconomic level is *not only economic in origin. Other factors also contribute to status, such as family history, occupation, influence of the person or family in the community of res-idence, reliance on tradition, age, gender, and personal endowment.*

Religious culture also influences the person, for a *religion con-stitutes a way of believing, living, and behaving, and therefore is a kind of culture.* **Religious influences** on values, attitudes, and be-havior are discussed in Chapter 7. ∞

Family culture *refers to family life, which is part of the cultural system. It consists of ways of living and thinking that constitute the family and sexual aspects of group life,* as discussed in **Tables 5-4** and **5-5**, Chapter 6, ∞ and throughout the text. The family is the medium through which the larger cultural heritage is transmitted to the child. The family gives the child status and a reputation. The family name gives the child a social position as well as an identity. Family status has a great deal to do with health and behavior throughout life because of its effect on self-concept.

Family rituals are the collective way of working out household routines, using time, handling family crises, and celebrating events. They are indicators of family values. **Ritual** *is a system of definitely prescribed behaviors and procedures. It provides exactness in daily tasks of living and has a sense of rightness about it.* Rituals de-velop in family life as a result of the intimacy of relationships and the repetition of certain interactions. Rituals change from one life cycle to another, for example, at marriage, before and after child-birth, when children go to school, and when children leave home. *Rituals are important in child development for other reasons,* includ-ing to promote family cohesion, identity, and harmony (2, 9, 104).

All cultures and subcultures possess certain values, customs, and practices common to every other culture; share certain values, customs, and practices with some other cultures; and have certain values, customs, and practices unique only to that group of peo-ple. Cultures can best be studied from an **emic approach** *by exam-ining each culture based on the adaptiveness of behavior within its own perspective or frame of reference.* In the past, studies have tended to take an **etic approach** *with a cross-cultural or comparative per-spective and conducted by someone from outside the group* (69).

Characteristics of Culture

Culture has three basic characteristics: (a) culture is learned, (b) cul-ture is stable but changing, and (c) it is composed of certain com-ponents or patterns universally. Use the following information in assessment and intervention for culturally competent care.

CULTURE IS LEARNED

People function physiologically in much the same way throughout the world, but their *culture, values, and behavior are learned* and are therefore relatively diverse. A **value** refers to a *learned social prin-ciple, goal, or standard held as acceptable or worthy of esteem.* These principles, goals, or standards are chosen, affirmed, and demon-strated consistently in various ways. A **value system** *is the overall concept of how a group of people should live and behave in various sit-uations and the goals to be pursued.* The value system of the domi-nant culture and of other cultural groups may conflict at times. Further, in the United States or other Westernized countries, peo-ple may change their economic level, but their original value sys-tem may be maintained. Children learn the values of their group and their group's attitudes toward people in another group. Be-cause of culture, a child is ascribed or acquires a certain **status** or *position in the group.* The child also learns or assumes certain **roles**, *patterns or related behaviors expected by others, and later by the self, that define behavior and adjustment to a given group.* What the per-son learns during development is of great significance (3, 9, 36). **Table 5-2** lists basic cultural values and questions, the range of be-liefs derived from these questions, and examples of groups adher-ing to these beliefs (53, 54).

Understanding the characteristics of culture will help you better understand and work with people from various cultures. What the person has learned from the culture determines how and what you will be able to teach him or her, as well as your approach during care. Interactions between you and the client are also influenced by the cultural influences each of you have experienced.

TABLE 5-2

Basic Values of Cultures with Selected Cultural Examples

Value	Range of Beliefs	Example of Cultural or Subcultural Group Adhering to Value
Human Nature (What is the innate nature of man?)	The person is basically *evil but capable of achieving goodness* with self-control and effort.	Puritan ancestors. Protestants of Pentecostal or Fundamentalist background. Appalachian subculture.
	The person is a *combination of good and evil,* with self-control necessary but lapses in behavior understood.	Most people in the United States.
	The person is basically *good.*	Some religious groups, such as Society of Friends. Some philosophical groups, such as humanistic psychologists and members of ethical society.
Person–nature (What is the relation of person to nature or supernatural?)	The person is *subjugated* to *nature* and cannot change whatever is destined to happen.	Spanish-speaking cultures. Appalachian subculture. Japanese and other Asian cultures.
	The person is to gain *mastery* over *nature;* all natural forces can be overcome.	Middle- and upper-class and highly educated people in the United States.
Time (What is the temporal focus of human life?)	*Past time* is given preference; most important events to guide life have happened in the past.	Historic China.
	Present time is the main focus; people pay little attention to the past and regard the future as vague.	Spanish-speaking cultures. Appalachian subculture.
	Future is the main emphasis, seen as bigger and better; people are not content with the present.	Educated, professional, and middle-class people in the United States.
Activity (What is the main purpose in life?)	*Being orientation.* The person is important just because he or she is and may spontaneously express impulses and desires.	Appalachian subculture. Although no culture allows complete expression of impulses and all cultures must have some work done, the Mexican fiesta and Mardi Gras in New Orleans are manifestations of this value.
	Becoming-in-being orientation. The person is important for what he or she is, but must continue to develop.	Most religious cultures. American Indian subcultures. Greek culture.
	Doing orientation. The person is important when active or accomplishing something.	Most people in the United States.
Relational (What is one's relation to other people?)	*Individualistic relations.* These emphasize autonomy; the person does not have to fully submit to authority. Individual goals have primacy over group goals.	Most *Gemeinschaft* societies, such as folk or rural cultures. Yankee and Appalachian subcultures. Middle-class America, with emphasis on nuclear family.
	Collateral relations. These emphasize that the person is part of a social and family order and does not live just for the self. Group or family goals have primacy.	Most European American ethnic groups, especially Italian American, Spanish-speaking cultures. American Indian tribal subcultures. Most cultures adhere somewhat through sibling relations in family.
	Lineal relations. These emphasize the extended family and biological and cultural relationships through time. Group goals have primacy.	Cultures that emphasize hereditary lines. Upper-class America. Asian cultures. Middle East cultures. British culture.
	Relations are impersonal, focused on role behavior.	Business interactions, upper-middle class, and those moving up the social ladder.

Adapted from references 53–54.

CULTURE IS STABLE BUT CHANGING

The second characteristic of culture is that *it is subject to and capable of change although it is basically a stable entity. The culture of a society, like a human body, is dynamic but maintained at a steady state by self-regulating devices. Stabilizing features are traditions, group pressure, and the ready-made solutions to life's problems that are provided for the group to regulate life. Everyone within the same culture does not behave in the same way.* In the United States and Westernized countries throughout the world, there is often much overt change occurring. Yet underneath the manifested lifestyle changes, certain basic values of people within some groups undergo less change. *Norms and customs that persist may have a negative influence on the group* (104). Food taboos during illness and pregnancy, pica, a diet high in animal fat, and crowding of people into a common dwelling that provides an apt incubator for spread of contagious disease are examples.

A culture makes change, stability, or adaptation possible through its ideas, inventions, and customs. Humans, for example, are able to live in a wide variety of climates because the body has adjusted gradually to permit survival. We have constructed a variety of lifestyles and patterns of social relationships to guarantee our survival and free ourselves from limits of the physical environment. Yet, how a culture uses natural resources and prevents or creates environmental problems influences survival of the culture (30).

Another stabilizing aspect of culture is **linguistics,** *the structure and use of language and the rules of verbal and nonverbal communication. Use of words and behaviors to construct messages varies from culture to culture* (37). *Use of language and the meanings of words and concepts change over time.* Learning cultural and family language is done primarily by ear. In addition, use of language is determined considerably by age and sex, for example, baby talk, child talk, adult talk, girl talk, and boy talk. Families and people from various geographic areas or from various ethnic or racial backgrounds differ in conversational conventions. Some of the conventions that might vary by cultural group include permitted topics of conversation, proper situations for discussing certain topics (such as during mealtime or before bedtime), level of vocabulary used, reaction to new words used, number of interruptions permitted, who can be interrupted, and who talks the most.

The meeting ground between cultures is in language and **dialect,** *a variety of a language spoken by a distinct group of people in a definite place.* In most countries, a national language as well as various dialects are spoken (37). In the United States, English is the national language, but for many people who have more recently entered the country, English is the second language. Some people regularly speak their native language as a way to maintain cultural identity. For example, American Indian elders are now striving to teach their children their specific native language, which was forbidden in this country in the past, in order to strengthen national or tribal identity (113). Coastal Carolina educators are also focusing on preserving the language and customs of the Gullah culture (113). Children in school often become interpreters for the family who relies on a dialect. Classes are available to assist people who have English as a second language. In any language, choice of words, pace, syntax, intonation, and level

of emotion in speech all convey meanings that, if understood, will avoid communication, relationship, employment, and life skill problems (37). Some cultural groups have more dependence on the ear (listening to the spoken word) than eye (reading the written word). Some groups are more spontaneous in communications; language is free-flowing and consistent with body gestures and movements. Other groups are more restrained in speech and body expression (82).

Use of nonverbal language also varies by cultural background. For example, Asian Americans and Haitians may smile and nod in agreement when they do not understand what is being said. People born in Vietnam may avoid eye contact with health professionals as a sign of respect. Mexican Americans may also interpret prolonged eye contact as disrespectful (2, 37).

Language emphasizes the values of a culture. For example, Americans use complex, abstract, fragmentary descriptions and emphasize time (37). The Hopi language describes events based on "fact"—memory, expectations, and customs—rather than on historical time. The Navajo language makes little mention of clock time but emphasizes activity, movement, or duration. Countries that use English tend to describe nonspatial relationships with spatial words, such as "long" or "short" for duration, "rise" and "fall" for trends, or "heavy" and "light" for intensity. In the Hopi language, psychological metaphors are used to name mental processes; for example, "heart" can be used for "think" or "remember." The Native Eskimos have numerous words to describe variations of space, different kinds of snow, and whaling activities in the spring. In all cultures, new words are being added and traditionally used words are disappearing with the increased use of technology and changing behaviors and activities.

Cultural **norms,** the *usual rules for living,* change to meet the group's needs as new life challenges arise. *Cultures change for various reasons, including* (2, 37, 112) (a) technologic change or innovation; (b) competition among groups for geographic regions or resources; (c) use of another culture's inventions, art forms, or lifeways; (d) education of the group/population; (e) change in political leadership; (f) increased scientific and industrial complexity; (g) increased or decreased population growth; and (h) promotion of values, lifestyles, and products through mass media and electronic programming and advertisements.

Culture is continually shaped by forces and people outside of our awareness. The United States is a **postindustrial/postmodern society,** *where there are few universal criteria or moral standards to guide or stabilize a culture.* Yet there is also an emphasis on conformity or normalization. *Some of the forces affecting current society and values and, in turn, health care, are* (30) (a) emphasis on an information society, (b) greater expectations of society's resources and seeking multiple options, (c) cultural diversity and power struggles between groups, (d) increased life expectancy and use of self-help practices, (e) changing values and lifeways, with little understanding of the culture's history, and (f) high-technology versus high-touch care and decentralization of services.

Adaptational breakdown and illness are likely to occur unless people come to grips with rapid social change. A **transient culture,** *one that focuses on disposable objects and transitory relationships,* makes it difficult for people to establish roots or pass on culture as a guideline to future generations. Not all people have adjusted to the continual rapid change (30, 104). *Risk of illness can be predicted from the amount of change.* If a person is continually in the equivalent of the Alarm Stage of the General Adaptation Syndrome, body defenses weaken, as described in Chapter 2. ∞ Extreme examples of persons caught in rapidly changing environments are the combat soldier, the disaster victim, the homeless person, and the migrant worker. Other examples of change include people who have moved to an unfamiliar location within the United States or who have come as an immigrant or refugee.

During assessment of and intervention with the client, utilize the content discussed in this section. Develop **linguistic competence:** *Realize that language differences and resistance to cultural or health care changes can give a false impression of the physical and mental status or intelligence of a person and contribute to health care disparities.* Some people have difficulty switching from their native language or dialect to standard American English. People from non-Western cultures may learn differently and at a different pace because of their cultural upbringing and value orientations and consequent meaning of various words or gestures in their language and perceptual skills. Listen carefully and be accepting of their language skills. Validate words and concepts as necessary. Adapt ways of speaking to and teaching the client. Learn from the client while also learning about the use of language and the ability to keep up with changes in our culture.

CULTURE IS COMPOSED OF CERTAIN COMPONENTS AND PATTERNS

The third characteristic of culture is that certain components or patterns are present in every culture, regardless of how "primitive" or "advanced" it may be. All cultural components and patterns influence and are influenced by adaptation to climate, use of natural resources, geography, sanitation facilities, diet, group biological and genetic factors, and disease conditions and health practices. **Table 5-3** describes components of all cultures and gives examples (2, 30, 37, 104).

Understanding these components of a culture will help you understand yourself, your clients, and their environment, and the health care system. Integrate this knowledge into assessment, care planning, intervention, and **evaluation** of care.

Comparison of Selected Cultures

Knowledge of cultural values is essential for providing culturally sensitive care as you interact, assess, teach, and intervene with people from various cultures. Basic values of all cultures are summarized in **Table 5-2.**

CULTURAL VALUES IN THE UNITED STATES

Perhaps the best indicator of what we really are and value is to observe what we watch in the media (e.g., television, videos, movies, the Internet), whom we consider to be our heroes, how we spend our money, and how we use our time. Values also are influenced by the historical time in which a person was reared (the decade of childhood) and, thus, the person's age, as well as religion or philosophy, socioeconomic level, and ethnic or racial background.

Many cultural groups make up the U.S. population and have contributed to the value system. Over the years, many ethnic or national groups have resettled in the United States and obtained citizenship. From the late 1700s through the 1940s, numerous people emigrated from Europe to North America in search of religious or political freedom, to expand educational and employment opportunities or for economic reasons, as refugees, and as a result of wars. Approximately 50 million Americans are directly descended from German immigrants (89, 99, 100). The next largest European immigrant groups are the Irish, English, and Italians (9, 81). Thus, European values and lifeways have seeped into all of American life, contributing to the mainstream value system (89). More recently there has also been a large influx of refugees and immigrants from other countries.

Several orientations and value systems may be simultaneously present in a given society or culture, but usually only one orientation dominates over a given period. Both **traditional** (*mainstream*)

TABLE 5-3

Components of All Cultures

Component of the Culture	Purpose or Meaning	Examples
Provision of physical welfare; feeding, clothing, and shelter patterns	Survival and maintenance of population. Health promotion.	Production and processing of food, shelter, clothing. Personal and health care patterns. Production and use of tools. Manufacturing, industrialization. Change of land terrain for home building, farming, industry. Health care services.
Communication systems	Basis for interaction and cohesion. Vehicle for transmission and preservation of the culture. Distinguishes groups from each other.	Language and dialects. Vocabulary and word taboos. Nonverbal behavior. Voice tone, rhythm, speed, pronunciation. Facial expressions, gestures, symbols. Mass media. Computers. Music. Art. Satellites.

TABLE 5-3

Components of All Cultures—continued

Component of the Culture	Purpose or Meaning	Examples
Exchange of goods and services	Production and distribution of goods and services. Work roles. Payment. Obtain at least necessities or luxury, depending on culture.	Barter. Trade. Commerce. Financial institutions. Economic policies. Regulatory mechanisms. Health care institutions and services.
Travel and transportation	Provision for obtaining goods and services. Mobility within and across cultures, societies, nations.	Walk. Use of animals, such as dog, llama, horse, oxen. System of car, truck, railway, air travel transport.
Social controls; institutions of government	Maintenance of order. Organization of people, society, government. Regulation of time and activity. Power systems.	**Mores,** *morally binding attitudes.* **Customs,** *long-established practices having force of unwritten laws.* Value systems. Laws. Policies. Regulations. Public or group opinion. Political offices; kingships; dictators.
Forms of property	Necessities to maintain survival. May contribute to person's worth, status, social position.	Personal belongings. Personal property. Real estate. Financial institutions and systems.
Human response patterns	Family relationships structure other relationships and "taken-for-granted" activities to maintain the group. Values, beliefs, attitudes taught for socialization of person into culture. Ready-made solutions to life problems and goal achievements. Relationships structured by age, sex, status, wealth, power, number of kin, wisdom.	Rules for all social interaction, handling competition, conflict, cooperation, and games. Intimate habits of daily living personally and in groups. Manner in which one's body, home, property perceived. Daily "taken-for-granted" activities and interactions. Use of time and space. Health care roles and practices.
Family and sexual patterns	Maintain structure for care and support of others. Regulate relationships for survival, harmony, generational longevity.	Wedding ceremonies. Birth, childbearing practices. Family division of labor. Roles assigned to men, women, children. Inheritance rights. Care of elderly. Guardianships. Forms of kinship. Divorce proceedings, or removal of undesired member, such as infanticide, burial of woman with husband, or elders leaving tribe to die. Use of time and space.
Knowledge	Survival and expansion of group and desired practices. Contributes to improved living standards through inventions, products, practices, services. Technologic innovation, mobility to higher social status.	Reasoning process. Education system, informal and local, formal and national. Skills. Values. **Science,** *systematized knowledge based on observation, study, experimentation.* Traditions. Folklore. Folk and scientific medical, nursing, and health care practices.
Belief system	Guides behavior of individuals and group during daily life, at special events, occasions, celebrations. Provides meaning to life and death. Indicates priorities. Guides health and illness behavior.	Religion. Ethical codes. Magical ideas and practices. Taboos. Rituals. Methodology. Philosophy. Organized institution of the church. Values and norms.
Artistic and aesthetic expression	Expression of meaning in life and death, feelings ranging from joy to sorrow, depending on situation. Spiritual expression. Expression of individual talents. Health promotion. Therapy and rehabilitation in illness.	Painting. Music. Dance. Architecture. Sculpture. Literature. Aesthetic expression also in body adornment. Use and decoration of space and surrounding environment, such as floral gardens.
Recreation and leisure activities	Socialization. Use of leisure time. Travel to other cultures.	Play activities and tools. Games. Organized sports. Leisure activities depend on climate, terrain, available time, resources.

and **current** (*changing*) *values*, however, are seen in the United States among ethnic populations as well as among Caucasians. **Table 5-4** lists both traditional and current values. Some values show conflict between ideal and manifested values and behavior, based on values held by different generations and the erosion of some basic values over the years (3, 8, 9, 36, 47, 57, 104).

Adapt your assessment, care plans, and intervention to accommodate elderly and middle-aged people and people from some religious groups or regions who adhere primarily to traditional values. Be as accepting of this group as you are of clients who demonstrate behaviors that are based on current value systems. *No one person embodies all the statements in* **Table 5-4**. The culture and values of U.S. families are also presented in Chapter 6. ∞

African American cultural values differ from the dominant cultural values in several ways, as shown in **Table 5-5**. No one person is embodied by all the statements listed in **Table 5-5** (2, 4, 6, 39, 81, 104, 112, 127). *Variations of African American values arise because of geographic location, degree of acculturation and assimilation, socioeconomic status, educational level, and occupation or profession.*

Validate with African American clients to determine values that are basic to assessment, planning of care, and intervention. Listen to the person, question to clarify, and modify nursing care measures to foster cultural comfort in the client.

American Indians and Alaskan Native people *have values and behaviors or lifestyles that are in conflict with some values of U.S. society and the health care system.* For example, they value nature; many people in the United States believe that environmental resources are to be used for self-benefit. A persistent sense of family responsibility is traditional to American Indians, in contrast to mainstream U.S. society. Although family members leave the reservation to find work, they are expected to return to visit relatives or for emergencies and life cycle or tribal rituals. When cultural values of sharing, cooperation, and mutual dependence conflict with the demands of a job, American Indians face a difficult choice. If the call to attend a funeral or help a sick relative comes when a worker cannot take time off, the decision may be to give up the job. Employers are not always understanding of the values underlying the behavior (2, 15, 35, 37, 71, 121). The health care appointment will be forgotten and personal health care measures may be neglected in order to meet family obligations.

American Indian values, such as assistance to others, family harmony, gentleness to and love of the natural environment, inclusion in community, respect for group members, care of the elderly, and cooperation instead of competition, are useful values for all of our society to learn and practice. In contrast to the movies, myths, and legends about the *American Indian,* early settlers survived because of the good will and assistance of various Native people. In some tribal nations such as the Iroquois and Hopi, women consistently have had a central role in community and governmental affairs (2, 15, 35, 37, 71). Health care workers must work with the elders and leaders to present health promotion services.

Second- and third-generation Latino or Spanish-speaking Americans have strong values of loyalty to the family and the larger kin group that act as support networks. Yet, educational and socioeconomic advances have paralleled a reduction in the size of their households and the development of individual and family, rather than community, orientation. Just as for American Indian students, the competitiveness against others that is part of the educational system is avoided, and children may not make the high

TABLE 5-4

Values of Dominant or Mainstream Culture in the United States

Traditional Values Practiced by Elders and Adults from Diverse U.S. Cultures and Conservative Religions	Current Values Practiced by Adolescents, Young Adults, and Baby Boomers
1. Marriage and children. Family stability; try to resolve or live with issues. Patriarchal.	1. Variety of alternative lifestyles. Marriage not considered permanent or only way of life. Divorce, a way out of issues or if lack of satisfaction in relationship.
2. Sexual activity in relationships if there is affection and commitment. Heterogeneous relationships.	2. Sexual relationships for self-satisfaction. Same-sex and bisexual relationships acceptable.
3. Willingness to sacrifice for good of family members and children. Role of parents/family to discipline and guide children, help children find answers. "Children seen, not heard."	3. Smaller families. Children are the center of attention in activities. Children expected to solve problems for self; given less discipline.
4. Socialization of child used to develop social conscience.	4. Mass media, information systems, electronic games, and computer technology used for education, personal enhancement, and to influence masses.
5. Work ethic, follow directions. Goal of work is to provide for life, status, success. Loyal to employer. Quality workmanship given to and appreciated by employer.	5. Decreasing work ethic. Increasing emphasis on leisure, recreation, and time to indulge self. Work should be enjoyable and creative. Loyalty to self and technology. Less loyalty between employer and employees.

TABLE 5-4

Values of Dominant or Mainstream Culture in the United States—continued

Traditional Values Practiced by Elders and Adults from Diverse U.S. Cultures and Conservative Religions	Current Values Practiced by Adolescents, Young Adults, and Baby Boomers
6. Rules of conduct, etiquette, socially acceptable behavior. Honest responses may be blunt. Tries to be sensitive to effect of behavior on others.	6. Decreased emphasis on etiquette. Informal approach; disregard rules of behavior. Don't care about effect of behavior on others. Self-absorbed. Less gentleness. Societal focus with sex, alternative lifestyles, and experimentation.
7. Materialistic. Thrifty. Economic security for present and future. Upward mobility important.	7. Materialistic consumerism for present excitement, enjoyment, prestige. Money and things taken for granted. Sense of entitlement.
8. Equality of people an ideal. Recognize differences. Inequality accepted, believed to be related to personal abilities or background.	8. Equal opportunity for people. Differences accepted and diversity expected. More freedom for personal choices. Respect for ability to perform. Desire to reduce inequality the ideal.
9. Rugged individualism but also cooperation with group on larger projects.	9. "Do your own thing" emphasized. Group conformity and peer relations during school and teen years, while seeking individual identity.
10. Emphasis on individual and competition, achievement, success. Conscious of social status.	10. Competition, emphasis on team sports. Aggressive and violent behavior accepted. Manipulate others to be successful. Disrespect for social status of others.
11. Authoritarian outlook. Respect for the offices of institutional and political leadership. Patriotic. Efforts maintain democracy and freedom.	11. Question all leadership and institutions. Apathy to or disrespect for leaders. Renewal of patriotism in some people.
12. Self-reliance. Responsible behavior. Gender-based division of labor. Self-sufficiency. Long-range planning.	12. Lack of long-range planning. Use others in system. Irresponsible behavior acceptable. More flexibility in division of labor.
13. Youth and beauty. Health, strength, and activity.	13. Youthful appearance, stylish. Health is a goal.
14. Future orientation. Interest in long-term goals. Willing to defer immediate satisfaction.	14. Present outcome emphasized. Immediate answers and satisfaction expected.
15. Education for social, geographic, economic, occupational stability. Science a focus. May keep same job a number of years.	15. Education for immediate goals and job changer. Mass and electronic media as an education tool; used to manipulate ideas and values, create desire for products, or change behavior.
16. Problem oriented; systematic in approach to life. Thoughtfulness valued; time for thinking and making good choices.	16. Concerned about outcomes and their evidence. Contemplation not valued. Status oriented.
17. Use of practical or functional goods or products. Keep objects considered valuable or sentimental. Maintain basic knowledge and skills.	17. New products. Utilize technology, automation, and disposable products. Recycle items for environment or for book fairs. Constant updating of knowledge and skills. Frequent job changes.
18. Speed. Change. Progress. Efficiency. Time important, scheduled.	18. Increasing demand for immediate output. Change even more rapid. Sense of hurry and no sense of control over time or schedules. A sense of "Hurry up and wait" at times.
19. Maintain or change the environment. Use environmental resources for societal and own needs.	19. Effort to save environment and resources in conflict with demand for products. Waste of resources.
20. Volunteerism, sense of humanitarianism, concern for others in trouble or disaster. Continued caretaking. Active in community organizations and activities.	20. Generosity to people in acute trouble. Robot or machine-like performance by people is expected. Concern about effects on self from helping others (legal or codependency) but also sense of volunteerism in some.

TABLE 5-5

Comparison of Selected African American Values and Dominant Cultural Values in the United States

Value	African American Culture	Dominant U.S. Culture
Psychological connections	Individual secondary to family and group. Individuality cannot be separated from group, concern for "brothers and sisters." Progress of group and younger people more important than that of self-involved individual. Members of group may share disappointments or concerns of group. Sense of connectedness and concern about neighborhood may be decreased if more socialized into dominant culture.	Primacy of the individual. Each person master of own destiny. Each citizen to carry own weight and be rewarded according to abilities and effort expended. Person esteemed for achievements. Group benefits from combined efforts of individual members; person feels less accountable for group's faults.
Openness to feelings and emotions	Emotions acknowledged; a natural flow of emotional release. Emotions expressed; all actions; song, dance, poetry, drama, sculpture, speech patterns. Engage in emotionality, such behavior is "real."	Emotional feelings expressed less spontaneously. Behavior cognitively examined for motives to understand another or self. Behavior governed by cognitive emphasis.
Social values	Home, family, and faith are centers of values rather than workplace. Presence, being with another is important.	Workplace, achievement, and material innovation valued as highly as home and family.
Time perspective	Time divided into natural units—day and night, seasons. Spontaneous use of time. Meetings and get-togethers scheduled around natural cycles. Emphasis on time is not a behavior of choice, but clock time is followed as necessary daily living. Exactness about time not expected or required. Time not artificially planned.	Time dissected into seconds, minutes, hours. Activities and meetings scheduled. Exactness about time expected and often required.
Direct experience	Person experiences reality through direct involvement; learning constantly occurs in interaction with environment. Learning not confined to classroom but gained through life experience. Book knowledge not as important as being able to put knowledge "to the test" of experience. Analogies often used and based on real experience.	Knowledge from electronic media, experience and books valued. Abstract learning and problem solving emphasized.
Oral tradition	Themes in the language are (1) emotional content, (2) realness, (3) resilience, (4) interrelatedness, (5) value of direct experience, and (6) distrust and deception. Black English provides organization to communicate unique cultural ideas. Careful about use of words and how expressed in order to be understood and accurate. Use body language and gestures instead of words.	Standard English follows different grammatical rules and syntax. Less attention to covert meanings of words.
Spirituality	Reality of the spiritual acknowledged and accepted as a basic part of self and central to life. Religion highly valued. Each person expected to know God personally. Many have a strong attachment to religion. Prayer and supernatural forces often seen as cause of events.	Religion as value varies with group. Spirituality often overlooked by mainstream psychological thought. Often less open expression about spirituality even if person has deep faith. More openly discussed than previously.
Creative improvisation	A group may perform as an act while each member also does creative improvisation. More spontaneous. Everything is part of a larger process, functionally connected.	Creativity appreciated. Performances may be more structured, less improvisation.

TABLE 5-5

Comparison of Selected African American Values and Dominant Cultural Values
in the United States—continued

Value	African American Culture	Dominant U.S. Culture
Family	Strong, close bond and loyalty to family, including elders, and extended family. Intricate family bonds include more than blood relatives. "Mixed" or "blended" family rather than "stepfamily." Members may speak for each other.	Focus on nuclear family, but include extended family. Stepparent family may create complex network with ambiguous bonds of support.
Education	Education emphasized as way to improve self and social status and to gain success.	Education valued as way to improve self, social status, and achieve success.
Privacy issues	Talk about financial status more openly. Sexuality less openly discussed.	Talk about sexuality more openly. Financial status less openly discussed.

grades in school that are likely to ensure continued educational and employment success (2, 37, 121).

The traditional Southern Appalachian population may have a value system that is almost on the opposite end of the continuum from the upper-middle-class professional in the urban U.S. culture, as shown in **Table 5-2** (53, 54). If the person moves from the traditional Appalachian culture to an educational institution or workplace in the dominant society, cultural value conflicts may be experienced.

Spanish-speaking, Middle-Eastern American, American Indian, and Asian American groups value indirect communication, modesty, cooperation with the team, and conformity to the group rather than the U.S. values of assertiveness and independence of the individual. Young adults may be discouraged from abruptly leaving home or striving for independence. Consideration for family elders is more important than desires to pursue personal goals (2, 37, 81). *Education or counseling that is counter to these values and behaviors will be ignored.*

Use of time varies with the culture and historical era. For example, in the Western world, time is seen as a progression of events, of new beginnings. Timetables are important. Appointments are to be kept by patients. Mass transportation and mass media have timetables. Currently in the United States, people are often hasty, impatient, and not attentive; they want things to be quickly and easily acquired. Many cultures do not emphasize promptness, hurry, or time schedules (2, 37, 81). These clients do not feel comfortable with the time orientation of the health care system, which may interfere with obtaining health care services.

COMPARISON OF CULTURAL PATTERNS: LATINO, JAPANESE, AND MIDDLE EASTERN
Focus: Latino and Japanese Cultures

Tables C5-1 through C5-7 on the Companion Website contrast and summarize Spanish-speaking American cultures in the south-

western United States and Japanese culture (2, 7, 37, 81, 83, 104). These tables are presented to focus on major values and related behaviors of each group. *The tables are not meant to be all-inclusive for the groups discussed.* Although many nationality groups fit under the Spanish-speaking category, each has its *unique values* and customs. The values, norms, customs, and behaviors described in the tables are *generally applicable* to people who have a Spanish/ Latino/or Japanese background. *Variations in expression of these values depend on where the person or family with a Latin background lives. Values may be expressed differently if the person resides in Spain, Mexico, or Japan rather than the United States.*

Assess and intervene with clients and their families according to the values and characteristics presented in these tables in the Companion Website. *The information is neither a comprehensive study nor a stereotype of everyone in these cultures.* In your culturally competent intervention, it is important to understand that these cultural patterns will be followed by different persons in each culture to varying degrees, ignored by some, and not identified yet taken for granted by others.

Focus: Middle Eastern Culture

The information presented in the Companion Website does not cover every Middle Eastern country but is applicable to Lebanon, Syria, Jordan, Arabia, Egypt, Central Asia, Turkey, Afghanistan, Iran, and Palestine. Refer to the Companion Website for information pertinent to assessment and health promotion for the individual and family system (1, 2, 37, 58, 82, 85).

BELIEFS ABOUT HEALTH AND ILLNESS

How health is defined, physically and emotionally, varies from culture to culture, as do ideas about the factors related to health and disease. Definitions generally used in the United States are presented in Chapter 2. ∞ The following discussion compares the beliefs of U.S. residents about health and illness with the corresponding beliefs of people who are from African American, Latino, or Japanese cultures.

Dominant or Mainstream U.S. Culture

Beliefs in the United States toward health influence your work as a health care professional; beliefs and attitudes are influenced considerably by society's emphasis on mastery of the environment as opposed to adjustment to it. Illness is perceived as a challenge to be met by mobilizing resources: research, science, funds, institutions, and people. Because independence is highly valued, clients are expected to help themselves as much as possible. Self-care is emphasized. A person is evaluated on productivity or "doing well." Because the ability to be productive depends in part on health, individual health is highly valued. Health in the broadest sense is considered necessary for successful interaction with others, educational accomplishment, ability to work, leadership, child rearing, and capacity to use opportunities. Medical, nursing, and other health sciences and technology are considered important. The physical cause of illness is generally accepted. More and more, the psychological and sociocultural causes of disease are also being emphasized.

The United States boasts of its medical research, technologically advanced medical care, and well-educated health care professionals. It devotes a high share of national income to medical care. Yet, it is more economical, more effective, and easier to keep people healthy than it is to cure disease. Doctors, researchers, and medical care facilities have little effect on general health if the population lacks basic disease prevention and health promotion measures (94). *There is increasing focus on* (a) advanced technology in health care; (b) interdisciplinary care, coordination, and integration of services; (c) use of complementary and alternative therapies; (d) wellness and prevention programs; (e) awareness and reduction of risk factors; (f) intensive use of information, including electronic; (g) consumer or client evaluation of services; (h) evidence-based outcomes of intervention rather than process of intervention; and (i) emphasis on same or better care, with fewer resources, as a result of Medicare, Medicaid, and welfare reform.

African American Culture

Beliefs about health and illness generally stem from the African belief that life is a process rather than a state. Beliefs in the African American population about illness and health care vary, depending on educational and occupational background, experience with the effects of poverty, accessibility to health care services, discriminatory practices toward the ill person, and the extent to which traditional healing methods have been effective to prevent and treat illness. Beliefs in some clients may reflect a combination of African heritage maintained through the days of slavery and incorporate American Indian and White colonial life patterns. Or, beliefs may reflect the latest scientific knowledge (37, 112).

African Americans believe all things influence each other, whether living or dead. Health incorporates mind, body, and spirit; illness results when these are not in harmony or balance. Thus, natural or supernatural causes, including evil spirits or demons, may result in disease or an illness experience (112).

Health is maintained or restored and illness treated through a variety of practices: extra rest, prayer and laying on of hands;

certain foods, herbs or roots, laxatives; massage, application of a poultice made from a combination of substances, heat or cold applications; or magical practices such as voodoo. Some practices may have been handed down for generations and may be the same as used by people for traditional healing in the dominant culture, such as poultices, massage, heat or cold, or herbs. Faith in God, the church or community healer, and the healing practices is a key factor; healing may occur despite scientific odds against recovery. Expectations about outcomes are a major influence. If the person believes in a negative prediction or that he or she has been placed under a spell, hex, or evil spirit, recovery may not occur. Early death may occur despite medical intervention (37, 112).

African Americans who are Muslims follow the beliefs and practices of the Islam religion described in the Companion Website in the section Middle East culture and Chapter 7 ∞ of the text. Lifestyle is strictly regulated; self-discipline is emphasized. No pork foods or products and many of the "soul foods" are not consumed; they are considered unclean. Muslims believe "you are what you eat" and the food eaten affects behavior. Alcohol beverages and tobacco are usually avoided (112).

Leading causes of death are the same for African Americans and Caucasians: diseases of the heart, malignant neoplasms, and cerebrovascular diseases. Infant mortality, though declining, is higher for the African American population. Death rates caused by diabetes, HIV/AIDS, and homicide are also higher, although death from suicide is lower except for young adult African American males. Some clients may experience cultural illnesses, such as **"falling out,"** *a sudden collapse without warning that is preceded by a feeling of dizziness or "swimming" in the head,* or a **"spell,"** *a trance-like state in which the person may be observed communicating with a deceased relative or a spirit* (2, 37, 112). African Americans are more likely to have lactose intolerance, sickle-cell anemia, tooth decay, and periodontal disease (112). A higher incidence of HIV/AIDS and sexually transmitted diseases, especially syphilis, has been found in African American recruits for the Armed Forces than in Caucasian recruits (112).

Latino Culture

Beliefs and attitudes may be traditional, based on the person's country of origin, or may combine traditional and dominant culture beliefs and behaviors, depending on the person's acculturation. Use the following information to give care that is culturally relevant for the person who has a Latino background.

Spanish-speaking people consider the self to be a whole person; thus, "better health" has no meaning. Good health is associated with the ability to work and fulfill normal roles, for one gains and maintains respect by meeting one's responsibilities. Criteria of health are a sturdy body, ability to maintain normal physical activity, and absence of pain. A person does not have to have perfect health; as long as the family is around, he or she is all right. Thus, preventive measures are not highly valued. Caring for self, however, occurs through moderation in eating, drinking, work, recreation, and sleep, and by leading a good life (104).

Latinos who retain Spanish as their first language and who do not know English or follow American norms and values are much less likely than their more assimilated counterparts to use health services. Attitudes and feelings toward access to services and screening processes, values about privacy, and sociodemographic factors are strong determinants of Latino health practices (2, 10, 37, 81, 83).

Latino people believe that hardship and suffering are part of destiny and that the reward for being submissive to God's will and for doing good comes in the next life. Ill health is accepted as part of life and is thought to be caused by an unknown external event or object, such as natural forces of cold, heat, storms, and water, or as the result of sinning—acting against God's will. Preventive measures are perceived as being unfaithful to God. One cause of illness is thought to be bad air, especially night air, which enters through a cavity or opening in the body. Thus, a raisin may be placed on the cord stump of the newborn, and surgery is avoided if possible, to prevent air from entering the body. Avoiding drafts, keeping windows closed at night, keeping the head covered, and following certain postpartum practices have the same basis. Other causes of disease, according to traditional beliefs, include overwork, poor food, excess worry or emotional strain, undue exposure to weather, uneven wetting of the body, taking a drink when overheated, and giving blood for transfusion. Underlying this thinking is the concept **yin** or "*cold*" and **yang** or "*hot*" or the *hot and cold theory of disease* (2, 37, 83).

The **hot and cold theory of disease** *does not always refer to the physical temperature of foodstuff, but also to the effects that certain substances have or are thought to have on the body.* Basically all diseases are classified as hot or cold. Arthritis, pregnancy, the postpartum period, cancer, pneumonia, colds, headaches, earaches, and teething are cold diseases or conditions. Hot diseases are fever, infections, diarrhea, rashes, ulcers, and constipation. It is considered dangerous to be outdoors at night if one's body is warm. Beliefs about which foods are warm and cold vary from one geographic region and culture to another. For example, prenatal vitamins may be a hot food and will not be taken during pregnancy (a hot condition) unless swallowed with fruit juice (a cold food). All foods, herbs, and medicines are classified as hot or cold. Avocado, fresh vegetables, dairy products, fish, and chicken are cold foods. Aspirin, cornmeal, eggs, beef, waterfowl, cereal grains, and chili peppers are considered hot. A goal is to balance the body; a hot disease is cured with a cold food and a cold disease is cured with a hot food, herb, or medication. Thus, aspirin could be taken for arthritis, which also fits into the Western medical system (2, 37).

The person goes to bed when too ill to work or move. Treatment from a folk healer is sought if family care does not help. A physician is called only when the person is gravely ill. The sick person does not withdraw from the group; doing so would only make him or her feel worse. *Acceptance of fate* (**fatalism**) amounts to saying, "If the Lord intends for me to die, I'll die." The discomfort of the present is considered, but not in terms of future complications. Communicable diseases are hard to control, for resistance to isolation is based on the idea that family members, relatives, and familiar objects cannot contaminate or cause illness. Taking home remedies, wearing special articles, and performing special ceremonies are accepted ways of getting and staying well. The person feels he or she will keep well by observing the ritual calendar, being brotherly, and being a good Catholic and member of the community. Any procedure, such as a diagnostic x-ray, is considered to be the treatment and hence the person believes he or she should be cured (2, 37, 81, 83, 112).

Accidents are feared because they disrupt the wholeness of the person. In addition, Latinos fear surgery, the impersonality of the hospital and nurses, and any infringement on modesty. The hospital represents death and isolation from family or friends. Several authors describe specific health care practices of Spanish-speaking people and families and nursing implications, including those for childbirth, childrearing, and prevention of communicable diseases. They also discuss customs related to use of folk medicine, use of surnames, and customs of interaction (2, 37, 112).

A common illness in this culture, **susto**, with *symptoms of agitation and depression, results from traumatic, frightening experiences and may result in death.* **Empacho** *is a gastrointestinal disease that results from eating food that is disliked, from overeating, or from eating hot bread.* **Caida de mollera** (*fallen fontanel*) *is caused by a child falling or someone pulling the nipple out of the mouth too quickly, and results in crying, vomiting, diarrhea, fever, restlessness, sunken eyes, and inability to grasp the nipple.* Hydration is essential in treatment. **Resfriado** (*chilled*) *results from getting wet and not changing to dry clothes.* In turn, **catarro constipado** (*head cold or sinusitis*) *may result.* Disease may also result from organs or parts of the body moving from the normal position. Little attention is paid to colds, minor aches, or common gastrointestinal disorders. **Mal ojo, "evil eye,"** *is a disease that is believed to result when a person looks admiringly at the child of another. Symptoms include headaches, fever, crying, diarrhea, vomiting, weight loss, insomnia, and sunken eyes* (2, 37, 112).

Avoid casting an "evil eye." Do not openly admire a child. Any such statements or actions must be accompanied by patting the child on the head or giving a light slap to prevent illness.

The role of the family is important in time of illness. The head of the house, the male, determines whether illness exists and what treatment is to be given. Obtaining assessment data, planning of care, and intervention must be directed to the male head of household. The "professional" (Anglo) approach is regarded as showing indifference to needs and the cause of anxiety and discomfort.

Japanese Culture

Use the following information to give care that is culturally relevant to the person of Japanese descent. Some of the concepts are applicable to clients from other Asian cultures. Attitudes in Japan toward health strongly reflect the belief in a body–mind–spirit interrelationship. Spiritual and temporal affairs in life are closely integrated; thus, health practices and religion are closely intertwined, influenced considerably by the magicoreligious practices of Shinto, Japan's ancient religion. Bathing customs stem from Shinto purification rites; for example, baths are taken in the evening before eating, not only for cleanliness but for ceremony and relaxation as well (2, 37).

There is strong emphasis on healthy diet (low fat, low sugar), physical fitness and strength, an intact body, determination, family and group relationships, and long life. Self-discipline in daily habits is highly valued, as are the mental, spiritual, and aesthetic aspects of the person. All of these values promote health and remain equally important to the sick person to promote recovery (2, 37).

As a child, the individual is taught to minimize reactions to injury and illness. Hence to the Westerner a sick person may appear **stoic**, *calm and reserved in expressing emotion and pain.* This behavior is also influenced by childrearing and interaction practices, which emphasize correct behavior, suppression of emotion, and independence. However, because of the 21st-century issues of crime and terrorism, parents are becoming more concerned about teaching young children to be self-sufficient by commuting unattended to school (75). The sick person, as much as one who is well, expects to be treated with respect and resents being addressed abruptly or informally by first name. The person also resents people entering the hospital room without knocking. The Japanese man resents being dominated by women, and he may feel uncomfortable with an American female health care professional because he interprets her behavior as overbearing. The person is eager to cooperate with the medical care program and wishes to be included in planning and decisions regarding care. The so-called professional approach of the average U.S. health care provider is likely to insult the average Japanese person, although he or she may be too polite to say so (2, 37, 81).

Socioeconomic Level Subculture

Research about social stratification indicates that *a person's class or caste position is influenced by economic and social status and political power of the family, which in turn affects formation of values, attitudes, lifestyle, and health* (104). Socioeconomic level is not determined only by income but also by educational level, residential area, and occupation of the head of household. It includes associated advantages and disadvantages, opportunities and limitations, past and future prospects, as well as present status of a group (104). Each income level in any country tends to have a more or less specified set of values and role expectations regarding practically every area of human activity. Social class includes a group consciousness. Yet, in the United States, economic level is not always a clear-cut distinction. People can be anywhere on the continuum and move along the continuum (104). However, the lower the educational level and occupational preparation and skills, the less likely the person is to move upward on the continuum. Further, people may be objectively placed within a certain class, but they are sometimes accorded a different status by others around them. Or, they may see themselves at yet a different status level, based on race, gender, religion, ancestry, ethnic origin, education, or wealth in material goods (104). The income of the person may rise significantly while

Practice Point

As you gain general knowledge about values, beliefs, and lifestyles of people in various economic levels, realize that no one person encompasses all that the literature describes. Knowledge about socioeconomic levels and lifestyles is essential to your assessment, planning, interventions, and evaluation of effectiveness. Avoid stereotyping people because of this knowledge but be aware of differences so that you give culturally competent care at all levels of prevention.

values, norms, patterns of thought and social interaction, and health practices may remain the same. To move from one economic level to another means giving up familiar relationships and patterns while assuming new ones (104).

The American ideal is upward mobility. For example, many African Americans, through education and effort, are now members of the upper, as well as other, economic levels (21). Upward mobility occurs in other cultural groups also.

THE UPPER-UPPER, AFFLUENT, OR CORPORATE LEVEL

The **upper-upper economic group** *consists of a relatively small number of people (about 1%) who own a disproportionate share of personal wealth and whose income is largely derived from ownership of investments, business, and property. Their work, profession, or business and family connections provide prestige, status, honor, wealth, and power.* Members of this level include the **very rich** *who have accumulated great fortunes—multimillions and billions—and the associated economic opportunities and advantages* (21, 104). According to a national survey, of these approximately 3 million people in the United States, about 338,400 households were worth at least $10 million (21). They include the **corporate rich** *who accumulate and retain high incomes with fringe benefits, and enjoy corporate and taxation privileges that are part of the newer system of the incorporated U.S. economy* (21). In turn, they maintain loyalty to and stay anchored in the specific corporation to maintain their benefits, including after retirement (3, 104). This group has both money and power, and it can control how its assets are used as well as various other financial, business, commercial, legal, and political aspects of society. The decisions made by this group affect everyone else (21, 42, 104).

These individuals *have had family lineage, inherited wealth, and power for several generations.* They are acknowledged by the general public and themselves as influential and leaders locally, nationally, and internationally. They feel obliged to tend their own financial and material resources well, obtain the best possible education, demonstrate impeccable tastes, and take care of their health so that they can meet their philanthropic and social obligations (104). The affluent family has many connections, belongs to elite clubs or organizations, and also participates in and contributes considerably to the community and society as a whole through financial contributions and volunteer activities. Yet, the very rich remain anonymous to most Americans, unless for some reason they are given media coverage (57, 104).

This person or family lives in an exclusive residential area in a house where the atmosphere is spatial, elegant, and formal and affords privacy from the masses. This person or family may own several estates in different areas of the country (or world), in the best locations, furnished with family heirlooms and works of art, and used in different seasons or for different purposes. The family may have a number of people to help maintain its lifestyle, such as a maid, butler, gardener, and other staff members (21, 104).

The children are reared by a governess, a nanny, or a maid, as well as the parents. The mother usually is selective in her teaching, guiding, and care. Certain aspects of rearing are done only by the mother, others only by the nanny or governess. The children may

TABLE 5-6

Comparison of Values of Persons in Upper and Upper-Middle Economic Levels

Upper-Level Values	Upper-Middle-Level Values
Family name, lineage, traditions, position, home, adult oriented. Entitled to privileged lifestyle.*	Family stability and prestige, future plans, child oriented.
Privacy, seclusion (person is prey to publicity, slander), but connections to right people important.	Friendliness, sociability, pleasantness, patience in relationships, honesty, interpersonal sensitivity.
Education, knowledge in breadth and depth respected, knowledge for knowledge's sake.	Education, creativity, problem solving, concepts, and abstractions used and enjoyed.
Philanthropy with the arts, civic causes, societal projects for improvement.* Includes international focus.	Service and financial contributions to one or several social causes, locally, nationally.
Professional/career achievements, success, choices.*	Professional/career success, achievement.
Service to and leadership of others, the wider community, civic events, nationally and even internationally; altruism, volunteerism.	Community involvement and leadership; local or regional focus, compassion for less fortunate.
High expectations and goals for family; initiative, sense of responsibility.	High goals; being responsible; initiative, plan for future.
Influence; power; prestige; patriotism.*	Democracy; patriotism.
Economic achievements, limitless abundance, acquire financial and material resources for future.*	Upward economic and social mobility; economic security.
Being strong; willpower; control or discipline over emotions, appearance, actions. Being self-directed but flexible; responsible.	Ability to withstand stress; spontaneous in emotions and actions. Appearance influenced by societal trends.
Excellence of performance; competence, success in activities, including leisure activities.*	Hard work; competence; success; postpone immediate gratification for highly desirable goal.
Traditional patterns in lifestyle, choice of educational institutions and business pursuits.	Change, societal progress.
Possession of cultural artifacts and art pieces; consumption of material goods. Designer clothes.*	Material comfort; consumption of material goods; value objects gained by hard work. Quality of good important.
Travel widely to seek intellectually stimulating experiences; wide association with others.*	Leisure activity; travel for enjoyment and educational opportunity.

*Values of the Lower-Upper Level.

feel closer to the parent surrogates than to the parents. They are educated in schools with fine reputations. They, like the parents, live with choices. They have many opportunities to follow the arts, learn certain sports, and travel worldwide. The children know the importance and value of the possessions and opportunities that surround them. They recognize the importance of self-control, of following family wishes, and of upholding the family name. They seek privacy and disciplined activity even though in the public view. They expect, and are expected, to be responsible, competent, and successful at their chosen academic, recreational, and social pursuits (57, 104).

Although the upper economic level is adult oriented, children know at an early age that they are special. Parents try to instill a feeling that the children must do well because they have special responsibilities to society upon reaching adulthood. Both adults and children are confident that life will be rewarding. Even crisis, such as illness or surgery, can be made into something basically pleasant, for the best of specialized health care professionals and comprehensive facilities can be obtained, and convalescence frequently involves a trip to and rest at a secluded place (104). **Tables 5-4** and

5-6 list values that are commonly held by people who are in the upper economic level in the United States (3, 36, 42, 57).

THE LOWER-UPPER, OR NEWLY RICH LEVEL

The **lower-upper economic group** *consists of people whose wealth is more recently acquired and who have become well known and influential. They have publicity, national recognition, and a lifestyle of their own but borrow considerably from the ways of the established upper class while living current values* described in **Table 5-4**. They are the new industrialists, the executives of major manufacturing firms or banking systems, business owners, developers and contractors, or prominent tradespeople who use their wealth to generate, competitively, more wealth. Men and women in this group are the currently well-known mass media professionals, commentators, journalists, movie stars, and television entertainers; chairpersons of technology and data information systems; famous doctors or lawyers; and well-known athletes. Or they may be less famous, such as stock and insurance investors and brokers, manufacturers, international business executives, or employees who have benefited from their company's stock options. They have large incomes, grand homes, and opulent lifestyles that show off their money. These individuals, who are billionaires and millionaires, have accumulated wealth through the stock market and technology rather than by traditional methods, such as manufacturing (21, 104). *Members of the lower-upper level have social position because of what they do* and may slide down into middle-level anonymity if wealth is lost (104).

The person or family has an abundance of possessions and opportunity but may be less humble or more self-conscious about it than the upper-upper-level person. Although this person or family may live in the same secluded community, attend the same activities, travel to the same areas, or send children to the same schools as the upper-upper-level family, this person or family is seen by the long-established wealthy as being different (21, 104). Children are not groomed for philanthropy in the same way as in the upper-upper level; the sense of leisure and entitlement is more apparent (104).

Often a fine line separates old and new wealth in a community; such intangibles as social charm or likeability, family background, religion, area and value of residence, and schools attended make the difference. Females, as well as males, work and are involved in community service. Or females may do consultant work to feel worthwhile, to provide structure to the day, or to avoid being important only through the spouse. These families, like the upper-upper-level members, fund foundations; such foundations rival governmental sources of money and have a tremendous impact on society. Some values of members in this economic level are listed in **Table 5-6** and are indicated by an asterisk (*) (21, 36, 57, 104).

THE POWER-ELITE LEVEL

In the United States, a new social class grouping is emerging: the **power elite**. *These very rich people occupy pivotal positions, have power and reputation just as the upper-upper and lower-upper levels, and may belong to one or the other level. In some ways, their lifestyle is different.* With access to centralized global information, their decisions, or lack of decisions, carry major consequences for the daily life of everyone. They command the major hierarchy of the 200 to 300 largest corporations and social organizations and have positions in the social structure and institutions of state and military establishment. They set up jobs for many thousands of workers. They create consumer and societal demands and cause others to meet them. They shape educational, religious, and family institutions. The lifestyles of these individuals are not confined by ordinary family responsibilities. Global travel takes them to many hotels and mansions; they are not bound to any specific community. They transcend ordinary environments and people. Yet, they do not operate alone. Advisors, consultants, spokespersons, and opinion makers often contribute to decisions, including personal health care practices (86).

THE CREATIVE LEVEL

The U.S. economy has been built on manufacturing (the upper-class executive level) and on service (the middle and lower economic levels). However, the economy has been changing; a new class is emerging (34). The **creative-class level** is *made up of about 30 million people who make their living principally by being mentally creative. Members include scientists, engineers, artists in all talent areas, musicians, computer program experts, and knowledge-based professionals.* They may be in either the lower-upper or upper-middle economic levels. This nearly 33% of the workforce generates considerable wealth, earning, on the average, twice that of workers in manufacturing or service jobs (34).

Human creativity is not limited to the people in this level. Everyone is creative in some way on the job, as they handle tasks or people, or make suggestions for workplace improvements. However, people in this group integrate traditional and current values described in **Tables 5-4 and 5-5** differently than do other groups (34).

Values, attitudes, and norms of the creative-class members include the following (34):

1. **Individuality and autonomy**–resistance to following group-related norms or conforming to organizational or institutional directions; willingness to take risks.
2. **Meritocracy**–desire to achieve through effort and excellent finality of work and production, and to be recognized accordingly.
3. **Diversity and openness**–an acceptance and enjoyment of people who differ from the self and who are nonstandard in approach to life.
4. **Self-expression**–freedom to focus on expressing ideas, talents, and creativity rather than to focus on survival or the routine.
5. **Responsibility**–responding to challenges and expectations of the workplace.
6. **Flexibility and autonomy in the workplace**–not being constrained by a time schedule, adjusting schedule to fit the work to be done.
7. **Time**–to balance work demands, life responsibilities, and leisure activities.
8. **Professional development**–continuing to learn and generate ideas.
9. **Seeking stimulating people to work with**–feeling esteem for and esteemed by colleagues and the managerial level.
10. **Exciting job content**–opportunity to solve interesting and intellectual problems.
11. **Comfortable organizational job culture**–"good people to work with," feeling "at home" when at work, feeling valued and supported.
12. **Stability in the work environment**–job compensation and benefits that offer job security for mental or creative productivity; job culture more important than salary.

The rise of the creative class and economy is occurring throughout nations of the Western world, as well as in some developing nations. These individuals are less likely to link identity or self-worth to the employer but more to their own interests and achievements. Members of this group are also likely to hire members of the service class to do routine or menial tasks related to living (34).

Stress levels rise as performance, production, and outcomes are rooted in creativity and mental labor. New kinds of social institutions and policies are needed to deal with the societal and value system transformation (34). Health problems may arise from the stress and changes.

THE UPPER-MIDDLE LEVEL

This group, the **top 15% of the middle class,** *is described as those who are well off and are considered to be the backbone of the community.* Income is high but varies ($80,000 to $140,000 average), depending on occupation and geographic area, and accumulating property and investments is important. Each spouse is college-educated and at least one is a professional—doctor, dentist, engineer, business manager, or lawyer. This group is increasingly diverse, made up of Caucasians, African Americans, Asian Americans, and Latinos (21, 36, 79). Their main work is intellectual instead of manual, requires professional training, and offers upward mobility. The workplace is as important to the spouse as to the employed member (2, 3, 21, 104).

They may begin family life in an apartment, but when financially able, they move to a large house in a better part of town or a suburb. Property and investments are gradually accumulated. They may have a maid, a gardener, and several vehicles. They may travel nationally and abroad. They may belong to a semi-elite country club and send their children to private schools and colleges. Family stability and community leadership are valued. They often play a role in local civic and political affairs. The children have a number of opportunities educationally and culturally; in return, they are expected to be successful academically and socially. The children are often involved in a number of prestigious out-of-home activities and organizations, as are the parents, and the children may actually have fewer home responsibilities than the child in an upper-class family. Child rearing is permissive; children are given explanations instead of punishment. These parents exert more direct influence on the child's schooling than parents of the middle or working class. The work ethic is different from the work ethic of the rich. Thus, children may do tasks to earn an allowance and may work at various jobs, such as babysitting, lawn mowing, or in retail or fast-food service, in the teen years to earn extra money. In contrast, parents at higher economic levels do not expect their children to work while attending school. This group has a lifestyle that may involve creative and leisure activities, indoor or outdoor sports, dancing, theater, museums, and travel or educational experiences. There may be an emphasis on acquiring a deeper self-knowledge and remaining youthful (2, 3, 37, 57, 79, 104). **Table 5-6** lists commonly held values of the upper-middle economic level (2, 3, 36, 42, 57, 79).

Some members of the upper-middle level are referred to as "**relos**" *because they frequently relocate (every 2 to 4 years) due to business and economic trends, job relocations, and demands on the husband or wife as the company expands across the country or internationally.* The relocation, typically a paid move, offers salary and benefit increases, and a home in a master-planned community with adjacent parks and upscale shops. These employees may be electronic engineers, information technology managers, pharmaceutical sales executives, data analysts for plant managers, or regional vice presidents. These are the middle elite in lifestyle, the new itinerant white-collar workers. They experience different stresses from the middle-class worker who experiences forced job change. Changing addresses may help the family and children to be more flexible if there is a strong family cohesion and identity. Or, the family may feel they have no roots, especially the at-home parent and children. They do not know a hometown. In the transition, there may be loss of friends, familiarity, finances, and sometimes treasured belongings. There are no consistent faith, community, or educational systems; no hometown shops; and no long-term neighbors or health care providers. Family members may feel a sense of **anomie,** *being isolated, alone and unknown, with a changing identity shaped by the surroundings* (9, 21).

THE MIDDLE LEVEL

About 42% of the middle economic level place themselves in the **middle-middle economic group,** according to a national survey (21). *The people in this group live a comfortable lifestyle and may purchase material comforts considered in the past to be for the upper class.* Generally, they have less influence in the community than the upper-level members, although they have a professional or specialized education beyond high school. Members of this group are directors of local agencies or organizations, elected officials, newspaper owners, teachers, clergy, health care professionals, artists, skilled workers, office personnel, or sales workers. They may own small or medium-sized businesses. They have a special status because of education and occupation and often work with people, but they do not have much wealth. They collaborate in strategic decision making and coordination of community events, often in liaison with more influential local leaders who have developed the major policies and procedures. People in this group usually own a nicely furnished home in a pleasant residential section and two or three cars or a van. They eat out regularly and vacation annually. They pursue sports or other leisure activities as a family unit as much as possible, but also go to activities separately (2, 3, 21, 36, 79, 104).

Recently, members of this economic level have experienced being forced out of jobs that have been changed, downsized, or eliminated. Those with a college education, even with job loss, are more likely to find a new job or develop a new niche for themselves. Sometimes they reenter the workforce through a more manual job, earning less and forfeiting benefits. Consequently, the family loses health insurance, dwindling savings must be spent, and house and car ownership may be jeopardized. Lifestyle change for family members may be drastic, and plans for the children or family activities may be altered (21).

Parents in the middle economic level are child oriented; family life often revolves around children and their interests. Families (single- or two-parent) have high aspirations for children and take pride in their accomplishments (104). Parents live and teach many of the traditional values described in **Table 5-4** to ensure their children's future success. They also acknowledge and practice some of the identified current values described in **Table 5-4**, often at their children's urging. They discuss childrearing practices with neighbors, friends, the physician, the nurse, or the child's teacher. Parents are consistently concerned about the child's feelings, try to understand the dynamics of the child's behavior, and mix discipline with permissiveness. Discipline is often in the form of withdrawal of privileges or of disapproval, threats, or appeals to reason (2, 3, 36, 79, 104). Overall, the people in this group use the internist, family-practice physician, pediatrician, and nurse practitioner for routine health care, but the services of specialists are used when indicated. They respect health professionals and want thorough and scientific diagnosis and treatment. They see themselves as knowledgeable about health and appreciate and try to use additional information. These parents are typically responsive to the advice of health care and educational experts (2, 21).

THE LOWER-MIDDLE, WORKING OR SERVICE LEVEL

The **lower-middle level** *is often perceived as those who are just getting by.* Generally both spouses have graduated from high school and may attend community college. They both have jobs as industrial or blue-collar workers, clerical or service workers, agricultural wage earners, technicians, or skilled or semiskilled workers. Many of this group work with machines or tools. Chances for advancement are minimal unless the person pursues further education. Job security is threatened by the effects of automation in the workplace. Many workers who are a part of this economic level are proud of their work, do it very well, and know that *they make an important contribution to society.* Society must have carpenters, plumbers, secretaries, farmers, garbage collectors, and all of the other workers who are in this group. These individuals are stable breadwinners, churchgoers, voters, and family men and women. They may have two jobs and little leisure. Many do not like their jobs but fear not finding another; therefore, they keep the job because of family responsibilities and the hold on respectability that the job brings. What they want most is a decent standard of living, but they are finding it more difficult to support their families (3, 21, 33, 36, 42, 57, 79, 104).

The family either rents or buys a small home with two or three bedrooms or rents an apartment and carefully maintains the home and belongings, including an older car. They have some conveniences but may not own many luxuries. The family depends on the extended family instead of social agencies for economic and emotional support and may be active in church but not in the PTA or other community organizations. In the nuclear family, the man is typically head of the house, and the woman is considered responsible for the home and child care. The family enjoys recreational activities as a family unit (3, 36, 42, 57, 79, 104). The single-parent family, often in this economic level, is described in Chapter 6. ∞ The members of this group have watched and feel concern about the steady erosion of values and customs they consider essential to their perception of a real America. They tend to have the traditional values listed in **Table 5-4.**

Child rearing is taken for granted and is not perceived as something that you do with a preset plan, nor as something that is problematic or to be discussed with others. These parents retain traditional methods of parenting and keep the same goals they were taught as children. Desirable characteristics in the child, according to the parent, include neatness, cleanliness, honesty, obedience, respect for others, trustworthiness, and conformity to externally imposed standards (33, 36, 104).

In this level, work and social roles and the roles of mother and father are more sharply differentiated, and the man and woman may lead separate social lives. The mother is the more supportive parent. Frequently, the father views himself as the economic provider but sees no reason to help shoulder the responsibility of child rearing. If children have the opportunity of education and to move into the middle level, they may slowly change their values and childrearing practices as they outwardly imitate other middle-class parents around them. Yet very often, values do not change and even overt behavior is nearer to that of their parents than that of their newly found middle-class friends (3, 4, 36, 104).

Health care is sought when a person is too sick to work—the group's definition of illness. Prevention is emphasized less than in the foregoing economic levels. People may try home or folk remedies first and then seek medical care. The neighborhood health center will be used if one exists. Dental care is more likely to be neglected than other medical care. Individuals and families in this level respond well to an approach that is respectful, personable, prompt, and thorough. They do not understand why health care should be so costly; most have no health insurance. They may omit very expensive treatments or drugs whenever possible (2).

The **service level** *is a group of people who work alongside members of the creative class to provide necessary services and to do the routine tasks and take care of family functions for which members of the creative class have no time or interest.* They are similar to members of the working class except they are not limited to traditional working-class jobs in manufacturing, construction, and transportation industries (34). This is the largest group in the new economic order. They have influence because of their numbers, the essential work they do, and the people for whom they work. However, they lack autonomy and flexibility typical of the upper, upper-middle, and creative levels (34). Some will leave this level as they pursue education.

The Case Situation depicts a family with traditional and current values and who engage in a lifestyle that combines the creative and service levels.

THE UPPER-LOWER LEVEL

Members of the **upper-lower level** *are those who are having a really hard time. The family is often only one step away from poverty and welfare.* An individual has fewer chances of acquiring education. Members of this group work at menial tasks, usually in nonunion jobs; they are proud to be working. Wages and job benefits are a concern. Individuals may work as domestics, gardeners, hospital or school maintenance or cafeteria workers, garbage collectors, or street cleaners. Often neither husband nor wife has completed high school. The family lives in a substandard apartment in an older building (usually with an absentee landlord), in a mobile home park, or in a small rental home. The family is patriarchal; the woman works but also has all house and child responsibilities. Children are an asset; they leave school early and help support the family. The family enjoys picnics in the park and other free diversions. The family's only long trips are typically for funerals of relatives. Often the family had its beginning in lack of motivation for education, resulting in dropping out of high school because of pregnancy or lack of academic success, early parent-

Case Situation

Melding of Cultures: Rural and Urban, Traditional and Current Values, Creative and Service Levels

Ian, 25 years old, completed a master's degree at Southern Illinois University–Carbondale and then moved from his small rural town to St. Louis. He found employment as a "computer geek" (creative class) in a large corporation known to have a friendly work culture and offer "good benefits." Leisure time was spent in "the Loop" in University City, an area where people of all ages congregate to meet other people, converse, and enjoy food, music, and theaters that represent diverse cultures. There he met Lucy, born in St. Louis and a graduate student in human resources at a nearby university, who was working as a waitress (service class). Courtship and marriage followed. After

a few months in his apartment, they purchased a home in a suburb adjacent to the city, near his workplace and the university to avoid a long commute. The house, about 40 years old, was well built, needed minimal remodeling, and provided the yard and space for a garden that they wanted. The neighborhood "would be perfect for raising a small family," with the private, tree-lined streets, walking and biking trails, and a garden to grow organic herbs and some of their own vegetables. They live modestly, and have returned to the Loop for leisure time with friends. They admit to combining both traditional and current values in their lifestyle.

Contributed by Ruth Murray, EdD, MSN, N-NAP, FAAN.

hood, a poor first job, a rapid succession of children, and an early separation or divorce. As life progresses, the chance to advance becomes less likely (3, 36, 104).

Values of individuals in this level are similar to the traditional values of the lower-middle level, with greater emphasis on thrift and conformity to external authority. Refer to **Table 5-4.**

THE LOWER ECONOMIC LEVEL— POVERTY LEVEL

Vulnerable Populations

In the **lower economic level***, people are vulnerable to life stressors and crises and health problems. They are poor, discriminated against, marginalized, or disenfranchised. They have low social status and lack power in social and political relationships. They experience relatively more illness, premature death, and lower quality of life overall than comparable groups. Misfortunes are related to lack of resources and increased exposure to risk.* Vulnerable populations, such as the homeless, various rural populations, migrant families, undocumented and documented immigrants, and refugees or asylees, typically lack health insurance and access to health care (55). Others often included in vulnerable populations are children, pregnant teens, adolescent mothers, the chronically ill, unemployed persons, divorced women, elders, people of diverse ethnicity, individuals with HIV/AIDS, abused women, individuals with dementia and their caregivers, and gay men and women. Youth, ages 17 to 25, who have been in the custody of the Division of Family Services and have no job or place to live, and ex-offenders released from prison are also among the vulnerable population. Vulnerability is increased for those who do not speak English well enough to be integrated into American life. Some of these populations are viewed as a threat to job security of others, and any one of the vulnerable population groups may become the target of violence (9, 36, 93, 112).

The number of people who are poor in the world's richest country is an international disgrace! The overall poverty rate in the United States is 13% of the population—40 million people, almost 8 million families. Of this population, 18% are children under the age of 18 years; 20% of children under 5 years of age live in poverty. The percentage of children in poverty according to race/ethnicity is as follows: African American, 34%; American Indian, 32%; Latino/Hispanic, 30%; Caucasian, 14%; and Asian, 13% (91, 115).

In 2004, the U.S. poverty line was an income of $18,850 for a family of four. In comparison, the median annual household income in the United States was $43,318, and 15% of U.S. households earned more than $100,000 (93).

Definitions

Poverty has several definitions. Poverty is *having inadequate pretax money or source of income to purchase a minimum amount of goods and services.* Poverty is *also a power issue. It is the relative lack of an individual's access to and control over environmental resources.* Poverty *reflects class and racial stratification and hopelessness and is seen in increasing homelessness and health problems* that result from the conditions of poverty (9, 93, 112). The person or family in **acute poverty** *has reduced economic means for a limited time because of given circumstances but anticipates being able to return to work and a better lifestyle.* The person or family in **chronic poverty** *has a long family history of being unemployed or underemployed and without adequate economic means and is unlikely to see much opportunity for improvement.* Life is worsened by lack of access to affordable housing or health benefits (93). **Near poverty** *is defined as families with incomes between 100% and 185% of the federal poverty line ($15,141 to $28,001).* **Extreme poverty** *is defined as families with income of less than half of the poverty line* (21, 93).

Generational poverty *is defined as people living in poverty for two or more generations.* **Situational poverty** *is of shorter duration;*

people have lost their economic resources because of situational crises, such as divorce, death, or illness (93). When economists discuss the **poverty threshold,** *they are referring to pretax income, excluding capital gains, and value of noncash benefits such as employer-provided health insurance, food stamps, or Medicaid* (112).

One of the fastest growing segments of the poor population is the **working poor,** *people from every ethnic/racial population whose job earnings (27% of all jobs) are not sufficient to support an adequate living for the family.* They may experience generational or situational poverty. Or they may be considered poor because their earnings are less than half of the national median income. They may be in **absolute poverty,** *unable to afford the basic necessities of life.* For example, in the United States in a given year, 10 million people experience hunger as a result of financial constraints; 3 million of these people are children (47, 115). Or they may experience **relative poverty,** *able to afford some necessities but not the goods or services that are considered normal for people in our society* (40, 93). The Website *Realities of Poverty,* www.nccbusec.org presents more information.

Causes of Poverty

Poverty has multiple causations; sometimes they are interrelated (40, 91, 93, 102, 104). However, poor people are often strong psychologically, physically healthy, and successful in various ways (92, 102). Often the negative effects of poverty are related to the cycle of poverty (102, 112). See **Table 5-7** for a summary.

The **cycle of poverty** *involves a home environment and parenting that affects physical and intellectual development and contributes to lack of opportunity or inability to progress.* Jobs (sometimes more than one) with low salaries and no health benefits contribute to unhealthy and unsafe housing, poor nutrition, limited health care, and sometimes eventual homelessness. The family members feel a lack of control over their lives. Parents are fatigued; feel anxious, depressed, and hopeless; and are inconsistent in child care and discipline. Children, neither monitored for school performance nor reinforced for good behavior, lack self-confidence, have difficulty with peer relationships at school, and may engage in activities that get them into trouble socially and legally. The family, usually matriarchal, turns to relatives for support and assistance, who themselves may be in dire straits. Parents and children suffer; getting out of the cycle is difficult (91, 93, 102).

The cycle of poverty reflects some of the values typically held by poor people. People in other economic levels may be critical of the values and consequent adaptive behaviors that have to be made for survival and sense of self. The most highly valued "possession" is *people,* not money. People stay with you while money is spent on that which brings a form of satisfaction or helps one to appear in a higher status. A *sense of humor* is highly valued; it's a way to cope with sad aspects of the life situation. People and sex are often the objects of humor and laughter. *Present time* is the most important; decisions are made on what is important for survival or on feelings. The future is unpredictable. **Fatalism,** *the belief that one cannot do much to change the situation or future,* affects motivation about *pursuit of education and job advancement,* which are *valued but not viewed as realistic goals.* The driving forces are survival, relationships, and entertainment (93).

TABLE 5-7

Causation of Poverty

1. Choices, behaviors, or situations in the life of the individual or family:
   a. Single parenthood, domestic violence, family breakup.
   b. Lack of planning, language, cognitive, or work skills.
   c. Chronic mental or physical illness, addictions.
   d. Dependence on welfare, lack of commitment to achievement.
   e. Participation in criminal activity.
2. Lack of resources available to individuals, families, or communities:
   a. Poor quality or lack of education.
   b. Lack of availability of jobs for skill set; lack of well-paying jobs.
   c. Lack of availability for child care, especially for one-parent household.
   d. City and regional planning and zoning, related to industrialization and housing.
3. Exploitation of individual or family because they are poor:
   a. Temporary employment; sweatshops.
   b. Cash-advance and subprime lenders take advantage economically.
   c. Drug trade; gambling in hope of winning fortune; Internet scams.
4. Political and economic structures in society:
   a. Job loss, deindustrialization; decline of unions.
   b. Economic disparity; lack of job benefits; and taxation patterns.
   c. Loss of financial assistance, such as welfare benefits and Medicaid.
   d. Immigration patterns; use of migrant workers.

People can be helped to move out of poverty through education, supportive relationships, monitoring, assistance with developing skills and pursuing a goal, and encouragement to make changes (93). Advocacy and program development by faith-based agencies in collaboration with and funding assistance by local, state, and regional governments or foundations is the current trend.

Who Is Poor?

Males and females of any age, race, or ethnic group may be poor. Children and adolescents, the elderly, people who are homeless, migrant people in the United States, immigrants, refugees, and asylees are examples. Because of unemployment cycles, people who were in the middle economic level may become economically classified as poor. For example, a single parent raising several children, although middle class by birth, may become acutely poor when a job is not available or a prolonged illness or other crisis occurs.

Children, *those under 18 to 21 years of age, may be poor.* Regardless of race or ethnicity, poor children are more likely than nonpoor children to suffer developmental delay, drop out of school, and give birth during the teen years without prenatal care. The baby is more likely to be born prematurely and with low birth weight; children born into poverty are more likely to die before age 18. They are also more likely to live in a one-parent family and be victims of abuse or neglect than are children of higher socioeconomic status. Children under age 6 living in a female-headed household, no male present, experience a poverty rate of 53.7%, in contrast to 9.7% for children in a married family (21, 26, 93).

Elderly people, *those over age 65,* continue to be at risk for poverty because of legislative and economic trends in the United States. *Elderly people in rural areas* are more likely to be poor than are urban elderly persons, and the poverty increases with age. Many elderly people have had less pension or insurance coverage and less lifetime earnings; therefore, they have less accumulated economic resources and lower Social Security benefits. Older women are particularly dependent on the marital union for economic well-being. To prevent poverty in future elderly people, employment prospects and strategies for retirement planning for today's young adults and middle-agers are key. Policies related to death and divorce benefits are also critical (9, 92, 103, 104).

Homeless people, *those who lack a fixed permanent nighttime residence and utilize public or private places temporarily for sleeping accommodations* (108), are poor, sometimes acutely or newly poor. The duration of homelessness varies from a short time to many years, depending on the cause and the type of social services and assistance available to the person. People of all ages and all walks of life are among the homeless. It is not unusual that someone who was middle class loses a job, remains unemployed, and then loses a home. Becoming a single parent or working at low-paying jobs adds to the risk, especially if living with family members is not an alternative. The homeless population is becoming younger and better educated; there are an increasing number of women with children and even entire family units. The homeless are represented by all racial groups and geographic areas. About 25% are chronically mentally ill, about 33% are chemically dependent, and some have co-occurring conditions as well as physical illness. However, being homeless for some time also brings stressors that contribute to a decline in both physical and mental health (88, 91).

Rural, or *nonurban, populations are experiencing increasing rates of poverty,* especially in the South and Midwest of the United States. Poverty is prevalent because of past employment experience, education, and life situations (5). Poverty occurs more among rural females than males, especially among female-headed households. Children in rural areas are more likely to live in poverty (21). Because of the economic losses of farmers during the past decade, an increasing number now also work off the farm at least part-time. Some farmers have lost money because of weather conditions and consequent poor crops, falling prices for grain and livestock, and increasing costs for machinery, land, seed, and fertilizer. The farm family may not be able to provide for basic needs as it once did. In fact, the family may suddenly lose the farm land and home and everything in it. Homelessness may follow. In a rural area, economic losses to farmers in turn affect the businesses in small towns. The circle of poverty grows larger. On Indian reser-

vations, in some areas of Appalachia, or in the Ozarks in southern Missouri, poverty may be at the extreme level.

Migrants *are people who temporarily move to another country or to another region of the country of residence for occupational reasons, not intending to stay.* The **migrant family** *is one with children under the age of compulsory school attendance that moves from one geographic region to another for the purpose of working in agricultural production and the harvest of tree and field crops and that receives 50% of its income from this activity.* Migrant workers and their families suffer poverty and its effects. Migrant laborers and their families may be citizens of the United States or foreign born. *There are three migrant streams* (35, 78, 116):

1. East Coast states, traveled mostly by persons of African American descent who make their home in Florida
2. Midwestern and Western states, traveled mostly by persons of Mexican descent
3. West Coast states, traveled by people of Mexican and Asian descent

Of the approximately 3.5 million migrant workers, it is estimated that 80% are Hispanic, 33% are under 35 years, and 25% are young children. Because more Spanish-speaking migrants are traveling as units in cars, vans, and pickup trucks, an increased number of children are exposed to the stresses of migrant life. Work crews without family are more common in the Eastern states and are composed of primarily African American workers (35, 116).

These workers and families (66% are parents with children) are deprived of safety and sanitation in their living quarters and work setting and do not receive livable wages or adequate health care. Yet, the U.S. agricultural industry relies heavily on this labor, and this group is vital to the food supply, the economy, and the overall wealth of the nation. **Box 5-1**, Characteristics of the Migrant Laborer and Family, summarizes pertinent information to be considered by health care providers, policy makers, and planners (16, 31, 35, 78, 93, 97, 104, 116).

Immigrants, *people with an international origin, choose to come to a specific location with the intention of taking up permanent residence and citizenship, reunification with family, and employment.* In the United States, approximately 30 million people are foreign born. Some immigrants are children being adopted and brought to a new home. Twenty percent of children under age 5 are estimated to have at least one foreign-born parent (93). Some children are born after the mother arrives and are natural-born citizens.

Various events in the country of origin may cause the adult to move (2, 93, 116), including (a) multiple natural disasters and famines; (b) failure of national economic policies; (c) political upheavals or war; (d) religious strife; (e) ethnic conflict or humanitarian crises; (f) warring criminal factions, such as drug cartel conflicts in some South American and Caribbean countries; or (g) knowing someone in the new country who has achieved a better life.

Immigrant groups are not homogeneous. For example, Mexican, Cuban, and Puerto Rican immigrants are all Latinos, but they are not alike. Immigrants come to the United States for different reasons and from varying socioeconomic backgrounds in their countries. They usually link up with others of their ethnicity and experience different rates of acculturation and employment. *They*

BOX 5-1 **Characteristics of the Migrant Laborer and Family**

MOBILITY

Travel from one work place to another, often across states, in older cars, trucks, or company buses.

The average migrant farmworker does 6 months of seasonal work, does 8 weeks of nonagricultural work, travels for 8 weeks, and is unemployed for 10 weeks.

EARNINGS

About $5,000 annually, half of the U.S. poverty threshold.

LIFESTYLE FACTORS THAT THREATEN PHYSICAL AND MENTAL HEALTH

1. Long work days, performing heavy or tiring tasks
2. Overexposure to sun and weather conditions
3. Lack of adequate housing—space, sanitation, water facilities, and safety
4. Improper nutrition related to poverty
5. Exposure to herbicides and insecticides
6. Frequent relocation, causing social isolation, limited education
7. Family abuse and violence resulting from crowded housing, little control over employment conditions, unstable incomes, hostile communities, and consequent anger and fear
8. Children who suffer homelessness, lack of friends, schooling interruptions, and developmental risks

LIFESTYLE FACTORS THAT SUSTAIN HEALTH

1. Sense of community based on cultural ethnicity, language, and religion
2. Promoting family structure through food, music, and social interactions
3. Beneficial folk health practices

LIFE EXPECTANCY

49 years, compared to national average of 75 years

INFANT MORTALITY

25 times higher than national average

COMMON HEALTH PROBLEMS

1. Malnutrition higher than for any other subpopulation
2. Parasitic infection 11 to 59 times higher than in general population
3. Influenza, pneumonia, and tuberculosis deaths 25% higher than in general population
4. Respiratory diseases and allergic reactions caused by chemical used on the land and housing conditions
5. Typhoid or other diseases from contaminated water in migrant laborers' camps
6. Anemia, hypertension, diabetes, and dental disease common, resulting from poor health care access (day appointments; lack of transportation, funds, and child care)
7. Communicable diseases caused by inadequate immunization
8. Higher than normal rates of accidental injuries
9. Skin diseases caused by lack of hygiene and exposure to chemicals used on the land
10. Injuries, depression, and hopelessness caused by family violence and abuse
11. High-risk pregnancies and low-birth-weight babies because of malnutrition, work schedules, lack of sanitation, lack of prenatal care

---

often experience stressors related to (a) language barriers, (b) dislocation and changed living conditions, (c) separation from support systems, (d) dual struggle to preserve ethnic identity and to acculturate, (e) problems with employment, and (f) changes in socioeconomic status (2, 93, 122). Depending upon the reason for arrival to the United States, immigrants may have economic problems but are less likely to be in poverty than refugees. Yet, even fourth-generation Mexicans in the United States trail behind other Americans in education, household income, and home ownership (2, 21, 97, 116).

Family structure and functions also change with immigration. The parent generation experiences additional stress because of intergenerational value discrepancies. Family obligations are more endorsed by the parents than by the youth; the values discrepancy increases with time lived in the United States (16). Parents and youth are likely to be at different stages of acculturation, which produces value conflicts (16). For example, more accultur-

ated Latino and Asian immigrant youth are more likely to experience higher rates of conduct problems, substance abuse, and risky sexual behavior (97). Depending on nation of origin, some immigrants are more accustomed to American culture, such as music, food, and movies, before they immigrate. However, impersonal and fast-moving people, fragmented events, and sensory stimulation typical of America may be challenging, even overwhelming. Culture shock results from the rapid changes, disorganization in personal and family life, and adjustment to a different social system (12, 97, 118). Consequently, the stressful life events increase susceptibility to physical and mental illnesses. See Chapter 2, ∞ which describes General Adaptation Syndrome. *Coping with the stressors is influenced by* (a) personal factors, such as perception of events and sense of mastery; and (b) environmental factors, such as social support, living conditions, employment status, network provided by ethnic churches, and other available resources (50, 51).

People who immigrate to the United States bring with them different coping skills. A study comparing Chinese, Korean, and Japanese immigrants revealed that all national groups relied heavily on social support from family and friends to cope with difficulties related to immigration. Koreans were more likely to find creative activities as an outlet and to seek religious help. The Japanese were more likely to decide to endure problems. The Chinese were more likely to keep to themselves (122).

Typically immigrants across ethnic groups are healthier than longtime U.S. immigrant residents of the same age and ethnicity. *Several factors may explain this health difference* (9):

1. Self-selection; only the hardiest people emigrate.
2. Health habits, particularly with regard to alcohol, drugs, diet, and exercise.
3. Optimism; a hopeful attitude fosters healthy living and longevity.
4. Family communication and support.
5. Early socioeconomic status; the person was often raised in a relatively wealthy family, having the drive, education, and income to emigrate. A healthy childhood attributed to better health in adulthood even though socioeconomic status declined.

Some immigrants come illegally or without legal or appropriate documentation, primarily across the Mexican-American border. They come to work in low-paying jobs that nevertheless pay more than they could earn in their native country. Their plan is to send money home and eventually to return home. They live in the shadow of society, doing work the Americans do not want to do. They dream of a better life, but have no language skills or legal papers that would permit opportunities for progression. They have no advocate, no rights or security, and no path to a better future. They are an exception to the classic immigrant's story of successful work and assimilation to become a citizen (21, 97, 116).

Health status varies. Health care providers should screen for parasites, tuberculosis, infectious diseases such as hepatitis, female genital mutilation, HIV infection and other untreated sexually transmitted diseases, cancer, trauma, malnutrition, and dental problems. The local health department is a resource. Depression and post-traumatic stress disorder should be included in the screening for stressors and coping mechanisms (94). The following Abstract for Evidence-Based Practice presents factors related to depression and mental health and the difficulty in assessment of mental status.

Refugees and asylees are poor. A **refugee** is *a person who is involuntarily living outside the country of origin or nationality to escape persecution because of race, religion, ethnicity, social group membership, or political opinion* (2). An **asylee** is *a person seeking asylum outside the country of origin to avoid political persecution* (2). Both may flee to several countries before finally entering the United States. Both the refugee and asylee continue to practice traditional cultural values and gender roles to maintain a sense of security. Both are likely to face limited employment opportunities and income in the host country. The person may have difficulty learning the English language, which slows acculturation (2, 27, 28). Because of life experiences, the refugee may develop a variety of phys-ical health problems; traditional health practices may delay seeking treatment (70). Anxiety, depression, and post-traumatic stress disorder may be experienced for decades after coming to the United States because of persecution and losses suffered in the country of origin, fleeing warfare, living in refugee camps, and torture experiences. Culture shock and scapegoating on arrival in the United States and thereafter compounds mental health problems (2, 52, 70, 81). Social problems relate to language and employment barriers, few economic resources, and traumatic life experiences that affect interpersonal relationships. Coping abilities are likely to be overwhelmed (2, 70, 108). Refugees, like immigrants, may have Social Security as their only source of income. Those who fail to become citizens within 7 years lose their eligibility to receive public benefits. To become citizens, they must pass their written examination and interview and participate in a swearing-in ceremony (51). Both refugee and immigrant families may keep their children home from school because of fear, scapegoating, and language difficulties or to act as interpreters. It is illegal in most states to keep a child out of school to act as an interpreter for the family (2).

Relationships in Poor Families

Patterns of child rearing and family relationships of the long-term or very poor affect the children, the next generation of parents. *These patterns may include the following* (2, 11, 26, 81, 92, 93, 103):

1. Mother, rather than father, is the chief child care agent. The milieu of the home is authoritarian.
2. Lack of belief in long-range goals or success exists because immediate needs must be met first.
3. Children are often given adult responsibilities early; they are not the focus of the family in the way that middle-class children are. They must fend for themselves.
4. Unmet needs in the parent cause the parent to have difficulty meeting the child's dependency needs.
5. Misbehavior is regarded in terms of overt outcome; reasons for behavior are infrequently considered.
6. Communication between family members is more physical than verbal. Explanations may not be given to the child, affecting curiosity and learning, although a loving attachment exists.
7. Discipline appears harsh, is inconsistent and physical, is based on whether the child's behavior annoys the parent, and is aimed to develop toughness and self-sufficiency for survival.
8. Aggressive behavior is alternately encouraged and restrained, depending on the circumstances. The child learns how to get away with certain behavior.

A study of European Americans, African Americans, and Latinos revealed that poverty was a more powerful indicator of the type of home environment than race or ethnicity. Children growing up in nonpoor homes were more likely to have response to their speech; to be provided with toys, interesting activities, and books; and to see their fathers on a daily basis. They were also less likely to be slapped or spanked for discipline (11).

Most ethnic cultures value the emotional, social, and economic support that the extended family provides, in contrast to dominant middle-class America, which values individualism and

Abstract For Evidence-Based Practice

Factors Associated with Depression in Immigrants from Korea Populations

Kim, M.T., Han, H., Shin, H.S., Kim, K.B., & Lee, H.B. (2005). Factors associated with depression experience of immigrant populations: A study of Korean immigrants. *Archives of Psychiatric Nursing, 19*(5), 217–225.

KEYWORDS

Korean, immigrant, depression, acculturation.

Purpose ➤ Identify factors influencing depression in Korean immigrants.

Conceptual Framework ➤ Lazarus and Folkman's Stress-Coping Theory was adapted to incorporate immigrant-specific literature.

Sample/Setting ➤ A purposive sample of 154 Korean Americans participated. They were born of Korean parents, over age 18 years, able to read and write Korean or English, and had no terminal condition or cognitive impairment. The sample consisted mostly of married women with at least a high school education. They had lived in the United States an average of 15 years; 22% were unemployed.

Method ➤ Network (snowball) sampling was used to recruit participants. Instruments used were back-translated, and functional and conceptual equivalence were analyzed. The Global Assessment of Recent Stress Scale, an 8-item Likert-type instrument, measured magnitude of daily stress. Sense of Mastery, a 7-item Likert-type scale, indicated belief in personal ability to overcome stressors. The Personal Resource Questionnaire Part 2, a 25-item Likert scale, assessed the person's perceived social support. The Center for Epidemiological Studies Depression (CES-D) Scale was used to measure depression. Demographic data were also collected.

Findings ➤ Level of reported stress was strongly correlated with depression. Sense of mastery and social support had buffering effects and were important to mental health and social adjustment. Acculturation status and socioeconomic status did not buffer the effects of stress or prevent depression.

Implications ➤ Instruments utilized in research with immigrants may reflect Western concepts and not be understood by non-Western participants. The concept of sense of mastery, that changes in an individual's environment are the result of personal initiatives or control, may have different meanings to non-Westerners. Further, non-Western people are more reluctant to discuss mental illness; thus, research results may be biased. Cultural sensitivity in collecting data is essential; avoid narrow interpretation of results. More research with different immigrant populations is needed in order to give culturally competent care.

independence. Much visiting goes on between relatives in the lower and working levels; assistance is sought and appreciated. All get along better by sharing meager resources or by working together to gain resources. The grandmother (and grandfather, if living) is valued as carrier of the culture and as caretaker for the child if the mother works. The grandparent also benefits from being valued as a person (2, 37).

Impaired verbal communication and problem-solving ability may be present, not because the poor person is cognitively deficient but for other reasons. Many ethnic groups speak a native language or dialect in the home, which may cause difficulty understanding standard English or being understood. Essentially the child must become bilingual to be successful in school. The poor person speaks directly and to the point with short sentences and little elaboration of meaning, which may create problems at school and work.

Most poor parents repeatedly emphasize that their children must get an education so that they can surpass the parents in achievement. Poor parents often lack the education, energy, time, or resources to help their children advance educationally. The further behind a child is in school, the less the likelihood of ever catching up with cognitive skills. Yet most poor parents are receptive to suggestions on how to make the best possible use of their limited resources or what specific measures to follow to enhance child development (9).

A poor person knows the value of work. Illness is being unable to work for days or weeks; folk or home remedies or a cultural healer are used for illness. Reluctantly, and only when absolutely necessary, does he or she enter the scientific health care system. A person in chronic poverty may not go for professional, scientific care at all because of lack of knowledge, money, and transportation; child care problems; fear of the medical system; or an inadequate sense of self-worth. A poor person is suspicious of health care professionals or feels that there is a distance between the practitioner and self (2, 37).

When caring for these clients, use a gentle, respectful, courteous, prompt approach and straightforward speech. Establish rapport and trust. Be empathic to the life situation; meet the immediate needs of the person and family. Refer to easily available community resources. These clients may be unfamiliar with or unlikely to use community agencies without assistance. Because they often do not have the resources to practice preventive physical or dental care, they may be very ill—even irreversibly—on entry into the health care system (2, 37, 112).

Influences of Culture on Health

CONCEPTS OF ILLNESS

Many cultures explain the cause of and treatment for illness in one or several of the following categories (2, 14, 37, 112):

1. **Natural:** *Weather changes, bad food, or contaminated water cause illness.*
2. **Supernatural:** *The gods, demons, or spirits cause illness as punishment for faulty behavior, violation of the religious or ethical code, or an act of omission to a deity; or as a result of black magic, voodoo, or evil incantation of an enemy or sorcerer.*
3. **Metaphysical:** *Health is maintained when nature and the body operate within a delicate balance* between two opposites, such as Am and Duong (Vietnamese), yin and yang (Chinese), dark and light, hot and cold, hard and soft, or male and female. An excess or shortage of elements in either direction causes discomfort and illness.

Because every culture is complex, it can be difficult to determine whether health and illness are the result of cultural or other elements, such as physiologic or psychological factors. Yet there are numerous accounts of the presence or absence of certain diseases in certain cultural groups and reactions to illness that are culturally determined.

Culture-bound illness or syndrome *refers to disorders restricted to a particular culture because of certain psychosocial characteristics of the people in the group or because of cultural reactions to the malfunctioning biological or psychological processes (2, 37, 112).* See **Table 5-8** for examples (2, 14, 37, 112). Culture and climate influence food availability, dietary taboos, and methods of hygiene, which in turn affect health, as do cultural folkways.

TABLE 5-8

Culture-Bound Illness or Behaviors

1. **Amok.** Asian and Southeast Asian males, Puerto Ricans, Navajos. Period of brooding followed by violent outbursts at people or objects, precipitated by insult, with persecutory ideas, amnesia, exhaustion, and return to premorbid state.
2. **Ataque de nervios.** Latinos. Uncontrollable shouting, crying, trembling, feeling heat, verbal or physical aggression, sense of being out of control precipitated by stressful family events. Resembles adjustment, anxiety, depressive, dissociative, or psychotic disorders.
3. **Belis, Colera, Muina.** Latinos. Acute nervous tension, headache, screaming, stomach disorder, fatigue caused by anger or rage. Resembles brief psychotic disorder. Chronic fatigue syndrome may result.
4. **Bouffee delirantes.** French, West Africans, Haitians. Sudden outburst of aggressive behavior; confusion; suspicion; dream state; hallucinations. Resembles brief psychosis disorder with elements of trance state.
5. **Bulimia.** North American European-Americans, mostly females. Food binging is followed by self-induced vomiting. Sometimes associated with other conditions, such as depression, anorexia, and substance abuse.
6. **"Falling out."** African Americans and Blacks in the Caribbean, Sudden collapse and paralysis and inability to see or speak; hearing and understanding intact.
7. **Ghost sickness.** American Indian. Preoccupation with death and deceased, bad dreams, feelings of danger, fainting, dizziness, anxiety, confusion, hallucinations, sense of suffocation, loss of consciousness.
8. **Grisi siknis.** Miskito Indians of Nicaragua. Headache, anxiety, irrational anger toward people nearby, aimless running, and falling down.
9. **Involutional paraphrenia.** Spanish and Germans. A midlife condition with paranoid features; "paraphrenia" distinct from schizophrenia and depression but contains elements of both.
10. **Latah.** Southeast Asian women. Minimal stimuli elicit an exaggerated startle response, often with swearing. This is also reported among the Ainu of Japan, the Bantu of Africa, and French-Canadians.
11. **Locura.** Latinos in U.S., Latin Americans. Caused by inherited vulnerability and multiple life difficulties. Agitation, hallucinations, unpredictable or violent behavior. Severe form of chronic psychosis.
12. **Maldicion, Voodoo, Hex.** Spanish-speaking, American Indians, African Americans, Jamaicans, Haitians, and Cajuns, as well as various Caucasian groups. Cause of illness or death is pronounced or cast upon the person. Victim develops symptoms accordingly with great sense of helplessness. Death may result from stimulation of sympathetic and parasympathetic nervous system response.
13. **Qi gong psychotic reaction.** Chinese or persons who are overparticipating in qi gong (exercise of vital energy). Acute, time-limited dissociative, paranoid, psychotic or nonpsychotic symptoms.
14. **Shinkeisbitsu.** Japanese. A syndrome marked by obsessions, perfectionism, ambivalence, social withdrawal, neurasthenia, and hypochondriasis.
15. **Susto (soul loss).** Spanish-speaking societies. An expression of emotional stress, helplessness, and role conflict; caused by a frightening experience; consists of anorexia, listlessness, apathy, depression, and withdrawal.
16. **Zar.** North African and Middle Eastern countries. Spirits possess person, who experiences dissociative episodes, shouting, laughing, hitting head, weeping, refusing to eat or do daily tasks. May develop long-term relationship with spirit. Not considered pathological locally.

SUSCEPTIBILITY TO DISEASE: HEALTH PROMOTION ISSUES

Differences exist among cultural populations and people from different races, ethnic groups, and socioeconomic levels with respect to occupation, lifestyle, decisions about health care, risk for disease, and incidence of disease and death. Biological differences—for example, body structure and weight, genetic makeup, and skin color—contribute to susceptibility to illness in various groups. Fair-skinned individuals have a higher risk of cutaneous and ocular melanomas than do dark-skinned people, because of the protective effect of melanin in darker skin tones against sun exposure. However, both fair-skinned and dark-skinned people have similar rates of visceral melanoma (2, 37). Income level affects health care. Members of the upper class have the best access to health promotion practices and illness treatment. They live longer and in better health, generally, than members of other classes. And this fact trickles down for each class (21). *Living in poverty takes its toll physically, emotionally, and mentally. Poverty and ill health are related.* Long-term ill health may contribute to poverty. Poverty predisposes to certain illnesses or causes a person to suffer adverse consequences of illness. As income level drops, health status declines. The ill child who is poor is more likely to miss school. Poor people have higher infant and maternal mortality rates and a higher number of deaths from accidents. Preventive measures are less likely to be carried out in the family; children are less likely to be immunized (2, 37, 46, 112).

The *African American population* demonstrates, overall, a decline in health. The most disadvantaged person in the nation in terms of health is the African American male, whose life expectancy is declining. Health risks to the male include smoking, high blood pressure, high cholesterol levels, alcohol and other drug intake, excess weight, and diabetes—health problems often associated with lower income and stressful life circumstances (2, 37, 94). A risk factor for African Americans of all ages is diet; the preferred foods for many include pork products, fried and salty foods, and baked goods. Obesity, chemical dependency, and exposure to violence are risk factors for disease and death (94). Inadequate prenatal care is a major risk factor; the mortality rate for African American babies before the first birthday is higher than for White babies (94). The leading cause of death for African Americans, as for the entire U.S. population, is cardiovascular disease. Hypertension is more common among both genders of this population than for the total U.S. population. Cancer incidence and mortality has continued to increase. Sickle-cell anemia is the most common genetic disorder in the United States and occurs predominantly in this population (37).

American Indian populations have higher incidence rates compared to the general U.S. population for tuberculosis, diabetes, alcoholism, pneumonia, influenza, and complications from these diseases. Leading causes of death are diseases of the circulatory system, accidents, homicide and violence, diseases of the digestive and respiratory systems, and cancer. Risk factors include poor living conditions and environmental hazards, emotional stress, chemical use, family abuse and violence, and cigarette smoking. Because of the location of reservation lands, geographic tempera-ture changes (extreme heat or cold) contribute to illness and death. In some areas, mining has resulted not only in land damage but arsenic contamination of water and uranium radiation poisoning. Logging has damaged land, removed food sources and home building resources, and contaminated water supplies. Reservation land has been used for toxic waste dumps. The elderly and children are especially at risk for **morbidity** *(illness)* and **mortality** *(death).* Living conditions are an obstacle to both physical and emotional health (2, 37). Community leaders and health care providers, both Indian and Caucasian, work to foster education, health, better living conditions, and hope, especially in the children and youth.

Health and disease patterns among *Asian Americans* differ by generation, immigration dates, and country of origin. New immigrants differ from the general population in many social and health-related issues. Incidence rate for cancer is high, especially for stomach, lung, and liver. Tuberculosis and hepatitis B viral infections are common. Japanese Americans have twice the rate of diabetes as White Americans and four times that of Japanese in Japan. Post-traumatic stress disorder, depression, and general anxiety are high among Asian refugees and recent immigrants (2, 37). Risks include situational stress, low socioeconomic status, limited English proficiency, rigid adherence to certain cultural beliefs, diet, and consumption of alcohol and smoking in some groups (94).

A major health problem for *Latinos* is diabetes. Diabetes is the third leading cause of death in Mexican Americans; the incidence rate is five times higher than for the general U.S. population. In contrast, incidence rates for cardiovascular disease and for lung, breast, prostate, and colorectal cancer are lower than for non-Latinos. The most marked increase in tuberculosis incidence is in Hispanics. Risk behaviors include cigarette smoking, alcohol consumption, and obesity (2, 37, 94).

Variations in dietary practices among ethnic groups may explain some differences in morbidity and mortality. Research suggests that dietary practices and nutrient intake of Mexican American women may protect them against lung and breast cancer. Dietary practices may also explain their low rates of low-birth-weight babies, despite low income and education. Dietary behaviors are sensitive to cultural changes that occur with migration. With acculturation, food choices begin to resemble those of White non-Latinos. Further, alcohol and tobacco consumption increases. These changes may be responsible for the increasing number of low-birth-weight babies being born to acculturated Mexican American women (2).

Occupations held by certain cultural groups predispose the people to illness. For example, in the United States, migrant farm workers of all races are at risk for many diseases. See **Box 5-1**, Characteristics of the Migrant Laborer and Family. Refer also to Chapter 4 ∞ for more information about the effects of various pollutants encountered by rural and migrant workers.

The *Journal of Transcultural Nursing* and the Websites listed in **Table 5-9** are excellent references for in-depth information about influences of culture on health and risks for morbidity and mortality. The **Webliography,** a *multilingual resource manual about maternal-child topics, is useful to provide care and health education to clients with limited or no English-speaking proficiency* (98).

TABLE 5-9

Websites Related to Transcultural Care

Transcultural Nursing Society (Madeleine Leininger)	http://www.tcns.org
Transcultural C.A.R.E. Associates (Josepha Campinha-Bacote)	http://www.transculturalcare.net
National Rural Health Association	http://www.nrharural.org
Minority Nursing Associations (A comprehensive list of minority nursing and health associations. Includes all the associations listed below.)	http://www.minoritynurse.com/associations/
National Coalition of Ethnic Minority Nurse Associations	http://www.ncemna.org
National Association of Hispanic Nurses	http://thehispanicnurses.org
National Black Nurses Association	http://www.nbna.org
National Alaska Native/American Indian Nurses Association	http://www.nanaina.com
Asian & Pacific Islander Nurses Association	http://www.aapina.org
Healthy People 2010 Objectives	http://www.healthypeople.gov
Tracking of *Healthy People 2010* Objectives	http://www.healthypeople.gov

Health Promotion and Nursing Applications

IMPORTANCE OF CULTURAL CONCEPTS AND THEORY IN CLIENT CARE

Many U.S. health care consumers are voicing a preference for caring behaviors and cultural practices. Especially the poor, middle to lower socioeconomic groups, rural populations, and ethnic or racial populations find medical care too complex, too questionable, too difficult to understand and attain, and too expensive. Further, human dignity and normal developmental processes may be sacrificed, and there is concern about lack of privacy for self, family, and health records. The response to what is perceived as poor or indifferent health care or inhumane treatment is to stay away (64, 114). Often the person relies first on various family and cultural remedies and folk healers, as described in **Table 2-9** ∞ and **Table 5-10**. Most people want a therapeutic relationship and a holistic approach in care, not just medical techniques.

The need for providing care to diverse cultural populations was recognized in the United States in the late 1800s, and earlier by Florence Nightingale when teaching British nurses to work in India. Madeline Leininger developed the concept of transcultural nursing in the United States in the 1950s, fusing nursing and anthropology (68). She developed the first formal definition, theory, and care practices of transcultural nursing (67, 68). In her **theory of Culture Care Diversity and Universality**, *Leininger uses worldview, social structures, language, ethnohistory, environmental context, and the generic (folk) and professional care systems to provide a comprehensive and holistic view of influences in culture care* (59, 63, 69). *Three modes of nursing decisions and actions are explained in the intervention section* (63). *The theory and the Sunrise Model can be used with individuals, families, groups, communities, and institutions* (59, 62, 66, 69).

Transcultural nursing *is the humanistic and scientific study and comparative analysis of different cultures and subcultures throughout the world in relation to differences and similarities in caring, health, illness, beliefs, values, lifeways, and practices, so that this knowledge can be used in practice to provide culture-specific and cultural-universal nursing care to people. The goal is to help people maintain or regain health and face disability or death in holistic, culturally competent, and beneficial ways of caring* (59, 62–65). Leininger has further developed *general principles to guide transcultural practice, education, and research* (65, 69). Now the concept of cultural competence in nursing also includes the providers, especially nurses who migrate from other countries (23) and who may be in cultural shock. You will have opportunities to be culturally sensitive to migrant (foreign) nurses or nurses who are from different backgrounds. Cowan and Norman describe strategies used by the United Kingdom to address needs of both native and migrant (foreign) nurses (23).

Cultural competence *is a set of congruent behaviors, practices, attitudes, and policies related to embracing cultural differences that are integrated into a system or agency, so that health care providers function effectively and contribute to a culturally competent system. Adaptations are made in service delivery that reflect understanding of cultural diversity, holistic care, and unique needs of the cultural population* (2, 23, 60–65, 69, 82). **Culturally competent care** *is being sensitive, during client contacts and care, to the differences of individuals' life experiences, values, beliefs, and behavior due to heritage and cultural background. Diversity is valued;* there is mutual respect (2, 13, 23, 60, 63, 64, 69, 73). **Culturally competent health care providers** (13, 71, 74, 77, 82) (a) *understand their own value system;* (b) *are not threatened by differences;* (c) *do not tolerate inequity, racism, prejudice, and stereotyping; and* (d) *advocate for the marginalized.* Human rights and ethical considerations are related to cultural care (64).

Culturally competent care often focuses on acute care for physical illness and status. Chronic illness and mental health needs may be overlooked. Mental health services are typically developed for the dominant U.S. culture and are seen as undesirable or ineffective for people from other cultures. *Mental illness is poorly understood*

TABLE 5-10

Folk Healers and Their Practice

Healer	Practice
African or Black American	
"Old Lady"	Older woman knowledgeable about and consulted for child care and folk remedies.
Spiritualist	Person called by God to help others with financial, personal, spiritual, or physical problems.
Voodoo Priest	Man or woman uses communication techniques to establish therapeutic milieu. Uses herbs, voodoo, and interpretation of signs and omens to treat.
Asian American	
Herbalist	Person uses interviewing, inspection, and auscultation to diagnose and herbal remedies to treat.
Spanish-Speaking American	
Curandero(a)	Person treats most traditional illnesses with herbs, diet, massage, and rituals.
Espiritualista (Spiritualist)	Person born with special gifts from God to analyze dreams, predict events, and use prayers, medals, or amulets to prevent or treat illness.
Yerbero	Person grows and prescribes herbs for traditional and Western illnesses.
Saboden	Person uses massage and manipulation of bones and muscles to treat traditional and nontraditional illnesses, especially musculoskeletal.

and carries great stigma in many cultural groups. For example, depression may be explained as physical illness; the person is expected to be strong, not show vulnerability, and regain composure (2, 20, 37, 52). Treatment is sought only when the family can no longer manage the person's behavior or the person's behavior is bringing disgrace to the family (5, 20, 52, 83, 105, 124). *Chronic illness, physical or mental, may not be a concept to some ethnic groups;* how the person feels day to day may be considered the norm. Thus, some ethnic populations, especially immigrants or refugees, do not seek treatment for chronic conditions, which would prevent complications (47, 52, 105).

IMPORTANCE OF CULTURAL CONCEPTS IN THE HEALTH CARE AGENCY

The health care workplace is a microcosm of the changing demographic social pattern. The diversity among nurses and other members of the health team can pose challenges and opportunities in the multicultural work setting (2, 77, 110). Diversity among the people in the work setting includes many variables. Most settings, including home health care agencies, have a mix of variables (77, 110). Getting along with colleagues and getting work done becomes a challenge. For some workers, to be a health care provider offers challenge, upper social mobility, and status. For others, such work is a divine calling or religious vocation. In contrast, in the Middle East, such as in Kuwait or Saudi Arabia, in some Asian countries, and in Russia, to be a nurse is considered an undignified job for lower-class workers (23).

How workers view each other and the work they do is determined by cultural, religious, and geographic background. Conflict, religious and geographic, can arise in a work group that is culturally diverse (2, 13, 77, 112). In the multicultural workplace, it is essential to maintain the value of **collectivism**, *to maintain group harmony rather than the U.S. value on individualism and the*

partisan interests of subgroups (2, 13, 121). For example, staff members who are Amish, Mennonite, Asian, Latino, or of American Indian heritage are likely to emphasize collectivism as a value. The meaning of work in a **collectivism culture** *is to enjoy working together; there is a commitment to relationships with others, a gentleness and cooperation, and use of indirect communication* (2, 13, 121). Nurses and other professionals in health care leadership positions must recognize and respect the basic value system of all staff members, understand the influence on behavior, and educate staff about diversity as necessary (2). Glittenberg has proposed a Transdisciplinary, Transcultural Model for Health Care to promote cultural education, client care, and research to foster an alliance among a number of related disciplines (38).

ATTITUDES RELATED TO CULTURALLY COMPETENT CARE

Essential to practice is the concept of **cultural relativity**—*behavior that is appropriate or right in one culture may not be so defined in another culture.* Avoid **ethnocentrism,** *behavior based on the belief that one's own group and behavior is superior.* For example, emphasizing daily bathing to a group that has a severely limited water supply is useless, because the water is needed for survival. Recognize that your patterns of life and language are peculiar to your culture; your judgment of another group may be inaccurate.

All people have some **prejudice,** *inaccurate, unfavorable, intolerant, injurious, preconceived ideas formed without adequate knowledge* (2). It emerges in such expressions as "Those upper-crust people always . . ." or "Those welfare people never . . ." Examine your thinking for unconscious prejudice, understand your own class background, and distinguish your values from those held by people for whom you care. Try to withhold value judgments that interfere with your relationship with the patient and with objective care. *There are too many unknown factors in people's lives to set*

Practice Point

In the United States, you are working in a **diverse or plu-ralistic society** *in which members of various ethnic, racial, religious, and social groups maintain distinct lifestyles and adhere to certain values within the confines of a larger culture or civilization.* Knowledge of other cultures helps you ex-amine your own cultural foundations, values, and beliefs, which, in turn, promotes increased self-understanding. However, *see the uniqueness of people in any culture; do not generalize knowledge.* Avoid **racism**, *assumptions that a certain group is inferior.* Avoid **stereotyping**, *fixed beliefs that do not permit an individual view of a person or group.* Accept people as they are. Perceive the world through the client's eyes during client care.

BOX 5-2 Self-Assessment of Cultural Attitudes

To become more aware of your attitudes toward and feel-ings about people of other racial and ethnic backgrounds, ask yourself the following questions:

1. What is your cultural or subcultural background?
2. What is your earliest memory of racial or ethnic differ-ences?
3. What messages have you received in your life about Caucasians of various nationality backgrounds? About non-Caucasians?
4. How much experience did you have with any person from a racial or ethnic minority group different from your own while you were growing up?
5. In what way have these experiences affected your be-havior toward people from the group(s)?
6. Describe people from other racial or ethnic minority groups with whom you have felt comfortable or uncom-fortable.
7. What features or characteristics are dominant in people from other racial or ethnic minority groups with whom you have had contact?
8. What have you observed about the racial or ethnic com-position of your community?
9. Do you consider yourself to be nonracist or racist? (A member of any race can be a racist against a different racial group.)
10. What do you plan to do to increase your understanding of a person different from you?

---

up *stereotyped categories.* If you feel you are stooping by helping poor people, you may be labeled a "do gooder" and be ineffective. Recognize the behavior of people who are poor not as pathologic but as adaptive for their needs. Realize, too, that *not only a poor person needs your help. A rich person also may need a great deal of help with care, health teaching, or counseling.* Having money does not necessarily mean one is knowledgeable about preventive health measures, nutrition, and disease processes. *Persons of all economic levels deserve competent care, clear explanations, and a helpful attitude.*

The misinterpretation of behavior typical of a social class or ethnic group does not always go in one direction, from upper to lower, or from Caucasian to ethnic people of color. For example, suppose that the nurse has a working-class background, and the patient is a 50-year-old corporate president who is a member of the newly rich class. The patient is admitted for coronary disease and seems obsessed with finding out when professional duties can be resumed, exactly how many hours can be worked daily, and what the chances are for a recurrence. An understanding of socioeco-nomic position, along with possible motives, values, and status (which this individual feels must be maintained), will enable the nurse to work with the seeming obsession rather than simply label the client as an "impossible patient."

Many cultural groups do not respond like the average middle-class American. For example, Caucasian health professionals may label Asian parents as noncompliant because they are not as forceful as Caucasian parents in having the chronically ill child carry out pre-scribed exercises when the exercises cause pain. Health profession-als are often unaware of the complex factors that influence client responses to treatment and care. Clients may not follow the treat-ment plan because they have different priorities (2, 37). Another example is the American Indian population, who value coopera-tion and patience, and respond quietly, even passively. Do not mis-interpret this behavior as apathy about health or health care. They believe each living thing follows a cycle; illness is defined in rela-tion to a personal inner cycle and seasonal cycles, in contrast to the emphasis on germ theory by the health care system. Thus, the medicine man is seen as more helpful than the physician (2, 15, 31, 35, 37).

Learning about another's cultural background can promote feelings of respect and humility as well as enhance understanding of the person and the family—needs, likes and dislikes, behavior, attitudes, care and treatment approaches, and sociocultural causes of disease. **Box 5-2**, Self-Assessment of Cultural Attitudes, is a questionnaire that can help you assess your own cultural attitudes and perceptions. The Cultural Self-Efficacy Scale is also available to measure the nurse's confidence in caring for people from non-Caucasian cultures (19). Cultural sensitivity training is effective in improving the health care provider's knowledge about, attitudes toward, and caring of patients from different cultural backgrounds (74).

Culture Shock

Culture shock *refers to feelings of bewilderment, confusion, disor-ganization, frustration, and stupidity, and the inability to adapt to differences in language and word meaning, activities, time, and cus-toms that are part of the new culture* (12, 118). These feelings oc-cur in various intensity to anyone who moves to live in a culture different from the culture of origin. The move may be to a dif-ferent geographic area. Or the move may be as an employee en-tering a different health care system that has clients from diverse cultures.

Brink and Saunders describe four phases of culture shock (12):

1. **Honeymoon phase:** *This stage is characterized by excitement, exploration, and pleasure. This phase may be experienced by a short-term visitor to a new area, by a geographic move to a different location, or during initial employment in a different health care agency.*

2. **Disenchanted phase:** *The person feels stuck, depressed, irritated, and that the environment is unpredictable and no longer exotic. The normal cues for social intercourse are absent and the person is cut adrift. The person may become physically ill.*

3. **Beginning resolution phase:** *New cultural behavior patterns are adopted. Friends are found. Life becomes easier and more predictable.*

4. **Effective function phase:** *The person has become almost bicultural and may experience reverse culture shock on return home after living abroad or when transferring to a different health care agency.*

An *antidote for culture shock* is to look for similarities between the native and the new culture. To adapt to a new culture, be interested in the culture and be prepared to ask questions tactfully and to give up some of your own habits. Learn the language, customs, beliefs, and values to the greatest extent possible. Seek a support system—someone with whom you can be yourself, validate your ideas, and help you to adapt (12, 118). Leininger (69) and Weiss (118) give a number of specific suggestions for adapting to another culture.

Culture shock also occurs in those who are immigrants or refugees to the United States. Deng (28) describes the culture shock, difficulties with adjustment, and feelings experienced as a refugee from Sudan, as well as the experiences in Sudan prior to being chosen by the Office of the United Nations Commission for Rescue Committee. He describes how people from the International Rescue Committee assisted him and directed him to education about the basics of U.S. life, language, cultural differences, social customs, computers, and employment preparation. He describes the difficulty of interacting with people or feeling emotionally close even to friendly people, which continued for several years.

CLIENT ASSESSMENT

Translate your knowledge of the health care system and need for assessment data into terms that match the client's concepts. Your approach and communication methods are critical in assessment.

When assessing a client, your questions may seem intrusive. For example, for some American Indians, a question carries with it assumptions and obligations. If the person is asked a question, it implies that he or she has the answer and that the answer is needed. Otherwise, there is no reason to ask the question. If the person does not know the answer, the person starts to talk about something else to maintain the cultural practice and to save face and dignity. You may be able to obtain information by more indirect means, without putting the person on the spot. It may also be necessary to use an interpreter. **Table 5-11** presents guidelines for working with an interpreter (2, 37, 76).

Assessment must consider the complexity and coherence between (a) the individual life span, (b) development and aging, (c) biological and physiologic factors, (d) contextual and interactional models of intellectual functioning, (e) personality development and expression, (f) social interaction, and (g) family and social support systems in relation to racial, ethnic, and cultural status and spiritual, religious, and philosophic beliefs and values. Various racial or ethnic groups may experience a very different process of development and aging and manifestation of illness. Variability within racial or ethnic groups and between men and women is also apparent. There is still limited research data on normative development, mental health characteristics over the life course, and manifestation of physical and psychiatric symptoms among various racial and ethnic groups.

Assessment Tools

A thorough cultural assessment guide would include the following components (2, 37, 69, 112):

1. *Values* about health, human nature, relationships between the person and nature, time, activity, relations, and others.
2. *Beliefs* about health, health maintenance, cause and treatment of illness, religion, and other practices.
3. *Customs* about communication (verbal and nonverbal), decision making, diet, grief, dying, religion, family roles, and role of the patient.
4. *Social structure*, including family lines of authority, education, ethnic affiliation, physical environment, religion, use of economic resources and health care facilities, use of art and history, and cultural change.
5. *Preferences* about the health care situation.

Leininger described seven major components to consider while doing a cultural assessment (60, 65, 69): (a) families and kinship groups; (b) social life and daily routines; (c) political systems; (d) language and traditions; (e) worldview and ethnocentric tendencies, values, and cultural norms; (f) religion; and (g) health and life care rituals, practices, and rites of passage to maintain health, folk and professional health-illness systems that are used, and methods of caring for self and others in regaining health.

The Transcultural Assessment Model by Giger and Davidhizar (37) focuses on (a) the person as a unique cultural individual; (b) communication patterns, including language use, use of silence, and nonverbal communication; (c) biological variation, such as body structures, skin and hair color, enzymatic and genetic risks for disease, nutritional preferences, and psychological characteristics; (d) social orientation, including culture, family, work, leisure, church, friends, and social support; (e) environmental control of events, health practices, values, beliefs, and definitions; (f) preferred space or distance between person and others; and (g) time orientation and use (41). During assessment, the model encourages discussion to determine how well the person is assimilated into or has become part of the mainstream culture and use of specific cultural practices related to health, food, religious belief, and general lifestyle (37). The assessment model is applicable to children (37).

Other models for assessment are presented by Spector (112), Purnell (95, 96), and Andrews and Boyle (2). Spector developed

TABLE 5-11

Guidelines for Using a Language Interpreter

1. Hospital translators, in contrast to family members, may not be as familiar with a particular dialect, but may be more neutral and better at interpreting technical aspects of health care.

2. Patients and family members may be embarrassed to answer some questions or reveal some information in the presence of each other but would be willing to talk with an interpreter. Clients may request a specific translator or bring their own.

3. Family members, in contrast to an interpreter, have knowledge of the patient and may be able to insert additional information in context, but may be guarded with personal information.

4. Family members, in contrast to an interpreter, may have issues about what is meant, how much is translated, and how much is condensed or omitted.

5. Plan what you want to say ahead of time. Avoid *confusing the interpreter* by backing up, inserting a proviso, rephrasing, or hesitating. Be patient.

6. Address the person or family directly. Avoid directing all comments to and through the interpreter.

7. Assure the person or family and interpreter of confidentiality.

8. Use short questions and comments. Technical terminology and professional jargon (e.g., "like psychotropic medication") should be reduced to plain English.

9. When lengthy explanations are necessary, break them up and have them interpreted piece by piece in straightforward, concrete terms in the foreign language by the interpreter.

10. Use language and explanations the interpreter can handle.

11. Make allowances for terms that do not exist in the target language.

12. Try to avoid ambiguous statements and questions.

13. Avoid abstractions, idiomatic expressions, similes, and metaphors. It is useful to learn about the use of these grammatical elements in the target language.

14. Avoid indefinite phrases using "would," "could," "if," and "maybe." These can be mistaken for actual agreements or firm approval of a course of action.

15. Ask the interpreter to comment on the client's word content and action.

16. Invite correction and induce the discussion of alternatives: "Correct me if I'm wrong. I understand it this way . . . Do you see it some other way?"

17. Pursue seemingly unconnected issues raised by the client. These issues may lead to crucial information or may uncover difficulties with the interpretation.

18. Return to an issue if you suspect a problem and get a negative response. Be certain the interpreter knows what you want. Use related questions, change the wording, and come at the issue indirectly.

19. Provide instructions in list format. Ask clients to outline their understanding of the plans. If alternatives exist, spell each one out. Check the quality of translated health-related materials by having them back-translated.

20. Clarify your nursing limitations. The willingness to talk about an issue may be viewed as evidence of "understanding" it or the ability to "fix" it.

---

the *HEALTH Traditions Model*, which focuses on the interrelationships of body, mind, and spirit, and identifies what people do to maintain and protect health, prevent illness, and restore health (112). Refer also to Kikuchi's article, which is an overview of cultural theories (49).

Specific Assessment Variables

Culture-Bound Illness Consider the presence of a culture-bound syndrome of illness during assessment when the client's explanation does not match scientific explanation of the symptoms. Refer to **Table 5-8** for examples. Listen carefully and validate meaning of the illness. The client may not be able to describe symptoms in precise terms expected by Western care providers (2, 37, 112). A person's behavior during illness is influenced by *cultural definitions of how he or she should act, the meaning of illness, and effective treatment.* Understanding this situation and seeking reasons for behavior help to avoid stereotyping and labeling a person as uncooperative and resistant just because the behavior is different.

Economic Level Variations In the assessment of clients, be mindful of their perceived and ascribed socioeconomic status. Adapt your approach. Members of the upper-upper, lower-upper, and power-elite levels place a high value on their power, celebrity, wealth, and privacy. Because of these values and lifestyle, their health status may be difficult to assess. The family and individual will determine who will give information, how much, to whom, and their interaction with the health care providers. Their sense of status may be a major consideration in treatment and rehabilitation measures. Further, the person may face the crisis of major lifestyle changes related to the illness process. Having money helps the person and family gain the best possible quality of care. However, it does not necessarily mean one is knowledgeable about preventive health measures, nutrition, and disease processes. In assessment of members of the upper-middle and creative-class levels, seek not only the usual information but also explore information about life stresses related to employment and conditions of the work environment. Refer to **Box 5-1**, Characteristics of the Migrant Laborer and Family, for assistance in assessing migrant workers, representative of people who are poor.

Immigrants and Refugees Cultural differences should be anticipated not only for immigrants, refugees, and first-generation immigrants, but also for persons even further removed in time from their country of origin and for persons from other regions within the

United States. The crisis of immigration appears to be manifested as follows (2, 29, 81):

1. **First year.** Sense of relief and happiness mixed with general anxiety, culture shock.
2. **Second year.** Culture shock, dissatisfaction, high levels of depression and unhappiness.
3. **Third year.** Increased adaptability, higher life satisfaction, emotional improvement.

Utilize Leininger's components of cultural assessment with immigrants, refugees, and asylees (69). Refer also to Giger and Davidhizar (37) and Spector (112), as they describe values, characteristics, needs, biological variations, and health care implications for people who have migrated from many countries to the United States.

Appointments Knowledge about socioeconomic levels and cultural groups may help explain late or broken appointments that result from fear, feelings of inferiority, lack of transportation, or not having someone to care for the children at home, rather than from lack of interest in health. A reservation American Indian, poor African American, or recent immigrant, for instance, may not be accustomed to keeping a strict time schedule or appointments if unemployed, because a strict clock-time orientation is not valued as highly as in the industrialized workforce. By taking time to talk with the person, you will learn of fears, problems, aspirations, and concerns for health and family and human warmth.

Use of Language *Assessment involves observing, listening, and talking with the client and, frequently, the family. Some people communicate best in their first (or native) language when they are ill.* Further, the elderly person from a nationality group may have never learned English. There is currently an emphasis on a group maintaining its national language, because language maintains cultural identity and provides the strength and connectedness of a community. Yet, it is helpful if people also know the English language. Because of the diversity of cultures found in the United States and the number of people for whom English is not the first language, you may need to use an interpreter to assist with assessment, care planning, and intervention. Become acquainted with people in the community who speak another language fluently and can be interpreters or translators for health care professionals. See **Table 5-11** for guidelines about utilization of interpreters. Learn key words of the client's language. Use language dictionaries or a card file of key words. Breach the language barrier so that the assessment is more accurate and care measures will be understood by the person.

Physical Assessment As you assess clients and do physical assessments, it is important to remember that people differ not only culturally but also biologically. See **Table 5-12** for examples. Studies on biological baselines for growth and development or normal characteristics have usually been done on Caucasian populations. These norms may not be applicable to non-Whites. For example, *African American* infants and young children demonstrate advanced neurologic and musculoskeletal function until puberty, at which time children of all races are comparable. Both genders have longer legs and shorter trunks than Caucasians. Heavier bone density lowers incidence of osteoporosis in African American elders. In contrast, people of *Asian* heritage are markedly shorter, weigh less, and have smaller body frames than their Caucasian counterparts. Weight norms vary with the cultural group in relation to body build. For example, *Mexican Americans* weigh more in relation to height than non-Hispanic Caucasians because of differences in truncal fat patterns. Aging is accompanied by skin wrinkling in all cultures; however, *Anglo Americans* wrinkle earlier in life than their counterparts in other races, unless the person is overweight (2, 37). Body odor, which can be indicative of disease, also varies with racial groups. Most *Asians* and *American Indians* have mild to absent body odor, in contrast to stronger body odor in Caucasians and African Americans, because of differences in apocrine and eccrine sweat glands, fluid balance, and thermoregulation (2). Thus, body odor in an Asian or American Indian client may be a disease indication.

Biological features such as skin color, body size and shape, and presence of enzymes are the result of genetically transmitted biological adjustments made by ancestors to the environment in which they originated (2, 37, 112). Cultural differences occur in the results from laboratory tests. **Mongolian spots** (*hyperpigmented, bluish-black discoloration*) *are normal for many Asians, American Indians, and African Americans.* Pelvic shape of the woman, shape of teeth and tongue, fingerprint pattern, blood type, keloid formation, and presence of the enzyme lactase vary among groups.

Adults who have **lactose intolerance** are *missing lactase, the enzyme for digestion and metabolism of lactose in milk and milk products; they become ill on ingestion of these foods.* This condition occurs in 90% of adult African Blacks; about 80% of African Americans, American Indians, and people of Asian descent; 66% of Mexican Americans; and 60% of Jewish descent Caucasians. The intolerance is caused by dietary habits (little lactose intake after infancy) and a deficiency of the enzyme glucose-6-phosphate dehydrogenase (G-6-PD). Symptoms include flatulence, distention, abdominal cramping, diarrhea, and colitis. Only people of Northern European Caucasian extraction and members of two African tribes tolerate lactose indefinitely; even some elderly Caucasians have lactose deficiency (2, 37, 112). Refer to Chapter 14 ∞ for more information.

Other biological variations exist. Susceptibility to disease varies with blood type. Rh-negative blood type is common in *Caucasians*, rarer in other groups, and absent in Alaskan Natives. Myopia is more common in *Chinese* people; color blindness is more common in *Europeans* and *East Indian* persons. Nose size and shape correlate with ancestral homeland. Small noses (seen in *Asians* or *Eskimos*) are common in cold regions; high-bridged noses (seen in *Iranians* and some *American Indian* natives) are common in dry areas; and the flat, broad noses characteristic of some *African American* persons are adaptive in moist, warm climates (2, 37, 112).

Susceptibility to illness varies with racial groups. For example, *African Americans* primarily have sickle-cell anemia, the most common genetic disorder in the United States. Hypertension, both primary and malignant, is more common in African Americans of all age groups than in other racial groups. G-6-PD, a hematological disease, occurs in 35% of African Americans; a fluorescent spot test screens for the deficiency that causes G-6-PD. Blood transfu-

TABLE 5-12

Clinical Assessment of Skin Color

Characteristic	White or Light-skinned Person	Dark-skinned Person
Pallor Vasoconstriction present	Skin takes on white hue, which is color of collagen fibers in subcutaneous connective tissue.	Skin loses underlying red tones. Brown-skinned person appears yellow-brown. Black-skinned person appears ashen gray. Mucous membranes, lips, and nailbeds are pale or gray.
Erythema, Inflammation Cutaneous vasodilation	Skin is red.	Palpate for increased warmth of skin, edema, tightness, or induration of skin. Streaking and redness are difficult to assess.
Cyanosis Hypoxia of tissue	Skin, especially in earlobes, as well as in lips, oral mucosa, and nailbeds, has bluish tinge.	Lips, tongue, conjunctiva, palms, soles of feet are pale or ashen gray. Apply light pressure to create pallor; in cyanosis, tissue color returns slowly by spreading from periphery to the center.
Ecchymosis Deoxygenated blood seeps from broken blood vessel into subcutaneous tissue	Skin changes from purple-blue to yellow-green to yellow.	Oral mucous membrane or conjunctiva show color changes from purple-blue to yellow-green to yellow. Obtain history of trauma and discomfort. Note swelling and induration.
Petechiae Intradermal or submucosal bleeding	Round, pinpoint purplish red spots are present on skin.	Oral mucosa or conjunctiva show purplish red spots if person has black skin.
Jaundice Accumulated bilirubin in tissues	Skin, mucosa membranes, and sclera of eyes are yellow. Light-colored stools and dark urine often occur.	Sclera of eyes, oral mucosa membranes, palms of hand, and soles of feet have yellow discoloration.

sions for African Americans, including infants, should contain this component (2, 37).

Pain assessment must consider cultural factors: *Different population groups have about the same physical thresholds of pain*, although there is individual variation in each group. However, *how different populations express pain varies* according to whether the individuals were taught to speak about or give evidence of their pain (physical and emotional). It is necessary to look for subtle cues of pain among Northern European, Asian, and American Indian populations and not to overmedicate patients who tend to be more expressive, such as Latino or Jewish people. Family members may also react differently when they see the patient in pain. Families of Eastern European groups tend to be proactive and assertive on behalf of the patient. Patients also respond differently when family members are present. In some cultures, for example, Anglo American, the patient is not expected to talk about the pain to the family (2, 24, 61, 125).

Spiritual and Religious Assessment Learn about the significant religious practices and their influences on everyday patterns of hygiene, types of foods eaten, sleeping, elimination, use of space, and various rituals that are a part of the person's culture. Because the client and the practitioner may have different perspectives of health and illness, *you may ask any of the following questions, which can enhance understanding about the client's viewpoint:*

1. What do you think caused your problem? Is it related to your religious beliefs?
2. Why do you think it started when it did?
3. What do you think this illness does to you? What problems has it caused for you?
4. What do you fear most about your illness? Its outcome?
5. How severe is your illness? What helps you bear the symptoms and illness?
6. What kind of treatment have you already tried? What else would help? Should spiritual or folk healers be contacted?
7. What would you like for health care providers to do for you? What results do you want or expect from treatment?

NURSING DIAGNOSES

The nursing diagnoses in the Box titled Nursing Diagnoses Related to Transcultural Nursing may be applicable to working with people from various cultures (90). Leininger discusses the importance of not focusing on Anglo-American Western cultural values in the North American Nursing Diagnosis Association (NANDA) taxonomy (66). It is important to use wellness nursing diagnoses to help the person focus on health, progress, and strengths, and not focus only on problems. *Wellness diagnoses could include* (66, 90) (a) gaining new information, (b) learning new skills, (c) acquiring new roles, and (d) achieving developmental tasks.

Nursing Diagnoses Related to Transcultural Nursing

Anxiety
Impaired Verbal **C**ommunication
Decisional **C**onflict
Fatigue
Grief
Ineffective Health **M**aintenance
Deficient **K**nowledge

Risk for **L**oneliness
Post-Trauma Response
Powerlessness
Relocation Stress Syndrome
Ineffective **R**ole Performance
Situational Low **S**elf-esteem
Social **I**solation

Source: Reference 90.

CONCEPTS OF CULTURALLY BASED INTERVENTION

Caring *involves assistive, supportive, or facilitative actions toward another person or group with evident or anticipated needs to ameliorate or improve a human condition or lifeway* (59). Nurses in different cultures tend to know and emphasize different care constructs, such as support, comfort, and touch. *Caucasian nurses in the United States* generally believe that care involves use of technologic aids, medicines, psychophysiologic comfort measures, and promoting self-care. Generally, Caucasian and some non-Caucasian clients agree. In several non-Western cultures, nurses and clients perceive care as protective with a sociocultural emphasis. For example, *nurses in Middle Eastern countries and Israel* emphasize restorative caring functions because of war activities. *Samoan caregivers* are expected to protect the person from breaking cultural or social rules to prevent illness or harm. *Chinese nurses* perceive surveillance and protection as dominant caring modes. Depending on the culture, Leininger states the concept of *care can have a number of meanings,* including some behaviors not frequently considered: tenderness, agape love, stimulation, presence, succorance, surveillance, and maintenance of well-being (59, 62, 69).

Client therapy goals should be congruent with cultural values, beliefs, and lifeways. The Anglo-American and Western European cultural values of individualism, autonomy, independence, self-reliance, self-control, and self-care may be in conflict with non-Western values. In non-Western cultures throughout the world and among some people in the United States (Mexican American, African American, Asian American, Polynesian, and American Indian), the value is **other-care,** *to retain the role of caring for family members,* rather than emphasizing *self-care* (60). Thus, the role reflects caring values such as interdependence, interconnectedness, understanding, presence, and being responsible for others. *Other-care* values are essential for survival of extended families, subclans, clans, and tribes (60).

Cultural care congruence, *a concept developed by Leininger, explains and predicts outcomes. Three principles for client therapy goals are defined as follows* (59, 63, 65, 66, 69):

1. **Cultural care preservation** *refers to assistive, facilitative, or enabling acts that preserve cultural values and lifeways viewed as beneficial to the client.*

2. **Cultural care accommodation** *refers to assistive, facilitative, or enabling acts that reflect ways to adapt or adjust health care services to fit the client's needs, values, beliefs, and practices.*

3. **Cultural care repatterning** *refers to altered designs to help clients change health or life patterns that are meaningful; it also refers to recognition of different attributes and features of a culture so new patterns of care can be learned and incorporated and for retention or preservation of selected values, beliefs, or practices of the culture.*

Cultural competence *is the ability of a health care provider, agency, or system to acknowledge the importance of culture on all levels—client, provider, administration, and policy—for incorporation into health care.* It is not necessary to know everything about the person's culture to competently treat or give care. *Cultural competence is an educational process that includes self-awareness, cultural knowledge, and the ability to develop working relationships across lines of difference, to be flexible, and to use intercultural communication skills.* It acknowledges that the patient/client and family may not want a health care worker from the same country of origin, in case that person would know the patient or family.

Evaluate your approaches to cultural care. *Be willing to compare approaches with the client.* Do not ridicule the person who has gone the nontraditional route. Above all, this person needs your listening ear and understanding guidance. Remember that people think in terms of having symptoms and eradicating them. If the latter takes place to their satisfaction, they will place their trust in the health care provider who was responsible for their improvement, regardless of his or her credentials. What one person calls a *hoax* others may call *hope.* Refer people who have been a victim of maltreatment or a quack to their local Better Business Bureau, medical society, and nursing organization.

SPECIFIC CULTURALLY BASED INTERVENTIONS

This section summarizes intervention approaches for some cultural groups. Refer to the *Journal of Transcultural Nursing* and the Websites in **Table 5-9** for more in-depth information about the groups presented in this chapter, about well-known populations in countries around the world, and for other less well-known groups, such as Amish, Hmong, Hondurans, Hutterites, Roma (Gypsies), and Aboriginese in Australia. Conceptual frameworks for nursing care and promoting health and development and cultural research methodology are also presented in these resources.

Communication Principles

The following communication principles are applicable as you intervene with any person from any culture. Specific communication approaches are also described. Your *approach to* and *way of speaking to the client* will set the tone for how the client reacts to you and everyone else on the team.

Call the person by title and last name until the person states that he or she would like to be called by his or her first name. Calling a client by first name may suggest a subservient role.

Be sensitive to terms used when speaking about the person. People of *Spanish descent* may prefer the terms Latino, Hispanic, Puerto Rican, or Cuban American. *American Indians* may prefer to be called Indian or by their nation or tribal name (e.g., Hopi, Lakota, or Nez Perce) rather than Native American. *People of African descent* may prefer the term African American or Black, depending upon age and geographic location. *Residents from the Caribbean* may refer to themselves by the island of birth (e.g., Belize, Jamaican, or Haitian American).

As you intervene, teach, or counsel, it is important to adjust your communication approach and behavior. Although you *may be communicating in a way that is natural to you, someone from another culture may perceive that behavior as too forward or aggressive, too passive, or unempathic.* While you cannot assume a different mask for each person you interact with, be aware that the client may misinterpret your well-intentioned behavior. Use general knowledge about a culture; while you simultaneously see individual, unique differences of people. The client who uses English as a second language may not understand English adequately. Assess, teach, or intervene in other ways.

Avoid use of the term "you people" or "these people" when speaking to anyone, especially to any member of an ethnic group. Those terms are considered disrespectful and stereotyping.

Be aware that *some topics may be taboo as you assess, intervene, or educate,* especially topics related to intimate sexual behavior or sexual organs, or topics related to conflictual relationships. If these topics must be presented, explain the reasons related to the client's well-being. Avoid "rapid-fire," probing questions. Establish rapport; convey warmth and interest. Speak to the implied feeling, "I realize this may be difficult for you to answer."

Learn what the client has as a priority in care. Include the person's ideas in planning and giving care. Often a nurse may have to negotiate with the individual or family to carry out the essential medical treatments and nursing care, as well as include the cultural practices, the medicine man or spiritualist, or spiritual healing rituals they hold most dear.

Some clients or families will not be expressive emotionally or verbally. Respect this pattern, recognizing that *nonverbal behavior is also significant.* The *meaning of a gesture* differs from country to country. A friendly wave of the hand may be an insult, depending on hand position. Be sure the gesture or touch you use conveys the message you intend. If you are unsure, it is best to avoid, to the extent possible, gestures, touch, or standing too close. Be aware, too, that *word meanings may vary considerably from culture to culture.* The client may have difficulty understanding you and vice versa.

For some clients, the hurrying behavior of the nurse or other health care providers is distressing; it conveys a lack of concern and lack of time to give adequate care. In turn, the person expresses guilt feelings when it is necessary to ask for help. Although you may look very efficient when scurrying, he or she is likely to miss many observations, cues, and hidden meanings in what the person or family says. *Examine your own attitude about busyness and leisure* to help others consider activity or exercise and leisure as part of life. The disabled person, whose inability to work carries a stigma, may seek your help to resolve conflicts about leisure.

In male-dominated households (Latino, Asian, Middle Eastern, and some religious groups), the male head of household must be included in all decisions and health teaching in order to solicit cooperation. In most such families, and *African American* and *Jewish* families, there is also an older female relative, such as an aunt, mother-in-law, or grandmother, who is the designated health care provider for that family. She must also be included in decision making and health teaching. Speaking to the important family elder with respect will gain you a staunch ally; the desired behavior change is almost certain to be assured (2, 37). Relations between the client and the family may at times seem offensive or disharmonious to you. Differentiate carefully between patterns of behavior that are culturally induced and expected and those that are unhealthy for the persons involved.

Holistic Care

Holistic nursing *is nursing practice that has healing the whole person as its goal.* **Holism** *involves understanding relationships among the biological, psychological, sociocultural, and spiritual dimensions of the person and that the person is an integrated whole interacting with internal and external environments* (2, 13, 37, 94). Holistic care is not new. It has been practiced since the time of ancient China (120).

Knowledge of different cultures will enable you to practice **holistic care**. *The nurse-client relationship is the key to holistic nursing care, for the person expects a caring interaction from the healer.* Holistic healing practices combine the best of two worlds: the wisdom and sensitivity of the East and the technology and precision of the West. The focus is on prevention and overall fitness and the individual taking responsibility for personal health and well-being. Multiple techniques as described in **Table 2-10** ∞ are used to restore and maintain the balance of body energy. Include the clergy or spiritual leader, local folk or traditional healer, tribal leader, matriarch/patriarch of the family, or trusted family advocate in intervention and education. For example, the African American client may rely heavily on the clergy or spiritual leader to validate use of prescribed treatments. Spanish-speaking clients may want to validate with the curandera.

Adapt Care to Daily Life Patterns

Interference with normal living patterns or practices adds to the stress of being ill. *Respect the person's need for privacy or need to have others continually around.* You will encounter and need to *adapt care and health education to various customs,* such as drinking tea instead of coffee with meals, eating the main meal at midday instead of in the evening, refusing to undress before a strange person, doing special hair care, avoiding use of the bedpan because someone else must handle its contents, maintaining special religious customs, refusing to bathe daily, refusing a pelvic exam by a male doctor, moaning loudly when in pain, and showing unreserved demonstrations of grief when a loved one dies.

A client with a *strict time orientation* must take medicines and receive treatments on time or will feel neglected. You are expected to give prompt and efficient, but compassionate, service to the patient and family. Time orientation also affects making appointments for the clinic, plans for medication routines, plans to return to work after discharge, and a person's ideas about how quickly he or she should get well. Clients with *little future-time orientation have difficulty planning a future clinic appointment or a long-range medication schedule.* They cannot predict now how they will feel at a later date and may think that clinic visits or medicines are unnecessary if they feel all right at the moment.

If the person or group is from a culture that strongly values stoicism, counseling about emotional status or feelings is likely to be felt as uncomfortable, unnecessary, unhealthy, immature, or embarrassing. The person may feel like a traitor to the family. For some groups, such as *Cherokee Indians* (71) or *people of German descent* (89, 99, 100), the values of self-reliance and being responsible are a way of life that influence health practices, delay seeking medical treatment, and enable the person to get through disastrous times.

Reinforce client and family strengths and how well they implement the treatment measures. Acknowledge that seeking help is a sign of strength and maturity. For example, to the *Cherokee Indian,* being as healthy as possible means the person can live the worldview that talents and abilities are a resource that benefit not only the self but also the family, community, and tribe or nation (87). People in other cultures also have this worldview.

Adapt Care to Culture-Bound Illness

Culture-bound illnesses may be treated by combining folk, alternative, or complementary methods, and Western diagnostic and treatment measures. Some methods may conflict with the Western models. Work *patiently* with the individual, family, and local or folk healer to resolve the conflict for the client's well-being. The recommended care will not be followed if the encounter with providers is perceived as hostile or negative. See **Table 2-10** ∞ and **Table 5-8** for more information (2, 37).

Based on the client's definition of causation, treatment varies. Treatment for diseases with a *naturalistic cause* involves medicinal herbs, therapeutic diets, and hygiene measures. Treatment for diseases with a *supernatural cause* involves having the local healer or shaman cast out the evil and call forth return of good spirits. Treatment of diseases with a *metaphysical causation* involves using foods, herbs, or medications, classified as hot or cold, or opposites on a continuum, so that the treatment is opposite to the causative factor. For example, "hot" food and medications are used to balance the need in "cold" diseases and vice versa. Use of these treatments is complex and varies with cultural definitions of the conditions that cause disharmony and the appropriate treatment (37).

Adapt Care to Physiologic Status

Screen for carriers of diseases and treat as necessary. Many immigrants find jobs as food workers when they first come to the United States. They should be in good health.

Culturally competent care involves **ethnopharmacology,** *use of knowledge of how race and ethnicity affect response to medications.* Genetic or cultural factors often influence **pharmacokinetics,** *medication absorption, metabolism, distribution, and elimination* and **pharmacodynamics,** *action and effects of the medication at its target site.* Nurses are in a key position to prevent adverse drug reactions in clients from different ethnic backgrounds. Response to medication varies because of ethnic genetic variations in producing certain enzymes that are responsible for drug metabolism. *There are also enzymatic variations within each ethnic group.* Thus, the medication may be metabolized and eliminated too quickly (giving ineffective action) or too slowly (causing cumulative effects and toxicity) (56, 87, 107). To *maintain current ethnopharmacology knowledge, refer to the following Websites:*

1. Center for Cross-Cultural Research, www.wwu.edu
2. Cross-Cultural Health Care Program, www.xculture.org
3. Diversity Rx, www.diversityrx.org
4. National Center for Cultural Competence, www.gucchd.georgetown.edu
5. Transcultural C.A.R.E. Associates, www.transculturalcare.net

Lactose intolerance may exist. Do not automatically teach everyone to drink milk. Calcium can be obtained in other ways: seafood and fish cooked to yield edible bones, dark leafy vegetables, yogurt, buttermilk, aged cheese (lactose has been changed to lactic acid during aging), foods cooked with milk, or homemade soup (add vinegar or fresh tomatoes to the water when cooking a soup bone to help decalcify the bone). Most ethnic groups have adapted ways of cooking to ensure calcium intake from nondairy sources; listen carefully to their dietary descriptions. If the lactase-deficient person wishes to ingest considerable milk foods, an enzyme product to add to milk may be purchased from drug or health food stores. An acidophilus milk (Lactaid), which contains a controlled culture of *Lactobacillus acidophilus* bacteria, is also easily digested. Children who are lactose deficient can drink a soybean-based milk substitute and should take calcium and vitamin supplements. Pregnant and lactating women must take calcium and vitamin/mineral supplements and eat foods high in calcium (37).

Adapt Care to Socioeconomic Level

Health promotion and education about health care must account for the socioeconomic level and lifestyle of the person. Review principles of communication and crisis intervention, described in Chapter 2. ∞ When caring for members of the upper-upper, lower-upper, power-elite, upper-middle, and creative economic levels, accommodate the approach to education and counseling methods. They will expect considerable client participation in decision making and treatment planning, rehabilitation, and future preventive measures. Focus on health promotion. Be flexible. Accept unique responses from the client who highly values individuality, autonomy, self-expression, and excellent performance. The concept of evidence-based practice will be understood by these clients. However, realize the person who is always on the "fast track," such as the creative-class or upper-middle-class worker, may welcome slowing down and expect more assistance and less participation. Members of the middle and lower-middle economic levels who arrive for care in the emergency department because they have no health care benefits respond well to a prompt, respectful, personable, and thorough approach. They are likely to be receptive to and follow well-explained suggestions. The communication principles discussed earlier are especially important with clients who are poor, immigrants, refugees, or asylees, as they often mistrust and are fearful of the health care system and professionals and feel a sense of stigma and discrimination related to lack of health insurance and poverty.

Adapt Care to African American Clients

Information about the African American population presented in **Table 5-5** and the earlier sections on African American culture will be useful. The communication principles and emphasis on holistic care described in this section are applicable to African American clients. Call the adult by title and proper name. Avoid a condescending attitude, which can be conveyed by abrupt commands, brusque behavior, or a hurrying approach. Listen carefully if Black dialect or Black English is used; do not mimic or correct. If necessary, state that you do not understand what is being said, but that you want to. Restate and clarify as necessary if the client does not appear to understand medical terminology or treatment plans. Use visual aids when necessary (37).

Accept that the African American may use space differently. The person may sit closer, touch more, and use torso movements and gestures. The person may be more passive as you speak; the person may feel he or she is being demeaned by the way you speak and may "suffer in silence" rather than comment on an insulting approach. Your ability to demonstrate empathy and foster trust is key to overcoming obstacles in health promotion or treatment methods.

The African American family is often matrifocal. Incorporate the client's grandmother and mother in the treatment plan and rehabilitation or follow-up care. Include other support persons as well in the holistic care.

Determine if a traditional or spiritual healer has been utilized prior to seeking health care services. If so, incorporate the person into the care and treatment plan if the person is accessible. Such a person can be especially helpful if the client is suffering from a culture-bound illness and also to encourage necessary scientific medical treatment and rehabilitation that does not conflict with traditional healing that has been effective.

Skin and hair care should follow the client's usual patterns to the extent possible. Observation of the mucous membrane and skin condition and coloration is important, especially if injury has occurred or anemia is present.

African Americans traditionally perceive time as flexible or elastic. It is necessary, unless the person is educated or in a profession or work that emphasizes time, to teach the client the importance of taking medication on time and the importance of timed treatments or keeping scheduled appointments (43).

Religious beliefs are likely to set the foundation for use of time, family life and roles, and health care. The church community, clergy, and spiritual faith are a foundation for all life patterns.

Adapt Care to Latino Clients

When caring for Latino clients, you are caring for the family. The information about Spanish-speaking populations in **Tables C5-1** through C5-7 on the Companion Website, and the earlier section on Latino culture will be useful. Further, note the degree of acculturation, as decision-making patterns in some Cuban American and migrant farm worker families are evolving to be more equal between husbands and wives. Respectful or deferential behavior is expected toward others on the basis of age, sex, social position, economic status, and position of authority. Health care providers are respected but are also expected to be respectful. Avoiding conflict and achieving harmony is important; *a trusting therapeutic relationship is essential.* Clients prefer more physical and interpersonal closeness than do Anglo Americans. *Personal relationships are more important than institutional relationships; talk with the person about family and daily life events.* Incorporate language preference of the person, who may be unwilling to speak about a problem if he or she cannot describe it in the native language, even though the person speaks English as well. Communication strategies listed in the next section, including the Interventions for Health Promotion box, would also be applicable (2, 7, 8, 10, 13). If a translator is necessary, an adult of the same sex as the client is preferred. *Avoid using a child in the family as an interpreter because that places the child in a superior position, which is unacceptable.* Parents are unlikely to expose family problems to the child or expect the child to assume responsibility for family difficulties. This client often expresses a sense of **fatalism,** *that he or she has no control over health outcomes of the life situation.* Thus, to engage in preventive measures is being unfaithful to God or is unnecessary because God or fate determines what will happen (2, 10, 13, 37, 83, 112).

Adapt Care to Selected Traditional Populations: American Indians, Appalachians, or Rural Clients

It is possible to incorporate indigenous folk medicine and practitioners into professional and scientific health care practices. The two are not automatically exclusive. **Table 5-10** describes folk healing practices. For example, in one *Navajo* nursing care service, the medicine man is an active participant, and Navajo mothers are encouraged to use their infant cradle boards and to be home for the blessing ceremonies. Having an Indian corn ceremony, where corn is ritualistically deposited around the patient's bed in the hospital, meets a cultural need and is not difficult for housekeeping to clean up later.

When caring for clients from different cultures, be aware of barriers to accessibility or receptivity to health care services. For example, *barriers to health care, including prenatal care, in a rural community may include the following:* (a) heavy work schedule, (b) economic difficulties, (c) lack of health insurance coverage or high deductibles, (d) lack of accessible health care services or long distances to services, (e) negative attitudes toward health care services, (f) lack of information about prevention, health maintenance, or warning signs of disease, (g) less attention to or care for chronic illnesses, and (h) value of self-reliance and risk-taking behaviors.

Adapt Care to Immigrants and Refugees

Immigrants and refugees who have recently arrived in the United States are likely to need health care. Be aware that newcomers to this country may be suspicious about the screening process; extra time must be spent in explaining why each component is necessary.

INTERVENTIONS FOR HEALTH PROMOTION

When you *care for individuals and families who come from a more traditional background, the following approaches are useful.* **Traditional populations** *include American Indians* (2, 25, 37, 43, 71, 112, 124), *people who live in Appalachia* (2, 37, 111), *and people who live in rural areas* (44, 55, 72, 84, 101, 106):

1. Begin initial assessment and intervention by showing interest in the family, daily life activities, the weather, or difficulties finding the care site. Social talk helps to build trust. To "sit a spell," for a few minutes, is important.

2. Realize that by the time the person seeks professional help, considerable time may have been lost to preventive care because of use of home remedies or other healers.

3. Take time to learn their perception of the problem or diagnosis and what remedies have been or would be used at home. If your recommended intervention is unacceptable, it will not be used.

4. Be prepared to interact with the entire family unit. The family is considered a support and often accompanies the person. In the home visit, the family is likely to remain in the same room while you care for the person.

5. Solicit advice and opinions from the person or family members before taking action. Use indirect questions. Give hints or suggestions rather than direct orders. Seek agreement with your ideas; it may come slowly. Being less direct builds rapport and self-esteem.

6. Maintain a friendly, cooperative, neutral approach; avoid aggressiveness and domination. Too much direct eye contact is considered intrusive and aggressive. To avoid conflict is important.

7. Listen carefully to their language and use their phrases when possible, for example, "running off" for diarrhea, "nerve trouble" for mental illness.

8. Realize that what you call "assessment" or "education" they may call "interference." Explain why you are asking a question or seeking information, because they will not answer unless it is necessary. Thus, it may be very difficult to obtain information about any kind of abuse, because it is believed that how the family members treat each other is their own business. Health teaching is ignored if it doesn't fit the person's worldview.

9. Realize they may tell you what they think you want to hear to get your approval or to shorten the interaction time.

10. Explain intervention to the whole family, for it is the family unit who determines whether it fits their ideas and is implemented.

11. Specify appointment times, but be aware that they are less important than in mainstream culture. If the person arrives late for an appointment, do not be judgmental, critical, or turn the person away, because such behavior is likely to result in quiet anger, a sense of neglect, and an unwillingness to follow your suggestions or to keep future appointments. Realize that being late may be caused by transportation, child care, or other problems.

12. Tell the person and family that you appreciate that they followed the prescribed interventions, especially if your interventions are contrary to (or "don't fit") their ideas. Praise is likely to motivate further care seeking.

13. Explain ideas and interventions as simply and directly as possible. Give specific examples rather than using broad generalizations. Explain printed literature or directions. Even if the person is literate, learning may be more hearing oriented than vision based, and written directions may seem confusing. In contrast to some groups, storytelling and humor can be useful to include with intervention for the American Indian (25).

14. Determine the family's use of other healers; convey that you desire to cooperate with them.

You may need to use an interpreter. **Table 5-11** gives guidelines for use of an interpreter. This population experiences stress related to cultural, language, and economic barriers; loss and grief from geographic translocation and change in life events; and a sense of powerlessness. There may be little social support and many challenges related to acculturation, inadequate housing, poverty, racism, and social and educational issues. They may experience acute stress, the General Adaptation Syndrome and phases of crisis as described in Chapter 2. ∞ Post-traumatic stress disorder, with nightmares, frightening memories, and flashbacks to prior traumatic events, is common, especially among refugees or people seeking asylum. Access to health care and medical services is difficult because of health policies and fragmented delivery systems. Utilize references for information about intervention (2, 29, 70, 78, 97, 105, 108, 122).

Community health workers can be teamed with nurses to implement community-based health promotion programs that include home visits, health education, outreach activities for ambulatory care sites, needs assessment, and referral to social services (80). A study (45) of 13 parents and 16 children from nine Taiwanese immigrant families revealed that learning computer technology can foster adaptation to life in the United States. Demands related to language proficiency, economic survival, loss of social networks, and social discrimination were handled through strategies learned in computer classes. The immigrants also gained knowledge about their health and health care (45).

Adapt Care to Asian Clients

The traditional Asian view of health does not separate mind and body. Any mental illness, such as depression, is reported as somatic symptoms (fatigue, indigestion). An initial focus on physical symptoms is more acceptable and lays the foundation for assessment and intervention with mental illness (7, 37, 41).

Folk medicine practices help people gain a sense of control over their fate. Often the practice does no real harm but can be misinterpreted (2, 37). In one example, a *Vietnamese* mother used the ancient Chinese practice of **cao gio** (*"scratching the wind"*) to care for her child's cold. In this practice, the child's chest or back is covered with mentholated oil and then rubbed with a coin or hard object. The striations left on the child's skin, although causing no harm or injury, were interpreted by a health care provider as signs of child abuse. The health care provider reported the family, as required by law, based on her perceptions. The parents were charged, and the father, in fear of a jail term and in humiliation, hanged himself. *Be aware of possible folk medicine practices and their terminology, and explore these practices before making conclusions about the client.*

Culturally, many Asian clients acknowledge a belief in a supernatural or magical cause of their illness and consult regularly with indigenous healers. Nearly all display evidence of healing methods such as **cupping** (*applying a heated jar to the skin to form a vacuum to suction out illness*) and **coinage** (*rubbing a coin or spoon over the skin to rub out illness*) for physical symptoms. Polypharmacy is the norm. They use substances from many sources: herbal medications, over-the-counter and prescription drugs from the United States as well as other countries, and remedies sent by relatives in Southeast Asia and other parts of the world. Use of prescription drugs ranges from total noncompliance to self-regulated drug use (2, 37). Some recent immigrants may adhere closely to traditional practices. Others may not. Your care cannot be based on assumption or stereotype. Immigrants may combine traditional cultural and Western practices.

Many *Chinese Americans* practice Western-oriented activities of exercise, religious practices, lifestyle, and illness behavior activities. In dietary practices and sick behavior measures, use of a mixture of Chinese and Western practices has been reported by more than 50% of Chinese Americans. They described using more Western practices the longer they lived in the United States. *Four influencing variables are significant in their described health beliefs, dietary practices, and sick behavior measures* (123): (a) the familiarity of the participant with Western health care systems, (b) language, (c) occupation, and (d) religion.

INTERVENTIONS FOR HEALTH PROMOTION

Yep (123) and Barrett (7) share information on *how nurses can better* **care for clients from an Asian culture**. *These guidelines are pertinent to people in other cultures as well.*

1. Talk to the person in a way that shows respect. Avoid overbearing posture. Call the person by title and last name. Do not talk down to the person or family.
2. Older people may not be fluent in English, even if they have lived in the United States for many years. Speak slowly and use simple language. Invite the family to help interpret to the client and communicate feelings or questions to the health professional. The client is unlikely to admit that he or she is not understanding and may smile and nod the head "yes."
3. Generally, clients value care that reflects silence, patience, smooth relationships, and protecting self-esteem. To avoid conflict is essential.
4. Asian clients probably will not want to bother the practitioners with their complaints and problems. Most Asians believe suffering is part of life and must be accepted; however, the client is likely to complain to family members. Include family in your assessment, and question the client repeatedly and in several different ways to assess pain and provide pain relief.
5. Illness may be viewed as the result of an imbalance between *yin* and *yang*, an evil spirit, improper food, or something bad in the family. Utilize this concept in intervention.
6. Have the family bring familiar foods to make the hospital stay more comfortable for the Asian client. Some are accustomed to having rice at every meal.
7. Most Asians highly respect and even fear authority; doctors and nurses represent authority. Thus, the client expects a formal relationship and may become confused by an informal approach. They expect the professional to be in appropriate attire, prepared for the appointment, and able to arrive at a diagnosis on the initial visit.
8. Older Asian people may associate hospitals with death; it's the last place to go. On the other hand, hospitals also represent power and dominion. Hospital routines may not be understood. For example, an Asian person views his or her blood as finite in supply, as vital energy, and a life source; thus, repeated blood samples may cause much fear.
9. Asian adults do not touch people readily and are not usually demonstrative about affection. A smile conveys caring much better than a touch, as does performing little extras for the client without being asked, such as filling the water pitcher or placing needed objects nearby.
10. The family should also be given the explanations so they can clarify for the client, if necessary.
11. Use the family as an important resource. Accept that they visit frequently and for long hours, if they desire. They can assist in care; in fact, the client may expect them to. Cooperation with treatment and care routines will be fostered through communication with and involvement of the family.
12. Resilience, flexibility, and cultural relativism are valued by Japanese and other Asians, which in turn encourages adaptation to diverse social situations. Acknowledge these characteristics and how they enhance health.

Among the Southeast Asian Vietnamese, Hmong, Cambodian, and Laotian refugees in the United States, adjustment difficulties are manifested in anxiety, family abuse, post-traumatic stress disorder, intergenerational conflict, psychotic episodes, suicidal threats, substance abuse, and other antisocial behaviors. These problems may be masked by physical symptoms. High levels of dysfunction occur for the first and second years, often into the third year of resettlement. If culturally focused health care is given, with appropriate psychotherapeutic intervention and low doses of antidepressant medication, emotional health shows improvement in the third or fourth year (2, 7, 37).

Mental illness carries shame and stigma in the Asian community as well as in many ethnic groups. Social support systems tend to disappear as the person becomes less manageable. Hospitalization is often for threatened or attempted suicide. Barriers to health care, in addition to cultural and family attitudes, include lack of transportation to or inaccessibility of services, job schedules, family demands, lack of professionals fluent in Asian languages, and financial limitations. A culturally appropriate mental status examination is necessary to determine effects of folk beliefs and healing modalities (7, 81).

Some cultures, such as the *traditional Philippine culture*, believe that illness is the result of evil forces and that treatment involves protection from or removal of these evil forces. For example, the body is viewed as a container that collects debris, so flushing it out involves stimulating perspiration, vomiting, flatus, or menstrual bleeding to remove evil forces from the body. Use of heat and control of cold through herbs, teas, water, and fire help maintain a balanced internal temperature. Protection involves a gatekeeping system against the invasion of natural and supernatural forces. Mental illness may be thought to be the result of a witch casting a spell. Carrying an oval stone or wearing a cross, if the person is a Christian, will act as an antidote or protection. Using direct eye contact with the sick person is also believed to remove a witch's spell (14, 81, 112).

HEALTH PROMOTION EDUCATION

The changing society may cause families of many ethnic groups to have a variety of problems. Be a supportive listener. Validate realistic ideas. Prepare the family to adapt to a new or changing environment. Be aware of community agencies or resources that can provide additional help. See **Table 5-13** for guidelines on making referrals. When a client has no family nearby and seems alone and friendless, you may provide significant support. The health care provider who develops a personal philosophy that promotes a feeling of stability can, in turn, assist the client and family to explore feelings and formulate a philosophy for coping with change.

Health teaching is one way to have a lasting effect on the health practices of a cultural group. Health education specifically (a) transmits information, (b) motivates the inner resource of the person, and (c) helps people adopt and maintain healthful practices and lifestyles. Outsiders cannot make decisions for others, but people should be given sufficient knowledge concerning alternative behavior so that they can make intelligent choices themselves.

Various pressures interfere with attempts at health teaching. Behind poor health habits lies more than ignorance, economic pressure, or selfish desires. Motivation plays a great part in continuing

---

TABLE 5-13

Guidelines for Making a Referral

1. Know the available community resources and the services offered.
2. Recognize when you are unable to further assist or work with the client; be honest about your own limits and your perceived need for a referral. Avoid implying rejection of the client.
3. Explore client readiness for referral. The client may also have ideas about referrals and sources of help or may be unwilling to use community agencies.
4. Determine which other professionals had contact with the client and confer with them about the possibility of referral. Various ethnic and racial groups prefer using the extended family or church.
5. Discuss the possibility of referral with a specific person at the selected agency before referral.
6. Inform parents of your recommendations and obtain their consent and cooperation if the client is a minor.
7. Be honest in explaining services of the referral agency. Do not make false promises about another agency's services or roles.
8. Describe specifics about location, how to get to the referral place or person, where to park and enter, and what to expect on arrival.
9. Have the client (or parent) make the initial appointment for the new service if he or she is willing to do so; some people may prefer you to make the initial contact. Tell the person that you have called the agency and that he or she is expected.
10. Do not release information to the referral agency or person without written permission from the client (or parent).
11. Ask the client to give you feedback about the referral agency or person to help you evaluate your decision and to help you make a satisfactory referral selection if needed for future needy individuals or families.

---

certain practices. Motivation, moreover, is influenced by a person's culture, by status and role in that culture, and by social pressures for conformity. *Starting programs of prevention can be difficult when people* (a) place a low value on health, (b) cannot recognize cause-and-effect relationships in disease, (c) lack future-time orientation, or (d) are confused about the existence of preventive measures in their culture. Thus preventive programs or innovations in health care must be shaped to fit the cultural and health profiles of the population. Long-range prevention goals stand a better chance of implementation if they are combined with measures to meet immediate needs. For example, a mother is more likely to heed your advice about how to prevent further illness in her sick child if you give the child immediate attention.

Health protection involves risk-reduction behaviors and changing threatening environmental and social conditions. This can be difficult for people from any culture. Screening and immunizations continue to be important, but changing personal health behaviors of people before the clinical disease develops is essential. Frequency and specific facets of the periodic health examination should be tailored to the unique health risks, age, and gender of the individual patient or client. Counseling and education that help the person, family, or group assume greater responsibility for health may be of more value than screenings every year.

EVALUATION GUIDELINES

Develop culturally relevant **evaluation** methods and tools; seek input from the group to whom care is being given for ideas about how to best evaluate their perspectives. Give feedback to the client group about efforts being made to improve services. Develop materials that are tailored to the educational and linguistic capabilities of the specific client group. Back-translation will be important.

Develop methods that do not rely on written surveys; some ethnic groups and older ethnic clients have difficulty with test-taking skills. Be familiar with the cultural values, beliefs, practices, and indicators of effective care held by ethnic clients or the ethnic group. Approaches and outcomes that are considered effective by Western standards may be perceived as aggressive, impersonal, impractical, or ineffective by non-Westernized clients.

Summary

1. You will encounter diverse cultural value systems and customs as you engage in health promotion and client care.
2. Cultural background has a major influence on development, health, and worldview.
3. Continue to learn more about your own cultural background and values that influence your behavior as a foundation for better understanding clients and avoiding ethnocentrism.
4. People from the *same* culture share values, beliefs, and customs, but they are also uniquely different from each other.
5. People from *different* cultural backgrounds share similarities as well as differences in various values, life patterns, and health care practices.
6. Enjoy interactions with people, including clients, from diverse cultures, and learn from each contact as well as from information presented in literature and the media.
7. You can practice principles of cultural care, based on information presented in this chapter, in every health care setting and with all clients.
8. Culturally competent care considers the client's acculturation level related to being first, second, third, or fourth generation in the United States. Acculturation processes affect the individual and group in different ways.
9. Communication approaches and methods described in this chapter and in **Table 2-10** ∞ will be useful as you work with clients from any culture or with people in community services, engage in advocacy, or assume leadership roles in the community with a diverse population.
10. Evaluate your client care in order to become more culturally sensitive and to give more culturally competent care.

Review Questions

1. The nurse is visiting a client who is a second-generation American, and who lives in a neighborhood populated by individuals from the same country of origin. Many of the dietary, religious, and lifestyle practices in this neighborhood were brought to the United States by the parents of the neighborhood residents. This group can be defined as a/an:
   1. Culture
   2. Manifest culture
   3. Ideal culture
   4. Subculture
2. The nurse is concerned that an elderly immigrant client is not eating the food that is served on her meal tray. In order to adequately assess this situation the nurse should:
   1. Help the client to select food choices from the diet menu.
   2. Request that a dietitian visit the client.
   3. Ask the client about specific food practices or tastes and determine if those preferences can be accommodated.
   4. Notify the physician that the client has a loss of appetite.
3. The nurse in an obstetrics and gynecology clinic is working with a client of Iranian descent who is having difficulty conceiving a child. Which characteristic of this culture should the nurse keep in mind when working with this client?
   1. Childbearing is a source of self-esteem for the women.
   2. This group rejects cultural practices regarding childbirth when immigrating to the United States.
   3. Child rearing is a shared responsibility of husband and wife.
   4. Birth control practices are widely accepted by this culture.
4. The home health nurse arrives for a scheduled appointment to be told by a neighbor that the client left to attend a religious service. What is the best action for the nurse to take?
   1. Send the client a letter about the importance of scheduled appointments.
   2. Call the client to reschedule the appointment, then call and confirm immediately prior to arrival.
   3. Call the supervisor and request that the client be informed of agency rules regarding keeping scheduled appointments.
   4. Charge the client for the missed appointment and request that the client arrange for another appointment.

References

1. Al Shahri, M. Z. (2002). Culturally sensitive caring for Saudi patients. *Journal of Transcultural Nursing, 13*(2), 133–138.

2. Andrews, M., & Boyle, J. (2003). *Transcultural concepts in nursing care* (4th ed.). Philadelphia: J. B. Lippincott.

3. Appelbaum, R., Duneier, M., & Giddens, A. (2003). *Introduction to sociology* (4th ed.). New York: W.W. Norton.

4. Bailey, H., Briscoe, D., Clift, E., Drooney, J., Skipp, C., & Rend, J. (2006, April 10). Americas divided. *Newsweek, 28–38.*

5. Barbee, E. (2002). Racism and mental health. *Journal of American Psychiatric Nurses Association, 8*, 194–199.

6. Baughman, E. (1996). *Black Americans* (2nd ed.). London: Academic Press.

7. Barrett, S. (2006). Interviewing techniques for the Asian-American population. *Journal of Psychosocial Nursing, 44*(5), 29–34.

8. Bent, K. (2003). Culturally interpreting environment as determinant and experience. *Journal of Transcultural Nursing, 14*(5), 305–312.

9. Berger, K. (2005). *The developing person through the life span* (6th ed.). New York: Worth.

10. Boschert, S. (2005). Access critical for Hispanic patients. *Clinical Psychiatry News, 35*(10), 1, 11.

11. Bradley, P. H., Corwyn, R. F., MeAdoo, H. P., & Coll, C. G. (2001). The home environment of children in the United States: Part I. Variations in age, ethnicity, and poverty status. *Child Development, 72*, 1844–1867.

12. Brink, P., & Saunders, J. (1978). Culture shock: Theoretical and applied. In P. Brink (Ed.), *Transcultural nursing: A book of readings* (pp. 128–138). Englewood Cliffs, NJ: Prentice Hall.

13. Campinha-Bacote, J. (2002). The process of cultural competence in the delivery of healthcare services: A model of care. *Journal of Transcultural Nursing, 13*, 181–184.

14. Campinha-Bacote, J. (1992). Voodoo illness. *Perspectives in Psychiatric Care, 28*(1), 11–17.

15. Cantore, J. (2001, Winter). Earth, wind, fire, and water. *Minority Nurse,* 24–29. Retrieved from http://www.MinorityNurse.com

16. Center for Law and Social Policy. (2004). The future of immigrant children. *CLASP Update, 17*(10/11), 1–8.

17. Clark, M. (2008). *Community health nursing: Advocacy for population health* (5th ed.). Upper Saddle River, NJ: Pearson Prentice Hall.

18. Coburn, A., MacKinney, A., McBride, T., Mueller, K., Slifkin, M., & Wakefield, M., (2007, March). Choosing rural definitions for health policy. *Issue Brief #2, Rural Policy Research Institute Health Panel.* Retrieved July 20, 2007, from http://www.rapri.org/ruralhealth

19. Coffman, M., Shellman, J., & Bernal, H. (2004). An integrative review of American nurses' perceived cultural self-efficacy. *Journal of Nursing Scholarship, 36*, 180–185.

20. Conrad, M., & Pacquiao, D. (2005). Manifestation, attribution, and coping with depression among Asian Indians from the perspectives of health care practitioners. *Journal of Transcultural Nursing, 16*, 32–40.

21. Correspondents of *The New York Times.* (2005). *Class matters.* New York: Times Books, Henry Holt and Company.

22. Courtney, B. (1995, February 13). Freedom from choice. *Newsweek,* 16.

23. Cowan, D., & Norman, I. (2006). Cultural competence in nursing: New meanings. *Journal of Transcultural Nursing, 17*(1), 82–88.

24. Davitz, L., Sameshima, Y., & Davita, J. (1976). Suffering as viewed in six different cultures. *American Journal of Nursing, 76*(8), 1296–1297.

25. Dean, R. (2003). Native American humor: Implications for transcultural care. *Journal of Transcultural Nursing, 14*(1), 62–65.

26. Dearing, E., McCartney, K., & Taylor, B. (2001). Change in family income-to-needs matters more for children with less. *Child Development, 72,* 1779–1793.

27. DeLeal, A., & Radtke, B. (2006). *Living as a refugee: Mohamed's story.* London: Ticktock Limited of Great Britain.

28. Deng, A. (2005, October 31). I have had to learn to live with peace. *Newsweek,* 16.

29. DeSantis, L. (1997). Building healthy communities with immigrants and refugees. *Journal of Transcultural Nursing, 9*(1), 20–31.

30. Diamond, J. (2005). *Collapse: How societies choose to fail or succeed.* New York: Penguin.

31. Dodgson, J., & Struthers, R. (2005). Indigenous women's voices: Marginalization and health. *Journal of Transcultural Nursing, 16*(2), 339–346.

32. Farrell, S., & McKinnon, C. (2003). Technology and rural mental health. *Archives of Psychiatric Nursing, 17*(1), 20–26.

33. Felski, R. (2002). Lower middle class is vital to understanding beliefs, values, and experiences of ordinary individuals and tells public about how class is lived in contemporary America. *Chronicle of Higher Education, 48,* 24.

34. Florida, R. (2002). *The rise of the creative class.* New York: Perseus Books.

35. Formichelli, L. (2001, Summer). A harvest of hope. *Minority Nurse,* 37–44.

36. Giddens, A., Duneier, M., & Applebaum, R. (2003). *Introduction to sociology.* New York: W.W. Norton.

37. Giger, J., & Davidhizar, R. (2004). *Transcultural nursing: Assessment and intervention* (4th ed.). St. Louis, MO: Mosby.

38. Glittenberg, J. (2004). A transdisciplinary, transcultural model for health care. *Journal of Transcultural Nursing, 15,* 6–10.

39. Hahn, S. (2003). *A nation under our feet: Black political struggles in the rural South from slavery to the great migration.* Cambridge, MA: Harvard University Press.

40. Heiner, R. (2002). *Social problems: An introduction to critical constructionism.* New York: Oxford University Press.

41. Helsel, D., Mochel, M., & Bauer, R. (2005). Chronic illness and Hmong shamans. *Journal of Transcultural Nursing, 16,* 150–154.

42. Henslin, J. B. (2005). *Sociology: A down-to-earth approach.* Boston: Allyn & Bacon.

43. Hodge, F., Marquez, C., & Geishert-Cantrell, B. (2002). Utilizing traditional storytelling to promote wellness in American Indian communities. *Journal of Transcultural Nursing, 13*(1), 6–11.

44. Hostetler, J. (1993). *Amish society* (4th ed.). Baltimore: Johns Hopkins University Press.

45. Hsin-Chun Tsai, J. (2006). Use of computer technology to enhance immigrant families' adaptation. *Journal of Nursing Scholarship, 38*(1), 87–93.

46. Jones, P., Zhang, X. E., & Meleis, A. (2003). Transforming vulnerability. *Western Journal of Nursing Research, 25,* 835–853.

47. Kalins, D. (2006, March 26). Design of the times. *Newsweek,* 54–63.

48. Kenney, G. (1998). Native Hawaiian health. *Reflections* (4th quarter), 21.

49. Kikuchi, J. (2005). Cultural theories of nursing responsive to human needs and values. *Journal of Nursing Scholarship, 37,* 302–307.

50. Kilgore, C. (2005). PTSD symptoms persist in refugees for decades. *Clinical Psychiatry News, 33*(9), 39.

51. Kim, E. (2006, April 21). Older immigrants, refugees can get help with citizenship. *St. Louis Post-Dispatch,* PC-10.

52. Kim, M. T., Hun, H., Shin, H. S., Kim, K. A., & Lee, H. B. (2005). Factors associated with depression experiences of immigrant populations: A study of Korean immigrants. *Archives of Psychiatric Nursing, 19*(5), 217–225.

53. Kluckhorn, F. (1958, February–March). Family diagnosis: Variations of basic values of family systems. *Social Casework, 32,* 63–72.

54. Kluckhorn, F., & Strodtbeck, E. (1961). *Variations in value orientations.* New York: Row, Petersen.

55. Kraybill, D. (2001). *The riddle of Amish culture* (Rev. ed.). Baltimore: Johns Hopkins University Press.

56. Kudzma, E. (1999). Culturally competent drug administration. *American Journal of Nursing, 99*(8), 46–51.

57. Lappe, F. (1999). *Rediscovering America's values.* New York: Ballantine Books.

58. Lawrence, P., & Rozmus, C. (2001). Culturally sensitive care of the Muslim patient. *Journal of Transcultural Nursing, 12*(3), 228–233.

59. Leininger, M. (2002). Culture care theory: A major contribution to advance transcultural nursing knowledge and practices. *Journal of Transcultural Nursing, 13*(3), 188–192.

60. Leininger, M. (1999). What is transcultural nursing and culturally competent care? *Journal of Transcultural Nursing, 10*(1), 5.

61. Leininger, M. (1997). Understanding cultural pain for improved health care. *Journal of Transcultural Nursing, 9*(1), 32–35.

62. Leininger, M. (1992). Self-care ideology and cultural incongruities: Some critical issues. *Journal of Transcultural Nursing, 4*(1), 2–4.

63. Leininger, M. (1991). *Culture care diversity and universality: A theory of nursing.* New York: National League for Nursing.

64. Leininger, M. (1991). Transcultural care principles, human rights, and ethical considerations. *Journal of Transcultural Nursing, 3*(1), 21–22.

65. Leininger, M. (1990). The significance of cultural concepts in nursing. *Journal of Transcultural Nursing, 2*(1), 52–59.

66. Leininger, M. (1990). Issues, questions, and concerns related to the nursing diagnosis cultural movement from a transcultural nursing perspective. *Journal of Transcultural Nursing, 2*(1), 23–32.

67. Leininger, M. (1979). *Transcultural nursing.* New York: Masson.

68. Leininger, M. (1970). *Nursing and anthropology: Two worlds to blend.* New York: John Wiley & Sons.

69. Leininger, M., & McFarland, M.R. (2002). *Transcultural nursing: Concepts, theories, research and practices* (3rd ed.). New York: McGraw-Hill.

70. Lipson, J., Weinstein, J., Gladstone, E., & Sarnoff, R. (2003). Bosnian and Soviet refugees' experiences with health care. *Western Journal of Nursing Research, 25,* 854–871.

71. Lowe, J. (2002). Cherokee self-reliance. *Journal of Transcultural Nursing, 13*(4), 287–295.

72. MacAvoy, S., & Lippman, D. (2001). Teaching culturally competent care: Nursing students' experiences in rural Appalachia. *Journal of Transcultural Nursing, 13*(4), 221–227.

73. Mahoney, D. (2005, May). Cultural sensitivity is essential. *Clinical Psychiatric News, 33*(5), 64.

74. Majumbar, B., Browne, G., Roberts, J., & Carpio, B. (2004). Effects of cultural sensitivity training on health care provider attitudes and patient outcomes. *Journal of Nursing Scholarship, 36,* 161–168.

75. Makihara, K. (2005, August 15). Are they too young to ride the trains alone? *Newsweek,* 11.

76. Maltby, H. (1999). Interpreters: A double-edged sword in nursing practice. *Journal of Transcultural Nursing, 10,* 248–254.

77. Mannix, E., & Neale, M. (2005). What differences make a difference? The promise and reality of diverse teams in organizations. *Psychological sciences in the public interest: A supplement to Psychological Science, 6*(2), 31–55.

78. Marshall, E., & Martin, J. (2002). Transcultural nursing among migrant workers. *Journal of Christian Nursing, 19*(1), 12–14.

79. May, R. (2001). *The United States middle class: Social life and customs.* New York: New York University Press.

80. McElmurry, B., Park, C., & Busch, A. (2003). The nurse-community advocate team for urban immigrant primary health care. *Journal of Nursing Scholarship, 35*(3), 275–281.

81. McGoldrick, M., Giordano, J., & Garcio-Preto, N. (2005). *Ethnicity and family therapy* (3rd ed.). New York: Guilford.

82. Meleis, A. (1999). Culturally competent care. *Journal of Transcultural Nursing, 10*(1), 12.

83. Mendelson, C. (2002). Health perceptions of Mexican American women. *Journal of Transcultural Nursing, 31,* 210–217.

84. Meyer, S., Huster, V., Rathbun, L., Armstrong, V., Anna, S., Ronyak, J., & Savrin, C. (2003). A look into the Amish culture: What should we learn? *Journal of Transcultural Nursing, 14,* 139–145.

85. Miller, J., & Petro-Nustas, W. (2002). Context of care for Jordanian women. *Journal of Transcultural Nursing, 13,* 228–236.

86. Mills, C. W. (2001). *The power elite.* New York: Oxford University Press.

87. Munoz, C., & Hilgenberg, C. (2005). Ethnopharmacology. *American Journal of Nursing, 105*(8), 40–48.

88. Murray, R., Yakimo, R., & Baier, M. (2008). Care of people who are homeless and mentally ill. In M. Boyd, *Psychiatric nursing: Contemporary practice* (4th ed., pp. 740–755). Philadelphia: Lippincott Williams & Wilkins.

89. Nagel, P. (2002). *The German migration to Missouri.* Kansas City, MO: Kansas City Star Books.

90. NANDA International. (2007). *NANDA nursing diagnoses: Definitions & classifications 2007–2008.* Philadelphia: Author.

91. National Coalition for the Homeless. (2005, June). *Why are people homeless: NCH fact sheet #1.* Washington, DC: Author. Retrieved May 16, 2006, from http://www.nationalhomeless.org

92. Papalia, D., Olds, S., & Feldman, R. (2004). *Human development* (4th ed.). Boston: McGraw-Hill.

93. Payne, R. (2005). *A framework for understanding poverty* (4th ed. rev.). Highlands, TX: Aha Process.

94. Pender, N., Murdaugh, C., & Parsons, M. (2006). *Health promotion in nursing practice* (5th ed.). Upper Saddle River, NJ: Pearson Prentice Hall.

95. Purnell, L. (2002). The Purnell model for cultural competence. *Journal of Transcultural Nursing, 13*(3), 193–195.

96. Purnell, L. (1998). *Transcultural health care: A culturally competent approach.* Philadelphia: F.A. Davis.

97. Ramos, J. (2004). *The other face of America: Chronicles of the immigrants shaping our future.* New York: Harper Collins.

98. Ridley, R., Nabor, J., Florea, F., & Gumenski, D. (2004). Development of a multilingual resource manual. *Journal of Transcultural Nursing, 15,* 231–241.

99. Rippley, L. J. (1970). *Of German ways.* New York: Barnes & Noble.

100. Rippley, L. J. (1976). *The German-Americans.* Boston: Twayne Publishers, Division of G.K. Hall.

101. Ryan-Nicholls, K., Racher, F., & Robinson, R. (2003). Providers' perceptions of how rural consumers access and use mental health service. *Journal of Psychosocial Nursing, 41*(6), 34–43.

102. Sachs, J. (2006). *The end of poverty. Economic possibilities for our times.* New York: Penguin Books.

103. Santrock, J. (2004). *Life-span development* (9th ed.). Boston: McGraw-Hill.

104. Schaefer, E. H. (2001). *Cultural sociology.* Malden, MA: Blackwell.

105. Schreiber, R., Stern, P., & Wilson, C. (2000). Being strong: How Black West Indian Canadian women manage depression and its stigma. *Journal of Nursing Scholarship, 32*(1), 39–45.

106. Schwarz, T. (2002). Making it safer down on the farm. *American Journal of Nursing, 102*(3), 114–115.

107. Sherman, C. (2005). Factor ethnicity into drug treatment: Part 2. *Clinical Psychiatry News, 33*(8), 42.

108. Simich, L., Beiser, M., & Mawani, F. (2003). Social support and the significance of shared experience in refugee migration and resettlement. *Western Journal of Nursing Research, 25,* 872–891.

109. Smith, A. (2003). Soul wound: The legacy of Native American schools. *Amnesty International, 29*(2), 14–17.

110. Smoyak, S. (2006). Diversity: What differences make a difference? *Journal of Psychosocial Nursing, 44*(4), 4–6.

111. Soderlind, L. (2006). Adirondack nurse. *American Journal of Nursing, 106*(4), 81–84.

112. Spector, R. (2003). *Cultural diversity in health and illness* (6th ed.). Upper Saddle River, NJ: Prentice Hall Health.

113. Swope, D. (2004, Spring). Let the mainland hear the word. *Teaching Tolerance,* Issue 25, 14–17.

114. Thies, K., & Travers, J. (2006). *Handbook of human development for health care professionals.* Boston: Jones and Bartlett.

115. United States Bureau of the Census. (2006). *Statistical abstract of the United States: 2006.* Washington, DC: Government Printing Office.

116. Urrea, L. A. (2004). *The devil's highway.* New York: Back Bay Books, Little, Brown & Co.

117. Ward, L. (2003). Race as a variable in cross-cultural research. *Nursing Outlook, 51*(5), 120–125.

118. Weiss, O. (1973). Cultural shock. *Nursing Outlook, 19*(1), 40–43.

119. Whaley, A. (2005, November 14). Once unique: Soon a place like any other. *Newsweek,* 13.

120. Wong, T., & Pung, S. (2000). Holism and caring: Nursing in the Chinese health care culture. *Holistic Nurse Practitioner, 15*(11), 12–21.

121. Wood, D. L. (2001, Summer). Mentors to the max. *Minority Nurse,* 52–57.

122. Yeh, C., & Inose, M. (2002). Difficulties and coping strategies of Chinese, Japanese, and Korean immigrant students. *Adolescents, 37*(145), 69–82.

123. Yep, J. (1991). An Asian patient. How does culture affect care? A family member responds. *Journal of Christian Nursing, 6*(5), 5–8.

124. Yurkovich, E., Clairmont, J., & Grandbois, D. (2002). Mental health care provider's perception of giving culturally responsive care to American Indians. *Perspectives in Psychiatric Nursing, 38*(4), 147–156.

125. Zborowski, M. (1960). Cultural components in response to pain. In D. Apple (Ed.), *Sociological studies of health and sickness* (pp. 118–133). New York: McGraw-Hill.

Interviews

126. Jordan, V. B.A. Social Work, St. Louis, Missouri, May 1, 2006. (African American Values)

127. Talley, P. MSN, CNS-BC, CSAC II, St. Louis, Missouri, May 2, 2006. (African American Values)

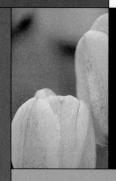

The Family: Basic Influences

OBJECTIVES

Study of this chapter will enable you to:

1. Describe the purposes, tasks, roles, functions, and adaptive mechanisms of the family system and their relationship to the development and health of its members.

2. Relate the developmental tasks to each stage of family life.

3. Analyze variables affecting the relationship between parent and child and general family interaction, including feelings about self and childhood experiences.

4. Discuss the influence of sociocultural changes on family life and parenting practices in the United States and other countries.

5. Assess a family, constructing a genogram and using criteria listed in the chapter.

6. Discuss your role in helping the family achieve its developmental tasks and in promoting physical and emotional health of a family in various situations.

MediaLink www.prenhall.com/murray

Go to the Companion Website for interactive resources that accompany this chapter.

Glossary	Critical Thinking
Review Questions	Tools
Challenge Your Knowledge	Media Link Applications
Learning Activities	Media Links

The family, the basic social unit, can so strongly affect our development and health that we may live successfully or unsuccessfully because of its influence. Loving, coping, and the various aspects of life are first learned in the family unit. Thus *Healthy People 2010* presents objectives and goals to promote prenatal care, provide quality child care, and reduce family lifestyle behaviors that are risks to health, such as smoking tobacco and alcohol and drug abuse. Goals include to increase the quality and length of a healthy life and to eliminate health care disparities for family members (61).

Some form of family exists in all human societies. Culture, not biology, determines family organization (49). Between society and the individual person, the family exists as a primary system and social group; most people share many of life's experiences with the family. The family has a major role in shaping the person, and it is a basic unit of growth, experience, adaptation, health, or illness.

The traditional family is challenged, with the fragility of marriage, the high incidence of divorce (and remarriage), the many styles of family life, the diversity of roles held by members, and the increasing number of homeless families. Today's children are being shaped differently—sometimes negatively—by the family unit. For many children, the pain of family life, a changing family scene, having no permanent home, and being separated from other family members are compounded by poverty and neglect.

This chapter is an overview of the various forms, stages, and functions of contemporary American families and how you can use this knowledge. Although various aspects of the family are discussed separately, family purposes, stages of development, developmental tasks, and patterns of interaction are all closely interrelated. Families are influenced by historical foundations and continually evolve into new forms. The family should be viewed as a system, affected by the culture, the environment, religious-spiritual dimensions, and other variables, which in turn affect the person and society.

Definitions

Families are defined in many ways. Families may have difficulty in maintaining the characteristics proposed in these definitions.

FAMILY

The **family** *is a small social system and primary reference group made up of two or more persons living together who are related by blood, marriage, or adoption or who are living together by agreement.* The family unit is *characterized by face-to-face contact; bonds of affection, love, loyalty, and emotional and financial commitment; harmony; and simultaneous competition and mutual concern. Families provide continuity of past, present, and future; share values, goals, and identity; and engage in behaviors and rituals unique to their specific unit* (11, 13).

The family may also be defined as *domestic partners, people who have chosen to share each other's life in an intimate and committed relationship of mutual caring.* This definition permits the extension of legal benefits (insurance, pensions, property rights, employment benefits) to homosexual or same-sex families or unmarried partners.

Family may be defined differently by different cultures. Latino families are an extended system, including blood relations and *godparents* (**compadres**) and *adopted children* (**hijos de crianza**). **Compadrazgo** *is a ritual kinship with mutual obligations for financial assistance, encouragement, and discipline* (32).

Family structure and function differ based on socioeconomic status, ethnicity and culture, history, and life cycle changes (13, 20). Sometimes families live together daily. Sometimes the adult partners are employed in different geographic areas, or one member is hospitalized or in prison. They maintain contact by telephone, correspondence, and visits. In the two-career family, the partners share the same residence on weekends or on a consistent basis. These families carry out their functions and characteristics in their own unique way.

Healthy families are characterized by (66) (a) a sense of relationship among members; (b) clear boundaries allowing for interchange between the family and the outside world; (c) clear social roles; (d) a clear hierarchy of power, with adults having more power than children; (e) warm, joyful, and comforting interactions; (f) negotiating skills; and (g) ability to accept change and loss.

FAMILY COMPOSITION

The family takes many forms, including traditional and nontraditional compositions. **Table 6-1** defines types of families. The nuclear family with two married parents and children living in one household makes up only 27% of households in the United States.

Same-sex families, including gay and lesbian couples, make up 17% of American families. Same-sex families may be childless, have custody of biological children, or have adopted children. A lesbian woman may choose to become pregnant through artificial insemination or one-time contact with a selected man and give birth to a child. Her partner takes on the parenting role with the understanding that she is not the mother. The gay male couple may contract with a woman to carry a baby to term for them. Gay and lesbian couples who have biological children are now more frequently exerting their rights and responsibilities with the child after establishment of the same-sex relationship (3, 24, 44, 51).

The family may comprise a childless couple; siblings living together in middle or late life; friends in a commune; or a man and woman living together without being married, with or without children. The family may also be a series of separate but interrelated families. Grandparents may be raising their children and grandchildren simultaneously. Middle-aged parents may be helping their young adult children live independently while caring for increasingly dependent parents, grandparents, or older relatives. More information is presented in Chapters 9 through 16. ∞

The family group may be a **psychologically extended family** in which *people who are not biologically related consider themselves as siblings, "adopted" parent, child, aunt, uncle, or grandparent-in-spirit.* Similarly, related or unrelated family members may not live in the same household. The family member who is no longer present because of divorce, death, or absence may remain a significant influence on the family and be acknowledged on special occasions. The family may be **symbolically duplicated** *in the work setting for an employee: A woman may be perceived and responded to as mother,*

TABLE 6-1

Types of Family Composition

Nuclear family: *Husband and wife and their biological children.*

Extended family: *Three or more generations of biologically related individuals.*

Single-parent family: *Mother or father, never married or now divorced, and his or her biological or adopted children.*

Stepparent family: *One divorced or widowed adult with all or some of his or her children and a new spouse with all or some of his or her children, and also any children born to this union so that parents, stepparents, children, and stepchildren (or stepsiblings) live together.*

Blended family: *One parent with all or some of his or her children and a new spouse with all or some of his or her children, and any children the parents have together.*

Adoptive family: *One or more nonbiological children raised by a single adult or couple.*

Grandparent family: *Children living in their grandparents' home, with their parents (extended family) or without them (grandparents alone).*

Gay/lesbian family: *Gay or lesbian partners and the biological or adopted children of one or both partners.*

Single state: *Never married, separated, divorced, or widowed.*

Patrifocal/patriarchal family: *Man has main authority and decision-making power.*

Matrifocal/matriarchal family: *Woman has main authority and decision-making power.*

---

grandmother, or sister, or a man as father, grandfather, or brother. Such relationships depend on emotional needs, age, or cultural factors and may contribute to harmony or conflict in the workplace.

The extended family affects thoughts and actions, provides sustenance, and contributes to identity. Present-day mobility of people, ease of long-distance communication, and ease of transportation allow families in the United States to be geographically distant yet emotionally close and involved in each other's lives. Today's families have freedom to evolve and think independently and develop in ways less restricted by strong or rigid ethnic or cultural mores.

The mass media presents a picture of family life dissolving in the United States. Media report that only 56% of all adults are now married compared to 75% 30 years ago. More than half of all marriages end in divorce; 60% of second marriages end in divorce (12, 60). Despite the grim statistics, there is also evidence that commitment to family life is increasing. Although the divorce rate is high, most divorced people remarry. Because of longer life expectancy and the young age at which some people marry, the young couples of today enter and may remain in marriage longer than did their grandparents. People are beginning to realize that divorce does not necessarily improve life. The allure of creativity, growth, and expanding oneself emotionally through divorce is not necessarily realistic. Some families try harder and resolve to stay committed to each other despite conflicts.

Family Theoretical Approaches

Many theoretical approaches have been used to study families. Refer to references at the end of the chapter for more extensive explanation of these theories (8, 20, 41, 67).

Developmental Theory *defines the family as a series of complex interacting positions with prescribed roles for each position. The family is studied in terms of role behaviors for each life cycle stage.*

Using this theory, focus on each member's changing roles and consider the cultural influences on each stage of the family life cycle. A family is in several developmental stages.

Structural-Functional Theory *sees the family as a system that is influenced by external forces. Each person is studied in relation to his or her roles within the social system.*

Focus on how family patterns and functions are related to the external social systems. The client's placement in the family structure affects care.

Interactional Theory *defines family members as interacting personalities with little relation to outside influences. Interactions among members have multiple meanings, and study is focused on interaction roles*, problem solving, decision making, and teaching effective communication methods.

Always analyze family interaction patterns while doing client care. They are crucial to healthy development and life patterns.

Role Theory *emphasizes each member's ascribed or assumed role and its contribution to social position, group interaction, and family norms.* A person can experience **role reciprocity** (*mutual exchange*), **role complementarity** (*differentiation*), or **role strain** (*conflict or overload*).

Client care would consider role interactions and analyze the type of roles displayed. The client's role in the family changes during illness.

Family Systems Theory *sees the family as a societal unit composed of interdependent and interacting members.* A person is seen as a member of a system and subsystem, but the family is seen as a whole unit, greater than the sum of its parts.

Analyze exchanges between subsystems in the family organization. The client's interaction in the family system changes during illness and may have also been a contributing factor to the illness. Chapter 1 and Figure 1-1 ∞ offer more information related to Systems Theory and family systems.

Crisis Theory *assumes that the family members individually experience and are affected by harmful events.* Chapter 2 ∞ presents information on Crisis Theory and its application.

Explore how a client's illness is a crisis for all family members. Assess each member's coping skills, suggest alternatives if needed, and provide strategies to handle future crises.

Purposes, Tasks, Roles, and Functions of the Family

The U.S. family has passed through major transitions. The family was once a relatively self-contained, cohesive domestic work unit. It has become a group of persons dispersed among various educational and work settings. Various agencies have absorbed many purposes once handled solely by the family group. Schools educate, hospitals care for the sick, mortuaries prepare the dead for burial, churches give religious training, government and private organizations erect recreational facilities, and nursing homes care for the aged. In addition, the home-cooked family meal is a rarity with fast-food takeout and prepackaged, precooked food readily available. Ready-made clothes have replaced home sewing.

Knowledge of the following sections will enhance assessment, health promotion intervention, teaching, referral, and advocacy. Family structure, roles, and responsibilities have been influenced by technology and the resulting social changes, which affects client care. But technologic advances alone do not determine family structure and function. Family systems are endlessly adaptive and very resistant to outside pressure or even professional education. In a society in which objects are often disposable and people feel dispensable, individuals seek secure relationships; the family can be a source of security. However, for some people, the family is a source of strain and conflict, with long-term detrimental consequences. The family, however structured, is your client as much as the individual.

PURPOSES AND TASKS OF THE FAMILY

The family is still considered responsible for the child's growth and development and behavioral outcomes and is a cornerstone for the child's development. Because the family is strongly influenced by its surrounding environment and by the child itself, the family should not bear full blame for what the child is or becomes. Few parents deliberately set out to raise a disturbed, handicapped, or delinquent child, although such situations occur. The family is expected to perform many tasks. These tasks may be the same for most types of family composition, but how they are manifested often is related to the type of family structure. Culture of the family group (racial, ethnic, geographic, socioeconomic, religious) also influences how tasks are achieved.

Basic tasks are as follows (17, 46, 65, 66):

1. Control reproductive function and ensure continuation of the species.
2. Provide for the physical, emotional, cognitive, social, and spiritual development of children and adults.
3. Provide for basic needs of food, shelter, clothing, and other resources to enhance human development.
4. Provide a sense of belonging, personal and social identity, and meaning and direction for life.
5. Foster a value system built on spiritual and philosophic beliefs and the cultural and social system that is part of the identity.
6. Teach members basic life skills, social roles, and to communicate effectively their needs, ideas, and feelings.
7. Provide protective care and support for young, ill, disabled, or otherwise vulnerable members.

8. Provide relationships and experience within and without the family that foster security, support, encouragement, motivation, morale, and creativity.
9. Maintain authority and decision making, with the parents representing society to the family and the family unit to society.
10. Release family members into the larger society—school, church, organizations, employment, and other systems.
11. Maintain constructive and responsible ties with the neighborhood and broader community.

The family often has difficulty in meeting these tasks and needs assistance from external resources. The family's ability to meet its tasks depends on the maturity of the adult members and the support given by the social system—health care, educational, employment, religious, social, welfare, governmental, and leisure institutions. The family that is most successful as a unit has a working philosophy and value system that is understood and lived, uses healthy adaptive patterns most of the time, can ask for help and use the community services available, and develops linkages with nonfamily units and organizations (2, 65).

ROLES OF THE FAMILY

Family roles are *patterns of behavior assigned to each member that fulfill family functions and needs.* Along with roles come social and family expectations about how the roles should be fulfilled. Parents are expected to teach and discipline their children, and children are expected to cooperate and respect their parents. **Instrumental roles** *are concerned with fulfilling physical needs such as food, clothing, and shelter.* **Affective roles** *fulfill emotional needs and provide emotional support and encouragement.* Members may fill more than one role. The fewer people there are to fulfill these roles, as in the nuclear family, the greater the number of demands placed on one person. If a member leaves home, someone else takes up his or her role. Any member of the family can satisfactorily fulfill any role in either category unless he or she is uncomfortable in that role. The male who is sure of his masculinity will have no problem providing emotional support to his teenage daughter. The female who is sure of her femininity will have no trouble gardening or taking the car for repair. Today many males and females no longer are restricted to carrying out only traditional gender-specific roles. They enjoy sharing roles, working together to complete family tasks without worrying about what is "man's" or "woman's" work (6, 45, 66).

The emotional response of a person to the role he or she fulfills should be considered. Someone may perform the job competently and yet dread doing it. The male may be a carpenter because his father taught him the trade, although he wants to be a music teacher. Changes in performance roles also necessitate emotional changes (e.g., in the male who takes over household duties when his wife becomes incapacitated).

The child learns about emotional response to roles in the family while imitating adults. The child experiments with various roles in play. The more pressure put on the child by the parents to respond in a particular way, the more likely that child is to learn only one role and be uncomfortable in others. For example, a star athlete may be a social misfit. With rigid roles, the child becomes less adaptive socially and within the family.

Exercising a capacity for a variety of roles, either in actuality or in fantasy, is healthy. The healthy family establishes clear roles, allows for flexibility of roles, allocates roles fairly, and takes responsibility for assigned roles.

FUNCTIONS OF THE FAMILY AS A SOCIAL SYSTEM

The family meets the criteria of a system because it functions as a unit to fulfill the previously described tasks and roles. See Table 1-1 for more information. ∞ The family is a group of interdependent individuals and their patterns of relationships. The family comprises two critical components: structure and function (66). **Family structure** *includes how a family is legally constructed and how its members are genetically connected* (4, 6, 65). Internal and external structures exist in a family. **Internal structure** *includes family composition, rank order, subsystems, and boundaries.* **External structure** *includes culture, religion, social class status and mobility, environment, and extended family* (13, 14, 20, 69). **Instrumental function** *refers to how routine activities of daily living are handled.* **Expressive function** *refers to nonverbal and verbal communication patterns, problem-solving roles, control aspects, beliefs, alliances, and coalitions.*

The organization of a family system is **hierarchical**, *built on kinship, power, status, and privilege relationships that may be related to individual characteristics of age, sex, education, personality, and health* (44). We can infer a hierarchy by observing each person's behavior and communication. For instance: Who talks first? Last? Longest? Who talks to whom? When? Where? About what? If one family member consistently approaches the health care staff about the client's health care, he or she probably holds an upper position in the family and has the task of being "expert." Your attempt to communicate with family members may meet with resistance if the communication inadvertently violates the family communication hierarchy.

Hierarchical relations in the family system determine the role behavior of family members. These hierarchical role relationships typically have great stability, and ordinarily family members can be counted on to behave congruently with their roles. Differences in behavior from situation to situation may be in response to the family's expectations for that particular situation (44). Families develop a system of balanced relationships. When one member leaves the family or experiences a change such as illness, other family members also must adapt. Roles and relationships are based on reciprocal interaction, with each member of the family contributing to the total unit in a unique and functional way. If a member should fail to meet the expectations of the roles established by his or her position in the hierarchy for the moment, the remaining members of the family generally react by using pressure (e.g., persuasion, punishment, argument, being ignored) on the rebellious person (44).

Family functions *cover the physical, affectionate or emotional, social, and spiritual dimensions.* Most families agree generally with the functions.

Physical functions of the family are met by the *parents' providing food, clothing, shelter, protection against danger, provision for*

body repairs after fatigue or illness, and reproduction. In some societies these physical needs are the dominant concern. In Western societies many families take them for granted (14).

Affectional functions *include meeting emotional needs and promoting adaptation and adjustment.* The family is the primary unit in which the child tests emotional reactions. Learning how to react and maintain emotional equilibrium within the family enables him or her to repeat the pattern in later life situations. The child who feels loved is likely to contract fewer physical illnesses, learn more quickly, and generally have an easier time growing up and adapting to society (2, 36).

A healthy family has several dominant characteristics (2, 8, 36):

1. Members know they are part of a larger group.
2. There is allowance for interactions within its borders and interchanges outside its borders.
3. Parents assist children in accepting role limitations by presenting clarity in generational boundaries.
4. A clear hierarchy of power exists, with adult shared leadership.
5. Joyful and comforting relationships and interactions occur regularly.
6. Shared tasks by input from all members are completed.
7. Members learn to accept change and loss.

Social functions of the modern family include *providing social togetherness, fostering self-esteem and a personal identity tied to family identity, providing opportunities for observing and learning social and sexual roles, accepting responsibility for behavior, and supporting individual creativity and initiative.* The family gives a name to the infant and hence indicates a social position or status in relation to the immediate and kinship-group families. Simultaneously, each family begins to transmit its own version of the cultural heritage and its own family culture to the child. Because the culture is too vast and comprehensive to transmit to the child in its entirety and all at once, the family selects what will be transmitted. In addition, the family interprets and evaluates what is transmitted. Through this process, the child learns to share family values (36).

Socialization is a primary task of the parents. They teach the child about the body, peers, family, community, age-appropriate roles, language, perceptions, social values, and ethics. The family also teaches about the different standards of responsibility society demands from various social groups. There is also a difference in the type of contact that society allows to a particular group. For example, a mail carrier does not enter the home, but an exterminator may access every room of a home.

The **spiritual function** to *raise the child to be a moral person with a belief system of some kind* is now discussed less frequently in texts. The authors believe parents have such a responsibility. Chapter 7 ∞ describes a number of belief systems.

The **cognitive or educational function** *involves the parent generation educating through internal* instruction and by serving as models. *Thus the child's **personality**, a product of all the influences that have been and are impinging on him or her,* is greatly influenced by the parents (51).

Family functions are achieved through a variety of behaviors over time. They are dependent upon the historical era, cultural background, family size and membership, and family support systems. Health promotion measures described throughout the text help the family achieve the physical, affectional or emotional, social, spiritual, and cognitive functions.

Family Adaptation

Adaptive responses in the family *represent the means by which it maintains an internal equilibrium so that it can fulfill purposes and tasks, deal with internal and external stress and crises, and allow for growth of individual members.* Some capacity for functioning may be sacrificed to control conflict and aid work as a unit. But the best functioning family keeps anxiety and conflict within tolerable limits and maintains a balance between effects of the past and new experiences. The family system must adapt similarly to other social systems (8, 20, 66).

Ideally, the family achieves equilibrium by talking over problems and finding solutions together. Humor, problem solving, flexibility, play, shared work, and leisure all help relieve tension. The family members know that certain freedoms exist within their confines that are not available elsewhere.

Successful and happy people define their first priority as their spouse, partner, or significant others and their family; their business or career comes second. Each spouse, partner, or significant person is a supportive and committed comforter, listener, companion, and counselor to the other. They may wish to set aside one night a week, or a month, to be only with each other, sharing uninterrupted time and activity. Each parent may wish to have a day date with each child monthly, spending time together at lunch, shopping, or in some mutually favorite activity.

Occasionally, even the healthiest family uses adaptive coping mechanisms that cause more stress, especially when faced with multiple stressors. However, over time, healthy families recover from their losses, access support resources, and help each other master ongoing challenges (6, 66).

ADAPTIVE MECHANISMS IN FAMILY LIFE

Various types of internal family coping strategies have been discussed. *Strategies that extend outside the family include* (a) seeking information, (b) maintaining links with the extended family or with people or agencies in the community, (c) using self-help groups or informal or formal support networks, and (d) seeking spiritual support (6, 20, 36, 66).

Ineffective coping strategies used by families during stressful times include denial of problems, exploitation or manipulation of one or more family members, violence toward children or adult members, and use of authoritarianism or threats. Family members might also cope with stress by changing to ineffective traditions or family myths, using alcohol or drugs, or abandoning the family through separation, divorce, or suicide (20). Family response to stressors and conflict between the spouses or the parents and children affect the personality development and behavior of children and adolescents and may contribute to physical illness, emotional problems, or behavioral disorders such as hyperactivity (6).

Emotional conflicts in the family may be avoided, minimized, or resolved in the following ways (36):

1. **Scapegoating or blaming:** *Labeling one member as the cause of the family troubles.* One member may offer self as a scapegoat to end an argument. Such labeling controls the conflict and reduces anxiety but stereotypes the person and prevents communication and resolution.

2. **Coalitions or alliances:** *Interacting so some family members side together against other members.* Antagonisms and anger result. Eventually the losing party tries to get control or may withdraw from interaction.

3. **Withdrawal of emotional ties:** *Reducing communication and seeking affections outside the family.*

4. **Repetitive fighting:** *Using verbal abuse, physical battles, loud complaints, curses, or accusations.* The fight may have the same theme each time stress hits the family. Some "blowing up" is a release from everyday frustrations, but every minor incident or temporary disagreement is not a major case.

5. **Family myths or traditional beliefs:** *Using repeatedly the same statements to overcome anxieties and maintain control over others.* "Children are seen, not heard." "We can't survive if you leave home." "Talking about feelings will cause loss of love."

6. **Reaction formation:** *Repressing traumatic ideas and transforming them into the opposite behavior so that there is superficial harmony or togetherness.* Great tension is felt because true feelings are not expressed.

7. **Resignation or compromise:** *Giving up or suppressing the need for assertion, affection, or emotional expression to keep peace or temporary harmony.*

8. **Designation of one person as family healer:** *Using a "wise one" (most often in the extended family) or an "umpire," such as a minister, storekeeper, bartender, or druggist, to arrange a reconciliation between dissenting parties.* The helper or referee may get great satisfaction from finding someone worse off than self. The family "protector" takes on all the stresses to save other members stress or conflict, and fights the battles for everyone else in the family.

Two or more of these mechanisms may be used within the same family. If these mechanisms are used exclusively, however, they become defensive and are unlikely to promote resolution of the conflict, so that the same issue arises repeatedly (41). Usually one member is designated as the one who must maintain a specific pattern of negative or unhealthy behavior to keep all other family members comfortable. If the designated member tries to change behavior and becomes more independent, he or she receives no support and is seen as disrupting the status quo. Other family members are uncomfortable. Ineffective behavior is maintained at the expense of the development of the designated person and of the family (8).

INEFFECTIVE ADAPTATION

Signs of strained or destructive family relationships or signs of emotional abuse in the family include the following (2, 6, 8, 21, 44):

1. Lack of understanding, communication, and helpfulness between members, resulting in unclear roles and conflict.
2. Lack of family decision making and lines of authority.
3. Harassment or ignoring the other family members.
4. Derogatory remarks by children to parents or vice versa.

5. Pattern of scapegoating or blaming each other for difficulties.
6. Possessive behavior toward the children or the mate.
7. Extreme closeness between husband/wife and his/her mother or family.
8. Lack of individuality, being too close or enmeshed or too distant with each other.
9. Parent being domineering about performance of household tasks.
10. Few outside friends for parents or children.
11. High level of anxiety or insecurity present in the home.
12. Lack of creativity and stability.
13. Pattern of immature or regressive behavior in parents or children.
14. Boundaries between generations not maintained; children carrying out parental roles because of parent's inability to function, illness, or abandonment.

You may find yourself in the role of family healer. If this happens, help the family to develop harmonious ways of coping and avoid the protector or omnipotent role. Several references give in-depth information pertinent to assessment of and intervention with families (8, 20, 23, 44, 51, 69).

Stages of Family Development

Like an individual, the family has a developmental history marked by predictable crises. The developmental crises are normal, but they are also challenging because each life stage is a new experience. The natural history of the family is on a continuum from single adults leaving home to families in later life. The nurturing of spouse, partner, or children goes on simultaneously with a multitude of other activities: working at a job or profession, managing a household, participating in church and community groups, pursuing leisure and hobbies, and maintaining friendships and family ties. Family stages may differ due to family structure, education, and socioeconomic status, and these differences are highlighted in the following discussion.

Table 6-2 summarizes the main stages of the family and major concerns or tasks for each stage (2, 5, 11, 17, 35, 37, 48, 51, 69). These tasks are also discussed in Chapters 9 through 16. ∞

You have a critical role in assisting families to prepare for and work through the tasks of each family stage. Often during client care, a family is working through tasks of several stages.

SINGLE YOUNG ADULT LEAVING HOME

During this initial stage, *young adults establish their independence, begin jobs or careers, and establish intimate relationships*. During this **stage of leaving home**, *separation between children and their parents is one of the primary developmental tasks of young adulthood*, as summarized in **Table 6-2**. For gay men and lesbians, young adulthood may be a time of "coming out" to their families, and this event may cause major family conflicts.

BECOMING A COUPLE THROUGH MARRIAGE OR COMMITMENT

In the **Establishment Stage**, *the couple establishes an identity and a home of its own*. The main psychological tie is no longer with the

family of origin, as summarized in **Table 6-2**. Readiness for marriage in U.S. society is discussed in relation to young adulthood in Chapter 14. ∞ Some couples cut off relationships in order to avoid conflicts, other couples are totally absorbed or enmeshed in the partner's family, or there may be a balance between closeness and distance. Sometimes couple divorce and remarry, as described in the Case Situation. Families may have difficulty accepting gay and lesbian relationships or acknowledging the two partners as a couple.

If and when to become parents is a crucial task during this stage. Today's families may choose to have no children, have one child and adopt others, or have two or three children instead of a larger family. Some females believe that motherhood is not necessary for fulfillment. Certainly the male's chief fulfillment is not necessarily from fatherhood. Children do not automatically bring happiness to a marriage. Children bring happiness to parents who want them and who are selfless enough to become involved in the adventure of raising them. Children bring trauma to a troubled marriage or partnership. Gay and lesbian couples who want to have children may choose to adopt, to have artificial insemination from donor sperm, or to find a surrogate mother (47, 69).

BECOMING PARENTS

The **Expectant Stage**, or *pregnancy, is a developmental crisis; many domestic and social adjustments must be made*, as listed in **Table 6-2**. The couple, or the single mother and her significant other, are learning new roles and gaining new status in the community. Attitudes toward pregnancy and the physical and emotional status of the mother and father (and of significant others) affect parenting abilities. Now the couple thinks in terms of family instead of a couple. As the pregnancy progresses, most women adapt to their new role as a mother and accept the pregnancy. The man experiences a variety of feelings throughout the pregnancy as the reality of the pregnancy increases. Concerns identified by expectant fathers are health of the mother and baby, finances, caring for the infant, adequacy as a father, and the baby's effect on the marital dyad (38, 44, 51, 69).

Early, comprehensive prenatal care for the pregnant woman is essential. Both the woman and her partner may experience similar physical and emotional symptoms, such as nausea, indigestion, backache, abdominal distention, irritability, and depression. Symptoms may result from hormonal changes or feelings about the pregnancy in the woman. In the father or partner, they are part of the **couvade syndrome**, *which may be a reaction based on identification with or sympathy for the pregnant woman, ambivalence or hostility toward the pregnancy, or envy of the woman's childbearing ability*. The symptoms of couvade syndrome are symbolically a means for the partner to participate in the child's development and birth and a means of affording the pregnant woman and new infant protection (20, 69). The physical symptoms, complex feelings, and changes in body image that accompany pregnancy are described by several authors (6, 35, 39, 44, 48, 51, 69).

*The partner must be prepared for fathering or co-parenting just as the woman is for mothering. Fathers also go through the **five operations*** (*mimicry, role play, fantasy, introjection–projection–rejection, and grief work*) *identified by Rubin (48).*

TABLE 6-2

Stages of the Family Life Cycle

Single Young Adults Leaving Home

Accept responsibility for self.

Differentiate from family of origin.

Develop friendships and intimate relationships outside of family of origin.

Establish career or job and financial independence, using parents for support and as role models.

Courtship and Engagement

Become better acquainted with partner.

Contend with pressures from parents or relatives about partner selection.

Resolve to mutually give up some autonomy and retain some independence.

Become free of parental domination.

Prepare for marriage, including mutually satisfying sexual patterns.

Establishment of Family

Commit self to the partner, usually through marriage.

Establish own home and life patterns, including extended family.

Focus psychological tie and lifestyle with partner.

Work out differences in expectations and patterns of communication, daily living, sexual relations.

Work on establishing philosophy of life for the family unit that incorporates each partner's personal philosophy.

Determine whether or not to have children (biological or adopted) and desired number and spacing of children.

Expectant Stage of Family

Woman is pregnant; prenatal care begun.

Couple incorporate idea of baby into thinking and planning for future and learn new roles.

Couple resolve feelings about pregnancy (desired, expected, not desired, unexpected).

Woman experiences changing emotions and physical changes.

Man works through feelings related to partner's pregnancy, childbirth, and fatherhood.

Couple rework sexual relationship.

Couple make decisions about attending childbirth education classes and labor and delivery experience.

Couple prepare for parenting by discussing parenting issues and seeking support from family.

Couple discuss childrearing and discipline plans, resolve differences of opinion.

Family with Young Children

Birth, adoption, or foster care creates status of parent.

Adjust to changes in lifestyle; less freedom for own pursuits; 24-hour responsibility.

Work through tasks of becoming a parent with birth of each child.

Realign relationships with extended family (grandparents, aunts, uncles).

Parents active in development, socialization, and education of each child.

Participate in community, school, and church activities.

Family with Adolescents

Increase flexibility of family boundaries to allow for adolescent independence.

Adapt parent-child relationship to permit adolescent to move in and out of family.

Refocus on midlife marital and career issues.

Begin caring for older generation.

Launching Stage: Contraction of Family

Change in parent-child family; let go of responsibilities; children move out of home.

Make readjustments if offspring return home for a time, with or without partner and children.

Encourage and assist autonomy and independence in children/stepchildren.

New focus on couple unit and time for each other.

Rework self-concept as person, parent, and grandparent.

Assume new roles, responsibilities, and leisure activities.

Woman may enter workforce if not previously employed.

Deal with disabilities and death of parents (grandparents).

**Family in Later Life:
Contraction and Disengagement Stage**

Engage in retirement planning and rework lifestyle and activities.

Prepare for death of spouse and self.

Resolve deaths, losses, and changes that occur in extended family and friends.

Role reversal with children as "parents" and parents needing assistance with life tasks.

For additional information about prenatal influences on the mother and baby, see Chapters 8 and 9. ∞ Information about parenting and developmental tasks for the expectancy phase is also presented in Chapter 14. ∞ Several authors give further information on the father's reactions and responsibilities (44, 51). The family that prepares for adoption of a child does not have the tasks associated with the physical aspects of pregnancy, but it does have to accomplish the other tasks of readiness.

PARENTHOOD WITH YOUNG CHILDREN

In this **Parenthood Stage**, *there is birth or adoption of a child, and the couple assumes a lifetime status of "parent" as they become caretakers of a younger generation*, as listed in **Table 6-2**. The couple may reject the idea of parenthood but genuinely love the baby who was unplanned. Often couples have difficulty because the romanticized ideal of pregnancy, childbirth, and parenting differs considerably from the reality of 24-hour responsibility and submersion of personal desires. The ups and downs of the early months of parenthood are shocking to most new parents. Individuals with fewer romanticized and exaggerated ideas about parenthood eventually become happier with their new role than individuals who have exaggerated or unrealistic expectations.

Some parents exert excessive power over a child and attempt to create an image of themselves. These parents believe they have the right to dictate the terms of their child's life. The parents' rigid control over their child's behavior is greater than their real love for the child. As a result, too much pressure is placed on the growing child, disturbing his or her emotional development. On the other extreme are the parents who show little interest or affection to their child and exert no influence over their child's life. These parents rarely spend time with the child, and the child may spend considerable time watching television, with electronic media, or with peers. Children who spend most of their time with peers may be more influenced by lack of the parents' presence, attention, and concern than by the attractiveness of the peer group (5).

Other parents invest themselves in the creative potentialities of their children. They see the child as a lamp to light rather than a vessel to fill. Their involvement in the child's life is empathic: being involved for the sake of the child, not themselves. These parents' demands on their children are flexible, not rigid, depending on the context of the situation (5, 37).

Lesbian and gay parents differ from heterosexual parents in that they (10):

1. Make the effort to include male/female role models.
2. Work to build unbiased support networks and community relationships.
3. Invent family rituals for every occasion.
4. Avoid gender-assigned roles/chores.
5. Attend to legal matters, such as inheritance, and documents.

PARENTHOOD WITH ADOLESCENTS

The **Adolescent Stage of Parenthood** *often includes many changes, conflicts, and upheavals. The parents' roles as provider and nurturer of their young children change to allow for more independence of their maturing children.* See **Table 6-2** for a summary. As the children mature and leave home, the parents must rework their self-concepts as parents and people. The mother may consider employment outside the home because her children no longer require constant supervision. During this stage when teenagers want more freedom, aging relatives may require more support and physical care (5, 69).

DISENGAGEMENT OR CONTRACTION STAGE

The **Disengagement or Contraction Stage** extends through midlife and the elder years and *occurs when children leave home. The partners must rework their separateness.* **Table 6-2** lists some of the major tasks. This is often a time for maximum contact between the partners, especially when retirement occurs. Retirement planning and preparation for eventual death must be done. Bereavement, loneliness, and further role changes and losses are inevitable.

Sometimes, however, this stage does not last too long. The young adult who is unemployed, a college dropout, or divorced may return home to live with the parents. Sometimes teenage or young adult offspring with children of their own return because of divorce, economic problems, or other crises, so that grandparents may become involved in raising the grandchildren. The aged parents or other relatives may be unable to continue to live independently and are included in the household of their middle-aged offspring. Consequently, the tasks, functions, roles, and hierarchical relationships of the family must be reworked. Space and other resources must be reallocated. Time schedules for daily activities

Case Situation

Divorce and Remarriage

Mart and Janice divorced after 15 years of marriage and two children, John and Jenna. Janice found Mart difficult to live with and initiated the divorce. Mart remarried 2 years later; Nellene was the perfect loving partner and loved by Mart's family. She was a good "household manager" for Mart and a nurturing but firm mother surrogate to the adolescent children, who chose to live with their dad and Nellene. Nellene and Mart became nurturing grandparents after John and Jenna married and had families of their own. Both Mart and Nellene had diabetes and hypertension, which were poorly controlled because they visited their physicians only in times of emergency, such as when Nellene was diagnosed with chronic renal disease. The doctor's recommendations for health promotion and illness prevention went unheeded by both, as were suggestions from relatives.

Six years ago Nellene died suddenly from a massive myocardial infarction while visiting her family; Mart and her family were present. Mart was in shock! He felt deep grief, loneliness, and helplessness.

Three days after the funeral, Janice called Mart, suggesting she come to "visit" and "help" him. Mart readily agreed. Shortly thereafter Janice moved in saying, "I regretted so often divorcing him." Six months later they remarried.

Their second marriage appears happy; Janice has become "household manager." The children and grandchildren are "glad Mother and Dad are back together," as they had seen less of Janice during the prior years. Mart needed Janice's help, and Janice felt secure. Janice and Mart admit they are unusual; most divorced couples do not remarry. They are both happy they did.

Contributed by Ruth Murray, EdD, MSN, N-NAP, FAAN.

Client Education

1. Parents should not be expected to drastically change their household and life routines; disruption in family routines may be frustrating.
2. Everyone involved should remember the house belongs to the parents.
3. The families should talk about resentments and discuss problems.
4. Adult children should contribute to family finances and chores.
5. Parents cannot expect to exert the same authority with a 30- or 40-year-old as with a child.
6. When grandchildren are involved, set rules about who is the primary disciplinarian and the parental roles.
7. Household chores should be shared without upsetting the parents' preferred responsibilities (cooking, decorating, home repairs).
8. The families should maintain privacy and separate living spaces for the parents and their children to the extent possible.
9. Parents should resist meddling in their adult children's affairs and vice versa.
10. Parents should set limits on the stay, making it clear that this is a temporary arrangement and assisting in plans for the separation.

may be reworked. Privacy in communication, use of possessions, and emotional space must be ensured. Old parent-child conflicts and ideas about who is in charge, how rules are set, and how discipline is accomplished may resurface and should be discussed and worked through. The middle-aged family is more fully discussed in Chapter 15. ∞

Families can benefit from counseling; your guidance and teaching may be crucial. The Client Education **Box** lists suggestions to adult children and their parents to make living together more harmonious (11). Use these suggestions to educate the family.

Family Interaction and Parenting Practices

Family interaction is a *unique form of social interaction based on a set of intimate and continuing relationships. It is the sum total of all the family roles being played within a family at a given time* (64). Families function and carry out their tasks and lifestyles through this process.

Family therapists, psychiatrists, and nurses are giving increased attention to the emotional balance in family dyads or paired role positions, such as husband and wife or mother and child. They have noted that a shift in the balance of one member of the pair (or one pair) alters the balance of the other member (or pair). The birth of a child is the classic example (67). Dyads and emotional balance also shift in single-parent and stepparent families (24, 62).

Interaction of the husband and wife or of the adult members living under one roof is basic to the mental, and sometimes physical, health of the adults and to the eventual health of the children. *Various factors influence this interaction* (5, 22): (a) the sense of self-esteem or self-love of each family member, (b) childhood socialization, (c) parental maturity, (d) ordinal position of the child, (e) number of children in the family, (f) gender of child, and (g) whether the child was adopted or is a stepchild.

Educate the family about the importance of family interaction to health. Foster a positive influence on interactions.

IMPORTANCE OF SELF-ESTEEM

A basic life task for each person—to feel a sense of self-esteem, to love the self and have a positive self-image—evolves through interaction with the parents from the time of birth onward. In turn, self-esteem affects how the person interacts in later life with others, including spouse and offspring.

The adult who lacks self-acceptance and self-respect probably will not be a loving spouse or parent. Behavior will betray feelings about self and others because he or she *perceives* no acceptance and little love from others in the family. Because perception of an event is the person's reality, the person in turn reacts in ways designed to defend self from rejection. He or she may criticize, get angry, brag, demand perfection from others, or withdraw. In this way, the self is built up; the emotional reasoning being: "I may not be much, but others are worse." Such behavior is corrosive to any relationship but particularly one as intimate as in the family. Because of overt behavior, those intimate with him or her are not likely to appreciate or respond to the person's basic needs for love, acceptance, and respect. To remain open and giving in such situations is difficult for the mate but may be the only way to elevate the other's self-esteem. Perhaps only then can the other reciprocate loving behavior (5, 29, 30, 43, 51, 69).

Demonstrate support and acceptance to the person with low self-esteem. Demonstrate support, empathy, and encouragement to the family members and help them understand the emotional dynamics. Reinforce that positive self-esteem is essential for emotional or mental health promotion and can be a factor in physical health status as well.

INFLUENCE OF CHILDHOOD SOCIALIZATION

Gender differences in the socialization processes are a crucial influence on interaction between adults in the family. These differences exist, even in modern mainstream society. In some cultural groups, the differences are more noticeable. Traditionally, girls have been socialized to foster strong relationships, to be caretakers, and to provide emotional security. Traditional feminine qualities include nurturance, emotionality, dependence, and selflessness. Boys have been traditionally socialized to be a provider for the future family. Traditional masculine qualities include independence, aggressiveness, and stoicism. Recognition and acceptance are given to individuals who comply with traditional gender roles. However, some families expect similar behavior from both sons and daughters. Difficulties and conflicts may occur if individuals act counter to their expected gender roles (5, 11, 23, 44, 69).

Gender roles are compounded by the shift in balance between the male and female found in modern marriages. The husband often labors under the illusion that he enjoys the rights and responsibilities inherent in a patriarchal family system. Yet he must recognize his wife's qualifications and drive for independence. Even though a wife may be employed outside of the home, the majority of child care duties and household tasks still fall on her.

Explore gender expectations and roles with the family members—parents and children. Help the adults openly discuss their expectations of each other and the children. Encourage parents to be flexible in expectations of their children's gender roles, in preparation for later societal expectations about roles.

PARENTAL MATURITY

Parental maturity is challenged by each period in the child's development and reminds the parent of past developmental experiences. Demands made on the parent vary with the child's age. The infant needs almost total and constant nurturance. Some parents thrive during this period and depend on each other for support. Other parents feel overwhelmed by the infant's dependency because their own dependent needs are stimulated but unmet. The baby's cry and behavior evoke feelings of helplessness, dependency, and anger associated with their unacceptable dependency needs and feelings and then guilt and fatigue. The toddler and preschooler struggles with individuality, autonomy, and initiative, exploring and vacillating between dependency and independency. At this stage the child is intense and often unreasonable in demands and refusal to obey commands. The parents may enjoy this explorative, independent behavior of the child, even though it leaves them feeling tired and frustrated. Parents may do very well with the independent preschooler, schoolchild, or adolescent, or the reverse may be true.

The child's spontaneity can evoke in the adult fresh ways of looking at life long buried under habit and routine. The child says, "It's too loud, but my earlids won't stay down" or "I want one of those little red olives with the green around" or "Give me that eraser with the handle," when pointing to a pencil. The child can also re-create for the adult the difficulty of the learning process: "Is it today, tomorrow, or yesterday? You said when I woke up it would be tomorrow, but now you call it today."

Parents tend to identify with their children and to treat them according to how they were treated as children. A parent can identify best with the child who matches his or her own sibling position. A male from a family of boys may not know how to interact with a daughter and may not empathize with her. In the process of identifying with the parent, the child picks up many of the parent's

characteristics, especially if the child is the oldest or lone child. For example, the oldest boy may be dependent instead of independent if his father was the youngest sibling and retained his dependent behavior into adulthood.

Reinforce the parents' mature behavior. Be accepting and empathic toward their fears and frustrations. Encourage them to discuss feelings and to seek assistance or counseling as needed. Each parent you interact with will demonstrate his or her unique level of maturity. Your behavior can be a role model for mature behavior in others.

ORDINAL POSITION OF THE CHILD

Birth order is important to development. **Table 6-3** lists characteristics of children in first, middle, and last ordinal positions, as well as of the only child (25, 31, 59). Siblings, both same and opposite sex, have an important influence on each other as buddies, bullies, or heroes, and the early relationship often affects the adult relationship. Whether the child has male or female siblings also affects personality development. For example, secondborn boys with an older sister are more feminine or empathic and nurturing than those with an older brother. If two siblings are more than 6 years apart, they tend to grow up like only children (25, 31, 36, 59).

Children are the logical targets for fulfilling many of the parents' frustrated ambitions and needs. In a large family these yearnings and aspirations can be parceled out among a number of children. The only child, in contrast, must learn multiple roles. Further, the only child may be a peacemaker if he or she is inadvertently brought into the parents' conflicts and is forced to help maintain harmony and preserve equilibrium in the household (31, 59). However, research shows a more positive side to the only child. An only child can be achievement oriented and display a friendly personality. Leman describes features of each child in a family, based on sex and ordinal position, how the child feels about and interacts with people, and which ordinal position spouse he or she will most happily marry (31).

Counsel parents who plan for or have only one child about the child's need for peer activity and the danger of too much early responsibility and pressure. Educate parents about the effects of ordinal position on the child and on their parenting. Refer to **Table 6-3** for research-based information about ordinal position.

SMALL FAMILY SYSTEM

Most children in the United States are members of a **small family system**, *including three children or less.* Some couples choose to have no children and to pursue careers or leisure interests instead of having children. Others make this choice because they believe the current world situation is not one into which to bring children.

The small family system with one to three children has the following features (44, 49):

1. Emphasis is on planning the number and the frequency of births, the objectives of parenting, and educational possibilities.
2. Parenthood is intensive rather than extensive; great concern is evidenced from pregnancy through every phase of parenting for each child.

TABLE 6-3

Influence of Ordinal Position on Child

First Born

1. Is subject to greater parental expectations for achievement.
2. Identifies more with parents/elders than peers.
3. Takes charge and knows what to do.
4. Commands respect; others want to follow his or her leadership.
5. Is cooperative, easy to work with, good team player.
6. Does things right and thoroughly; strong superego or conscience.
7. Has everything under control; strong self-discipline.
8. Is ambitious, enterprising, energetic.
9. Plans thoroughly; sets goals and reaches them.
10. Is known as straight thinker and problem solver.
11. Loves to read and accumulate facts.

Middle Child

1. Holds variety of positions/roles in family.
2. Receives less of parents' time, generally.
3. Is unspoiled and realistic in problem solving.
4. Makes friends and keeps them; relationships are very important.
5. Is willing to take risks and strikes out on own; may be rebellious at times.
6. Knows how to get along with others; learns to compromise.
7. Is skilled mediator and negotiator.
8. Knows how to keep secrets and can be trusted with sensitive information.

Last Born

1. Benefits from parents' experience with parenting.
2. Tends to identify more with siblings and peers than parents.
3. Is likable, fun to be around, easy to talk to.
4. Knows how to work well with others in small groups and social settings.
5. Is persistent; may not take "no" for an answer.
6. Is affectionate and engaging, caring and lovable.
7. Is relaxed, genuine, and trustworthy.
8. Knows how to get noticed; is entertaining and funny.

Only Child

1. Resembles firstborn child in behavior.
2. Learns to fill many roles because fewer family members.
3. Feels pressure to assume roles prematurely.
4. Is able to entertain self; finds satisfaction in personal pursuits.
5. Learns less about close interactions with opposite- or same-sex peers, but is friendly to either gender.
6. Is not afraid to make decisions but may be self-centered.
7. Is a perfectionist; always wants to do things right; assertive.
8. Is ambitious and puts self under pressure to be successful.
9. Makes lists, plans, and sets goals.
10. Is logical thinker; peacemaker.
11. Is scholarly, serious, good problem solver; achievement oriented.

3. Group actions are usually more democratic.
4. Greater freedom is allowed individual members.

The child in a small family usually enjoys advantages beyond those available to children in large families of corresponding economic and social level, including more individual attention. On the other hand, these children may retain emotional dependence on their parents, grow up with extreme pressure for performance, and retain an exaggerated notion of self-importance.

LARGE FAMILY SYSTEM

The **large family** *is generally thought of as one with four or more children.* Emphasis is on the group rather than on the individual, but there is still plenty of love for each child. Conformity and cooperation are valued above self-expression. There is a high degree of organization in the activities of daily living (19, 22, 63). The large family is less common today than in the past. The lastborn child may be less wanted than the first or middle child, although parents feel more skilled and self-confident in raising the younger children. Parents must divide their attention among more children. Large families have advantages for the children. Of necessity, the children learn thrift and conservation of resources and mate-

rial goods. Members know the hot water supply is not unlimited, that food is not to be wasted, and that toys and clothing can be recycled. Children learn to share time, space, and possessions. The children learn responsibility by taking care of themselves and each other. In a loving home, they have not only their parents' love but also that of siblings. There is always someone with a listening ear, respect, support, compassion, and help. If the parent does not have time to read to the 3-year-old, the older sibling does. The older sibling gains more experience in reading, gains increased self-esteem from being helpful, and learns responsibility and caring. Each child learns cooperation, compromise, tolerance, and how to handle peer pressure. The effort, work, expense, and self-denial of having a large family can be offset by the rewards of watching children grow and develop and by a sense of contribution to the generations to come (19, 22, 60).

MULTIPLE BIRTHS

The incidence of twins and other multiples has increased dramatically over the past 20 years because of infertility treatments such as *in vitro* fertilization. Twins or other multiple births affect family interactions differently than birth of a single baby. *Multiples create parental challenges:* (a) health of mother and babies, (b) financial strain, (c) ethical decisions if some embryos cannot survive *in utero*, and (d) family relationships.

Because multiple births are often premature, the first 4 or 5 months are very demanding on the parents. Often these parents lack emotional and financial support and sufficient help with child care and household tasks. Lack of sleep, lack of time for other children and spouses, mood fluctuations, and financial strain are some of the most frequent problems expressed by parents of twins. Postpartum depression is more frequent in mothers of multiples. Parents require help with child care and household tasks (57).

Parents may find it challenging to interact individually with each infant. Encourage parents of twins or other multiples to celebrate the unique qualities of each baby and to individualize child care routines as much as possible. Some parents prefer to treat their multiples as one unit: taking care of them collectively, giving them similar-sounding names, dressing them alike, and expecting them to behave alike. This approach may still provide opportunities to develop an individual relationship with each child.

Multiple-birth children usually are closer than ordinary siblings because they are connected intimately before birth. Their experiences are different from those of siblings with varying ages. Identical twins meet the world as a pair; it is difficult to imagine life without each other. During adolescence and young adulthood, it takes longer to separate emotionally or physically. Each tends to seek multiple-birth persons as friends or mates. Although parents may socialize one twin to be older and one to be younger in behavior, it is difficult for twins to adapt because they are on the same level developmentally. With fraternal twins, gender preference of parents may determine whether the girl or the boy is perceived as older (2).

Twins soon learn how to take advantage of their special birth status by acting "in collusion" or solving family conflicts by acting as a team. Interaction between them and roles are often complementary: one twin may be dominant and the other submissive. Each learns from reinforcement of his or her experiences about the advantages of the particular role chosen.

Multiples usually are more detached from other siblings or parents than they are from each other. Multiple-birth children may each receive less parental affection and communication because parents have less time to devote to each child. Thus, they are often slower to talk and many have slower intellectual growth unless parents work to prevent it (2, 37, 44). Yet the bond between multiples can have positive effects on development as well. Interpersonal relationships are enhanced by a sense of security and identity, a strong ability to share, unique empathy, and role flexibility (2, 37, 44).

Intervention is key to health promotion. Your suggestions and support in engaging health care providers, relatives, friends, and neighbors to assist the family can influence how well the parents cope with their overwhelming responsibilities. The study cited in the Abstract for Evidence-Based Practice presents information to share about the experience of coping with parenting of multiple births. Twins and triplets can be breastfed successfully, but mothers will need extra support and education to manage the feeding schedule to avoid becoming completely exhausted or feeling like a milk machine. You can suggest ways to streamline daily routines in order to get adequate rest and have more time for infant care. Al-

Abstract for Evidence-Based Practice

Psychosocial Challenges of Mothering Multiple Births

Tatano Beck, C. (2002). Releasing the pause button: Mothering twins during the first year of life. *Qualitative Health Research, 12*, 593–608.

KEYWORDS

mothering, twins, infancy, multiple births.

Purpose ➤ This grounded theory study explored psychosocial challenges of mothering multiple births during the first year of life and unique coping strategies used by mothers.

Conceptual Framework ➤ Symbolic Interactionism, which focuses on the nature of social interaction, was the study framework.

Sample/Setting ➤ Sixteen married mothers of twins participated in at-home unstructured interviews. Field notes were also collected from Parents of Multiples support group meetings.

Method ➤ Data were simultaneously collected, coded, and analyzed, using the construct comparative method.

Findings ➤ Life-on-hold was the basic psychosocial challenge faced by mothers of twins during their first year of life.

Releasing the pause button was the coping strategy used by mothers, which involved four phases: (a) draining power, related to many demands on the mother's time and energy during the first 3 months; (b) pausing own life, living through the blur of days and nights and putting own life on hold for the twins; (c) striving to reset, shifting priorities and establishing a routine, asking for help, solving problems, and venturing into society; and (d) resuming own life, recognizing positive aspects of mothering twins as life became more manageable and resuming personal life patterns.

Implications ➤ Nurses can use study results to provide realistic, knowledgeable guidance to mothers of multiples, especially during infancy. Education on innovative coping strategies can be used to reduce risk of depression and help mothers manage challenges the first year and beyond.

though multiples are extremely challenging during the early months, by a year of age most parents are able to shift their priorities, establish a routine, and begin to reap the many benefits of parenting multiples. Tell parents about support groups such as Mothers of Twins, Twins Club Association (U.K.), and Mothers of Multiples. These organizations provide education and advocacy for parents and places where parents can share feelings and ideas and get practical suggestions. (57).

GENDER OF THE CHILD

Gender also influences development within the family. In most cultures, a higher value is placed on male than on female children. Actually, in some cultures only a boy's birth is welcomed or celebrated, and the family's status is partially measured by the number of sons. A family with several girls and no boys may perceive another baby girl as a disappointment. The girl may discover this attitude in later years from overhearing adult conversations. She may try to gain parental affection and esteem by engaging in "tomboy behavior" and later assuming traditional masculine roles, if the culture permits (5).

If a boy arrives in a family that hoped for a girl, he may receive pressure to be feminine. He may even be dressed and socialized in a feminine manner. If the boy arrives after a family has two or three girls, he may receive much attention or indulgence but also the jealousy of his sisters. Often he will grow up with three or four "mothering" figures (some may be unkind) and in a family more attuned to feminine than to masculine behavior. Developing a masculine identity may be more difficult for him, especially if there is no male in the family with whom to relate. In spite of being pampered, he may be expected by his family to be independent. The boy may feel envious of his sisters' positions and their freedom from such expectations (5).

The girl who arrives in a family with a number of boys may also receive considerable attention, but she may have to become tomboyish to compete with her brothers and receive their esteem. Feminine identity may be difficult for her.

ADOPTED CHILD

The adopted child may have to work through feelings about rejection and abandonment by the biological parents versus being wanted and loved by the adoptive parents. *Adopted children feel their losses on several levels.* **Overt loss** *includes changing relationships and familiar environments.* **Covert loss** *refers to low self-esteem from being given up by their birth parents.* **Status loss** *comes from being labeled as "nonbiological" ("not one of us") by family members and society.* It is often difficult for adopted children to attach to their adoptive families because of fear of another abandonment and rejection (42).

Adoptive parents also may feel a sense of loss if their decision to adopt occurred after attempts to have a biological child failed. Infertile couples need time to mourn their loss, but this process may be curtailed if the adoption occurs before grieving is complete. Consequently, the adopted child may sense the emotional distress and act out with negative behaviors (42).

The child should be told as early as possible that he or she is adopted, even though the disclosure may result in painful emo-

tions that last for many years. As a preschooler, he or she can begin to understand the idea of being adopted. Explanations will have to be repeated frequently and expanded upon over time. A child usually does not fully understand the concept of being adopted until age 8 or 9 (56).

It is not unusual for the adopted child to seek his or her biological parents in late adolescence or young adulthood, especially if the child was old enough to remember both parents when adopted. Some adopted children want to know not only the parents but also the family background and possible genetic disease risks. The search may be a threat to adoptive parents, or they may feel secure enough to assist their child with the search. The adopted child is likely to always consider the adoptive parents the "real parents," even if a relationship is established with the biological mother.

Major determinants of the child's adjustment and development are the preadoption circumstances, the age of the child at the time of adoption, and the child's ability to make friends. Other factors influencing successful adoption include the adoptive parents' personal qualifications, their marital harmony, their love of the child, their ability to communicate with the child about the adoptive process, and their acceptance of the child.

The definition of "suitable" adoptive parents has been liberalized. Adoption agency requirements for age, marital status, race, and mother's employment status are more flexible. The adoptive parent may be a man, a homosexual couple, an infertile couple, or a relative. Additionally, today's couples consider adoption even if they have their own children. Others are single or older persons who want to offer love and security to a child. However, adoptive parents now face legal precedent that the biological parent may seek to restore the parental rights and remove the child from the adoptive parents. This may occur even after 3 or 4 years, when the child has established attachment to the adoptive parents.

Social and legal changes have affected the kinds of children available for adoption (27, 28, 33, 42, 52). Earlier adoption agencies served mainly unmarried Caucasian mothers who saw adoption as the only alternative for their babies. Today there is greater social acceptance of single parenting, and more single mothers choose to keep and raise their babies. Contraceptives and abortions have also reduced the number of available infants. The number of adoptable **special-needs children** has increased. *These children have at least one of the following characteristics: disabilities (mental, physical, or emotional); age over 5 years; minority race, especially males; sibling groups (two or more); or at risk (exposed to drugs or alcohol).* Extra help and financial support is given to parents who choose to adopt children with special needs. Increasingly, state legislatures terminate parental rights in cases of children in long-term foster care who have been abandoned by their biological parents and when the likelihood of the child returning to his or her own home is minimal. Legislation has also allowed abused children to become eligible for adoption (28, 42).

Because of fewer available children in the United States, more families are considering international adoption. **International adoption** *is a cultural and political process involving many hardships, yet many benefits, for both child and parents.* Children from foreign countries have often lived in orphanages or foster homes. It takes time and a variety of services to overcome the lack of love and affection and other negative effects of these environments. In general, families who choose international adoption want to provide a nurturing, loving environment for children in spite of the difficulties (27, 28, 33, 42, 52, 56). Additional information is available from A Helping Hand Adoption Agency, www.worldadoptions.org.

Stresses to adoptive families include the following (27, 42, 52, 56):

1. Parents may worry about the child's heredity and prenatal exposure to drugs and alcohol.
2. Parents invest considerable expense and time.
3. Parents have difficulty setting limits and are oversensitive to problems in the child.
4. Infertile couples may have feelings of hostility or inferiority that are projected on the child who is a constant reminder of their inability to conceive.
5. Parents may think normal developmental problems are a result of adoption.
6. Competition may occur between biological children and adopted children.
7. Adoptive parents may receive little emotional support or public recognition.
8. The community or school may distinguish between "real" and "adopted" children.

What was once viewed as a process that ended when the adoption decree was granted is now recognized as a condition that affects those involved throughout their lives. It is a permanent change in legal status. Adoption is a unique way of building families. Adopted children bring their own genetic makeup, birth experiences, biological family ties, and life history to their adoptive family. The adoptive family is not the same as a biological family. Adoptive family dynamics are also different. Sometimes these differences generate problems within a family, and sometimes the adoption becomes the focus of other conflicts or unresolved family issues. Both adoptive parents and adopted children tend to feel that they have less control over their situation than other families. If the adoption was biracial or international, cultural differences must be acknowledged. The adopted child must be given opportunities to learn about his or her cultural background.

STEPCHILD

The number of stepchildren is increasing because of the high divorce and remarriage rates in the United States. Often a second marriage also ends in divorce, and another remarriage creates another stepfamily. Children experience loss, disruption, and changed life patterns and roles with each restructuring cycle of the family. The major issues for stepchildren in a stepfamily are loss, loyalty, and lack of control (64). A major loss is losing attention of the primary parent who remarries. The stepchild may feel rejected by the remarried natural parent and perceive the stepparent as a rival for the parent's attention. Jealousy, conflict, and hate may be dominant feelings toward stepsiblings, if present. The stepchild mourns loss of the familiar lifestyle at the loss of a biological parent from death or divorce; divorce adds to the grief because of problems associated with integration into a new family unit. Conflicting loyalties are felt when parents argue about the children af-

ter remarriage. The stepchild may believe acceptance of the stepparent is rejection of the biological parent. Lack of control is felt when the biological parent tries to impose stricter rules than the remarried parent in order to be considered the "good parent." Conflicts between parents are internalized and create problematic relationships; often emotional and behavioral maladjustments occur in the child (3, 18, 24, 50, 55, 63).

The child's response to being a stepchild varies by age and gender. Young children become anxious and fearful and may believe they are responsible for their parents' problems. School-age children may become angry and depressed at the time of remarriage and may view one parent as "wrong" and the other parent as "right." Adolescents often choose to move to a different parent's household when a remarriage occurs. Males are more likely to be affected with disturbed emotions and behavior from high-conflict divorce. Court-ordered joint physical custody and frequent visitation arrangements in high-conflict divorce are associated with poorer child outcomes, especially for girls (50, 64).

Other Family Lifestyles

There is no single type of contemporary U.S. family. The lifestyles of many vary with the factors discussed in this section, including family structure, family cultural pattern, and the impact of the 21st century. These factors, in addition to those already discussed, influence family interaction.

SINGLE-PARENT FAMILY

The number of single-parent families has steadily increased during the last 10 years in the United States, mainly because of the increasing divorce rate and the increased number of children born to single parents (18, 26). If the parents are divorced, the family may have experienced considerable disruption before the breakup. Sometimes the single-parent family is a planned event. A woman wanting to be a mother may choose to have a child by artificial insemination. A single man or woman may choose to adopt a child. Financial strain is especially apparent for single mothers because of wage inequities, difficulty with divorce settlements and child support, or lack of preparation financially in the case of a partner's death.

In many healthy persons, emotional attachment to a deceased or divorced spouse, with recurrent episodes of painful grief, may remain for many years. Mourning in later life may be qualitatively different from that in earlier life; it may be more prolonged and more difficult to complete. The long-lasting attachment for the spouse, lost through either divorce or death, may be unknown to even the closest friends or family of the survivor. Yet most mourners resolve their loss, become involved in life in new ways and with new people, and begin to see it as an opportunity for personal development (49).

In the single-parent family, the children may experience grief for the absent parent, guilt for their real or imagined part in the loss, shame for the change in their family structure, and fear about what changes the future may bring. Roles are changed, and each person may need to assume additional responsibilities and tasks. Parents may change their lifestyles. For example, Mother may go to work or school; Father may move into an apartment; or both parents may begin dating. An adolescent may serve as a parent substitute to younger siblings, or other children may assume new household tasks. Inappropriate social behavior, difficulty with identity formation, depression, and poorer school performance may be manifested by the children after a divorce. If there are frequent changes, children are more likely to quit school, leave home, and use drugs (4, 18, 26, 49).

Some researchers have found positive aspects of single-parent families. Children living in the single-parent household often exhibit more adaptability, responsibility, and maturity than children in two-parent families. Single-parent families have more role flexibility and fewer power struggles than two-parent families. Ford-Gilboe reported three family strengths in families after divorce: enjoying each other, strong family bonds, and shared family power. In another study, the same amounts of cohesion, teamwork, optimism, and togetherness were found in single-parent families as in two-parent families. The increased and varied responsibilities given to children in single-parent families lead to higher levels of independence, responsibility, self-esteem, and personal goals (18).

Help the single-parent family after divorce to accept this family structure as a workable option. Often an open discussion of the lifestyle, along with support from relatives, friends, and other single-parent families, enhances problem solving. Professional help may be needed if symptoms of more extreme dysfunction or grieving occur. Give information about various community resources for singles and single parents. Acknowledge the strengths and capabilities to create a nurturing healthy environment for each other (17).

STEPPARENT FAMILY

Today, more than a million children each year experience the divorce of their parents, and at least one of every three children will have a stepparent before they reach the age of 18. It is estimated that 50% to 60% of first marriages will end in divorce (34, 46). A **stepfamily** is formed when *a divorced, single, or widowed parent with children marries. When the marriage combines two sets of single parents with children*, it is considered a **blended family**. The new husband or wife becomes an instant stepparent. This addition of children to a couple's life differs from the situation of first-marriage couples, whose children are added at a slower pace. The remarried couple may then decide to have children of its own. In-laws and several sets of grandparents complete the picture. These relationships may not be an official remarriage, but the divorced parent living with another adult creates a living arrangement with a similar impact on the child.

Family interaction in stepparent and blended families can become increasingly complex. Because remarriages are fragile, 50% to 60% of second marriages end in divorce, creating more loss and devastation (34). If a third marriage or unmarried partnership occurs, there are more upheavals and changes and more layers of relatives. An unanswered question is whether the current generation of stepchildren or other steprelatives will care for stepparents in old age.

The common belief that familial love occurs via the marriage ceremony is a myth. Adjustment to a new, unique family unit is the major task of the stepfamily, and it is a lengthy, stressful process. *Stepfamilies benefit from education about the following stages of development and integration* (64):

1. **Fantasy.** *The adults expect the newly formed family to quickly adjust and live together in harmony*, but this fantasy ends soon after everyone moves together into one household.
2. **Immersion.** *Family members are immersed in frequent conflicts, and tensions are high.*
3. **Awareness.** *There is growing awareness by the parents that changes are needed to restore order and bring about a new cohesiveness.*
4. **Mobilization.** *Couples take action to make change*, such as seeking professional help, in order to resume closeness to their children and stepchildren.
5. **Action.** *The couple begins to work as a team to deal with their children's needs and conflicts.* It may take 3 to 4 years to reach this stage.
6. **Contact.** *All family members become familiar with and accept the family's routines and patterns of behavior.*
7. **Resolution.** *Security and cooperation exist within the family and with outside family members.* There is still less cohesion but more flexibility in stepfamilies than in first-marriage families.

Table 6-4 summarizes the unique characteristics of the stepfamily structure that makes their adjustments more difficult than first-marriage families, and the tasks needed to integrate the stepfamily (16, 64). New members cannot be assimilated within an existing family; instead a new family unit is formed. New rules, customs, and activities must be developed. Conflictual values and family ghosts must be resolved. All members of this new family bring a history of life experiences, relationships, and expectations to the stepfamily. Conflict often occurs when the values and rules of the two combined families or individuals differ. Conflicts about raising stepchildren can be the most explosive issue in remarriages. Initially, parents may take sides and favor their biological children, or they may be overly affectionate to their stepchildren in an effort to win them over. However, these strategies often cause the biological child to feel jealous toward the stepsibling and further alienated from his or her own parent. Eventually parents learn to present a united front and consistent approach to family discipline and treat each other's children and their own with love and respect. This process takes years to accomplish (16, 64). In time, stepfamily members work through their differences and resolve conflicts more amicably. They reach consensus about such matters as where to go to church, when to eat dinner, and how to celebrate birthdays, holidays, and other major family events.

In addition to adjusting in the family, stepfamilies must adjust to expectations of the outside world. Often differences in the stepparent family are ignored because the family appears intact. Feelings of frustration, inadequacy, and isolation in family members stem from expectations that they should feel as close to one another as blood relatives. The absent parent may still be an active influence in the original family. For instance, a divorced father may still contribute to his children's support and spend time with them on a regular basis, but they may be living with a stepfather. A deceased parent may be vividly remembered and compared unfairly

TABLE 6-4

Stepfamily Characteristics and Tasks

Characteristics	Tasks
Begins after many losses and changes	Dealing with losses and changes
Incongruent individual, marital, and family life cycles and needs	Negotiating different developmental needs
Children and adults have values and expectations from previous families	Establishing new traditions, expectations, values, roles
Parent-child relationships predate the new couple	Developing a solid couple bond and forming new relationships
Biological parent in another location or in memory	Creating a "parenting coalition," working on own union first
Children are members of two households	Accepting continual shifts in household composition
No legal relationship between stepparent and stepchildren	Risking involvement despite little societal support

to the stepparent. The child's ability to work through these feelings is influenced by age, gender, level of development, adaptive capabilities, and the understanding and support received from significant adults. The child may need professional help to work through the difficulties of integration into a new family structure.

The stepfamily is a potentially stressful situation that requires flexibility and adaptability of its members. This family offers many opportunities for growth and friendship through the differing experiences of its members; yet studies show that children in stepfamilies generally do not fare better than children in single-parent families (39).

Despite the old adage that children are flexible and can "bounce back," the trauma of divorce is second only to death. Often the problems that arise in the second marriage are more devastating than earlier ones. The children know that the original parent will not return, and they are faced with a new parent whom they often initially neither want nor accept emotionally (19).

Stepfamilies will benefit from education about typical stages of development and integration and related tasks. See **Table 6-4** for a summary. Encourage open communication between members that will foster acceptance of the family structure, decisions that are acceptable to all members, coping strategies, and conflict resolution. The children and adults may need professional help to work through difficulties. You may initiate and lead groups in churches, schools, or the community for children from single-parent and stepparent families. Refer families to relevant community resources, including support groups such as the Stepfamily Association of America, www.saafamilies.org.

SINGLE-PERSON FAMILY

In the United States, there has been a dramatic rise in the number of single adults (never married, separated, divorced, widowed) in the past 30 years. It is no longer considered necessary to marry and bear children to be fulfilled and accomplished. *The single state can promote individual development of creativity, extended emotional and social ties, and healthy self-care through the following* (49):

1. Time to make decisions about one's life course
2. Time to develop personal resources to meet goals
3. Freedom to make autonomous decisions
4. Freedom to pursue one's own schedule and interests
5. Opportunity to travel and try new things
6. Privacy

Yet solitary life is not always happy for the single person. Absence of intimate relationships may lead to loneliness and depression. Society is marriage oriented, and single adults may be unable to find a place for themselves in a couple-dominated world (49). There can be too much space and freedom and the inability to make decisions. The silence of the home when entering from a day's work may be overwhelming. There is no one readily available with whom to talk and share both the joys and stresses and the daily routine events. There may be financial concerns or unwise use of money because of lack of opportunity or experience with financial affairs. The person is a nonentity until someone needs something, and then the single person is seen as always available to help, because he or she "has no family or obligations." The single person may have difficulty receiving help in return or even asking for it, because society expects the single person to manage everything alone. The single person may be taken advantage of by home repairmen, by businesses, or by acquaintances. There may be places the single person cannot go because of cultural restrictions. Special holidays and anniversary dates can be especially painful if the person is alone and forgotten by friends who are busy with their families. Even in a crowd of merrymakers, despite a smiling face, the person may feel isolated and alone.

Some single people may have few biological relatives. Instead, they have a "psychologically extended" family of close friends, and are godparents or substitute "relatives" to their friends' children. They have learned to implement family tasks and all family roles. They have learned to go places alone, do repairs or know who to call for help, cope with stressors, and reach out to others. Their emotional and social needs are met through supportive people and relevant organizations, activities, or being part of a church faith family. They can be helpful friends as well as contributing through a career or profession.

The single person may need to vent feelings or seek assistance or support. Use communication and crisis intervention principles, as described in Chapter 2. ∞ Be empathic if the single, childless female describes a sense of grief *and* loss because she has no children. Reinforce her strengths and what she has contributed to the lives of other children and families.

STEPGENERATION FAMILY

The **stepgeneration family** *develops when grandparents raise their grandchildren or great-grandchildren because the parents are unable or choose not to raise their children.* More than a million children live in households that are headed by one or both grandparents or great-grandparents (9). The phenomenon of families headed by grandparents transcends culture, age, race, geographic location, and economic level. Grandparents provide a home to their grandchildren when the parent is addicted to drugs, and in cases of child abuse, neglect and abandonment, teenage pregnancy, death, joblessness, divorce, incarceration, illness, and parental death.

How well the situation works depends on the degree of respect, love, and communication shown; how clearly rules are set and enforced in the home; and who takes responsibility for child care and home maintenance tasks. The demands of raising grandchildren can have negative effects on grandparents' physical and mental health. Some problems reported in the literature include developing chronic conditions, worsening of preexisting chronic conditions, depression, anxiety, feeling overwhelmed, lost relationships with peers, and financial strains. In contrast, grandparents report many benefits to raising their grandchildren. These include developing a closer relationship with the parent, taking pride in their accomplishments, being able to provide love and affection, and having a better relationship with their spouse (9, 44, 51, 68).

Help grandparents seek support groups as a way to feel less isolated and to combine resources. Be an attentive listener. **Box 6-1**, National Organizations for Grandparent Caregivers, lists major organizations that offer assistance to grandparent caregivers.

BOX 6-1	**National Organizations for Grandparent Caregivers**

AARP Grandparent Information Center
601 East Street Northwest
Washington, DC 20049
202-434-2296

Grandparents As Parents (GAP)
PO Box 964
Lakewood, CA 90714
310-924-3996

Grandparents United for Children's Rights National
   Coalition of Grandparents
137 Larkin Street
Madison, WI 53705
608-238-8751

R.O.C.K.I.N.G. (Raising Our Children's Kids: An
   Intergenerational Network of Grandparents, Inc.)
PO Box 96
Niles, MI 49120
616-683-9038

FAMILY CULTURAL PATTERN

The ways of living and thinking that constitute the intimate aspects of family group life constitute the **family cultural pattern** (32). The family transmits the cultural pattern of its own ethnic background and social class to the child, together with parents' attitudes toward others. Refer to Chapter 5 for more information. ∞

Within the national cultural pattern of the United States, significant variations have been found in family cultural patterns and social systems (32). In Millstadt, Illinois, the German farm family provides a distinctive social system, with cultural features distinct from its Italian neighbors across the river in St. Louis. People from Maine and North Carolina may speak the same language, but the meanings of the words used may be quite different because of regional variables. How families raise their children depends on ethnicity, social class, geographic region, nationality, and historical period.

Influence of Societal Changes

TRENDS RELATED TO LIVING IN A COMPLEX INDUSTRIAL SOCIETY

Families live primarily in urban or metropolitan areas; more families than ever are homeless or at risk for homelessness. More women work outside the home. The woman who stays home today concentrates more on "mothering," and she may receive considerable criticism (22, 35, 44, 49). Her outside activities may include volunteer work so she can make significant contributions outside the family unit, control her hours, and feel she has prime time at home. The father may be the houseparent because he has an office in the home or is the unemployed member who thereby assumes child and home care responsibilities.

PARENTING PRACTICES IN THE UNITED STATES

Rapid change in all areas of society, including families, is a fact of life. Educate parents that research continues to show that children who experience consistent love, attention, and security will grow up to be adults who can better survive change and stressors with self-reliance, optimism, and identity intact (4, 5, 32, 44, 49). Despite the constant state of change in the family, current research shows that children can survive and thrive in many types of family environments if they are given adequate emotional support (2, 6, 14, 44, 54).

FATHER'S ROLE

Fathers are taking a more active role in caring for their children (3, 5, 23, 29, 30, 49, 51, 58). Seventeen percent of preschool children are cared for by their fathers while their mothers are at work, and 5% of children are raised solely by their fathers (4). In addition, shared custody arrangements have become more common for divorced couples. Good fathering involves changes in behavior, cognition, and emotions. It has developmental consequences for both fathers and their children. Initially, the father may be in a relationship with the child's mother, but changes in the relationship with the mother often bring about changes in the father-child relationship. Active fathering involves relating to the children or stepchildren, taking responsibility for them, planning for their future, and helping them develop into mature adults. Involved fathers reap many benefits, including improved health, happiness, and personal development (43). Unfortunately, some types of involved fathers can also be a threat to their children's development and safety. Children sometimes have to overcome the effects of fathers who are physically or sexually abusive or have unpredictable behavior.

Most literature shows that fathers' positive involvement with their children is good for the children, for the mother, and for the marriage. Interactions with fathers can help children deal with stress, improve their emotional health, and contribute positively to cognitive development. A father's involvement can have a positive effect on his son's success in school and later on in his marriage. In essence, good fathering has positive outcomes for everyone: children, partners, families, and communities (43).

RENEWED FOCUS ON THE FAMILY

Certainly, the health of a nation, and the world, depends on the health of the family.

The American family has changed, and family life has changed in many countries of the world because of war, natural disasters, famine, and the resulting poverty and its consequences. However, families dissolve by choice at a greater rate in the United States than in any other major industrialized country, and the United States leads the world in father absence from the home (3). The poverty rate for children in single-parent homes is more than 10 times that for children in two-parent homes. Divorce plunges many women and their children into poverty or near poverty (4). Children are left with less time and less moral guidance from parents than ever before (4). The key is for families to make sacrifices in their economic lifestyle to make time for each other and their children. To maintain a marriage and raise children takes time and commitment (50).

Society can promote the family. Businesses can promote family values by providing opportunities for flex-time and using the home as the workplace when it is feasible, and by providing paternity as well as maternity leave. The father who is at home for 1 or 2 weeks with the new mother and baby provides necessary nurturing and help to the mother with child care and household tasks. There must be more media and cultural emphasis on the real freedom that comes from fulfilling duties to the spouse and children, rather than from pursuing economic gains and work demands.

Family Life Around the World

In **Canada there is a wide range of cultures, but the family is the basic societal unit.** Most Canadian families have been shaped by Catholicism, by language, by family and work, and by their rural roots. Large families, conservative family traditions, and religious family rituals play an important part in Canadian culture. French language and ancestry dominate the Eastern Canadian population; Western Canadian populations include people with American Indian ancestry. Rural families and older family members cling to their French roots and still prefer to speak French. Although there is openness to new experience, there are strongly held beliefs about traditional gender roles. More families are leaving farming and lumberjack lifestyles to pursue big-city lifestyles, abandoning their Catholic beliefs. Canadian families seek help from health care providers when a crisis such as substance abuse, depression, or other illness requires treatment (1, 6, 21, 32). Government payment of health care fosters accessibility.

In **African American families** the grandmother is often the most powerful person. The extended family is a system of blood relatives and people who are informally adopted into the system through marriage and other relationships. Three- or four-generation families are common and provide a source of strength and support. There is variation in the amount of commitment African American males make to their families. Some are very active in child rearing; others are not involved in their children's lives. The divorce rate is higher among African American families than White families, but poverty may contribute to the uneven divorce rate. African Americans place a high value on the spiritual dimension and religious faith, which is incorporated into family life and child rearing (1, 4, 21, 32).

Latino families include people from diverse countries, including nations of South America, Central America, and the Caribbean. Most share a common language—Spanish—and a common religion—Roman Catholicism. **Machismo** *defines the role of the male as providing financial support for older parents, younger siblings, nieces, and nephews.* **Marianismo**, *stemming from the Virgin Mary, glorifies the role of motherhood.* **Hembrismo** *refers to the female's ability to be strong and survive adversity.* Latinos value individualism, but they strongly value family unity, welfare, and honor. Latino families are larger than either African American or White families. The family protects its individuals and helps those having problems. The extended family includes blood relatives, *godparents* (**compadres**), and *adopted children* (**hijos de crianza**). **Compadrazco** *is a system of ritual kinship with binding mutual obligations for economic assistance, encouragement, and personal correction.* Latinos view health holistically, place spiritual goals above materialistic goals, and prefer help from a spiritual healer rather than other health care providers or mental health professionals (1, 15, 21, 34).

Asian families value the family unit, from one generation to the next, through family rituals and the family genealogies. Traditional families are guided primarily by the teachings of Confucianism, Taoism, and Buddhism. The individual is not emphasized but rather seen as on a continuum from one generation to the next. Marriages are arranged by parents or grandparents; divorce is uncommon. The male is head of the family, and the female's role is to preserve the family name by bearing sons. In communication, silence is used to emphasize what was said and that the listener should be thoughtful in the answer. The child-parent attachment is stronger than the husband-wife relationship, and parental respect is demanded. Many Asian families have endured great hardships during war or political unrest and view this trauma in different ways. Chinese families see traumatic events as a matter of fate. South Asian families view hardship as part of life and something to be endured (*karma*). Japanese associate hardships (*gamman*) with maturity (1, 15, 21, 32).

In **Asian Indian families,** relationships within and across generations are influenced by the caste system. Males and their mothers are the most prominent family members in both Hindu and Christian Asian Indian families. Karma also influences intergenerational relationships. Asian Indians believe that today's problems are the result of bad behavior in a past life. Fasting and praying change the karma, and move the person ahead to a better life. Education of male children is necessary to fulfill the economic needs for the whole family. Females are expected to marry at age 18 to 22 years; the family selects the mate (1, 15, 21, 32).

For **Irish people,** the Catholic church is more important than the family. Irish families do not generally value the extended family system to the same extent as do some other cultures. They do not share their family problems outside the nuclear family. Irish place less emphasis on the importance of marriage than other cultures and accept women remaining single. Irish parents demand respect and conformity from their children and express a more traditional, authoritarian parenting approach. Irish mothers are the center of the family. Fathers are not as committed to family relationships, especially the extended family. For this reason children rarely speak disrespectfully about their mothers. Irish parents may frequently belittle, tease, and ridicule their children, making it difficult to develop loving parent-child relationships. Alcoholism is a common problem in Irish families because traditionally the pub has been the family gathering place rather than the dinner table (1, 15, 32).

In the **Jewish family,** marriage and having children, grandchildren, and great-grandchildren are central to life's meaning and are seen as a religious and social obligation. The recent trends of later marriages, divorce, and singlehood threaten these values. Jewish families emphasize education and nurturing of their children, most often from the mother. Family conflicts occur because of intermarriage (marrying outside the Jewish faith) and maintaining religious observances. Rituals are an important part of family life and include the **bris** (*circumcision*) and **bat** and **bar mitzvah** (*when a girl or boy reaches 12 or 13 years of age*). Jewish parents value education and professional achievement; Jewish children are strongly urged to attend college and pursue professional lives. The importance of charity and philanthropy in Jewish family life evolves from the belief that we are obligated to make the world a better place. Verbal debate and problem solving is highly regarded in Jewish families, even in children (1, 15, 21, 32).

Traditionally, the basic unit of **Slavic countries (Poland, Czech Republic, Slovak Republic, Ukraine, Belarus, Russia, Bulgaria, Slovenia, Croatia, Bosnia, and Macedonia) is a large extended family, or clan.** These families live communally, sharing property, homes, cattle, and money. The father is the head of the home, makes all the important decisions, and demands respect from other family members. The mother is her husband's helper, and grandparents often help in raising children. Communication involves silence, which is considered agreement (1, 15, 21, 32).

Africans place great importance on the family, which traditionally includes kin relationships that extend beyond ties of blood or marriage to include other individuals, especially members of the tribe or clan. One is born in a tribe and remains part of it. The clan is a subdivision of the tribe and is composed of several families who share a heritage through their mother or father.

Clans are named after animals, plants, or rocks (totems) that are a symbol of their strengths, hopes, and dreams. Males are the heads of their families, and their sons inherit their position. Females take care of children and the elderly, tend the house, and do the hard physical labor. As female roles have changed, males may feel threatened by their independence and domestic abuse is increasing. Important family events such as deaths and births are observed by elaborate ceremonies with songs, dances, drums, and other music. Spirituality is an important part of Africans' lives (1, 11, 15, 21, 32). Because of the AIDS epidemic in parts of Africa, many children are orphaned and cared for by other children or by their grandparents. In war-torn countries, soldiers (including school-age and adolescent boys forced into service) may rape women or force them into slavery.

In the past 20 years, **Britain's families have struggled with increasing rates of divorce, remarriage, lone parenting, mobility, and cohabitation.** Often both parents work. In some areas state education begins early, but older family members or private institutional care are typically used for young children of working parents. Even afternoon tea, designed for family time, is gradually disappearing. English persons may use silence out of respect for another's privacy. Marriage seminars and literature and films supporting family life are popular as young families work to commit themselves to each other and their children (1, 7, 15).

In the multicultural society of **Australia, marriages and children are valued, although families are experiencing an increasing rate of divorce.** The church has dropped some of the strong moral stands it took in the 1950s and 1960s. Home schooling, typical in the Outback, is increasing in urban areas. Children are disciplined but also encouraged to be independent. Teens are becoming more unsettled and more Westernized in behavior. Conflicts between generations over the old and new ways are common. Family life in urban areas differs considerably from family life in sparsely settled rural areas, on the huge ranches in the Outback, or for the Aborigines. Yet amidst the harshness of the sunburnt country is seen a gentleness in families (15, 53).

Health Promotion and Nursing Applications

FAMILY ASSESSMENT

Use prior information to assess how the family carries out its purposes, tasks, roles, stage of development, effective and ineffective

Practice Point

Support families you work with to affirm them as the basic unit for the developing person and health. You will frequently encounter the entire family as your client in the health care system, regardless of the setting. Increasingly, the emphasis is on health promotion of the family (6, 20, 67, 69). Yet you will not be able to care for the family even minimally unless you understand the family system and the dynamics of family living presented in this chapter.

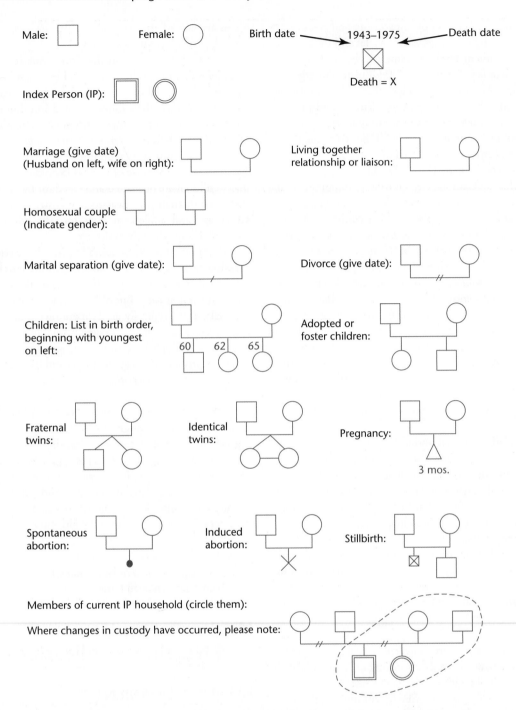

FIGURE ▪ 6-1 Genogram format. Symbols describe basic family membership and structure (include on genogram significant others who lived with or cared for family members; place them on the right side of the genogram with a notation about who they are). Religion, education, or ethnic origin can be written in by oldest generation or other units. Health problems noted by person.

patterns, and parenting practices. Find out about the family's internal and external structures by developing a **genogram**, *a diagram of family members, their characteristics, and their interrelationships*, such as depicted in **Figure 6-1 ▪** (69). Also, determine communication patterns and relationships, family health, access to health care, occupational demands and hazards, religious be-

liefs and practices, parenting practices, participation in the community, and support systems. Use the family assessment tool in **Figure 6-2 ▪** to help assess the family's lifestyle and needs. Other information for assessment is presented in **Box 6-2,** Family Assessment Tool Utilizing Theory Approaches, and **Box 6-3,** Criteria for Assessing Healthy Families.

Meeting of Physical, Emotional, and Spiritual Needs of Members
- Ability to provide food and shelter
  Space management as regards living, sleeping, recreation, privacy
  Crowding if over 1.5 persons per room
  Territoriality or control of each member over lifespace
  Access to laundry, grocery, recreation facilities
  Sanitation, including disposal methods, source of water supply, control of rodents and insects
  Storage and refrigeration
  Available food supply
  Food preparation, including preserving and cooking methods, (stove, hotplate, oven)
  Use of food stamps and donated foods as well as eligibility for food stamps
  Education of each member as to food composition, balanced menus, special preparations or diets if required for a specific member
- Access to health care
  Regularity of health care
  Continuity of caregivers
  Closeness of facility and means of access such as car, bus, cab
  Access to helpful neighbors
  Access to phone
- Family health
  Longevity
  Major or chronic illnesses
  Familial or hereditary illnesses, such as rheumatic fever, gout, allergy, tuberculosis, renal disease, diabetes mellitus, cancer, emotional illness, epilepsy, migraine, other nervous disorders, hypertension, blood diseases, obesity, frequent accidents, drug intake, pica
  Emotional or stress-related illnesses
  Pollutants that members are chronically exposed to, such as air, water, soil, noise, or chemicals that are unsafe
- Neighborhood pride and loyalty
- Job access, energy output, shift changes
- Sensitivity, warmth, understanding between family members
  Demonstration of emotion
  Enjoyment of sexual relations
    Male: Impotence, premature or retarded ejaculation, hypersexuality
    Female: Frigidity (inability to achieve orgasm), enjoyment of sexual relations, feelings of disgust, shame, self-devaluation; fear of injury, painful coitus Menstrual history, including onset, duration, flow, missed periods and life situation at the time, pain, euphoria, depression, other difficulties
- Sharing of religious beliefs, values, doubts
  Formal membership in church and organizations
  Ethical framework and honesty
  Adaptability, response to reality
  Satisfaction with life
  Self-esteem

Childrearing Practices and Discipline
- Mutual responsibility
  Joint parenting
  Mutual respect for decision making
  Means of discipline and consistency
- Respect for individuality
- Fostering of self-discipline
- Attitudes toward education, reading, scholarly pursuit
- Attitudes toward imaginative play
- Attitudes toward involvement in sports
- Promotion of gender stereotypes

Communication
- Expression of a wide range of emotion and feeling
- Expression of ideas, concepts, beliefs, values, interests
- Openness
- Verbal expression and sensitive listening
- Consensual decision making

Support, Security, Encouragement
- Balance in activity
- Humor
- Dependency and dominance patterns
- Life support groups of each member
- Social relationship of couple: go out together or separately; change since marriage mutually satisfying; effect of sociability patterns on children

Growth-Producing Relationships and Experiences Within and Without the Family
- Creative play activities
- Planned growth experiences
- Focus of life and activity of each member
- Friendships

Responsible Community Relationships
- Organizations, including involvement, membership, active participation
- Knowledge of and friendship with neighbors

Growing With and Through Children
- Hope and plans for children
- Emulation of own parents and its influence on relationship with children
- Relationship patterns: authoritarian, patriarchal, matriarchal
- Necessity to relive (make up for) own childhood through children

Unity, Loyalty, and Cooperation
Positive interacting of members toward each other

Self-Help and Acceptance of Outside Help in Family Crisis

FIGURE ■ 6-2 Family assessment tool.

BOX 6-2   Family Assessment Tool Utilizing Theory Approach

STRUCTURAL FAMILY ASSESSMENT

Internal Structure

Family composition (nuclear, stepfamily, grandparent family, blended family)—includes all family members, biologically related and by kinship, and those not living at home

Gender—ideas about masculinity and femininity, expected behaviors

Rank order—birth order, gender, and distance in age

Subsystems—dyads, small groups within the large family unit

Boundary—who participates and how

External Structure

Extended family—family of origin, present generation, in-laws and steprelatives

Larger systems—work systems, public welfare, child welfare, clinics, health care

Context—Background Relevant to Event or Personality

Ethnicity—a combination of cultural history and religion

Race

Social class—upper-upper, lower-upper, upper-middle, lower-middle, upper-lower, lower-lower, education, income, occupation

Religion—organized church affiliation, local church, temple, or synagogue

Environment—larger community, community services, the neighborhood, and the home

Tools

Genogram

Ecomap

DEVELOPMENTAL FAMILY ASSESSMENT

Middle-Class North American Family Life Cycle

Launching of the single young adult

Marriage: The joining of families

Families with young children

Families with adolescents

Launching children and moving on

Families in later life

Divorce and Postdivorce Family Life Cycle

Deciding to divorce

Planning the breakup of the system

Separation

Divorce

Single-parent custodial

Single-parent noncustodial

Remarried Family Life Cycle

Entering the new relationship

Planning the new family

Remarriage

FUNCTIONAL FAMILY ASSESSMENT

Instrumental functioning—routine activities of daily living

Expressive functioning—communication, problem solving, roles, influence, beliefs, alliances and coalitions

Adapted from references 5, 69.

BOX 6-3   Criteria for Assessing Healthy Families

1. Ability to provide for the physical, emotional, social, and spiritual needs of the family
2. Ability to be sensitive to the needs of family members
3. Ability to listen and communicate effectively
4. Ability to provide trust, support, security, affirmation, and encouragement
5. Ability to initiate and maintain growth-producing relationships and experiences inside and outside the family
6. Demonstration of mutual respect for family and others
7. Commitment to teach and demonstrate moral code
8. Concern for family unity, loyalty, and interfamily cooperation
9. Capacity to use humor and to share leisure time with each other, to enjoy each other
10. Commitment to strong sense of family where rituals and traditions abound
11. Ability to perform roles flexibly and share responsibility
12. Ability to maintain balance of interaction and privacy among the members
13. Ability for self-help and helping other family members, when appropriate
14. Ability to use crisis or seemingly injurious experience as a means of growth
15. Ability to grow with and through children
16. Capacity to maintain and create constructive and responsible community relationships in the neighborhood, school, town, and local and state governments and to value service to others

Taken from references 2, 6, 20, 69.

FORMULATION OF NURSING DIAGNOSES

In a health care setting where the nurse is including the family unit as part of client care, nursing diagnoses may be general, or family issues may be included in the client's nursing diagnoses. See the **Box** Nursing Diagnoses Related to Family, which presents commonly derived nursing diagnoses (40). The nurse will also formulate nursing diagnoses related to physical, emotional, and social health of family members.

Examples of a nursing diagnosis may be derived from some of the material presented earlier in the chapter. Using Family Systems Theory, state nursing diagnoses in the following manner:

1. Family system insufficiently open to internal (or external) environment related to inability of members to express feelings (or impaired ability to interact with neighbors)
2. Impaired communication processes in family system related to power struggles
3. Unmet family goals and functions related to disorganized family lifestyle patterns
4. Dysfunctional family system related to ineffective communication among family members, including extended family
5. Impairment in fulfilling family functions and activities related to inadequate material resources
6. Disruptive family interpersonal relationships related to power conflicts and lack of closeness
7. Altered family coping (tension between partners) related to work stress and disagreements about parental discipline

Using a genogram, state nursing diagnoses as follows:

1. Altered family relationships related to death, divorce, or remarriage
2. Unachieved family goals related to inability to use family resources

INTERVENTION WITH THE FAMILY

Help families understand processes and dynamics underlying interaction so that they, in turn, learn to respect the uniqueness of the self and of each other. Certainly members in the family need not always agree with each other. Instead, they can learn to listen to the other person describe feelings and accept each person's impression as real for the self. This attitude becomes the basis for mutual respect, honest communication, encouragement of individual fulfillment, and freedom to be. There is then no need to prove or defend the self. Help the person work through problems stemming from low self-esteem. Utilize the principles of communication presented in Chapter 2. ∞

Validate with families about the forces pulling them apart. Reinforce that people need one place—their home—where they can act without self-consciousness, where the pretenses and roles demanded in jobs, school, or social situations can be put aside. Emphasize that the family home should be a place where communication takes place with ease, each knows what to expect from the other, a cohesiveness exists that is based on nonverbal messages more than verbal, and each person is accepted.

Once the attitude "we are all important people in this family" is established, conflicts can be dealt with openly and constructively. Name calling and belittling are out of place. Families need to structure time together; otherwise individual schedules will allow them less and less time to meet. Parents need to send consistent messages to their children. For example, to say "don't smoke" while immediately lighting a cigarette is hardly effective.

Times of communication are especially necessary when children are feeling peer pressure. Children should be praised for what they do right rather than reprimanded for what they do wrong. Children need structure but should be told the reason for the structure if they are old enough to comprehend. As you help family members achieve positive feelings toward and with each another, they are better equipped to fulfill their tasks, roles, and functions. Review the adaptive mechanisms of families described in this chapter.

The person's health problems, especially emotional ones, may well be the result of the interaction patterns in childhood or in the present family. Teach about variables influencing family interaction—parents' self-esteem and upbringing, number of siblings, person's ordinal position in the family, cultural norms, and family rituals. Assist the person in talking through feelings related to past and present conflicts. Sometimes helping the person understand the effect of socialization and gender expectations in relation to the spouse's upbringing and behavior can be the first step in overcoming current marital problems. In turn, overcoming negative effects helps the parents avoid repeating them in parenting. With intervention, support, and teaching, the parent may be able to resolve personal conflicts and more effectively work with the developing child. Each stage of development is a crisis to resolve. See Chapter 2 for communication principles. ∞

You may help families explore and resolve ethical dilemmas related to their decisions about use of newer technology for getting pregnant. Technology that allows infertile couples to become

---

Nursing Diagnoses Related to Family

Caregiver Role Strain	Disabled Family **C**oping
Risk for **C**aregiver Role Strain	Readiness for Enhanced Family **C**oping
Parental Role **C**onflict	Readiness for Enhanced **S**elf-Concept
Ineffective **C**oping	Chronic Low **S**elf-Esteem
Compromised Family **C**oping	

Source: Reference 40.

Practice Point

To help families explore values (see Tables 5-4 and 5-5) ∞ and ethical principles, you must first explore and resolve these issues within yourself. You cannot give another person the answer, but you can use therapeutic communication skills to enable clients to find their own answers.

pregnant with *in vitro* fertilization may also cause parents to face major ethical dilemmas as they determine which of the fertilized embryos should be transplanted into the uterus and which should be frozen for future use. Another difficult decision is whether to hire a surrogate mother to become pregnant and bear the baby for the family. Exploration of feelings and implications is essential.

Other decisions may not be as difficult but are key to future family development and relationships. For example, help adoptive parents relate with their child. Or review with the homosexual family how to explain "coming out." Parents must be prepared to explain the child's origins when the child asks and to help the child understand that there are many kinds of families in the United States. We do not yet know the long-term consequences, developmentally and emotionally, for children who are raised without guidance from the opposite gender or who are raised by only one parent. Your assessment, exploration, and teaching with such families are important.

You may assist families to cope with crises or various unexpected disorganizing events, such as illness and natural disasters. **Table 6-5** presents guidelines to assist families to cope with crises. You are not a specialized family counselor; advanced educational preparation is required to do family therapy. But you can often sense lack of communication in a family. Through use of an empathic relationship and effective communication, teaching, and crisis therapy, encourage family members to talk about their feelings with one another and assist in the resolution of their conflicts. Help them become aware of the need to work for family cohesiveness, just as they would work at a job or important project. Your

listening, counseling, and education may help them work through not only the current crises but also past unresolved crises, or several crises occurring simultaneously. Families often experience a cumulative effect from multiple crises, which can impair physical, emotional, and social health. Refer them to a family counseling service if the problems are beyond your scope. Your work with the family should also help them better use other community resources, such as private family or psychiatric counseling or family and children's services.

One family self-help resource can be the formation of a group of four or five complete family units (including stepfamily, single-parent, cohabitation, or traditional units) who contract to meet together over an extended period for shared educational experiences that concern relationships within their families. This setting provides a positive approach and affirms family members because a commitment is made for all persons—no matter what their age—to have both power and input into the group.

ROLE OF THE NURSE IN WELL-BABY CARE

You may care for well babies and mothers in a variety of settings—clinic, hospital, home, or doctor's office. Well-baby care includes assessment for growth and development patterns, feeding patterns, and neurologic development; immunizations; and testing for abnormalities such as hearing tests and vision screening. Refer to Chapter 9 for more information. ∞

PRENATAL CARE

Prenatal assessments include uterine growth, weight, blood pressure, and screening for sexually transmitted infections and other diseases such as diabetes and hepatitis B. Refer to a text on maternity nursing for in-depth information. Teach the pregnant female during these assessments about the importance of the care of baby through her self-care.

Give information about healthy eating and adequate nutrition; abstaining from smoking, drugs, and alcohol; and avoiding exposure to environmental hazards. Listen to both partners vent frustrations or share fears, provide counseling and encour-

TABLE 6-5

Family Crisis Intervention to Assist Families with Coping

1. Encourage each family member to identify the stressor or hazardous life event.
2. Assess each family member's interpretation of the event and its real impact.
3. Determine family's usual and current coping abilities and resources to handle the event.
4. Assess family's level of functioning as a whole and function of individual members.
5. Assist family members in communicating with each other.
6. Encourage all family members to be involved in finding a solution or resources.
7. Be supportive but encourage the family to mobilize its own resources and extended family or community resources.
8. Empower families by indicating their strengths, reinforcing positive behavior, helping them make sense of the event, and promoting a sense of being normal.
9. Explore how to prevent and cope with future stressful experiences.
10. Teach coping strategies, ways to prevent or minimize future stressors, stress management, and lifestyle alterations.
11. Recognize members at risk for violence and intervene as necessary.
12. Either continue longer-term therapy, if needed, with the family unit or members or refer them to ongoing therapy as necessary.

agement during periods of depression or uncertainty, and encourage sharing of happy feelings about becoming parents. Many couples attend prenatal classes conducted by nurses to learn about the physical and psychological changes during pregnancy, adequate nutrition, preparing for childbirth, breastfeeding, and parenting. There are also prenatal classes for special situations such as teen pregnancy, adoption, cesarean section, multiples, and grandparenting. A maternity nursing text will provide more information.

Single parents need special attention. The father's involvement needs to be assessed. Some mothers refuse the father's help for safety reasons, but it is usually best for all if the father can be involved in the pregnancy and parenting. The single father needs help in talking about his feelings about becoming a single parent; he often feels proud because he has proven his masculinity (44). All parenting options should be thoroughly explored with and by both partners. These options include marriage, adoption, and parenting alone or with help from parents and grandparents. The majority of single mothers choose to keep and raise their babies alone or with help from their partners or parents.

Teen parents have special needs. Although teenagers are aware of the benefits of using contraceptives, they frequently do not use them; hence most teen pregnancies are unplanned and may be unwanted. Teens need help in developing their support systems within the family or in the community. Educate the parents of the single teen father to communicate their feelings and support directly to their son, and to assert themselves in helping the young man take responsibility for his actions. During the postpartum period, provide teaching about consistent contraceptive use so as to avoid another pregnancy (20).

Advocate to prevent single pregnancies, improve or strengthen family life, and develop a better respect for the father's role in the family. Fathers can help adolescent sons by talking with and listening to them, by being slow to judge, by taking them to the work site so they can see how the father earns a living, and by being a role model in relating maturely to the spouse and other females. Fathers can create an atmosphere in which the sons will want to talk about emerging sexual feelings and experiences (20). If the adolescent son comes from a home where no father is present, the mother can work at listening to and discussing problems and feelings with the son. She may also be able to foster a bond between the son and another male member of the family.

CHILDBIRTH EDUCATION CLASSES

Try to interview each couple early in the pregnancy, to observe their relationship and determine their responses to the pregnancy. During prenatal classes, include opportunities for both men and women to talk about their unique feelings or problems. Provide anticipatory guidance about the couvade syndrome. Avoid pushing the father into participation and provide support for him. Focus childbirth education on the known benefits to the baby and parents and not on overromanticized and dramatic statements about improved marital relationships. Educate both parents about family planning so that future pregnancies can be mutually planned. Refer either partner, or both, to psychological counseling when necessary, especially if antisocial behavior is seen or if there has been fetal loss (5).

LABOR AND DELIVERY

During labor and delivery, the nurse gives necessary physical care, may act as a coach for the mother, or may support the father as he assists his partner. Flexibility in hospital routines for obstetric patients is usually possible and contributes to the parents' sense of control. The physician and nurse, or nurse-midwife, work as a team with the expectant couple and their families. In some facilities the nurse-midwife assumes primary responsibility for the family unit. Wherever a mother delivers, she has the right to capable, safe care by qualified caretakers. Home deliveries can be carefully planned and safe for mothers without obstetric complications. Hospital deliveries can be more homelike. Maternity centers now provide families with a homelike setting with all medical equipment hidden but readily available. Labor and delivery rooms are designed to accommodate the coach and other family members. Lights can be dimmed for a more relaxing atmosphere before and after the birth. The newborn can remain with the mother, and the newborn's physical examination can be done with the family present. New mothers usually stay in the hospital for 1 to 2 days for a vaginal birth or 3 to 4 days for cesarean-section birth. Follow-up phone calls and postpartum home visits by public health nurses are effective (39). Refer to community agencies as needed.

Childbirth should be a positive, maturing experience for the couple. Expectant parents have the right and responsibility to be involved in planning their care with the health team and to know what is happening. Cultural beliefs should be recognized, respected, and accommodated whenever possible. A positive childbearing experience contributes to a healthy family unit (1, 21, 39). You can be instrumental in continuing new trends in care to make the hospital or clinic environment more homelike, while providing safe, modern care.

POSTPARTUM PERIOD

Realize that various cultural groups may have specific traditional rituals that will be implemented during this period. *Mexican Americans and Asian Americans may carry out practices related to the hot and cold theory or concepts of yin and yang.* See Chapter 5 for a summary. ∞ The postpartum period is considered a cold, or yin, period (39).

Educate the family member who will be caring for the new mother and baby. Additional care may be given by a nurse in the home. In the immediate postpartum period, focus on the mother's physical needs and recovery. Mothers need to be mothered to enhance attachment between mother and baby. After the mother's physical needs have been met, after the initial **"taking in" period** *of having received special care and attention,* the mother moves to the **"taking hold" stage,** *in which she is able to focus her attention on learning about the care of the baby* (39, 48). Listen to the parents' concerns, answer questions, and support maternal and paternal attachment behaviors. In a nonthreatening way, teach the parents how to respond to the baby's needs. Help them begin to see themselves as a family rather than as a couple and to see the positive aspects of being parents. If the mother is breastfeeding, teaching and assistance needs to include frequency of feeding, positioning for feeding, and how to handle common breastfeeding problems (39, 48).

The interaction between the infant and primary caretaker is crucial. The mothering person helps the baby feel secure and loved, fosters a sense of trust, provides stimulation, reinforces certain behavior, acts as a model for language development, and trains the baby in basic learning strategies. In turn, maternal behavior is influenced by the baby's cries, coos, smiles, activity, and gazes and by how well the baby's behavior meets the mother's expectations. Refer to Chapter 9 ∞ for information on neonate and infant assessment and care, including promotion of the parent-child relationship and health of the family.

CONTINUED CARE IN THE POSTPARTUM PERIOD

During the 6 to 8 weeks after delivery, the mother needs assistance with child care and an opportunity to regain her former self physically and emotionally. The father also needs support as he becomes involved in child care responsibilities. In the nuclear or single-parent family the parent may struggle alone. Continued visits by a home health nurse may be useful. Some communities have a crisis line for new parents. You may be able to suggest services or help the parent think of people who could be helpful.

Assessment of the mother's functioning should consider her physical and emotional energy, support systems, and current level of parenting activity. If she apparently is not caring adequately for the child, assess for anemia, pain, bleeding, infections, lack of food or sleep, drug use, or other medical conditions that would interfere with her activity level and feelings of caring. In **postpartum blues,** *caused by hormonal shifts and the crisis of parenthood, the mother may feel overwhelmed and cry frequently, but she is able to care for herself and her baby.* These typical blues last up to 2 weeks after the baby's birth. **Postpartum depression** is a *persistent feeling of sadness, helplessness, and hopelessness continuing for more than 2 weeks after birth. The mother is immobilized and is unable to provide basic care for herself and her baby.* Medications and psychotherapy are the most effective treatment for postpartum depression. Be aware of the differences between postpartum blues and postpartum depression and provide the appropriate care and referrals for each.

The mother's support system is crucial for her energy maintenance, both physical and emotional. If the baby is developing normally, focus on the mother's needs and concerns. Helping her stay in good physical and emotional health ensures better parenting. She needs direct support and assistance with daily tasks, plus moral support, a listener, a confidant. Support comes from personal and professional sources—the partner, parents, friends, other relatives, and the nurse, doctor, social worker, or pastor. Parenting skills and parent-infant attachment can be assessed by observing behaviors such as touching, cuddling, voice tone, and loving gazes. Additional information about parents' feelings and the parenting process is provided in Chapter 9. ∞

Because of their more active role in caretaking, fathers need to be included in the health care decisions regarding their children. This inclusion offers them support for their challenges and provides incentives for continuing their work as involved fathers (26, 29, 30, 42, 58).

Observe interactions and relationships between the parents or between the mother and other members of the family. It will be difficult for the mother to remain caring if she is abused. A father who is abusive to the mother—verbally, physically, or emotionally—may become abusive to the child at some point. Chapters 8, 9, and 10 and other references provide information (39, 44). ∞

CARE OF FAMILIES WITH A CHRONICALLY ILL OR SPECIAL-NEEDS CHILD

Families who have a child with chronic illness or a special-needs child with the challenges of developmental disabilities or chronic physical or emotional illness experience continuing stressors, including time demands; physical, emotional, and social burdens; and financial costs of continuing care. Parents may want collaboration and control but feel that they have no control over the care of and treatment consequences for their child, depending on the health care providers' approaches to the child and family. Parents experience a sense of loss, chronic sorrow, and ongoing grief and mourning related to the ideal or healthy child they expected, as they adapt their expectations to fit the real child they have. Ongoing physical care and guidance problems are constant reminders of developmental lag; the child will not achieve certain developmental tasks and will remain dependent on someone, perhaps for life. There are continual, lifelong adjustments to the child and care demands. Parents worry about the child's care and quality of life in the future when they are unable to continue care. Marital stress occurs as parents negotiate parental roles and responsibilities, time, energy, and finances, and reconcile career-versus-family demands. Career mobility, especially related to geographic moves, may occur because of dependence on a specific treatment agency or team or the employer's insurance plan. Divorce in families with special-needs children is not unusual.

Families with special-needs children need a social support system to maintain family stability and care adequately for the child. Social support may include an extended family, close friends, religious affiliation, parents of other children with special needs, empathetic professionals, and family support groups in the community or church. Extra effort is often needed to encourage these parents to participate in self-help or other groups, because they often do not develop or maintain social contacts and so become more isolated. **Table 6-6** lists toll-free telephone numbers and Websites of organizations that provide information for families with special-needs children. Share this information with families.

TEEN PARENT EDUCATION

To combat the problems associated with the high adolescent birth rate, some junior and senior high schools are establishing creative programs in parenthood education. Some hospitals and health clinics are initiating specialized prenatal and postnatal services to help adolescent mothers become more effective parents and avoid a cycle of repeated pregnancies, child neglect and abuse, and economic dependency.

Formation of a mothers' or parents' group, including women and men of various ethnic origins and income brackets, can provide parent education and support and foster talking about feelings. Educate parents about using community resources. Establish and refer parents to Parent Effectiveness Training groups. Initiate nontraditional programs in the community.

TABLE 6-6

Toll-Free Telephone Numbers and Websites for Special-Needs Information

National Association of People with AIDS	240-247-0880	www.napwa.org
American Cancer Society	800-227-2345	www.cancer.org
American Cleft Palate Educational Foundation	800-24-CLEFT	www.cleftline.org
American Council for the Blind	800-424-8666	www.ACB.org
American Diabetes Association	800-342-2383	www.diabetes.org
American Kidney Fund	800-638-8299	www.kidneyfund.org
American Liver Foundation	800-223-0179	www.liverfoundation.org
American Lung Association	800-LUNGUSA	www.lungusa.org
American SIDS Institute	800-232-7437	www.SIDS.org
American Speech and Hearing Association	800-638-TALK	www.asha.org
Association for Retarded Citizens	800-491-4445	www.thearc.org
Beginnings (Hearing)	800-541-HEAR	www.beginningssvcs.com
Child Abuse/Parents Anonymous	800-421-0353	www.parentsanonymous.org
Cystic Fibrosis Foundation	800-344-4823	www.cff.org
Epilepsy Information Service	800-332-1000	www.efa.org
International Dyslexia Association	800-222-3123	www.interdys.org
Juvenile Diabetes Foundation International	800-223-1138	www.jdrf.org
March of Dimes	800-663-4637	www.marchofdimes.com
National Center for Stuttering	800-221-2483	www.stuttering.com
National Dissemination Center for Children with Disabilities	800-695-0285	www.nichcy.org
National Down Syndrome Society	800-221-4602	www.ndss.org
National Hearing Aid Society	800-521-5247	www.healthatoz.com
National Organization for Rare Disorders	800-477-6673	www.raredisease.org
National Organization on Fetal Alcohol Syndrome	800-666-6327	www.nofas.org
National Reye's Syndrome Foundation	800-233-7393	www.reyessyndrome.org
Scoliosis Association	800-800-0669	www.scoliosis-assoc.org
Shriners Hospitals for Crippled Children	800-237-5055	www.shrinershq.org
Sickle Cell Disease Association	800-421-8453	www.sicklecelldisease.org
Spina Bifida Association of America	800-621-3141	www.sbaa.org

WORKING WITH ADOPTIVE FAMILIES

Educate adults about the opportunities and stresses involved in any adoption, including adopting an older child with special needs or international adoptions. Work with adoptive parents, who also have needs. Help parents understand that the attachment process may take many years, especially if the child was neglected or came from an abusive environment. Assure parents that attachment develops over time. Help them think through how and when to tell the child that he or she is adopted so that the child understands and is not traumatized. Help the parents anticipate how they will help the child cope when the child is taunted by peers about being adopted. Help them realize that the adopted child will probably seek answers to many questions when he or she gets older. Who were the parents? Their cultural, racial, or ethnic background? Their ages, occupations, interests, appearance? Why was he or she relinquished? What are the medical facts surrounding heredity and birth? Help parents realize that these questions do not mean that the child does not love them. Refer to prior information in this chapter. Various articles supply information on adoption procedures, stresses encountered, and how to make adoption a success

(27, 28, 33, 42, 54, 56). **Box 6-4**, Intervention Guidelines for Therapy with Adoptive Families, summarizes therapy considerations (28, 42, 52, 56).

WORKING WITH STEPFAMILIES

Intervention programs are essential for the parents and children (13, 64). There is great need to educate parents, family members, attorneys, and judges about the impact of divorce and remarriage on children. Children need to be cared for and nurtured in the midst of disruptions and chaos. Children need to be kept informed of any changes taking place in the family and to be a part of the decision-making processes. Public assistance programs and ensuring support from the father are critical to reduce the effects of poverty on divorced women who are awarded child custody (64).

The guidelines previously discussed will be useful in helping the single-parent family or stepfamily adjust to its situation. The single-parent family can be referred to a local chapter of Parents Without Partners if the person seeks support from peers. Do not rush in with answers for these families; it is important to understand their

BOX 6-4	Intervention Guidelines for Therapy with Adoptive Families

1. Conventional treatment may not work well with adoptive families.
2. Adoptive parents need validation as parents and of their decision to adopt.
3. Adoptive parents must be included in therapeutic interventions to empower them further and to reinforce the adoptive commitment.
4. In treating child-rooted problems, often the job will be to help parents modify their expectations.
5. A child cannot successfully mourn the past and integrate it into the present circumstances if preoccupied with emotional survival. Developing a sense of safety and security is of paramount importance.
6. Child-rooted barriers can come from unfinished emotional business, attachment disorders, or poor preparation for adoption.
7. Adult-rooted barriers may stem from unfinished business, marital problems, or individual pathologies.
8. Environmental barriers include lack of support or active disapproval from the extended family or the broader community.
9. Any assessment is useful only if the assessed family accepts it as valid.
10. In deciding to terminate an adoption that is not working, one must be committed to preserving the family's integrity, yet open to the removal of the child as a viable option.
11. When an adoption is terminated, avoid judgment about reasons for its failure. Plans for adoption of another child should not be made until grief over the loss is resolved.

unique problems. Acknowledge their strengths; help them formulate their own solutions. Often a few sessions of crisis therapy will be sufficient. Several references give further information (6, 44, 49, 64).

FAMILY CARE THROUGHOUT THE LIFE CYCLE

You may be called on to assist families as they meet various developmental crises throughout the life cycle. The goal is health promotion and primary disease prevention. *The care you give to young parents lays the foundation for their children's health.* You may also become an *advocate for families* in relation to state or federal legislation that affects families and child care (6).

Work to improve the family as an institution from within. Support parents' efforts to teach their children not just to get ahead but to serve, to cooperate, and to be kind. We can teach children to believe that family ties are the most rewarding values, that social, cultural, and community activities can be deeply satisfying, and that the gratification from income and jobs is not the main priority (5, 6, 8).

Educate parents about societal trends; validate their healthful decisions. Excessive competitiveness is being passed on to children as parents try to be a superfamily and produce "superkids." Misplaced educational pressure is likely to produce lopsided development and an aversion to schooling. Excessive competitiveness overlaps with excessive materialism. In most parts of the world, materialism is balanced by spiritual values (e.g., dedication to Allah in Islamic countries, dedication to the nation in Israel, dedication to the family in Greece). In contrast, in the United States many children get their values from television, video games, or the Internet. In turn, rates for violent crime are shockingly high. Advocate with parents as they demand good programs from media producers. Support parents as they forbid their children's watching television programs with excessive violence and sordid sex. Adolescents and young adults without strong values and moral beliefs may turn to drugs, alcohol, violent crimes, promiscuous sexual activity, and suicide (5, 6).

Reinforce that parents can make a profound difference by teaching spiritual values throughout childhood. These include helpfulness, cooperation, generosity, and love. Volunteering with parents in a homeless shelter or food pantry can give children a sense of accomplishment. Young children can be encouraged to do other helpful activities, such as offering to walk the elderly neighbor's dog. As children get older they can be encouraged to do more difficult volunteer tasks, such as raking leaves, shoveling snow, or cleaning house for an elderly or disabled neighbor.

Educate families to create a family atmosphere in which parents treat each other and their children with respect and affection. Using supportive and encouraging language instead of attacks on character and criticism can greatly improve family morale and children's behavior. Family meals together have been shown to improve older children's risky behaviors (5, 6, 50).

Educate parents to give careful attention to the topic of sexuality. We have done well to overcome the shame that used to surround sex. But in declaring sex more wholesome and natural, we have mistakenly ignored its tenderness, generosity, and intensely spiritual aspects. Children primarily learn the importance of male-female relationships within their families. Parents' behavior toward and commitment to each other and their admiration and respect for one another has a tremendous impact on children. Answers to questions about sexual matters by 2-, 3-, and 4-year-old children should emphasize the loving and caring aspects of sex and marriage. Joking and disparaging remarks about marriage should be avoided. Parents can suggest that if young people want to claim the right to sexual freedom, they should be aware of the responsibilities. If a youthful marriage soon ends in divorce, parents can point out that no marriage succeeds by itself but must be continually cultivated, like a garden. *Teach parents how* to look for openings to discuss these topics when children are 9, 10, or 11 years of age. When they are 13 years old and beyond, they think their parents are hopelessly old-fashioned and consider peer opinions as the only truth (6, 44).

You have a role as educator and advocate, as well as health care provider, to assist parents as they guide children toward meeting developmental needs and cooperation for the common good. You can assist adults to be mature parents who present a positive model for the future of the family and society.

Summary

1. There are various types of family structures and systems.
2. The family is the basic unit of health and health promotion.
3. You will care for clients who may come from a family background quite different from your own family system in structure and dynamic relationships.
4. All families, regardless of structure, share similar purposes, developmental tasks, roles, and functions.
5. Family relationships, use of adaptive mechanisms, and the extent to which developmental tasks are met within the family are a major influence on development and health.
6. Use of ineffective adaptive mechanisms in the family can interfere with achieving developmental tasks, roles, and functions.
7. Family interaction and parenting practices are influenced by a number of parental and current family variables.
8. The adopted child and stepchild influence and are influenced by family interaction and parenting practices.
9. Family lifestyles that differ from the traditional family include the single parent, stepparent, single person, and stepgeneration families.
10. Each family, whether in the United States or other countries around the world, has its own family culture.
11. Practice principles of family-centered care, based on concepts in this chapter, in every health care setting.
12. Engage in lifelong learning about your own and other family systems to assess, plan, and provide comprehensive care to the client and family.

Review Questions

1. A student nurse working on a pediatric unit asks the instructor why visitors are allowed to be in the unit with less restriction compared to other units in the hospital. The instructor should base the response to this student on the fact that:
   1. Family presence is important to the development of a child.
   2. Children will cooperate when visitors are present.
   3. Adults require more rest than children.
   4. Numerous visitors are less disturbing in a pediatric unit.

2. A young woman reports a positive home pregnancy test to the nurse in the student health clinic. The woman tells the nurse that she and her partner intend to marry and raise the baby in a family. Which stage of family development have this couple entered?
   1. Stage of leaving home
   2. Establishment stage
   3. Expectant stage
   4. Parenthood stage

3. A new mother confides in the nurse that she is unhappy with her role as a stay-at-home mother and she is eager to return to work. The client states that she is afraid to tell her husband about her desire to go back to work, because he places great value on his childhood experience with a stay-at-home mother. How should the nurse respond to this client?
   1. "Do you need to work for financial reasons?"
   2. "It is best to have a parent at home during a child's early years."
   3. "Perhaps joining a group or taking a class will be an alternative to going back to work."
   4. "How do you think your husband will respond to your desire to go back to work?"

4. The school nurse is working with the parents of an adopted child who is entering school. The father feels that the child should be told that he was adopted, but the mother feels that there is no purpose in revealing this information. How should the nurse respond to this couple?
   1. "What are your concerns about telling your child about his adoption?"
   2. "There may be serious health risks that accompany your decision to withhold this information from your child."
   3. "Children are very perceptive and on some level, your child may already know that he was adopted."
   4. "Your child will be very angry if this information is discovered accidentally."

References

1. Andrews, M., & Boyle, J. (2003). *Transcultural concepts in nursing care* (4th ed.). Philadelphia: Lippicott Williams & Wilkins.
2. Beavers, R., & Hampson, R. (2003). Measuring family competence: The Beavers systems model. In F. Walsh (Ed.), *Normal family process* (3rd ed.). New York: Guildford Press.
3. Bee, H., & Boyd, H. (2003). *Lifespan development* (3rd ed.). Boston: Allyn & Bacon.
4. Berger, K. (2005). *The developing person through the lifespan* (6th ed.). New York: Worth.
5. Bettelheim, B. (1988). *A good enough parent: A book on child-rearing.* New York: Knopf.
6. Bomar, P. J. (2004). *Promoting health in families: Applying family research and theory to nursing practice.* Philadelphia: Saunders.
7. Booth, J. (1995, July). British families: Loss of a stiff upper lip? *Focus on the Family,* 5.
8. Bowen, M. (2002). *Family therapy in clinical practice.* New York: Jason Aronson.

9. Butler, F. R., & Zakari, N. (2005). Grandparents parenting grandchildren. *Journal of Gerontological Nursing, 31*(3), 41–54.

10. Cano, A., & Vivian, D. (2003). Are life stressors associated with marital violence? *Journal of Family Psychology, 17*, 302–314.

11. Carter, B., & McGoldrick, M. (2005). *The expanded family life cycle: Individual, family, and social perspectives* (Classic ed.). Boston: Allyn and Bacon.

12. Centers for Disease Control and Prevention. (2005). Retrieved March 25, 2006, from http://www.cdc.gov

13. Crandell, S. (2005, September–October). Oh, baby. *AARP*, 108–117.

14. Cherlin, A. J. (2002). *Public and private families: An introduction*. New York: McGraw-Hill.

15. D'Avanzo, C., & Geissler, E. (2003). *Mosby's pocket guide series: Cultural health assessment* (3rd ed.). St. Louis, MO: Mosby.

16. Deal, R. (2006, March). Merge right: Ensure the successful journey of your future stepfamily. *Focus on the Family*, 22–23.

17. Duvall, E., & Miller, B. (1984). *Marriage and family development* (6th ed.). New York: Harper & Row.

18. Ford-Gilboe, M. (2000). Dispelling myths and creating opportunity: A comparison of the strengths of single-parent and two-parent families. *Advances in Nursing Science, 23*, 41–58.

19. Foundation for Large Families. (2005). *The large family: A blessing and a challenge*. Retrieved March 25, 2006, from http://www.foundationforlargefamilies.com

20. Friedman, M. M., Bowden, V. R., & Jones, E. (2003). *Family nursing: Research, theory, and practice* (5th ed.). Upper Saddle River, NJ: Prentice Hall.

21. Giger, J., & Davidhizar, R. (2004). *Transcultural nursing: Assessment and intervention* (4th ed.). St. Louis, MO: Mosby.

22. Greenberg, P. (1998, May). Stay-home moms need support, not bad mouthing. *American Family Association Journal*, 20.

23. Greene, M.F. (2001). The family mobile. *New York Times Magazine*. Retrieved March 25, 2006, from http://www.foundationforlargefamilies.com

24. Gormly, A. (1997). *Lifespan human development* (6th ed.). Fort Worth, TX: Harcourt Brace College.

25. Hooper, M., & Harper, J. (1987). *Birth order roles and sibling patterns in individual and family therapy*. Rockville, MD: Aspen.

26. Irwin, B., & Copen, K. (2006). The fatherless epidemic: Transforming tragedy to triumph. *Journal of Christian Nursing, 23*(2), 26–30.

27. Judge, S. (2004). Adoptive families: The effects of early relational deprivation in children adopted from Eastern European orphanages. *Journal of Family Nursing, 10*, 338–356.

28. Juffer, F., & van Ijzendoorn, M.H. (2005). Behavior problems and mental health referrals of international adoptees: A meta-analysis. *Journal of the American Medical Association, 293*, 2501–2515.

29. Lamb, M. (1986). *The father's role*. New York: John Wiley & Sons.

30. Lamb, M. (1987). The emergent American father. In M. Lamb (Ed.), *The father's role: Cross cultural perspectives*. Hillsdale, NJ: Erlbaum.

31. Leman, K. (2002). *The new birth order book*. Grand Rapids, MI: Fleming H. Revell.

32. McGoldrick, M., Giordano, J., & Garcia-Preto, N. (2005). *Ethnicity and family therapy* (3rd ed.). New York: Guilford.

33. McGuiness, T. M., Ryan, R., & Robinson, C. B. (2005). Protective influences of families for children adopted from the former Soviet Union. *Journal of Nursing Scholarship, 37*, 216–221.

34. McGuiness, T. M. (2006). Marriage, divorce, and children. *Journal of Psychosocial Nursing, 44*, 17–20.

35. Mercer, R. T. (1995). *Becoming a mother*. New York: Springer.

36. Messer, A. (1970). *The individual in his family: An adaptational study*. Springfield, IL: Charles C. Thomas.

37. Minuchin, S., & Nichols, M. P. (1998). *Family healing: Strategies for hope and understanding*. New York: Free Press.

38. Mulrine, A. (2004, September). Making babies. *U.S. News & World Report*, 61–63.

39. Murray, S. S., & McKinney, E. S. (2006). *Foundations of maternal-newborn nursing* (4th ed.). St. Louis, MO: Saunders.

40. NANDA International. (2005). *NANDA nursing diagnoses: Definitions and classification: 2005–2006*. Philadelphia: Author.

41. Nichols, M. P., & Schwartz, R. C. (2001). *The essentials of family therapy*. Boston: Allyn and Bacon.

42. Nickman, S. L., Rosenfeld, A., Fine, P., MacIntyre, J., Pilowsky, D., Howe, R., et al. (2005). Children in adoptive families: Overview and update. *Journal of the American Academy of Child and Adolescent Psychiatry, 44*, 987–995.

43. Palkovitz, R. (2002). *Involved fathering and men's adult development: Provisional balances*. Mahwah, NJ: Lawrence Erlbaum.

44. Papalia, D., Olds, S., & Feldman, R. (2004). *Human development* (9th ed.). Boston: McGraw-Hill.

45. Peterson, R., & Green, S. (1999). *Families first—keys to successful family functioning: Family roles*. Retrieved March 11, 2006, from http://www.ext.vt.edu/pubs/family/

46. Popenoe, D., & Whitehead, B. D. (2005, June). *The state of our unions, 2005: The social health of marriage in America*. The National Marriage Project, Rutgers State University of New Jersey. Retrieved March 3, 2006, from http://marriage.rutgers.edu

47. Rollin, B. (2003, July–August). Baby blues: How I stopped mourning the child who never was. *AARP*, 42–43.

48. Rubin, R. (1984). *Maternal identity and the maternal experience*. New York: Springer.

49. Santrock, J. W. (2004). *Life-span development* (9th ed.). Boston: McGraw-Hill.

50. Segrin, C., & Flora, J. (2005). *Family communication*. Mahwah, NJ: Lawrence Erlbaum.

51. Seifert, K., Hoffnung, R., & Hoffnung, M. (2000). *Lifespan development* (2nd ed.). Boston: Houghton Mifflin.

52. Shapiro, V. B., Shapiro, J. R., & Paret, I. H. (2001). *Complex adoption and assisted reproductive technology: A developmental approach to clinical practice*. New York: Guilford Press.

53. Shepherd, F. (1994, July). The multicultural families down under. *Focus on the Family*, 13.

54. Smalley, G. (1997, February). Advice you can bank on. *Focus on the Family*, 2–4.

55. Step Family Association of America Website. Retrieved March 21, 2006, from http://www.saafamilies.org

56. Sullivan, M. G. (2005). Children process adoption throughout early years. *Clinical Psychiatry News, 33* (12), 37.

57. Tatano Beck, C. (2002). Releasing the pause button: Mothering twins during the first year of life. *Qualitative Health Research, 12*, 593–608.

58. Tiedje, L. B., & Darling-Fisher, C. (2003). Promoting father-friendly healthcare. *Maternal Child Nursing, 28*, 350–357.

59. Toman, W. (1993). *Family constellation* (4th ed.). New York: Springer.

60. United States Census Bureau. (2005). *Provisional number of marriages and divorces: Each state, April 2004 and 2005*. Retrieved February 21, 2006, from http://factfinder.census.gov

61. United States Department of Health and Human Services. (2000). *Healthy people 2010: With understanding and improving health and objectives for improving health* (2nd ed.). 2 vols. Washington, DC: U.S. Government Printing Office.

62. Vaughan-Cole, B., Johnson, M. A., Malone, J. A., & Walker, B. L. (1998). *Family nursing practice*. Philadelphia: Saunders.

63. Vanderkam, L. (2002). Mega-families bring 'it takes a village to life.' *USA Today*. Retrieved March 25, 2006, from http://usatoday.com.

64. Visher, E. B., & Visher, J. S. (1996). *Therapy with stepfamilies*. New York: Bruner/Mazel.

65. Wallace, H. M., Green, G., Jaros, K. J., Paine, L. L., & Story, M. (2003). *Health and welfare for families in the 21st century*. Boston: Jones & Bartlett.

66. Walsh, F. (2003). *Normal family processes*. New York: Guildford Press.

67. Walsh, W. M., & McGraw, J. A. (2002). *Essentials of family therapy: A structured summary of nine approaches* (2nd ed.). Denver, CO: Love.

68. Woodworth, R. S., Dabelko, H., & Hollidge, M. (1998). *ARCH Factsheet 45*, May. Retrieved March 1, 2006, from http://www.archrespite.org/archfs45.htm

69. Wright, L., & Leahey, M. (2005). *Nursing families: A guide to family assessment and intervention* (4th ed.). Philadelphia: F.A. Davis.

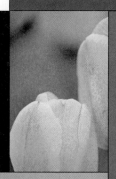

Spiritual and Religious Influences

OBJECTIVES

Study of this chapter will enable you to:

1. Define the terms *spiritual* and *religious* and the connotations of each.

2. Review research studies and client descriptions related to the spiritual and religious dimension.

3. Contrast the major tenets of the Hindu, Sikh, Buddhist, Jainist, Shinto, Confucian, Taoist, Islamic, Jewish, Christian, and North American Indian religions.

4. Compare the major tenets of the various branches of Christianity: Roman Catholicism, Eastern Orthodoxy, various Protestant denominations, and other Christian sects.

5. Examine how religious beliefs influence lifestyle and health status in the various religious groups and subgroups.

6. Discuss your role in meeting the spiritual needs of clients and families.

7. Relate the role of the parish nurse in the faith community and with the client.

MediaLink **www.prenhall.com/murray**

Go to the Companion Website for interactive resources that accompany this chapter.

Glossary
Review Questions
Challenge Your Knowledge
Learning Activities

Critical Thinking
Tools
Media Link Applications
Media Links

Current Perspectives

The earlier divisions between medical science and the spiritual dimension or religion are diminishing. Health care professionals are increasingly aware of and responsive to the client's expression of faith and religious belief, or lack of it, and of the broader spiritual dimension. For many people, including clients and providers, religious denominations pose less of a barrier between people than before. People worldwide are seeking serenity, peace, and the transcendental; it may or may not be sought in formal religion (25, 110). While the vitality of Christianity is less vigorous in some Western hemisphere countries, the center of Christianity is shifting to the developing world, especially Africa and India. People are embracing the faith in many different ways, so Christianity continues to evolve (38, 98). In most countries, the number of Muslims is increasing, as is their influence in their communities (125).

A self-report, national survey in the United States revealed that 78% of the respondents reported having faith in God as very important. However, only 29% attended religious services weekly and only 24% reported religion being extremely important in everyday life (20). We live in a **post-materialistic society**, *one in which people generally are spiritually oriented but rejecting of mainstream religious beliefs, and interested in personal development and relationships.* They have eclectic taste, enjoy foreign and exotic experiences, and verbalize higher priority to quality of life than "financial materialism." The person may believe God is everywhere; church support and attendance is not necessary (29, 56). They continue to ask why "bad things happen to good people" (54).

Places of worship also have a changing role in the community as they reach out to promote physical and social health services. They are also being changed by the surrounding culture. Traditionally, the cathedral, synagogue, mosque, or other worship places were considered safe from all but natural disasters. Increasingly, terrorist activities include all kinds of structures designated for worship. Safety and disaster plans for churches and health care agencies are now formulated for man-made as well as natural disasters (84).

Nursing's commitment to spiritual care is part of the concept of holistic care and dates back to Florence Nightingale's model for nursing education. Yet, nurses feel poorly prepared to give spiritual care (1). In her manuscript, "Suggestions for Thought," Nightingale attempted to integrate science and mysticism. She felt the universe was an incarnation of a divine intelligence that regulated all things through law (60). She recognized that humans have spiritual needs; spiritual care enables the person to be conscious of the presence of God, the creator and sustainer of the universe (60). Spiritual care has continued to be part of the nursing tradition that has biblical foundations (24).

Combining the spiritual dimension and religious beliefs with physical and mental care is now more acceptable (50, 113). In health care agencies, a team approach is emphasized. Even the American Psychiatric Association has acknowledged that psychological problems arising from religious or spiritual conflicts are not attributable to a mental disorder (2). The *Diagnostic and Statistical Manual of Mental Disorders* (4th ed.) (*DSM-IV*), Appendix I, encourages professionals who use the *DSM-IV* for psychiatric diagnoses to consider religion, spirituality, and culture in all aspects of the patient's identity, psychological environment, and manifestation of illness (2). The importance of addressing children's spiritual needs and giving care related to religious beliefs is also increasingly recognized and described (19, 76, 103).

Definitions

One definition for **religion** is defined on various levels: *It is a belief in a supernatural or divine force that has power over the universe and commands worship and obedience to a supernatural force. It is a personal and institutional system of beliefs; a comprehensive code of ethics or philosophy; a set of practices that are followed; a church affiliation.* Ameling defines religion *as an organized set of beliefs that attempt to answer life's questions, expressed in sacred texts, rituals, and practices, and through participation in a faith or believing community. It is related to but not synonymous with spirituality* (1). Primal religions are earth based, such as Wicca, traditional American Indian religions, and Shamanism (1).

In every human there seems to be a **spiritual dimension**, *a quality that goes beyond religious affiliation, that strives for inspiration, reverence, awe, meaning, and purpose even in those who do not believe in any god. The spiritual dimension permeates all of life and integrates values and beliefs. It involves harmony with the universe, strives for answers about the infinite, and especially comes into focus as a sustaining power when the person faces emotional stress, physical illness, or death. It goes outside a person's own power.* Spirituality is defined differently by various religions and cultures (3, 33, 57, 71).

In the midst of specialized health care, you have an opportunity to go beyond the dogma to bring together the biopsychospiritual being through the study of the religions and religious beliefs of clients. Those are world religions, not your personal religion or a country's basic religion. Mass media, rapid transportation, and cultural exchanges have nullified the provincial approach.

Related Research

More research is being done about the influence of spirituality and religion on health, health care outcomes, recovery, and illness prevention. Most research has been done on adult Christian patients, either European American or African American (108). Research has related the meaning of spirituality and the importance of spiritual care to the patient/client and family members (69, 108).

A qualitative descriptive study with well adults, ages 18 to 24 years, revealed *seven themes that indicate a strengthening spirituality* (14):

1. **Beliefs:** The framework in which life's choices are based, for example, following the Golden Rule, faith in God, hope, and transcending the physical domain—the spirit lives on after death.
2. **Connectedness:** A relationship formed with self, others, nature, the universe, and a higher power; reaching out to others even if others don't respond.
3. **Inner motivating factors:** A deep commitment and the beliefs that guide behavior, attitude, and existence; taking responsibility for one's personal life.

4. **Life events:** Incidents or occurrences that provoke a spiritual response, such as loss and grief, illness, or all of life's events.
5. **Understanding the mystery:** The meaning and purpose of life, the search for identity, and finding a reason for events.
6. **Walking through:** Using personal resources to get through life.
7. **Divine providence:** The ever-present and benevolent guidance of a higher power; God is everywhere.

These themes have been reflected in non-research-based writings throughout the centuries. *An integrative review of 73 articles about the concept of spirituality related to health sciences from 1990 to 2000 revealed the following themes* (17): (a) existential reality, (b) transcendence, (c) connectedness, and (d) power/force/energy. Several instruments were used to study spirituality, such as the Spiritual Well-Being Scale, Spiritual Orientation Inventory, and Spiritual Perspectives Scale. No consistent definition of spirituality was found in the reviewed articles (17). The spiritual dimension can be a very personal experience.

In a review of research, the *following themes indicated ways to foster spirituality* (108): (a) fostering connectedness, (b) affirming others with love and quality interpersonal nurse-client relationships, (c) enabling hope, (d) gaining transcendence over the present situation, (e) being present to the person, (f) fostering reconciliation, (g) sharing near-death mystical experiences, (h) supporting the patient's desire to either let go or to struggle to live, and (i) helping the family and patient prepare for death.

Case study descriptions have indicated the importance of spiritual care to the patient/client and family. Walker described the importance of a therapeutic relationship, grief therapy, and crisis intervention, as well as appropriate self-disclosure, as part of effective spiritual intervention (115). Case descriptive research with adults generally indicates the importance of faith, hope, and religious practices for healing (4, 14–16, 36, 59, 77, 96, 99, 115). Other studies show the importance of religion for mental, emotional, and spiritual comfort and peace (21, 26, 44, 86). Several research studies also indicate the importance of religious beliefs and spiritual care in fostering recovery and preventing mortality (52, 66, 78, 108). Church attendance, if positive, has been reported to add 7 years to the Caucasian's life span and 14 years to the life of African Americans, per actuarial predictions (16). Holding positive spiritual thoughts during illness appears to enhance recovery; negative thoughts about one's condition or recovery may increase the risk of death (78). This affirms earlier writings about the power of positive thinking (81, 82).

Stephenson and Wilson discussed their study of patients' experiences with spiritual care while in an acute care setting. Patients revealed in interviews their heightened spiritual needs during illness and the positive experience of having those needs addressed by the nurse. The nurse's sensitivity to spiritual needs, the ability to establish trust, and an attitude of openness fostered a calming effect in times of anxiety and promoted the patient's total well-being (104).

Furlow and O'Quinn discussed the importance of prayer and the difficulty of conducting research to determine whether prayer in the Judeo-Christian tradition affects the hospitalized patient's medical condition and recovery. Their study indicated that intercessory prayer has positive therapeutic effects. However, research replication with large samples and rigorous controls is necessary to support prayer and spiritual interventions as scientific health care therapy (31).

Neurotheology *is a new field of research that examines the biological basis of spirituality.* Brain imaging techniques pinpoint brain activity when people meditate, experience enlightenment, or have visions. Scientists are studying whether some people are predisposed by genetics, temperament, or environment to have mystical experiences (5). However, spirituality and religion are not the same. Doing the will of a divine being involves more than meditation, prayer, or certain traditions. To see the divine in any person, to really love and forgive one's enemy, requires insights that may not be apparent in brain studies. Believers of any faith are not likely to focus on brain circuits but on expressing their beliefs, influenced by environment, opportunity, and others' responses (124). The Abstract for Evidence-Based Practice presents a summary of another research study.

World Religions and Belief Systems

Use this information about world religions in assessment, intervention, and teaching of clients and family members. Understanding these beliefs will help you better understand and work with co-workers. The approaches to all levels of health promotion and client care are influenced by spiritual beliefs, or rejection of belief systems.

Studying world religions poses semantic difficulties. For example, an expression in the Chinese-based religion of Confucianism may have no equivalent in the English language. Thus, language has dictated what people think, how they act, and how their religious beliefs are carried out (7, 67). The section on linguistics in Chapter 5 ∞ discussed the issues related to language in any culture, including religious cultures. Concepts, however, are often basically the same but are rephrased in each religion's own linguistic style. The saying "Love one another as I have loved you" will appear to the Hindu as "This is the sum of religion, do not unto others what causes pain to you," to the Taoist as "Return goodness for hatred," and to the Muslim as "No one is a believer unless he desires for his brother what he desires for himself."

Each major religion also has other characteristics in common (7, 53, 67):

1. A worldview, a way of perceiving reality, a description of existence and life meaning, and assumptions about the universe and life
2. A basis of authority or source(s) of power
3. A portion of scripture or sacred word
4. An ethical code that defines right and wrong
5. A psychology and identity so that its adherents fit into a group and the world is defined by the religion
6. Aspirations or expectations
7. Some ideas about what follows death

See **Table 7-1** for key facts about eight major world religions. For additional information about philosophic and mystical aspects

Abstract for Evidence-Based Practice

Spirituality and Self-Transcendence in People with HIV/AIDS

Ramer, L., Johnson, D., Chan, L., & Barrett, M. (2006). The effect of HIV/AIDS disease progression on spirituality and self-transcendence in a multicultural population. *Journal of Transcultural Nursing, 17*(1), 280–289.

KEYWORDS

spirituality, multicultural, HIV/AIDS, Hispanic, California.

Purpose ➤ To examine the relationship of sociodemographic and clinical factors with spirituality and self-transcendence in people with HIV/AIDS.

Conceptual Frameworks ➤ Spirituality, a belief in and communication with a higher power, and Victor Frankl's concept of self-transcendence: finding meaning in life, beyond self, to promote hope and will to live.

Sample/Setting ➤ The sample was composed of 420 persons (83% male); ages 18 to 68 years (X=39 years); Hispanics (72%), Whites (14%), African Americans (12%), and Asians (0.5%). The majority (88.6%) were patients returning to a large, multicultural, university-based outpatient clinic for treatment for HIV/AIDS (95%) and substance abuse (61%).

Method ➤ The Spirituality Subscale of the Quality of Life Questionnaire, Self-Transcendence Questionnaire, Physical Functioning Scale, Acculturation Scale, and CES-Depression Scale were administered to all patients who were seen during a 2-week period. Data abstracted from the patients' charts included demographics, current medications, current and chronic disease processes, documentation of depression, and clinical data related to CD4 (T cells) and vRNA (viral) blood levels.

Findings ➤ Several statistically significant results were found. Hispanic and African American ethnicity was associated with spirituality. Hispanics scored higher than non-Hispanics. Individuals with lower levels of acculturation scored higher in spirituality. Depressed subjects scored lower on spirituality. No significant correlations were found between spirituality and other demographic characteristics or with clinical disease markers. African Americans scored higher for self-transcendence than other subjects; Hispanics scored lower than non-Hispanics. No significant correlations were found between other demographic data and spirituality or self-transcendence. Depression, energy level, and pain were associated with spirituality. Subjects with higher depression scores reported lower spirituality. As energy level increased, spirituality scores increased. No significant correlations were found between spirituality and other clinical variables. Subjects earning more than $30,000 per year, who identified family support, and who scored higher on acculturation and energy levels reported higher self-transcendence scores.

Implications ➤ Energy level, pain, and depression may be interactive; physiologic needs must be met before the person can meet higher level needs (Maslow's Theory of Hierarchy of Needs). The person cannot be assumed to feel well when CD4 and viral loads are normal or improving. Health care providers should assess patients who complain of fatigue, low energy, pain, and depression and the consequent effect on meeting spiritual needs, since clinical indicators of immune system function are not accurate indictors of well-being and ability to participate in the spiritual dimension of life.

of Hinduism, Buddhism, Islam, Taoism, and Sikhism, see the descriptions in this chapter and related references (7, 22, 72, 97).

The major world religions can be divided into categories in an attempt to group characteristics even further (7). The **alpha group** *includes Christianity, Judaism, and Islam. All adhere to a biblical revelation of a supernatural, monotheistic God.* People in these religions are "doers." They obey because God commands; they make covenants with God for protection; they have a historical fixed scripture that is canonized for public use, and they often proselytize. Included in the **gamma group** are *Taoism (pronounced "dowism"), Confucianism, and Shintoism. In these religions, people believe either that everything is in the being of God or that there is no personal God (still a definite belief).* These people try to be in harmony with the world around them. Their most immediate concern is in relationships with others. Scripture is a family affair. They can be characterized as simple in faith, spontaneous, and straightforward in feelings of affection for people, plants, and animals. The final grouping, the **beta group**, *includes Buddhism and Hinduism. These religions have their roots in Indian soil, their worldview is pantheistic, and they teach that everything is in the being of God.* Adherents are interested in "being" rather than "doing." They have a collective literature for private devotion. Control of mind and body is desired, as some of the yoga practices show. The beta and gamma groups do not define God as clearly as the alpha group. The beta and gamma groups look inside themselves for answers: common sense rather than commands from God determines good. Salladay (93) contrasts pantheistic with Christian beliefs.

The following discussion presents a more detailed insight into each major world religion through personality sketches. *Each person has a fictitious name and represents not a single person but a composite of knowledge gained from the authors' interviewing a number of people, reading, and personal experience.* Although these personalities are presented as acting and thinking in a certain way, remember that *the person's culture, family background, and personality affect how that person lives out a religious experience.* Thus, a particular Hindu and a given Roman Catholic may be

TABLE 7-1

Key Facts About Eight Major World Religions

Religion	Primary Location	Supreme Being	Founder and Date	Historical Leaders	Sacred Writings	Leadership	Holy Places	Some Holy Days
Hinduism	India Ceylon	Brahman All reality	No founder 3200 BC	Mahatma Gandhi Ramakrishna	Vedas Brahmanas Upanishads Great Epics	Sannyasis (holy men) Guru (preacher)	Benares (city) Ganges (river)	The Mela Holi Festival Dasera Divuli
Judaism	Israel Western Hemisphere	Yahweh (Jehovah or God)	Abraham 1300 BC	Moses Amos Micah Other prophets	Torah Talmud	Rabbis	Jerusalem	Rosh Hashanah Yom Kippur Hanukkah Purim Passover
Taoism	China	Jade Emperor Many folk gods	Lao-Tzu (or Lao-Tse) 604 BC	Lao-Tse Chuang-Tse 350–275 BC	Tao-Te-Ching	None	Kiangsi and many holy mountains	Birthdays of Gods Festival of Souls Autumn Festival
Confucianism	China Japan Korea	Confucius Shang-Ti	Confucius 557 BC	Yang Chu Moh Tih	NuChing Sau Shu	None	None	None
Buddhism	China Japan India Burma	108 different names	Gautama 560–480 BC	Gautama Amitabha	Dharma (Sutta) Vinaya Abhidhamma	Bhikkhus Monks Nuns Lamas	Sarnath Lumbini Buddh-Gaya Kusinara	Perahera Festival in Ceylon Wesak (Kason) in May
Christianity	Western Hemisphere	God	Jesus AD 30	John the Baptist, 12 disciples, 4 gospel writers, writers of epistles	Bible Old Testament New Testament	Priests Ministers Layman	Bethlehem Jerusalem Rome Nazareth	Christmas Good Friday Easter Pentecost
Shinto	Japan	Izanagil (Sky Father) Izanami (Earth Mother)	No founder AD 6th century	None	Nipongi Kojiki	None	Mt. Fujiyama	New Year Bon (Festival of Dead) Tenri-Kyo (January)
Islam	Middle East	Allah	Mohammed AD 570–632	Mohammed Husein (grandson) Abu Bakr Omar Othman Ali	Koran	None	Mecca Jerusalem	Ramadan (Sacred Month)

more in agreement religiously than two Lutherans. You cannot make generalizations about a religion from knowing an individual follower. **Table 7-1** summarizes information about the eight major world religions.

 # HINDUISM AND SIKHISM†

Rama, a young businessman, tells us that nothing is typically **Hindu** and that anyone who puts religion in neat packages will have difficulty comprehending his outlook. Rama is named after **Ramakrishna**, *the greatest saint of **Hinduism** of the 19th century.* The history of Rama's religion goes back to approximately 1500 B.C., when the **Vedas**—*divine revelations*—were written. His main religious texts are the **Upanishads**, or *scriptures*, and the **Bhagavad Gita**, *a summary of the former with additions. The most expressive and universal word of God is* **Om**, or **Aum**, providing the most important auditory and visual symbol in Rama's religion. He explains that *Om*, or *Aum*, *God*, and *Brahman* are synonymous and mean a *consciousness* or *awareness* rather than a personified being.

Rama speaks of some of the worship popular in India today: of the family and local deities and of the trinity—**Brahma**, *the creator*, **Vishnu**, *the preserver and god of love*, and **Shiva**, *the destroyer*.

Rama has a shrine in his home where, in the presence of various pictures of **incarnations** (*human forms of God*) and with incense burning, he meditates. He also thinks of Buddha, Muhammed, and Jesus as incarnations and sometimes reads from the scriptures inspired by their teachings, although they represent other major religions.

Despite this vast array of deities and the recognition that all religions are valid, Rama believes in one universal concept—**Brahman**, the *Divine Intelligence*, the *Supreme Reality*. Rama believes all paths lead to the understanding that this "reality" exists as part of all physical beings, especially humans. Rama's entire spiritual quest is directed toward uniting his *inner and real self*, the **atman**, with the concept of Brahman. So, although Rama has gone through several stages of desire—for pleasure, power, wealth, fame, and humanitarianism—the last stage, *his desire for freedom, for touching the infinite, is his main goal.* **Figure 7-1** ▢ expresses that journey.

Rama is interested in health and illness only as a guide to this goal. He feels that a self-centered focus on the body is a cause for illness. He says, for example, that we overeat and get a stomachache. He views the pain as a warning—in this case, to stop overeating. He does not oppose medical treatment if absolutely necessary, but he believes that medicine can sometimes dull the pain and then the person overeats again, thus perpetuating the cause of the problem. Medical or psychiatric help, Rama says, is at best transitory. The cause of the pain must be rooted out.

To avoid dwelling on physical concerns, Rama strives for moderation in eating and in other body functions. He considers only the atman as real and eternal and the body as unreal and finite. The body is a temple, a vehicle, no more. He tries to take care of it so that it will not scream at him because of overindulgence or underindulgence. Rama is a vegetarian. He believes that meat and intox-

† The symbol at the beginning of each of the following sections represents the religion under the heading.

GITA IS A WAY OF LIFE
a way of karma—
a way to Moksha

Like a lamp of a steady flame
Not overjoyed by achievements.
Nor dejected by calamities.
One observes the light
and darkness evenly.

Reigning the senses,
Within the reasonable limits
knowing that atma is eternal
unlike physical existence of self—
which changes from time to time,
bound by one's karmas and
controlled by the 'treacherous' mind

But the wise one
bows to the Lord in humility
in the 'wake' of humble surrender
offers karma without desire
For this can only be led by
'Gyana' the light
That enlightens by the practice of
uniting mind and body to a peaceful Omkar.

Unyielding to one's pride & passion
Persisting destructive thoughts,
undisillusioned by the illusions
of this world as 'Maya'.

Where—what is there is not there
But what doesn't seem to be there (atma) is very
much present
When the veil is unfurled by the light of 'Gyana'

One reaches the Lord even by the feel of His existence—
One opens the path of eternity
—a journey to an empty road
Where the tripti of the desired senses
Have evaporated in the air as the water takes the form
of vapor
It's then that one realizes . . . the blissful state of
atma
Vibrating OM ! OM !! OM !! chanting
'Om Namo Bhagawate Vasudevaya. Om!!'

FIGURE ▢ **7-1** Gita Is a Way of Life.
(Written by A. D. Desai, Boulder, Co.)

icants would excite his senses too much. Yet the Hindu diet pattern is flexible; definite rules are not set. If Rama is sick, he tries to bear his illness with resignation, knowing its temporary nature. He believes that the prayer of supplication for body cure is the lowest form of prayer, whereas the highest form is devotion to God. To him, death and rebirth are nearly synonymous, for the atman never changes and always remains pure. He compares the atman to the ocean: As ocean water can be put into various containers without changing its nature, so can the atman be put into various physical and human containers without changing its nature.

Thus if death is imminent, Rama believes that the body, mind, and senses weaken and become lifeless but that the never-changing atman is ready to enter into a new form of life, depending on the person's knowledge, deeds, and past experiences. Full acceptance of death is encouraged. Death is a friend to be faced bravely, calmly, and confidently.

Rama says that as a devotee of God he is following **yoga** as a *training course.* As a preliminary, however, he must establish certain moral qualifications. He must strive for self-control, self-discipline, cleanliness, and contentment. He must avoid injury, deceitfulness, and stealing. His overwhelming *desire to reach God can be implemented through one or a combination of the four yoga paths:* (a) **inana yoga** through *reading and absorbing knowledge,* (b) **bhakti yoga** through *the devotion of emotion and love,* (c) **karma yoga** through *work dedicated to God,* and (d) **raja yoga** through *psychological experiments on oneself.* Rama combines the first three by reading and memorizing portions of the ancient scriptures, by meditating daily at his shrine, and by dedicating the results of his professional work to God.

Rama mentions that various forms of yoga have spread around the world to form hybrid groups with varied purposes. One branch that has appeared in medical centers is **hatha yoga**, meaning *sun and moon, symbolizing an inner balance that is achieved through muscle and breathing exercises.* Ultimately the body is prepared for meditation through these exercises.

From the bhakti emphasis comes **Sikhism**, founded by Nanak, who was born in 1469. The Sikhs had nine other gurus, or spiritual mentors, who sequentially taught that God was the one and only reality. The fifth guru compiled the scripture. *There are three basic commandments* (7, 72): (a) meditate on God's name, (b) earn an honest living, and (c) share with others and treat everyone equally. Starting as a pacifist group, the Sikhs evolved to warriors. That emphasis has changed; modern-day Sikhs are building more **gurdwara** *worship halls,* to promote community.

Also from bhakti influence has come the **Hare Krishna** movement in the United States, starting in 1965 when A.C. Bhaktivedanta came to New York City. The first Krishna temple was established on the Lower East Side (7, 72).

For Rama, religion is not something to be picked up and put down according to a schedule or one's mood. It is a constant and all-pervading part of his life, every value and action, and the life of his country. India's literature and art are witness to this fact. It also influences family life and structure. Basically marriage is for life, and people usually marry someone in the same social level. The husband is treated with respect, and the mother is thought of as ideal. The family is patrifocal; the father usually has final authority. All family members are close. Elders are respected, cared for

when they are ill, and considered as experienced models; children and grandchildren seek their wisdom. Children have reverence for both father and mother, and disrespectful talk is unthinkable. Friends are to be treated as brothers and sisters, and visitors are always treated congenially.

Rama will be married soon and gives us some insight into the ceremony and meaning. The traditional Indian wedding customs were formulated more than 5,000 years ago. Each ceremony, each occasion, and each ritual has a deep philosophic meaning and purpose. The ceremony is performed in Sanskrit, the most ancient surviving language in the world. It is meant to unite two souls so firmly that after they are married, although their bodies remain separate, their souls merge and become spiritually one. Thus, divorce is unacceptable (127, 128). First, eight sacred blessings are given. Then the groom is welcomed amid recitations including the five elements. The bride follows the bridesmaids and groomsmen and is welcomed following an exchange of garlands between bride and groom. The couple declare their union and tie together the ends of scarves that each is wearing. The bride and groom then walk around a fire (purifier), taking seven sacred steps, each signifying vows and promises made to each other. Finally, the rings are exchanged (128).

Incorporate the beliefs of the client who is Hindu into health care practices to the extent possible. Many of the values, beliefs, and practices described by Rama will not conflict with Westernized health care approaches. Listen carefully to the client who is Hindu to avoid any conflicts generated by the Western approach.

 ## BUDDHISM, JAINISM, AND SHINTOISM

Umeko Sato is a member of the sect of **Buddhism** called **Soka Gakkai.** This sect is a powerful religion in Japan, with a government party, a university, and a grand temple representing it. This organization, known previously as a militant proselytizing group, has toned down this phase and is living more graciously with other sects and creeds. Based on the **Lotus Sutra**, *part of the Buddhist scriptures,* its doctrine advocates the three values of happiness: profit, goodness, and beauty. Umeko Sato is attracted by the practicality of the teaching, the mottoes that she can live by, the emphasis on small-group study, and the present world benefits, especially healing.

Although Umeko Sato's beliefs at some points seem in direct contrast to the original Buddhist teachings, she is happy to explain the rich multireligious tradition that her family has had for generations. She emphasizes that she is affected by the **Confucian** emphasis on the family unit, by Christianity's healing emphasis, by **Shintoism**, the state religion of Japan until 1945, and by Buddhism, which originated about 600 B.C. in India with a Hindu named Siddhartha Gautama.

Currently, most people in Japan adhere both to Buddhism and to Shintoism, although the nation has never been known as devout. Less than 1% are Christian. Another religion with a *fewer* number of people is **Jainism**. The "Jains" hark back to the 6th century B.C., about the same time as Buddha. Their fundamental tenet is **ahimsa**, *a refusal to injure any living thing.* Jains believe every living thing has a soul. There are two groups of Jains. A small group of approximately 100 are called *sky clad* because they wear no clothes. They renounce clothing and all earthly possessions. The other, larger group is called *white clad* because they wear white clothes. Together the groups contain monks, nuns, laymen, and laywomen who all take vows to guide them in all aspects of daily life. Although the Jains are found in Japan and other countries, including the United States, they probably are known best for their bird hospital in Old Delhi, India, which treats 20,000 birds each year.

Gautama, *shortly after a historic enlightenment experience during which he became the* **Buddha**, *preached a sermon to his followers and drew on the earth a wheel representing the continuous round of life and death and rebirth.* Later, eight spokes were added to illustrate the sermon and to provide the most explicit visual symbol of Buddhism today. Umeko Sato repeats *Buddha's four noble truths*: (a) life is disjointed or out of balance, especially in birth, old age, illness, and death; (b) the cause of this imbalance is ignorance of one's own true nature; (c) removal of this ignorance is attained by reaching **nirvana**, *the divine state of release, the ultimate reality, the perfect knowledge;* and (d) nirvana is reached via the eightfold path.

The *eight spokes of the wheel represent the eightfold path used to reach nirvana*: followers subscribe to (a) right knowledge, (b) right intentions, (c) right speech, (d) right conduct, (e) right means of livelihood, (f) right effort, (g) right mindfulness, and (h) concentration. From these concepts has arisen a moral code that, among other things, prohibits intoxicants, lying, and killing of any kind (which explains why Buddhists are often vegetarians). She further explains that the Mahayana branch of Buddhism took hold in Japan as opposed to the Theravada branch. The **Theravada branch** *emphasizes an intellectual approach through wisdom, people working by themselves through meditation and without ritual.* The **Mahayana branch** *emphasizes involvement with humankind, ritual, petitionary prayer, and concern for one's sibling.* Umeko Sato believes that the Mahayana branch provides the happier philosophy of the two, and she tells of the ritual of celebration of Gautama's birthday. But most Japanese believe in **Amitabha Buddha**, *a god rather than a historical figure,* who is replacing the austere image of Gautama as a glorious redeemer, one of infinite light. Also, the people worship **Kwannon**, *a goddess of compassion.*

Umeko Sato explains that she cannot omit mention of the *one austere movement within the Mahayana branch,* the **Zen sect**. Taking this example from Gautama's extended contemplation of a flower, Zen followers care little for discourse, books, or other symbolic interpretations and explanations of reality. Hours and years are devoted to meditation, contemplation of word puzzles, and consultation with a Zen master. In seeking absolute honesty and truthfulness through such simple acts as drinking tea or gardening, the Zen student hopes to experience enlightenment. In America, a version of Buddhism called *Buddhadharma* is emerging. Women and men are considered equal. This group provides meditations for the public on a CD-ROM.

Umeko Sato next turns to her former state religion, **Shintoism**. Whereas Buddhism produced a solemnizing effect on her country, Shintoism had an affirmative and joyous effect. Emperor, ancestor, ancient hero, and nature worship form its core. Those who follow Shintoism, she says, feel an intense loyalty and devotion to every lake, tree, and blossom in Japan and to the ancestral spirits abiding there. They also have a great concern for cleanliness, a carryover from early ideas surrounding dread of pollution in the dead.

Umeko Sato says that her parents have two god shelves in their home. One contains wooden tablets inscribed with the name of the household's patron deity and a symbolic form of the goddess of rice and other texts and objects of family significance. Here her family performs simple rites, such as offering a prayer or a food gift each day. In a family crisis, perhaps an illness, the family conducts more elaborate rites, such as lighting tapers or offering rice brandy. The other god shelf, in another room, is the Buddha shelf; if a family member dies, a Buddhist priest, the spiritual leader, performs specified rituals there.

Umeko Sato strongly emphasizes that if illness or impending death causes a family member to be hospitalized, another well family member will stay at the hospital to bathe, cook for, and give emotional support to the ill person. She believes that recovery depends largely on this family tie. The Buddhist doctrine teaches that death is a total nonfunction of the physical body and mind and that the life force is displaced and transformed to continue to function in another form. Every birth is a rebirth, much as in the Hindu teaching. The rebirth happens immediately after death, according to some Buddhists. Others believe that rebirth occurs 49 days after death, during which time the person is in an intermediary state. The difference in quality of death, birth, and existence depends on whether the person lived a disciplined or undisciplined life.

Buddhism teaches the living how to die well. The elderly, or feeble, are to prepare themselves mentally for a state that would be conducive for a good rebirth. The person is to remain watchful and alert in the face of death, to resist distraction and confusion, and to be lucid and calm. Distinct instructions are given in what to expect as life leaves the body, as the person enters an intermediary state, and as nirvana is about to occur. So, although Umeko Sato has grasped a new religious path for herself, her respect for tradition remains.

In giving care to a person with Umeko Sato's background, be aware of the varied religious influences on the person's life. The sect's emphasis on the here-and-now, rather than on the long road to nirvana, may place a high value on physical health so that the person can benefit from the joys and beauty of life. The person may readily voice impatience with the body's dysfunction. You can respond to the great concern for cleanliness, the desire to have family nearby, and the need for family rites that are offered for the sick member. Should a family member be dying, you may see some ambivalence. The family member may want to prepare himself or herself in the traditional way, but someone with Umeko Sato's background, with emphasis on present world benefits and healing, may deny that there is a valid preparation for death.

 CONFUCIANISM AND TAOISM

Wong Huieng is a young teacher in Taiwan simultaneously influenced by **Taoism**, the *romantic and mystical,* and **Confucianism**, the *practical and pragmatic.* Wong Huieng uses the **yin-yang**

symbol (although it is more representative of Taoism, it provides insights into both of these Chinese modes of thinking). The symbol is a circle, representing **Tao** or the *absolute*, in which two tear shapes fit perfectly into one another, each containing a small dot from the other. Generally **yang** is *light or red*, and **yin** is *dark*. Ancient Chinese tradition says that everything exists in these two interacting forces. Each represents a group of qualities. **Yang** is *positive or masculine—dry, hot, active, moving, and light.* **Yin** is *feminine or negative—wet, cold, passive, restful, and empty.* For example, fire is almost pure yang and water almost pure yin, but not quite. The *combination of yin and yang constitutes all the dualisms a person can imagine*: day-night, summer-winter, beauty-ugliness, illness-health, life-death. Both qualities are necessary for life in the universe; they are complementary and, if in harmony, good. Yang and yin energy forces are embodied in the body parts and affect food preferences and eating habits.

Wong Huieng translates this symbol into a relaxed philosophy of life: "If I am sick, I will get better. Life is like going up and down a mountain; sometimes I feel good and sometimes I feel bad. That's the way it is." Although educated, she is not interested in climbing up the job ladder, accumulating wealth, or conquering nature. Her goal is to help provide money to build an orphanage in a natural wooded setting.

Wong Huieng thinks of death as a natural part of life, as the peace that comes when the body is worn out. She admits, however, that when her father died, human grief took hold of her. Before his death, her mother went to the Taoist temple priest and got some incense to help cast the sickness from his body. After death, they kept his body in the house for the required time, 49 days. The priest executed a special ceremony every 7 days. Her mother could cry only one hour daily, from 2:00 until 3:00 in the morning. Now her mother talks through the priest to her father's ghost. Although Wong Huieng regards this practice as superstitious and thinks that painting a picture of a lake and mountain is a more fitting way to erase her grief, she wears a little yellow bag containing a blessing from the priest around her neck. She finds it comforting if not intellectually acceptable.

Now Wong Huieng turns to her practical side and talks about **Confucius**, the *first saint of the nation*. Although **Lao-tzu**, the *founder of Taoism*, is a semilegendary figure said to have vanished after he wrote **Tao-te-ching**, *the bible of Taoism*, Confucius has a well-documented existence.

Confucius, born in 551 B.C., wrote little. His disciples wrote the **Analects**, *short proverbs embodying his teachings*. He is revered as a teacher, not as a god. Wong Huieng does not ask him to bless her but tries to emulate him and his teachings, which she has heard since birth. The temple in his memory is a place for studying, not for praying. And on his birthday, a national holiday, people pay respect to their teachers in his memory.

Five important terms in Confucius' teaching are **Jen**, *a striving for goodness within*; **Chun-sui**, *establishing a gentlemanly or womanly approach with others*; **Li**, *knowing how relationships should be conducted and having respect for age*; **Te**, *leading by virtuous character rather than by force*; and **Wen**, *pursuing the arts as an adjunct to moral character*. Wong Huieng stresses that in **Li** are the directives for family relationships. So strongly did Confucius feel about the

family that he gave directives on proper attitudes between father and son, elder brother and junior brother, and husband and wife. Also, Wong Huieng believes she cannot harm her body because it was given to her by her parents. Her concept of immediate family includes grandparents, uncles, aunts, and cousins. Her language has more words for relationships between relatives than the English language does. Wong Huieng believes that in caring for her body, she cares for her family, the country, and the universe. Essentially, to her, all people are family.

Important in your understanding of a person with Wong Huieng's background is the dualism that exists in such thinking. Acceptance of the particular version of mysticism and practicality and of the yin and yang forces that are seen as operating within self will help in building a foundation of personalized care.

Address the person by the proper name. Do not use excessive touch signals unless they are invited. This person may be in awe of health care authority and may be intimidated. The person may have more respect for older than younger staff members and may respond well to teaching. There may be a strong desire to attain and maintain; wellness. These factors are directly related to the religious teaching, use them to enhance care. Additionally, talk slowly to the person if language is an issue. Rely on family members to help understand the person's feelings. Permit familiar foods; foods are divided into appropriate groups for types of illness.

☪ ISLAM

Omar Ali is Muslim, a member of **Islam**, the youngest of the major world religions. "There is no God but Allah; Mohammad or Muhammad is His Prophet" provides the key to Omar's beliefs. He must say this but once in his life as a requirement, but he will repeat it many times as an affirmation. Muslims believe in a final judgment day when everyone will be sent either to paradise or to the fire of hell, depending on how justly he or she lived life according to God's laws. They believe everyone, except children before the age of puberty, are responsible for their own good and bad actions and deeds and that no one can intercede on behalf of another (97).

Omar has also been influenced by 3,000-year-old **Zoroastrianism**, *which is a religion of pre-Islamic Iran* that flourishes in Mumbai today. Likewise, it was a monotheistic religion even though dualism was also espoused.

Omar is an Egyptian physician whose religious tradition was revealed through Muhammad, born approximately A.D. 571 in Mecca, then a trading point between India and Syria on the Arabian Peninsula. Hating polytheism and paganism in any form, Muhammad recited God's revelation to him as is documented in the **Qur'an** (or **Koran**) *scriptures*. Omar believes in the Old Testament prophets and Jesus as a prophet, but he calls Muhammad the greatest—the seal of Prophets.

Through the Qur'an and the **Hadith**, *the traditions*, Omar has guidelines for his thinking, devotional life, and social obligations. He believes he is a unique individual with an eternal soul. He believes in a heaven and hell, and while on earth he wants to walk the straight path.

To keep on this path, Omar prays five to seven times a day: generally on rising, at midday, in the afternoon, in the early evening, and before retiring. Articles needed are water and a prayer rug. Because the Qur'an emphasizes cleanliness of body, Omar performs a ritual washing with running water over the face, arms, top of head, and feet before each prayer. Omar explains that in the bedridden client this requirement can be accomplished by pouring water out of some sort of receptacle. If a Muslim's entire body is considered ritually unclean, he must wash the entire body. If water is unavailable or the person cannot bathe, clean soil may be used in place of the ritual washing. After this washing the Muslim needs either a ritually clean cloth or a prayer rug and a clean place to pray. He may not face a dirty area such as the bathroom when making his prayer, even if this area is in the line toward Mecca. The Muslim must physically readjust himself in this case to comply with Islamic regulations. Then, facing Mecca, he goes through a series of prescribed body motions and repeats various passages in praise and supplication.

Omar also observes **Ramadan**, *a fast month*,[†] that comes during the ninth lunar month of the Muslim year, always at a different time each year by the Western calendar, and sometimes spelled *Ramazan*. During this time he eats or drinks nothing from sunrise to sunset; after sunset he takes nourishment only in moderation. He explains **fasting** (*abstinence from eating*) as a discipline aiding him to understand those with little food and more importantly, as a submission to Allah. The sick, the very old, pregnant and lactating mothers, children, and Muslims who require the ingestion or injection of substances throughout the day hours are exempt without penalty from practice of this belief. At the end of Ramadan, he enters a festive period with feelings of goodwill and gift exchanges.

Omar has made one pilgrimage to Mecca, another requirement for all healthy and financially able Muslims. He believes the experience created a great sense of brotherhood, for all the pilgrims wore similar modest clothing, exchanged news of followers in various lands, and reviewed their mutual faith. The 12th day of the pilgrimage month is the **Feast of Sacrifice** (**Eida-Fita**), when all Muslim families kill a lamb in honor of Abraham's offering of his son to God.

In line with the Qur'an's teaching, Omar does not eat pork or pork products (including such items as bologna, which might contain partial pork products), gamble, drink intoxicants, use illicit drugs, or engage in religiously unlawful sexual practices such as premarital sex, homosexuality, and infidelity. The emphasis on strict moral upbringing—dating, dancing, drinking, and sexual relationships outside marriage are forbidden—puts the Muslim on a common ground with conservative Christians. Abstinence from drug use also eliminates many potential health and social problems.

Omar worships no images or pictures of Muhammad, for the prophet is not deified. Nor does he hang or display pictures of any prophet or any god or worship statues or religious symbols. He obeys **Zakat**, *an Islamic command to give alms to the poor* in order to be responsible to society; 2.5% of personal wealth is to be given to a committee or directly to the poor.

Omar points out that not all Arabs are Muslims and not all Muslims are Arabs. Arabs come from a number of nations stretching from Morocco to the Persian Gulf. Persons who are Arab Muslims speak Arabic and uphold the tenets of Islam. Omar emphasizes the importance of gaining specific knowledge about their complex social structure. The centrality of religion and the family are closely related and reflect many aspects of health care.

Omar mentions that parts of the basic Islam faith are used by a United States–based group commonly known as the **Black Muslims**. Known to have stringent, seclusionist rules, the Black Muslims seem to be moving away from orthodox Islam. Membership is especially appealing to young African American males who like the masculine focus, the structure, and the emphasis on self-help and self-esteem.

Omar outlines the ideas of his religion as it applies to his profession. He believes that he can make a significant contribution to health care but that essentially what happens is God's will. Submission and obedience to God is the very meaning of Islam. This belief produces a fluid feeling of time and sense of fatalism. Planning ahead for a Muslim is not a value as it is in Western culture; to defy God's will brings on the evil eye.

Muslim clients who are ill are excused from many, but not all, religious rules, but many will still want to follow them as closely as possible. Even though in a body cast and unable to get out of bed, a client may want to go through prayers symbolically. The person might also recite the first chapters of the Qur'an, centered on praise to Allah, which are often used in times of crises. Family is a great comfort in illness, and praying with a group is strengthening, but the Muslim has no priest. The relationship is directly with God. Some clients may seem fatalistic, completely resigned to death, whereas others, hoping it is God's will that they live, cooperate vigorously with the medical program. Muslims do not discuss death openly, because if they did, the client and family may lose all hope and the client could die as a result. Instead, Muslims tend to communicate grief in gradual stages rather than immediately and all at once. Further, they make it a point never to let the affected person lose hope. The family, even in the gravest of situations, will not attempt to prepare for the death even when it is imminent. After death, a body must be washed with running water by a Muslim and the hands folded in prayer. Muslims do not perform autopsies, embalm, or use caskets for burials. Instead, they wrap a white linen cloth around the dead person and place the body into the ground facing Mecca. Knowledge of these attitudes and traditions can greatly enhance your care (55). Refer also to **Table C7-1** in the Companion Website and to Chapter 5 for more information related to client health promotion and care. ∞

☰ JUDAISM

Seth Lieberman, strongly influenced by the emphasis on social concern in **Judaism**, is a psychiatrist. In the Jewish community each member is expected to contribute to others' needs according to his or her ability. Jews have traditionally considered their community as a whole responsible for feeding the hungry, helping the widowed and orphaned, rescuing the captured, and even burying the dead. Jewish retirement homes, senior citizens' centers, and medical centers are witnesses to this philosophy.

Seth cannot remember when his religious instruction began—it was always there. He went through the motions and felt the emotion of the Sabbath eve with its candles and cup of sanctification long before he could comprehend his father's explanations. Book learning followed, however, and he came to understand the fervency with which his people study and live the law as given in the **Torah**, *the first five books of the Bible*, and in the **Talmud**, *a commentary and enlargement of the Torah*. The **rabbi** *is his spiritual leader*. His *spiritual symbol* is the **menorah;** the seven-branched candelabrum stands for the creation of the universe in 7 days, the center light symbolizes the Sabbath, and the candlelight symbolizes the presence of God in the temple.

His own *entrance into a responsible religious life and manhood* was through the **bar mitzvah**, a ceremony which took place in the synagogue when he was 13 years old. Girls are also educated to live responsible religious lives, and congregations now have the **bat mitzvah**, *a similar ceremony for girls*.

Although raised in an Orthodox home, Seth and his family are now members of the Reform sect. He mentions another group, the Conservatives. The **Orthodox** *believe God gave the law*; it was written exactly as he gave it; *it should be followed precisely*. **Reform Jews** *believe the law was written by inspired men* at various times and therefore is *subject to reinterpretation*. Seth says he follows the traditions because they are traditions rather than because God demands it. **Conservatives** *are in the middle, taking some practices from both groups*. Overriding any differences in interpretation of ritual and tradition is the fundamental concept expressed in the prayer "Hear, O Israel, the Lord our God, the Lord is One." Not only is he one, he loves his creation, wants his people to live justly, and wants to bless their food, drink, and celebration. Judaism's double theme might be expressed as "Enjoy life now, and share it with God." Understandably then, Seth's religious emphasis is not on an afterlife, although some Jewish people believe in one. Although Jews have had a history of suffering, the inherent value of suffering or illness is not stressed. Through their observance of the law, the belief of their historical role as God's chosen people, and their hope for better days, Jews have survived seemingly insurmountable persecution.

Seth works with physically, emotionally, and spiritually depressed persons. He believes that often the spiritual depression is unnoticed, misunderstood, or ignored by professional workers. He cites instances in which mental attitudes have brightened as he shared a common bond of Judaism with a client.

He offers guidelines for working with a Jewish person in a hospital or nursing home. Although Jewish law can be suspended when a person is ill, the client will be most comfortable following as many practices as possible. This information is relevant to the care of the person who is of Jewish faith.

Every Jewish person observes the **Sabbath**, *a time for spiritual refreshment, from sundown on Friday to shortly after sundown on Saturday*. During this period Orthodox Jews may refuse freshly cooked food, medicine, treatment, surgery, and use of radio, television, and writing equipment lest the direction of their thinking be diverted on this special day. An Orthodox male may want to wear a **yarmulke** or *skullcap* continuously, use a *prayer book* called a **siddur**, and use **phylacteries**, *leather strips with boxes containing scriptures*, at weekday morning prayer. Also, the ultra-Orthodox male may refuse to use a razor because of the Levitical ban on shaving.

Some Orthodox Jewish females observe the rite of **mikvah**, *an ancient ritual of family purity*. From marriage to menopause (ex-

cept when pregnant) these females have no physical or sexual relations with their husbands from 24 hours before menstruation until 12 days later when a ritual immersion in water renders them ready to meet their husbands again.

Jewish dietary laws have been considered by some scholars as health measures: to enjoy life is to eat properly and in moderation. The Orthodox, however, obey them because God so commanded. Food is called **treyfe** (or *treyfah*) if it is *unfit* and **kosher** if it is *ritually correct*.

Foods forbidden are pig, horse, shrimp, lobster, crab, oyster, and fowl that are birds of prey. Meats approved are from those animals that are ruminants and have divided hooves. Fish approved must have both fins and scales. Also, the kosher animals must be healthy and slaughtered in a prescribed manner. Because of the biblical passage stating not to soak a young goat in its mother's milk, Jews do not eat meat products and milk products together. Neither are the utensils used to cook these products nor the dishes from which to eat these products ever intermixed.

Guidelines for a satisfactory diet for the Orthodox Jewish person are as follows:

1. Serve milk products first, meat second. Meat can be eaten a few minutes after milk, but milk cannot be taken for 6 hours after meat.
2. If a person completely refuses meat because of incorrect slaughter, encourage a vegetarian diet with protein supplements, such as fish and eggs, which are considered neutral unless prepared with milk or meat fat.
3. Buy frozen kosher products marked Ⓤ, K, or *pareve*.
4. Heat and serve food in the original container and use plastic utensils.

Two important holy days are Rosh Hashanah and Yom Kippur. **Rosh Hashanah**, *the Jewish New Year, is a time to meet with the family, give thanks to God for good health, and renew traditions*. **Yom Kippur**, *the day of atonement, a time for asking forgiveness of family members for wrongs done*, occurs 10 days later. On Yom Kippur, Jews fast for 24 hours, a symbolic act of self-denial, mourning, and petition. **Tishah-b'Ab**, the *day of lamentation*, recalling the destruction of both temples of Jerusalem, is another 24-hour fast period. **Pesach** or **Passover** (8 days for Orthodox and Conservative, 7 days for Reform) *celebrates the ancient Jews' deliverance from Egyptian bondage*. **Matzo**, *an unleavened bread*, replaces leavened bread during this period.

The Jewish person is preoccupied with health. Jews are future oriented and want to know the diagnosis, and how a disease will affect business, family life, and social life. The Jewish people as a whole are highly educated, and although they respect the doctor, they may obtain several medical opinions before carrying out a treatment plan.

Although family, friends, and rabbi may visit the ill, especially on or near holidays, they will also come at other times. Visiting the sick is a religious duty. And although death is final to many Jews except for living on in the memories of others or in memorials, guidelines exist for this time. When a Jewish person has suffered irreversible brain damage and can no longer say a **bracha**, *a blessing to praise God*, or perform a **mitzvah**, *an act to help a fellow*, he or she is considered in a vegetative state with nothing to save.

Prolonging the life by artificial means would not be recommended. But until then, the dying client must be treated as the complete person he or she always was, capable of conducting his or her own affairs and entering into relationships.

Jewish tradition says never to leave the bedside of the dying person, which is of value to the dying and the mourners. The dying soul should leave in the presence of people, and the mourner is shielded from the guilt of thinking that the person was alone at death or that more could have been done. The bedside vigil also serves as a time to encourage a personal confession by the dying, which is a *rite of passage* to another phase of existence (even though unknown). This type of confessional is said throughout the Jewish life cycle whenever one stage has been completed. Confessional on the deathbed is a recognition that one cycle is ending and that another cycle is beginning. Recitation of the Shema in the last moments before death helps the dying to affirm faith in God and focus on the most familiar rituals of life.

Death, being witnessed at the bedside, helps to reinforce the reality of the situation. **Tahara**, *the traditional purification ritual of preparing a body for burial*, is performed by the **chevra kadisha**, *the Jewish burial society*, at the Jewish mortuary (see also reference 39). Immediate burial and specified mourning rituals also help the remaining loved ones through the crisis period. (Note, however, that if a Jew dies on the Sabbath, he or she cannot be moved, except by a non-Jew, until sundown.) After the burial, the mourners are fed in *a meal of replenishment* called **se'udat havra'ah**. The step symbolizes the rallying of the community and the sustenance of life for the remaining. Also, Jews follow the custom of **sitting shiva**, or *visiting with remaining relatives for 1 week after the death.*

Judaism identifies a *year of mourning*. The first 3 days are of deep grief; clothes may be torn to symbolize the tearing of a life from others. Seven days of lesser mourning follow, leading to 30 days of gradual readjustment. The remainder of the year calls for remembrance and healing. During that year a prayer called the mourner's *kaddish* is recited in religious services. It helps convey the feeling of support for the mourner. At the annual anniversary of death, a candle is burned and special prayers are said.

Seth summarizes his faith as follows: From his circumcision on the eighth day after birth to his deathbed, just like from the days of the original menorah in the sanctuary in the wilderness until the present day, he and the followers of Judaism reenact their traditions. Many of these traditions remain an intrinsic part of the Jewish person's life. The traditions help the person to maintain or regain health and wellness. The preceding guidelines offer a foundation for knowledgeable care.

✝ CHRISTIANITY

Beth Meyer, a *Roman Catholic*; Demetrius Callas, an *Eastern Orthodox*; and Jean Taylor, a *Protestant*, are Christian American nurses representing the three major branches of Christianity. Although **Christianity** was divided into Eastern Orthodox and Roman Catholicism in A.D. 1054, and the Protestant Reformation provided a third division in the 16th century, these nurses share some basic beliefs, most importantly that Jesus Christ, as described in the Bible, is God's son. Jesus was born in Bethlehem; the change from "B.C." to "A.D." on the calendar is based upon his year of birth. The details of Jesus 33 years of life are few, but his deeds and words recorded in the Bible's New Testament show quiet authority, loving humility, forgiveness, and an ability to perform miracles and to visit easily with people in varied social positions (48, 101, 117).

The main symbol of Christianity is the cross, but it signifies more than a wooden structure on which Jesus was crucified. It also symbolizes the finished redemption—Christ rising from the dead and ascending to God the Father to rule with him and continuously pervade the personal lives of his followers. Christians observe **Christmas** as *Christ's birthday*; **Lent** as a *season of penitence and self-examination preceding* **Good Friday**, *Christ's crucifixion day*; and **Easter**, *Christ's resurrection day* (48, 101, 117).

Beth, Demetrius, and Jean rely on the New Testament as a guideline for their lives. They believe that Jesus was fully God and fully man at the same time, that their original sin (which they accept as a basic part of themselves) can be forgiven, and that they are acceptable to God because of Jesus Christ's life and death. They believe God is three persons—the Father, the Son, and the Holy Spirit (Holy Ghost), the last providing a spirit of love, truth, and counsel or guidance (48, 101, 117).

Beth, Demetrius, and Jean differ in some worship practices and theology, but all highly regard their individuality as children of God and hope for life with God after death. They feel responsible for their own souls, the spiritual dimension of themselves, and for aiding the spiritual needs of their patients.

Roman Catholic Church

Roman Catholicism, according to Beth, is a religion based on the dignity of the person as a social, intellectual, and spiritual being made in the image of God. She traces the teaching authority of the church through the scriptures: God sent his son to provide salvation and redemption from sin. Jesus established the church to continue his work after his ascension into heaven. Jesus chose apostles to preach, teach, and guide. He appointed Saint Peter as the church's head to preserve unity and to have authority over the apostles. The mission given by Jesus to Saint Peter and the apostles is the same that continues to the present through the pope and his bishops. Beth notes that women in the Roman Catholic Church, both nuns and laywomen, are speaking out more on issues and are gaining more recognition as God's spokespeople. **Priests**, *the spiritual leaders for the individual parish*, are more open to women participating in the worship service.

Beth believes that the seven **sacraments** are *grace-giving rites that give her a share in Christ's own life and help sustain her in her efforts to follow his example*. The sacraments that are received once in life are baptism, confirmation, holy orders, and usually matrimony.

Through **baptism**, Catholics believe the *soul is incorporated into the life of Christ and shares his divinity*. The healthy baby is baptized some time during the first weeks of life. Adults are also baptized when they convert to Catholicism and join the church.

Any infant in danger of death should be baptized, even an aborted fetus. If a priest is not available, a health care provider who believes or a non-believer can perform baptism by pouring water on the forehead and saying, "I baptize thee in the name of the Father, of the Son, and of the Holy Spirit."

Confirmation *is the sacrament in which the Holy Spirit is imparted in a fuller measure to help strengthen the individual in his or her spiritual life.* **Matrimony** *acknowledges the love and lifelong commitment between a man and a woman.* **Holy orders** *ordain deacons and priests.*

The sacraments that may be received more than once are **penance** (*confession*), the **Eucharist** (*Holy Communion*), and the **anointing of the sick** (*sacrament of the sick*). Beth believes that **penance**, *an acknowledgment and forgiveness of her sins in the presence of a priest*, should be received according to individual need, even though it is required only once a year by church law. The **Mass**, often called the **Eucharist**, is the *liturgical celebration whose core is the sacrament of the Holy Eucharist.* Bread and wine are consecrated and become the body and blood of Christ. The body and blood are then received in Holy Communion.

The Eucharist is celebrated daily, and all Roman Catholics are encouraged to participate as often as possible. They are required by church law to attend on Sundays (or late Saturdays) and specified holy days throughout the year unless prevented by illness or some other serious reason.

Beth is glad that the anointing of the sick has been modified and broadened, and she explains the rite to client and family to allay anxiety. Formerly known as extreme unction, or the last rites, this sacrament was reserved for those near death. Now **anointing of the sick**, *symbolic of Christ's healing love and the concern of the Christian community*, can provide spiritual strength to those less gravely ill. After anointing with oil, the priest offers prayers for forgiveness of sin and restoration of health. Whenever possible, the family should be present to join in the prayers.

If the client is dying, extraordinary artificial measures to maintain life are unnecessary. At the hour of death, the priest offers Communion to the dying person by means of a special formula. This *final Communion* is called **Viaticum**. In sudden deaths, the priest should be called and the anointing and Viaticum should be administered if possible. If the person is dead when the priest arrives, there is no anointing, but the priest leads the family in prayer for the person who just died.

Beth divides the Roman Catholic funeral into three phases: the **wake**, *a period of waiting or vigil during which the body is viewed and the family is sustained through visiting*; the **funeral Mass**, *a prayer service incorporated into the celebration of the Mass*; and the **burial**, *the final act of placing the person in the ground.* (This procedure may vary somewhat, for some Catholics are now choosing cremation.) The mourners retain the memory of the dead through a Month's Mind Mass, celebrated a month after death, and anniversary Masses. Finally, the priest integrates the liturgy for the dead with the whole parish liturgical life.

Beth is convinced that her religious practice contributes to her health. She believes that the body, mind, and spirit work together and that a spirit rid of guilt and grievances and fortified with the strength of Christ's life has positive effects on the body. She believes that suffering and illness are allowed by God because of our disobedience (original sin) but that they are not necessarily willed by God or given as punishment for personal sin.

While in the hospital, a Roman Catholic may want to attend Mass, have the priest visit, or receive the Eucharist at bedside. Fasting an hour before the sacrament is traditional, but in the case of physical illness, fasting is not necessary. Other symbols that might be comforting are a Bible, prayer book, holy water, lighted candle, crucifix, rosary, and various relics and medals.

Eastern Orthodox Church

The **Eastern Orthodox Church**, *the main denomination, is divided into groups by nationality.* The **Greek Eastern Orthodox faith** is discussed by Demetrius. Each group has the **Divine Liturgy**, the *Eucharistic service*, in the native language and sometimes in English also. Although similar in many respects to the Roman Catholic faith, the Eastern Orthodox faith has no pope. The seven sacraments are administered by the **priest**, *the spiritual leader*, with slight variations from those of the Roman Catholic church. Baptism is by triple immersion: The priest places the infant in a basin of water and pours water on the forehead three times. He then immediately confirms the infant by anointing with holy oil.

If death is imminent for a hospitalized infant and the parents or priest cannot be reached, the believer can baptize the infant by placing a small amount of water on the forehead three times. Even a symbolic baptism is acceptable, but only a living being should receive the sacrament. Adults who join the church are also baptized and confirmed.

The **unction of the sick** has never been practiced as a last rite by the Eastern Orthodox; it is a *blessing for the sick.* Confession at least once a year is a prerequisite to participation in the Eucharist, which is taken at least four times a year: at Christmas, at Easter, on the Feast Day of Saint Peter and Saint Paul (June 30), and on the day celebrating the Sleeping of the Virgin Mary (August 15).

Fasting from the last meal in the evening until after **Communion**, another term for the *Eucharist*, is the general rule. Other fast periods include each Wednesday, representing the seizure of Jesus; each Friday, representing Jesus' death; and two 40-day periods, the first before Christmas and the second before Easter.

Fasting, to Demetrius, means avoiding meat, dairy products, and olive oil. Its purpose is spiritual betterment, to avoid producing extra energy in the body, and instead to think of the spirit. Fasting is not necessary when ill. Religion should not harm one's health.

Demetrius retains the Eastern influence in his thinking. He envisions his soul as blending in with the spiritual cosmos and his actions as affecting the rest of creation. He is mystically inclined and believes insights can be gained directly from God. He tells of sharing such an experience with a patient, Mrs. A., also Greek Orthodox.

Mrs. A. had experienced surgery to build up deteriorating bones caused by rheumatoid arthritis. She faced another surgery. On the positive side, the surgery promised hope for walking; on the negative, it was a new and risky procedure. Possibly she would not walk; possibly she would not live. Demetrius saw Mrs. A. when he started working at 3:30 p.m. She was depressed, fearful, and crying. Later, at 6:30 p.m., he saw a changed person—fearless and calm, ready for surgery. She explained that she had seen Jesus in a vision, and that he said, "Go ahead with the surgery. You'll have positive results. But call your priest and take Communion first." Demetrius called the priest, who gave her Communion. She went into surgery the next day with supreme confidence. She now walks.

In addition to Communion, other helpful symbols are prayer books, lighted candles, and holy water. Especially helpful to the Orthodox are **icons**, *pictures of Jesus, Mary, or a revered saint.* Saints can intercede between God and the person. One of the most loved is *Saint Nicholas*, a 3rd-century teacher and father figure who gave his wealth to the poor and became an archbishop. He is honored on Saint Nicholas Day, December 6, and prayed to continuously for guidance and protection.

Every Sunday morning Demetrius participates in an hour-long liturgy. Sitting in an ornate sanctuary with figures and symbols on the windows, walls, and ceiling, facing the tabernacle containing the holy gifts and scripture, Demetrius finds renewal. He recites, "I believe in one God, the Father Almighty, Maker of Heaven and Earth, and of all things visible and invisible. And in one Lord Jesus Christ, the only begotten Son of God."

Protestantism

There are many Protestant denominations and sects. Jean Taylor is a member of the *Church of God* (Anderson, Indiana). She identifies the church by its headquarters because there are some 200 independent church groups in the United States using the phrase "Church of God" in their title. Her group evolved late in the 19th century because members of various churches felt that organization and ritual were taking precedence over direction from God. They banded together in a drive toward Christian unity, toward a recognition that any people who followed Christ's teachings were members of a universal Church of God and could worship freely together.

This example speaks of one of the chief characteristics of Protestantism: the insistence that God has not given any one person or group of persons sole authority to interpret his truth to others. Protestants use a freedom of spiritual searching and reinterpretation. Thus, new groups form as certain persons and their followers come to believe that they see God's teaching in a new and better light. Jean believes that reading the Bible for historical knowledge and guidance, having a minister to teach and counsel her, and relying on certain worship forms are all important aids. But discerning God's will for her life individually and following God's will are her ultimate religious goals.

Jean explains that she "accepted Christ into her life" when she was 8 years old. This identified her as personally following the church's teaching rather than just adhering to family religious tradition. A later experience, in which the *Holy Spirit gives the person more spiritual power and discernment*, is called **sanctification**.

Jean defines her corporate worship as free liturgical, with an emphasis on congregational singing, verbal prayer, and scripture reading. A sermon by the **minister**, *the spiritual leader*, may take half the worship period. As with many Protestant groups, *two sacraments or ordinances are observed:* (a) baptism (in this case, **believer's**, or **mature, baptism** by *total immersion into water*) and (b) **Communion**. To *Protestants, the bread and wine used in Communion are symbolic of Christ's body and blood rather than the actual elements.* One additional ordinance practiced in Jean's church and among some other groups is **foot washing**, *symbolic of Jesus' washing the disciples' feet.* These ordinances are practiced with varied frequencies.

Because of the **spectrum of beliefs and practices, defining Protestants** even within a single denomination or sect is almost impossible (122). See **Table C7-1** in the Companion Website for more information about many of the Protestant denominations as related to client health promotion and care. Some Protestant groups, retaining their initial emphasis on individual freedom, have allowed no written creed, but expect members to follow an unwritten code of behavior. Jean does suggest some guidelines, however. She lists some of *the main Protestant bodies* in the United States, beginning with the most formal liturgically and sacramentally, the *Protestant Episcopal* and *Lutheran* churches. Some denominations, such as the *Presbyterians, United Church of Christ, United Methodists*, and *Disciples of Christ (Christian Church)*, have less centralized formality and more autonomy as congregations. The liturgically freest and the least sacramental are the *Baptists* and *Pentecostals.* However, all denominations are responding to the changing societal trends in aspects of the worship service, social justice issues, and involvement in the community—local, national, and international.

Among the beliefs of Protestant denominations are various opposing doctrines and practices, such as living in sin versus living above sin, predestination versus free will, infant versus believer's baptism, and loose organization versus tightly knit organization. Some uphold **fundamental precepts**, *holding to the scriptures as infallible*, whereas others uphold **liberal precepts**, *using the scriptures as a guide, with various interpretations for current living.* Recently Christian groups have become even more divided by subjects such as abortion, same-sex relationships, and what constitutes morality.

With this infinite variety, Jean believes that asking the individual beliefs of her Protestant client is essential. When and if a client wants Communion, if an infant should be baptized, and what will be most helpful spiritually to the patient—these factors are learned by careful interviewing. Generally Jean believes that prayer, a scriptural motto such as "I can do all things through Christ who gives me strength" (Philippians 4:13), or a line from a hymn can give strength to a Protestant. Some patients will also want anointing with oil as a symbolic aid to healing.

Jean has discovered that there are wide differences in Protestantism, sometimes even within the same denomination, about why illness, crises, or bad events occur, and the theology and rituals of death. Some Protestant theologies have come to grips with the realities and meaning of death. Others block authentic expression of grief to life events and focus on "If you are a Christian, you won't be sad."

Some Protestants view death as penalty and punishment for sins. Others see death as a transition when the soul leaves the body for eternal reward; still others view death as an absolute end. All agree that death is a biological and spiritual event, a mystery not fully comprehended.

Rituals surrounding death vary widely. Some churches believe that the funeral service with a closed casket or memorial service with no casket present is more of a testimony to the joy and victory of Christian life than the open-casket service. Others believe that death is a reality to face instead of deny and that viewing the dead person promotes the grief process and confrontation with death in a Christian context.

Jean believes that, for most Protestants, the clergy represents friendship, love, acceptance, forgiveness, and understanding. His or her presence seems to help the dying face death with more ease. She also believes that Protestants are becoming more active in ministering to the bereaved through regularly scheduled visits during the 12 to 18 months after the funeral, although there are no formal rituals.

SPECIAL RELIGIOUS GROUPS OF INTEREST

Some religious groups are less well known than those just described. Practices or beliefs unique to certain groups should be part of every health provider's knowledge.

Seventh-Day Adventists *rely on Old Testament law more than do other Christian churches.* As in Jewish tradition, the Sabbath is from sundown Friday to sundown Saturday. Like the Orthodox Jew, the Seventh-Day Adventist may refuse medical treatment and use of secular items, such as television, during this period and prefer to read spiritual literature. Diet is also restricted. Pork, fish without both scales and fins, tea, and coffee are prohibited. Some Seventh-Day Adventists are **lacto-ovo-vegetarians:** *They eat milk and eggs but no meat.* Tobacco, alcoholic beverages, and narcotics are also avoided. Because Adventists view the body as the "temple of God," health reform is high on their list of priorities and they sponsor health institutes, cooking schools, and food-producing organizations. They are pioneers in making foods for vegetarians, including meatlike foods from vegetable sources. Worldwide they operate an extensive system of schools and medical institutions and are active medical missionaries. Much of their inspiration comes from Ellen G. White, a 19th-century prophetess who gave advice on diet and food and who stressed Christ's return to earth (7, 67).

The **Church of Jesus Christ of Latter-Day Saints (Mormon)** takes much of its inspiration from the **Book of Mormon**, *translated from golden tablets found in what is now the United States by the prophet Joseph Smith.* The Mormons believe that this book and two others supplement the Bible. Every Mormon is an official missionary. There is no official congregational leader, but a **seventy** and a **high priest** *represent successive steps upward in commitment and authority.*

The Articles of Faith of the Church of Jesus Christ of Latter-Day Saints include statements of belief in:

1. God and his Son, Jesus Christ, and the Holy Ghost.
2. Worship of God according to personal conscience while obeying the law of the land.
3. People being punished for their own sins and not for Adam's transgression.
4. All people being saved by repentance and obedience to the laws and ordinances of the Gospel.
5. Being honest, true, chaste, benevolent, virtuous, hopeful, persistent, and doing good to all people.

The family is highly valued. The church believes in a whole-being approach and provides education, recreation, and financial aid for its members. *A health and conduct code* called **Word of Wisdom** prohibits tobacco, alcohol, and caffeinated drinks (interpreted as tea and coffee) and recommends eating sparingly and with thankfulness, herbs, fruit, meat, fowl, and grain foods.

Mormons believe that disease comes from failure to obey the laws of health and from failure to keep the other commandments of God. However, they concur that righteous persons sometimes become ill simply because they have been exposed to microorganisms that cause disease. They also believe that by faith the righteous sometimes escape plagues that are sweeping the land and often, having become sick, the obedient are restored to full physical well-being by the gift of faith.

Statistics indicate that this population succumbs to cancer and diseases of the major body systems at a much lower rate than the general population in this country. Fewer members of the Church of Jesus Christ of Latter-Day Saints have diseases of the nervous, circulatory, and digestive systems; kidney diseases; and respiratory diseases. Mental illness occurs only half as often among Mormons as among the general population (61). An explanation for these differences from the norm might be that they literally believe the body is the temple of God. They have programs of diet, exercise, family life, and work to help that "temple" function at optimum level.

The two groups just discussed, the Seventh-Day Adventists and the Church of Jesus Christ of Latter-Day Saints, generally accept and promote modern medical practices. The next two groups, Jehovah's Witnesses and Church of Christ, Scientist, hold views that conflict with the medical field.

The first group, **Jehovah's Witnesses**, *refuses to accept blood transfusions.* Their refusal is based on the Levitical commandment, given by God to Moses, declaring that no one in the House of David should eat blood or he or she would be cut off from his or her people, and on a New Testament reference (in Acts) prohibiting the tasting of blood (Genesis 9:3–6, 1 Samuel 14:31–35; Acts 15:19–21, 28–29). Members meet in halls rather than in traditional churches, and they produce massive amounts of literature explaining their faith. Every Jehovah's Witness is a minister. Jehovah's Witnesses in need of surgery may be fortunate enough to be near a surgeon who uses no blood transfusions because of reduced operating time. Other surgeons are becoming more willing to do surgery without using blood, using intravenous fluids similar to the body's fluid composition instead. The new plasma expanders can also be used.

Wherever there is a Jehovah's Witness community, there will be a representative from their Hospital Liaison Committee to call if there are questions about care of a Jehovah's Witness patient.

Members of this committee are well-informed church members who can act as a link between physician or nurse and patient or family, explain use of acceptable alternatives to medical treatment, and help locate and arrange assistance from or referral to a center for bloodless surgery, if necessary.

The second group, **Church of Christ, Scientist (Christian Scientists)**, *turn wholly to spiritual means for healing*. They allow an orthopedist to set a broken bone if no medication is used. Parents do not allow their children to undergo a physical examination for school; to have eye, ear, or blood pressure screening; or to receive immunizations. In addition to the Bible, Christian Scientists use as their guide Mary Baker Eddy's *Science and Health with Key to the Scriptures*, originally published in 1875. The title of this work indicates an approach to wholeness, and those who follow its precepts think of God as Divine Mind, of spirit as real and eternal, of matter as unreal illusion. Sin, sickness, and death are unrealities or erring belief. Christian Scientists do not ignore their erring belief, however, for they have established nursing homes and sanatoriums, the latter recognized in the United States under the federal Medicare program and in insurance regulations. These facilities are operated by trained Christian Scientist nurses who give first-aid measures and spiritual assistance.

A Christian Scientist graduate nurse must complete a course of training at one of a number of accredited sanatoriums. The training includes, among other subjects, classes in basic nursing arts, care of the elderly, cooking, bandaging, nursing ethics, care of reportable diseases, and theory of obstetric nursing. The training is nonmedical, and in the work of a Christian Scientist nurse no medication is administered. The nurse supports the work of the **practitioner**, *who devotes full time to the public practice of Christian Science healing*. Healing is not thought of as miraculous but as the application of natural spiritual law.

The practitioner helps people apply natural spiritual law. Such a person is not a clergyman and does not necessarily hold special church office. Becoming a practitioner is attained largely through self-conducted study and a short course of intensive study from an authorized teacher of Christian Science, but daily study, prayer, application, and spiritual growth are the foundation of practice. The practitioner will treat anyone who comes for help and is supported by clients' payments.

A Christian Scientist who is in a medical hospital has undoubtedly tried Christian Science healing first, may have been put there by a non-Scientist relative, or may be at variance with sacred beliefs. If brought in while unconscious, the person would want to be given the minimum emergency care and treatment consistent with hospital policy. The person may also appreciate having a Christian Science practitioner called for treatment through prayer. Yet sometimes the Christian Scientist or family may feel so desperate about their own or a loved one's health status that they seek traditional medical care—sometimes too late.

Two more groups of special interest because of their positive personal and health emphasis are the **Society of Friends** and **Unity School of Christianity**. Their beliefs contrast with most Roman Catholics, who acknowledge the earthly spiritual author-

ity of the pope, and with most Protestants, who regard the Bible as their ultimate authority.

The **Society of Friends (Quakers)** *believe their authority lies in direct experience of God within the self*. A Friend obeys the **light within**, the **inner light**, or the **divine principle**; *this spiritual quality causes the Friend to esteem self and listen to inner direction*. All Friends are spiritual equals. Without a minister and without any symbols or religious decor, unprogrammed corporate worship consists of silent meditation, with each person seeking divine guidance. Toward the end of the meeting, people are free to share their inspiration. The meeting closes with handshaking. Always interested in world peace, Friends are pacifists and have been instrumental in establishing organizations that work toward human brotherhood and economic and social improvements resulting in better health. Friends have staffed hospitals, driven ambulances, and served in medical corps, among numerous other volunteer services.

The **Unity School of Christianity** *believes that health is natural and sickness is unnatural*. Followers think *illness is real, but they believe it can be overcome by concentrating on spiritual goals*. Late in the 19th century, Charles and Myrtle Fillmore started this group after studying, among other religions, Christian Science, Quakerism, and Hinduism. Thus it blends several established concepts in a new direction. Today Unity Village in Missouri has a publication center that publishes several inspirational periodicals, is beautifully landscaped and open for guests to share in the beauty, and houses its real force, Silent Unity. **Silent Unity** *consists of staff who are available on a 24-hour basis to answer telephone calls, telegrams, and letters from people seeking spiritual help*. They offer prayer and counseling to all faiths with no charge.

The following *religious groups have each retained a traditional lifestyle, geographic solidarity, and theological unity*. These groups, the Mennonites, Moravians, Waldenses, and Unitarian Universalists, originated in other countries and immigrated to America.

The **Mennonites**, some of whom settled in Pennsylvania, are part of a group called the Pennsylvania Dutch, but are of German, rather than Dutch, descent. The Mennonites generally emphasize plain ways of dressing, living, and worshipping. They do not believe in going to war, swearing oaths, or holding offices that require the use of force. Many of them farm the land or are inclined toward service professions. They are well known for their missionary efforts. Another group, the Amish, split from the Mennonite family, and are stricter but similar in life patterns to the Mennonites.

The **Moravians** are a group with northern headquarters in Bethlehem, Pennsylvania, and southern headquarters in Winston-Salem, North Carolina. This faith community has been noted for their missionary work. A restored Moravian village is open for touring in Winston-Salem, and during Christmas and Easter, special services are shared with non-Moravian friends.

The **Waldenses**, a Presbyterian group, have their headquarters in Rome but largely populate the town of Valdese, North Carolina. Each summer an outdoor drama portrays their pilgrimage to freedom.

Unitarian Universalists constitute yet another group of interest. The principal founder and leader in the early 19th century was William Ellery Channing. A Unitarian is considered a member of a universal church from which no person can be excommunicated except by the "death of goodness" in that person's heart. Freedom, democracy, positive faith, and saving the world from tyranny and oppression are major themes. Jesus is usually viewed by the members as a great prophet but not as part of a Trinity.

Neo-Pentecostalism is *another facet of Christianity in the United States.* This is not a group but a *trend* or phenomenon that *has gained support from groups in all major denominations*—some Roman Catholics, Presbyterians, and Lutherans—and from those churches traditionally closer to the Pentecostal spirit.

The heart of the Pentecostal spirit is an enthusiastic personal relationship with Christ. Those who are a part of this trend tell about leaving a dead organized religion or of leaving a religious tradition that no longer has meaning. They are anxious to share their insights. The hallmark of this experience is *"speaking in tongues"* or **glossolalia**. Christians trace this experience back to the 1st century A.D. In 1914, however, the phenomenon became institutionalized with the organization of the Pentecostal Assembly of God Church. This group placed its emphasis of a right relationship with God on glossolalia. The Case Situation describes the behavioral change that can result from belonging to a Neo-Pentecostal faith community.

Other Neo-Pentecostal denominations have come into being, such as Church of God (Cleveland, Tennessee), Foursquare, and United Evangelical Brethren.

Neo-Pentecostalism *is thought of as the renewed interest in glossolalia*; it is sometimes called the **Charismatic Movement**. Just what is *glossolalia*? Oral Roberts and Neo-Pentecostals describe it

as the *prayer language of the spirit; a release of thoughts so deep within the person that ordinary words do not suffice.* Sounds made by the person are not in any known language, and the conscious mind, through prayer, should interpret the glossolalia after the experience so that the person can use the gained insight in everyday living.

Followers of the Neo-Pentecostal phenomenon have sometimes remained as part of the mainline churches in which their experience originated. Others have formed new organizational fellowships that are evolving into new mainline churches. For example, followers of a certain television evangelist will go to that person's religious training center or college. In turn, that religiously trained person will start a congregation following the tenets of that leadership. Eventually all those congregations will bind together in an overall identity membership.

Included in the Neo-Pentecostal group are **evangelicals**, *who call themselves born-again Christians.* According to one national survey, 29% of Americans reported themselves in this category (20); in another national survey, 40% identified themselves as part of this group (110). The *current evangelism is a trend that represents people from diverse racial and ethnic faith traditions* (98, 110) *as well as mainline Protestant denominations such as Episcopalians and Presbyterians* (20). They seek a personal relationship with Jesus and God. The current evangelistic movement is a trend toward revival, personal and therapeutic relationship, and an entrepreneurial or megachurch. The commission is to bring "the good news" to others, as well as implement social service ministries (98, 110). An increasing number of people who attend evangelistic churches are from the higher socioeconomic level (20). The rising income pays

Case Situation

Spiritual Distress and Spiritual Development

Lew was 40 years old. He had a lovely wife, three beautiful children, and an excellent job. Why did he feel a nagging loneliness? Why did he find himself crying?

Lew had been raised in a mainline Protestant denomination. His parents were "pillars of the church." Lew had attended church until his teen years; then he became interested in activities other than church. His life was filled with his marriage and children, but the spiritual dimension was not acknowledged. His children were not receiving a spiritual foundation.

A co-worker asked Lew to accompany him to a 3-day spiritual retreat. Lew was reluctant, but thought, "It can't hurt." The retreat messages fit into Lew's sense of emptiness, and he returned home to celebrate his newfound spirituality with his wife. She wasn't interested. It took months of his urging before

she agreed to attend another retreat. She felt the same fulfillment Lew had found.

This family gained a new set of friends, although they kept former friends and introduced them to the new sense of spirituality. Now Lew and his family are involved in the business aspect of the church, teach a Sunday School class for children, and participate in two Bible study groups. Lew allows a brief time after his daily exercise regimen to read the Bible or other spirituality-focused materials.

Lew found in discussing his interest in the spiritual dimension that several friends of non-Christian religions had similar experiences as they approached midlife. They all agreed that many life situations are draining and distressing. Maturity involves spiritual development as well as physical, emotional, cognitive, and social changes.

Contributed by Judith Zentner, BS, MA, FNP-BC.

for construction of megachurches, national and international broadcasts of worship services, and a vast number of charitable and mission agencies (20, 110). The concern of some theologians is that the evangelicals' enthusiastic religion could place individual or worldly agendas, not God and theological principles, at the center of religious experiences. However, contemporary evangelical Christians are serious about their religion and the authenticity of their faith. They take examples of Jesus seriously (88, 110, 123). Some people are part of a worship group but avoid involvement in social, legislative, or political movements. Others in this group participate actively in social justice issues or political trends as an expression of faith (98, 110).

THE AFRICAN AMERICAN CHURCH*

In the United States, religion and spiritual involvement is as diverse as the cultures that make up the populations. Just as this is true for the country, the same religious diversity can be found within the African American population. Although African American memberships in Christian organizations may appear prevalent, the variety of religious or spiritual influences and practices vary. Religious and spiritual beliefs are a combination of formal institutions and cultural beliefs and practices. This intermingling of culture and religion is common among all nationalities and is not different for African Americans.

To understand the spiritual and religious beliefs and practices of African Americans, we must look at spirituality from a historical perspective. The African American religious experience in America was strongly influenced by the dominant religious culture of Christianity when they originally immigrated to America as indentured servants or were brought to America by slavery. For the enslaved African, induction into Christian practices was through strict discipline and prohibition of use or display of their African spiritual and cultural practices. The Africans were not Christians when they came to America. They were, however, a spiritual people in their native lands. This spirituality was a basic part of daily life. The Africans therefore brought their spirituality with them (40). Through the forced prohibition of their spiritual culture, the religion of the dominant culture was adopted and adapted to accommodate the spiritual needs of the enslaved African. This new spirituality was intertwined in their daily life experiences as it was in their homeland (40).

The adaptation of the religious practices of the dominant culture provided a means of viewing the world at large and a way to fulfill the psychological and social needs within the harshness of slavery. Religion was useful to the indentured African, as well, for solidarity and social cohesion. Thus the spirituality of African Americans had its growth and development rooted in the need to assimilate into a sometimes harsh and withholding dominant culture. This adaptation to the dominant culture's religious practices offered the Africans a means of assimilation and acceptance by this new culture and world. And as they recognized a need to develop an organized life, the church became an essential component in the creation of the African American communal life (40).

The church became a spiritual, social, and psychological source of support to the Black family and the community. It supported the father in a position of authority and was a source of support for the people in times of illness and death, for the widowed, the orphaned, and those in need of financial assistance within the community. The educational needs of the community were addressed and supported by the church. It was also the meeting place for the discussion of community issues. The church provided banking, an employment bureau, social clubs, and a whole range of social services. It was a place in which the community could combine its resources. Therefore, the wealth of the community was within the church. The church then and now continues to be a major voice in addressing the social needs of African Americans. Through the church they could replace and develop cultural norms stripped away by slavery (30).

Today, African Americans are members of numerous religious organizations and espouse a variety of spiritual practices. These organizations or ideals include, but are not limited to, the Nation of Islam or Black Muslims, Judaism, Buddhism, Hinduism, many forms of Christianity, and other spiritual rites and beliefs that are generally accepted in certain geographic locations within the United States. An example of this is voodooism in the southern United States (12). African American churches have provided their congregations with an opportunity for the development of leadership, self-determination, and self-esteem in a culture that denied them opportunities to meet these needs.

It is precisely for these reasons that there is an emergence of Islam in the African American community. Increasingly, all Islamic sects are challenging the African American Christian church for the mind and soul of its youth. The Muslim religion is attractive to an increasing number of young people because of the redefined roles of men and women in the home and in the religious life of the sect. There is a strong emphasis on the equality of individuals without regard for gender. But each gender is assigned a role considered proper for itself. This redefinition seems to meet self-esteem needs. However, this religious group makes up only approximately 11% of practicing religious African Americans. Refer to the Answering Islam Website for more information by Edgerly and Ellis about a Christian-Muslim dialogue, www.answering-islam.org.

National polls on religion have long shown that African Americans are more religious in thought and behavior than other Americans. The media have reported that 82% of African Americans say that religion is very important in their lives. The level of religious commitment among African Americans who described themselves as very or fairly religious according to the Surgeon General's Supplemental Report on Mental Health was almost 85% of the population. Prayer was the most commonly identified coping strategy (114). This collective use of religion or religious practices as a coping strategy, according to the study by Matoni and colleagues, was positively linked to the positive self-esteem of the African American youth when compared to Caucasian youth (64).

The practice of spiritualism's use of God or spirits as a form of help and healing is central to the African American experience. Spiritual powers are evident in the praying to God or a higher power, the calling on of forces seen and unseen, laying on of hands, and all other acts of spiritual beliefs.

*This section contributed by Sylvia Adams, MSN, CNS-BC and Pamela Talley, MSN, CNS-BC, CSAC II.

MediaLink Answering Islam

The influence of spiritual and religious leaders, communities, and social networks for psychological support often leads to a delay in seeking professional mental health services (6). Self-professed religious African American women were less likely to seek mental health services than those who did not identify themselves as religious (43). African Americans historically do not seek assistance from resources external to the family system for psychological support. However, the exception is the spiritual and religious connection. The African American church has helped African Americans cope with a harsh life through benevolent associations, mutual aid societies, and informal support networks (40).

Leininger's Theory of Cultural Care Diversity and Universality identifies the role of the nurse in performing an in-depth assessment of the client, which includes the patterns and lifestyle of the client. The theory especially emphasizes the cultural mores and norms (57). Several assessment tools may be helpful in assessing the African American client when religious and spiritual treatment planning is relevant. *Tools that show good validity and reliability are the* (a) Systems of Belief Inventory-Revised (SBI-15R), (b) Index of Core Spiritual Experiences (INSPIRIT), and (c) Brief RCOPE (99). A holistic approach will support goal achievement and therapeutic treatment outcomes. Peplau's Theory of Interpersonal Relations, described in Chapter 2, ∞ signifies the importance of the ability to interact and relate to the religious and spiritual factors that impact the well-being of the individual seeking mental health services, health promotion, or care during physical illness (83).

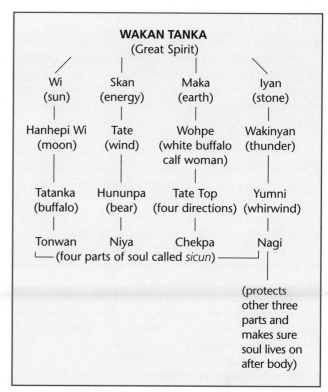

FIGURE ■ 7-2 Wakan Tanka (Great Spirit).

NORTH AMERICAN INDIAN RELIGIONS

The **North American Indian religions** developed for centuries with very little influence from outside the continent. Power, a supreme being, guardian spirits, totems, fasting, visions, **shamanism** (*belief in a priest who can influence good and evil spirits*), myth telling, and ritualism are all part of a varied belief system. The location of the tribal group influenced its belief system. Indians of the Far North, the Northeast Woodlands, the Southeast Woodlands, the Plains, the Northwest Coast, California, the Intermountain Region, and the Southwest make up the main tribal divisions.

Yet *all belief systems have certain features in common* (34): (a) a **spirit world**—*a dimension that permeates life but is different*; (b) a **supreme being**—*the God who represents other lesser deities*; (c) a **culture hero**—*a spirit who competes with the Great Spirit and who sometimes is a trickster*; (d) spirits and ghosts, such as atmospheric spirits (wind) or underworld powers (snakes); (e) guardian spirits acquired by visions seen during fasting; (f) medicine men and medicine societies; (g) ritual acts, such as the sun dance; and (h) prayers and offerings.

A direct descendant from the Oglala Sioux outlines the belief of the Makaha (34). The **Great Spirit**, or **Wakan Tanka**, *which is in all and throughout all, manifests itself in 16 powers.* See Figure 7-2■. Note that people (who have souls) rank at the bottom. This explains the reverence for aspects of nature and animals (44). Harmony or spiritual balance is what North American Indians want to achieve in their relations with the supernatural powers.

When caring for an American Indian, it is wise to obtain access to the spiritual leader from that particular region and his or her tribe nation. Many healing rituals are kept secret, so the health care provider can be most effective by making the appropriate connection, rather than by trying to intervene in the belief system. The medicine wheel is a holistic symbol that should be included in intervention (34).

OTHER SPIRITUAL MOVEMENTS
New Age

The **New Age** *is a current American spirituality movement. Belief is pantheistic and does not dwell on sin or evil. All humans are considered all good. God is in everything.* In contrast, Christianity believes humans are sinful and saved by God through Jesus. However, both approaches make use of optimism, holism, and synergism. The New Age movement, however, has a commitment to self and individualism, the future, and transformation of self and society (13, 75, 93). Despite the name, some of the philosophies and practices are generally old (41, 93) such as astrology, vision questing (41, 93), and use of positive thinking (81, 82). Inspiration is drawn from early European religions. New Agers do not imitate authentic American Indian religious traditions because of past tribal criticism for their imitations. Instead, **channeling**, *direct communication with spirits*, work with one's "inner child," or past, and a variety of other newer unconventional healing techniques are used. Biofeedback, meditation, and autosuggestion can be helpful adjuncts to healing (41, 75).

Holistic nursing or health care may incorporate some New Age practices even while using practices from other religions (75). Be aware of the philosophy base from which you he or she practice and the client's preferences and beliefs.

Neo-paganism

Neo-paganism *is another current movement in American spirituality: Pagan expressions revive pre-Christian forms of spirituality* as an antidote to the perceived rigidity of Christianity and its perceived disregard for the natural environment (9, 75). Group members seek spiritual meaning in ancient traditions. Specific identities include experience as Druids, Wiccans, witches, fairies, practitioners of the "craft," and worship of "the Goddess." Sometimes denominations are formed, for example the New Reformed Orthodox Order of the Golden Dawn. Neo-pagan worship is ritualistic, secretive, and connects with nature. In-depth information is available in the article by Michael Brown (9). He also cites other people who immersed themselves in neo-paganism in order to do research (9).

Your role is that of astute client assessment, consultation with other professionals during intervention as appropriate, and community educator. The client may or may not express these beliefs. Or the client's visitors in the hospital may make unusual-sounding requests related to their "interventions." Your role is patient or client safety, to be respectful toward the client, and to consult with other health care professionals as appropriate.

Agnosticism and Atheism

This chapter has concentrated so far on worship of God, the divine or other positive spirits, with an emphasis on traditional teaching. Some people live by ethical standards, considering themselves either **agnostic**, *incapable of knowing whether God exists*, or **atheistic**, *believing that God does not exist.*

Cults

Various *cults* have gained publicity since the 1970s. Some older cults are based on fundamental religions, but they are unique in their own way. The Snake People, for example, incorporate the holding of snakes into their services. Newer cults have arisen from communal groups whose goals are stated as religious. Some cults spring from the philosophy and schedule of a self-chosen leader who entices youth, in search of identity, from their parents and formalized church. Attention has focused on cults that are attracting not only the young but also the elders (67, 75, 100, 111). Sexual abuse of women and children in cults is a common story, both as

part of initiation into the cult and as part of their ongoing role. Cults are a phenomenon in many countries.

Singer gives a comprehensive description of cult life historically and currently (100). She defines **cult** as *any group that forms around a person who claims he or she has a special mission or knowledge, which will be shared by those who turn over their decision making to the self-appointed leader.* Cults vary in philosophy, purpose, power, and structure.

Cults have the following characteristics (67, 108, 111):

1. Rigid belief system that cannot be questioned.
2. Charismatic, authoritarian leader who claims to have a new vision or truth, and exercises total control, including physical, emotional, and sexual abuse.
3. Isolation of the person from family of origin and nonmembers, which is considered detrimental to the person's total obedience.
4. Demanding schedule, focus on group-centered activities, and extreme peer pressure and conformity.
5. Deceptive recruitment, extreme emotional manipulation, and abuse to recruit and retain members.
6. Privileges or material goods and comforts granted to the leader but denied the members.
7. Members are expected to relinquish all financial assets and personal property to the group.

Singer describes how cults work: how they recruit people, their physically and psychologically persuasive techniques, the thought reform that occurs, their intrusion into the workplace and general society, the difficulty in leaving a cult, and their harassment of critics, citizens, and even state and national governments (100). As a psychologist who has counseled thousands of people who experienced cult life, she describes at length how we can help survivors escape and recover. The effects of the abuse and forced neglect on the children and their parents and the guilt of adults about the behavior they participated in without choice, even when devastating, can be overcome. Exit counseling, deprogramming, support, love, and understanding—over time—are necessary. Postcult adjustment involves every aspect of life. Comprehensive health care is essential to help the person regain identity (100). Melton (68) also gives in-depth information.

INTERVENTIONS FOR HEALTH PROMOTION

Wright (126) discusses *ethical principles that must be practiced with all people as follows:*

1. **Beneficence:** *the duty to do no harm.* Give of self wholeheartedly in interactions with patients or clients because this positive action is beneficial.
2. **Nonmaleficence:** *constraint from doing harm to another.* Do not judge another's beliefs. However, you can share your beliefs in a nonjudgmental way as you provide care

in the spiritual dimension if deemed appropriate by the client.

3. **Autonomy:** *the right of patient or client self-determination.* Assess who desires spiritual care and avoid imposing your own ideas.
4. **Advocacy:** *actively assist the person in exercising autonomy,* to find meaning, hope, and clarification of personal beliefs and values.

Be aware of and teach parents the *behaviors or symptoms that indicate someone is under the influence of a cult* (68, 92, 100):

1. Personality changes that are not associated with normal development, extremely secretive
2. Extreme shifts in vocabulary, beliefs, and values, inability to make decisions (must consult the cult leader)
3. Extreme persistent dietary and sleep changes, refusal to attend family events, ignoring prior patterns
4. Violation of law or justification of antisocial acts (which further the cult's cause—the most dangerous sign)
5. Stockpiling of firearms, poisons, or weapons

A cult member may never come to a traditional health care setting. Yet, emergency services may be needed. It is problematic if the cult leader prevents necessary care or if manifestations of child abuse or neglect are observed. The policies of the health care agency and state laws must be followed. Protection for staff, other patients or clients, family members, and visitors must be implemented if the person is admitted to the care unit.

Devil or **Satan worship** is also practiced as a cult. The satanic bible was reportedly written by Anton Szandor LaVey, who was part of the Church of Satan in San Francisco. The basic beliefs encompass power or energy in souls and bodies of animals and humans that can be absorbed through rituals. Rituals can be nature oriented or sometimes macabre when they involve murder, dismembering body parts of animals and humans, and eating body organs. One young man spoke of how he became a precocious student of Satan. He read dozens of books on Satan as "Light-Bearer, the strongest and wisest angel in heaven, robbed of his rightful worship by a jealous God." He spoke of putting a hex on others, drinking ghoulish concoctions, and being obsessed with certain rites as he moved through the hierarchy to priesthood (100).

Signs associated with satanism are "666," an upside-down cross, the word *Satan*, a picture of a horned beast, skulls, hoods, goat heads, reversed words (*natas*), ashes, and obsession with black, such as a black room and black candles (100). Symbols and signs vary with the geographic area. Unusual visual presentations are a clue.

Adolescents are most likely to investigate satanism. Usually they are unsure of their identity, need a group to accept them, and can find a sense of power in the rituals. Occasionally a teenager or college student will appear to have one life of being an outgoing honor student and another life of occult satanism. Cults may be of temporary interest with imitation of hair and clothing (100).

Be aware of satanic signs or items when caring for patients or clients. Counselors, psychiatrists, and some ministers and priests have had to deal with devil possession in treating clients. Although professionals do not often speak in these terms in today's scientific age, devil possession is a recurring theme in clients' self-diagnosis and one that you should listen for, with the new wave of interest in psychic occultism and witchcraft and their various practices.

Voodoo

Voodoo, witchcraft, and magic *are integral to folk medicine.* **Voodoo** *is a religious cult practice that dates back to preslavery days in West Africa. A dominant belief is that the person is surrounded by a variety of powerful spirits* (good and bad). It is important to be

have in a way that maintains contact with good spirits and avoids contact with bad, evil, or demonic spirits. People of various ethnic groups as well as descendants of West Africa practice this belief system, especially residents of the rural Southern United States, the islands off the Georgia and South Carolina coasts, and Haiti, as well as Haitians living in the United States (3, 11, 12, 33).

Voodoo illness *involves the belief that illness or death may occur as a result of a supernatural force.* Various terms are used interchangeably with voodoo, including *rootwork, hex, black magic, witchcraft, spell,* and *conjuring.* **Rootwork** *is part of the voodoo system associated with putting a hex on a person so he or she has good or bad experiences.* There is a "misery hex" and a "lucky hex." Bags with dirt and roots may be hidden on a person's property. Mediating these experiences is a root doctor who can cast or remove spells (3, 11, 33, 40, 42). Several authors describe the history of voodoo illness, the nonacceptance of Western medicine by voodoo believers, how the nurse may assess for this cultural phenomenon, and relevant nursing interventions for these clients, who are usually of African Haitian, West African, or African American descent (3, 11, 12, 33).

Acknowledge the belief system, even if it seems illogical. Related practices may provide physical or emotional comfort. Take time to learn what the client has tried prior to coming to the health care facility, which is often an emergency or last-resort situation. Gently assist the client and family to build trust and to recognize how you can help the client become a "stronger" person. Explain what medical or nursing care practice may be used (instead of the apparently harmful one previously used) to help the client become "stronger" in this *specific situation.* Thus, you avoid confrontation about folk and scientific belief systems and apparent rejection of the person. Some practices can be retained, such as keeping nonpoisonous leaves inside the garment next to the body. Explain if they must be moved or removed because of an incision or infusion site or other treatments. Work with the cultural healer to avoid casting of bad hexes or spells on the client. Foster in the client a sense of strength, self-help, independence, and positive self-esteem. Work with staff to maintain culturally and spiritually sensitive care (3, 11, 33).

Health Promotion and Nursing Applications

Ideally, religion provides strength, an inner calm and faith with which to work through life's problems. But be prepared to see the negative aspect. To some, religion seems to add guilt, depression, and confusion. Some may blame God for making them ill, for letting them suffer, or for not healing them in a prescribed manner. One Protestant believed she had made a contract with God; if she lived the best Christian life she could, God would keep her relatively well and free from tragedy. When an incurable disease was diagnosed, she said. "What did I do to deserve this?" Another Protestant, during her illness, took the opposite view of her contract with God. She said, "I wasn't living as well as I should and God knocked me down to let me know I was backsliding." Other clients view disease as "something that happens to people" (54).

Healing, too, has varied meanings. Some will demand that God provide a quick and miraculous recovery, whereas others expect the

The foregoing information may help you define your personal spirituality and belief system. Even more basic as understanding these concepts is respecting your client as a person with spiritual needs who may or may not want them addressed specifically. Yet, during illness or times of crisis, the spiritual dimension may become a major focus, even if it's suppressed in daily life. You are not expected to be a professional spiritual leader, but your approach, interest, and willingness to talk about spirituality or religious beliefs may be comforting. Do not evangelize, overwhelm, or antagonize. Further, no one will respect your spiritual aid if you do not appear thoughtful and competent in your work. Take time to prepare yourself for encounters with the spiritual dimension through literature, media programs, peer discussions, and following a plan to clarify your beliefs, either within or outside of a specific religious denomination.

process to occur through the work of the health team. Still others combine God's touch, the health providers' skill, and their own emotional and physical cooperation. Some even consider death as the final form of healing.

Sometimes you must deal with your own negative reactions. Your medical background and knowledge may cause dismay at some religious practices. For instance, a postoperative Jehovah's Witness client might die because she has refused blood. Or you might believe that a Christian Scientist client should have sought medical help a month ago to avoid present complications. Here is an explanation given by a Christian Scientist nurse: "People can be ruined psychologically by going against a long-held belief. They may live and get better physically but will suffer depression, guilt, and failure in not holding to their standard." Basically the person may prefer to die. Should you dictate otherwise? Think through and discuss such situations with a spiritual leader.

ASSESSMENT

Utilize information related to specific religions from this chapter, **Table C7-1** on the Companion Website, and questions posed in **Table 7-2**. However, these are only a basis. Accept each client's individual spiritual development. *Assessment of spiritual needs should be done as part of the nursing history.* Depending on the physical or mental status of the patient or client, the assessment may need to be modified or delayed (91). Essential questions can be directed to a family member, if present, especially if the person is seriously injured or near death. *Spiritual needs are related to the individual, others, and the transcendental* (59, 105). *Needs related to the individual person include to* (a) find meaning and purpose, (b) feel useful, (c) have vision and hope, (d) be supported in coping with life transitions, (e) adapt to increasing dependency, (f) transcend life's challenges, (g) maintain personal dignity, (h) express feelings, (i) have fellowship with others, (j) love, serve, and be forgiven, (k) have continuity with the past, and (l) prepare for and accept death. *Needs related to others include to* (a) forgive others, (b) cope with loss of loved ones, (c) be responsible toward others, (d) know what and when to give and take, and (e) be respected. *Needs related to the transcendental include to* (a) know there is a God or an ultimate power, (b) believe God is loving and present, (c) serve and worship God, and (d) learn the scripture or sources inspired by God.

Spiritual need is defined as *lack of any factor necessary to establish or maintain a dynamic, personal relationship with God, or a higher being, as defined by the individual.* Four areas of concern can

TABLE 7-2

Questions for Spiritual Assessment

1. What is your concept of God? What is your God like? (Or, what is your religion? Tell me about it.)
2. Do you believe that God or someone is concerned for you?
3. Who is the most important person to you? Is that person available?
4. Has being sick (what has been happening to you) made any difference in your feelings about God? In the practice of your faith? If it has, could you explain how it has changed?
5. Do you believe that your faith is helpful to you? If it is, how? If it is not, why not?
6. Are there any religious beliefs, practices, or rituals that are important to you now? If there are, could you tell me about them? May I help you carry them out by showing you where the chapel is? By telling the dietary department about your vegetarian preference? By allowing you specific times for prayer or meditation?
7. Is there anything that would make your situation easier? (Such as a visit from the minister, priest, rabbi, or chaplain? Someone who would read to you? Time for reading your religious book or praying? Someone to pray with you?)
8. Is prayer important to you? (If so, has being sick made a difference in your practice of praying?) What happens when you pray?
9. Do you have available religious books or articles such as the Bible, prayer books, phylacteries, or a crucifix that mean something to you?
10. What are your ideas about illness? About life after death?
11. Is there anything especially frightening or meaningful to you right now?
12. If these questions have not uncovered your source of spiritual support, can you tell me where you do find support?

be covered later in the interview as part of assessment after the client feels safe with the nurse. *The following are assessment areas:*

1. Person's concept of God or deity
2. Person's source of strength and hope
3. Significance of religious practices and rituals
4. Perceived relationship between spiritual beliefs and current state of health

Espeland describes reflective questions to use in spiritual assessment that relate to several components of spirituality: meaning to life, relationship with a higher power, sense of hope, need for encouragement and caring, use of meditation, spiritual goals, and forgiveness (26).

During this part of the assessment, be prepared for any answer. The agnostic or atheist may answer with as much depth and meaning from his or her perspective as someone with a specific religious background. The person who is part of a formal religion may not answer freely, reserving such conversation for the spiritual leader or hesitating until the nurse is better known to the client.

Realize people may use the same words but have different meanings. For example, *saved, sanctified, fell out, slain by the Holy Spirit,* and *deathbed conversion* all connote religious experiences. Listen carefully. Clarify as necessary. In response to a question about religious preference, the client may say he or she attends a 12-step program with Alcoholics Anonymous (AA) to overcome addiction and build spiritual strength. Or the person may explain that the family of four attends four different denominations.

When *determining medical background,* such as drug or food allergies, ask about religious dietary laws, rituals, or restrictions that are important. Beliefs about work, money, family, child rearing, right and wrong, or political behavior may also convey spiritual beliefs or needs that are relevant to care and recovery.

In *primary care, the FICA approach can incorporate a spiritual history into assessment* (61, 62):

F—Faith: How important is faith, religion, or spirituality?

I—Influence: Does religious faith or spirituality influence health care practices?

C—Community: Is the person a part of any religious or spiritual community or congregation?

A—Address: Should religious or spiritual issues or concerns be addressed with the person?

Because your relationship with the person may be of short duration, it is important to *document well the results of this interview.* Later, assess for religious or spiritual needs that may be expressed through nonreligious language. Let the client know what options are open for spiritual help. If you hide behind busyness and procedures, you may lose a valuable opportunity to aid in health promotion and restoration.

The discussion of social class and cultural differences in Chapter 5 ∞ applies to some religious differences. For instance, a poor Protestant American who has grown up with the barest survival materials and who has no economic power, no money for recreation, no hope for significant gain, and no positive attitude about this life may center his or her whole being in the church. It provides as best it can for emotional, recreational, and spiritual needs. When the person sings about heaven in terms of having beautiful clothes, a crown, and a mansion, he or she is singing with a much different meaning than the wealthy Protestant American who is really more concerned about mansions here than over there.

Table 7-3 presents guidelines to assist you in assessment of the African American client. *The guidelines are useful for work with all people* (8, 40, 57, 115). The clergyman is a major leader in the African American community and is perceived as a community leader by other populations as well. This person can also assist you in assessment.

NURSING DIAGNOSIS

A major diagnostic category is **spiritual distress**, *the impaired ability to experience and integrate meaning and purpose in life through the person's connections with self, others, art, music, literature, nature, or a power greater than oneself* (73). *The person experiences or could experience a disturbance in the belief system that is usually a source of strength.* This problem may be related to not being able to practice spiritual rituals or may be caused by a conflict between spiritual beliefs and the health regimen. See the **Box** Nursing Diagnoses Related to the Spiritual Dimension (89).

INTERVENTION

Hospital accreditation requires that spiritual care be provided to all patients (126). The International Council of Nurses and the American Nurses Association have declared through their codes of ethics that nurses should promote an environment in which the values, customs, and spiritual beliefs of individuals be respected (126). Wright describes the ethical, professional, and legal responsibilities for spiritual care (126).

Spirituality is an integral part of holistic health care. Several authors write how prayer and faith enable them to better implement the nursing process and give holistic care—physical, emotional, sociocultural, and spiritual (61, 62, 92, 105). Fostering hope, acceptance, and self-transcendence is associated with a positive treatment outcome (37). Nurses can only cooperate in spiritual care; they cannot dictate it. *Spiritual needs will differ from person to person and from culture to culture* (3, 33, 49). Spiritual care must be personalized to meet spiritual needs and can be given within the brief time period of acute illness when such intervention is combined with routine care by a nurse who is comfortable with the spiritual dimension (23, 49, 104). Some spiritual interventions may not be desired or may be refused because they seem intrusive or conflict with beliefs (23, 108, 109). **Table 7-3** presents guidelines for spiritual care interventions for one group of believers, African American clients. These guidelines are applicable, to some extent, with all clients.

Spiritual care is presented and received in a context in which the recipient is physically and emotionally vulnerable and thereby receptive to the spiritual perspective. Spiritual care is part of giving culturally competent care because often the belief system is closely related to the person's culture, as described in Chapter 5. ∞ Establish a trusting relationship and show concern. *Sometimes spiritual care means to* (a) look into another person's

TABLE 7-3

Assessment and Intervention with the African American Client

1. Faith, tradition, experience, and current reality are intertwined for the religious or spiritual person. Let the person know you realize the importance of spiritual and religious experiences.
2. An open approach and environment allows the person to feel comfortable and encourages self-disclosure. Engage in small talk. Be genuine and friendly in your verbal and nonverbal behavior.
3. Call the adult person, especially someone older than you, by the appropriate title, Miss, Mrs., Ms., or Mr., and his or her last name until the client says you may use the first name.
4. Do not attempt to impress the person with how much you know or act "too professional." If the client questions your credentials, it may be an indication that you are perceived as unapproachable, noncaring, or not understanding, and the person is unlikely to respond to your questions or suggestions.
5. Inquire on how the church has been *important to the person* in meeting needs.
6. Be straightforward as you inquire about the worldviews based on religious or folk beliefs and practices. Listen for taboos, or what you consider superstitions or myths; realize these are part of the worldview.
7. Inquire about beliefs and practices. Expect to hear the spiritual person say that he or she prays to God and believes that God has healing power, which the health care system often does not.
8. Realize that religious and spiritual beliefs are not delusions and that lifestyle rituals that are frequently practiced are not obsessions. Do not evaluate the cultural and spiritual norm as pathology.
9. Do not challenge or argue with beliefs and practices. To do so causes a feeling of mistrust and diminishes or destroys the therapeutic relationship.
10. Demonstrate concern, assess, and provide treatment for the current problem; do not focus on past behaviors or individual and family history.
11. Ask about sources of help the person has used to solve past problems, and in a matter-of-fact way, use the words "spiritualism," "faith," "spirituality," or "spirits."
12. Ask if there is a phrase, motto, proverb, scripture, song, or religious teaching that helps the person determine how to live.
13. Inquire if there are family or friends who have qualities especially admired or whom the person uses as a role model for behavior. Ask for details about the qualities, as these are a clue to behaviors.
14. Ask what or who in the past helped most at the time when there was a physical or emotional problem.
15. Inquire if the person has ever been healed without the help of a doctor after praying or attending a religious church service.
16. If a trusting, caring relationship does not appear to be developing, a discussion about spiritual issues must take place immediately in the assessment or intervention.
17. Engage the person in problem identification, interventions, and goals of care. Seek consultation from people or sources that have helped the client in the past, including the persons's clergy or spiritual leader or the person's church.
18. Realize that if the client feels uneasy with your approach, questions, or suggestions, he or she believes you cannot help and will not keep the next appointment.
19. The African American may share responsibility with (or blame) the provider when treatment is not considered successful.
20. Assess your own attitude in relation to cultural preconceptions, beliefs contradictory to the client's beliefs, and disagreements in role perceptions. Don't act as if you understand or agree when you do not.
21. Seek resources in your community and from the literature to help understand the client's spiritual beliefs.
22. Cultural caring, using Leininger's Theory of Culture Care Diversity and Universality, should be the essence of the therapeutic relationship from the beginning to the end.
23. Assessment and intervention should focus on basic needs, using Maslow's Theory of Hierarchy of Needs.

This material was contributed by Sylvia Adams, MSN, CNS-BC, and Pamela Talley, MSN, CNS-BC, CSAC II.

eyes; (b) remain quiet; (c) convey empathy and deep caring by listening, touching a hand or arm, or giving a hug; (d) demonstrate a willingness to be with the other in their pain; and (e) show we "ache with them" as we give the best possible holistic care (23).

Be careful about sharing personal experiences or beliefs. It may be appropriate. Often it is not. The patient wants the nurse to be present and respectful. Most patients or clients appreciate having their spirituality supported by the caregiver, but on their own terms

(108, 109). For example, Deller (21) describes how she, a Christian nurse, was able to combine spiritual and physical care and comfort for a Muslim woman, for whom English was a second language, by saying a few Arabic words. One word, *Du'a*, is an Arabic word for a prayer asking for a blessing and comfort, for God/Allah to meet the person's needs and to strengthen and grant peace. Both nurse and patient understood the meaning of this prayer said by the nurse.

Nursing Diagnoses Related to the Spiritual Dimension

Anxiety
Decisional **C**onflict
Ineffective **C**oping
Fear
Grieving
Hopelessness
Risk for **L**oneliness

Powerlessness
Impaired **R**eligiosity
Social Isolation
Chronic **S**orrow
Spiritual Distress
Readiness for Enhanced **S**piritual Well-Being

Source: Reference 73.

Guidelines for Intervention to Promote Spiritual Health

Certain norms for providing spiritual care must be followed:

1. Do not impose personal beliefs on clients or families. A clinic or other health care agency, or a sickbed or deathbed is not a proper place or time for proselytizing.
2. Respond to the person out of his or her own background. Use knowledge about that background, but avoid acting on stereotypes. (For example, "all Catholics believe this" or "all Hindus do this.")
3. If you cannot give the spiritual support being asked for by the person, enlist someone who can.

The clergy, the person designated as family healer, a trusted friend, or even a nondenominational prayer telephone number or e-mail address may be referrals for the client and family. However, a phone line, Internet acquaintances, or a chat room may not take the place of direct contact with people.

Kumar describes spiritual care across cultures (53). *Validate the appropriateness of proposed interventions* with the client. For example, ask if the person wishes you to pray with him or her about the concerns that have been voiced. The person can then accept or reject your offer.

Spiritual support can be given to the *ill and dying* person in various ways. A warm, empathic, and caring human relationship is essential. Respect for the person's beliefs, willingness to discuss spiritual matters, and providing for rituals and sacraments of religion are important. Be open to others' religious and philosophic beliefs. *You may be uncomfortable discussing spiritual matters, yet it may be helpful for the client if you try to overcome personal reluctance to discuss spiritual concerns.* Often the intimacy of spiritual concerns is discussed by the client during the intimacy of physical care. Helping the person ask questions and seek solutions does not mean that you have to supply the answers.

With the dying client, the aspects of spiritual support considered most helpful are (a) calling the person directly by name, (b) talking directly to the person (realize everything may be heard by the dying person), and (c) supporting the family by staying with them as they say good-bye. Let family members know they can touch their dying loved one, offer condolences, and offer to help them in any appropriate way.

Spiritual care of the person with mental illness is often overlooked (47, 84, 87, 88, 95). Assessment must determine whether the person is describing a religious delusion, something most people would consider false, such as "I am Jesus Christ" or "I am Mohammed," or stating conflicts between religious beliefs and rituals and the current situation or feelings. Such statements may sound like and be labeled as delusions, but the *nursing diagnosis of spiritual distress* would be more appropriate. The spiritual components that you can address through listening and counseling are the person's sense of not being loved by others, of having no meaning or purpose in life, and of feeling unforgiven or not being able to forgive another. These issues take time to resolve. Referral to clergy may be indicated.

Be alert to subtle clues that indicate desire to talk about spiritual matters, need for expressions of love and hope, desire for your silent presence, and acceptance of behavior when the client labels self as bad. The client may have experienced anger, resentment, and guilt in relationships; these feelings may contribute to symptoms or illness. Help clients understand the *importance of and need for forgiveness.* Forgiveness involves renouncing the hold of anger, resentment, and grudges and increasing empathy for the other person (28, 38, 107). *Counseling and mental and spiritual methods can be combined* to help the client heal hurtful or traumatic memories, forgive self or others, work through unresolved grief, promote healing within self, and establish healthier relationships with others.

Communication and a team approach between health care providers and pastoral care representatives are essential. You can fill that gap. Such rapport can mean that the whole person is served.

Maintain a list of available spiritual leaders, know when to call them, and know how to prepare for their arrival. If a client cannot make the request, consult with the family. One woman said, "If my sister sees a priest, she will be sure she is dying." Once a health care provider took the initiative to call an Eastern Orthodox priest who, unfortunately, represented the wrong nationality; the client's main source of comfort was to have come from discussion and prayers in the native language.

Help the person maintain religious practices and worship. Prepare the client and the setting for a spiritual leader. Create an atmosphere that reflects more than sterile procedure. Privacy is important. Cheerful surroundings, such as sunshine, flowers, lighted candles, openness, and participation by family and staff, may be important.

INTERVENTIONS FOR HEALTH PROMOTION

Nine **combinations of client behavior that call for conferring with or referring to a spiritual leader,** *unless contraindicated by the care plan, are:*

1. Withdrawn, sullen, silent, depressed.
2. Restless, irritable, complaining.
3. Aggressive, excitable, garrulous, wants to talk a lot.
4. Shows, by word or other signs, undue curiosity, anxiety about self.
5. Becomes worse or critical, a terminal condition.
6. Shows conversational interest and curiosity in religious questions, issues; reads scripture.
7. Inquires specifically about chaplain, chapel worship, scripture.
8. Has few or no visitors; has no cards, flowers.
9. Has had, or faces, particularly traumatic or threatening surgical procedure.

Perhaps the client and spiritual leader could *meet outdoors in a garden area.* The *Shintoist and Taoist would especially benefit from the aesthetic exposure.* If the client is a *child* with a *prolonged hospitalization, a special area might be designated for religious instruction.* Assist in preparing the client for prayer time, a visit to a chapel or a chapel service, or the Sabbath ritual. Work with the health care team to provide the factors that are important to the client, such as rituals or diet; quiet and privacy; arranging flowers, prayer books, or relics; group work or visitors; reading materials; or family relationships. For some people, art, music, complementary therapies (presented in Chapter 2), ∞ or a walk in a garden (or gardening) can be part of a therapeutic milieu and meet spiritual needs.

Keep one or more calendars of various religious holidays. The Eastern Orthodox Easter usually does not coincide with the Roman Catholic and Protestant Easter. Jewish holidays usually do not fall on the same dates of the Western calendar in successive years. Remember, also, that holidays are family days and that ill people separated from the family at such times may be especially depressed.

Many will benefit from the sacraments, prayers, scripture reading, and counseling given by the spiritual leader and health care providers. However, some patients or clients will want to rely on their own direct communication with God. The *Zen Buddhist, Hindu, Muslim, and Friend might be in this category.* All may want reading material, however. Most will bring their sacred book with them, but if they express a desire for more literature, offer to get it. Some hospitals furnish daily and weekly meditations and a Bible.

Occasionally it may be helpful to give scripture references for various stated spiritual needs. For example, reference to love and relatedness can be found in Psalm 23, reference to forgiveness in Matthew 6:9–15, and reference to meaning and purpose in Acts 1:8. Or you may share books or magazines. A positive interfaith magazine is *Guideposts* (Guideposts Associates). Some novels and books for children, spiritually inspiring books, and journals, including *Journal of Christian Nursing,* are available for use by clients and health care providers. Some clients may prefer devotional literature from their therapy groups, such as Alcoholics (Narcotics, Overeaters, Gamblers) Anonymous (102).

Shared prayer, if it is accepted by the client, counteracts the loneliness of illness or dying by offering the person intimacy with a supreme being and another person without the need for confession. It can be a means of bringing both human and divine love. It

holds transcendent qualities and conveys both present and future hope. Prayer can focus on the conditions or emotions that the client is unable to talk about, allowing the person to handle the matter or vent in another way. Prayer should promote closeness, through closed eyes and hands that touch. Prayer should not strip the person of defenses. Nor should prayers be recited as a way to avoid the person or avoid questions raised by the person. Some health care providers express that when they pray with patients, they benefit as much as the patients.

Use of life review can foster developmental, emotional, and spiritual maturity (not only in the elder and dying person). Encourage the person to reminisce about past life experiences. Memories can be pleasurable or painful, but recalling them with a skilled listener can help resolve those ridden with shame, guilt, anger, or other feelings. Past sources of strength can also be identified, and sometimes they are useful in the present situation. Chapter 16 ∞ presents more information on reminiscence and life review. Music can also be used to lift depression, convey calm, stimulate hope and joy, and promote physical and mental healing.

Atheists should not be neglected because they do not profess a belief in God. They have the same need for respect and the transcendental as everyone else and may need someone to listen to fears and doubts. The person does need your understanding and ethical practices.

Various groups refuse medical or hospital treatment for illness, including members of *Fundamentalist or Holiness groups, Jehovah's*

Practice Point

If you feel comfortable doing so, you can at times say a prayer, read a scripture, or provide a statement of faith helpful to the client. If you do not feel comfortable in providing this kind of spiritual care, you can still meet the client's spiritual needs through respectful conversation, listening to the client talk about beliefs, referral to another staff member, or calling one of the client's friends who can bolster his or her faith. If spiritual leaders are not available, you could organize a group of health workers willing to counsel with or make referrals for clients of their own faiths.

Witnesses, Amish, and *Christian Scientists.* Realize that if adults refuse treatment for themselves or their children, they are not deliberately choosing death. They are rejecting something objectionable, based on their beliefs (58). *If at all possible, offer acceptable alternative treatments. Jehovah's Witnesses* accept intravenous normal saline solution and various other nonblood products. Members of *rural Fundamentalist sects and the Amish* are often willing to go to chiropractors and allow physicians to set fractures and suture lacerations. Nurses may teach nutritional therapy or various stress management or relaxation techniques. Sometimes parents accept the services of a home health nurse for their child, even though they refuse hospital and formal medical treatment.

Steen and Anderson (103) describe *specific care measures for children from various faiths.* Parents from different ethnic groups may request measures that reflect their belief systems. Requests should be accommodated when possible. Explanation is necessary if the measure is not safe for the child or if it must be modified (103). For example, the parent may request that the *shaman* give the child holy water to drink before surgery to foster healing. If the child is to receive no liquids orally, it may be acceptable to the parents and shaman to sponge holy water on the child to protect from evil spirits. A nursing concern may be related to placement of intravenous needles and a requested shaman practice (103).

Steen and Anderson describe faith practices and traditions for children from *Hmong, Orthodox Jewish, American Indian, Roman Catholic,* and *Muslim* families (103). They also describe the importance of the folk spiritual healer, such as a shaman or medicine man in any setting, including hospital, nursing home, hospice, school, industry, clinic, home, or other health center (103). Ott, Al-Khadhuri, and Al-Junalbi discuss Islamic health care issues pertinent to care of children (76).

Role of Faith Communities in Intervention*

Churches or faith communities contribute to health promotion. Churches have been a refuge for people of all faiths throughout the centuries, and they have been and still are a major center for health promotion.

Westberg (120) said, "The church is a healing community . . . engaged in keeping people well" (p. 189), which was accomplished by particular qualities found in a faith community that were not usually present in the modern scientific medical model of health services. The qualities were the power of group dynamics, inspirational experiences, and caring fellow humans. *Faith communities have contributed to health promotion in two ways* (46, 65, 100, 118): (a) by the generic nature of the faith community, and (b) by intentional, planned activities to address health issues in the faith community and in the larger community.

Atkins reported findings from four integrated qualitative case studies conducted in a community of 5,000 people in four mainstream Christian denominations. These churches did not have a parish nurse. Participants reported they experienced spiritual, mental, emotional, and physical health as a result of their church attendance, faith and prayer, friendships and fellowship, moral and religious teachings, youth groups, and community service. Members saw the need and shared the responsibility for

providing the healing community that was engaged in keeping people well (4).

Although most research addressing the role of churches in health promotion has studied adults, a significant study involved youth populations. The Search Institute surveyed nearly 47,000 sixth to twelfth graders in 111 U.S. communities (79, 94). Adolescents who reported a positive family life, positive school experiences, participation in structured youth activities, and a feeling of belonging to a church or synagogue were six times less likely to report drinking, riding with someone who was drinking, and participating in early sexual activities (94). Based on these findings, Search Institute identified 40 developmental assets for youth and tips for incorporating these assets into the congregation activities. More information is available at the Search Institute Website, wwwsearchinstitute.org.

A survey of 5,000 high school seniors indicated religious youth, compared to their peers, were less likely to engage in risky behaviors, such as carrying weapons, fighting, drinking and driving, and marijuana use. The relationship persisted after controlling for demographic variables, as well as over time (106). Some dimensions of religiousness in adolescent girls have been associated with sexually responsible behavior (64, 70). A survey of 1,098 African American and Caucasian adolescents suggested suicide risk was modified by commitment to core, lifesaving religious beliefs (35).

The modern role of the nurse in faith communities has been reported since the mid-1970s. In holistic church-based primary care clinics, nurses were key to the success of the clinics because the nurses could speak both the scientific and the religious language for patients (27, 44, 63, 121). These leaders concluded that nurses in churches would be a cost-effective way to implement holistic health practices. Thus began the modern movement of **parish nursing**. The first nurses were hired in 1985 (119). A guide to starting a parish nurse program was published by Granger Westberg (119). A text was published (116, 119), and articles began appearing in professional journals (18). In 2006, the key words *parish nursing* entered for a computer search of the *Cumulative Index of Nursing and Allied Health Literature* produced a list of 579 articles, attesting to parish nursing development.

King (51) analyzed 20 research reports. She concluded that the most beneficial activities of parish nurses were caring interactions, listening, being there with individual church members and family caregivers, health promotion, screenings, and education.

Palmer (77) discussed the evolving parish nurse services in Canada since the 1990s, based on the earlier establishment of the parish nurse role in the United States. *Primary functions of the parish nurse are* (74, 77): (a) integrator of faith and health, (b) health educator, (c) personal health counselor, (d) referral agent and liaison with congregational and community resources, (e) facilitator of volunteers, (f) developer of support groups, and (g) health advocate.

Quenstedt–Moe (89) described how the parish nurse can be instrumental in identifying the need for a home care nurse referral. However, a combined role of parish nurse and home health care nurse is often what is needed in practice, since a combined parish nurse/home care nurse would be both spiritually and medically focused. Health counseling and education, community referrals, and

---

*This section contributed by Frances Atkins, PhD, CNS-BC.

coordination of volunteers—roles of the parish nurse—could be conducted along with physical and functional assessment and skilled care services typically conducted as part of the home health care role (80, 89).

Instruments for continuous quality improvement for the parish nurse role are also necessary. A review of outcome-based literature for church-based health promotion programs reported the following *key elements as important for success* (85): (a) partnerships, (b) positive health values, (c) availability of services, (d) access to church facilities, (e) community-focused interventions, (f) health behavior change, and (g) supportive social relationships.

The role of parish nurse was formalized by the *Scope and Standards of Parish Nursing Practice*, jointly published by the Health Ministries Association and the American Nurses Association in June 1998: **Parish nursing** is a unique, specialized practice of professional nursing that focuses on health promotion within the context of the values, beliefs, and practices of a faith community, such as a church, synagogue, or mosque, and its mission and ministry to its members (families and individuals), and the community it serves (p. 1). *Using the acronym of HEALTH, the role of the parish nurse was described in the following way* (104, p. 15):

H –Health counselor

E –Educator of holistic health

A –Advocate/resource person

L –Liaison to community services

T –Teacher of volunteers/support groups

H –Healer—body, mind, and spirit

To augment the usual nursing assessments, a brief spiritual assessment guide, with suggested interventions (112) and more extensive spiritual needs protocols (65), and a comprehensive spiritual assessment instrument (32) have been developed. Ways to evaluate parish nursing continue to evolve (44, 46).

EVALUATION

Exactly what aspects of spiritual care can be evaluated is difficult to determine. *Barriers to nurses giving spiritual care include* (45, 108, 109): (a) insufficient time in the work schedule, (b) lack of education and confidence, (c) respect for patients' and clients' specific beliefs, (d) lack of privacy in talking with the person, (e) differences between the nurses' and clients' spiritual or religious beliefs, (f) neglect of personal spirituality, (g) belief that spiritual care is not a nursing activity, and (h) peer criticism. **Evaluation** of spiritual care interventions can best be analyzed by using both ob-

jective and subjective criteria, with spiritual well-being as the major criterion. *The following questions with positive answers indicate a direction toward that criterion. Does this intervention* (105):

1. Bring peace or unity?
2. Provide a source of help, comfort, relief, or strength?
3. Promote transcendent values such as meaning, purpose, love, relatedness, and God's forgiveness or forgiveness of self and others?
4. Decrease or alleviate symptoms, such as anxiety, withdrawal, helplessness, agitation, crying, hostility, guilt, shame, depression, and unforgiveness?
5. Bring integration to the personality?
6. Help the person to cope and solve problems?
7. Promote hardiness, hope, and intrinsic spiritual values?

The above would provide evidence of spiritual well-being. These questions can be measured on a continuum of 1 to 10 answered by both nurse and patient.

Outcomes to strive for are those that (a) enhance trust, (b) allow people to carry on spiritual practices not detrimental to health, (c) decrease feelings of anxiety and guilt, and (d) cause satisfaction with their spiritual condition (24). To ensure these responses, spiritual care should be considered part of quality assurance.

Rethemeyer and Wehling described the development of a questionnaire to determine attitudes and beliefs about parish nursing and the perceived role of the parish nurse in the congregation or community. Results indicated that the congregation benefited from the services offered by the parish nurse and that a number of health practices were improved by individuals (90). Blank, Mahmood, Fox, and Guterbock (6) compared mental health and social service in African American and White church congregations. Results indicated that Black churches provided more services than did White churches, regardless of rural or urban locations. Most of the churches had few linkages with formal health provider services. The church is central to the Black community; hence, it could be an important avenue for helping to reduce the stigma of mental illness and for ensuring accessible, effective health care for physical and mental conditions. In turn, the church in the White community could also better foster health care (6).

Evaluating effectiveness of spiritual care involves documentation. Burkhart describes electronic documentation, utilizing nursing diagnoses and the NIC (Nursing Interventions Classification) and NOC (Nursing Outcome Classification) systems (10). She also describes the parish nurse documentation system, *Integration*, available at their Website, www.parishnurses.org.

Summary

1. Spirituality and the spiritual dimensions are inherent in all people, regardless of the presence of beliefs.
2. You will care for clients who adhere to beliefs different from your own.
3. The major world religions are Hinduism, Sikhism, Buddhism, Jainism, Shintoism, Confucianism, Taoism, Islam, Judaism, and Christianity.

4. Other religious groups are Seventh-Day Adventists; Church of Jesus Christ of Latter-Day Saints (Mormon); Jehovah's Witnesses; Church of Christ, Scientist (Christian Scientist); Society of Friends (Quaker); Unity School of Christianity; Mennonites; Amish; Moravians; Waldenses; Unitarian Universalists; and Neo-Pentecostalists.

5. The African American church and North American Indian religions have each made a special contribution to our culture.
6. Other belief systems may be encountered, such as New Age, neo-pagan, agnostic, atheism, cult, and voodoo.
7. You can practice principles of spiritual care based on concepts in this chapter in every health care setting.
8. Engage in lifelong learning about your own and others' beliefs to assess, plan, and provide health promotion and holistic care to the client and family.

Review Questions

1. While interviewing a client upon admission to the agency, the nurse asks if the client has a religious affiliation. The client responds, "I do not practice a religion, but I am a spiritual person." The nurse understands that:
   1. Spirituality is a form of religion.
   2. Those who practice religion do not consider themselves to be spiritual.
   3. Religion and spirituality have no relationship.
   4. Spirituality is a quality that goes beyond religious affiliation.

2. A client tells the nurse about a journal article she read that explained that spirituality and beliefs might be programmed into a person's DNA. The nurse recognizes this as:
   1. A new area of research
   2. An ancient belief
   3. Not accepted by Christian faiths
   4. A common belief of Middle Eastern faiths

3. The nurse is reviewing the medical history of a client who was brought to the emergency room following a motor vehicle accident. The record reveals the client is a Christian Scientist. What effect can the nurse anticipate this religious affiliation will have on the client's care?
   1. There will be no conflict of religion and medical care.
   2. The client will likely accept medical care, but not medications.
   3. The client will reject the spiritual methods of healing.
   4. The client will only be treated by a physician of the same faith.

4. While working with a client at the end of life, the nurse inquires about funeral arrangements and if a clergy member should be notified. The client tells the nurse, "I am agnostic." How should the nurse interpret this statement?
   1. The client is a member of a New Age religious group.
   2. The client feels that one is incapable of knowing if God exists.
   3. The client believes that God does not exist.
   4. The client is a Christian.

References

1. Ameling, A., & Povilonis, M. (2001). Spirituality: Meaning, mental health, and nursing. *Journal of Psychosocial Nursing, 39*(4), 15–20.
2. American Psychiatric Association. (1994). *Diagnostic and statistical manual of mental disorders* (4th ed.). Washington, DC: Author.
3. Andrews, M., & Boyle, J. (2003). *Transcultural concepts in nursing care* (4th ed.). Philadelphia: Lippincott, Williams, & Wilkins.
4. Atkins, F. (1997). *Church members' views about healing and health promotion in their church: A multi-case study.* Unpublished doctoral dissertation, Saint Louis University, St. Louis, MO.
5. Begley, S. (2001, May 7). Religion and the brain, *Newsweek*, 50–55.
6. Blank, M., Mahmood, M., Fox, J., & Guterbock, T. (2002). Alternative mental health services: The role of the Black church in the South. *American Journal of Public Health, 92*(10), 1668–1672.
7. Braswell, G. J. (1994). *Understanding world religion* (rev.). Nashville, TN: Broadman & Holman.
8. Brisbane, S., & Womble, N. (1992). *Working with African-Americans. The professional handbook.* Chicago: HRDI, International Press.
9. Brown, M. (2004). American spirit. *National History, 113*(8), 46–49.
10. Burkhart, L. (2005). Documenting spiritual care. *Journal of Christian Nursing, 22*(1), 6–12.
11. Campinha-Bacote, J. (2003). Cultural desire: The spiritual key to cultural competence. *Journal of Christian Nursing, 20*(3), 20–22.
12. Campinha-Bacote, J. (1992). Voodoo illness. *Perspectives in Psychiatric Care, 28*(1), 11–12.
13. Carson, V. (1992). *Spiritual dimensions of nursing practice.* Philadelphia: Saunders.
14. Cavendish, R., Luise, B., Bauer, M., Gallo, M., Horne, K., Medefindt, J., & Russo, D. (2001). Recognizing opportunities for spiritual enhancement in young adults. *Nursing Diagnoses, 12*(3), 77–91.
15. Cavendish, R., Luise, B., Russo, D., Mitzeliotis, C., Bauer, M., Bajo, M., et al. (2004). Spiritual perspectives of nurses in the United States relevant for education and practice. *Western Journal of Nursing Research, 26*(2), 196–212.
16. Christiansen, G. (2001). Is religion good for your health? Faith and mental illness. *NAMI Advocate, 4*(1), 29.
17. Chiu, L., Emblem, J., Van Hofwegen, L., Sawatzky, R., & Meyerhoff, H. (2004). An integrative review of the concept of spirituality in the health sciences. *Western Journal of Nursing Research, 26*(4), 405–428.
18. Coenen, A., Weis, D. M., Schank, M. J., & Matheus, R. (1999). Describing parish nurse practice using the nursing minimum data set. *Public Health Nursing, 16*(6), 412–416.
19. Coels, R. (1991). *The spiritual life of children.* Boston: Houghton Mifflin.
20. Correspondents of the New York Times. (2005). *Class matters.* New York: Henry Holt.
21. Deller, K. (2001). A prayer for Sarah: Crossing cultures with a tender heart. *Journal of Christian Nursing, 20*(1), 18–19.
22. Diaman, D. A. (2007). *Living a Jewish life: Jewish traditions, customs, and values for today's families* (Updated rev. ed.). New York: Collins.
23. Diggins, K. (2007). Can caring spiritually mean remaining quiet? *Journal of Christian Nursing, 24*(3), 165.
24. Donley, Sister R. (1991). Spiritual dimensions of health care: Nursing's mission. *Nursing and Health Care, 12*(4), 178–183.
25. Eigo, F. (1999). *Religious values at the threshold of the third millennium.* Villanova, PA: Villanova University Press.
26. Espeland, K. (1999). Achieving spiritual wellness: Using reflective questions. *Journal of Psychiatric Nursing, 37*(1), 36–40.
27. Ferrell, S., & Rigney, D. (2005). From dream to reality. How a parish nurse program is born. *Journal of Christian Nursing, 22*(2), 34–37.
28. Five reasons to forgive. (2005). *Harvard Women's Health Watch, 12*(5), 1–3.

29. Florida, R. (2002). *The rise of the creative class*. New York: Basic Books/Perseus Books Group.

30. Frazier, F. (1963). *The Negro church in America*. New York: Schocken Books.

31. Furlow, L., & O'Quinn, J. L. (2002). Does prayer really help? *Journal of Christian Nursing, 19*(2), 31–34.

32. Galek, K., Flannelly, K. J., Vane, A., & Galek, R. M. (2005). Assessing a patient's spiritual needs: A comprehensive instrument. *Holistic Nursing Practice, 19*(2), 62–69.

33. Giger, J., & Davidhizar, R. (2004). *Transcultural nursing: Assessment and intervention* (4th ed.). St. Louis, MO: Mosby.

34. Gill, S. (1994). Native Americans and their religions. In S. Neusner (Ed.), *World religions in America: An introduction*. Louisville, KY: Westminster/John Knox Press.

35. Greening, L., & Stappelbein, L. (2002). Religiosity, attributional style, and social support as psychosocial buffers for African American and White adolescents' perceived risk for suicide. *Suicide Life Threatening Behavior, 32*(4), 404–417.

36. Groupman, J. (2003). *The anatomy of hope*. New York: Random House.

37. Haase, J., Britt, T., Coward, D., Leidy, N., & Penn, P. (1992). Simultaneous concept analysis of spiritual perspective, hope, acceptance, and self-transcendence. *IMAGE: Journal of Nursing Scholarship, 24*(2), 141–145.

38. Hallowell, E. (2003). *Dare to forgive*. Boston: Health Communications.

39. Halpern, L. (2006). Tahara: An ancient Jewish ritual for the dead. *American Journal of Nursing, 106*(4), 39.

40. Hatch, J., & Derthick, S. (1992). Empowering Black churches for health promotion. *Health Values, 16*(5), 3–8.

41. Hensley, D. E. (1991). Old or new? Understanding the New Age movement. *Vital Christianity, 111*(7), 21–23.

42. Hillard, J. R. (1982). Diagnosis and treatment of the rootwork victim. *Psychiatric Annals, 12*(7), 709–714.

43. Hines-Martin, V. P. (2002). African American consumers: What should we do to meet their mental health needs? *Journal of American Psychiatric Nurses Association, 8*(6), 189.

44. Hughes, C. B., Trofino, B., O'Brian, B. L., Mack, J., & Marrinan, B. (2001). Primary care parish nursing: Outcomes and implications. *Nursing Administration Quarterly, 26*(1), 45–59.

45. Hurley, J. (1999). Breaking the spiritual care barrier. *Journal of Christian Nursing, 16*(3), 8–13.

46. Hurley, J., & Mohnkem, S. (2004). Mobilize support groups to meet congregational needs. *Journal of Christian Nursing, 21*(4), 34–39.

47. JCN Resource Article. (2007). Religion and mental illness: Safe spirituality or risky religious intervention? *Journal of Christian Nursing, 24*(2), 71–74.

48. Jenkins, P. (2007). *The next Christendom: The coming of global Christianity*. Oxford University Press, New York.

49. Johanson, L. (2007). Cultural sensitivity: Beyond first impressions. *Journal of Christian Nursing, 24*(2), 96–98.

50. Kalb, C. (2003, November 10). Faith and healing. *Newsweek*, 44–55.

51. King, M. A. (2004). Review of research about parish nursing practice. Online *Brazilian Journal of Nursing* (OBJN-ISSN 1676-4285), *3*(1), 1–8. Retrieved February 17, 2006, from http://www.uff.br/nepae/objn301king.htm

52. Koenig, J. (1999). How does religious faith contribute to recovery from depression? *Harvard Mental Health Letter, 15*(8), 8.

53. Kumar, K. (2004). Spiritual care: What's worldview got to do with it? *Journal of Christian Nursing, 21*(1), 24–28.

54. Kushner, H. (1989). *When bad things happen to good people*. New York: Schocken Books.

55. Lawrence, P., & Rozmus, C. (2001). Culturally sensitive care of the Muslim patient. *Journal of Transcultural Nursing, 12*(3), 228–233.

56. Leardi, J. (2003, December 21). Religion is no longer faith of our fathers. *The Charlotte Observer*, p. 6H.

57. Leininger, M., & McFarland, M. R. (2002). *Transcultural nursing: Concepts, theories, research, and practices* (3rd ed.). New York: McGraw-Hill.

58. Linnard-Palmer, L. (2006). *When parents say no: Religious and cultural influences on pediatric health care treatment*. Indianapolis, IN: Sigma Theta Tau International.

59. Luna, L. J. (1989). Transcultural nursing care of Arab Muslims. *Journal of Transcultural Nursing, 1*(1), 22–26.

60. Macrae, J. (1995). Nightingale's spiritual philosophy and its significance for modern nursing. *IMAGE: Journal of Nursing Scholarship, 27*(1), 8–14.

61. Maddox, E. (2002). *Spiritual care: Nursing theory, research, and practice*. Upper Saddle River, NJ: Prentice Hall.

62. Maddox, M. (2002). Spiritual assessments in primary care. *Nurse Practitioner, 27*(2), 12–13.

63. Maddox, M. (2001). Circle of Christian caring: A model for parish nursing practice. *Journal of Christian Nursing, 18*(1), 11–12.

64. Matoni, K. I., Teti, D. M., Corns, K. M., Vieira-Coker, C. C., LaVine, J. N., Gouze, K. R., & Keating, D. P. (1996). Cultural specificity of support sources, correlates and context: Three studies of African-American and Caucasian youth. *American Journal of Community Psychology, 24*(4), 551–587.

65. Mayhugh, L., & Martens, K. (2001). What's a parish nurse to do? *Journal of Christian Nursing, 18*(3), 14–16.

66. McCullough, M., Hoyt, W. T., Larson, D. B., Koenig, H. G., & Thoreson, C. (2000). Religious involvement and mortality: A meta-analytic review. *Health Psychology, 19*(3), 211–222.

67. Mead, F., & Hill, S. (1990). *Handbook of denomination in the United States* (9th ed.). Nashville, TN: Abingdon Press.

68. Melton, J. (1992). *Encyclopedic handbook of cults in America*. New York: Garland.

69. Miller, L., & Gur, M. (2002a). Religiosity, depression, and physical maturation in adolescent girls. *Journal of the American Academy of Child and Adolescent Psychiatry, 41*(2), 206–214.

70. Miller, L., & Gur, M. (2002b). Religiosity and sexual responsibility in adolescent girls. *Journal of Adolescent Health, 31*(5), 401–406.

71. Mira, L. (2004). Spirituality in Korea: A fog of religion and culture. *Journal of Christian Nursing, 21*(1), 29–31.

72. Morgan, D. (2001). *The best guide to Eastern philosophy and religion*. New York: Renaissance Books.

73. NANDA International. (2007). *NANDA nursing diagnoses: Definitions & classification 2007–2008*. Philadelphia: Author.

74. Nist, J. A. (2003). Parish nursing programs. *Health Progress, 84*(1), 50–54.

75. Noonan, M. (2005). *Ransomed from darkness: The New Age Christian faith and battle for souls*. El Sobrante, CA: Northbay Books.

76. Ott, B., Al-Khadhuri, J., & Al-Junalbi, S. (2003). Preventing ethical dilemmas: Understanding Islamic health care practices. *Pediatric Nursing, 29*(3), 227–230.

77. Palmer, J. (2001). Parish nursing: Connecting faith and health. *Reflections on Nursing Leadership, 27*(1), 17–18.

78. Pargament, K., Koenig, H. G., Tarakeshwar, N., & Hahn, J. (2001). Religious struggle during illness may predict mortality. *Archives of Internal Medicine, 16*(15), 1881–1885.

79. Park, H.S., Bauer, S., & Oescher, J. (2001). Religiousness as a predictor of alcohol use in high school students. *Journal of Drug Education, 31*(3), 289–303.

80. Pattilo, M.M., Chesley, D., Castles, P., & Sutter, R. (2002). Faith community nursing: Parish nursing/health ministry collaboration model in Central Texas. *Family and Community Health, 25*(3), 41–51.

81. Peale, N. V. (1961). *Positive thinking for times like this*. Pawling, NY: Foundation for Christian Living.

82. Peale, N. V. (1982). *Imaging: The powerful way to change your life*. Carmel, NY: Guideposts.

83. Peplau, H. (1952/1991). *Interpersonal relations in nursing*. New York: Springer.

84. Peterson, S. (2002). Safe churches prepared to manage crisis. *Journal of Christian Nursing, 19*(4), 29–31.

85. Peterson, J., Atwood, J.R., & Yates, B. (2002). Key elements for church-based health promotion programs: Outcome-based literature review. *Public Health Nursing, 19*(6), 401–411.

86. Pincharcen, S., & Congden, J. (2003). Spirituality and health in older Thai persons in the United States. *Western Journal of Nursing Research, 25*(1), 93–108.

87. Plante, T. G., & Sharma, N. (2001). Religious faith and mental health outcomes. In T. G. Plante & A. C. Sherman (Eds.), *Faith and health: Psychological perspectives* (pp. 242–250). New York: Guilford Press.

88. Price, J. (2002). How faith helped my recovery: Faith and mental illness. *NAMI Advocate, 5*(4), 11.

89. Quenstedt-Moe, G. (2003). Parish nursing & home care: A blended role? *Journal of Christian Nursing, 20*(3), 26–30.

90. Rethemeyer, A., & Wehling, B. (2004). How are we doing? Measuring the effectiveness of parish nursing. *Journal of Christian Nursing, 21*(2), 10–12.

91. Richardson, S. (2001, December). Making a spiritual assessment. *Nursing Spectrum Metro Edition*, pp. 30–34.

92. Rubin, M. (1999). The healing power of prayer. *Journal of Christian Nursing, 16*(3), 4–7.

93. Salladay, S. A. (1991). World views apart: Nursing practice and New Age therapies. *Journal of Christian Nursing, 6*(4), 15–18.

94. Scales, R. (1991). *A portrait of young adolescents in the 1990s: Implications for promoting healthy growth and development.* Carrboro: Center for Early Adolescence, University of North Carolina.

95. Scharf, A. (2007). Good spiritual care: Befriending the mentally ill. *Journal of Christian Nursing, 24*(2), 74–76.

96. Sending prayers: Does it really help? (2002). *Harvard Health Letter, 27*(7), 7.

97. Shakir, M. H. (Translator). (2006). *The Qur'an translation* (16th ed.). New York: Tahrike Tussile Qur'an, Inc.

98. Sheler, J. (2004, May 3). Nearer my God to thee. *U.S. News and World Report*, 59–62, 65–66.

99. Sherman, A.C., & Simonton, S. (2001). Assessment of religiousness and spirituality in health research. In T. S. Plante & A. C. Sherman (Eds.), *Faith and health: Psychological perspectives* (pp. 139–157). New York: Guilford Press.

100. Singer, M. (1995). *Cults in our midst.* San Francisco: Jossey-Bass.

101. Speny, J. (2002). *A new Christianity in a new world.* San Francisco: Harper.

102. Stafford, T. (1991). The hidden gospel of the 12 steps. *Christianity Today, 35*(8), 14–19.

103. Steen, L., & Anderson, B. (2002). Caring for children of other faiths. *Journal of Christian Nursing, 19*(1), 14–21.

104. Stephenson, C., & Wilson, K. (2004). Does spiritual care really help? A study of patient perceptions. *Journal of Christian Nursing, 21*(2), 26–28.

105. Stoll, R. (1989). The essence of spirituality. In V. B. Carson (Ed.), *Spiritual dimensions of nursing practice* (pp. 4–33). Philadelphia: Saunders.

106. Striepe, J., King, J., & Scott, I. (1995). Nurses in the church: Profiles of caring. *Journal of Christian Nursing, 10*(1), 8–11.

107. Sweat, M. (2007). Is forgiveness important in spiritual care? *Journal of Christian Nursing, 24*(2), 103.

108. Taylor, E. J. (2005). What have we learned from spiritual care research? *Journal of Christian Nursing, 22*(1), 22–28.

109. Taylor, E. J. (2007). *What do I say? Talking with patients about spirituality.* West Conshohocken, PA: Templeton.

110. Tolson, J. (2003, December 6). The new old-time religion. *U.S. News & World Report*, 37–44.

111. Topper, A. (2002, December). The impact of cults on health. *Nursing Spectrum Midwestern Edition*, pp. 26–31.

112. Treloar, C. (1999). Spiritual care: Assessment and intervention. *Journal of Christian Nursing, 16*(1), 16–18.

113. Tuck, I., & Baliko, B. (2001). Why deliver health care with spirituality? *Reflections: Sigma Theta Tau International Honor Society of Nursing, 2*(3), 1, 4–5.

114. U.S. Department of Mental Health and Human Services, Public Health Service, Office of the Surgeon General. (2001). *Mental health: Culture, race, and ethnicity—A supplement to mental health: A report of the Surgeon General.* Rockville, MD: Author.

115. Walker, J. (2004). Journey into hope: A therapeutic relationship. *Journal of Christian Nursing, 21*(2), 19–22.

116. Wallace, J., Jr., & Forman, T. (1998). Religion's role in promoting health and reducing risk among American youth. *Health Education and Behavior, 25*, 721–741.

117. Ward, K. (2000). *Christianity: A short introduction.* New York: One World.

118. Weis, D. M., Schank, M. J., Coenen, A., & Matheus, R. (2002). Parish nurse practice with client aggregates. *Journal of Community Health Nursing, 19*(2), 105–113.

119. Westberg, J. (1990). A historical perspective: Holistic health and the parish nurse. In P. Solari-Twadell, A. Djupe, & M. McDermott (Eds.), *Parish nursing: The developing practice* (pp. 29–37). Park Ridge, IL: National Parish Nurse Resource Center.

120. Westberg, G. (1988). The church as "health place." *Dialog, 27*(3), 189–191.

121. Westberg, G. (1989). Parish nursing's pioneer: A *JCN* Interview. *Journal of Christian Nursing, 6*(1), 26–29.

122. Winslow, W. (2004, March). Is denominationalism dead? *United Church News*, 87.

123. Wolfe, A. (2003). *The transformation of American religion: How we actually live our faith.* New York: Free Press.

124. Woodward, K. (2001, May 7). Faith is more than a feeling. *Newsweek*, 56.

125. Woodward, K. (2001, April 16). The changing face of the church. *Newsweek*, 48–51.

126. Wright, K. (1998). Professional, ethical, and legal implications for spiritual care in nursing. *IMAGE: Journal of Nursing Scholarship, 30*(1), 81–83.

Interviews

127. Desai, A.D., Boulder, Colorado, November 26, 1998.

128. Desai, D., & A., Boulder, Colorado, May 17, 1997.

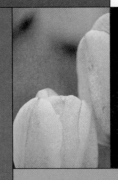

Prenatal and Other Developmental Influences

OBJECTIVES

Study of this chapter will enable you to:

1. Review and assess major physical developmental changes that occur during the 9 months of gestation.

2. Examine influences that affect the developing person during the prenatal period, during childbirth, and in early childhood.

3. Relate maternal and paternal variables and sociocultural factors that influence prenatal development.

4. Educate the pregnant woman, and partner if possible, about the normal changes that occur in the developing fetus and in the pregnant female.

5. Explore lifestyle variables with the pregnant female, and partner if possible, that are considered to have a negative or teratogenic effect on the embryo/fetus.

6. Analyze lifestyle changes that can be made (e.g., dietary, exercise, smoking, use of alcohol, as relevant) by the pregnant female and her partner to foster her health and health of the newborn.

7. Discuss variables following childbirth that will influence the infant's development, and encourage the couple in their planning.

MediaLink www.prenhall.com/murray

Go to the Companion Website for interactive resources that accompany this chapter.

Glossary	Critical Thinking
Review Questions	Tools
Challenge Your Knowledge	Media Link Applications
Learning Activities	Media Links

The Beginning

This chapter presents a brief overview of the prenatal period as the beginning of life. For in-depth study of the biological differences of the male and female, the reproductive process, including fertilization and development of the unborn child in utero, inheritance patterns, and the process of labor and delivery, refer to anatomy and physiology, developmental, and maternity nursing texts.

The cell, the basis for human life, is a complex unit. All body cells have 22 pairs of rod-shaped particles, nonsex **chromosomes** (*autosomes*), and a pair of sex chromosomes. The biological female has two X chromosomes; the biological male has one X and one Y chromosome. Each of the chromosomes contains approximately 30,000 **genes**, *the basic unit of heredity*. The genes are made up of deoxyribonucleic acid (DNA). DNA carries the biochemical instructions that tell the cells how to make the proteins that enable cells to carry out specific body functions. The genes play a major role in determining hereditary characteristics (34, 52). See Chapter 1 for general information related to genetics. ∞

The female reproductive cycle is more regular and is easier to observe and measure than is the male reproductive cycle. A newborn girl has approximately 400,000 immature ova in her ovaries; each is in a **follicle**, or *small sac*. **Ovulation**, *the expelling of an ovum from a mature follicle in one of the ovaries*, occurs approximately once every 28 days in a sexually mature female. In contrast to the normal ovulatory cycle, spermatogenesis normally occurs in cycles that continuously follow one another (34, 52).

Spermatozoa, much smaller and more active than the ovum, are produced in the testes of the mature male at the rate of several hundred million a day and are ejaculated in his semen at **orgasm**, *sexual climax*. For fertilization to occur, at least 20 million sperm cells must enter a woman's body at one time. They enter the vagina and try to swim through the **cervix** (*opening to the uterus*) and into the fallopian tube. Only a tiny fraction of those millions of sperm cells makes it that far. More than one may penetrate the ovum, but only one fertilizes it to create a new human. The sex of the baby is determined by the pair of sex chromosomes; the sperm may carry either an X or Y chromosome, resulting in either a girl (XX zygote) or a boy (XY zygote). Thus *the male determines the gender of the baby* (34, 52).

Spermatozoa maintain their ability to fertilize an egg for a span of 24 to 90 hours; ova can be fertilized for approximately 24 hours. Thus, there are approximately 24 to 90 hours during each menstrual cycle when conception can take place. If fertilization does not occur, the spermatozoa and ovum die. Sperm cells are devoured by white blood cells in the woman's body; the ovum passes through the uterus and vagina in the menstrual product (34, 52).

Approximately 14 days after the beginning of the menstrual period, **fertilization or conception** may occur in the outer third of the fallopian tube. *The sperm cell from a male penetrates and unites with an ovum (egg) from a female* to form a *single-cell* **zygote**. The sperm and ovum, known as **gametes** (*sex cells in half cells*), are produced in the reproductive system through **meiosis**, a *specialized process of cell division and chromosome reduction* (52). Artificially assisted reproduction is used when one or both prospective parents

are infertile, or if the lesbian wants to become pregnant. See Chapter 6 for information about the homosexual family. ∞

At conception, the zygote has all the biological information needed for development of the body. This happens through **mitosis**, a *process by which cells divide in half over and over*. Each new cell has the same DNA structure as the others. Genes become active when conditions call for information they can provide. Genetic action that triggers growth is often regulated by hormonal levels, which are affected by environmental factors such as nutrition and stress. From the beginning, heredity and environment are intertwined (34, 52).

Multiple births may occur. For example, with twins, two ova are released within a short time of each other; *if both ova are fertilized*, **fraternal** (*dizygotic*, or *two-egg*) **twins** will be born. Created by different eggs and different sperm cells, the twins are no more alike in their genetic makeup than other siblings. They may be of the same or different sex. If the *ovum divides in two after it has been fertilized*, **identical** (*monozygotic*, or *one-egg*) **twins** will be born. At birth, these twins share the same placenta. They are of the same gender and have exactly the same genetic heritage. Any differences they later exhibit are the result of the influences of environment, either before or after birth. Other multiple births—triplets, quadruplets, and so forth—result from either one or a combination of these two processes (34, 52).

Multiple births have become more frequent in recent years as a result of the administration of certain fertility drugs that spur ovulation and often cause the release of more than one egg. In vitro fertilization techniques have also increased the number of multiple births. The tendency to bear twins apparently is inherited and more common in some families and ethnic groups than in others. Twins have a limited intrauterine space and are more likely to be premature and of low birth weight. They therefore, overall, have a lower rate of survival at birth (34).

After either single or multiple fertilization, the zygote travels to the uterus for **implantation** or *embedding in the uterine wall* (about 6 days). The placenta is functioning a week later. Progesterone secretion has prepared the uterus for the possible reception of the fertilized ovum. The continued secretion of ovarian estrogen and progesterone develops the uterus for the 9-month nurturance of the developing embryo and fetus in pregnancy. Continued secretion of estrogen during this period increases the growth of the uterine muscles and eventually enlarges the vagina for the delivery of a child. Continued secretion of progesterone during pregnancy serves to keep the uterus from prematurely contracting and expelling the developing embryo before the proper time. In addition, progesterone prepares the breast cells in late pregnancy for future milk production (34).

Stages of Prenatal Development

Life in utero is usually divided into three stages of development: germinal, embryonic, and fetal. The **germinal stage** lasts *approximately 10 days to 2 weeks after fertilization*. This first stage is characterized by rapid cell division and subsequent increasing complexity of the organism and its implantation in the wall of the uterus. The **embryonic stage**, *from 2 to 8 weeks*, is the time of rapid growth and differentiation of major body systems and organs. The **fetal stage**, *from 8 weeks until birth*, is characterized by rapid growth and changes in body form caused by different rates of growth of different parts of the body (34).

The fetus is a very small but rapidly developing human being who is influenced by the maternal and external environment. The mother responds to the fetus, especially when fetal movement begins. **Table 8-1** summarizes some major physiologic milestones in the sequential development of the conceptus, the *new life that has been conceived* (34). **Table 8-2** summarizes major physiologic changes in the pregnant woman (34).

TABLE 8-1

Summary of the Sequence of Prenatal Development

Time Period After Fertilization	Developmental Event
Germinal Stage	
30 hours	First division or cleavage occurs.
40 hours	Four-cell stage occurs.
60 hours	**Morula,** *a solid mass of 12 to 16 cells;* total size of mass not changed because cells decrease in size with each cleavage to allow morula to pass through lumen of fallopian tube. Ectopic pregnancy within fallopian tube occurs if morula is wedged in lumen.
3 days	Zygote has divided into 32 cells; travels through fallopian tube to uterus.
4 days	Zygote contains 70 cells. Morula reaches uterus; forms a **blastocyst,** *a fluid-filled sphere.*
4 1/2–6 days	Blastocyst floats in utero. **Embryonic disc,** *thickened cell mass from which baby develops,* clusters on one edge of blastocyst. Mass of cells differentiates into two layers: (1) **ectoderm,** *outer layer of cells* that become the epidermis, nails, hair, tooth enamel, sensory organs, brain and spinal cord, cranial nerves, peripheral nervous system, upper pharynx, nasal passages, urethra, and mammary glands; (2) **endoderm,** *lower layer of cells* that develops into gastrointestinal system, liver, pancreas, salivary glands, respiratory system, urinary bladder, pharynx, thyroid, tonsils, lining of urethra, and ear.
6–7 days	**Nidation,** *implantation of zygote* into upper portion of uterine wall, occurs.
7–14 days	Remainder of blastocyst develops into the following: (1) **Placenta,** *a multipurpose organ connected to the embryo by the umbilical cord* that delivers oxygen and nourishment from the mother's body, absorbs the embryo's body wastes, combats internal infection, confers immunity to the unborn child, and produces the hormones that (a) support pregnancy, (b) prepare breasts for lactating, and (c) stimulate uterine contractions for delivery of the baby. Placenta circulation evidenced by 11 to 12 days. (2) **Umbilical cord,** *a structure that contains two umbilical arteries and an umbilical vein and connects embryo to placenta.* Approximately 20 inches long and ½ inch in diameter. Rapid cell differentiation occurs. (3) **Amniotic sac,** *a fluid-filled membrane that encases the developing baby,* protecting it and giving it room to move.
2–8 weeks	Period during which embryo firmly establishes uterus as home and undergoes rapid cellular differentiation, growth, and development of body systems. This is a *critical period when embryo is most vulnerable to deleterious prenatal influences.* All development birth defects occur during *first trimester (3 months)* of pregnancy. If embryo is unable to survive, a **miscarriage** or **spontaneous abortion,** *expulsion of conceptus from the uterus, occurs.*
Embryonic Stage	
15 days	Cranial end of elongated disk has begun to thicken.
16 days	**Mesoderm,** the *middle layer,* appears and develops into dermis, tooth dentin, connective tissue, cartilage, bones, muscles, spleen, blood, gonads, uterus, and excretory and circulatory systems. Yolk sac, which arises from ectoderm, assists transfer of nutrients from mother to embryo.
19–20 days	Neural fold and neural groove develop. Thyroid begins to develop.
21 days	Neural tube forms, becomes spinal cord and brain.
22 days	Heart, the first organ to function, initiates action. Eyes, ears, nose, cheeks, and upper jaw begin to form. Cleft palate may occur if development is defective.
26–27 days	Cephalic portion (brain) of nervous system formed. Leg and arm buds appear. Stubby tail of spinal cord appears.
28 days	Crown to rump length, 4–5 mm.

TABLE 8-1

Summary of the Sequence of Prenatal Development—continued

Time Period After Fertilization	Developmental Event
30 days	Rudimentary body parts formed. Limb buds appear. Cardiovascular system functioning. Heart beats 65 times per minute; blood flows through tiny arteries and veins. Lens vesicles, optic cups, and nasal pits forming. By end of first month, new life has grown more quickly than it will at any other time in life. Swelling in head where eyes, ears, mouth, and nose will be. Crown to rump length, 7–14 mm (¼ to ½ inch).
31 days	Eye and nasal pit developing. Primitive mouth present.
32 days	Paddle-shaped hands. Lens vesicles and optic cups formed.
34 days	Head is much larger relative to trunk. Digital rays present in hands. Feet are paddle-shaped. Crown to rump length, 11–14 mm.
35–38 days	Olfactory pit, eye, maxillary process, oral cavity, and mandibular process developing. Brain has divided into three parts. Limbs growing. Beginning of all major external and internal structures. Crown to rump length, 15–16 mm.
40 days	Elbows and knees apparent. Fingers and toes distinct but webbed. Yolk sac continues to (1) provide embryologic blood cells during third through sixth weeks until liver, spleen, and bone marrow assume function; (2) provide lining cells for respiratory and digestive tracts; (3) provide cells that migrate to gonads to become primordial germ cells.
42 days	Crown to rump length, 21–23 mm.
50 days	All internal and external structures present. External genitalia present but sex not discernible; yolk sac disappears, incorporated into embryo; limbs, hands, feet formed. Nerve cells in brain connected.
55–56 days	Eye, nostril, globular process, maxilla, and mandible almost completely formed. Ear beginning to develop.
8 weeks	Stubby end of spinal cord disappears. Distinct human characteristics. Head accounts for half of total embryo length. Brain impulses coordinate function of organ systems. Facial parts formed, with tongue and teeth buds. Stomach produces digestive juices. Liver produces blood cells. Kidney removes uric acid from blood. Some movement by limbs. Weight, 1 g. Length, 1–1½ inches (2.5–3.75 cm).
Fetal Stage	
9–40 weeks	Remainder of intrauterine period spent in growth and refinement of body tissues and organs.
9–12 weeks	Eyelids fused. Nail beds formed. Teeth and bones begin to appear. Ribs and vertebrae are cartilage. Kidneys function. Urinates occasionally. Some *respiratory*-like movements exhibited. Begins to swallow amniotic fluid. Grasp, sucking, and withdrawal reflexes present. Sucks fingers and toes in utero. Makes specialized responses to touch. Moves easily but movement not felt by mother. Reproduction organs have primitive egg or sperm cells. Sex distinguishable. Head one third of body length. Weight, 30 g (1 oz). Length, 3–3½ inches at 12 weeks.
13–16 weeks	Ova formed in female. Much spontaneous movement. Sex determination possible. **Quickening,** *fetal kicking or movement,* may be felt by mother. Moro reflex present. Rapid skeletal development. Meconium present. Uterine development in female fetus. **Lanugo,** *downy hair,* appears on body. Head one fourth of total length. Weight, 120–150 g (4–6 oz). Length, 8–10 inches. Fetus frowns, moves lips, turns head; hands grasp, feet kick. First hair appears. Umbilical cord as long as fetus. Placenta fully developed 16 weeks.
17–20 weeks	New cells exchanged for old, especially in skin. Quickening occurs by 17 weeks. Vernix caseosa appears. Eyebrows, eyelashes, and head hair appear. Sweat and sebaceous glands begin to function. Skeleton begins to harden. Grasp reflex present and strong. Permanent teeth buds appear. Fetal heart sounds can be heard with stethoscope. Weight, 360–450 g (12 oz–1 lb). Length, 12 inches.
21–24 weeks	Extrauterine life, life outside uterus, is possible but difficult because of immature respiratory system. Fetus looks like miniature baby. Mother may note jarring but *rhythmic* movements of infant, indicative of hiccups. Body becomes straight at times. Fingernails present. Skin has wrinkled, red appearance. Alternate periods of sleep and activity. May respond to external sounds. Weight, 720 g (1½ lb). Length, 14 inches.

continued

TABLE 8-1

Summary of the Sequence of Prenatal Development—continued

Time Period After Fertilization	Developmental Event
25–28 weeks	Jumps in utero in synchrony with loud noise. Eyes open and close with waking and sleeping cycles. Able to hear. Respiratory-like movements. Respiratory and central nervous systems sufficiently developed; some babies survive with excellent and intensive care. Assumes head-down position in uterus. Weight, 1,200 g (2 1/2 lb).
29–32 weeks	Begins to store fat and minerals. Testes descend into scrotal sac in male. Reflexes fully developed. Thumb-sucking present. Mother may note irregular, jerky, crying-like movements. Lanugo begins to disappear from face. Head hair continues to grow. Skin begins to lose reddish color. Can be conditioned to environmental sounds. Weight, 1,362–2,270 g (3–5 lb). Length, 16 inches.
33–36 weeks	Adipose tissue continues to be deposited over entire body. Body begins to round out. May become more or less active because of space constriction. Increased iron storage by liver. Increased lung development. Lanugo begins to disappear from body. Head lengthens. Brain cells number same as at birth. Weight, 2,800 g (6 lb). Length, 18–20 inches.
37–40 weeks Gestational age— 280 days in utero—266 days	Organ systems operating more efficiently. Heart rate increases. More wastes expelled. Lanugo and vernix caseosa disappear. Skin smooth and plump. High absorption of maternal hormones. Cerebral cortex well defined; brain wave patterns developed. Skull and other bones becoming more firm and mineralized. Continued storage of fat and minerals. Glands produce hormones that trigger labor. Ready for birth. Weight, 3,200–3,400 g (7–7 ½ lb). Length, 20–21 inches. Baby stops growing approximately 1 week before birth.

Prenatal Influences on Development

Maternal and prenatal health is a major goal of the *Healthy People 2010* Initiative in the United States. Refer to the **Box** *Healthy People 2010:* Examples of Objectives for Maternal and Prenatal Health Promotion (139).

This section summarizes major health risks to the embryo and fetus. More information is available in maternity nursing texts. *Preconception risk factors include the following diseases* (23): (a) diabetes onset before conception, (b) folic acid deficiency, (c) hepatitis B, (d) HIV/AIDS, (e) hypothyroidism, (f) maternal phenylketonuria (PKU), (g) obesity, and (h) sexually transmitted diseases such as *Chlamydia trachomatis* and gonorrhea. *Other preconception risk factors include* (23) (a) use of isotretinoins such as Accutane, (b) alcohol intake, (c) use of antineoplastic drugs, (d) folic acid deficiency, (e) oral anticoagulant use, and (f) smoking.

HEREDITY

Genetic information is transmitted from parents to the offspring through a complex series of processes. The gene is the basic unit of heredity. Relatively few people are born without abnormal chromosomes. Everyone carries abnormal genes that could produce serious diseases or handicaps in the next generation. These genes are usually recessive or additive. Most of the 7,000 known genetic disorders are dominant, since the effects of dominant genes are apparent in the person's phenotype (34). Refer to Chapter 1 for additional explanation. ∞

Congenital malformations are *physical or mental disabilities* that occur before birth for a variety of reasons. However, sometimes diseases or defects are **genetic**, *the result of dominant or recessive transmission of abnormalities in the genes or chromosomes.* An example is *Fragile X syndrome, which involves an abnormal fragile section of DNA at a specific location on the X chromosome.* This is a sex-linked inherited disorder. The female is usually a carrier, and the male is more likely to demonstrate the effects. It is estimated that 5% to 7% of all mental retardation is caused by this syndrome. Recessive genes may cause inherited diseases, such as cystic fibrosis, sickle-cell syndrome, muscular dystrophy, PKU disease, and Tay-Sachs disease (57).

An example of a congenital but not inherited disorder is **Down syndrome (trisomy 21)**, *in which the child has three of the chromosome 21 instead of the normal two.* Various factors contribute to the chromosomal break. The level of mental retardation varies. An inherited predisposition to a disorder may also interact with an environmental factor before or after birth and lead to expression of a disorder. Some abnormalities or diseases that are inherited appear months or years later (34, 57).

Hereditary factors do not by themselves fully determine what the person will become. **Reaction range**, *a range of potential expression of a trait* (for example, *weight*), *depends on environmental conditions.* Then, there are some traits, such as eye color, that are so strongly programmed by genes that they are **canalized**, *there is little variance in their expression* (57).

For example, diabetes mellitus has a familial (hereditary) or genetic etiology although other factors contribute to the cause. Incidence in African Americans, Hispanic Americans, and many

TABLE 8-2

Summary of Major Physiologic Changes in Woman During Pregnancy

Physiologic Characteristics	Change Related to Pregnancy
Weight	First trimester: increases by 2 to 4 pounds.
	Second and third trimester: increases by 0.8 to 1 pound per week.
Skin	Warmed by increased blood flow.
	Linea nigra: *dark vertical line from sternum to symphysis pubis.*
	Stretch marks on abdomen with increasing **chloasma:** *dark brown patches on face or over bridge of nose.*
Musculoskeletal System	Center of gravity changes, tilting pelvis forward, causing lower back pain.
	Fatigue and aches caused by increasing weight in abdomen and breasts.
Cardiovascular System	First trimester: blood volume increases gradually.
	6–8 weeks: may hear systolic ejection murmur on auscultation. Heart displaced upwards and to the left by rising diaphragm.
	Orthostatic hypotension during pregnancy because blood pools in lower limbs; varicose veins and hemorrhoids are common.
	14–20 weeks: pulse gradually increases by 10 to 15 beats per minute; cardiac output increases 30% to 50%.
	Last half of pregnancy: drop in colloid osmotic pressure shifts fluid into extravascular space, causing edema in lower limbs.
	32–34 weeks: blood volume increases to 40% to 50% above baseline; 40 weeks: blood volume gradually declines.
Respiratory System	Diaphragm rises and waistline expands even before enlarging uterus exerts much upward pressure.
	24th week: thoracic rather than abdominal breathing; mild dyspnea; nasal mucosa swells as a result of higher estrogen level; nasal stuffiness, epistaxis (nosebleeds) common.
	Costal ligaments relax because of rising estrogen levels; chest can expand and deeper breathing for increasing oxygen requirements.
	Respiratory rate increases slightly.
	Respiratory volume increases 26%, decreasing alveolar carbon dioxide concentration, compensated respiratory alkalosis.
	Alkalosis facilitates diffusion of nutrients to and wastes from the fetus through placenta.
Renal System	Kidneys excrete additional bicarbonate to compensate for drop in alveolar carbon dioxide concentration.
	Second trimester: increase in renal plasma flow (35%) and glomerular filtration rate (50%); both drop in late pregnancy.
	Urinary stasis caused by enlarging uterus and increasing blood volume.
Gastrointestinal System	First trimester nausea and vomiting resulting from increased human chorionic gonadotropin and estrogen.
	Gastric reflux as uterus enlarges and progesterone relaxes smooth muscle.
	Reduced bowel sounds; intestinal transit time increases, causing better nutrient absorption and constipation.
Hematologic System	Second trimester: physiologic anemia with hemoglobin level and hematocrit slightly lower, proportionate to increased plasma volume.
	White blood cell count: 10,000 to 12,000 during pregnancy; 25,000 during labor because of physiologic stress.
	Platelets remain normal.
Reproductive System	Uterus enlarges 20 times normal size to hold fetus, placenta, amniotic fluid. 12th week: uterus expands out of pelvis into abdominal cavity.
	16th week and after: supine position causes uterus to compress vena cava and iliac veins, decreasing blood flow to uterus and lower extremities (left lateral position recommended for sleeping).
	Vagina: pH more acid in mucus, which acts as barrier against infection to uterus. Breasts begin to feel full and tingly at second month; gradually enlarge as number and size of milk ducts and lobules increase; breast may leak colostrum.

1. Increase proportion of pregnant women who receive early and adequate prenatal care.

2. Reduce fetal deaths.

3. Reduce maternal deaths.

4. Increase proportion of pregnant women who attend a series of prepared childbirth classes.

5. Reduce maternal illness and complications due to pregnancy.

6. Increase proportion of very-low-birth-weight infants born in level III hospitals or subspecialty centers to reduce complications.

7. Reduce low and very low birth weights, especially for non-Caucasian women.

8. Decrease preterm births.

9. Decrease occurrence of developmental disability and neural tube defects, such as spina bifida in infants.

10. Increase proportion of mothers who achieve recommended weight gain during pregnancy, especially during second and third trimester.

11. Increase proportion of pregnancies begun with optimum maternal folic acid levels.

12. Increase abstinence from alcohol, cigarettes, and illicit drugs among pregnant women.

13. Decrease occurrence of fetal alcohol syndrome.

14. Increase the proportion of pregnant females screened for sexually transmitted diseases (including HIV infection and bacterial vaginosis) during prenatal health care visits, according to recognized standards.

Adapted from reference 139.

American Indian tribes is higher than in the U.S. population as a whole (9). However, diet is pivotal. Diabetes does not occur unless a person is genetically vulnerable and has more body fat than is considered ideal for a person of a specific age and height. Thus, nature and nurture interact (1, 57).

Genetic endowment with respect to any personality or cognitive trait may be compared to a rubber band. The rubber band may remain unstretched because of environmental influences and remain dormant. Or the rubber band may be stretched fully, causing the person to excel beyond what seems his or her potential. The person in later maturity, for example, has had many years of changing environmental influences; what he or she has become is no doubt an expression of innate genetic potential, environmental supports, and the wisdom to take advantage of both (19, 22, 57, 71).

Positive effects of nurture or environment have been found in research on shyness or inhibition to the unfamiliar. There is a genetic predisposition to shyness; however, the child can be helped to overcome this by parents who, in some cases, were also shy when they were young children. Nonparental caregivers during the first 2 years also help shy infants overcome their shyness (42, 62, 104). The parent can help the child face threatening situations, especially those involving people, and reduce anxiety. The child can be encouraged to interact with a variety of adults, play with children, and be around pets and other animals. If this is begun in infancy, by age 4 less than 20% of shy children are still shy. The competent parent can teach the child how to overcome the predisposition, and research over time shows that such children have become competent adults socially, often leaders. In a 4-year longitudinal study of 153 infants, those whose behavior patterns changed from shy to uninhibited (not shy) showed different brain activities (42, 62, 104).

Thus, judgments cannot be made at birth. Whatever the genetic background, the child deserves the opportunities to master the trait, turn the trait into an advantage, or learn how to cope with the trait. Experience strongly influences a child's personality traits by adulthood (19, 71, 96, 104).

PARENTAL AGE

More females are having children in their 30s or early 40s, often because early adult years are spent getting advanced education and establishing careers. Delay of pregnancy is more likely to cause complications due to diabetes, hypertension, or severe bleeding. After age 35 there is more chance of miscarriage or stillbirth, premature delivery, retarded fetal growth, and birth defects such as Down syndrome (34, 57).

Age of the mother and father and number of previous pregnancies affect the health of the fetus:

1. Pregnancy during the teen years, especially in poverty and before age 17, for the first birth is associated with prematurity, low birth weight, neurologic defects, higher mortality rates during the first year, and more developmental problems during preschool and school years. Pregnant teens are more likely to have inadequate income, poor diet, and inadequate prenatal care (19, 38, 53, 57, 138).

2. A baby born to a female who has had three or more pregnancies before age 20 is less likely to be healthy (38, 57, 138, 152).

3. Pregnancy after age 35 may increase the risk of delivery complications and problems in the neonate: prematurity, low birth weight, Down syndrome, and other birth defects. Fraternal twinning is also more common (34, 57, 58, 133).

4. The more pregnancies a female has had, the greater the risk to the infant. Maternal physiology cannot support many pregnancies in rapid succession, and as age increases, the ability to cope with the stresses of pregnancy decreases (34, 57, 145, 152).

5. When males are age 40 or older, they are at risk because sperm cells have divided so many times that there are more opportunities for errors. Anomalies linked to autosomal dominant mutations include Down syndrome, dwarfism, bone malformations, and Marfan syndrome (52, 57).

It is possible that the family situation following birth can offset some of the effects, especially in young childhood, associated with parental age. Disadvantaged maternal, and possibly paternal, background may explain some of the maternal age effects (34, 57, 138).

PRENATAL ENDOCRINE AND METABOLIC FUNCTIONS

Maternal endocrine function during pregnancy affects fetal growth and development. The placenta helps to provide necessary estrogens, progesterone, and gonadotropin to sustain pregnancy and trigger other endocrine adjustments that involve primarily the pituitary, adrenal cortex, and thyroid. Fetal endocrine function is regulated independently from the mother, but endocrine or hormonal drugs, such as birth control pills, progestin, diethylstilbestrol (DES), androgens, and synthetic estrogen, that are given to the mother may produce undesirable effects in the fetus (34, 52, 57).

The fetal period is the first critical period for sexual differentiation. Although the fetus has a chromosomal combination denoting male or female, the fetus must be exposed to corresponding hormones during pregnancy. If the male fetus is insensitive to androgen (a masculinizing hormone) and exposed to large amounts of estrogen (a feminizing hormone), the child may possess many female characteristics. Testicular inductor substance causes production of fetal androgens that suppress anatomic precursors of the oviducts and ovaries and, in turn, causes the male genital tract to develop during the seventh to twelfth weeks. The male embryo's testosterone offsets the maternal hormone influences. Unless androgens are present, the external genitalia of the fetus will appear female regardless of the chromosomal pattern. Estrogens are released in the genetically female embryo and are necessary for the fetus to develop female genitalia. Likewise, inspection of the external genitalia of a newborn female may show abnormal fusion of the labia and enlargement of the clitoris caused by an androgen agent taken by the mother early in her pregnancy (34).

The second critical period for sexual differentiation occurs just before or after birth, when sex typing of the brain may occur. Testosterone may influence the hypothalamus so that a noncyclic pattern for release of pituitary hormones, the gonadotropins, will occur in males and a cyclic pattern of gonadotropin release will occur in females (34, 52).

The mother's metabolic functions affect fetal and placental growth, nourishment, waste excretion, and total function (34, 52). For example, maternal hyperglycemia or diabetes promotes transfer of excessive glucose across the placenta to the fetus, stimulating fetal insulin secretion, a potent growth factor (34, 57). The mother with diabetes is at high risk, as is her fetus. Elevated levels of hemoglobin A_{1C} during the first trimester appear to be associated with higher incidence of congenital malformations, especially cardiac. High maternal blood glucose is a continual stimulus to insulin production by fetal islet cells (34, 52, 57). The sustained hyperglycemia causes excess growth, fat deposition, and **large for gestational age (LGA)**, *birth weight above the 90th percentile on the intrauterine growth curve* (34). When the newborn's glucose supply is removed abruptly at delivery, hypoglycemia soon occurs. The sudden glucose decrease can cause respiratory distress, neurologic damage, electrolyte imbalance, or death (57).

Infant survival is affected by the severity of maternal diabetes, duration of disease before pregnancy, age of onset, extent of vascular and renal complications, and abnormalities in the current pregnancy (1, 57).

Careful regulation of maternal glycemia by medical monitoring is essential during preconception and pregnancy. As most of the anomalies occur in the first few weeks of pregnancy, strict glycemic control beginning before conception is necessary to prevent long-range neurodevelopmental problems. Information for the mother is available from the local chapter of the American Diabetes Association.

MATERNAL NUTRITION

Requirements for most nutrients increase during pregnancy. Nutrition is one of the most important variables for fetal health and prevention of prenatal and intrapartal complications and long-term negative effects on the child. Normal gains are 25 to 35 pounds if the mother is of normal weight for height, 28 to 40 pounds if the mother is underweight, and 15 to 25 pounds if the mother is overweight. Desired weight gain depends on the female's weight-to-height ratio before pregnancy. Scientists know that at least 60 nutrients are basic to maintenance of healthy growth and development (39). *Lack of these nutrients may contribute to the following* (38, 57): (a) depressed appetite in the mother, (b) disease in the mother and in the baby, (c) low birth weight, (d) infant prematurity or stillbirth, (e) congenital malformation, (f) intrauterine growth retardation (IUGR), with consequent lower number of brain cells and mental retardation, and (g) infant mortality.

During the first 2 months of pregnancy, the developing embryo consists mostly of water. Later, more solids in the form of fat, nitrogen, and certain minerals are added. Because of the small amount of yolk in the human ovum, growth depends on nutrients obtained from the mother (38). During the first trimester, nutritional deprivations can negatively affect placental structure and the ultimate birth weight. For example, lack of vitamin A, as well as folate and iron, is linked to growth retardation, whereas supplements of calcium and magnesium may increase birth weight and length of gestation (34, 38). Malnutrition during pregnancy has long-term effects. People born during famine or wartime are more likely to die earlier than other people in the same country at other times (84, 91) or to demonstrate antisocial behavior (98). A link between fetal undernutrition and schizophrenia has been found (142).

Caloric and *protein intake* are of particular importance. Calories are needed for cell multiplication, and protein is believed to be primarily related to enlargement of these cells. Therefore, failure of the cells to receive sufficient protein and calories during critical periods of growth can lead to slowing down and ultimate cessation of the ability of these cells to enlarge, divide, and develop specialized functions. Lack of protein also affects later intellectual performance. Further, sufficient calories from fats and carbohydrates are needed so that protein is not used for energy (38).

Caloric requirements for the pregnant female are approximately 200 to 300 calories higher daily than for the nonpregnant female, starting the second trimester. If she has not gained at least 10 pounds by 5 months (20 weeks) of gestation, she is at risk for delivery of a child with intrauterine growth retardation, IUGR, or low birth weight for gestational age and prone to development delays. High weight gain during pregnancy increases the risk of an LGA infant large for gestational age and is associated with excess body fat during childhood. Further, the increase in maternal fat stores increases the risk of postpartum weight retention (38, 40, 57). The overweight female jeopardizes the fetus if she tries to lose weight during pregnancy. The effects of ketoacidosis, which results from calorie limitations, have been associated with neuropsychological defects in the infant (38, 57).

Educate about nutrition. Refer to the **Box** Client Education: Recommended Increases for Major Nutrients Needed by the Pregnant Woman, for major nutritional increases and the rationale related to function of the nutrient (38, 57). Educate about the need for a prenatal vitamin/mineral preparation daily during pregnancy, as well as other nutrient needs.

The recommended intake of phosphorus, sodium, zinc, iodine (via iodized salt), magnesium, potassium, and fluoride remains essentially unchanged during pregnancy. Substantial decreases in minerals can predispose the offspring to debilitating conditions. Most diets that supply sufficient calories for appropriate weight gain also supply adequate minerals and vitamins (38).

Educate that effects of inadequate nutrition are most severe for the pregnant adolescent, who herself has growth requirements, and for the mother with accumulated effects of several pregnancies, especially closely spaced ones. Nutritional deficiencies of the mother during her own fetal and childhood periods contribute to structural and physiologic difficulties in supporting a fetus. Improvement of the pregnant female's diet when she has previously been poorly nourished does not appreciably benefit the fetus. *The fetus apparently draws most of its raw materials for development from maternal body structure and lifetime reserves* (38, 57). Ultrasound assesses gestational age, fetal size, fetal structure, and fetal function (57).

Refer to **Appendix A**, Major Sources and Functions of Primary Nutrients, for information about nutrients. ∞ Education about a healthy diet should begin in childhood, since the nutritional status during pregnancy depends on prior nutritional status. You have a significant role in teaching proper nutrition to children and adolescents, as well as the pregnant woman. Emphasize the importance of water intake (8 glasses daily) and adequate fiber intake. Because caffeine is in so many drinks (coffee, tea, colas) and chocolate, emphasize the importance of limiting intake throughout life and pregnancy. Educate that *drinking more than eight cups of caffeine beverages daily during pregnancy is associated with increased risk of stillbirth* (38, 146).

We are advised to eat seafood, but there is a caveat. Mercury is a known teratogen and may be ingested when anyone, including the pregnant woman, unwittingly eats contaminated fish or water fowl, or wildlife that has eaten contaminated fish. Mercury enters the food chain when products containing it are incinerated, for example by hospitals and other health care or occupational settings. The mercury-laden waste products become airborne and settle in water, grass, and soil. It converts to methylmercury, a toxic form absorbed by living organisms in the food chain. In the fetus, mercury accumulates in the muscle tissue and is linked to neurologic and renal disorders. However, eating specially farmed fish or seafood carries less chance of mercury contamination (107, 118, 141).

Anemia

Effects of maternal anemia on the fetus are less clear than those on the mother. **Anemia** *denotes a decrease in the oxygen-carrying capability of the blood,* which is directly related to a reduction in hemoglobin concentration and number of red blood cells. Anemia, regardless of its cause, has been associated with spontaneous abortion, prematurity, low birth weight, and fetal death (34, 40, 57).

Iron deficiency anemia (*IDA*) accounts for most of the anemias diagnosed during pregnancy (38). Educate that extra iron requirements of pregnancy are needed for the fetus and placenta and to expand the maternal hemoglobin mass (38). IDA (as well as underweight and congenital defects) develops unless an adequate maternal iron replacement occurs. The developing fetus may not suffer severe ill effects of the mother's decreased iron supply if its own hemoglobin production is maintained at a normal level (i.e., if the placental source of iron is of sufficient amounts for the fetus to establish and maintain normal hemoglobin levels) (34).

Sickle-cell anemia syndrome in the mother is seen predominantly in the African American population and may show a number of negative effects on the developing fetus. Changes in the mother's pathophysiologic state may lead to IUGR, premature labor, a reduction in average birth weight, and even stillbirth, related to the "sickling" or clumping of malshaped erythrocytes within the placental vascular system (34, 57).

Pica

One nutritional tradition is **pica**, *a craving for and eating nonfood substances*, such as clay, unprocessed flour, cornstarch, laundry starch, coal, soap, toothpaste, mothballs, petrol, tar, paraffin, wood, plaster, soil, chalk, charcoal, cinders, baking powder, baking soda, powdered bricks, ice chips, and refrigerator frost scrapes. Pica is common in children and women of all cultures who are hungry, poor, and malnourished, and desire something to chew (9, 38, 40, 49, 50). Sometimes secrecy, folklore, or superstitious beliefs accompany this habit. Some African Americans in the southern part of the United States and their descendants believe that eating red and white clay overcomes the chances of disfigured offspring, may reduce nausea, and promotes a healthy baby or easy delivery. Pica is usually associated with iron deficiency; whether anemia is the cause or the effect is unknown (9, 38, 40).

Educate that pica interferes with normal nutrition by reducing appetite and can be harmful to baby and mother. Some clays interfere with the absorption of iron, zinc, and potassium (38).

Client Education

Recommended Increases for Major Nutrients Needed by the Pregnant Woman

Nutrient	Daily Requirement	Function
Protein	Increase 1.1 to 1.5 g/kg/day or 25 g over normal requirement.	Prevent maternal anemia, poor uterine muscle tone, spontaneous abortion, infection. Necessary for fetal growth and development of placenta, uterus, breasts, and increased maternal blood volume.
Folate/Folic acid	Increase from 400 to 600 mcg.	Build new cells and genetic material. Ensure 400 mcg intake 1 month before conception. Prevent neural birth defects (e.g., spina bifida), growth retardation, and anemia in fetus. Prevent maternal anemia.
Vitamin B_{12}	Increase from 1.3 to 1.9 mcg.	Interdependent with folate.
Niacin	Increase from 14 to 18 mcg.	Vitamin Bs needed in proportion to increased calories needed to use energy from food eaten. Needed for extra plasma of mother.
Thiamine and Riboflavin	Increase from 1.1 to 1.4 mg.	
Vitamin B_6	Increase 1.3 to 1.9 mg.	Involved in protein metabolism and body cell production.
Vitamin D	Maintain 400 IU or 5 mcgm.	Aid calcium absorption.
Calcium	1,000–1,300 mg.	Prevent or minimize depletion of maternal reserves. Fetal skeletal development, especially last month.
Iron	Increase 8–10 to 27–30 mg.	Protect maternal reserves; prevent iron deficiency anemia, which contributes to hemorrhage and preterm birth. One fourth of maternal iron transferred to placenta and fetus.
	Double from 30 to 60 mg with supplementation during last 3 to 4 months; take with 15 mg of zinc and 2 mg copper; iron interferes with absorption of these elements.	Maternal blood volume may double due to increases in plasma and erythrocytes. Secure fetal liver storage to sustain infants for 4 to 6 months.
Iodine	Consume through normal diet and use of iodized salt.	Prevent cretinism and neurodevelopmental anomalies.
Zinc	Increase 8 to 11–15 mg.	Prevent dwarfism, small head size, and lack of neuron/brain development in fetus.

MATERNAL EXERCISE AND PHYSICAL ACTIVITY

Moderate exercise does not endanger the fetus of healthy females. Regular exercise prevents constipation and improves respiration, circulation, muscle tone, and skin elasticity, which promotes a more comfortable pregnancy and safer delivery. Exercise in low-risk pregnancy should not raise the pulse above 140 beats per minute and should be tapered off—not stopped abruptly. Exercise that could cause abdominal trauma should be avoided (29, 34). Employment that involves strenuous and stressful working conditions, excess fatigue, and long working hours increases the risk of premature birth (8, 66, 67, 73, 76, 90, 93, 135, 149).

ENVIRONMENTAL HAZARDS TO THE FETUS: TERATOGENIC EFFECTS

Teratogens

A **teratogen** *is an agent or substance that causes cell death, malformation, growth retardation, or functional decline. The extent is determined by the type and dose or intensity of the agent and the vulnerability, the presence of a critical period, and the extent to which the environment can offset the negative effects* (34, 57, 132). **Teratogenesis** *is development of abnormal structures.* Teratogenesis is time-specific; the stimulus is nonspecific. Timing is more important than the nature of the insult or negative stimulus. *The first trimester is the most critical.* Development is characterized by a precise order. The timing, intensity, and duration of insult, injury, teratogen, or abnormal stimulus or event is important for the consequence. *Teratogenic agents affect genes in several ways* (34, 52, 57, 142): (a) genes cease protein production so that development ceases, (b) genes fail to complete development already begun, or (c) excess growth of part of the organism occurs.

Prominent environmental factors that have potential for damaging the fetus include (a) radiation, (b) chemical wastes, (c) contaminated water, (d) heavy metals such as lead, (e) some food additives, (f) various pollutants, (g) chemical interactions, (h) nicotine from smoking tobacco, (i) pica, (j) medicinal and nonmedicinal drugs, (k) alcohol, (l) maternal and paternal infections, and (m) maternal stress. The timing of fetal contact with a specific teratogen is a crucial factor, as depicted in Figures 8-1■ and 8-2■.

During the implantation period when the fertilized ovum lies free within the uterus and uses uterine secretions as its nutrition source, teratogens can cause spontaneous abortion of the embryo or severe birth defects. Once implantation has occurred (7 or 8 days after fertilization), the embryo undergoes very rapid and important transformations for the next 4 weeks. The sequence of embryonic events shows that each organ (brain, heart, eye, limbs, and genitalia) undergoes a critical stage of differentiation at precise times. For example, during the third week, teratogens can harm basic structures of the heart and central nervous system. Even during the third trimester, fetal cerebral vascular reaction to certain teratogens can be detrimental. Each teratogen acts on a selected aspect of cellular metabolism (34, 52, 141).

A complicated interplay exists among the father, mother, offspring, and teratogen. In addition to the critical period of developmental stage and genetic susceptibility, the *degree to which a teratogen causes abnormalities depends on the* (a) dosage, (b) absorption, (c) distribution, (d) metabolism, (e) physical state of the mother, and (f) excretion by the separate body systems of mother and fetus. A teratogen that enters a mother's system also enters the system of her developing child, meaning that the so-called *placental barrier is practically nonexistent* (34).

External Environmental Factors

Prenatally, environmental teratogens may interfere with the development of the embryo or fetus directly or may cause hormonal, circulatory, or nutritional changes in the mother that in turn damage the organism. Many teratogens are linked to gross malformations and growth retardation; some are linked to stillbirth, prematurity,

developmental delay, or even increased risk of malignancy in later life. Examples of teratogens are described in Chapter 4. ∞
Teratogens also include:

1. Excess heat, soaks in hot tubs, or sauna baths in early pregnancy, which may cause fetal neural tube defects (34, 96).
2. High levels of noise (34, 73).
3. Radiation from multiple sources at work (maternal or paternal) or from diagnostic tests (most procedures cause low-level fetal x-ray exposure if performed accurately, but the pregnant woman should inform diagnosticians) (34, 97, 105, 108, 109).
4. Ultraviolet light from excessive sun or a sunlamp (34, 40, 82, 141).
5. Air, water, and soil pollutants, including lead, mercury, and pesticides or chemicals (20, 64, 72, 137, 141).
6. Trace minerals or chemicals linked to the work setting (64, 99, 105, 141, 149).
7. Chemicals, hormones, and drugs in food or used in meat production (64, 98, 118).
8. Chemotherapeutic (antineoplastic) medications (23, 34, 45).

Occupational hazards include transfer of drugs and chemicals from the male to the female during intercourse—an action that later can negatively affect fertilization or implantation or, if she is already pregnant, can have teratogenic effects on the developing fetus. For example, decreased sperm count and infertility are related to paternal exposure to dibromochloropropane (DBCP). Paternal exposure to toxic agents is most likely to result in male infertility or spontaneous abortions. Anesthetic gases, vinyl chloride exposure, chloroprene, or other hydrocarbons have all been connected to spontaneous abortions. Lead present in the environment directly increases sperm abnormalities, induces male infertility, and facilitates spontaneous abortion through either affected sperm or indirect contamination (20, 64, 72, 105, 107). Persistent environmental contaminants, such as dioxin and polychlorobiphenyls (PCBs), alter the activities of several different hormones (20, 136, 141).

Occupational hazards may include the effects of physical effort or activity, such as exertion of high-speed performance, repeated bending or twisting, and lifting heavy objects. Such activity may contribute to preterm delivery and low birth weight (29, 73, 76, 78, 90, 93, 100, 135, 149). Nurses who have strenuous working conditions, occupation fatigue, and long working hours have greater risk of premature birth (73, 78, 141). Certain kinds of jobs may also predispose to spontaneous abortion because of contact with chemicals. Lead exposure at work is associated with lower birth weight, premature birth, or stillbirth (57). Radiation, even diagnostic x-ray within a year before conception, can cause low birth weight or slowed fetal growth (57, 109). Health care providers and their employers should be sensitive to the presence of occupational fatigue associated with workload during pregnancy.

Polyvinyl chloride (PVC) plastics are common in many products used in the United States and constitute about 25% of health care products and packaging. These products, including plastic food containers and toys, are problematic when incinerated, as dioxin is produced. **Dioxin,** *a highly toxic substance, is believed responsible for*

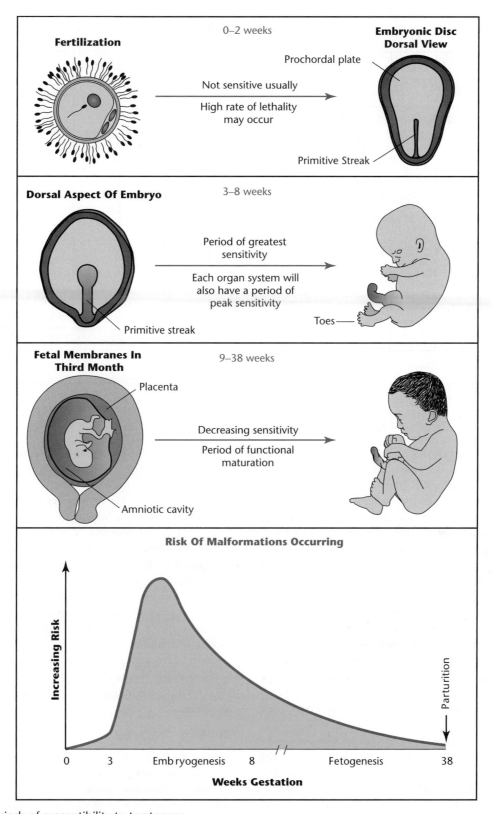

FIGURE ◼ **8-1** Periods of susceptibility to teratogens.

Source: Sadler, T.W. (1985). *Langman's Medical Embryology* (5th ed.). Baltimore: Lipincott, Williams & Wilkins. Used with permission.

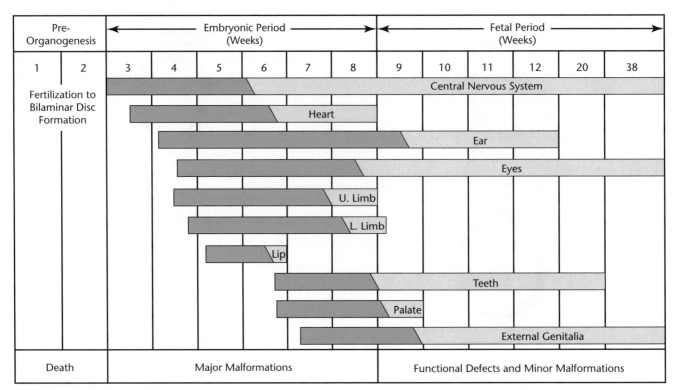

FIGURE ■ 8-2 Susceptibility of organ systems to teratogens. Solid bars denote highly sensitive periods.
Source: Sadler, T. W. (1985). *Langman's Medical Embryology* (5th ed.). Baltimore: Williams & Wilkins.

the many adverse effects of exposure to Agent Orange, a chemical widely sprayed during the 1970s in the Vietnam War. Vietnam veterans have experienced chloracne, latent extreme fatigue, liver damage, various cancers, and joint pain in back, hips, and fingers. Offspring of Vietnam veterans exposed to dioxin have experienced increases in spontaneous abortions and congenital malformations (spina bifida, cleft lip, and neoplasms) (20, 131, 136). *Dioxin is still with us,* due to the manufacture and disposal methods of products with PVC. Dioxin, the by-product, travels airborne across the landscape to affect the food chain. Grass-eating animals ingest it; dioxin is stored in animal fat, in cow's milk, and less so in human milk. Dioxin is carcinogenic when ingested over time (107, 136). Continued research is warranted because veterans of the Gulf War are also complaining of a variety of symptoms some time after return to the United States (54). Veterans of World War II who were involved in the atomic bombing of Japan also have evidenced similar long-term symptoms and illnesses that appear related to their proximity to radiation (54).

Contaminants that are passed from mother to baby during the prenatal period can alter a child's immune system, increasing the later risk of cancer, infectious disease, and autoimmune disorders. Exposure to *agricultural pesticides and industrial chemicals* may cause abnormalities in the reproductive system, causing later infertility. Playing in lead-contaminated dust can disrupt brain development, causing attention and learning disorders, and possibly aggressive and antisocial behavior (57). Studies of the effects of pesticides in agricultural regions show a higher rate of birth defects in the children of both farming and nonfarming families, and in the children of migrant workers (104, 141).

Mercury, like lead, has major implications for the health of the mother and offspring. Mercury-contaminated water results from medical wastes, industrial by-products, incinerator emissions, and dumpsite leakage. Inorganic mercury converts to the more harmful organic form, methylmercury, which is absorbed by fish and then consumed by humans. When ingested during pregnancy, nervous system impairment, compromised immune function, and a congenital syndrome similar to cerebral palsy may occur (141).

Educate clients about these teratogens. Discuss ways to limit or avoid contact with them. Encourage parents to avoid PVC plastic products for their homes and plastic toys for their children when possible. Educate families about organic food choices. Explore working conditions with clients and the possibility of workplace legislative advocacy. Health care consumers and professionals should work together so that hospitals and health care agencies use PVC-free equipment and supplies and limit contact with other teratogens.

Smoking Tobacco

Tobacco smoking is addictive; nicotine is the substance responsible for the addictive process.

Although data on smoking related to pregnancy are usually collected via self-report, a more accurate method is to measure the cotinine level in either maternal or umbilical serum (34). Females who continue to smoke during their pregnancy may cut down but have difficulty quitting the addiction. Many express a desire to quit, feeling guilty about not being able to do so, but report that smoking relaxes them and helps mood control. Based on the abundance of evidence pointing to the damaging effects of smoking to

INTERVENTIONS FOR HEALTH PROMOTION

Educate that smoking is associated with numerous detrimental effects:

1. Decreased maternal pulmonary function; increased carbon monoxide levels (34, 120).
2. Vasoconstriction in the mother, reducing blood flow to the fetus (34, 57).
3. Abnormal bleeding during pregnancy (34, 57).
4. Decreased fetal oxygen, lower oxygen tension, and fetal apnea or hypoxia from nicotine and cotinine transfer through the placenta (34, 57, 140).
5. Reduced fetal hemoglobin from carbon monoxide that crosses the placenta (34, 140).
6. Higher percentage of spontaneous abortions, stillbirths, and preterm or premature births (decreased gestational age) (7, 34, 140).
7. Lower birth weight (less than 2.5 kg, or 5.5 pounds) as number of cigarettes smoked daily increases (34, 140, 151).

8. Higher perinatal mortality for infants at every level of birth weight (34, 57, 140).
9. Increased possibility of sudden infant death syndrome (SIDS) (57, 104).
10. Later growth retardation in the child, related to carbon monoxide effects (34, 57, 140).
11. Increased respiratory disease, pneumonia, bronchitis, and allergy in infancy and childhood (34, 40, 57, 140).
12. Decreased physical and social development in young children of mothers who smoke 10 or more cigarettes daily (16, 41, 125, 127, 140).
13. Childhood cancer linked to prenatal smoking by mother or exposure to smoking by others (passive smoking) (69, 140).
14. Poor attention span, hyperactivity, slower perceptual-motor and linguistic development, learning difficulties (reading, mathematics), and minimal brain dysfunction in school-age children (19, 34, 57, 140).

both mother and fetus, total avoidance of smoking before and during pregnancy is a major medical and health promotion recommendation.

Health education for pregnant smokers increases the rate of quitting; counseling and information are effective and cost beneficial. Encourage smoking cessation programs, either self-help or structured interventions. Educate that a growing body of research links smoking with lowered birth weight as well as reduced sperm count and abnormal sperm shape.

DRUG HAZARDS TO THE FETUS: TERATOGENIC EFFECTS

Medications That Cross the Placenta

Many medications cross the placenta to the fetus from the mother's blood. The placenta acts like a sieve, not a barrier. Thus *no drug, whether obtained by prescription or over-the-counter, should be taken during pregnancy unless it is medically prescribed as necessary for the mother* (34, 79). With rare exception, any drug that exerts a systemic effect in the mother will cross the placenta to reach the embryo or fetus. If an essential drug is administered during pregnancy, the advantages to be gained must clearly outweigh any risks inherent in its use. A drug should be prescribed only if withholding it would cause a more serious consequence for the mother than its adverse effects on the fetus (40, 46).

Antidepressant medication use in pregnant women must be considered carefully for risk to the baby. Selective serotonin reuptake inhibitors (SSRIs), such as fluoxetine (Prozac) and sertraline (Zoloft), may not cause serious birth defects and may be considered acceptable treatment for the depressed pregnant woman (5, 46, 63, 79, 115, 147). However, if the mother takes an SSRI, the

baby at birth may suffer the neonatal serotonin syndrome (67) or temporary discontinuation syndrome, with abnormal movements and behavioral effects (80, 115, 148).

Lithium, a mood stabilizer, has serious teratogenic effects, causing risk of birth defects. However, bipolar mood swings during pregnancy may be so dangerous that medication is necessary (40, 46, 147). An alternative is to discontinue and then administer lithium near the delivery date (40, 46).

Psychotherapy alone is preferable to medication use in pregnant females who are depressed. Support groups can also be effective. Including the father-to-be in counseling sessions is ideal in order to explore feelings about the pregnancy, crisis and loss issues, anticipated as well as current role changes, and interpersonal and sexual difficulties (147).

Educate adolescents and females of childbearing age that many commonly used prescribed and over-the-counter medications have teratogenic effects. The first trimester is a critical period, but some medications are more teratogenic in the third trimester. Teach clients how to obtain information about hazardous drug effects, for example, by asking the pharmacist, physician, or nurse; reading labels or packaged inserts; using *reliable* sources on the Internet; or reading relevant texts or periodicals.

Drug Abuse and Addiction

During pregnancy, drug abuse and addiction continue to manifest themselves as major psychosocial and physical problems for both mother and child. Substances commonly abused during pregnancy, taken individually or in combination, are known to have multiple effects on the developing fetus, on the outcome of pregnancy, on neonatal neurobehavior, and on development in childhood and adolescence (40, 57). Infants exposed to addictive drugs *in utero* throughout pregnancy are at great risk for a higher rate of congenital malformations, obstetric complications, and perinatal mortality (34, 40, 46).

There are many addictive substances. Several will be discussed in this section. Drugs that act on the central nervous system are often lipophilic and have relatively low-molecular-weight characteristics, which facilitate crossing of the so-called placental–fetal blood–brain barrier (34). Some drugs can be metabolized by the fetal liver and placenta; however, these metabolites are water soluble (34).

MARIJUANA *When used by the mother, marijuana affects the embryo, the fetus, and the child after birth.* Low birth weight, premature delivery, small size for gestational age, neurologic disturbances (e.g., tremors), and various malformations, including chromosomal abnormalities, occur more often than the norm. At birth, the baby is likely to have a depressed Apgar score and neuromuscular abnormalities. Following birth, weight loss is accelerated. There has been a linkage found with acute lymphoblastic leukemia in the young child (7, 44, 57). Cancer-causing mutations have been found in blood samples from the umbilical cord, indicating increased risk for cancer (7). At age 4, poor verbal and memory development has been found (7, 19).

COCAINE AND OPIATES *Addictive drugs, such as cocaine, heroin, morphine, and codeine, affect the mother and baby because they* (21, 65, 121) (a) affect the mother's overall health and nutrition, (b) often interfere with motivation to obtain prenatal care, and (c) interfere with blood flow to the placenta by means of vasoconstriction and increasing uterine contractibility. Cocaine, the number-one illicit drug in the United States, acts peripherally to inhibit nerve conduction and prevent norepinephrine uptake at nerve terminals, increasing norepinephrine levels, with subsequent vasoconstriction and abrupt rise in blood pressure. This effect is greater than with use of opiates. *The drugs cause a high incidence of maternal complications including* (a) hypertension, (b) spontaneous abortion, (c) lack of sufficient maternal weight gain, (d) intrauterine growth retardation, (e) toxemia, (f) abruptio placentae, (g) shorter gestation period and premature birth, (h) stillbirth, (i) breech delivery, and (j) postpartum hemorrhage (13, 21, 24, 65, 121, 150).

Addiction to narcotics, such as heroin, morphine, or codeine, creates another problem: fetal addiction. Withdrawing the drug from the addicted female before delivery causes the fetus to experience withdrawal distress as a result of visceral vasoconstriction and reduced circulation to the uterus. Intrauterine death may occur. However, when addiction continues, the infant is born with drug addiction (92). The addicted newborn is twice as likely to die soon after birth than the nonaddicted baby. If the newborn does not die, it will experience withdrawal in 2 to 4 days. This is the *acute* period. The baby will require treatment during the *withdrawal* period (92). The limited ability of the newborn to metabolize and eliminate these fat-soluble drugs may be responsible for postponement of early withdrawal symptoms. However, the withdrawal does not end the problems (92). Babies born addicted to opiates may suffer effects of the addiction until at least age 6 years (57).

The Brazelton Neonatal Behavioral Assessment Scale can be used to evaluate normality of responses to environmental stimuli (57). Finnegan's Neonatal Narcotic Abstinence Syndrome Scale is useful for assessing neonatal narcotic withdrawal (121). *The specific pattern of symptoms is dependent on* (a) the type, amount, and combination of drugs used by the mother; (b) the length of time between drug exposure and delivery; and (c) the fetal ability to metabolize the drug. See **Box 8-1**, Neonatal Narcotic Abstinence Syndrome, for a list of the symptoms and signs that are typically observed in the neonate who has been addicted during pregnancy to cocaine, heroin, or another narcotic and suddenly suffers withdrawal (24, 25, 70, 92, 121).

The effects of addictive drugs on the child extend beyond the neonatal and infancy periods. In early childhood, babies who were addicted may weigh less and be shorter than the norm, and overall be less well adjusted. They show slowed psychomotor development at 1 year of age. These children score lower on perceptual and learning ability tests, are more anxious, and do not perform as well in school (12, 34, 43, 44, 57, 110).

Clinical assessment during pregnancy for substance abuse should include evaluation of physical appearance, since demeanor and hygiene may give clues; a thorough history and physical examination; and a substance abuse interview to determine multiple drug use or exposure to more than one teratogen. Urine samples of mothers also screen for ingestion of illicit drugs.

Be aware that a more recent addictive teratogen is affecting the fetus. Pregnant females who are addicted to *inhalants*, such as solvents, glue, or aerosols, create risks for the fetus with continued use. The newborn typically manifests crossed eyes, microencephaly, and other signs of brain damage (19). Assess for signs of

---

INTERVENTIONS FOR HEALTH PROMOTION

Educate the public and families that cocaine and opiates cause a high incidence of the following complications at birth and in the **neonatal** *(newborn) period* (13, 24, 25, 57, 65, 70, 112):

1. Fetal growth retardation; premature delivery.
2. Lower birth weight.
3. Shorter body length.
4. Smaller head circumference.
5. Cardiopulmonary abnormalities.

6. Tachycardia and hypertension, causing cerebrovascular hemorrhage; computed tomographic (CT) scan of the neonate can confirm presence of acute focal cerebral infarction.
7. Impaired neurologic development.
8. Learning problems the first years of life.
9. Perceptual and motor impairments that continue long term to affect the child's learning.

INTERVENTIONS FOR HEALTH PROMOTION

Educate the public and families that children exposed to cocaine or "crack" in the fetal state have an abnormally high incidence of later severe physical, neurologic, and emotional problems, including the following (12, 43, 65, 104, 110, 112):

1. Brain shrinkage or cerebral atrophy.
2. Learning difficulties; impaired attention span for at least 5 years.
3. Impaired orientation; decreased ability to orient to auditory and visual stimuli.
4. Growth retardation.
5. Severe impairments in motor movements, including simple movements such as eating, dressing, and nonnutritive sucking into early childhood, and tremors.
6. Irritability; impulsivity.
7. Extreme sensitivity to sounds.
8. Disrupted rapid eye movement (REM) sleep patterns, affecting personality.
9. Various social and personality difficulties.
10. Permanent physical and mental damage as a result of fetal anoxia or fetal or neonatal cerebrovascular hemorrhage.

this addiction, and encourage treatment. Refer the females to appropriate treatment resources.

Explain to the pregnant female that *effects of drug use on the fetus, neonate, and child depend on the type of drug ingested, dose, duration of drug use before and during pregnancy, and state of maternal nutrition. There are fewer infant symptoms when the pregnant female stops drug use in the first trimester of pregnancy than if drug use continues.* Thus, it is imperative to prevent drug use, to support the mother's efforts to stop drug use, and to encourage adequate prenatal care and nutrition. Prenatal care must include increased surveillance for drug-related complications. Prenatal rehabilitation and support efforts should continue after delivery and address issues that lead to and maintain patterns of abuse.

METHAMPHETAMINE The easily manufactured **methamphetamine** or **"meth"** *is a powerful nervous system stimulant that quickly becomes powerfully addictive related to a massive release of dopamine in the brain.* It is snorted, smoked, swallowed, or ingested by mouth. The person experiences a short and intense euphoria, increased alertness, self-confidence, and sexual stimulation, and is

BOX 8-1 Neonatal Narcotic Abstinence Syndrome: Manifestations of Narcotic Withdrawal

CENTRAL NERVOUS SYSTEM (SIGNS APPEAR WITH FIRST 24 HOURS)

1. Hyperirritability
2. Hyperactivity: hard to hold; failure to mold to mother's body
3. Restlessness
4. Incessant shrill cry
5. Inability to sleep, disturbed REM sleep
6. Hypertonia of muscles
7. Hyperactive reflexes
8. Stretching
9. Tremors
10. Poor temperature regulation; fever
11. Possible generalized convulsions

RESPIRATORY SYSTEM

1. Rapid irregular breathing
2. Yawning
3. Sneezing
4. Nasal stuffiness, congestion
5. Excessive secretions
6. Intermittent cyanosis
7. Respiratory alkalosis
8. Periods of apnea

CARDIOVASCULAR SYSTEM

1. Tachycardia

GASTROINTESTINAL SYSTEM

1. Frantic sucking of hands; disorganized sucking behavior
2. Difficulty sucking and feeding; poor closure of lips around nipple
3. Appearance of being very hungry
4. Sensitive gag reflex
5. Regurgitation
6. Vomiting
7. Diarrhea
8. Progressive weight loss

SKIN

1. Pallor
2. Sweating
3. Excoriation

MUSCULOSKELETAL SYSTEM

1. Small head size
2. Short length

unlikely to stop use. Long-term use causes extensive adverse physical, emotional, cognitive, and social effects that are teratogenic (27, 32, 60, 81, 113).

Use during pregnancy is associated with maternal hypertension, placenta abruptio, fetal hypoxia and distress, and premature delivery. Effects on the fetus include microencephaly, intrauterine growth retardation, cerebral infarcts, cardiac defects, cleft lip, eye deformities, biliary atresia, and small for gestational age at birth. Effects on the newborn are more extensive with three trimesters of exposure and are dose related. Some of the effects may be a result of maternal malnutrition and body rhythm disturbance due to insomnia. Some users also smoke tobacco or marijuana; either agent could contribute to teratogenesis. At birth, the infant is likely to be quiet and withdrawn. In early childhood, neurophysical and developmental problems are manifested: difficulty with motor skills, poor visual recognition memory, delay in language and other cognitive skill acquisition, and aggressive behavior (27, 32, 60, 81, 113).

Care of the female and child is intensive. Rehabilitation of the addicted female and partner is difficult because of mental, emotional, and social effects of drug use. Follow-up of the child is necessary to determine abuse or neglect. Follow-up is also difficult because of the lifestyle and geographic mobility of the user. Colyar and Schmidt present information about medical care of the patient who is abusing meth (27).

ALCOHOL *Alcohol ingested before or during pregnancy serves as another common cause of abnormal changes in the fetus and may increase perinatal mortality (34, 144). Every time a mother-to-be drinks, the unborn baby drinks in a matter of minutes.* Alcohol circulates to every tissue and through the placenta. The *blood alcohol concentration (BAC) in the female is influenced by* (a) amount ingested, (b) duration of drinking, (c) body size, (d) health status, (e) when food was last eaten, (f) body metabolism, and (g) genetic makeup. The BAC is the same in the fetus as in the mother. Alcohol is cleared from the mother's body in 1 to 1 1/2 hours; it takes about 8 to 12 hours to be eliminated from the fetus. Both the first and third trimesters are critical periods (34, 144).

First-trimester exposure to alcohol has the potential to affect total development of the fetus, including physical deformities, major cognitive impairment, and diminished growth (3, 57). Fetal alcohol exposure during the third trimester negatively affects the child's higher brain functions, including attention and behavioral deficits, in contrast to effects of alcohol exposure during the first and second trimesters (2, 15, 57). The timing of prenatal alcohol exposure is critical for outcomes to the child, according to a study that prospectively tracked African American females' substance abuse throughout pregnancy and followed the children 6 to 7 years (124). Effects of alcohol exposure during the third trimester are more readily assessed during the school years, outweighing environmental influences (95, 124, 126). Thus, at any point in pregnancy it will benefit the child if the female reduces alcohol intake or quits (3). Ethanol acts as a teratogen, as an inhibitor in the conversion of vitamin A to a molecule (retinoic acid), which is needed for normal nervous system and limb development (34). It affects production and release of hormones and neurotransmitters, which

in turn may affect later cognitive skills and behavior (2, 14, 17, 57, 124, 127).

Alcoholic beverages should be avoided by the couple. Drinking as little as 3 oz of liquor daily increases the chances of congenital defects, low birth weight, preterm delivery, stillbirth, abruptio placentae, and spontaneous abortion (38). The central nervous system develops through the entire gestational period and is thereby vulnerable to alcohol exposure at any time during pregnancy, particularly the third trimester (38). Alcoholism in the father may inhibit spermatogenesis and also act as a teratogen that contributes to chromosomal breaks or damaged genes, resulting in spontaneous abortion or birth defects (57, 144).

Fetal alcohol syndrome (FAS) or alcohol-related birth defects (ARBD) is the diagnosis when alcohol ingestion by the pregnant female causes a number of deformities usually seen in the child, including (3, 26, 57, 86, 87, 122, 128, 130, 144):

1. Eye and face malformation, short palpebral fissures, thin upper lip, flattened philtrum, flat midface features, and extra digits (these features occur with alcohol intake during the first 2 months).
2. Cardiac malformation (occurs with alcohol exposure during the first trimester).
3. Decreased brain weight and microencephaly, defective neuronal migration, delayed myelinization of fetal brain, and hippocampal and cerebellar cell loss.
4. Impaired fine motor skills, poor tandem gait and eye-hand coordination, neurosensory hearing loss, and disturbed sleep patterns.
5. Growth deficiency, low birth weight, lack of weight gain, and disproportionately low weight to height over time, into school age.

Fetal alcohol effects (FAE) *is the diagnosis when the person is significantly, adversely affected by prenatal alcohol exposure but does not demonstrate completely the criteria for FAS.* Facial structure deformity may not be as apparent but the central nervous system has been compromised, which affects physical and cognitive development negatively (3, 87, 144).

Heavy prenatal alcohol exposure (a case of beer or a fifth of hard liquor daily) has psychiatric and behavioral consequences by mid-childhood and adolescence (17, 123). Diagnoses include attention deficit/hyperactivity disorder (ADHD), oppositional defiant disorder (ODD), conduct disorder, tic disorders, and mood disorders by age 8 to 14 years (17, 126). Impairments in social problem-solving skills and executive functions are found in adolescents who were exposed to alcohol *in utero*. No child or adolescent, matched by age and socioeconomic status in the control group (no prenatal alcohol exposure), has met the criteria for these disorders (17, 95, 123, 126).

In a sample of 43 alcohol-exposed and 23 nonexposed children, 42 of 43 exposed and 1 of 22 nonexposed subjects met the criteria for ADHD. Almost 33% (13 of 43) of exposed and 1 nonexposed met the criteria for ODD. Mood disorders were found in 8, tic disorders in 4, and conduct disorders in 5. No child in the control group had these disorders. Social problem-solving deficits were found in 24 of 43 adolescents. They approached problems with a pessimistic orientation and low frustration tolerance. They were less effective at identifying problems, generating solutions, making decisions, and implementing or verifying a chosen solution (17).

Educate females to abstain from drinking from the time of conception, or when planning conception. Otherwise, she should stop drinking at the point she knows she is pregnant. If the female is addicted, she is unlikely to be able to stop abruptly. Thus, females of childbearing age should be screened for alcohol problems and educated about the risks of alcohol use prior to and during pregnancy. Referral to agencies and professionals that specialize in counseling and addiction is recommended. Infants born with FAS or ARBD should be medically monitored and referred to specialized care, as should their parents. If the mother has sought or completed addiction treatment, give support for her abstinence or reduced intake. The partner also needs support and education. Relatives or foster parents unfamiliar with FAS or ARBD should be educated; realistic expectations of the child must be established. The child needs a calm environment, adequate care, and appropriate opportunities to achieve maximal potential.

EFFECTS OF FOLKLORE

Folklore can be defined as *strong beliefs about certain facets of or influences on basic aspects of life.* Most cultures, especially those that adhere less to scientific thinking, define certain desirable or forbidden activities for the pregnant female. Folklore may be believed, feared, or unconsciously practiced even by well-educated or professional people, although they might not openly admit it. The commonly experienced fear of giving birth to an abnormal infant causes the pregnant female, or even the father-to-be, to act in ways that would otherwise be rejected or opposed. The more tightly the female is bound by her culture, the more she follows the rules or taboos surrounding food, hygiene, activity, and contacts with other people. Many cultures emphasize that she should look at pleasant sights, think positive thoughts, eat certain foods, and pursue certain leisure activities to ensure a healthy, happy, talented child. Many cultures emphasize that unhappy thoughts, aggressive actions, certain foods, unpleasant sights, or unusual or strenuous activity should be avoided to prevent bearing a sick, deformed, or dead baby. Often folklore practices do not interfere with scientific practices. Therefore, you should not ridicule or try to convince the mother to drop these practices, since the resulting conflict she feels internally or from her culture may have adverse health effects. Further, folklore often evolves so that the pregnant female is protected from hazards or given extra care that, in turn, meets her needs emotionally and physically (9, 50, 114).

MATERNAL INFECTIONS: HAZARDOUS INFLUENCE ON THE FETUS

The pregnant female is more susceptible to infections. The placenta cannot screen out all infectious organisms; therefore, infectious diseases in the vaginal region can travel up to the amniotic sac and penetrate its walls and infect the amniotic fluid. Viral, bacterial, and parasitic diseases that have a mild effect on the mother may have a profound effect on the development of the fetus, depending on gestational age (34). *Viruses causing other infections, such as mumps, chickenpox, smallpox, scarlet fever, and viral hepatitis, may be related to formation of anomalies in utero, and during the last month of pregnancy, they may cause a life-threatening fetal infection and major consequences to the infact* (34, 57, 68).

Rubella and Rubeola

Rubella (*German measles*) *can manifest as a maternal infection that may occur during the first trimester with harmful effects.* Rubella may go unnoticed by the mother, but it can cause severe effects, Congenital Rubella Syndrome, and even death (40). Amniocentesis can be used to detect the presence of rubella *in utero* (34). The fetus suffers an abnormal decrease in the absolute number of cells in most organs because of the viral interference with cell multiplication. The virus also causes adverse changes in the small blood vessels of the developing fetus and does profuse damage to the placental vascular system, thus interfering with fetal blood flow and oxygenation. **Rubeola** (*"long measles"*) is also associated with congenital defects (34, 57).

Human Immunodeficiency Viral Disease

HIV and AIDS in males and females is a worldwide concern because of transmission between heterosexual and homosexual partners and in nonpartnered sexual relationships. The number of HIV-infected females of childbearing age is rising worldwide. However, the overall number of HIV-infected females giving birth has declined in the United States. Because of the long incubation period (at least 5 years), the pregnant female may be unaware that she has the virus. Females who are intravenous drug users are at high risk, as are their babies. One of the 28 focus areas for research and practice and widespread education in *Healthy People 2010* is human immunodeficiency virus (139). There is considerable focus on decreasing HIV/AIDS among various cultural groups, educating people about prevention, and avoiding a fatalistic attitude among people at risk or infected. Not all infants born to HIV-infected females become infected. Transmission appears more likely when the mother has full-blown AIDS than when she is HIV-positive but not yet experiencing AIDS symptoms. Infection may depend on the strain of virus to which the fetus is exposed. Infant consequences may be severe.

The typical life expectancy of the child born with AIDS is as yet unknown. The medical and psychological consequences are devastating. The child faces physical deterioration, social isolation and stigma, early death, and the deterioration and death of his or her mother and possibly other family members or friends.

To protect the health care provider, the Centers for Disease Control and Prevention (CDC) emphasizes the consistent use of blood and body fluid universal precautions with all patients to avoid contact with secretions during all patient or client care.

The CDC mandates testing of infants born in the United States for certain congenital diseases, such as PKU and thyroid disease. In 1988, the HIV antibody test was added to this panel. The

MediaLink Centers for Disease Control and Prevention

purpose was to identify trends of HIV infection in childbearing females, because the presence of antibodies in the newborn reveals the HIV status of the mother. Some states mandate this testing because an HIV-positive child can be treated, reducing the risk of AIDS. However, it takes 4 to 6 weeks for test results to be obtained, and follow-up of HIV-positive mothers and infants for treatment purposes may be difficult. Often, these mothers cannot be located; they do not return for well-baby or postpartal checkups (40, 57, 74).

An interdisciplinary team approach is essential to address the complex medical, psychological, social, and economic problems of persons with AIDS. Research on prevention, treatment, and eventual eradication of the disease, for all age groups, is essential.

Maternal Syphilis, Chlamydia, and Gonorrhea

Maternal syphilis should be identified and treated before or early in pregnancy to prevent devastating consequences for the neonate and child. Treatment of the mother also ensures treatment of the ill fetus because penicillin or erythromycin readily crosses the placenta (40, 57).

Chlamydia trachomatis **and gonorrhea are two genital infections that are easily transmitted and can produce pelvic inflammatory disease (PID) and affect the fetus and neonate.** Younger females (ages 15 to 24) are the group most affected. Tubal adhesions resulting from PID are an important factor in the occurrence of ectopic pregnancies. Sexual partners should be tested and treated with appropriate antibiotics (34, 40, 57).

Genital Herpes Simplex

The incidence of **herpes simplex virus (HSV),** *an infection of the genital area,* is increasing. Thus, the prevention and treatment of perinatal herpes simplex (type 2) is of great public concern. Primary and recurrent genital herpes can range from severe extensive ulceration to asymptomatic virus shedding.

Unlike rubella, which readily crosses the placenta, the potential hazards of herpes simplex generally await the fetus in the maternal cervix or lower genital tract. The herpes simplex virus invades the uterus following the rupture of membranes or during the normal vaginal birth descent. Vaginal delivery may mean the development of systemic lesions. The primary source is maternal; genital herpes infections are sexually transmitted. The majority of genital infec-

tions are asymptomatic and difficult to recognize on clinical examination, thus making the identification of a mother whose fetus is in jeopardy very difficult (34, 40, 57).

Cytomegalovirus Disease

Cytomegalovirus (CMV), *another dangerous virus, causes infection similar to one of the herpes viruses.* Sixty percent of all females have CMV antibodies; the disease occurs in 1% to 3% of pregnant females and approximately half of their babies. CMV may go undetected in the mother and in the young child because the disease is asymptomatic, but the virus is transmitted via urine, saliva, tears, semen, and breast milk. Laboratory analysis of infant cord blood detects the virus. CMV is now thought to be the single most important known infectious cause of congenital mental retardation and deafness.

Toxoplasmosis

Toxoplasmosis *is an infection caused by a parasite harbored in the bodies of cattle, sheep, and pigs and the intestinal tracts of cats.* It is contracted by eating infected meat or eggs that are raw or undercooked or through contact with the feces of an infected cat. Should the mother become infected during pregnancy, there is a good possibility that the parasite will cross the placental barrier. Flulike symptoms can be mild in adults.

Hepatitis B virus infection and **varicella (chickenpox)** *are other infections transmitted from the pregnant woman to the fetus* and have serious consequences.

IMMUNOLOGIC FACTORS

The fetus is immunologically foreign to the mother's immune system, yet the fetus is sustained. Selected antibodies of measles, chickenpox, hepatitis, poliomyelitis, whooping cough, and diphtheria are transferred to the fetus. The resulting immunity lasts for several months after birth. Antibodies to dust, pollen, and common allergens do not transfer across the placenta (34). *Incompatibility between maternal and infant blood factors* is the most commonly encountered interference with fetal development, resulting in various degrees of circulatory difficulty for the baby. When fetal blood contains a protein substance, the Rh factor (Rh-positive blood), but the mother's blood does not (Rh-negative

---

INTERVENTIONS FOR HEALTH PROMOTION

Educate the public and expectant families about the following:

1. Prevention of fetal infections begins with both partners maintaining health prior to conception.
2. Maintenance of up-to-date immunizations is essential, especially for females.
3. Prevention and early treatment of all infections, especially of the urinary tract, male genital tract, vagina, and female reproductive system, is essential for health during preconception and pregnancy.

4. Utilization of safe sex practices prevents sexually transmitted infections to the female before and during pregnancy and to the fetus and child.
5. Prevention and health promotion measures for specific infections are described in the table, Effects of Material Infection and Disease, which is found on the Companion Website.

blood), antibodies in the mother's blood may attack the fetus and possibly cause spontaneous abortion, stillbirth, jaundice, anemia, heart defects, mental retardation, or death. Usually the first Rh-positive baby is not affected adversely, but with each succeeding pregnancy the risk becomes greater. A vaccine can be given to the Rh-negative mother within 3 days of childbirth or abortion that will prevent her body from making Rh antibodies. Babies affected by the Rh syndrome can be treated with repeated blood transfusions (34, 57). In-depth information can be attained from a physiology, obstetrics, or pediatrics text.

MATERNAL EMOTIONS

During pregnancy, many factors combine to affect emotional status. These include maternal age and hormonal changes, current and past life situations, social support or lack of it, perceptions of self and role changes, adaptability in meeting developmental tasks, and family and job responsibilities.

Anxiety and fear, resulting from physical abuse, worries about the current living situation or finances, or violence in the neighborhood or community, produce a variety of physiologic changes in the person. See Chapter 2 for the effects of stress. ∞ Hyperactivity of the fetus occurs because increased maternal cortisone is secreted and enters the blood circulation, crossing the placenta to the fetus (34, 36, 37, 56, 57). Fetal circulatory and nutritional processes are affected, interfering with intrauterine development and contributing to preterm delivery, low birth weight, and microencephaly (56, 57, 59, 60). The fetus may also experience the same sensations as the mother experiences with fear and anxiety (59). The fetus does respond to loud environmental noises with increased activity (104).

Job stress may occur. The pregnant female who works outside of the home may experience considerable stress on the job. Work schedules, such as extended or rotating shifts, or mandated overtime and strenuous working conditions, can contribute to risks for the pregnant female and fetus. The emotional environment and social support, or lack of it, either add to or diminish stress. Some jobs bring the risk of violence to the worker, such as police officers or personnel who work in emergency departments or psychiatric units. Fear of assault or being assaulted are emotional and physical stressors. Actual assault can cause direct injury to the pregnant female and may be associated with stillbirth, abruptio placentae, or premature delivery (8, 135, 137).

Physical and emotional abuse during pregnancy has been associated with unemployment, substance abuse and addiction, poverty, and family dysfunction that may be both past and current. Thus, it is difficult to determine the relative contribution of each of these risks. *Domestic violence is a severe and common stressor for the pregnant female.* Physical abuse or battering and verbal abuse involve fear, anxiety, and other feelings related to emotional abuse.

Maternal anxiety reactions are also related to physiologic responses of pregnancy, such as nausea and vomiting, backaches, and headaches, which in turn affect the fetus. The female who begins pregnancy with fewer psychic reserves is especially vulnerable to the stresses and conflicting moods that accompany pregnancy. Maternal anxiety and stress response in early pregnancy have been found to affect infant temperament in relation to attention and interest in the outside world at 3 and 8 months (59). It is unclear

if genetic vulnerability factors in the mother contributed to her emotional responses and were passed on to the infant. Regardless, the risk of even mild prenatal stress on infant temperamental variations may enhance the risk of later behavior problems in the child (59). The Abstract for Evidenced-Based Practice presents research about the importance of avoiding stress and anxiety during pregnancy.

BIRTH DEFECTS TRANSMITTED BY THE FATHER

Genes of both the mother and father and the prenatal maternal environment may cause birth defects. Genetic mutations or abnormalities in sperm are being formed in an increasingly greater percent of the population. More male than female cells undergo mutation, for example, by exposure to irradiation, infection, drugs, and chemicals. These mutations occur more frequently in the male over 45 years of age and may be responsible for various inborn disorders and congenital anomalies. See **Box 8-2**, Causes of Paternal Contributions to Birth Defects in the Child, and other sources for information (4, 6, 19, 34, 54, 57, 61, 105, 109, 134, 151).

Variables Related to Childbirth that Affect the Baby

MEDICATIONS

Analgesics and general anesthetics given during childbirth cross the placental barrier, affecting the newborn for days after delivery. Respirations, circulation, and motor skills after birth are negatively affected; the **Apgar score** will be low. Refer to Chapter 9 for more information about the newborn. ∞

Thus, **analgesics** (*drugs to reduce pain*) and sedatives (mild tranquilizers to reduce anxiety) are given in early labor, usually by epidural block, one form of local anesthesia. However, all drugs and local anesthetics also indirectly affect the fetus by reducing blood flow to the uterus, thus affecting the fetal heart rate. Drugs given during labor remain in the infant's bloodstream for a few days (34, 57).

Childbirth without drugs was first introduced in 1914 by Grantly Dick Read. He was followed by Dr. Fernand Lamaze. The **natural or prepared childbirth method** *teaches voluntary or learned physical responses to the sensations of uterine contractions, which reduce fear and pain responses.* The preparatory classes are popular with both mothers and fathers because they can both actively participate in the birth of their child. During classes the mother and father (or partner) learn about the physiology of pregnancy and childbirth, exercises that strengthen the mother's abdominal and perineal muscles, and techniques of breathing and relaxation during labor and delivery. The father or partner acts as encourager and coach throughout the prenatal classes and during labor and delivery so that the birth experience is shared between the couple. Equally of benefit is the child who comes into the world without any ill effects from medication. Refer to literature from the American Society for Psychoprophylaxis in Obstetrics and obstetric nursing texts for more information on prepared childbirth.

Abstract for Evidence-Based Practice

Pregnancy Beliefs and Practices of Mexican American Childbearing Women

Lagana, K. (2003). *Come Bien, Camina y No Se Preocupe*—Eat right, walk, and do not worry: Selective biculturalism during pregnancy in a Mexican American community. *Journal of Transcultural Nursing, 14*(2), 117–124.

KEYWORDS

pregnancy, Mexican American, health promotion, stress, acculturation, social support.

Purpose ➤ Examine the influence of acculturation in pregnancy beliefs and practices of Mexican American childbearing women.

Conceptual Framework ➤ Biculturalism and acculturation theories guided the study. Mexican American women gave birth to large, healthy babies, although they have sociodemographic profiles associated with low-birth-weight babies (e.g., young maternal age, less prenatal care, lower levels of education and socioeconomic status). **Selective biculturalism** *exists when an individual from one cultural group interacts regularly with another cultural group and selectively takes on, maintains, or abandons certain cultural components.* Through the process of acculturation to U.S. lifestyle, certain traditional protective practices during pregnancy may be lost.

Sample/Setting ➤ Twenty-nine women who attended a Catholic Pastoral Center in southern California were participants. Purposeful sampling and the snowball technique were used to have approximately equal numbers of U.S.-born and Mexican-born women who were permanent residents of the area. Ages ranged from 17 to 60 years. Participants spoke either English or Spanish; education ranged from 1 to 18 years (X 11.5 years). No one had diabetes, which can contribute to larger birth weights.

Method ➤ The ethnographic study collected data by audiotaped interviews in the preferred language. Women also completed the Acculturation Rating Scale for Mexican-Americans; Likert scores indicated either an Anglo or Mexican cultural influence. Additional data were collected from prenatal care provider interviews, participant observation, and birth and population records.

Findings ➤ Qualitative analysis revealed pertinent data. Many pregnancy beliefs of the 1970s and 1980s were still held by Mexican American women. As women became more educated, they demonstrated more biculturalism. All Mexican Americans reported that motherhood was a desired role, in contrast to U.S. women, who reported the work role to be highly rewarding. Mexican American women were willing to give up multirole and employment lifestyles to ensure good pregnancy outcomes and for child care after birth. During pregnancy, all women became more present-time oriented; too much focus on the future was stressful (*"no se preocupe"*).

Regardless of level of acculturation, pregnant Mexican American women returned to traditional pregnancy beliefs and practices, as taught by the maternal grandmother: "Eat right" (*come bien*), "walk" (*camina*), and "don't worry" (*no se preocupe*). Diet was low fat, high protein, nutritious, and natural, or homemade. A fuller figure was ideal. Failure to walk and maintain physical activity daily could result in **pego**, *a condition in which the fetus sticks to the inside of the uterus, making delivery difficult.* Women gave up more rigorous exercise, such as aerobics or running. Lifting, bending, or standing an extended time were seen as harmful. Emphasis was on protecting the pregnant woman from upsetting news, worry, stress, and job conflict. Family members who upset her were sharply criticized. Family social support and chamomile tea were calming.

Prenatal care was widely utilized by Mexican American women, but excess education by the health care provider was considered stressful. In contrast, U.S. women wanted considerable information.

Implications ➤ The maternal mother and grandmother, other female family members, and the curandera should be incorporated into prenatal care of the Mexican American woman. Male partners should be reinforced for being loving and not controlling. Traditional health practices by the woman should be reinforced as effective. Written information should be offered but may not be taken. Accept biculturalism behavior.

INADEQUATE OXYGENATION

Anoxia, *decreased oxygen supply*, and increased carbon dioxide levels may result during delivery. Some degree almost routinely occurs from compression of the umbilical cord, reduced blood flow to the uterus, or placental separation. Fortunately, newborn babies are better able to withstand periods of low oxygenation than are adults. Other causes of asphyxia, however, such as drug-induced respiratory depression or apnea, kinks in the umbilical cord, wrapping of the cord around the neck, very long labor, and malpresentation of the fetus during birth, have more serious effects (35). Longitudinal studies of anoxic newborns revealed lower performance scores on tests of sensorimotor and cognitive-intellectual skills and personality measures than for children with minimal anoxia at birth. Anoxia is also the principal cause of perinatal death and a common cause of mental retardation and cerebral palsy (34, 57).

BOX 8-2   Causes of Paternal Contributions to Birth Defects in the Child

DIRECT (OCCUR AT CONCEPTION)

1. Damage to spermatozoa caused by exposure to fumigants, solvents, vinyl chloride, methylmercury, hypothermia, lead, radiation, pesticides, diethylstilbestrol (DES), alcohol, lack of vitamin C, marijuana and tobacco smoking.
2. Factor or agent affects chromosomes or cytogenic apparatus in sperm cells or their precursors, e.g., cocaine, lead, mercury.
3. Drugs, alcohol, and chemicals cross into testes and male accessory reproductive organs for secretion in semen.

EXAMPLES OF PATERNAL CONTRIBUTIONS TO FETAL AND EARLY CHILDHOOD RISKS

1. Down syndrome (trisomy 21): paternal nondisjunction and extra chromosome; 20% to 30% of cases occur when father is 55 years or older at time of conception.
2. Sex chromosome disorders in child.
3. Adverse outcomes such as spontaneous abortion and perinatal death (stillbirth) due to methadone, morphine,

or heroin dependency and chemicals such as fumigants, solvents, and vinyl chloride.
4. Hemophilia: coagulation disorder in child; deficiency of factor VIII.
5. Marfan syndrome: connective tissue disorder with elongated extremities, hands.
6. Progeria: premature aging, growth deficiency.
7. Decreased neonatal survival due to methadone, morphine, and heroin dependency.
8. Birth defects if father is epileptic, taking phenytoin; or if father is exposed to lead, anesthetic gases, Agent Orange, or dioxin.
9. Tumors of nervous system if father is miner, printer, pulp or paper mill worker, electrical worker, or auto mechanic.
10. Low birth weight linked to nonsmoking pregnant woman's exposure to secondhand smoke from male partner; cancer development in childhood.

PREMATURE OR PRETERM BIRTH AND LOW BIRTH WEIGHT

Prematurity may have long-term consequences for the child. **Premature or preterm birth** is defined as *birth at a gestational age of 37 weeks or earlier, regardless of birth weight.* The **low-birth-weight infant** *weighs less than 5.5 pounds or 2,500 g* regardless of gestational age. The baby may have completed the 38th week in utero. The **very-low-birth-weight (VLBW)** *baby weighs less than 1,500 grams (3.3 pounds).* The **extremely low-birth-weight (ELBW)** *baby weighs less than 1,000 grams (a little over 2 pounds).* Both the VLBW and ELBW baby will be of low gestational age or premature (34, 57). The **small-for-gestational-age (SGA)** or **small-for-date newborn**, as a result of **slow intrauterine growth**,

has a birth weight less than the 10th percentile in the intrauterine growth curve (*weighs less than 90% of all babies of the same gestational age*). Low birth weight is the major factor associated with death of the infant during the first 4 weeks of life (57). Later developmental and behavioral problems, such as physical and cognitive retardation or hyperactivity, may also result (53). Females who are physically abused during pregnancy are more likely to deliver low-birth-weight infants, compared with unabused pregnant females. Being physically abused also doubles the chance of having a miscarriage. Abuse, physical and emotional, may be one of the most frequent problems in pregnancy (57).

If low-birth-weight babies survive the dangerous early days, and more do, there is concern about their development. SGA infants

INTERVENTIONS FOR HEALTH PROMOTION

Educate that the following *maternal factors contribute to a higher risk of low-birth-weight babies* (34, 38, 57, 152):

1. Underweight before pregnancy, or less than 21 pounds gained during pregnancy.
2. Inadequate prenatal care.
3. Age of 17 years or younger, or over 40 years.
4. History of hypertension.
5. Low socioeconomic level.
6. Smoking cigarettes or use of addictive drugs or alcohol during pregnancy.

7. Exposure to toxic substances or chemicals.
8. Complications during pregnancy, poor health status, vaginal bleeding, or exposure to infections.
9. High stress levels, including physical or emotional abuse.
10. Previous low-birth-weight infants or multiple miscarriages.
11. Having given birth less than 6 months or 10 or more years before. A safe interval between pregnancies is a minimum of 18 to 23 months.
12. Many of these factors are interrelated and affected by low socioeconomic level (19, 51, 96, 104).

are more likely to develop neurologic and cognitive impairment than premature infants whose weight was appropriate for gestational age (77).

The VLBW newborns have less promising prognoses; they tend to have more language, cognitive, behavioral, and social problems into the school years and adolescence (102, 103). However, some overcome the early deficits and have a productive adulthood (53, 57).

Early Childhood Variables that Affect the Person

NUTRITION

Nutrition exerts an important influence on growth and development, especially if nutritional deficiency diseases occur. As many as 30% of the brain's neurons may never be formed if protein intake is inadequate during the second trimester of pregnancy or the first 6 months of life (34). Children who suffer starvation do not catch up with growth norms for their group, although later in life adequate nutrition and socioemotional support help to offset the differences (38).

Breast milk is considered the food of choice for the newborn and infant. Yet, breastfeeding is not completely safe. Many substances and drugs ingested by the mother are excreted in human milk. The infant is susceptible to foreign substances because the body's principal detoxifying mechanisms are not functional, the enzyme system is immature, and kidney function is incompletely developed (34, 38). Pesticides in food and other environmental pollutants unknowingly ingested by the mother are excreted in human milk, as discussed in Chapter 4. ∞

If the child is fed a **vegetarian or macrobiotic diet**, the diet must be nutrient and calorie dense, and not high in fiber. Because an infant's stomach capacity is less than an adult's, the volume of food that can be consumed is limited. *Growth retardation is the major visible marker for an inadequate diet. There must be enough calories to support adequate growth, so that protein consumed is not used primarily for energy, instead of growth and repair* (38).

The diet may be low in fat because it lacks animal products. Plant foods must be combined in such a way to supply essential amino acids in the proportions needed for growth. Legumes, cereals, nuts, seeds, avocados, and olives are nutrient dense, but they must be prepared and cooked so they can be eaten by the infant and young child. Infant cereal can be given to the age of 18 months, since it is fortified with iron. Fortified soy milk and mineral supplementation can be given through the childhood years to ensure adequate calcium intake if dairy products are not eaten. Tofu, green leafy vegetables, legumes, almonds, and sesame seeds help supply calcium. To prevent rickets, which have been seen in children on macrobiotic diets, vitamin D supplementation, sunlight, and cod-liver oil should be supplied. Vitamin B_{12} has no practical plant food source; without supplementation there is likely to be a deficiency after one year of age and even in breastfed infants. Vitamin B_{12} deficiency causes fretfulness, apathy, decreased responsiveness, and loss of motor control. Neurologic damage may be permanent. Iron deficiency is common in vegetarian children; the usual meat sources are not eaten. A good source

of ascorbic acid at each meal will improve absorption of whatever iron is ingested. Zinc deficiency may occur unless sufficient legumes, nuts, seeds, tofu, hard cheese, and eggs are eaten. Some vegetarians refuse supplementation. They must select a diet carefully for themselves and their children (38). Nutritional needs of the child are discussed in Chapters 9 through 12. ∞

STRESS

Stress comes in various forms to young children as well as to individuals of any age. There may be illness and hospitalization; neglect, abuse, or abandonment by parents; emotional and sensory deprivation; natural disasters; and wars. The environment up to age 3 is especially critical. Adverse and harsh or stressful living environments or life experiences cause a heightened sympathetic system activity and can alter the structure of the brain. The young child is especially vulnerable. Brain neurotransmitters also appear to be affected long term. In turn, reduced functioning of the neurotransmitter serotonin can increase risks for ill health. Animal studies reveal that insufficient maternal care reduces serotonin function, causing increased aggression and reduced ability to respond to or give affection (96, 104). These findings are similar to the studies decades ago by Spitz (116, 117) and to other studies about the effects of emotional and social hurts during the first years of life (57, 104). A steady flood of stress chemicals in the brain alters the brain's system of response, causing depression, a shutting down emotionally, unresponsiveness to stimuli, withdrawal, and intermittent impulsiveness and acting out (18, 52, 147). Neurobiological research findings add to the emotional, social, and spiritual reasons for giving children adequate nurturing, attention, love, support, and guidance. Only then can they develop, learn, cope, and be healthy.

ENDOCRINE FUNCTION

Mediation of hormones is crucial to the child and person throughout life. A **hormone** is a *chemical substance produced by an endocrine gland and carried by the bloodstream to another part of the body (the target organ) where it controls some function of the target organ.* The major functions of hormones include integrative action, regulation, and morphogenesis. **Integration**, *permitting the body to act as a whole unit in response to stimuli, results from hormones traveling throughout the body and reaching all cells of the body.* For example, the response of the body to epinephrine during fright is generalized. Estrogen, although more specific in its action, affects overall body function. **Regulation**, *maintaining a constant internal environment or homeostasis*, results from all the hormones. The regulation of salt and water balance, metabolism, and growth are examples. In **morphogenesis**, the *rate and type of growth of the organism*, some hormones play an important part (34, 52).

Growth hormone (GH) or somatotropic hormone (STH), secreted by the anterior pituitary gland and regulated by a substance called *growth hormone–releasing factor (GHF)*, produced in the hypothalamus, affects morphogenesis. It promotes development and enlargement of all body tissues that are capable of growing. *Growth hormone has three basic effects on the metabolic processes of the body* (52): (a) protein synthesis is increased, (b) carbohydrate conservation is increased, and (c) use of fat stores for energy is increased.

Case Situation

A Well-Prepared Pregnancy

Casey, age 32, and Matthew, age 34, are young Caucasian adults with two daughters, ages 2 and 4 years. Matthew was an engineer; he has just entered a second career of nursing. Casey was an elementary school teacher; she is now a stay-at-home mother. Casey is 6 months pregnant. Like the other two, the third child was intentionally planned. Casey has consistently, as a vegetarian, maintained good nutrition and exercise between and during pregnancies, and both daughters are healthy, energetic, and gifted. Matthew, even while engaged in nursing studies, remained helpful and attentive to Casey and the children. Both manage the usual life hassles and stressors with a calm approach. They state their life philosophy and religious beliefs and practices give them a solid foundation for a loving, communicative marriage and a desire to give their children every possible opportunity. Casey and Matthew each came from a home that was verbally abusive; they intentionally avoid any language to each other or their daughters that would be perceived as abusive. Their consistent patience, realistic limit setting, behavioral guidance, and encouragement of the children's autonomy and initiative are obvious. Casey and Matthew are active in church; interaction with people of all ages in their faith community is friendly. Likewise, their daughters approach various adults for interaction and play with their peers. Casey's pregnancy has progressed with no complications. She plans to breastfeed the third child for a year, as she has the other two children. She shares information readily with other females of childbearing age about her physical care practices and diet for a healthy pregnancy and breastfeeding. The couple emphasize the importance of handling stress and communicating openly with each other to handle problems.

Contributed by Ruth Murray, EdD, MSN, N-NAP, FAAN.

Growth hormone is secreted in spurts instead of at a relatively constant rate. The lowest concentrations of plasma GH are found in the morning after arising; the highest concentrations occur between 60 and 90 minutes after falling asleep at night. The peak of GH is clearly related to sleep. Enough sleep in infancy and early childhood is essential for growth and healing (52).

ENVIRONMENTAL POLLUTION

Children are especially affected by environmental pollution. *The five worst environmental hazards to children in the United States are lead, drinking water contamination, pesticides, air pollution, and tobacco.* Children are exposed to more toxic chemicals because they ingest more food, water, and air than their parents, pound for pound. The life of a child is exploration on hands and knees. They encounter pesticides, lead, and other poisons lurking in soil, house dust, and carpets, which they swallow while sucking on their hands or thumbs (19, 96, 104, 141). These contaminants are more toxic to children than adults and are more likely to cause permanent damage. The child is not fully developed at birth; the brain and the neurologic, immune, endocrine, and reproductive systems pass through numerous critical periods when they are especially vulnerable. Damage from even minor exposure can last a lifetime (19, 57, 141).

There has been a decline in blood lead levels in the past 20 years, but it remains a top environmental hazard because learning difficulties, lower IQ, hyperactivity, neurologic impairment, and increased aggression occur in children with blood levels as low as 8 to 10 ug/dL of blood (57). Excessive lead, although eliminated from gasoline and house paint, remains in a large number of older houses and is ingested through contact with painted surfaces and house dust. Other sources of lead are contaminated water from lead pipes or pottery, factory emissions, and lead-containing batteries (57).

Asthma is caused in part, and attacks are prolonged, by air pollution. However, the main causative factors are allergens that are inhaled because today's children spend more time in tightly sealed buildings, where they have greater exposure to mold, dust mites, animal dander, and cockroach droppings. Children with asthma have an underlying immune system dysfunction, making them overreactive to substances in the environment (57). The child's early experience can change the relative proportion of T cells and development of the immune system (34). Contaminant exposure before birth has been linked to altered T cells; the higher the mother's level of PCBs and dioxin, the greater the change in the T cells. The result can be immune suppression, allergy, or autoimmunity (34, 141).

Many hazards can occur during pregnancy. However, pregnancy can be an intentionally developmental task and a safe time for the mother and the developing baby. Refer to the Case Situation.

Sociocultural Factors that Influence the Developing Person

CULTURAL AND DEMOGRAPHIC VARIABLES

Culture, social class, race, and ethnicity of the parents, as discussed in Chapter 5, affect the child's development and health. ∞ Foods eaten by the pregnant woman, prenatal care and childbirth practices, childrearing methods, work and lifestlye patterns, development of language and thought processes—all variously affect the person from the moment of conception (9, 50, 114).

Many cultural groups have beliefs especially related to pregnancy, labor and delivery, and postpartal care (50). For example, the Hmong people were part of the second wave of Southeast

Asian refugees who fled to the United States because of the Vietnam War. The lives of people in this preliterate, agrarian, animistic culture were forever changed as they left their slash-and-burn farming techniques to be immigrants in the industrialized United States. California is home to most of the Hmong people; some have emigrated to the central states and North Carolina in search of jobs. The Hmong practices and beliefs related to reproductive health, contraception, child spacing, prenatal care, and route of delivery are best implemented by combining culturally competent Western care with animistic ceremonies and herbal remedies. For example, Western health care providers have accommodated Hmong patients' wishes regarding placental disposal/burial. The Hmong believe that the placenta is the infant's first "clothing"; the soul of the deceased must return to the place his or her placenta was buried to retrieve the afterlife "garment." Only by wearing the placental "jacket" can the soul find safe passage to the spirit world and be reunited with ancestors (55). Helping the family carry out their cultural traditions is important for future mental and spiritual health.

The health care given to the child by the parents is related to sociocultural status. For example, *in urban areas parents of children who are adequately immunized and given well-child care are likely to have the following characteristics* (31): (a) they perceive childhood diseases as serious; (b) they know about the effectiveness of vaccination; (c) they are older in age; (d) they are better educated; (e) they have smaller family size (number of children); and (f) they read newspapers, listen to radio or television promotions of immunizations, and respond to community educational efforts. Inadequately immunized children in urban areas are found in families in which the parents are young, poor, and minimally educated, and have a large number of children. The parents do not perceive childhood diseases as serious, do not know about the effectiveness of vaccines, or do not pay attention to health education in the mass media (31).

Response to personal traumatic events and natural and man-made disasters varies with the culture. Cultural values and norms promote healing. Meaningful social relationships can protect members from overwhelming stress and are essential to assist children through the situation. Repeated childhood trauma injures the child's adaptive processes (10).

Educate the public, health care providers, and families about the connection between cultural practices and health. Health promotion includes culturally competent care by health care providers and implementing guidelines discussed in Chapters 5 and 7. ∞

SOCIALIZATION PROCESSES

Socialization is the *process by which the child is transformed into a member of a particular society and learns the values, standards, habits, skills, and roles appropriate to sex, social class, and ethnic group or subculture to become a responsible, productive member of society* (19, 96, 104). You have a major role in healthy socialization processes in client care.

All humans experience socialization, the shaping of the person into a socially acceptable form, especially during the early years of life. Thus heritage and culture are perpetuated. The newborn is a biological organism with physical needs and inherited characteristics, which will be socialized or shaped along a number of dimensions: emotional, social, cognitive, intellectual, perceptual, behavioral, and expressive. During childhood socialization, various skills, knowledge, attitudes, values, motives, habits, beliefs, needs, interests, and ideals are learned, demonstrated, and reinforced. Various people are key agents in the socialization process: parents, siblings, relatives, peers, teachers, and other adults. Certain forces, including the external environment and nature (11), will impinge on the person and interact with all the individual is and learns. Forces include culture, social class, religion, race or ethnicity, the community, the educational system, mass media, and various organizations. Integration of all the various individual and socializing forces will form the adult character, personality traits, role preferences, goals, and behavioral mode. Refer to Vygotsky's Sociocultural Theory, Chapter 1. ∞

The success of the socialization process is measured by the person's ability to perform in the roles he or she attempts and to respond to rapid social change and a succession of life tasks. The life cycle is seen as a succession of roles or transitions and changing role constellations. Certain order and predictability of behavior occur over time as the person moves through the given succession of roles. The person learns to think and behave in ways consonant with the roles to be played. Your health care roles will always involve a social dimension.

COMMUNITY SUPPORT SYSTEM

Community relationships influence primarily the parents, but they also influence the child. An emotional support system for the parents, physical and health care resources in the community, and social and learning opportunities that exist outside the home promote the child's development and prepare him or her for later independence and citizenry roles. If the parents are unable to meet the child's needs adequately, other people or organizations in the community may make the difference between bare survival and eventual physical and emotional normalcy and well-being.

Cultures vary in the degree to which the new mother is given help (9, 50, 114). For example, in India the mother traditionally is assisted with child care and is allowed to do nothing except care for her baby for 40 days after delivery. Several decades ago mothers in the United States were hospitalized for 10 to 12 days, and the family helped at home for another couple of weeks or so. Now the mother is sent home after 24 to 48 hours, often to assume total child care. Physical health of the baby and emotional health of the mother in the months following delivery depend in part on whether she had assistance with infant care and a support system during the first month after delivery. Ongoing support is essential for healthy development and life.

The mother's emotional expression to the child, related to her own feelings of family satisfaction, can affect parenting. Mothers who feel secure and satisfied with family relationships are more likely to be warm and positive and less likely to be critical or hostile when interacting with their children, including high-risk children who were premature and low birth weight (119).

FAMILY FACTORS

The family structure, developmental level and roles of family members, their health and financial status, their perception of the baby, and community resources for the family influence the child's development and well-being, before birth and afterwards. Social and environmental factors that produce low birth weight, for instance, are likely to continue to operate on the infant and child as well. Refer to Chapter 6 ∞ for in-depth information about how the family influences the infant and childhood development. Refer also to Chapter 5 ∞ for cultural influences on the family and, in turn, the child.

The mother has traditionally been credited with having the most effect on the child, whether the outcome was good or bad. Researchers now acknowledge the importance of the father and the effect of the father's presence or absence on the developing child. Refer to Chapter 6. ∞

VULNERABLE AND RESILIENT CHILDREN

Both vulnerable and resilient children develop within the same family system. Siblings brought up under the same chaotic situations, with alcoholic or drug-using parents, or in impoverished circumstances do not all develop the same personality traits. One becomes physically or emotionally ill, whereas a sibling thrives. The resilient child appears different from a vulnerable sibling from birth. Children who are exposed to more than one adverse factor or long-term crisis or who do not have a consistent caring adult are less able to offset the negative effects of stress and maintain resiliency (96).

Resilience *is characterized by a healthy personality and effective behavioral outcomes in spite of serious threats to adaptation or development* (83). **Resilient children** *appear to be endowed with innate characteristics that insulate them from the pain of their families, allow them to reach out to some adult who provides crucial emotional support, and enable them to bounce back from circumstances.* For example, Garmezy (48) found in the African American community that the church was the child's strongest support. At least one competent adult as role model, such as minister, youth leader, teacher, or coach, was especially important to boys and girls to remain resilient and overcome vulnerability.

Characteristics of these resilient children include the ability to (48, 75, 96, 143):

1. Use some talent or personality traits to draw some adult to them as a substitute parent and to have compensating experiences.
2. Recover quickly from stressors, and be adaptable, resourceful, creative, and socially competent.
3. Be more alert to their surroundings from birth.
4. Establish trust with the parent or with a parent surrogate.
5. Be more independent, easygoing, friendly, enthusiastic for activities, and better able to tolerate frustration by age 2.
6. Be more cheerful, flexible, and persistent in the face of failure; seek help from adults by age 3 1/2; and be well liked.
7. Be sensitive to others and responsive to peers and adults.
8. Feel that they can exert some control over life and have a positive self-concept.
9. Demonstrate good school performances and good problem-solving skills.

Vulnerable children *are closest emotionally to the distressed parent and are most likely to show signs of distress and later psychiatric disorders* (48). These children are more likely to be self-

derogatory, anxious, depressed, and physically ill. *Risk factors associated with psychiatric disorders in vulnerable youth include* (10, 48, 57) (a) discord in the parental relationship; (b) nonsupportive milieu—boundaries, roles, and expectations not clear; (c) low socioeconomic status; (d) large family crowded into a small space; (e) parental disorders, such as father in jail or mother with psychiatric diagnosis; and (f) removal of child from home and placement in foster care.

However, these vulnerable children at risk for deviant behavior in adolescence, can develop into competent adults. Even apparently well-adjusted, successful, resilient children may pay a subtle psychological cost. In adolescence they are more likely to cling to a moralistic outlook. In intimate relationships they are apt to be disagreeable and judgmental. They tend to be constricted and overcontrolled. If the disturbed parent is of the opposite sex, the resilient person is often emotionally distant in intimate relationships, breaking off relationships as they become more intimate. Some seek partners with problems, with the idea of rescuing or curing them (57).

CHILD MALTREATMENT

Being a parent in the 21st century is challenging, even overwhelming at times. The parent may not have had good parental role models, which adds to the problem.

Child maltreatment *is a broad term including all intentional harm or avoidable endangerment of anyone under 18 years of age. It includes all forms of child abuse and neglect, abandonment, and failure to thrive caused by nonorganic or psychosocial causes* (47, 57, 83). Children from any race, creed, ethnic origin, or economic level may be victims of maltreatment from parents, foster parents, caretakers, relatives, or family friends.

Child Abuse

Child abuse *is a pattern of abnormal parent-child interactions and attacks over a period that results in nonaccidental injuries to the child physically, emotionally, or sexually or from neglect.* Abused children range in age from neonate through adolescence (47, 57, 83). Child abuse is a major health problem and a negative influence on the developing person. Children are suffering more serious and brutal injuries than ever before (57, 83). **Nonaccidental physical injury or physical abuse** *includes many types of assault*: multiple bruises or fractures from severe beatings, poisonings or overmedication, burns from immersion in hot water or from lighted cigarettes, excessive use of laxatives or enemas, and human bites (83). The trauma to the child is often great enough to cause permanent blindness, scars on the skin, neurologic damage, subdural hematoma, and permanent brain damage or death. **Sexual molestation or abuse**, *exploitation of the child for the adult's sexual gratification*, includes rape, incest, exhibitionism to the child, or fondling of the child's genitals. **Emotional abuse** *includes excessively aggressive or unreasonable parental behavior to the child, deliberate attempts to destroy self-esteem or competence*, placing unreasonable demands on the child to perform above his or her capacities, verbally attacking or constantly belittling or teasing the child, or withdrawing love, support, or guidance (57, 83). **Neglect** *includes failure to provide the child with basic necessities of life* (food, shelter, clothing, hygiene, or medical care), *adequate mothering, or emotional, moral, or* *social care* (57, 83). The parents' lack of concern is usually obvious. The parents, the people who should provide love and protection, do not, which makes the behavior especially hurtful to the child.

Abandonment *may occur. In all forms of abuse, the child frequently acts fearful of the parents or adults in general. The child is usually too fearful to tell how he or she was injured.*

There are a number of characteristics of the potentially or actually abusive parent. Typically the abuser (19, 47, 57, 83, 96, 104):

1. Is young in age.
2. Is emotionally unstable and unable to cope with the stress of life or even usual personal problems.
3. Is lonely, has few social contacts, and is isolated from people.
4. Is unable to ask for help; lacks friends or family who can help with child care.
5. Does not understand the development or care needs of children.
6. Is living through a very stressful time, such as unemployment, spousal abuse, or poverty.
7. Has personal emotional needs previously unmet; has difficulty in trusting others.
8. May have been abused or raised in an abusive or rejecting home.
9. Is angered easily; has negative self-image and low self-esteem.
10. Has no one from whom to receive emotional support, including partner.
11. Expects the child to be perfect and to cause no inconvenience.
12. May perceive the child as different, too active, or too passive, even if the child is normal or only mildly different.

Practice Point

Your role with the child-abusing parent and the abused child is a significant one. To help parents and child, you must first cope with your own feelings as you give necessary physical care to the child or assist parents in getting proper care for the child. Often parents who feel unable to cope with the stresses of child rearing will repeatedly bring the child to the emergency room for a variety of complaints of minor, vague illnesses or injuries.

Sometimes the child has mild neurologic dysfunction and is irritable, tense, and difficult to hold or cuddle. The child may have been the result of an unwanted pregnancy, may have been premature, or may have a birth defect. Usually only one child in a family becomes the scapegoat for parental anger, tension, rejection, and hate. The child who does not react in a way to make the parent feel good about his or her parenting behavior will be the abused one (57, 83, 132).

Cooperate with legal, medical, and social agencies to help abusive parents and to prevent further child abuse—and possible death or permanent impairment of the child. Child abuse is against the law in every state, and every state has at least one statewide agency to receive and investigate suspected cases of child abuse. Any citizen or health worker can anonymously report a case of child abuse to authorities without fear of recrimination from the

INTERVENTIONS FOR HEALTH PROMOTION

Certain health promotion interventions are useful:

1. Be alert to the subtle message; talk with the parent about himself or herself, the management of the child, feelings about parenting and the child, and who helps in times of stress.
2. Establish rapport, act like a helpful friend, and convey a feeling of respect for the parent as a person (which may be difficult if you feel that the child abuser is a monster).
3. Avoid asking probing questions too quickly.
4. Do not lecture or scold the parent about his or her child-rearing methods.
5. Help the parent to feel confident and competent in any way possible.
6. Form a "cool mothering" relationship with the parent (i.e., make yourself consistently available but do not push too close emotionally). Often the mother responds well to having a grandmotherly person (usually a volunteer) spend time with her. This person could go to the home, where she could mother the mother, assist with a variety of household chores, and give the mother time to spend with her baby while unharried by demands of other children or household tasks.

7. Be a model on how to approach, cuddle, and discipline the child; the parent may expect the 6-month-old baby to obey commands.
8. Convey that consistency of care is important. Realize that the parent will need long-term help in overcoming the abusive pattern.
9. Use the principles of therapeutic communication and crisis intervention (see Chapter 2) ∞ to avoid driving the parent away from potential help or becoming more abusive to the child.
10. Intervene sensibly with the parent and the child to avoid further harm and to avoid disrupting any positive feelings that might exist between parent and child. Foster home care is not necessarily the answer; foster parents are sometimes abusive, too. Rapid court action may antagonize abusive parents to the point of murdering the child or moving to a different geographic location where they cannot receive help.
11. Refer the parent to Parents Anonymous, a self-help parents' group that exists in some large cities, or to other local self-help crisis groups.

abuser. An investigation by designated authorities of the danger to the child is carried out shortly after reporting; the child may be placed in a foster home or institution by court order if the child's life is threatened. The goal of legal intervention is to help the parents and child, not to punish (83). Unless the problem of child abuse can be curbed, many of today's children will become the next generation of abusing parents. Primary prevention is essential. Mothers and children constitute approximately 66% of the population in any society. They are worth caring for physically and emotionally because of their worth to the future of the society. You are their advocate.

Additional information about child and adolescent maltreatment and abuse is found in Chapters 9 through 13. ∞

Failure to Thrive

Failure to thrive *is the term used to describe infants who are unable to obtain or use calories and other nutrients required for growth. Weight and often height are below the 5th percentile for the child's age. Causative categories for lack of weight gain include the following* (57, 83):

1. **Organic**–*Physical causes*, such as congenital cardiac, neurologic, or endocrine anomalies; microencephaly; malabsorption syndrome; chronic renal or gastric disease; cystic fibrosis; AIDS; or addiction created by parental addiction prenatally or after return to the parental home. Sensory deprivation or inability to respond to auditory, tactile, and vestibular stimuli may also contribute to failure to thrive.

2. **Nonorganic**–*Psychosocial causes*, such as deficient maternal care or maternal neglect, disturbed mother-child bonding or attachment, lack of attention from an addicted mother, and lack of knowledge about feeding and nutritional needs for the infant or young child.

Children may starve in front of their parents/foster care parents and not be noticed. Parental attitudes about the child and responsibilities of child care, parental chronic mental illness or substance abuse/addiction, lack of or poor parenting skills, and lack of social support are major factors in being unable to recognize or empathize with the child's distress or imminent death.

The child may not be fed, even if physically able to eat, for a variety of reasons related to (57, 83):

1. Poverty and lack of funds for food.
2. Parental health beliefs based on fads or religion, or ideas about obesity prevention.
3. Parental cognitive impairment or mental retardation, or lack of knowledge about infant and child feeding and nutritional needs.
4. Lack of maternal attachment or bonding to the child.
5. Family stress, such as care of a large number of children or chronically ill children, parental substance use/abuse, dysfunctional marital situation, employment demands, family illness, or maternal depression.
6. Feeding resistance by the infant because of prematurity or neonatal congenital defects of the mouth, lips, or gastrointestinal tract; the treatment methods; or delayed oral feeding.

The following manifestations are common; the child may not readily demonstrate all of these signs and symptoms. Astute assessment and follow-up home visits may be necessary in order to hospitalize and treat the child and place him or her in safe custody.

Obvious signs and symptoms include (a) thin, emaciated, potbelly, limp or weak muscles; (b) cold, dull, pale, splotchy skin, appears dehydrated; (c) insensitive to pain, may have self-inflicted injuries, tense; (d) feeding or eating difficulties; (e) episodes of diarrhea; and (f) insomnia or disrupted sleep, which bothers the parents (40, 57, 83).

Emotionally, the child may demonstrate apathy, avoidance of personal contact when approached, lack of emotional or verbal response, and avoidance of eye contact. Parents may report that the child roams the house at night (probably looking for food) or will eat or drink inappropriate substances from the garbage can, toilet bowl, or dish for feeding the cat or dog (47, 83).

Astute assessment for causation, sometimes interrelated, is essential for legal reporting, relevant diagnostic procedures, and therapy. The goal is to provide enough calories to support "catch-up" growth. Growth may not occur if psychosocial or home environmental problems are not corrected. Medical problems will be more easily treated. A multidisciplinary team approach is necessary. Prognosis is related to the cause. You will need to work with the parents (or foster care parents), as well as the child, over time. Teaching parents about long-term parenting skills and ways to foster attachment is as important as teaching about nutrition and feeding.

Although damage to the child from maternal deprivation may be severe, not every deprived child becomes a problem adolescent or adult. Some infants who have lacked their mother's love appear to suffer little permanent damage. The age of the child when deprived or abused, the length of separation or duration of abuse, the parent-child relationship before separation or in later childhood, care of the child by other adults during separation from the parents, and the stress produced by the separation or abuse all affect the long-range outcome.

SPIRITUAL FACTORS

Religious, spiritual, philosophic, and moral insights and practices of the parents (and of the overall society) influence how the child is perceived, cared for, and taught. These early underpinnings—or their lack—will continue to affect the person's self-concept, behavior, and health as an adult, even when he or she purposefully tries to disregard these early teachings.

Incorporate the client's spiritual and religious beliefs into health promotion practices and education with the client to the extent possible. For example, the placenta can be sent home with the family to be buried. The nursing unit and health care system can incorporate color, art, music, or symbols that are important to the spiritual and cultural background and age of the clients served. Clients will probably share ideas, if asked, about what is pleasing or appropriate. An example is the American Indian **medicine wheel**, *a symbol meaning holism, relationship, and the cyclic aspects of life.* The medicine wheel can be used as a guide for teaching and interventions that convey individualized care (35).

Taylor (129) describes spiritual care that contributes to the health of various groups. Refer to Chapter 7 ∞ for information specific to various religious beliefs. Spiritual, religious, and moral development for the family and person in each life era is also discussed in Chapters 9 through 16. ∞

MACROENVIRONMENTAL FACTORS THAT INFLUENCE THE DEVELOPING PERSON

The home environment and the overall environment of the nation or region in which the person lives affect development and health. Variables include (a) the climate the person learns to tolerate, (b) water and food availability, (c) emphasis on cleanliness, (d) demands for physical and motor competency, (e) social relationships, (f) opportunities for leisure, and (g) inherent hazards. These depend on whether the child lives on a farm or in the city, on the seacoast or in a semiarid region, in the cold North or sunny South, or in a mining town or a mountain resort area. *Added to these effects are the hazards from environmental pollution that affect all societies,* whether it is excrement from freely roaming cattle or particles from industrial smokestacks. No part of the world is any longer uncontaminated by pesticides; all parts have disease related to problems of waste control. On a more immediate level, the size, space, noise, cleanliness, and safety within the home will affect the person's behavior and health and the home environment he or she will eventually build. **In the local and national community, the media also constitute the macroenvironment**. Effects of the media are discussed in Chapters 12 and 13. ∞

Part of the macroenvironment is the health care system. The newborn who is small for gestational age, low birth weight, or premature, or who has a congenital anomaly, has benefited from the research and advances in medical care. The costs and benefits of such care to the family, society, and health care system have been studied (33).

Current issues in the broader health care, political, or national arena may at some point influence the development and health of a person who suffered teratogenic effects. Stem cell research is one of those issues. A **stem** *is an undifferentiated human cell that is able to copy itself and can be maintained in large numbers (called stem cell lines) indefinitely within laboratory settings.* Although the stem cell is undifferentiated, it has the capacity to be guided by scientists to produce specialized tissues such as heart, liver, or nerve cells (28). There are two types of stem cells: embryonic and adult. **Embryonic stem cells** *can be found in a cluster of cells called a blastocyte, which is a developing microscopic embryo.* These stem cells are more capable of becoming any type of cell in the human body than other stem cells. *Embryonic stem cells obtained from children or adults can only produce limited tissue types.* **Adult stem cells** *exist in the bone marrow, blood, skin, and other organs.* Many are dividing and becoming new cells in the body. The best known example of the **use of adult stem cells** *is the bone marrow transplant in which cells that are the precursors of blood and immune system cells can be transferred from a healthy individual to someone who is ill* (30, 88).

Stem cells have the potential to manufacture new healthy tissue for individuals whose organs were damaged by injury or illness. They may also be used to gain knowledge of how genetic processes in early cell development lead to abnormalities such as birth defects or cancer. The specialized tissues created by stem cells may also prove helpful in the early testing of new medications for adverse and side effects. This drug testing would take place on the tissue level, before human participants are involved (89).

Opponents of the use of embryonic stem cells maintain that a fertilized egg or fetus is a human being with rights that require protection. In this view, the end of helping someone with a disease does not justify the means of ending a life. Supporters of stem cell research maintain that aborted fetuses and fertilized eggs not needed for in vitro fertilization (IVF) are a reality; they will be discarded anyway and thus should be used to help those who are ill. At this time, federal funding for stem cell research is confined to stem cell lines that have already been established; no money will be appropriated for new lines to be developed. It is expected that research related to and the use of stem cells will be a continuing debate (94).

Further discussion of the effects of the macroenvironment on the person's health can be found in Chapter 4. ∞

Health Promotion and Nursing Applications

HOLISTIC CARE

Health promotion measures have been presented throughout the chapter, as relevant to the childbearing family and developing fetus and young child. The Centers for Disease Control and Prevention (CDC) has generated recommendations for improvement in preconception health. The full CDC report is found on its Website, www.cdc.gov.

Preconception care *refers to strategies to improve the health of women, children, and families, and to prevent or manage risks to healthy pregnancies. Recommendations for improvement include the following* (23, 106):

1. Each woman, man, and couple should have a reproductive life plan about whether and when they might have children.
2. Schools and public health agencies should present information about preconception health.
3. Preconception care for all women should be integrated into primary care services.
4. Evidence-based strategies should be identified and implemented in relation to known risk factors, and research should continue to identify other potential risk factors.
5. Special care should be given to pregnant women who had prior poor pregnancy outcomes.
6. Women and couples who are planning pregnancy should have at least one prepregnancy visit with a primary care provider.
7. Low-income women of childbearing age should have increased access to health care coverage.
8. Public health programs should include preconception education and care.
9. More research should be conducted on the effectiveness of interventions, the value of better service integration, and the potential cost-benefit ratio of preconception care.
10. Public health surveillance should monitor improvements in preconception care.

Nursing Diagnoses Related to Developmental Influences

Risk for Delayed **D**evelopment
Delayed Growth and **D**evelopment
Risk for Disproportionate **G**rowth

Deficient **K**nowledge
Readiness for Enhanced **K**nowledge
Ineffective **P**rotection

Source: Reference 85.

Incorporation of preconception care into medical, nursing, and public health services will further contribute to holistic care. **Holistic care** *has as its goal the whole person, biopsychosociocultural and spiritual dimensions, with consideration of the environment and social systems context. These dimensions and the surrounding context are integrated into a wholeness and are interdependent; none can be managed in isolation.* Holistic care is a foundational concept in nursing.

ASSESSMENT

Previously presented content will be useful in assessment. Some general guidelines are as follows:

1. Assess the pregnant female to determine whether there is risk because of negative influencing factors or teratogens.
2. Consider the sociocultural and religious background and the lifestyle of the person to prevent overlooking or misinterpreting factors that are significant to the pregnant female and her family.
3. Determine what the pregnant female who is at risk has done to get necessary care to prevent fetal damage and maternal illness; consider family factors.
4. Be aware of community services, such as genetic screening and counseling, family planning, nutritional programs, prenatal classes, counseling for prevention of child abuse, and medical services.

NURSING DIAGNOSIS

Refer to the **Box**, Nursing Diagnoses Related to Developmental Influences (85). Other nursing diagnoses would be formulated, depending upon the medical and emotional status of the pregnant female, the status of the fetus, and any concurrent diseases.

INTERVENTION

Your support, assistance, and teaching with the pregnant woman and her significant support system will contribute to more nurturing parenting. Interventions specific to certain situations or conditions and ways to prevent or overcome teratogens have been integrated throughout the chapter. Refer also to use of therapeutic relationships and communication principles and guidelines described in Chapter 2. ∞ Pregnancy is a developmental crisis. Crisis intervention principles and methods are applicable and are presented in Chapter 2. ∞

Teach potential parents about the many factors discussed in this and following chapters that can influence the health of the mother, offspring, and family. Refer clients to community services as needed. Join with other professionals and citizens to advocate for better control of teratogenic agents and to reverse environmental and child maltreatment hazards.

A number of factors contribute toward premature birth and the potential adverse consequences to the child and the family, as well as economic costs to the family and society (33). Your advocacy for prenatal care for every childbearing female and couple and your participation in community education will help to reduce the costs associated with unplanned pregnancy, lack of prenatal care, and limitations in ongoing primary care for the infant and family (33).

EVALUATION

Based on CDC recommendations and the emphasis in each profession on evaluation and evidence-based practice, more research about developmental influences will be generated related to prevention, management, and long-term consequences. Research is important (101). Equally important is that findings from current and future research will be utilized by the staff member in any setting who works with the childbearing and developing family.

Summary

1. Each stage of prenatal development has potential risks that can interfere with the normal prenatal processes.
2. Prenatal influences on development include heredity, various physiologic processes, and age, health, and nutritional status of the mother and father.
3. Environmental hazards, drugs, alcohol, infections, and other conditions are teratogens that may adversely affect the developing organism, especially during the critical period of the first trimester.
4. Certain variables, such as medication in the mother, may negatively affect the fetus during labor and delivery.
5. Early childhood variables that affect the developing person include nurturance from the parents, nutrition, stressors, physiologic functions in the infant, and various sociocultural and family characteristics.
6. Holistic care during the preconception, prenatal, and postpartum periods is essential to ensure the health status of the present and future generations.

Review Questions

1. The nurse is assessing a woman at 15 weeks of pregnancy who has gained 20 pounds. When discussing the weight gain with the client, the nurse should base instructions on the fact that:
   1. This is an expected weight gain at this point in the pregnancy.
   2. High weight gain during pregnancy will result in a healthy baby at birth.
   3. Calorie intake at this point should only be about 200 to 300 calories more than the nonpregnant intake.
   4. Higher weight gain is a more favorable situation than not gaining sufficiently.
2. A recently diagnosed pregnant client tells the nurse that she is a vegetarian and plans to continue this lifestyle during pregnancy. How can the nurse best advise this client?
   1. Inform the client that a vegetarian diet is contraindicated during pregnancy.
   2. Ensure that the diet includes 100 mcg of folate.
   3. Avoid dairy products and eggs.
   4. Many fish and seafoods can pose problems during pregnancy.
3. The nurse is advising a couple who are planning to conceive about the importance of a diet adequate in folate. The couple asks why this nutrient is important to include in the woman's diet even before conception. The nurse should base the response to this couple on the fact that:
   1. Good nutrition is vital throughout the life span, not just when planning to conceive.
   2. Changing diet before pregnancy will support good nutrition habits throughout life.
   3. Neural tube development begins soon after fertilization and continues into the embryonic stage.
   4. Folate supplements are not widely available.
4. A client in the third trimester of pregnancy tells the nurse that she feels bloated and has had some abdominal discomfort. The nurse assesses the client and finds diminished bowel sounds. How should the nurse interpret this finding?
   1. This is a usual change in a pregnant woman's physiologic function associated with the hormonal environment of pregnancy.
   2. This is an abnormal finding and should be reported to the physician.
   3. This finding is likely a result of poor nutritional intake and requires intravenous fluids.
   4. The client likely has a bowel obstruction and should be sent to the emergency department.

References

1. Acton, K., Burrows, N. R., Moore, K., Queree, L., Geiss, L., & Engelgau, M. (2002). Trends in diabetes prevalence among American Indian and Alaska Native children, adolescents, and young adults. *American Journal of Public Health, 92,* 1485–1490.
2. Alcohol exposure in third trimester may affect children's higher order functions. (2005). *Clinical Psychiatry News, 33*(10), 52.
3. American Academy of Pediatrics (AAP). (2000). Fetal alcohol syndrome and alcohol related neurodevelopmental disorders. *Pediatrics, 106,* 358.
4. American Academy of Pediatrics Committee on Drugs. (1994). The transfer of drugs and other chemicals into human milk. *Pediatrics, 93,* 137–150.
5. American Academy of Pediatrics Committee on Drugs. (2000). Use of psychoactive medication during pregnancy and possible effects on the fetus and newborn. *Pediatrics, 105,* 880–887.
6. American Academy of Pediatrics Committee on Substance Abuse. (2001). Tobacco's toll: Implications for the pediatrician. *Pediatrics, 107,* 794–798.
7. Ammenheuser, M., Berenson, A., Babiak, A., Singleton, C., & Whorton, E. (1998). Frequencies of hrpt mutant lymphocytes in marijuana smoking. *Mutation Research, 403,* 55–64.
8. Anderson, C., & Parish, M. (2003). Report of workplace violence by Hispanic nurses. *Journal of Transcultural Nursing, 14*(3), 237–243.
9. Andrews, M., & Boyle, J. (2003). *Transcultural concepts in nursing care* (4th ed.). Philadelphia: Lippincott Williams & Wilkins.
10. Antai-Otong, D. (2002). Culture and traumatic events. *Journal of the American Psychiatric Nurses Association, 8,* 203–208.
11. Antonioli, C., & Reveley, M. (2006, January). A look at "biophilia." How does nature impact physical and mental health? *NeuroPsychiatric Review,* 10–11.
12. Arendt, R., Angeloporios, J., Salvator, A., & Singer, L. (1999). Motor development of cocaine exposed children at age two years. *Pediatrics, 103,* 86–92.
13. Askin, D., & Diehl-Jones, B. (2001). Cocaine: Effects of *in utero* exposure on the fetus and neonate. *Journal of Perinatal & Neonatal Nursing, 14*(4), 83–102.
14. Baer, J., Sampson, P., Barr, H., Connor, P., & Streissguth, A. (2003). A 21-year longitudinal analysis of the effects of prenatal alcohol exposure on young adult drinking. *Clinical Psychiatry, 60*(4), 337–383.
15. Bailey, B. (2005). Alcohol exposure in third trimester may affect children's higher functions. *Clinical Psychiatry News, 33*(10), 52.
16. Barr, H., Streissguth, A., Darby, B., & Sampson, P. (1990). Prenatal exposure to alcohol, caffeine, tobacco, and aspirin: Effects on fine and gross motor performances in 4-year-old children. *Developmental Psychology, 26,* 339–348.
17. Bates, B. (2005). Heavy prenatal alcohol linked to behavioral ills. *Clinical Psychiatry News, 33*(10), 41.
18. Beck, C. (1995). The effects of postpartum depression on maternal-infant interaction: A meta-analysis. *Nursing Research, 44,* 298–303.
19. Berger, K. (2005). *The developing person through the lifespan* (6th ed.). New York: Worth Publishers.
20. Birnbaum, L. (1994). Endocrine effects of prenatal exposure to PCBs, dioxins, and other xenobiotics: Implications for policy and future research. *Environmental Health Perspectives, 102*(8), 678–679.
21. Blatt, R., Megrici, N., & Church, C. (2000). Prenatal cocaine: What's known about outcomes. *Contemporary Pediatrics, 17*(5), 43–57.
22. Brown, R. (1999). Optimizing expression of the common human genome for child development. *Current Directions in Psychological Sciences, 8*(2), 37–41.
23. Centers for Disease Control and Prevention. (2007). *Preconception care questions and answers. Professionals.* Retrieved August 25, 2007, from www.cdc.gov/ncbddd/preconception/QandA_providers.htm
24. Chasnoff, I. (1990). Prenatal cocaine exposure is associated with respiratory pattern abnormalities. *American Journal of Public Health, 84*(3), 411–414.
25. Chasnoff, I., & Griffith, D. (1989). Cocaine: Clinical studies of pregnancy and the newborn. *Annals of the New York Academy of Sciences, 562,* 260–266.
26. Coakley, L. (2007). Preventable birth defects: A golden teaching opportunity. *Journal of Christian Nursing, 24*(3), 126–132.

27. Colyar, M., & Call-Schmidt, T. (2006). Methamphetamine abuse in the primary care patient. *Clinician Reviews, 16*(3), 55–60.

28. Committee on the Biological and Biomedical Applications of Stem Cell Research. (2002). *Stem cells and the future of regenerative medicine.* Washington, DC: National Research Council.

29. Committee on Obstetric Practice. (2002). ACOG Committee opinion: Exercise during pregnancy and the postpartum period. *International Journal of Gynecology & Obstetrics, 77*(1), 79–81.

30. Cookson, C. (2005, July). Mother of all cells. *Scientific American, 293*(1), A6–A11.

31. Correspondents of *The New York Times.* (2005). *Class matters.* New York: Henry Holt.

32. Cricken, E. (2005). Meth's burning issues. *Newsweek, 6*(8), 22–23.

33. Cuevas, K., Silver, P., Brooten, D., Youngblut, J., & Bobo, J. (2005). The cost of prematurity: Hospital charges at birth and frequency of rehospitalization and acute care visits over the first year of life. *American Journal of Nursing, 105*(7), 56–64.

34. Cunningham, F., MacDonald, P., & Gant, N. (2005). *Williams obstetrics* (22nd ed.). Upper Saddle River, NJ: Prentice Hall.

35. Dapice, A. (2006). The medicine wheel. *Journal of Transcultural Nursing, 17*(3), 251–260.

36. Dietek, J., Field, T., Hernandez-Reif, M., Jones, N., Lecanuet, J., Salmon, F., & Redzepi, M. (2001). Maternal depression and increased fetal activity. *Journal of Obstetrics and Gynecology, 21*, 468–473.

37. Dunkel-Schetter, C. (1998). Maternal stress and preterm delivery. *Prenatal and Neonatal Medicine, 3*, 39–42.

38. Duyff, R. (2006). *American Dietetic Association complete food and nutrition guide* (Revised and updated 3rd ed.). Hoboken, NJ: John Wiley & Sons.

39. Ekwo, E. E., & Moawad, A. (2000). Maternal age and preterm births in a Black population. *Pediatric Perinatal Epidemiology, 2*, 145–151.

40. Fenstermacher, K., & Hudson, B.T. (2004). *Practice guidelines for family practitioners* (3rd ed.). Philadelphia: W.B. Saunders.

41. Ferguson, D., Horwood, L., & Lynskey, M. (1993). Maternal smoking before and after pregnancy: Effects on behavioral outcomes in middle childhood. *Pediatrics, 92*, 815–822.

42. Fox, N. A., Henderson, H. A., Rubin, K. H., Calkins, S. D., & Schmidt, L. A. (2001). Continuity and discontinuity of behavioral inhibition and exuberance: Psychophysiological and behavioral influences across the first four years of life. *Child Development, 72*, 1–21.

43. Frank, D., Augustyn, M., Knight, W., Pell, T., & Zuckerman, B. (2001). Growth, development and behavior in early childhood following prenatal cocaine exposure. *Journal of the American Medical Association, 285*, 1613–1625.

44. Fried, P. A., & Smith, A. M. (2001). A literature review of the consequences of prenatal marijuana exposure. An emerging theme of a deficiency in executive function. *Neurotoxicology and Teratology, 23*, 1–11.

45. Frome, M. R. (2003). Work-family balance. In J. C. Quick & L. E. Tetrick (Eds.), *Handbook of occupational health psychology* (pp. 143–162). Washington, DC: American Psychological Association.

46. Fuller, M., & Sajativic, M. (2005). *Lexi-Comp's drug information handbook for psychiatry* (5th ed.). Hudson, OH: Lexicomp.

47. Garbarino, J., Dubrow, K., Korteling, K., & Parde, C. (1992). *Children in danger: Coping with consequences of community violence.* San Francisco: Jossey-Bass.

48. Garmezy, N. (1985). Stress resistant children: The search for protective factors. In J.E. Stevenson (Ed.), *Recent research in developmental psychopathology* (pp. 215–233). Oxford, England: Pergamon Press.

49. Geissler, E. (1998). *Cultural assessment* (2nd ed.). St. Louis, MO: Mosby.

50. Giger, J., & Davidhizar, R. (2004). *Transcultural nursing: Assessment and intervention* (4th ed.). St. Louis, MO: Mosby.

51. Greene, M. (2002). Outcomes of very low-birth-weight in young adults. *New England Journal of Medicine, 346*(3), 146–149.

52. Guyton, A., & Hall, J. (2006). *Textbook of medical physiology* (11th ed.). Philadelphia: Elsevier.

53. Hack, M., Flunnery, D., Schluchter, M., Carter, L., Borawski, E., & Klein, M. (2002). Outcomes in young adulthood for very low-birth-weight infants. *New England Journal of Medicine, 346*(3), 149–157.

54. Hanson, D., & Shriner, C. (2005). Unanswered questions: The legacy of atomic veterans. *Health Physics, 89*(2), 155–163.

55. Helsel, D., & Mochel, M. (2002). Afterbirths in the afterlife: Cultural meaning of placental disposal in a Hmong American community. *Journal of Transcultural Nursing, 13*(4), 282–286.

56. Hobel, C., Dunkel-Schetler, C., Roesch, S., Castro, L., & Anora, C. (1999). Maternal plasma corticotrophin-releasing hormone associated with stress at 20 weeks gestation in pregnancies ending in preterm delivery. *American Journal of Obstetrics and Gynecology, 180*, 257–263.

57. Hockenberry, M., & Wilson, D. (2007). *Wong's nursing care of infants and children* (8th ed.). St. Louis, MO: Mosby.

58. Holding, S. (2002). Current state of screening for Down syndrome. *Annals of Clinical Biochemistry, 39*, 1–11.

59. Huizink, A., Robles de Medina, P., Mulder, E., Visser, G., & Buttelaar, J. (2002). Psychological measures of prenatal stress as predictors of infant temperament. *Journal of the American Academy of Child and Adolescent Psychiatry, 41*(9), 1078–1085.

60. Jefferson, D. (2005, August 8). America's most dangerous drug. *Newsweek,* 41–48.

61. Ji, B.T., Shu, X.O., Linet, M.S., Zheng, W., Wacholder, S., Gao, Y.T., et al. (1997). Paternal cigarette smoking and the risk of childhood cancer among offspring of nonsmoking mothers. *Journal of the National Cancer Institute, 89*, 238–244.

62. Kagan, J. (1997). Temperament and the reactions to unfamiliarity. *Child Development, 68*, 139–143.

63. Keltner, N. (2005). Neonatal serotonin syndrome. *Perspectives in Psychiatric Care, 41*(2), 88–91.

64. Kennedy, M. (2005). Pregnancy and chemicals don't mix. *American Journal of Nursing, 185*(2), 19.

65. Kearney, M. (1996). Crack cocaine and pregnancy. *American Journal of Nursing, 96*(3), 17–19.

66. Kindy, D., Petersen, S., & Parkhurst, P. (2005). Perilous work: Nurses' experiences in psychiatric units with high risks of assault. *Archives of Psychiatric Nursing, 19*(4), 167–175.

67. Kovner, C., Brewer, C., Wu, Y.W., Cheng, Y., & Suzuki, M. (2006). Factors associated with work satisfaction of registered nurses. *Journal of Nursing Scholarship, 38*(1), 71–79.

68. Kravetz, J., & Federman, D. (2002). Cat-associated zoonoses. *Archives of Internal Medicine, 162*, 1945–1952.

69. Lackmann, G.W., Salzberger, U., Tollner, U., Chen, M., Carmella, S., & Heckt, S. (1999). Metabolites of a tobacco specific carcinogen in the urine of newborns. *Journal of the National Cancer Institute, 92*, 859–865.

70. Lester, B. (2003). The Maternal Lifestyle Study (MLS). Effects of prenatal cocaine and/or opiate exposure on auditory brain response at one month. *Journal of Pediatrics, 142*(3), 279–285.

71. Little, P. (2002). *Genetic destinies.* Oxford, England: Oxford University Press.

72. Longnecker, M., Klebanoff, M., Zhou, H., & Brock, J. (2001). Association between maternal serum concentration of the DDT metabolite DDE and preterm and small-for-gestational-age babies at birth. *Lancet, 358*, 110–114.

73. Luke, B., Mamelle, N., Keith, I., Munoz, E., Minogue, J., Papiernik, E., et al. (1995). The association between occupational factors and preterm birth. A United States nurses' study. *American Journal of Obstetrics and Gynecology, 173*, 849–862.

74. Macmillan, C., Magder, L., Bronwere, P., Chase, C., Hittleman, C., Lusky, T., et al. (2001). Head growth and neurodevelopment of infants born to HIV-infected drug-using women. *Neurology, 57*, 1402–1411.

75. Martin, A.S. (2001). Ordinary magic: Resilience processes in development. *American Psychologist, 56*, 227–228.

76. Mason, D., & Kany, K. (2005). The state of the science: Focus on work environments. *American Journal of Nursing, 105*(3), 33–34.

77. McGrath, M., Sullivan, M., Lester, B., & Oh, W. (2000). Longitudinal neurologic follow-up in neonatal intensive care unit survivors with various neonatal morbidities. *Pediatrics, 106*(6), 1397–1405.

78. McNeely, E. (2005). The consequences of job stress for nurses' health: Time for a check-up. *Nursing Outlook, 53*, 291–299.

79. Mechcatie, E. (2005). SSRI use tied to reports of neonatal withdrawal symptoms. *Clinical Psychiatry News, 33*(7), 7.

80. Melville, N. (2005). New data on pregnancy, SSRIs need perspective. *Clinical Psychiatry News, 33*(10), 30.

81. Meth epidemic having communities straining health care resources. (2005). *Clinician News, 9*(10), 1, 21–22.

82. Metules, T. (2001). Protect your eyes. *RN, 64*(10), 69–70.

83. Monteleone, J. (1998). *A parent's & teacher's handbook on identifying and preventing child abuse.* St. Louis, MO: G.W. Medical Publishing.

84. Moore, S. E., Cole, T., Poskins, E., Sonko, B., Whitehead, R., McGregor, I., & Prentice, A. (1997). Season of birth predicts mortality in rural Gambia. *Nature, 388*, 434.

85. NANDA International. (2007). *NANDA-I nursing diagnoses: Definitions & classifications 2007–2008.* Philadelphia: Author.

86. National Institute on Alcohol Abuse and Alcoholism (NIAAA). (1999). *Identification and care of fetal-alcohol-exposed children: A guide for primary care providers* (*Vol. 99–4369*). Rockville, MD: National Institutes of Health.

87. National Institute on Alcohol Abuse and Alcoholism (NIAAA). (2000). Prenatal exposure to alcohol. *Alcohol Research & Health, 24*, 32–41.

88. National Institutes of Health. (2001). *Stem cells: Scientific progress and future research directions.* Washington, DC: Department of Health and Human Services.

89. National Institutes of Health. (2006). *Stem cell information: The official National Institutes of Health resource for stem cell research.* Retrieved July 31, 2006, from http://stemcells.nih.gov/

90. Nelson, A., Fragata, G., & Menzet, N. (2003). Myths and facts about back injuries in nursing. *American Journal of Nursing, 103*(2), 32–39.

91. Neugebauer, R., Moore, J. W., & Lowe, J. C. (1985). Prenatal exposure to wartime famine and development of antisocial personality disorder in early adulthood. *Journal of the American Medical Association, 282*, 455–462.

92. O'Brien, C. M., & Jeffrey, H. E. (2002). Sleep deprivation, disorganization, and fragmentation during opiate withdrawal in newborns. *Pediatric Child Health, 38*, 66–71.

93. O'Brien-Pallos, L., Shamian, J., Thomson, D., Alksnis, C., Koehorn, M., Kerr, M., & Bruce, S. (2003). Work related disability in Canadian nurses. *Journal of Nursing Scholarship, 36*(4), 352–357.

94. Okie, S. (2005). Stem cell research—signposts and roadblocks. *New England Journal of Medicine, 353*, 1–5.

95. Olson, H., Sampson, P., Barz, H., Streissguth, A., & Bookstein, E. (1992). Prenatal exposure to alcohol and school problems in late childhood: A longitudinal prospective study. *Development and Psychopathology, 4*, 341–359.

96. Papalia, D., Olds, S., & Feldman, R. (2004). *Human development* (9th ed.). New York: McGraw-Hill.

97. Parker, L., Pearce, M. S., Dickinson, H. O., Aitkin, M., & Craft, A. W. (1999). Stillbirths among offspring of male radiation workers at Sellafield nuclear reprocessing plant. *Lancet, 354*, 1407–1414.

98. Parver, M. (2005). New report finds dangerous toxins in baby products. *Missouri Public Interest Research Group (MOPIRG), 6*(1), 1.

99. Paskawicz, J. (2005). Latex allergy revisited. *Clinician Reviews, 15*(11), 66–75.

100. Peipins, L., Burnett, C., Alterman, T., & Lalich, N. (1995). *Mortality patterns among nurses: 28-state study (1984–1990).* American Public Health Association 123rd Annual meeting, San Diego, CA, October 29–November 2.

101. Pender, N., Murdaugh, C., & Parsons, M. (2006). *Health promotion in nursing practice* (5th ed.). Upper Saddle River, NJ: Pearson Prentice Hall.

102. Saigal, S., Hoult, I., Streiner, D., Stoskopf, B., & Rosenbaum, B. (2000). School difficulties at adolescence in a regional cohort of children who were extremely low birth weight. *Pediatrics, 105*, 325–331.

103. Saigal, S., Stoskopf, B., Streiner, D., & Burrows, E. (2001). Physical growth and current health status of infants who were of extremely low birth weight and controls at adolescence. *Pediatrics, 108*(2), 407–415.

104. Santrock, J. (2004). *Life-span development* (9th ed.). Boston: McGraw-Hill.

105. Schrag, S. G., & Dixon, R. L. (1985). Occupational exposure associated with male reproductive dysfunction. *Annual Review of Pharmacology and Toxicology, 25*, 467–592.

106. Secor, M. (2006). Preconception health care: Recommendations from the CDC. *American Journal of Nursing, 106*(7), 46–50.

107. Shaner, H., & Botter, M. (2003). Pollution: Health care's unintended legacy. *American Journal of Nursing, 103*(3), 79–84.

108. Shaw, G.M. (2001). Adverse human reproductive outcomes and electromagnetic fields. *Bioelectromagnetics, 5*(Suppl.), S5–S18.

109. Shea, K. M., Little, R. F., & The ALSPAC Study Team. (1997). Is there an association between preconceptual paternal x-ray exposure and birth outcome? *American Journal of Epidemiology, 145*, 546–551.

110. Singer, L.T. and others. (2002). Cognitive and motor outcomes of cocaine-exposed infants. *Journal of the American Medical Association, 287*(15), 1952–1960.

111. Sirgo, C., & Coeling, H. (2005). Work group culture and the new graduate. *American Journal of Nursing, 105*(2), 85–86.

112. Smith, L., Chang, L., Vonchura, M., Gilbride, K., Kuo, J., Poland, R., et al. (2001). Brain proton magnetic resonance spectroscopy and imaging in children exposed to cocaine in utero. *Pediatrics, 107*, 227.

113. Smith, L., Yonekura, M., Wallace, T., Berman, N., Kuo, J., & Berkowitz, C. (2003). Effects of prenatal methamphetamine exposure in fetal growth and drug withdrawal symptoms in infants born at term. *Journal of Developmental & Behavioral Pediatrics, 24*(1), 17–23.

114. Spector, R. (2000). *Cultural diversity in health & illness* (5th ed.). Upper Saddle River, NJ: Prentice Hall Health.

115. Spittler, K. (2006). Risks associated with antidepressant use during pregnancy. *Neuropsychiatry, 7*(3), 1, 18.

116. Spitz, R. (1975). Hospitalism: The genesis of psychiatric conditions in early childhood. In W. Sze (Ed.), *Human life cycle* (pp. 29–43). New York: Jason Aronson.

117. Spitz, R., & Wolf, K. M. (1946). Anaclitic depression: An inquiry into the genesis of psychiatric conditions in early childhood. In *The psychoanalytic study of the child* (Vol. 2, pp. 313–342). New York: International University Press.

118. Springer, K. (2006, February 27). Food mercury rises. *Newsweek*, 64.

119. St. John-Seed, M., & Weiss, S. (2006). Maternal state of mind and expressed emotion: Impact of mother's mental health, stress, and family satisfaction. *Journal of the American Psychiatric Nurses Association, 11*(3), 135–143.

120. Stick, S. M., Barton, P. R., Gurrin, I., Sly, P. D., & LeSonef, P. N. (1996). Effects of maternal smoking during pregnancy and a family history of asthma on respiratory function in newborn infants. *Lancet, 348*, 1060–1064.

121. Strachan-Lindenberg, C., McDaniel, A., Gendrop, S., Nencioli, M., and Williams, D. (1991). A review of the literature on cocaine abuse in pregnancy. *Nursing Research, 40*(2), 69–75.

122. Streissguth, A. (1997). *Fetal alcohol syndrome. A guide for families and communities.* Baltimore: Paul H. Brookes.

123. Streissguth, A., Aase, J., Cairren, S., Kandels, S., LaDue, R., & Smith, D. (1991). Fetal alcohol syndrome in adolescents and adults. *Journal of the American Medical Association, 265*, 1961–1967.

124. Streissguth, A., Barr, H., & Sampson, P. (1990). Moderate prenatal alcohol exposure: Effects on child IQ and learning problems at age 7 1/2 years. *Alcoholism: Clinical and Experimental Research, 14*, 662–669.

125. Streissguth, A., Barr, H., Sampson, P., Derby, B., & Martin, D. (1989). IQ at age 4 in relation to maternal alcohol use and smoking through pregnancy. *Developmental Psychology, 25*, 3–11.

126. Streissguth, A., Bookstein, F., Sampson, P., & Bau, H. (1995). Attention, prenatal alcohol, and continuities of vigilance and retentional problems from 4 through 14 years. *Development and Psychopathology, 7*, 415–446.

127. Streissguth, A., Martin, D., Barr, H., Sandman, B., Kirchner, G., & Darby, B. (1984). Intrauterine alcohol and nicotine exposure: Attention and reaction time in 4-year-old children. *Developmental Psychology, 20*, 533–541.

128. Swayze, V.W., 2nd, Johnson, V.P., Hanson, J.W., Piven, J., Seto, Y., Giedd, J., et al. (1997). Magnetic resonance imaging of brain anomalies in fetal alcohol syndrome. *Pediatrics, 99*, 232–240.

129. Taylor, E. (2002). *Spiritual care: Nursing theory, research, and practice.* Upper Saddle River, NJ: Prentice Hall.

130. Thackray, H., & Tiftt, C. (2001). Fetal alcohol syndrome. *Pediatrics in Review, 22*(2), 47–55.

131. Theiler, P. (1984, November–December). Vietnam aftermath. *Common Cause Magazine*, 29–34.

132. Thies, K., & Travers, J. (2006). *Handbook of human development for health care professionals.* Boston: Jones and Bartlett.

133. Tough, S. C., Newburn-Cook, C., Johnston, D. W., Svenson, I. W., Rose, S., & Belik, J. (2002). Delayed childbearing and its impact on population rate

changes in lower birth weight, multiple birth, and preterm delivery. *Pediatrics, 109*, 399–403.

134. Trasler, J. (2000). Paternal exposure: Altered sex ratios. *Teratology, 62*, 6–7.

135. Trinkoff, A., Geiger-Brown, J., Brady, B., Lipscomb, J., & Muntaner, C. (2006). How long and how much are nurses working? *American Journal of Nursing, 106*(4), 60–71.

136. Trossman, S. (1999). RN explores Agent Orange's lasting effect on women vets. *American Nurse, 31*(3), 24.

137. Trossman, S. (2005). Who you work with matters. *American Nurse, 37*(4), 1, 8, 9.

138. Turley, R. (2003). Are children of young mothers disadvantaged because of their mother's age or family background? *Child Development, 74*(2), 465–474.

139. United States Department of Health and Human Services. (2000). *Healthy People 2010: Understanding and improving health* (2nd ed.). 2 Vol. Washington, DC: U.S. Government Printing Office.

140. United States Department of Health and Human Services. (1989). *The health consequences of smoking: Nicotine addiction. A report of the Surgeon General.* Bethesda, MD: Centers for Disease Control.

141. Van Dongen, C. (1998). Environmental health risks. *American Journal of Nursing, 98*(9), 16B–16E.

142. Wahlbeck, K., Forsen, T., Osmond, C., Barker, D., & Erikson, J. (2001). Association of schizophrenia with low maternal body mass index, small size of birth, and thinness during childhood. *Archives of General Psychiatry, 58*, 48–55.

143. Werner, E. E. (1990). *Protective factors and individual resistance.* In S. Meisels & J. Shonkoff (Eds.), *Handbook of early childhood intervention* (pp. 97–116). New York: Cambridge Press.

144. West, J. B., & Goodlett, C. R. (1990). Teratogenic effects of alcohol on brain development. *Annals of Medicine, 22*, 319–325.

145. Wilcox, A. J., Weinberg, C. R., & Baird, D. D. (1995). Timing of sexual intercourse in relation to ovulation. Effects of the probability of conception, survival of pregnancy, and sex of the baby. *New England Journal of Medicine, 333*, 1563–1565.

146. Wisborg, K., Kesmodel, U., Beck, B. H., Hedegaard, M., & Henriksen, T. B. (2003). Maternal consumption of coffee during pregnancy and still-birth and infant deaths in first year of life: A prospective study. *British Medical Journal, 326*, 420–426.

147. Women and depression. (2004). *Harvard Mental Health Letter, 20*(11), 1–3.

148. Worcaster, S. (2005). Use of SSRI's linked with birth defects. *Clinical Psychiatry News, 33*(9), 10.

149. Worthington, K. (1998, February). Workplace hazards: The effects on nurses as women. *American Nurse, 15.*

150. Yazigi, R., Odem, R., & Polakoski, K. (1991). Demonstration of specific binding of cocaine to human spermatozoa. *Journal of the American Medical Association, 266*, 1956–1959.

151. Zhang, J., & Ratcliffe, J. (1993). Paternal smoking and birth-weight in Shanghai. *American Journal of Public Health, 83*(2), 207–210.

152. Zhu, B., Rolfs, R., Nangle, B., & Horen, J. (1999). Effect of the interval between pregnancies on perinatal outcomes. *New England Journal of Medicine, 340*, 589–594.

UNIT III

The Developing Person and Family Unit:
Infancy Through Adolescence

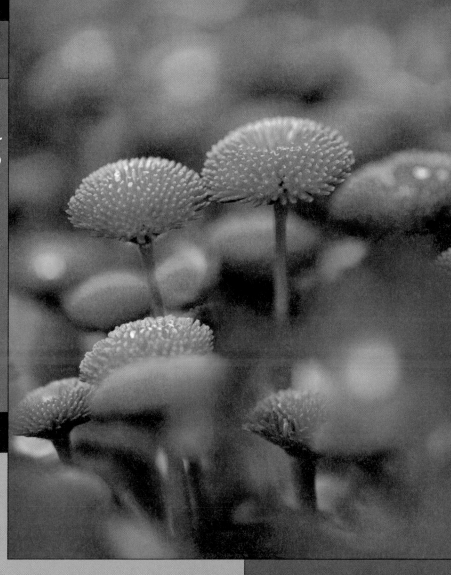

CHAPTERS

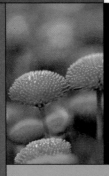

CHAPTER 9

The Infant: Basic Assessment and Health Promotion

OBJECTIVES

Study of this chapter will enable you to:

1. Define terms and give examples of basic developmental principles pertinent to the neonate and infant.

2. Discuss the crisis of birth for the family, factors that influence parental bonding and attachment, and your role in assisting the family to adapt and meet their developmental tasks.

3. Describe the adaptive physiologic changes in the newborn that occur at birth.

4. Assess the neonate's physical characteristics and the manner in which psychosocial needs begin to be filled.

5. Contrast and assess the physiologic, motor, cognitive, linguistic, emotional, and social characteristics and adaptive mechanisms of the infant.

6. Interpret the immunization schedule and other safety and health promotion measures for a parent.

7. Examine your role in assisting parents to foster the development of trust, promote parental attachment and a positive self-concept, and nurture the infant physically.

8. Relate the developmental tasks for the infant and behavior that indicates that these tasks are being met.

9. Compare parental behavior toward the infant who thrives with parental behavior toward the infant who is maltreated.

10. Plan, with guidance, intervention measures with parents and baby after delivery and during the first year of life.

MediaLink www.prenhall.com/murray

Go to the Companion Website for interactive resources that accompany this chapter.

Glossary	Critical Thinking
Review Questions	Tools
Challenge Your Knowledge	Media Link Applications
Learning Activities	Media Links

This chapter discusses the growth and developmental patterns of the baby during the first year of life, the baby's effect on the family, and the family's influence on the baby. It builds on prior information and focuses on the developmental tasks of the infant and family after birth. Measures to promote the infant's welfare that are useful in health promotion and nursing practice and that can be taught to parents are described throughout the chapter. Refer to an embryology and obstetric nursing textbook for detailed information on fetal development, prenatal changes, and the process of labor and delivery.

The term **neonate**, or **newborn**, refers to the *first 30 days or 4 weeks of life;* **infant** refers to the *first 12 months* (in some texts, 15, 18, or up to 24 months is defined as infancy). In most Asian cultures, the child is considered 1-year-old at birth. Traditional Chinese custom adds 1 year to an infant's age on January 1, regardless of the birthday (4). **Mother** or **parent(s)** is the term used to *denote the person(s) responsible for the child's care and long-term welfare.* **Couple** *refers to the mother and father or person in the fathering or complementary role with the mother.*

The authors are aware that some characteristics and developmental tasks of the infant and family described here reflect the United States or Westernized countries and may differ in other countries. Certainly the infant will be slower to develop some characteristics if he or she is born where there is famine, economic deprivation, political unrest or war, or devastation from natural disaster. For example, for the child born in a refugee camp or between bombings, the parents have survival as the main task.

In 1959, the United Nations (UN) Commission in Human Rights drafted the nonbinding Declaration of the Rights of the Child. It was adopted by the General Assembly of the UN on November 20, 1959. In November 1989, the UN General Assembly adopted the International Convention on the Rights of the Child, to which 176 nations have become "state parties" to the binding treaty. The emphasis is on importance of motherhood and childhood and need for special care, assistance, opportunities, and protection from harm physically, mentally, and socially (56). However, the plight of mothers and children around the world is evidence that much work is necessary to implement the treaty's intent.

Family Development and Relationships

The coming of the child is a developmental and sometimes situational **crisis**, a *turning point in the couple's life in which old patterns of living must be changed for new ways of living and new values* (8, 57). The crisis may first be felt by the female as she recognizes body changes and new emotional responses, and considers how long she can work if she is in a career or profession and whether she can balance working and child rearing. Other challenges are spatial changes in the home, possibly moving to a new home to accommodate the baby, and balancing the budget to meet additional expenses. The crisis will be less if the baby is wanted than if the couple had planned on having no children. But having a baby is always a crisis—a change.

The crisis is greater when the baby is not planned for or wanted. Do not assume that either the female or her partner is happy about the pregnancy. She may not deliberately seek an abortion, but she may not eat or may exercise vigorously in an effort to maintain a slim figure. Sometimes the male fears becoming a father, the consequent responsibility, and loss of freedom. As the pregnancy progresses, as she looks more pregnant and activity must be curtailed, the male may withdraw emotionally. He may be apathetic about the baby; spend more time with male friends, work associates, or other females; and avoid preparation for the baby's arrival. In turn, the female spends more time alone and feels increasingly rejected, abandoned, depressed, and angry. She may challenge the male's behavior, and tension, resentment, and verbal (and sometimes physical) fighting or abuse may occur in the relationship.

"Your life will never be the same again." An expectant couple often hears this phrase. What do these words really imply? With the advent of parenthood, a couple is embarking on a journey from which there is no return. To put it simply, parents cannot quit. An "I'll-try-it" attitude cannot be assumed toward parenthood. The child's birth brings a finality to many privileges and a permanence of responsibilities. The baby's needs and demands may call for massive changes in lifestyle. The "childhood" of parents comes to a screeching halt.

Going to work, to visit friends, or even to shop is no easy task. Even a few hours away from home means taking along everything the baby needs—bottle, food, pacifier, a few toys, a clothing change, and more than enough diapers. In addition to this armful, an infant seat or stroller must also be packed. By the time the baby is dressed and everything is packed, the mother may want a nap more than anything else. Making sure the baby is wearing a dry diaper before the final exit through the door becomes more important than the finishing touches of makeup or putting on the special jewelry for the outfit. If there are several small children to care for in addition to the baby, the planning and effort are compounded. Older brothers and sisters can help with various tasks only to a certain point. As each child comes into the family unit, the process is worked through again.

If pregnancy and parenting create a crisis for a couple who want a baby, they are even more stressful and a greater crisis for the adolescent or for the woman who is a single parent, left to face pregnancy, birth, and child rearing alone. This adolescent or woman needs the support of and help from at least one other person during this period. A parent, relative, or friend can be a resource. Often the support and help of a number of people are needed.

You may be the primary source of support. The couple may need help to admit and work through their feelings and recommit their love for each other. It is important that such assistance be given—for the future health and well-being of both the baby and the parents. Your empathetic listening, acceptance, practical hints for better self-care and baby care, and general availability can make a real difference in the outcome of the pregnancy and in the mother's and father's ability to parent and to handle future crises. Referral to other resources and self-help groups or to a counselor may also be of great help.

GROWTH AND DEVELOPMENT OF PARENTS

Parenting is an inexact science. An increasing number of people are not prepared either intellectually or emotionally for family life because of the lack of nurturing or the difficult family life they experienced in childhood. Creating and maintaining a family unit is difficult in today's society. Many occupations demand travel, frequent change of residence, and working on Sundays and holidays, the traditional family days. The rapid pace of life and available opportunities interfere with family functions. Expectations for self and others have increased. For example, the woman may be striving for success in a career and as a mother. Children demand that parents become other-centered instead of self-centered.

Pregnancy is preparation for the birth event. Parenting is a process that continues for many years. Becoming a parent involves grieving the loss of one's own childhood and former lifestyle. The person must be able to work through feelings of loss before he or she can adapt and move on to a higher level of maturation. Being aware of the tremendous influence of parents on their children's development, parents may feel challenged to become the best persons they are capable of being. New parents may need to develop a confidence that they do not feel, an integrity that has been easy to let slide, and values that can tolerate being scrutinized. To grow and develop as a parent, the person needs to make peace with his or her past so that unresolved conflicts are not inflicted on the child.

Sexual relationships usually decrease during pregnancy, childbirth, and the postpartum period. By 6 weeks after birth the woman's pelvis is back to normal, lochia has ceased, involution is complete, and physically she is ready for an active sex life. But the mother may be so absorbed in and fatigued by challenges and responsibilities of motherhood that the father is pushed into the background. He may feel in competition with the baby, resenting both the baby and his partner. Either one may take initiative in renewing the role of lover and being sexually attractive to the other. The woman can strengthen flabby perineal muscles through prescribed exercise. Patience on the man's part is necessary. If an episiotomy was done before delivery, healing continues for some time, and the memory of pain in the area may cause the woman involuntarily to tense the perineal muscles and wish to forgo intercourse. Couples who have a sound philosophy and communication system soon work out such problems, including the fact that the baby's needs will sometimes interrupt intimacy. If the earlier sex life was unsatisfactory and the couple does not work together as a team, such problems may be hard to surmount. The mother may prolong nursing, or complain of fatigue, ill health, or pain. The father may find other outlets.

Encourage the couple to work at effective communication. They can share the feelings of pride, joy, anxiety, insecurity, and frustration of early parenthood, and understand the involvement of their multiple roles of mate, parents, and persons. Your support, suggestions, and assistance in helping the couple seek and accept help from family and friends foster their ability to manage. Explore with parents ways to reestablish a mutually satisfying sexual relationship, which is not a simple process but has intricate psychological overtones for males and females. You may also need to address the couple's desire for family planning; educate that the female may become pregnant while nursing. See Table 13-3 for information on contraceptive measures. ∞

The following stress indicators may be used in the assessment to predict the likelihood of postpartum difficulties (57, 73, 75, 78):

1. The female is a **primipara** *having her first baby.*
2. No relatives are available to help with baby care; the woman's mother is dead.

3. Complications occurred during pregnancy; the female was ill on bed rest during pregnancy, and the male partner was not supportive.
4. The female is ill apart from pregnancy or experienced depression.
5. The female has a distant relationship or conflict with own mother.
6. The male partner is often away from home or not involved with pregnancy or child rearing.
7. The female has no previous experience with babies.
8. The female is an adolescent or has suffered child abuse, especially sexual abuse or incest.

The more past and present stresses, the more difficulty the female has in coping with the postpartum experience.

Parenting is a risky process. It involves facing the unknown with faith because no one can predict the outcome when the intricacies of human relationships are involved. Parents grow and develop by taking themselves and their child one day at a time and by realizing the joy that can be part of those hectic early weeks and months. The feelings of joy and involvement increase as the parent-child attachment is cemented. Because establishing this attachment is crucial to long-term nurturing of the child, the process is explored in-depth to assist you in assessment and intervention.

INFANT-PARENT ATTACHMENT

Attachment *is an emotional tie between two persons, a human phenomenon characterized by certain behaviors.* It is a *close, reciprocal relationship between two people that involves contact with and proximity to one another and that endures over time.* Bowlby (19) *believed that human babies are predisposed to behaviors that promote and maintain proximity to caregivers.* It is only when these behaviors are directed to one or a few persons rather than to many persons that the behaviors indicate attachment (see **Figure 9-1■**). Health care professionals often use the term attachment to describe *interactive behaviors between caregivers and their infants and their larger environment.* Ainsworth et al. (1) and Main and Solomon (72) described patterns of attachment as secure, anxious-resistant, or anxious-avoidant, or sometimes as disorganized-disoriented. Authors often use the term attachment interchangeably with the term bonding. **Bonding** *refers to the initial maternal emotional tie to the newborn immediately following delivery.* Early contact between parents and infants is beneficial because it is thought to begin the relationship, but it is not absolutely critical. **Engrossment** *is the term to describe the father's initial paternal response to the baby.* This concept of the father-infant dyad developed along with the concept of maternal-infant bonding (1, 22, 34, 38, 54, 61, 62).

When considering infant behavior, temperament is a concept frequently linked with attachment. **Temperament** *is a behavioral style, a characteristic way of thinking, behaving, or reacting in a given situation.* It is believed that from birth children are predisposed to respond to the environment in different ways, which influences the way others respond to them and their needs. Temperament influences the dynamic interactions, including attachment behaviors, between children and other people in their environment (26, 32, 38).

Rubin describes the beginning of the mother-child relationship as similar to the beginning of any new relationship (98). Be-

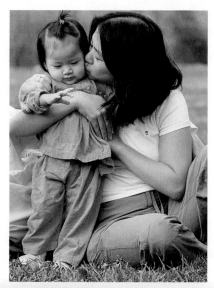

FIGURE □ **9-1** Mother-infant attachment develops mutually over the first year of life.

fore any interaction begins, certain information is obtained to identify the other person in the relationship, for example, sex, condition, and size. Introductory information is sought before any interaction occurs (91). **Table 9-1** outlines some behaviors of the infant, mother, and father in the typical order of progression in establishing this initial relationship (1, 19–22, 54, 91, 93–98, 104, 105).

Some research shows that **not** *all mothers initially follow the sequence of handling the newborn that is described in most of the literature and in* **Table 9-1**. Some mothers initially use palms or arms to handle the infant and then their fingers to explore the infant. Often mothers simultaneously use fingers and palms and then arms and trunk to explore and hold the baby. Some mothers may be initially hesitant or awkward in touching or holding the baby. Others may hold the baby differently than most mothers, and yet feel very maternal. These differences should be considered in assessment of maternal bonding and attachment (106). Realize also that there are cultural differences in expression of attachment. In some cultures, the parents of the mother or the father take care of the newborn and mother for a designated time. Further, out of respect for the elderly, the new parents will comply with their parents' wishes, regardless of what professionals tell the young parents (6, 53).

The behavior of the infant is a strong predictor of the relative frequency with which fathers display interactive, affectionate, and comforting behavior toward the infant. Very young crying infants are comforted or shown affectionate behavior. Fathers are more likely to stimulate by touching infants who are awake but not crying. Fathers are as likely to talk in a stimulating manner to crying as noncrying infants and to sleeping as awake infants. Research shows new fathers begin early to respond to infant cues (68).

Studies in bonding and attachment have included primarily middle-class, reasonably well-educated Caucasians. Bonding and attachment behaviors, especially for the male, could be different in other racial and cultural groups. Some cultures emphasize the

TABLE 9-1

Infant-Parent Attachment Behaviors

Infant	Mother	Father
Reflexively looks into mother's face, *establishes eye-to-eye contact* or *"face tie"*; molds body to mother's body when held	*Reaches* for baby; *holds high against breast-chest-shoulder area;* handles baby smoothly	Has great *interest in baby's face and notes eyes*
Vocalizes, cries, and *stretches out arms* in response to mother's voice; responds to mother's voice with *"dance"* or *rhythmic movements*	Talks softly in *high-pitched voice* and with intense interest to baby; puts baby face-to-face with her (*en face position*); eye contact gives baby sense of identity to mother	*Desires to touch, pick up, and hold baby;* cradles baby securely; shows fingertip touching and smiling to male baby; has more eye contact with infant delivered by forceps or cesarean section
Roots, licks, then *sucks* mother's nipple if in contact with mother's breast, cries, smiles	*Touches* baby's extremities; examines, strokes, massages, and kisses baby shortly after delivery; puts baby to breast if permitted; oxytocin and prolactin released	*Looks for distinct features;* thinks newborn resembles self; perceives baby as beautiful in spite of newborn characteristics
Reflexively embraces, clambers, clings, using hands, feet, head, and mouth to maintain body contact	*Calls baby by name;* notes desirable traits; *expresses pleasure* toward baby; *attentive* to reflex actions of grunts and sneezes	*Feels elated,* bigger, proud after birth; has strong *desire to protect and care for child*
Odor of mother distinguished by breastfeeding baby by fifth day	*Recognizes odor* of own child by third or fourth day	

Note: Similar behaviors are seen with a premature baby but the timing will vary.

mother as caretaker of the infant; the bond or attachment between father and child is less overt and may be emphasized later in childhood (6, 36, 51, 53).

The first hour after birth is a critical time for stimulating attachment feelings and bonding in the parents, because the baby tends to have eyes open, gaze around, have stronger sucking reflexes, cry more, and show more physical activity than in subsequent hours. Research indicates that attachment begins when the infant is first held, regardless of how long after delivery the holding occurred (54, 75, 92).

Some authors believe that in addition to causing increased alertness in the baby, *effective maternal-infant bonding can promote the baby's physical health in the following ways* (56, 61): (a) transference of maternal nasal and respiratory flora to the baby may prevent acquiring hospital strains of infectious organisms; (b) maternal body heat is a reliable source of heat for the newborn; and (c) regular breastfeedings can pass on the antibodies IgA and T- and B-lymphocytes to the baby to protect against enteric pathogens.

Binding-in is the term Rubin (93–98) uses to describe the *maternal-child relationship as a process that is active, intermittent, and cumulative over a period of 12 to 15 months.* Maternal identity is essential for the binding-in process, and both maternal identity and binding-in are either enhanced or inhibited by the infant's behavior and society. Maternal binding-in is stimulated and augmented by fetal movement during pregnancy and the physical needs of the newborn. After birth, fantasies about the child are replaced by the actual child, who can be seen, touched, heard, smelled, and cared for. This organizes maternal behavior and attitudes. Gender, size, and condition of the infant are critical to the maternal response.

The binding-in process involves (97, 98):

1. **Identification of the infant** by the *mother as part of self and belonging to self.* **Complete identification** occurs when the *mother knows by looking, touching, hearing, or smelling that the child is well or unwell, satisfied or hungry, or comfortable or in distress.*
2. **Claiming the child as her own** emotionally and physically. **Claiming** *occurs with the mother's commitment to the child in labor and delivery and is seen in the pleasure with the birth of the child.* Claiming also occurs by association with significant others in the social environment who claim the infant and mother.
3. **Polarization**, *or separating the infant from the unity of mother's self and fetus, begins with labor and delivery.*

Gradually the mother realizes the baby is not inside of her. The infant is held, nurtured, and compared to self and family members but is increasingly seen as a separate, unique individual and less as an extension of self and her own body image. Family life is reorganized; the baby is included in family activities. Over the period of the first year the mother can let go of the child as he or she gains motor, social, and emotional competence. The psychological loosening allows the mother also to give the child more physical space (93–98).

Development of attachment between parent and baby continues through infancy, as depicted in **Figure 9-1 ■**. *It involves emotional, cognitive, and socialization processes:* loving through cuddling, touching, stroking, kissing, cooing and talking to, laughing and playing with, and reinforcing and teaching the baby. Such contact should be consistent and done while caring physically for the baby. The touching, cooing, talking, and laughing can also be focused on the baby while the mother (or father) is preparing a meal, doing a household task, or waiting in a grocery line. The parent's voice across the room can also soothe and promote attachment. The infant, in turn, promotes proximity by smiling, babbling, crying, holding on, and rooting and sucking reflexes. Further, just as the parent may need to learn to respond to the infant, sometimes the child needs prompting to be responsive to the parent and to signal needs and not just wait for every need to be automatically met (19, 34).

Observe for maternal-child attachment. Educating the mother prenatally, such as by videotape about infant behaviors, developmental norms, and communication cues, facilitates a more positive mother-infant interaction in the postpartum period. The infant develops effective reciprocal interactions with the caregiver when the caregiver is responsive to the infant. Education could continue in maternal-child home visits. Observations and communication about quality of caregiving during the home visit would be effective for prevention of parenting problems and health promotion of the child and mother.

FACTORS INFLUENCING MATERNAL ATTACHMENT

Motherly feelings do not necessarily accompany biological motherhood. Various factors affect the mother's attachment and caretaking. *Variables that are difficult or impossible to change include* (24, 56, 61, 62, 95, 96) (a) the mother's level of emotional maturity, (b) how she was reared, (c) what her culture encourages her to do, (d) relationship with her family and partner, (e) experience with previous pregnancies, and (f) planning for and events experienced during the course of this pregnancy.

Deterrents to adequate mothering include (a) the mother's own immaturity or lack of mothering, (b) stress situations, (c) fear of rejection from significant people, (d) loss of a loved one, (e) financial worries, (f) lack of a supportive partner, and (g) the gender and appearance of the child. Separating mother and infant in the first few days of life, depersonalized care by professionals, rigid hospital routines, and the current practice of early discharge from the hospital without adequate help also interfere with establishing attachment and maternal behaviors (11, 18, 56).

Parenting skills can be manifested in various ways. Although eye contact, touch, and cuddling are important, love can be shown by a tender, soft voice and loving gazes. *Other indications of warm parenting feelings include* (a) calling the baby by name, (b) expressing enjoyment of the baby and indicating that the baby is attractive or has other positive characteristics, (c) looking at the baby and into baby's eyes, (d) talking to the baby in a loving voice, (e) taking safety precautions for the baby, and (f) responding to the baby's cues for attention or physical care.

The mother's health and well-being is critical. Nurturing will be essential for the mother who returns home within the 24- to 48-hour period after delivery. She will be exhausted, sore, and possibly overwhelmed with emotion and responsibility. The home health nurse is one support system; relatives or friends will also be needed for help. The nurse's assessment regarding the mother's physical and emotional status and need for information about child care is essential and helps to determine status of the newborn. The first 72 hours of the baby's life is a significant period of transition and stabilization and also a time when malformations or cardiorespiratory or feeding problems are evidenced. Infection in both the mother and baby may occur in this initial period.

Assess for deterrents to mothering as well as the physical condition of the baby and mother. Your nurturing of the mother and helping her seek additional help may offset the negative impact of these factors.

FACTORS INFLUENCING PATERNAL ATTACHMENT

Fatherly feelings do not necessarily accompany fatherhood. Bonding and attachment feelings in the father appear related to various factors: (a) general level of education, (b) participation in prenatal classes, (c) gender of infant, (d) role concept, (e) attendance at delivery, (f) type of delivery, (g) early contact, and (h) feeding method for baby (54, 86, 104, 105).

Support from the expectant mother is most effective in reducing stress levels in the expectant father; support from others is critical only if she cannot be supportive. This may be because intimacy and self-disclosure for males are maintained primarily in the partner relationship. For the expectant female, support from both the partner and others is critical in coping with stress, perhaps because females are socialized to value and depend on social relations to a greater extent than males (28).

The father is increasingly recognized as an important person to the infant and young child, not only as a breadwinner but also as a nurturer. In turn, the father needs a support system from family, friends, work colleagues, and males in church or other organizations in order to be a support system to the mother. Lack of a father figure can cause developmental difficulties for the child. Just as the mother is not necessarily endowed with nurturing feelings, the father is not necessarily lacking nurturing feelings. Some fathers seem to respond better to this role than mothers (22, 48, 68, 69, 75, 87, 104).

Include the father or father figure in your attention and nurturing care. Help the single mother determine who can be a father figure for the child. You contribute to family health when you promote paternal attachment. Refer to the Abstract for Evidence-Based Practice in relation to the father's needs.

Abstract for Evidence-Based Practice

What Fathers Need

Buckelow, S., Pierrie, H., & Chabra, A. (2006). What fathers need. A countywide assessment of the needs of fathers of young children. *Maternal and Child Health Journal, 10*(3), 285–291.

KEYWORDS

fatherhood, family involvement, needs assessment, MCH programs, county MCH services.

Purpose ➤ To determine personal and service needs of fathers of young children to improve services for families in a designated county.

Conceptual Framework ➤ Information about father's role.

Sample/Setting ➤ A convenience sample in San Mateo, California, of about 1,200 males in 16 agencies and community-based organizations and all male employees who had added a newborn child to their insurance plans in the prior 5 years. The county is geographically, culturally, and socioeconomically diverse.

Method ➤ A survey, written in both English and Spanish, that took 15 to 30 minutes to complete, was sent to the male participants. A total of 240 surveys were returned (20% return rate); 204 were usable. Surveys were completed in either English (94%) or Spanish (6%). Qualitative data were obtained through nine focus groups (n=80) conducted throughout the county. Key themes were summarized.

Findings ➤ All major racial/ethnic groups were represented in the response. Most of the fathers (79%) were married and had one or two children (80%). Half of the fathers had a college degree. Almost half (44%) were from 30 to 38 years; 22% were under 30 years; 33% were over 39 years. In this sample, 82% had private insurance. The highest current needs reported by fathers were finances (61%); health care (37%); housing (35%); food (34%); employment training, family planning, and legal assistance (each 6%); child support assistance and child custody assistance (each 5%); smoking cessation classes (4%), and alcohol or drug abuse counseling (1%). Focus group themes included the need to provide sex education to boys before they became sexually active, concerns about low social expectations of fathers, and negative stereotypes portrayed in the media about fathers. Ideas were generated for improving county services.

Implications ➤ Geographic regions should define and clarify needs of fathers of young children in order to improve programs. More research with fathers is needed to improve services. Advocacy for increasing public awareness and favorable media presentations related to the role of fathers are needed.

BEHAVIORAL CHARACTERISTICS OF PARENTAL DIFFICULTY IN ESTABLISHING ATTACHMENT

Parents tend to project their own feelings onto their child, turning the child into a figure from their own past. Negative feelings in the parent can create a dysfunctional relationship with the child.

Assess the *methods of relating to and holding the infant that would indicate the parent's difficulty in establishing attachment* (24, 56, 61, 62, 68–70, 75, 86, 92, 94, 95):

1. Maintains little or no eye contact with baby.
2. Does not touch baby, or picks up baby at times to meet own needs.
3. Does not support baby's head.
4. Holds baby at a distance, at arm's length after initial visits, loosely, or not at all.
5. Appears disinterested in baby, is preoccupied with something else when baby is present, and has a flat, fixed facial expression or unconvincing smile in response to your enthusiasm about baby.
6. Perceives baby as unattractive or looking like someone who is disliked.
7. Talks or coos to baby little or not at all.
8. Has passive response to baby; allows baby to be placed in arms rather than reaching out to baby.
9. Calls baby "it" rather than saying "my baby" or calling baby by name.
10. Notes defects or undesirable traits in baby, even if baby is normal, or is convinced baby is abnormal.
11. Avoids talking about baby, even when someone else initiates the topic.
12. Expresses dissatisfaction with or revulsion about care of baby.
13. Ignores baby's communications of cries, grunts, sneezes, and yawns.
14. Gets upset when baby's secretions, feces, or urine touch body or clothes; perceives care of baby as revolting.
15. Readily gives baby to someone else.
16. Does not take adequate safety precautions with baby (e.g., in relation to diapering, feeding, covering baby, or baby's movements).
17. Handles baby roughly, even after baby has eaten or vomited.
18. Gives inappropriate responses to baby's needs, such as overfeeding or underfeeding, or underhandling.
19. Thinks baby does not love him or her.
20. Expresses dislike of self, finds attribute in baby that is disliked in self.
21. Complains of being too tired to take care of baby.
22. Expresses fears that baby might die of a minor illness.

You may not observe all these behaviors in the mother initially, or in the mother or father later, *but a combination of several behaviors should alert you to actual or potential difficulty with being a parent.* You may educate and counsel, or you may refer to a family counselor to resolve any difficulties.

Several instruments that measure maternal-infant interactions, based on sound theoretical foundations and empirical evidence, are useful for practice and research (58). **Evaluating** the mother's ability to relate to her infant when the child exhibits behavioral problems is extremely important, as is documentation of observations. Fostering a healthy maternal-infant relationship, especially in at-risk situations, may help to prevent subsequent childhood developmental, behavioral, and mental health problems. Further, *interaction problems may be amenable to interpersonal, cognitive, behavioral, and psychoeducational treatment strategies which include* (a) your interest and support, (b) demonstration of ways to interact with the child, (c) education about the child's needs, (d) attention to parents' needs, and (e) fostering a support system.

CHILD MALTREATMENT, ABUSE, AND NEGLECT

A common area of concern for the nurse who cares for infants and their families is **child maltreatment** (*child abuse and neglect*). Because the spectrum of child maltreatment is so broad, professionals spend considerable time trying to decide what constitutes child maltreatment. *Child maltreatment is both demonstrable harm and child endangerment (i.e., the child who has suffered harm or is in danger of being harmed).* This specifically includes the *child whose health and well-being is endangered through acts that are nonaccidental, avoidable, and committed by a parent or parent substitute, another adult, or adolescent caretakers.*

Abuse is classified based on the nature of the abusive acts or neglectful omissions into six major types: physical abuse, sexual abuse, emotional abuse, physical neglect, emotional neglect, and educational neglect. With the exception of physical abuse, each of these categories is broken down into subtypes (50, 81, 82). The Child Abuse Prevention and Treatment Act (CAPTA) as amended and reauthorized in October 1996 (Public Law 104-235, Section 111; 42USC 5100g) defines **child abuse** and **neglect** as *any act or failure to act that results in risk for serious physical or emotional harm, sexual abuse, exploitation, or death of a child or youth under age 18* (56). See Chapter 8 for other definitions and information. ∞ **The professional is mandated to report child maltreatment.** *Each state has a central agency to follow up reported cases.*

Whenever the developing person and family and influences on development and behavior are considered, the microsystem, exosystem, and macrosystem are all contributors. Each of these components is discussed in relation to maltreatment, child abuse, and neglect (26, 27, 87).

The **microsystem** *consists of the family. Maltreatment, abuse, or neglect of the child is a symptom of extreme disturbance in the family* (26, 27). *Parents who have themselves been abused or did not receive good parenting are more likely to be abusive.* **Abusing parents or parent surrogates** *are angry and anxious, have poor impulse control and low self-esteem, are under great stress, and are lonely and depressed.* In general, they cannot cope with the demands of child rearing. They do not understand normal child development; they become enraged because the child does not meet their expectations for behavior to not cry or to stay clean. They are highly stressed by behavior most parents take in stride. Some of these parents are emotionally ill or have antisocial personalities. They are less effective in resolving problems with their children or with the spouse or other family members. Often these parents are lonely and isolated, cut off from any support system. As children are abused, some become more aggressive, which causes even more abuse from the parent. Or, the child may be unwanted, hyperactive, ill, disabled, or difficult to parent. In contrast, **neglectful parents** *tend to be apathetic, incompetent in relationships, irresponsible, and emotionally withdrawn* (26, 27, 56, 81–83, 87).

The **exosystem**—*the outside world*—can be a contributor. Poverty, unemployment, job dissatisfaction, social isolation, and lack of assistance from others all contribute to stress, rage, and withdrawal. The low-income neighborhood that experiences no sense of community, criminal activity, lack of facilities or resources, inadequate safety overall, and poor political leadership affects families and their ability to cope and care for themselves. A neighborhood may be poor, but if there are strong social support networks and a sense of community, there is less child abuse (26, 27, 87).

The **macrosystem**—*cultural values and patterns of punishment*—is key. The United States has a high rate of violence in various forms, including the media. Child abuse rates are high. In countries where violent crime is less frequent, child abuse is rare (26, 27, 87).

Shaken baby syndrome (SBS) *is a form of child abuse that is caused by vigorous shaking, sharply and quickly, back and forth, with or without impact. It produces acceleration and deceleration forces in the head and consequent damage, with little or no evidence of intracranial trauma.* The infant fears loss of support, sudden or unexpected motion, and looming objects, especially with loud noise or bright lights. Thus, shaking the baby can constitute psychological as well as physical abuse. Head trauma is the leading cause of death of abused children; shaking is involved in many of these cases. The majority of perpetrators are males. Many survivors of SBS suffer brain damage from ruptured blood vessels in the brain and broken neural connections, resulting in lifelong impairments. The victims of SBS are usually less than 1 year of age, with the majority under the age of 6 months (14, 56, 81, 82). Children as old as age 5 are vulnerable to SBS, but children 2 to 4 months old are especially at risk (81, 82).

Box 9-1, Shaken Baby Syndrome, summarizes risk factors, manifestations, and prevention strategies (56, 81, 82). Utilize the information in your assessment and intervention.

Factitious disorders by proxy, formerly called **Munchausen syndrome by proxy**, *is another form of abuse, usually physical. The parent, usually the mother, induces or fabricates illness about the neonate or infant.* The illness appears dramatic in onset and has multiple manifestations that are difficult to document. Repeated visits to multiple health care providers result in numerous diagnostic tests or therapies. The parent (the proxy) appears very attentive to the child but actually seeks attention, for self more than for the child, from medical personnel. The child may suffer real illness or injury, or the mother may describe a history of apnea, seizures, blood in the urine or feces, vomiting, and diarrhea. There is likely to be a discrepancy between the history and clinical findings, and

---

BOX 9-1   Shaken Baby Syndrome

THOSE AT RISK

Infants and small children because of physical characteristics: heavy head, weak neck muscles, soft and rapidly growing brain, thin skull wall, lack of control over head and neck, lack of mobility

CLINICAL PRESENTATION

1. Mild form may be mistaken for viral illness
2. Rigidity
3. Unexplained seizures
4. Vomiting, associated with drowsiness, lethargy, or feeding problems
5. Irritability
6. Listlessness, lethargy
7. Bradycardia
8. Hypothermia
9. Unexplained bulging or full fontanels or large head circumference
10. Apnea, dyspnea
11. Coma or altered consciousness
12. Retinal hemorrhage, blindness
13. Subdural hematoma, subarachnoid hemorrhage
14. Permanent brain damage, developmental delay
15. Speech and learning difficulties
16. Paralysis
17. Cardiac arrest
18. Death

RISK FACTORS

1. Behavioral difficulties of parent; unconscious desire for role reversal when parent expects child to provide love and nurture
2. Immaturity or illness in parent, inability to manage normal crying and colic, other than with anger and abuse
3. Addiction in mother, resulting in drug-addicted baby who is more irritable and difficult to manage
4. Lack of knowledge about child behavior, how to handle baby, and danger of shaking
5. Male caregiver at time of incident, may or may not be related to baby, commonly father or mother's boyfriend

PREVENTION

1. Education about appropriate expectations of child
2. Education about parenting, and infant and child care
3. Education about dangers of shaking child
4. Stress management education and counseling; anger management strategies
5. Prenatal classes, support groups after baby is born
6. Education of boys and men (e.g., schools, Scouts, YMCA, church youth and adult groups)

the illness is unresponsive to treatment. Often the parent tells the medical personnel what should be done and is reluctant to leave the emergency room or hospital. Consequences to the infant, or child of any age, can be serious physically and emotionally. Suspected cases should be reported and handled the same as any abused child case (5).

Garbarino, Guttmann, and Seeley (50) describe types of **psychological abuse, battering, or maltreatment**, which are a *deliberate pattern of attack by a parent or an adult on a child's developmental status, sense of self, or social competence.* See **Box 9-2**, Parental Behaviors Characteristic of Psychological Maltreatment of the Infant. As a result, the child becomes vulnerable to negative forces in the broader social environment, does not develop a sense of trust, and becomes emotionally, socially, and sometimes physically ill (50). Utilize the information for assessment. Strategies and tools for identification and intervention with the family, individual child, and institutional network of social services are further discussed by the authors (50) and in this chapter.

Teach parents, both mother and father (or stepparent or boyfriend, if involved), to better understand normal infant behavior and how to manage their frustrations to avoid abusive behavior. If the parent feels angry, he or she should avoid touching the baby, step back, and leave the room to calm down. Teach parents to consider causes for crying: the child may be hungry, soiled, teething, tired, ill, injured, or frightened. The need behind the crying must be addressed by the parent, and you can be a role model in responding to the infant's expression of needs.

INTERVENTIONS TO PROMOTE ATTACHMENT AND HEALTH

Incorporate the parents' cultural beliefs, values, and attitudes into your nursing care and modern health care practices whenever possible (6, 51, 53, 56, 65, 84, 92, 101). Observe and listen to the parental behavior. Ask what specific behaviors on your part will make the parents or family more comfortable with your care. Maintaining important cultural traditions is one way to individualize care. Your scientific knowledge and practices can usually be

---

BOX 9-2	**Parental Behaviors Characteristic of Psychological Maltreatment of the Infant**

REJECTING

1. Refuses to accept the child's attachment behavior or spontaneous overtures
2. Refuses to return smiles and vocalizations

ISOLATING

1. Denies child the experience of enduring patterns of interaction
2. Leaves the child in his or her room unattended for long periods
3. Denies access to the child by interested others

TERRORIZING

1. Exposes the child consistently and deliberatly to intense stimuli or frequent change of routine
2. Teases, scares, or gives extreme or unpredictable response to child's behavior

IGNORING

1. Fails to respond to infant's spontaneous behavior that forms basis for attachment
2. Does not respond to infant's smiles, vocalizations, or developing competence and changing skill levels

CORRUPTING

1. Reinforces bizarre habits
2. Creates alcohol or drug addictions
3. Reinforces the child for oral sexual contact

Source: Adapted from Garbarino, J., Guttmann, E., & Seeley, J. (1987). *The psychologically battered child: Strategies for identification, assessment, and intervention.* San Francisco: Jossey-Bass. Copyright 1986. Adapted by permission of Jossey-Bass, Inc., a subsidiary of John Wiley & Sons, Inc.

INTERVENTIONS FOR HEALTH PROMOTION

The following interventions directed to the parents will assist them to develop attachment with the infant:

1. Call the child, mother, and father by their names during your care.
2. Inquire about the mother's well-being; too often all the focus is on the baby. She is in a receptive state and must be emotionally and physically cared for.
3. Encourage parents to unwrap the baby and inspect the hands, fingers, toes, and body. This inspection will foster identification and attachment.
4. Position the newborn in an en-face (face-to-face) position and describe the infant's visual abilities.

5. Model behaviors (holding, talking to, making eye contact with newborn).
6. Nurture the father to help him be caring and helpful to the mother and baby.
7. Make favorable comments about the infant's progress.
8. Compliment the mother on her intentions or ability to comfort, feed, or identify her baby's needs. Speak of the pleasure the baby shows in response to the parent's ministrations.
9. Reassure the parents that positive changes in the baby are a result of their care, and avoid judgmental attitudes or statements that foster guilt.

INTERVENTIONS FOR HEALTH PROMOTION

The following interventions support, teach, and counsel parents about how they can promote attachment, give optimum infant stimulation, and promote holistic health include:

1. Encourage both parents to cuddle, look at, and talk to the baby; if necessary, demonstrate how to stroke, caress, and rock baby.
2. Encourage parents to be prompt and consistent in answering the infant's cry.
3. Assist parents in gaining confidence in responding effectively to baby's cry through recognizing the meaning of the cry, meeting the child's needs, and using soothing measures such as rocking, redundant sounds, and swaddling.
4. Explain the infant's interactive abilities, and help the parents develop awareness of their own initial effective responses to the newborn's behavior.
5. Explain the basis of early infant learning as the discovery of associations, connections, and relationships between self and repeated occurrences. Explore how to provide a gradually increasing variety of stimuli. Sights, sounds, smells, movements, positions, temperatures, and pressure all provide opportunities for learning and for emotional, perceptual, social, and physical development.
6. Call attention to the baby's behaviors that indicate developmental responsiveness, such as reflex movements, visual following, smiling, raising chin off bed, rolling over,

and sitting alone. Pupil dilation in the presence of the parent begins at approximately 4 weeks of age. During the first few weeks of life, babies prefer the human face to other visual images.
7. Explain contact stimulation present in fetal life that continues after birth. Pressure and touch sensation is present *in utero* a few months before birth, thus the newborn responds well to touch and gentle pressure. Rooting and hand-mouth activity occur in fetal life and are major adaptive activities after birth.
8. Encourage mutual eye contact between parent and baby and talking to the baby. All of the infant's efforts to vocalize and develop social behaviors should be reinforced. Eye contact between the parent and baby increases during the first 3 months of life and is soon accompanied by other social responses—smiling and vocalization.
9. Encourage regular periods of affectionate play when the infant is alert and responsive. Mother and father may pick up and hold the baby close, encourage visual following and smiling, and talk to the infant, repeating sounds. Rhythm and repetition are enjoyed. Often baby is most alert after a daytime feeding.
10. Promote awareness in other family members of the baby's competencies so that they can also respond to and reinforce the infant.

---

safely adapted. Specific traditions may extend to naming or bathing the baby, prenatal and postnatal care of the mother, how to hold or dress the baby, inclusion or exclusion of the father from the delivery, and roles of various family members. Be sensitive to the preferences of clients who represent a culture different from your own. Listen to and try to follow their requests. Listen to what is said and implied. Suggest rather than advise or direct when you teach.

Listen attentively for information and signs that give you clues about the parents' feelings about themselves, where they are in their own developmental growth, who they rely on for strength, their ideas about child discipline, and their expectations of the new child. As you see gaps in necessary information, you can present information. If your approach is gentle, the parents will recognize you as a helpful friend. Mothers are receptive to information and to your reinforcement of mothering skills.

Help parents realize that soon the complete focus on mother, father, and new baby will be gone. Other roles will be reestablished: husband, wife, employer or employee, student, daughter, son, friend, and so on. The new parents will have to allow for all aspects of their personalities to function again. The baby will fit in the family. Refer to Chapter 6 and Table 6-2 ∞ to incorporate information about family development tasks when the couple assumes parenthood.

BABY'S INFLUENCE ON PARENTS

Some babies have a high activity level and a temperament to warm up easily to the parent. Some are quiet and withdrawn, with a low activity level. Various other mixtures of activity level and temperament exist. The infant's dominant reaction pattern to new situations manifests an innate temperament, and the temperament affects the reactions of others, especially the parents. They, in turn, will mold the baby's reaction pattern (23, 24, 32, 87, 103).

It is easy to love a lovable baby, but parents have to work harder with babies who are not highly responsive. Assess the reactions between the baby and parents, as the style of child care that will develop has its basis here. A highly active mother who expects an intense reaction may have a hard time mothering a low-activity, quiet baby because she may misinterpret the baby's behavior, feel rejected, and in turn reject the child. The baby may be denied the stimulation necessary for development. If the mother is withdrawn, quiet, and unexpressive and has a high-activity baby, she may punish the baby for normal energetic or assertive behavior and ignore the bids for affection and stimulation. The child needs to feel his or her behavior will produce an effect that meets the child's needs.

Help parents understand the *mutual response* between the baby and themselves. Teach them to read the baby's signals and to give consistent signals to the baby. Help parents feel competent even if at times they are unable to understand the child's cues and meet needs.

Point out positive behaviors that you observe. If self-confidence is consistently lacking, the parent's despair may turn to anger, rejection, and abuse. Give information and support that builds self-confidence and self-esteem.

EXPANSION OF INTRAFAMILY RELATIONSHIPS

Grandparents-to-be and other relatives frequently become more involved with the parents-to-be, bringing more gifts and advice than is necessarily desired. Yet their gifts and supportive presence can be a real help if the grandparents respect the independence of the couple, if the couple has resolved their earlier adolescent rebellion and dependency conflicts, and if the grandparents' advice does not conflict with the couple's philosophy or professional advice. The couple and grandparents should collaborate rather than compete. In some cultures, the maternal grandmother has a major role in care of the pregnant and postpartum daughter and in care of the infant (6, 36, 51, 53). The grandmother may give advice about nutrition, self-care, or baby care to the daughter; however, the advice may be contrary to scientific and medical knowledge and practices. Suggest that grandparents not take over the situation. The couple's autonomy should be encouraged in that they can listen to the various pieces of advice, evaluate the statements, and then as a unit make their own decision. New parents should refrain from expecting the grandparents to be built-in babysitters and to rescue them from every problem. Grandparents usually enjoy brief rather than prolonged contact with baby care. For the single parent, the grandparents or other relatives can be a major source of emotional and financial help and can provide child care assistance.

You may assist the parent(s) in working with grandparents, resolving feelings of either being controlled or not adequately helped, understanding grandparents' feelings, accepting help, and avoiding excessive demands. The parent(s) may also need encouragement in resolving issues with other family members. Establish rapport with both the grandmother and the mother or mother-to-be. Respect the role of the grandmother. Often the advice she gives is culturally based—the practices have maintained the group for centuries. The practices may be carried out along with modern-day health and medical practices. If the advice is truly harmful to the mother or baby, your rapport, nonjudgmental approach, and well-timed, low-key teaching of the grandmother may help her to accept the teaching you direct to the mother. Indeed, if either or both grandparents are considered the head of the household, direct attention initially to them and direct your teaching to them. Initial or exclusive focus on their daughter is likely to alienate them, so that they discontinue coming for care, become resistant, and not allow their daughter to carry out your teaching. Health promotion includes these considerations.

Physiologic Concepts: Physical Characteristics of the Neonate

The **neonatal period of infancy** *includes the critical transition from intrauterine fetal existence through the first 30 days of life.* The normal newborn is described in the following section. Transition begins at birth with the first cry. Air is sucked in to inflate the lungs. Complex chemical changes are initiated in the cardiopulmonary system so that the baby's heart and lungs can assume the burden of oxygenating the body. The foramen ovale closes during the first 24 hours; the ductus arteriosus closes after several days. For the first time, the baby experiences light, gravity, cold, and firm touch. The newborn is relatively resistant to the stress of anoxia and can survive longer in an oxygen-free atmosphere than an adult. The reason is unknown, as are the long-term effects of *mild* oxygen deprivation (13, 35, 56).

GENERAL APPEARANCE

The newborn appearance does not match the baby ads and may be a shock to new parents. The misshapen head, flat nose, puffy eyelids and often undistinguished eye color, discolored skin, large tongue and undersized lower jaw, short neck and small sloping shoulders, short limbs and large rounded abdomen with protruding umbilical stump that remains until 3 weeks, and bowed skinny legs may prove very disappointing if the parents are unprepared for the sight of a newborn. *The head, which accounts for 25% of the total body size, appears large in relation to the body.* Refer to Cephalocaudal Principle in Chapter 3. ∞

The **anterior fontanel**, *a diamond-shaped area at the top of the front of the head,* and the **posterior fontanel**, *a triangular-shaped area at the center back of the head,* are often called **soft spots**. These *unossified areas of the skull bones,* along with the suture lines of the bones, allow the bones to overlap during delivery and also allow for expansion of the brain as they gradually fill in with bone cells. The posterior fontanel closes by 2 or 3 months; the anterior fontanel closes between 8 and 18 months. These soft spots may add to the parents' impression that the newborn is too fragile to handle (13, 65, 84, 111).

The baby's characteristic position during this period is one of flexion, closely imitating the fetal position, with fists tightly closed and arms and legs drawn up against the body. The baby is aware of disturbances in equilibrium and will change position, reacting with the Moro reflex described in **Table 9-3**.

Reassure the parents that the newborn, although in need of tender, gentle care, is also resilient and adaptable. The head and fontanels can be gently touched without harm, although strong pressure or direct injury should be avoided. Reassure them also that the baby will soon take on the features of the family members and look more as they expected.

APGAR SCORING SYSTEM

The physical status of the newborn, a measure of the newborn's successful transition to extrauterine life, is determined with the **Apgar tool***.* The Apgar assessment is made 1 minute after birth and again 5 minutes later. The newborn's respirations, heart rate, muscle tone, reflex activities, and color are observed. A maximum score of 2 is given to each sign, so that the Apgar score could range from 0 to 10, as indicated in **Table 9-2** (7). A score of less than 7 means that the newborn is having difficulty adapting, needs even closer observation than usual, and may need lifesaving intervention (7).

Caucasian norms may lead to erroneous conclusions or be meaningless at times. For example, to receive a 2 for color on the Apgar scoring system, the newborn's upper body must be pink,

TABLE 9-2

Assessment of the Newborn: Apgar Scoring System

Sign	0	1	2
Heart rate	Absent	Less than 100 beats/min	More than 100 beats/min
Respirations	Absent	Slow, irregular	Cry; regular rate
Muscle tone	Flaccid	Some flexion of extremities	Active movements
Reflex irritability	None	Grimace	Cry
Color	Body cyanotic or pale	Body pink; extremities cyanotic	Body completely pink

Source: Adapted from Apgar, V. (1966, August). The newborn (Apgar) scoring system, reflections, and advice. *Pediatric Clinics of North America, 13,* 645.

which is unlikely to be seen in the newborn who is of African American, Asian, American Indian, or even Latino descent (53). A cultural practice to determine the true color of a newborn is to look at the ears, which tend to be darker at birth than the rest of the body. The range of coloring for the lips may vary from pink to plum. Palmar and plantar surfaces may vary from light to dark pink to brown, depending on the amount of pigmentation (53).

GESTATIONAL AGE ASSESSMENT

In addition to using the Apgar score, assessment includes estimating **gestational age**, *using parameters other than weight to assess an infant's level of maturity.* By considering *both birth weight* and *gestational age,* you can categorize infants into one of several groupings. Problems can then be anticipated and, if present, be identified and treated early. Assessment can be done as early as the first day of life and should be done no later than the fifth day of life because external criteria, such as hip abduction, dorsiflexion of foot, and size of breast nodules change after 5 to 6 days of life. If the neonate is examined on the first day of life, he or she should be examined again before the fifth day to detect neurologic changes. Neonate status can be affected by asphyxia or maternal anesthesia.

To assess gestational age, several scales can be used. The **Classification of Newborns by Intrauterine Growth and Gestational Age Scale** *uses weight, length, and head circumference to determine gestational age.* **Figure 9-2**◻ depicts this classification (10). **The Dubowitz Guide to Gestational Age Assessment** *examines 10 neurologic and 11 external signs* (40). Ballard et al. modified the Dubowitz scale. The **Ballard Gestational Age Assessment** *determines neuromuscular and physical maturity in relation to gestational age* (9). **Figure 9-3**◻ depicts this assessment (9), *which will place the infant in one of nine categories based on age and weight* (17, 42, 65). The **Brazelton Neonatal Behavioral Assessment Scale (BNBAS)** *assesses the neonate's response in relation to habituation, orientation, motor performance,* **range of state** (*general arousal level*), *regulation of state or response when aroused, autonomic stability or signs of stress, and reflexes* (25).

SKIN

The skin is thin, delicate, and usually mottled, varies from pink to reddish, and becomes very ruddy or reddish when the baby cries. **Acrocyanosis,** *bluish color of the hands and feet,* is the result of the

sluggish peripheral circulation that occurs normally only for a few days after birth. **Lanugo,** *fine, downy hair of fetal life,* most evident on shoulders, back extremities, forehead, and temples, is lost after a few months and is replaced by other hair growth. **Vernix caseosa,** *the gray-white cheeselike substance, lubricates and protects the skin* of the fetus and newborn. It rubs off in a few days. **Milia,** *tiny whitish-yellow papules,* are small collections of sebaceous secretions. Milia are sprinkled on the forehead, nose, cheeks, and chin and should not be squeezed or picked as they are not pimples. They will resolve spontaneously within the first few weeks after birth. **Epstein's pearls,** the oral counterpart of facial milia, appear on the palate. **Desquamation,** *peeling of skin,* occurs in 2 to 4 weeks. **Hemangiomas,** *vascular lesions* on the upper eyelids, between the eyebrows, and on the nose, upper lip, or back may or may not be permanent (13, 17, 33, 65, 84, 112). **Mongolian spots** are *flat, slate-gray, bluish black-colored areas on the buttocks, lower back, thighs, ankles, and arms of children of color,* especially African American (90%), Asian American, and American Indian (80%) children. In contrast, only about 9% of Caucasian children have Mongolian spots (6). The dark areas should not be mistaken for a sign of abuse; they usually disappear by the end of the first year.

If a birthmark is present, parents should be assured it is not their fault. **Jaundice,** *yellowish discoloration of skin and sclera,* should be noted. If it occurs during the first 24 hours of life, it is usually caused by blood incompatibility between mother and baby and requires medical investigation and possibly treatment. **Physiologic jaundice** *normally appears on the third or fourth day of life because the excess number of red blood cells present in fetal life that are no longer needed are undergoing hemolysis, which in turn causes high levels of bilirubin (a bile pigment) in the bloodstream.* The jaundice usually disappears in approximately 1 week when the baby's liver has developed the ability to metabolize the bilirubin. If bilirubin levels are excessively high, the neonate is exposed to **phototherapy,** *high-intensity light to promote bilirubin breakdown.* Phototherapy can be provided when the newborn is placed under full-spectrum lights or a fiber-optic blanket, on a fiber-optic mattress, or by a combination of these methods. The baby's eyes must be covered during phototherapy provided by a bank of lights (56). In some agencies, the neonate's gonads are also covered.

Parents should be reassured about conditions of the skin that normally occur and if phototherapy is needed. Foot or hand prints are made for identification, as these lines remain permanently.

Classification Of Newborns (both Sexes)
by Intrauterine Growth And Gestational Age[1,2]

Name _____ Date Of Birth _____ Birth Weight _____

Hospital No. _____ Date Of Exam _____ Length _____

Race _____ Sex _____ Head Circ. _____

Gestational Age _____

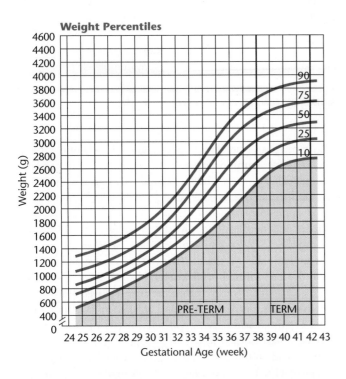

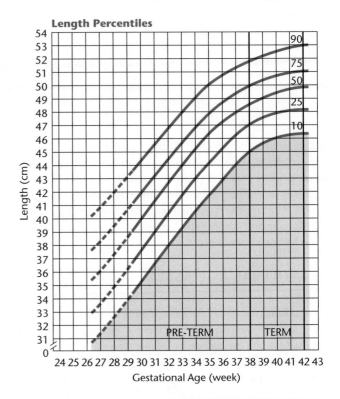

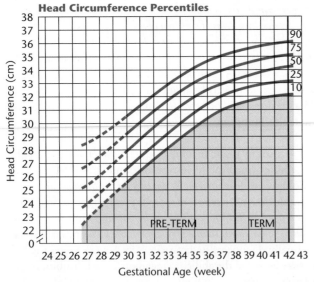

Classification Of Infant*	Weight	Length	Head Circ.
Large for Gestational Age (LGA) (>90th Percentile)			
Appropriate for Gestational Age (AGA) (10th to 90th percentile)			
Small for Gestational Age (SGA) (<10th percentile)			

*Place an "X" in the appropriate box (LGA, AGA, SGA) for weight, for length and for head circumference.

FIGURE ■ 9-2 Classification of newborns (both sexes) by intrauterine growth and gestational age.

Source: From Battaglia, F., & Lubeheco, L. (1967). A Practical Classification of Newborn Infants by Weight and Gestational Age. *Journal of Pediatrics,* 71, 159–163.

Gestational Age Assessment (Ballard)

Name _____   Date/Time Of Birth_____   Birth Weight _____
Hospital No. _____   Date/Time Of Exam _____   Length _____
_____   Age When Examined _____   Head Circ. _____
Race _____   Sex _____   Examiner_____
Apgar Score: 1 Minute _____   5 Minutes _____

Score
Neuromuscular_____
Physical_____
Total_____

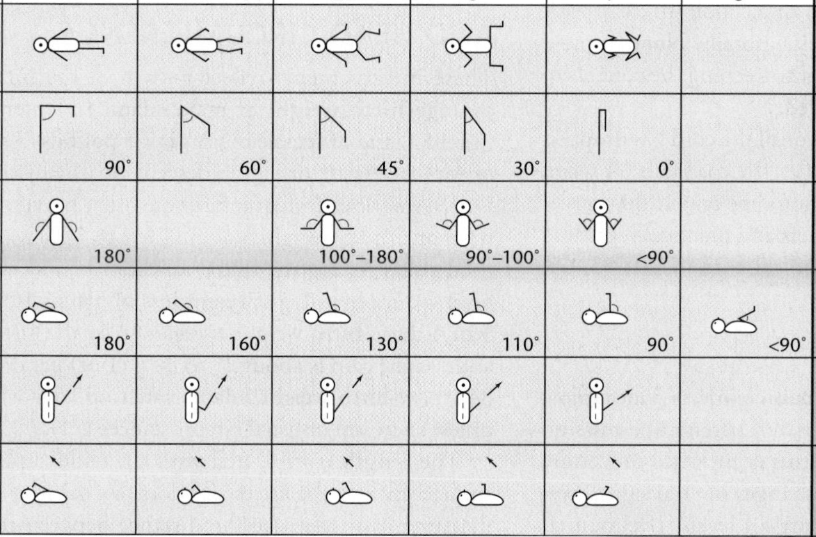

Neuromuscular Maturity

Neuromuscular Maturity Sign	Score						Record Score Here
	0	1	2	3	4	5	
Posture							
Square Window (Wrist)	90°	60°	45°	30°	0°		
Arm Recoil	180°		100°–180°	90°–100°	<90°		
Popliteal Angle	180°	160°	130°	110°	90°	<90°	
Scarf Sign							
Heel To Ear							

Total Neuromuscular Maturity Score

Maturity Rating

Total Maturity Score	Gestational Age (Weeks)
5	26
10	28
15	30
20	32
25	34
30	36
35	38
40	40
45	42
50	44

Physical Maturity

Physical Maturity Sign	Score						Record Score Here
	0	1	2	3	4	5	
Skin	gelantinous red, transparent	smooth pink, visible veins	superficial peeling, &/or rash few veins	cracking pale area rare veins	parchment deep cracking no vessels	leathery cracked wrinkled	
Lanugo	none	abundant	thinning	bald areas	mostly bald		
Plantar Creases	no crease	faint red marks	anterior transverse crease only	creases ant. 2/3	creases cover entire sole		
Breast	barely percept.	flat areola no bud	stippled areola 1–2mm bud	raised areola 3–4mm bud	full areola 5–10mm bud		
Ear	pinna flat, stays folded	sl. curved pinna; soft with slow recoil	well–curv. pinna; soft but ready recoil	formed & firm with instant recoil	thick cartilage ear stiff		
Genitals (Male)	scrotum empty no rugae		testes descending, few rugae	testes down good rugae	testes pendulous deep rugae		
Genitals (Female)	prominent clitoris & labia minora		majora & minora equally prominent	majora large, minora small	clitoris & minora completely covered		

Total Physical Maturity Score

Gestational Age (weeks)
By dates _____
By ultrasound _____
By score _____

FIGURE 9-3 Gestational age assessment.

Source: From Ballard, J., Novek, K., & Driver, M. (1979). A Simplified Score for Assessment of Fetal Maturation in Newly Born Infants. *Journal of Pediatrics, 95,* 769–774.

UMBILICAL CORD

The *bluish-white, gelatinous structure that transports maternal blood from placenta to fetus* is the **umbilical cord**. Because of the high water content, the stump of the cord dries and shrinks rapidly, losing its flexibility by 24 hours after birth. By the second day, it is a very hard, shriveled, yellow or black (blood) tab on the skin. Slight oozing where the cord joins the abdominal wall is common and offers an excellent medium for bacterial growth.

Cord care policy differs at different agencies: (a) treat the area with triple-dye solution, antibiotic ointment, or alcohol; (b) clean with a mild soap solution; or (c) allow to dry naturally. None of these treatments has been found to be superior to keeping the cord clean and dry, and using water to clean if soiled.

Cord care is given several times daily until the cord has dropped off (7 to 14 days) and for 2 or 3 days after the cord falls off when the area is completely healed. Parents should be taught this procedure. There are a variety of cultural beliefs and practices regarding cord care. Some cultures keep the umbilical cord (6, 51, 53, 65, 84, 101).

CIRCUMCISION

The *surgical removal of the foreskin*, **circumcision**, is done almost automatically on newborn males. However, parental permission is necessary. In contrast to past belief, this is a painful procedure for the baby, as evidenced by the cry, changes in vital signs, oxygen saturation levels, and increased cortisol levels. If circumcision is performed, analgesia should be provided. Scientific evidence suggests several potential medical benefits associated with newborn male circumcision, but the medical community is divided. Some think evidence is insufficient to recommend routine neonatal circumcision. Others argue that existing data support potential medical benefits. It is currently recommended that parents should make the determination in the best interest of their child (56).

Reasons to do circumcision include: (a) sign of manhood, (b) cultural norms, (c) social concern (look like father or peers), (d) sexual concerns, (e) hygienic, cosmetic, or comfort concerns, (f) biblical or religious mandate, (g) prevention of later genitourinary problems, and (h) medical advice. *Reasons not to do circumcision include:* (a) traumatic or dangerous procedure, (b) painful for baby, and (c) decreased sexual pleasure later in life. The same reasons may be given to either do or not do circumcision.

In order for parents to make an informed choice, they must be given accurate and unbiased information on circumcision and an opportunity to discuss this decision. Share that the American Academy of Pediatrics states there are no medical indications for circumcision (4). Urologists report that a small percentage of uncircumcised males develop genitourinary infections, inflammation of the glands, or phimosis (35, 65, 84).

Some parents choose circumcision for cultural, religious, or social reasons. The main difference among various cultural groups related to circumcision is the issue of pain (6, 51, 53, 101). Cultures vary in their beliefs about this practice. Although ritual circumcision is frequently practiced in Judaism, other families have the male circumcised to facilitate hygiene of the penis and to decrease the risk of penile and cervical cancer.

Although there are risks to circumcision, *complications occur infrequently.* Irritation and infection can occur. Hemorrhage and local infection are the most common complications, requiring sutures or pressure dressings that can cause scarring, deformity, or **phimosis**, *tightening of the foreskin.* If the physician is not skilled, various surgical mishaps may occur. Good hygiene provides the same medical benefits without the risk of surgery and the pain (35, 65, 84).

WEIGHT, LENGTH, AND HEAD CIRCUMFERENCE

These measurements reflect growth of the infant *in utero.* The **average birth weight** of male infants in America is 7.8 pounds (3,530 g) and of female infants is 7.5 pounds (3,400 g). Newborns of African, Asian, or Latino descent are usually smaller at full-term birth; American Indian infants are often heavier (65). Because the newborn's body weight is about 70% to 75% water and because of fluid shifts during the initial newborn period, the full-term newborn has a physiologic weight loss of 5% to 10% during the first 3 or 4 days. Birth weight is regained by the 10th to the 14th day and weight gain is about 25 to 30 g (1 oz) per day (31, 35, 42, 65, 84). Low-birth-weight infants catch up later with other children unless there are unusual circumstances (71).

The **length** is measured with the child supine on a flat, hard surface. Extend the knees and dorsiflex the foot to ensure accurate measurement. Measure the distance between the vertex (top) of the head and the soles of the feet. The **average length** of American infants at birth is 21 in. (53 cm). Males range from 20 to 24 in. (52 to 60 cm); females average slightly less. The bones are soft, consisting chiefly of cartilage. The back is straight and curves with sitting. The muscles feel hard and are slightly resistant to pressure (31, 33, 35, 65, 84).

Body mass index (BMI), *the relationship between height and weight*, provides a guideline for health care providers to use to determine the healthy weight (whether overweight or underweight) of an individual based on height. These charts are age- and gender-specific. An individual with a BMI at or above the 85th percentile is at risk for overweight (33, 35, 41, 56). The most important tools for assessing somatic growth are growth charts. Expected growth patterns in children by age and gender can be found on the Website for the Centers for Disease Control and Prevention, www.cdc.gov.

Measurement of **head circumference** *assesses the growth of the head, which reflects growth of the cranium and the brain.* This measurement detects whether any abnormalities, such as too rapid or too slow growth, are present. The measurement is taken just above the eyebrows and ears and across the posterior occipital protuberance. Head circumference measures 12.5 to 15.5 in. (32 to 38.4 cm) at birth, but variations of one-half inch are common. The chest circumference is approximately 1 inch (2 to 3 cm) less than head circumference at birth (31, 33, 35, 42, 56, 60).

Parents should be prepared for the appearance of the neonate's head. Molding of the skull occurs during vaginal delivery. **Molding** *refers to changes in the shape of the head that allow it to pass through the birth canal.* It is caused when the bones of the skull overlap during labor and delivery. **Caput succedaneum**, *irregular* *edema of the scalp*, disappears approximately the third day of life. **Cephalohematoma**, *a collection of blood between the periosteum and the skull bones, occurs from pressure during birth*. These lesions absorb within a few weeks to months (65, 84).

Despite widespread poverty and lack of access to medical care, Latinos in the United States, especially Mexican Americans, have less risk of a low-birth-weight baby and less infant mortality than do Caucasians or African Americans. In Latin cultures the prevalence of traditional family values, better prenatal diets, fewer single mothers, strong extended families, and lower smoking rates may account for the difference. Health practices of Mexican Americans deteriorate the longer they live in the United States as they become more likely to eat fast foods, smoke, and drink alcohol, activities that have serious health effects (6, 53, 66).

OTHER NEONATE CHARACTERISTICS

Several other characteristics are also normal and resolve themselves shortly after birth: swollen (engorged) breasts in males and females, swollen genitalia with undescended testicles in the male, and vaginal secretions in the female. These characteristics are caused by maternal hormones. Genital size varies for males and females. Urine is present in the bladder, and the baby voids at birth. Obstruction of the nasolacrimal duct is also common, and excessive tearing and pus accumulation usually clear up when the duct opens spontaneously in a few months (56).

VITAL SIGNS

In the newborn, vital signs are not stable. Physiology is summarized in the following discussion.

Respiratory Efforts

Respiratory efforts at birth are critical, and immediate adaptations must occur to counter the decreasing oxygen level and increasing carbon dioxide level in the blood. *Causes of respiratory initiation include* (a) cutting of the umbilical cord, which causes hypoxia, resulting in carbon dioxide accumulation; (b) physical stimulation of the birth process; (c) the sudden change in the baby's environment at birth; (d) the exposure to firm touch; and (e) the cool air. If the mother was medicated during labor or if the baby is premature, the respiratory center of the brain is less operative, and the baby will have more difficulty with breathing. In the normal newborn, respirations range from 30 to 60 breaths per minute. Respirations are rapid, shallow, and diaphragmatic, with an irregular pattern and depth. This **periodic breathing pattern** *is characterized by intermittent 5- to 15-second pauses* (13, 31, 65, 84). **Surfactant** *is a thin lipoprotein film produced by the alveoli that reduces surface tension of the alveoli, allows them to expand, and allows some air to remain in the alveoli at the end of expiration.* Thus it takes less effort to reexpand the lungs (56).

Body Temperature

Body temperature ranges from 97.7 °F to 99.7 °F (36.5 °C to 37.7° C) because (a) the heat-regulating mechanism in the hypothalamus is not fully developed, (b) the large surface area facilitates heat loss to the environment, (c) shivering to produce heat does not occur, (d) there is less subcutaneous fat, and (e) heat is lost to the environment by evaporation, conduction, convection, and radiation (35, 56, 65, 84).

At birth, amniotic fluid increases temperature loss by evaporation from the skin; thus, diligent efforts to dry the skin are necessary. The wet newborn can lose heat about four times as fast as adults, causing a loss of calories per minute. If the room is cool and the baby is placed in contact with cold objects, heat loss also occurs. Excessive heat loss or cold may lead to apnea, respiratory depression, and hypoglycemia (35, 56).

Several mechanisms occur to help the newborn conserve heat (35, 56, 65):

1. Vasoconstriction, by which constricted blood vessels maintain heat in the inner body.
2. Flexion of the body to reduce total amount of exposed skin (the premature baby does not assume flexion of the extremities onto the body).
3. Increased metabolic rate, which causes increased heat production.
4. Metabolism of adipose tissue that has been stored during the eighth month of gestation.

Body temperature of the baby normally drops 1 to 2 degrees (Fahrenheit) immediately after birth, but in a warm environment it begins to rise slowly. Prevention of heat loss through environmental temperature control and skin contact with the mother is crucial to adaptation to extrauterine life. Axillary temperature should be taken for 5 minutes. Insertion of a thermometer into the rectum determines anal patency but may cause perforation of the rectum. Gentle insertion of the thermometer is essential. A tympanic thermometer probe may be inserted into the auditory canal. Temperatures taken at different sites may vary slightly (56, 65, 84).

This **adipose tissue** is called **brown adipose tissue (BAT)** because it is *brown in color from a rich supply of blood vessels and nerves. It is unique in that it aids adaptation to the stress of cooling.* Brown fat, located between the scapulae around the neck, behind the sternum, and around the kidneys and adrenal glands, accounts for 2% to 6% of the neonate's body weight and is metabolized quickly (56, 65, 84).

Heart Rate

Heart rate ranges at birth from 120 to 160 beats per minute because of the immature cardiac regulatory mechanism in the medulla. The heart rate may increase to 180 beats per minute when the newborn cries and drop to 80 to 100 beats per minute during sleep. The pulse rate gradually decreases during the first and subsequent years (56, 65, 84). Count the heartbeat for a full minute when the baby is quiet, especially if the rate is irregular.

Blood Pressure

Blood pressure (BP) may range from 65 to 78 mm Hg systolic and 50 to 62 mm Hg diastolic. Newborn blood pressure varies with activity, gestational age, and size. Further, it varies depending on cuff size of the instrument used for measurement. By the end of the first month, blood pressure averages 80/40 mm Hg. It increases slowly the first year and remains under 90/60 mm Hg (56, 65, 84). Blood pressure is not routinely assessed at birth.

MECONIUM

Meconium, *the first fecal material, is thick and sticky, odorless, and tarry black or dark green in appearance,* and is composed of byproducts of *in utero* metabolism. It usually is passed from 8 to 24 hours and almost always within 48 hours of birth. Transitional stools, thin brown to green, are a combination of meconium and milk stools. These stools last for a few days and are followed by milk stools. The breastfed infant's stools are seedy in consistency, pale yellow (some are pasty green), and looser than in the formula-fed infant. The breastfed infant generally has at least three stools per day. The formula-fed infant may excrete several stools or only one or two daily (65, 84, 91).

REFLEX ACTIVITY

Reflex activity is innate or built in through the process of evolution. It is a genetically endowed survival mechanism that develops while the baby is *in utero*. A **reflex**, an *involuntary, unlearned response elicited by certain stimuli, indicates neurologic status or function*. Individual differences in the newborn's responses to stimulation are apparent at birth. Some respond vigorously to the slightest stimulation, others respond slowly, and some are in between. Several types of reflexes exist in the neonate and young infant: consummatory, avoidant, exploratory, social, and attentional. **Consummatory reflexes**, such as rooting, sucking, and swallowing, *promote survival through feeding*. Other reflexes that aid feeding include crying when hungry and spitting up when too much has been swallowed too quickly. **Avoidant reflexes** *are elicited by potentially harmful stimuli* and include the Moro, withdrawing, knee jerk, sneezing, blinking, gagging, and coughing reflexes. **Exploratory reflexes** *occur when infants are wide awake and are held upright so that their arms move without restraint*. The visual object at eye level elicits both reaching and grasping reflexes. **Social reflexes**, *such as smiling, promote affectionate interactions between parents and infants* and thus have a survival value. *Examples of innate reflexes that can be modified by experience and that persist throughout life include* (a) crying in response to painful stimuli, loud noise, food deprivation, or loss of support; (b) quieting in response to touch, low soft tones, or food; and (c) smiling in response to changes in brightness, comforting stimuli, or escape from uncomfortable stimuli. **Attentional reflexes**, including orienting and attending, *determine the nature of the baby's response to stimuli* and have continuing importance throughout development (14, 15, 38, 65, 84, 87, 99).

The nervous system of the newborn is both anatomically and physiologically immature, and reflexes should be observed for their presence, strength, and symmetry. Reflexes are described in **Table 9-3** (14, 15, 38, 39, 65, 84, 87, 99).

SENSORY ABILITIES

The newborn has more highly developed sensory abilities than was once supposed. Apparently a **moderately enriched environment**, *one without stimulus bombardment or deprivation*, is best suited for sensory motor development. The infant's use of the senses, innate abilities, and environment lays the groundwork for intellectual development, which is discussed later.

Touch

The newborn is very sensitive to touch, especially around the mouth and on the palms and soles, and to vestibular stimuli, such as rocking or holding upright. Sensitivity to touch is more fully developed at birth than the other senses. The reflexes are an indication that the newborn responds to touch. Infants use touch to gather information about the world around them. Connecting information from vision with information from touch occurs during the first year of life (38, 56). Females are more responsive to touch than males. Cutaneous and postural stimulation is necessary for development of the nervous system (23, 63, 80). Moderate, gentle kinesthetic stimulation daily results in a baby who is quieter, gains weight faster, and shows improved socioemotional function. Earlier studies indicated that 20 minutes of extra handling a day of premature infants would result in earlier exploring and grasping behavior by the infant (63). The baby needs to feel the father's large hands as well as the smaller, more gentle hands of the mother. However, premature babies, if not given additional stimulation, will catch up developmentally by the toddler period (38).

Kangaroo care, or *skin-to-skin contact, is the practice of holding the neonate's skin next to the parent's skin*. The infant wears only a diaper and hat and is placed next to the parent's skin. Both are covered with a blanket to ensure warmth. This gentle stimulation provides opportunities for the parent to be close to the infant—to touch, hold, talk to, and care for the neonate. Thus, it promotes parental attachment.

Teach parents that the first impressions of life, security, warmth, love, pleasure, or lack of them come to the infant through touch. Knowledge of the people around him or her, initially of the mother and then of the father, is gradually built from the manner in which the baby is handled and talked to. He or she soon learns to sense mother's self-confidence and pleasure as well as her anxiety, lack of confidence, anger, or rejection. These early touch experiences and the infant's feelings through them apparently lay the foundation for feelings about people throughout life.

Sensitivity to Pain, Pressure, and Temperature

Sensitivity to pain, pressure, and temperature extremes is present at 26 weeks' gestational age; pain is shown by a distinct cry, facial expression, and muscle tension (56, 84). The newborn reacts diffusely to pain, as he or she has little ability to localize the discomfort because of incomplete myelination of the spinal tracts and cerebral cortex. Females are more sensitive to pain than males. The baby's response to pain increases each day in the neonatal period. Visceral sensations of discomfort, such as hunger, overdistention of the stomach, passage of gas and stool, extremes of temperature, and overstimulation, apparently account for much of the newborn's crying. At first the cry, the infant's means of communicating with the world, is simply a primitive discharge mechanism that calls for help. He or she wails with equal force regardless of stimulus. In a few weeks the baby's subtle modifications in the cry provide clues to the attentive parent about the nature of the discomfort, so that response can be adjusted to the baby's need. Distinct crying patterns for hunger, discomfort or pain, upset or anger, fatigue, boredom, frustration, and tension discharge have been reported (14, 15, 23, 38, 52, 84, 99).

TABLE 9-3

Assessment of Infant Reflexes

Reflex	Description	Appearance/Disappearance
Rooting	Touching baby's cheek causes head to turn toward the side touched.	Present in utero at 24 weeks; disappears 3–4 months; may persist in sleep 9–12 months
Sucking	Touching lips or placing something in baby's mouth causes baby to draw liquid into mouth by creating vacuum with lips, cheeks, and tongue.	Present in utero at 28 weeks; persists through early childhood, especially during sleep
Bite	Touching gums, teeth, or tongue causes baby to open and close mouth.	Disappears at 3–5 months when biting is voluntary, but seen throughout adult years in comatose person
Babkin	Pressure applied to palm causes baby to open mouth, close eyes.	Present at birth; disappears in 2 or 4 months
Pupillary response	Flashing light across baby's eyes or face causes constriction of pupils.	Present at 32 weeks of gestation; persists throughout life
Blink	Baby closes both eyes.	Remains throughout life
Moro or startle	Making a loud noise or changing baby's position causes baby to extend both arms outward with fingers spread, then bring them together in a tense, quivery embrace	Present at 28 weeks of gestation; disappears at 4–7 months
Withdrawing	Baby removes hand or foot from painful stimuli.	Present at birth; persists throughout life
Colliding	Baby moves arms up and face to side when object is in collision course with face.	Present at birth or shortly after; persists in modified form throughout life
Palmar grasp	Placing object or finger in baby's palm causes his or her fingers to close tightly around object.	Present at 32 weeks of gestation; disappears at 3–4 months, replaced by voluntary grasp at 4–5 months
Plantar grasp	Placing object or finger beneath toes causes curling of toes around object.	Present at 32 weeks of gestation; disappears at 9–12 months
Tonic neck or fencing (TNR)	Postural reflex is seen when infant lies on back with head turned to one side; arm and leg on the side toward which he or she is looking are extended while opposite limbs are flexed.	Present at birth; disappears at approximately 4 months
Stepping, walking, dancing	Holding baby upright with feet touching flat surface causes legs to prance up and down as if baby were walking or dancing.	Present at birth; disappears at approximately 2–4 months; with daily practice of reflex, infant may walk alone at 10 months
Reaching	Hand closes as it reaches toward and grasps at object at eye level.	Present shortly after birth if baby is upright; comes under voluntary control in several months
Orienting	Head and eyes turn toward stimulus of noise, accompanied by cessation of other activity, heartbeat change, and vascular constriction.	Present at birth; comes under voluntary control later; persists throughout life
Attending	Eyes fix on a stimulus that changes brightness, movement, or shape.	Present shortly after birth; comes under voluntary control later; persists throughout life
Swimming	Placing baby horizontally, supporting him or her under abdomen, causes baby to make crawling motions with his or her arms and legs while lifting head from surface as if he or she were swimming.	Present after 3 or 4 days; disappears at approximately 4 months; may persist with practice
Trunk incurvation	Stroking one side of spinal column while baby is on his or her abdomen causes crawling motions with legs, lifting head from surface, and incurvature of trunk on the side stroked.	Present in utero; then seen at approximately third or fourth day; persists 2–3 months

continued

TABLE 9-3

Assessment of Infant Reflexes—continued

Reflex	Description	Appearance/Disappearance
Babinski	Stroking bottom of foot causes big toe to raise while other toes fan out and curl downward.	Present at birth; disappears at approximately 9 or 10 months: presence of reflex later may indicate disease
Landau	Suspending infant in horizontal, prone position and flexing head against trunk causes legs to flex against trunk.	Appears at approximately 3 months; disappears at approximately 12–24 months
Parachute	Sudden thrusting of infant downward from horizontal position causes hands and fingers to extend forward and spread as if to protect self from a fall.	Appears at approximately 7–9 months; persists indefinitely
Biceps	Tap on tendon of biceps causes biceps to contract quickly.	Brisk in first few days, then slightly diminished; permanent
Knee jerk	Tap on tendon below patella or on patella causes leg to extend quickly.	More pronounced first 2 days; permanent

Data from references 38, 56, 91.

Vision

Vision is the least well-developed sense at birth. In utero, the fetus has little to look at, and thus, the connection between the eyes and the visual cortex does not develop until after birth. The eyes of the newborn are smaller than of the adult. Retinal structures are immature, muscles of the lens are weak, and the optic nerve is underdeveloped. Initial vision is blurred. The visual abilities change from birth to 4 months of age. As these structures mature and the newborn has visual experiences, visual ability improves (15, 56). Tear glands do not begin to function until 2 to 4 weeks of age (15, 56, 87).

The following are characteristics of newborn vision (13, 15, 31, 38, 56, 91):

1. **Acuity:** *Clarity of vision begins within the first day* but is initially blurred. Later, 8 to 20 inches are necessary for focus. Visual acuity can be measured at 20/100 to 20/400.
2. **Fixation:** *The newborn directs both eyes to the same point in space for a specific limited time* (4 to 18 seconds), *focuses briefly on objects, and follows to midline.* The ability to fixate or coordinate eye movements is greater in the first hours of life than during several succeeding days.
3. **Tracking:** *The baby follows visually large moving objects,* beginning a day after birth.
4. **Discrimination:** *The baby demonstrates preference for particular sizes and shapes* (large circles, dots, or squares); large pictures or objects; contrasts of black and white patterns (concentric circles, bull's-eye); and medium (yellow, pink, green) over dim (blue) or bright (orange, red) colors. Less complex stimuli and reflecting objects over dull surfaces are preferred.
5. **Conjugation:** *The baby moves the eyes together;* refixation is more frequent.
6. **Sensitivity to light:** *Reaction to light is equal to that of adults.*
7. **Scanning:** *The newborn is able to move his or her eyes over the visual field and focus briefly on a satisfying image,* and prefers to scan edges and contours of complex shapes. Peripheral vision is narrow.
8. **Accommodation:** *The baby is able to adjust the eyes for distance.* The preferred distance is 8 inches for infants up to 1 month in age.
9. **Visual preference:** *The baby varies amount of time spent looking at different sights* in the environment.

The infant maintains contact with the environment through visual fixation, scanning, and tracking and pays more attention to stimuli from the face than to other stimuli as depicted in **Figure 9-4■**. The newborn looks at the mother's face while feeding and while sitting upright and prefers a human face to a mobile toy. The newborn follows the path of an object, crying or pulling backward if it comes too close to his or her face. By the age of 1 month, the baby has a pupillary reflex, can distinguish between the face of the mother and a stranger, and differentiates between brightness and darkness. Bright lights cause discomfort.

Teach parents that a baby needs eye contact and the opportunity to see the human face and a variety of changing scenes and colors. Providing a mirror or chrome plate that reflects light and objects and rotating the bed help the baby use both eyes, avoiding one-sided vision. Hang cardboard black and white mobiles, especially those that make sound, and have them within reach of the baby's kicking feet. Later the infant enjoys other colors and designs that are within grasp. By age 2 months, the baby can see the ceiling and decorations on it. As the baby grows older the crib should be low enough for him or her to see beyond the crib.

Parents should be reassured that the antibiotic ointment correctly placed in the baby's eyes at birth will not damage vision but

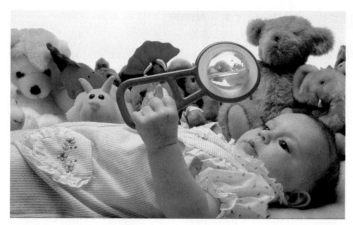 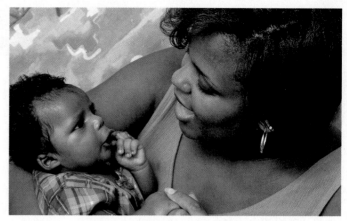

FIGURE □ 9-4 A. The newborn demonstrates increasing visual ability. B. The newborn has the ability to fix on the mother's face. (A: Mike Malyszko, Stock Boston, B: Laura Dwight, Creative Eye/MIRA.com)

prevents blindness if the mother should have an undetected gonorrheal infection (56, 65, 84).

Hearing

Hearing is developed in utero as demonstrated by sensitivity to sound in the fetus at about 26 to 28 weeks of gestation. This occurs when the fetus is exposed to internal sounds of the mother's body, such as the heartbeat and abdominal rumbles (heard at 5 months), and external sounds, such as voices, music, and a cymbal clap (heard at 7 months). Hearing is blurred the first few days of life because fluid is retained in the middle ear, but hearing loss can be tested as early as the first day. The sound must be louder to be heard by the newborn than by an adult. *The neonate cannot hear whispers but can respond to voice pitch changes.* Infants hear high pitches better than lower pitches. A low pitch quiets and decreases motor activity and crying, whereas a high pitch increases alertness. An infant turns the head toward the source of a sound and responds best to the mother's voice, to sounds directly in front of his or her face, and to sounds experienced during gestation. Newborns startle to sudden or loud sounds, are soothed and may fall asleep upon listening to rhythmic sounds, quiet upon hearing their mother's voice, and momentarily cease activity when sound is presented at a conversational level (14, 15, 38, 56). A baby often sleeps better with background songs or a tape recording of the mother's heartbeat. The newborn prefers the sound of the human voice to other sounds in the environment. The neonate discriminates between the voice of the mother and another female. A 1-month-old can discriminate between the syllables "ba" and "pa." Differentiation of sounds and perception of their source take time to develop, but there are startle reactions. The baby withdraws from loud noise (14, 15, 38, 56, 87, 91).

The presence of **congenital hearing loss** (*born deaf*) is more common than ordinarily understood. It is believed that newborn hearing loss is approximately 1 to 2 per 1,000 live births. **Box 9-3,** Checklist to Detect Presence of Hearing in Infancy, is a guide for parents and health care professionals to check for hearing ability in the neonate and infant. The Joint Committee on Infant Hearing, American Academy of Pediatrics, recommends that all infants be screened for hearing problems before discharge from the birthing hospital (4).

Taste and Smell

The newborn's senses of taste and smell develop in utero. These senses are more fully developed than their senses of hearing and vision. The infant reacts to strong odors by facial expressions, turning the head away, and using other avoidant behaviors. A newborn turns the head toward a milk source, whether breast or bottle. Breastfed infants are able to differentiate the odor of their mother's milk from that of another mother. Infants can discriminate the smell of their mother's body from other bodies or objects and can sense the odors that adults can sense. Newborns are sensitive to sweet, sour, and bitter tastes, but sensitivity to salty tastes develops over the first 4 to 6 months of age. Breathing rhythm is altered in response to fragrance, showing some ability to smell (15, 38, 56, 65).

SPECIAL CONSIDERATIONS IN PHYSICAL ASSESSMENT OF THE NEONATE

Neonates differ in their appearance, size, and response. Females are more developmentally advanced than males, and African Americans are more developmentally advanced than Caucasians. The most accurate assessment is made by comparing the neonate against norms for the same gender and race (6, 17, 47, 53, 56).

When a newborn is examined, the primary concerns are neurologic status, congenital deformities, and metabolic disturbances. History of hereditary diseases and the pregnancy and delivery information are essential. Reflex status indicates neurologic development and some congenital deformities. The following are particular aspects to check when physically assessing the neonate (47, 56).

A *small chin*, called **micrognathia**, means that the neonate may experience breathing difficulties, because the tongue can fall back and obstruct the nasopharynx.

Ear position is important because there is a strong association between low-set ears and numerous syndromes, renal malformation, internal organ abnormalities, or a chromosomal anomaly such as Down syndrome. The top of the ear should be in alignment with the inner and outer canthi of the eyes. The Eustachian tube is shorter and wider than in the adult. Occasionally, small skin tags may be seen in front of the ears (47, 56, 65, 84).

| **BOX 9-3** | **Checklist to Detect Presence of Hearing in Infancy** |

FROM BIRTH TO 2 WEEKS DOES BABY:

1. Jump or blink when there is a sudden loud sound
2. Stop crying when you start to talk
3. Seem aware of your voice
4. Stir in sleep when there is continuous noise close by
5. Jump or blink when there is a sudden soft click such as a light switch or a camera click when the noise is otherwise quiet
6. Stop sucking momentarily when there is a noise or when you start to talk
7. Look up from sucking or try to open eyes when there is a sudden noise

FROM 2 TO 10 WEEKS DOES BABY:

1. Stop crying when you talk to him or her
2. Stop movements when you enter the room
3. Seem aware of your voice
4. Sleep regardless of noises
5. Waken when the crib or bassinet is touched
6. Respond to comforting only when held against mother or familiar caretaker

7. Cry at sudden loud noises
8. Blink or jerk at sudden loud noises

FROM 2½ TO 6 MONTHS DOES BABY:

1. Always coo with pleasure when you start to talk
2. Turn eyes to the speaker
3. Know when father comes home and wriggle in welcome (if awake)
4. Startle when you bend over the crib after awakening
5. Seem to enjoy a soft musical toy (e.g., a crib musical toy)
6. Cry when exposed to sudden, loud, unexpected noise
7. Stop movements when a new sound is introduced
8. Try to turn in the direction of a new sound or a person who starts to talk
9. Make many different babbling sounds when alone
10. Try to "talk back" when you talk
11. Start wriggling in anticipation of a bottle when you start preparing it (if the baby is awake and the preparation is out of sight, such as the refrigerator door opening, and so on)
12. Know own name (smiles, turns, or otherwise gives an indication)

Note: If the child is hearing-impaired or deaf, a source of information about treatment facilities and other educational materials for parents can be obtained from Galludet College, Washington, DC.

Discharges from the eye may result from **chemical** or **infectious conjunctivitis**. A lateral upward slant of the eyes with an inner epicanthal fold in a Caucasian infant may suggest a chromosome abnormality. Observe for symmetry and **hypertelorism**, *an abnormally wide space between the eyes.* **Ptosis** (*drooping*) of the eyelids should be a cause for concern. Drooping eyelids reduce the amount of light entering the retina and can decrease development of sight. **Subconjunctival hemorrhage**, *manifested by red streaks in the eye*, caused by changes in tension and pressure during birth, is usually of no significance. An infant lid retractor may be used to view the fundus if the muscles of the newborn keep the eyelids closed (47, 56, 65, 84).

Since the newborn is an obligatory nose breather, the *nose* should be patent. If breathing seems difficult, blockage of one or both nostrils should be considered. The newborn clears the nose by sneezing. Flaring of the nostrils or presence of nasal mucus usually represents respiratory distress (47, 56, 65, 84). A thick bloody discharge from the nose suggests congenital syphilis (47). A bulb syringe is used to remove thick nasal discharges.

Asymmetry of the face or mouth may indicate facial palsy. The mouth should be inspected for cleft lip and cleft palate. Although spitting up is common in the newborn, projectile vomiting is not. The newborn should have very little saliva, and tonsil tissue should not be present at birth. If the frenulum is too short the infant may be tongue-tied (47, 56, 65, 84).

The *neck* is quite short at this time. Webbing of the neck or excess of tissue may be indicative of chromosomal abnormalities (47, 56, 65, 84).

The *chest and abdomen* are considered a unit in the newborn. The anteroposterior diameter is usually equal to the transverse diameter. Because of the large structures of the thorax, large abdomen, weak intercostal muscles, horizontal rib position, and increased airway resistance, there is decreased space available for lung expansion. Thus respiratory distress is more prevalent. Wide-set nipples may indicate Turner syndrome, a genetic disorder. Smaller breasts that contain liquid are not uncommon in both male and female. The breath sounds in the infant are bronchovesicular. Depending on the type, heart murmurs may be heard at various locations over the heart, but are heard best over the base of the heart rather than over the apex (47, 56, 65, 84).

The *umbilical cord* should have two arteries and one vein. *Auscultation of bowel sounds* should precede palpation for masses, an extremely important procedure in the newborn (47).

The *genitalia* are examined for deformities. Only the external genitalia are examined in children. The penis is inspected. In uncircumcised males up to 3 months of age, the foreskin should not be retracted to avoid tearing the membrane. The testes should be palpated in the scrotum, although sometimes they are still undescended. A **hydrocele**, *a collection of watery fluid in the scrotum or along the spermatic cord*, and **hernia**, *a protrusion of part of the intestine through the abdominal muscles*, are common findings in males (47).

A *bloody or mucous vaginal discharge* (**pseudomenstruation**) may be present in females. It is the result of the abrupt decrease in maternal hormones at birth. Fused labia are a serious anomaly, but simple adhesion may be due to inflammation (47).

The *anus* should be examined for proper location and patency. A very gentle rectal exam should be performed if anal stenosis is suspected (47, 65, 84).

The *spine* should be palpated for **spina bifida**, a *congenital neural tube defect characterized by anomaly in the posterior vertebral arch.* Refer to several references for in-depth information on appearance (56, 84, 91). Observation for symmetric bilateral muscle movements of the hips and knees is essential. The *hips* should be examined for dislocation by rotating the thighs with the knees flexed.

Extremities should be noted for the right number of fingers and toes and bilateral movements. Position of hands and feet should be checked for symmetry and normal appearance.

Signs of prematurity include low birth weight and small size, thick lanugo, excess vernix, slow or absent reflexes, undescended testicles in the male, and nipples not visible (47, 56, 65, 84).

Physiologic Concepts: Physical Characteristics of the Infant

GENERAL APPEARANCE

The growing infant changes in appearance as he or she changes size and proportion (47, 56, 84, 91). The face grows rapidly, trunk and limbs lengthen, back and limb muscles develop, and coordination improves. By 1 month the baby can lift the head slightly when prone and hold the head up briefly when the back is supported. By 2 months the head is held erect, but it bobs when he or she is sitting unsupported (*cephalocaudal development*).

Skull enlargement occurs almost as rapidly as total body growth during the first year and is determined mainly by the rate of brain expansion. From birth to 4 weeks, the head size increases to 14.75 in. (37.5 cm); at 3 months to 15.75 in. (39.5 cm); at 20 weeks to 16.5 in. (41 cm); and at 30 weeks to 17 in. (43 cm). By the end of the first year the head will be 66% of adult size (47, 56, 84, 91).

PHYSICAL GROWTH

Physical growth and development of psychosocial areas of learning are concurrent, interrelated, and rapid in the first year. The first year of life is one of the two periods of rapid physical growth after birth. (The other period is prepuberty through postpuberty.) The baby gains two-thirds of an ounce per day in the first 5 months and one-half ounce per day for the next 7 months. Birth weight doubles by 5 to 6 months and triples by 12 months. The baby grows approximately 12 inches in the first year. The skeletal system should be assessed for any orthopedic problems (47, 56). *Physical and motor abilities are heavily influenced by* (47, 56, 87, 93, 99): (a) genetic, biological, and cultural factors; (b) maturation of the central nervous system; (c) skeletal formation; (d) overall physical health status and nutrition; (e) environmental conditions; (f) appropriate sensory-motor stimulation; and (g) consistent loving care.

Ethnic differences for weight, length, head circumference, and other measurements have been noted in Anglo and Mexican American children ages 48 to 56 weeks. The Mexican American child has shorter stature and greater weight for length than the Anglo child, with greater chest circumference, subscapular skinfolds, and estimated body fat, with no difference by gender. Head circumference is greater for males than females in both ethnic groups but is greater in Anglo than Mexican American children. Thigh circumference is greater in Mexican Americans than Anglos and in females than in males (6, 51, 53). African American infants mature ahead of Caucasian infants in motor skills, bone ossification, and walking. This is apparently caused by genetic factors (14, 53).

Table 9-4 divides further developmental sequences into 3-month periods for specific assessment (6, 14, 39, 52, 56, 87, 99). *It is only a guide,* not an absolute standard. Great individual differences occur among infants, depending on their physical growth and emotional, social, and neuromuscular responses. Girls usually develop more rapidly than boys, although the activity level is generally higher for boys. Even with these cautions, Table 9-4 can be a useful tool to observe overall behavior patterns rather than isolated characteristics.

NEUROLOGIC SYSTEM

Babies are born with most of the brain cells they need. The neurologic system continues to develop neurons and functional capacity rapidly. Neurons form **synapses**, or *connections*, rapidly in the first 15 months. Without synapses, neurons cannot communicate. *Dendrites spread to connect with each other* (**branching or blooming**). If these neurons are used, they continue development. The infant brain makes more neurons and synapses than it needs. Later *those not used or needed are removed or* **pruned** (55, 56).

Development of the neurologic and sensory systems, among the first to develop, and *myelination of the nervous system follow the* Cephalocaudal and Proximodistal Principles described in Chapter 3. ∞ **Myelination**, *the process of encasing the axons with a myelin or fat cell coating or insulation,* begins prenatally and continues after birth. Myelination of the visual pathways is complete by 6 months. Myelination of other nerve pathways is completed at various times, and continues in adolescence, in middle age, and up to age 70. During this time, there is also a rapid increase in the development of connections between neurons. Myelin, produced by glial cells, speeds the conduction of impulses and increases ability of the brain to take on new functions (15, 38, 55, 84, 99).

The *brain stem*, which controls the basic body functions and reflexes, is completely developed at birth. The *cerebellum* begins to control muscle tone and balance and to coordinate basic sensory and motor activity. The *cerebrum* constitutes about 70% of the weight of the nervous system and begins basic cognitive functions. These and all other brain structures will become increasingly complex in growth and function (35, 55).

Teach parents that consistent stimulation of the nervous system is necessary to maintain growth and development, or function is lost and cannot be regained (14, 56, 87, 91, 99). Explore ways to enhance visual and auditory development, for example through attachment behaviors previously discussed and through play, discussed later. Encourage parents to stroke, massage, and cuddle baby; to talk and sing to baby; and to provide toys that have primary colors, different textures, and movement. These are basic health promotion measures.

TABLE 9-4

Assessment of Physical Characteristics of the Infant

1–3 Months	3–6 Months	6–9 Months	9–12 Months
Many characteristics of newborn, but more stable physiologically	Most neonatal reflexes gone Temperature stabilizes at 99.4°F (37.5°C)		Temperature averages 99.7°F (37.7°C)
Heartbeat steadies at about 120–130 beats/min		Pulse about 115/min; gradually decreases	Pulse about 100–110/min; resting–awake range of 80–150/min
Blood pressure about 80/40; gradually increases		Blood pressure about 90/60	Blood pressure 100/54 girls; 98/52 boys
Respirations more regular at 30–40/min; gradually decrease		Respirations about 32/min	Respirations 20–30/min
Appearance of salivation and tears			
Weight gain of 5–7 oz (141.75–198.45 g) per week	Weight gain of 3–5 oz (85.05–141.75 g) per week		Weight gain of 3–5 oz (85.05–141.75 g) per week
Weight at 8–13 lb (3,629–5,897 g)	Weight at 15–16 lb (6.8–7.3 kg) by 6 months	Birth weight doubled by 6 months	Birth weight tripled; average 22 lb (10 kg)
Head circumference increases 1 in. up to 16 in. (40 cm)	Head size increases 1 in. (2.54 cm)	Head size 17.8 in. (43.21 cm)	Head size increases slightly more, about ½ in. (18.3 in. or 45–46 cm)
Chest circumference 16 in. (40 cm)	Chest size increases more than 1 in. (17.3 in. or 43–44 cm)	Chest circumference increases ½ in. (17.8 in. or 44–45 cm)	Chest circumference increases about ½ in. (18.3 in. or 45–46 cm)
Body length: Growth of 1 in. (2.54 cm) monthly	Growth of ½ in. (1.27 cm) monthly	Growth of ½ in. (1.27 cm) monthly	Growth of ½ in. monthly; height 29–30 in. (72.5–75 cm), increased by 50% since birth
Tonic neck and Moro reflexes rapidly diminishing	Most neonatal reflexes gone Palmar reflex diminishing		
Arms and legs found in bilaterally symmetrical position			
Limbs used simultaneously, but not separately	Movements more symmetric		
Hands and fingers played with			
Clenched fists giving way to open hands that bat at objects			
Reaches for objects	Reaches for objects with accurate aim and flexed fingers	Palmar grasp developed Picks up objects with both hands; bangs toys	Throws objects
Plays with hands	Objects transferred from one hand to another by 6 months	Holds bottle with hands; holds own cookie	Puts toys in and out of container

TABLE 9-4

Assessment of Physical Characteristics of the Infant—continued

1–3 Months	3–6 Months	6–9 Months	9–12 Months
	Bangs with objects held in one hand Scoops objects with hands	Preference for use of one hand	
	Begins to use fingers separately	Probes with index finger Thumb opposition to finger (prehension) by 7 months	Points with finger Brings hands and thumb and index finger together at will to pick up small objects Releases objects at will
Can follow moving objects with eyes when supine; begins to use both eyes together at about 2 months	Binocular depth perception by about 5 months Looks for objects when they are dropped	Explores, feels, pulls, inspects, tastes, and tests objects	Makes mark on paper
	Improving eye–hand coordination	Hand–mouth coordination Feeds self cracker and other finger foods	Eats with fingers; holds cup, spoon
	Eruption of one or two lower incisors	Begins weaning process	Has 6 teeth, central and lateral incisors; eruption of first molars at about 12 months
Attends to voices Raises chin while lying on stomach at 1 month Raises chest while lying on stomach at 2 months; raises head and chest 45° to 50° off bed, supporting weight on arms Holds head in alignment when prone at 2 months; holds head erect in prone position at 3 months	Biaural hearing present Turns head to sound	Turns to sounds behind self	
Supports self on forearms when on stomach at 3 months	Rolls over completely by 6 months		Rolls easily from back to stomach
Sits if supported	Sits with support at 4 months Holds head steady while sitting Pulls self to sitting position Begins to sit alone for short periods Plays with feet Kicks vigorously Begins to hitch (scoot) backward while sitting Bears portion of own weight when held in standing position	Sits erect unsupported by 7 months Creeps or crawls by 8 or 9 months Pulls self to stand by holding onto support	Sits alone steadily Pivots when seated Puts feet in mouth Hitches with backward locomotion while sitting Sits from standing position without help

continued

TABLE 9-4

Assessment of Physical Characteristics of the Infant—continued

1–3 Months	3–6 Months	6–9 Months	9–12 Months
	Pushes feet against hard surface to move by 3 or 4 months	Cruises (walking sideways while holding onto object with both hands) by 10 months	Stands alone for a minute
			Walks when led by 11 months
		Begins to walk with help	Walks with help by 12–14 months
			Lumbar and dorsal curves developed while learning to walk
			Turning of feet and bowing of legs normal
			Beginning to show regular bladder and bowel patterns; has one or two stools per day; interval of dry diaper does not exceed 1 to 2 hours
			Not ready for toilet training
Smiles at comforting person reflexly	Smiles at person deliberately during interaction	Experiences separation anxiety by about 7–9 months	Attachment to caregiver
	Displays joy, frustration, rage	Engages in social play; elicits response from others	Sociable increasingly with others
Coos, chuckles, laughs	Babbles; plays with sounds		Begins to cooperate in dressing; puts arm through sleeve; takes off socks
			Improves previously acquired skills throughout this period

Vision

The infant demonstrates increasing visual ability, as depicted by **Figure 9-4**. *By 2 months of age, the infant can* (14, 47, 56, 87, 91, 99):

1. Focus both eyes on an object steadily.
2. Look longer at colors of medium intensity (yellow, green, pink) than at bright (red, orange, blue) or dim (gray, beige) colors.
3. Distinguish red from green.
4. Accommodate better; the lenses have become more flexible.
5. Use broader peripheral vision, which has doubled since birth.
6. Follow path of an object.
7. Notice and imitate facial movements.

By 4 months of age, the infant can (14, 47, 56, 85, 99):

1. Distinguish between red, green, blue, and yellow, and prefers red and blue.

2. Use binocular vision (both eyes focus), which allows perception of depth and distance and ability to distinguish stripes and edges.
3. Accommodate on an adult level.

At this time, tear glands begin to function.

Under 3 to 4 months of age, the baby does not look for an object hidden after seeing it, and when the same object reappears, it is as if the object were a new object. The infant has no knowledge that objects have a continuous existence; the object ceases to exist when it is not seen (84, 87, 89). The baby coordinates both eyes and attends to and prefers novel stimuli. *At 4 months,* he or she can focus for any distance and perceive shape constancy when the object is rotated at different angles. Infants look longer at patterned stimuli of less complexity than at stimuli that have very complex designs or no lines or contours, and can detect change of pattern. The infant prefers faces but is attracted by checkerboard designs, geometric shapes, and large pictures (circles, dots, and squares at least

3 in. high and with angles rather than contours). Full depth perception develops at approximately *8 to 9 months* when the images received in the central nervous system from the macula of each eye are integrated, and may be related to experiences with crawling (14, 84, 99, 109).

Visual stimulation of both eyes simultaneously is necessary for the baby to develop binocular vision. Otherwise **amblyopia** (*lazy eye*), *which is a gradual loss of the ability to see in one eye because of lack of stimulation of visual nerve pathways,* develops without damage to the retina or other eye structures. If visual stimulation is not lacking for too many weeks, the condition reverses itself. If one eye continues to do all the work for several months, blindness results in the other eye (47).

Hearing

Babies are neurologically prepared to respond to the sounds of any human voice. The fetus hears *in utero*. The newborn recognizes and responds to the pattern and time of sounds heard *in utero*, for example, music or being read, sung, or talked to consistently. The young infant sucks more rapidly on a nipple in order to listen to some sounds rather than others. For example, classical music of Beethoven is preferred to rock music. At *2 to 3 months*, the baby turns head to side when sound is made at ear level. By 4 months, the baby locates sounds by turning head to sound and looking the same direction. By *8 to 10 months*, the baby turns head diagonally toward sound. By 1 year, the baby knows several words heard regularly and their meaning, such as "no," and names of family members (14, 56, 88, 99).

Touch

The *haptic system* is that body system pertaining to tactile stimulation. *There are different neural receptors for heat, warmth, cold, dull pain, sharp pain, deep pressure, vibration, and light touch.* At birth, all humans possess central nervous system ability to register and associate sensory impressions received through receptor organs in the skin and from kinesthetic stimuli that originate with contact with other humans. Sensory pathways subserving kinesthetic and tactile activities are the first to complete myelination in infancy, followed by auditory and visual pathways (14, 80, 84, 100).

Touching the infant from birth on provides the basis for higher-order operations in the neurologic, perceptual, muscular, skeletal, and cognitive systems. Each tactile act carries a physiologic impact with psychological and sociocultural meaning. Much information is gained through discriminating one physical stimulus from another, with the form or quality of touch changing the perception of the tactile experience. Tactile stimulation is essential for both beginning body image development and other learning (56, 80).

Vital Signs

During infancy, vital signs (temperature, pulse, respirations, and blood pressure) stabilize, as shown in **Table 9-4** (35, 56). Variations occur based on size, activity, and physical status. Changes from the child's usual measurements should be investigated to determine illness (35, 56).

RESPIRATORY SYSTEM

Babies are obligatory nose breathers during the first few months of life. The structures of the upper respiratory tract remain small and relatively delicate and provide inadequate protection against infectious agents. *Close proximity of the middle ear, wide horizontal eustachian tube, throat, short and narrow trachea, and bronchi results in rapid spread of infection from one structure to the other.* Mucous membranes are less able to produce mucus, causing less air humidification and warming, which also increases susceptibility to infection. The *chest shape is almost circular;* transverse diameter exceeds anteroposterior diameter, causing an increased respiratory rate. The rounded thorax, limited alveolar surface for gas exchange, and amount of anatomic dead air space in the lungs or portion of the tracheobronchial tree where inspired air does not participate in gas exchange means that more air must be moved in and out per minute than later in childhood. *By age 1 year*, the lining of the airway resembles that of the adult. *Respiratory rate at rest decreases gradually during the first year* (35, 56).

ENDOCRINE SYSTEM

The endocrine system *is functionally immature.* Change in one gland has a major effect on any other gland. The child is very susceptible to stress, which affects fluid and electrolyte imbalance, glucose concentration, and amino acid metabolism. *During the first 18 months, the pituitary gland, adrenal cortex, and pancreas do not function well together.* The pituitary gland continues to secrete growth hormone and thyroid-stimulating hormone (begun in fetal life), which influence growth and metabolism (76). Plasma electrolyte concentrations do not vary much among infants, small children, and adults. Blood levels of calcium, sodium, magnesium, and potassium are low immediately after birth and should be monitored to ensure that they approach normal levels (44, 76).

GASTROINTESTINAL SYSTEM

At birth, the full-term infant adapts to extrauterine nutrition, which includes coordinated sucking and swallowing, gastric emptying and intestinal motility, regulation of digestive secretions and enzymes, efficient digestion and absorption, and excretion of waste products. Swallowing is an automatic reflex for 3 months (44).

The *gastrointestinal system matures somewhat after 2 to 3 months,* when the baby can voluntarily chew, hold, or spit out food. The tongue size is proportional to mouth size. When the tongue is touched or depressed, the baby responds by thrusting it outward. Thus, the extrusion reflex protects the infant from ingesting undigestible foods or objects. At *2 to 3 months*, the sucking reflex is replaced by *voluntary swallowing*. Saliva secretion increases and composition becomes more adultlike. **Box 9-4**, Stomach Capacity of Infant, depicts capacity by age. The stomach's emptying time changes from 2.5 to 3 hours and 3 to 6 hours. Gastric hydrochloric acid and pepsinogen secretion are low and increase levels at 3 months (13, 44, 47, 55, 65).

Tooth eruption begins at approximately *6 months* and stimulates saliva flow and chewing. Once primary teeth erupt, cleaning should begin (56).

BOX 9-4	Stomach Capacity of Infant
Newborn	10–20 mL
1-week-old	30–90 mL
2- to 3-week-old	60–90 mL
1-month-old	90–120 mL
3-month-old	150–200 mL
1-year-old	210–360 mL

The *small intestine* is proportionally longer than it is in an adult; the *large intestine* is proportionally shorter. Peristaltic waves mature by slowing down and reversing less after approximately 8 months; then stools are more formed and the baby spits up or vomits less. **Colic**, a term that indicates *daily periods of distress, refers to paroxysmal abdominal pain or cramping with rapid peristaltic movements and gas pressure on the rectum,* as shown by x-ray films. *It usually occurs between 2 to 3 weeks and 2 to 3 months.* These movements are normally set off by a few sucking movements. Causes may include allergy to formula or cow's milk, too rapid feeding or overeating, swallowing excess air, improper position or burping (bubbling) during feeding, and emotional tension between parent and child. Some mothers find that changing formula and giving plain, low-fat yogurt or chamomile tea, changing baby's position, and gentle pressure to the abdomen may help reduce the pains (44, 56). When small yogurt feedings do not help, vitamin A and E supplements have been found effective. Apparently colic disappears as digestive enzymes become more complex, and normal bacterial flora accumulate as the baby ingests a larger variety of food.

By *2 months*, the baby usually averages two **stools** (*bowel movements*) daily; source of nutrition causes a variance. By *4 months* there is a predictable interval of time between feeding and bowel movements. Breastfed babies usually have soft, semiliquid stools that are light yellow. Breastfed babies may vary more in the bowel movement pattern. The baby may have three or four watery stools a day or may go several days without a bowel movement. The stools of the formula-fed baby are more brown and formed (44, 56).

The *liver* occupies a larger part of the abdominal cavity than does an adult's liver and remains functionally immature until age 1 year. Glyconeogenesis and glycogen and vitamin storage is less effective than it is later in life (44, 55). Bilirubin conjugation and bile secretion develops during the neonatal period (56).

As the autonomic nervous system and gastrointestinal tract mature, interconnections form between higher mental functions and the autonomic nervous system. *The infant's gastrointestinal tract responds to emotional states in self or someone close to him or her* (47, 56).

MUSCULAR TISSUE

At birth muscular tissue is almost completely formed. Growth results from increasing size of the already existing fibers under the influence of growth hormone, thyroxine, and insulin. As muscle size increases, strength increases in childhood. *Muscle fibers need continual stimulation to develop to full function and strength* (47, 55). *Ossification of the skeletal system develops over the first year* (56).

SKIN

Structures typical of adult skin are present, but they are functionally immature; thus the baby is more prone to skin disorders. The epidermal layers are very permeable, causing greater loss of fluid from the body. Dry, intact skin is the greatest deterrent to bacterial invasion. *Sebaceous glands,* which produce sebum, are very active in late fetal life and early infancy, causing milia and cradle cap, which go away at approximately 6 weeks. Production of sebum decreases during infancy and remains minimal during childhood until puberty (56).

Eccrine (sweat) glands are functional in response to heat and emotional stimuli at birth. By 3 weeks, palmar sweating on crying occurs and can be a way to assess pain. The inability of the skin to contract and shiver in response to cold or perspire in response to heat causes *ineffective thermal regulation in the newborn, but it develops during infancy* (56).

RENAL SYSTEM

Renal structural components are present at birth. By *5 months* tubules have adultlike proportions in size and shape. The ureters are relatively short, and the bladder lies close to the abdominal wall. *Renal function,* however, is *not mature until approximately 2 years;* therefore, the child is unable to handle increased intake of proteins, which are ingested if cow's milk is given too early (41, 44, 56, 65, 84). The kidneys have a limited concentrating ability and require more water to excrete a given amount of solute. Thus, the infant has difficulty conserving body water. The infant also has difficulty excreting an excess fluid volume. Infants have difficulty adapting to too much or too little fluid; they can tolerate disturbances for only a few hours (76).

Total *urinary output* is about 200 to 300 ml per 24 hours by the end of the first week of life. The first voiding should be within 24 hours after birth. Thereafter, the bladder involuntarily empties when stretched by 15 ml. There may be as many as 20 voidings a day (56).

IMMUNE SYSTEM

Components of the immune system are present or show beginning development. The *phagocytosis process is mature, but the inflammatory response is inefficient and unable to localize infections.* The ability to produce antibodies is limited; much of the antibody protection is acquired from the mother during fetal life. The newborn receives maternal immunoglobulin G (IgC), which gives immunity for about 3 months, when the infant begins synthesis of IgC. By 1 year, the infant synthesizes 40% of the IgC. Production of IgM, IgA, IgD, and IgE is more gradual; maximum levels are not reached until early childhood. Development of immunologic function depends on the infant's gradual exposure to foreign bodies and infectious agents (35, 56, 65, 84).

RED BLOOD CELL AND HEMOGLOBIN LEVELS

High at birth, *red blood cell (RBC) and hemoglobin levels drop after 2 or 3 months. Maternal iron stores are present about 5 to 6 months;* the gradual decrease in the infant accounts for lower hemoglobin until erythropoietin is stimulated (56). *Iron deficiency anemia becomes apparent around 6 months of age if the physiologic system does not function adequately to sustain red blood cell and hemoglobin levels.* By the *end of infancy, the level of white blood cells,* high at birth, *declines to reach adult levels.* Red blood cell and hemoglobin levels reach adult norms in late childhood (41, 55, 56).

SEXUALITY DEVELOPMENT

Sexuality may be defined as a *deep, pervasive aspect of the total person and the sum total of one's feelings and behavior as a male or female, the expression of which goes beyond genital response.* Sexuality includes the attitudes that are necessary to maintain a stable and intimate relationship with another person. Sexuality culminates in adulthood, but it begins to develop in infancy (87, 99).

Gender is determined at the moment of fertilization. Chromosome combination and hormonal influences affect sexual development prenatally. Sometimes mothers respond to the fetus in a sex-differentiated way. An active fetus is interpreted as a boy, a quiet one as a girl. Prenatal position, according to folklore, relates to gender; boys are supposedly carried high, and girls are carried low.

Gender or sex assignment occurs at birth. The parents' first question, unless they already know, is usually "Is it a boy or a girl?" The answer to this question often stimulates a set of adjectives to describe the newborn: soft, fine-featured, little, passive, weak girl, or robust, big, strong, active boy, regardless of size or weight. The name given to the baby also reflects the parents' attitudes toward the baby's gender and may reflect their ideas about the child's eventual role in life. Mothers, however, engage in less gender-typing stereotypes than fathers (87). The stereotypes about sex do have some basis in fact, because at birth males usually are larger and have more muscle mass, are more active, and are more irritable than girls. Females are more sensitive to auditory, tactile, and painful stimuli. Newborn boys and girls react differently to stress, possibly because of genetic, hormonal, or innate temperament differences (37). At 3 weeks of age, males are still more irritable and are sleeping less than females (87).

Occasionally external genitalia are ambiguous in appearance, neither distinctly male nor distinctly female. When this occurs, parents should be given as much support and information as possible to cope with the crisis. Gender assignment based on chromosomal studies or appearance should be made as soon as possible (56).

According to research, mothers seem to respond initially more to male infants than to female infants (perhaps because male infants have traditionally been more highly valued). But by 3 months this reverses, and mothers are thought to have more touch and conversational contact with female infants, even when they are irritable. This reverse may occur because mothers are generally more successful in calming irritable daughters than irritable sons (16, 87).

By *5 months* the baby responds differently to male and female voices, and by 6 months he or she distinguishes mother from father and as distinct people. At 6 months the female infant has a longer attention span for visual stimuli and better fixation on a human face, is more responsive to social stimuli, and prefers complex stimuli. The male infant has a better fixation response to a helix of light and is more attentive to an intermittent tone than is a female (16, 87).

Research indicates that when babies are *6 months old,* mothers imitate the verbal sounds of their daughters more than their sons, and mothers continue to touch, talk to, and handle their daughters more than their sons. Throughout infancy and childhood, female children talk to and touch their mothers more, whereas boys are encouraged to be more independent, exploratory, and vigorous in gross motor activity (16, 64, 87).

The father tends to treat the baby girl more softly and the baby boy more roughly during the last 6 months of infancy. At *9 months,* a baby girl behaves differently with her mother than with her father. She will be rougher and more attention seeking with her father (16, 68). By *9 to 12 months,* the baby responds to his or her name, an important link to gender and role. Research indicates that female babies are more dependent and less exploratory by 1 year than males because of different parental expectations (16, 87). **Gender typing,** *the process by which the child learns* what is expected of him or her, begins early in some families and varies by culture (87).

Infants receive stimulation of their erogenous zones through maternal care. The mouth and lower face are the main erogenous zones initially, providing pleasure, warmth, and satisfaction through sucking. Both genders explore their genitalia during infancy. Erection in the male and lubrication in the female occur (16, 87).

Explore sexuality development with parents. Help them be aware of the importance of their tone of voice, touch, behavior, and feelings toward the boy or girl for sexuality development. Help them develop ways to relate optimally to and promote trust and well-being in the child.

Nutritional Needs

The feeding time is crucial for baby and mother: a time to strengthen attachment, a time for baby to feel love and security, a time for mother and baby to learn about self and each other, and a time for baby to learn about the environment. Either breastfeeding or formula feeding can be effective and satisfying. In poor nations, breastfeeding is crucial protection against malnutrition. Further, formula is expensive and often prepared in unsterile bottles with unsterile water, thereby causing illness. Both methods will be discussed in this section. **Table 9-5** summarizes the changing schedule and amount of food during the first year of life (41, 44).

BREASTFEEDING: PREPARATION, BENEFITS, AND PROCESS

Breastfeeding of infants has come in and out of fashion. The American Academy of Pediatrics *recommends exclusive breastfeeding for the first 6 months and that infants receive breast milk for at least the first 12 months of life* (4). Children as old as 2 years can benefit from the antibodies and folic acid in mother's milk (41, 44). *Healthy People 2010* presents the goal of increasing the proportion of mothers who breastfeed their babies (108).

Preparation for breastfeeding begins during pregnancy. The mother's decision about infant feeding should be made during

TABLE 9-5

Feeding Schedules and Amounts During the First Year of Life

Age of Infant	Schedule for Milk and Food	Amount of Milk Each Feeding
1 week	Every 2–4 hours (six to eight feedings)	60–90 mL (2–3 oz)
2–4 weeks	Every 4 hours (six feedings)	90–120 mL (3–4 oz)
1 month	Every 4 hours (six feedings)	90–120 mL (3–4 oz)
2–3 months	Five feedings	120–180 mL (4–6 oz)
	Sleeps through night	
	May add rice cereal (fewest allergic reactions)	
4–5 months	Five to six feedings	150–210 mL (5–7 oz)
	May add iron-fortified cereals; cooked, strained, pureed vegetables; and meat	Average serving size for food, 1–2 tablespoons
6–7 months	Four to five feedings	210–240 mL (6–8 oz)
	Enjoys finger foods	Serving size, 2 tablespoons
	May add foods with eggs, fruits, oven-dried toast, and soy or wheat flour	
	Ready to eat solid foods, not just thickened feedings	
8–9 months	Three to four feedings	240 mL (8 oz)
	Eats iregular food, mashed or chopped; follows eating pattern of family	Needs additional fluids during days
	Will accept variety of foods	
9–12 months	Three feedings	Whole milk added at 12 months
	May add juice by cup	

Adapted from references 41, 44.

pregnancy and is influenced by her obstetrician, pediatrician, nurse, husband, mother, and friends. Or there may be no decision. It may be assumed the mother will feed one way or the other, related to family upbringing, religious or regional culture, societal pressures, or personal preference. An adequate diet during pregnancy is important not only for fetal development; it is an initial step toward successful lactation and breastfeeding (41, 44).

Any mother is physiologically able to nurse her baby, with rare exceptions (35). But childbirth, breastfeeding, and child rearing are sexual experiences for the woman. Breastfeeding may be a sexual experience for the male partner. Her success in breastfeeding is related to other aspects of her psychosexual identity. She may choose not to breastfeed or to limit the lactation period because of personal preference, illness, or employment in a place where she cannot take her baby with her. In cultures in which breastfeeding is accepted, women breastfeed without difficulty. A positive social support system is essential for the woman who breastfeeds because fear of failure, embarrassment, anxiety, exhaustion, frustration, anger, or any stress-producing situation can prevent the effect of oxytocin and block the flow of milk. The pregnant woman's level of information and motivation for achievement are positively related to successful breastfeeding (41, 44).

Explore with the woman and partner, as appropriate, any feelings and questions about breastfeeding. Teach about the advantages and challenges of both breastfeeding and bottle feeding, and the importance of preparation nutritionally and of breast care. Refer the mother to the La Leche League and encourage her to seek out other women who have breastfed to gain a variety of perspec-

tives. Identify early any problems with breastfeeding and offer one-to-one support so that it is a positive experience.

Human milk is considered ideal. Even in undernourished women, the composition of breast milk is adequate, although vitamin content depends on the mother's diet. Breast milk is all that a baby needs the first 6 months of life (41, 44).

Breast milk has about 200 components. Major components include the following (3, 41, 44):

1. *Protein* provides 4% to 5% of total calories, enough to promote growth without causing excess renal solute load. Most of the protein is easily digested whey.
2. *Fat,* 55% to 60% of the total calories, is easily digested because of the digestive enzymes in the milk. The fatty acid, linoleic acid, is high. Polyunsaturated fatty acids and an omega-3 fatty acid promote optimal central nervous system development. The high cholesterol level helps develop enzyme systems capable of handling cholesterol in adulthood.
3. *Carbohydrate* provides 35% to 40% of total calories. The higher level of lactose stimulates growth of normal gastrointestinal bacterial flora and promotes calcium absorption. Amylase, a starch-digesting enzyme, promotes starch digestion since pancreatic amylase is low.
4. *Minerals* are adequate for growth but not excessive, which would burden kidneys with a high renal solute load. Iron absorption is approximately 50%, compared to 4% from iron-fortified formulas. Zinc absorption is better than from formula or cow's milk. Low sodium keeps renal solute load low.

5. *Vitamins* are supplied in totality but the content varies with the mother's diet. Vitamins D and B_{12} are of concern in vegan mothers. Vitamin D content varies with diet and exposure to sun, but generally it is low in breast milk. All infants should consume 20 IU of vitamin D to prevent rickets. If the breast-feeding mother is a complete vegan, a vitamin B_{12} supplement is essential.

6. *Other components include* (a) antibodies; (b) anti-infective factors; (c) the resistive bifidus factor, which promotes growth of normal gastrointestinal bacteria; (d) enzymes; (e) insulin, thyroid, and adrenal hormones and hormone-like substances such as melatonin; and (f) estrogen and prostaglandins (41).

Good nutrition starts with mother's milk. **Colostrum** *is a thick (yellow) high-caloric fluid secreted by the woman's breasts at birth and for about 3 to 4 days* (44). Colostrum has higher levels of antibodies than the later milk; is rich in carbohydrates, which the newborn needs; and serves as a laxative in cleaning out the gastrointestinal tract. Colostrum fed immediately after birth protects against infection because it triggers antibody production. Depending on how soon and how often the mother nurses, **true milk**, *less concentrated, comes in the first few days* (41, 44). The baby should be put to breast immediately after delivery and fed within hours after birth to reduce hypoglycemia and hyperbilirubinemia (56). *Even a brief period of breastfeeding, particularly the 3 or so days of colostrum, gives immunologic and other benefits* to the infant, including the preterm baby (35). However, in some cultures colostrum is considered unhealthy. Breastfeeding does not begin until true milk is produced (35, 41, 51). The mother should not automatically receive medication to stop lactation, and the baby should not be fed in the nursery between breastfeedings.

If a *mother nurses after delivery*, the pituitary gland secretes prolactin. The high levels of estrogen from the placenta that inhibited milk secretion during pregnancy are gone. As the baby sucks, the nipple is in the back of the mouth, and the jaws and tongue compress the milk sinuses. These tactile sensations trigger the release of the hormone oxytocin from the pituitary gland, which, in turn, causes the "let-down" response. The sinuses refill immediately, and milk flows with very little effort to the baby. This is the crucial time for baby to learn breastfeeding. Oxytocin also causes a powerful contraction of the uterus, lessening the danger of hemorrhage after delivery (3, 47). The mother needs an encouraging partner or family member, knowledgeable and supportive nursing and medical personnel to assist, and hospital and home routines that allow the baby to be with her for feeding when the baby is hungry and her breasts are full.

The *mother who works outside the home* can breastfeed when at home. Some work sites allow her to bring the baby to work so breastfeeding can continue. Or, she may express breast milk into a bottle that can be given to the baby by the caretaker while she is at work. The La Leche League offers helpful suggestions (56).

Teach the mother the *breastfeeding technique*. If needed, help her get the baby latched on to the nipple. Build her self-confidence, and foster a comfortable position. The first feeding should be within 20 to 30 minutes after birth; the baby will nurse about 10 minutes. Explain the baby's signals for hunger and how a schedule will be established that is essentially on-demand. Frequent breastfeeding (every 2 to 3 hours) will establish the milk supply and prevent the breasts from becoming hard and swollen. It's recommended to offer both breasts at each feeding. The baby may nurse 10 to 20 minutes on each breast. The last portion, called **"hind milk,"** *is higher in fat and helps the baby feel satisfied* (41, 44). The baby should be **burped** (*bubbling or gently patting baby's back*) after each ounce when very young. Later, the baby should be burped halfway through feeding, when the breasts are changed, and at the end of the feeding. More specific information is available from the La Leche League lactation specialists, booklets prepared by formula companies, and maternity nursing texts. The mother may also benefit from talking with another mother who successfully breastfed.

Teach the breastfeeding mother to increase her fluid intake and meet the increased recommended dietary allowances for lactating women. She should avoid smoking, drinking alcoholic beverages, ingesting or using addictive drugs, or taking over-the-counter or herbal medications. All pass into the bloodstream and into mother's milk. Breastfeeding may be contraindicated in these

INTERVENTIONS FOR HEALTH PROMOTION

Teach mothers that the benefits of breastfeeding to the infant are substantial. Mother's milk (35, 41, 44):

1. Is a natural food and easily digestible. It contains no artificial colorings, flavorings, preservatives, or additives.
2. Is always sterile, available, and at body temperature.
3. Contains more iron, vitamins A and C, and other nutrients than cow's or goat's milk.
4. Contains specific fats and sugars that are needed and that are more easily digested than is formula.
5. Fosters appropriate weight gain; overfeeding is not as likely.

6. Prevents or reduces risk of food allergies, diarrhea, respiratory diseases, bacterial infections, urinary tract diseases, and otitis media.
7. Promotes growth of denser bones in childhood and adulthood.
8. Promotes better jaw and tooth development because the infant has to suck harder than on a bottle nipple.
9. Fosters better neurologic and cognitive development and visual acuity. Breast milk has growth-promoting substances not found in formula or cow's milk.

INTERVENTIONS FOR HEALTH PROMOTION

Teach the mother that she also benefits from breastfeeding (41, 44, 56):

1. The maternal-infant bond is strengthened.
2. Breast milk is readily available. There is no need to purchase, measure, mix, or warm formula and no bottles to clean. Disposable bottles do not add to surface waste, as discussed in Chapter 4. ∞
3. Breastfeeding is economical. Formula costs are substantial, plus the cost of bottles.
4. During breastfeeding, the mother can sit and relax. A break every few hours is a helpful change in the schedule. The baby may nurse for 15 to 30 minutes.

5. Breastfeeding helps the mother regain the preconception figure because nursing stimulates release of **oxytocin**, *a hormone that promotes uterine contraction and shrinking.* The fat pads deposited during pregnancy in the hips and thighs as fuel for milk production disappear. Gradual weight loss during breastfeeding does not affect milk production.
6. Breastfeeding lowers risk of developing premenopausal breast cancer, ovarian cancer, and osteoporosis.
7. During breastfeeding, menstruation may not occur for several months. However, ovulation can occur.

---

situations. The mother who does smoke or drink alcohol in moderation should not do so right before breastfeeding. Secondhand smoke predisposes the infant to sinus infections, other respiratory diseases, colic, irritable behavior, and possible risk of sudden infant death syndrome (SIDS) (44, 56).

There are *situations when the mother should not breastfeed.* Refer to **Box 9-5** (2, 3, 14, 41, 47, 99). In-depth information is available at the American Academy of Pediatrics Website, www.policyapplications.org, which lists 170 medications that are either compatible with breastfeeding or that cause negative effects in the mother or infant.

BOX 9-5 — Reasons Mother Should Not Breastfeed

1. Is HIV positive or AIDS-infected, or has another infection; the virus is transmitted through mother's milk.
2. Has active untreated tuberculosis.
3. Is taking any medication, including antidepressants, that would not be safe for baby.
4. Uses toxic drugs or addictive substances.
5. Has high level of exposure to toxic chemicals or pesticides.
6. Has child with inborn error of metabolism, such as galactosemia, as special formula may be necessary.
7. Was diagnosed with breast cancer during pregnancy.
8. Is pregnant with the next child; pregnancy and lactation combined place too much demand and stress on body.
9. Is uncomfortable and highly anxious with breastfeeding.
10. Is unable to produce enough milk to satisfy baby.
11. Partner or significant family members want to take turns feeding baby, or mother prefers father or another person feeding baby during her hours of sleep.

BOTTLE FEEDING— COMMERCIAL FORMULAS

Infants can be adequately nourished by formula (41, 44, 47). In many developed countries, about half the babies are breastfed for a month, but bottle feeding is more convenient when the mother goes back to work. *Soy and rice milk are not formulas and should not be used.* They lack nutrients found in fortified formula and cow's milk, and can cause severe vitamin D and protein deficiencies. They are also low in fat and cholesterol; both are needed.

Commercial formulas are similar to each other and to human milk, but they are not exactly the same as human milk. Most have a slightly higher renal solute load than does breast milk. Higher protein intake from formula produces a higher blood urea nitrogen level and serum or urine level of amino acids (except taurine). If the osmolality is too high, water is drawn from the tissue, causing dehydration (41, 44). Too high a sodium level in the formula may cause transient elevation of blood pressure in neonates (41, 44). Special formulas are available to meet the needs of infants who are born preterm, have malabsorption or other health problems, are allergic to regular formula or cow's milk, or are born into vegan families. Soy protein substitute used by the vegan family must be supplemented with the amino acid methionine in the formula. Normal growth and development are possible without breastfeeding; however, formula feeding causes greater deposits of subcutaneous fat (41, 44). *Infants should receive supplemental iron by 4 months of age and preterm babies by 2 months.* Iron-fortified formulas are the best source for formula-fed babies.

Teach parents that it is not essential to heat formula. Formula should *never* be heated in the microwave. The bottle, nipple, and milk all become too hot and will cause oropharyngeal and esophageal burns. Further, the formula-filled disposable plastic liner of a commercial nurser may explode after removal of the heated bottle from the microwave, causing body burns.

Teach parents and other family members about sitting comfortably during bottle-feeding time and to hold the baby with head slightly raised so that he or she can comfortably suck and swallow. Angle the bottle to prevent the baby swallowing too much air. *The bottle should never be propped. The baby could aspirate formula and choke, and holding formula in the mouth promotes baby-bottle mouth and tooth decay.* If the baby falls asleep while feeding or when the bottle is empty, the bottle should be promptly removed to prevent air bubbles in the stomach.

COW'S MILK

Cow's milk is designed for another animal; thus, it is not surprising that it varies considerably in composition from human milk. *Cow's milk is unsuitable for the infant less than 6 months of age* (3) Cow's milk contains from two to three times as much protein. More of the protein is casein, which produces a large, difficult-to-digest curd. It is higher in saturated fats and lower in cholesterol than is human milk. Cow's milk contains half as much total lactose as human milk and also has galactose and glucose. It contains more sodium, potassium, magnesium, sulfur, and phosphorus than human milk and is a relatively poor source of vitamins C and D and iron. Cow's milk contains more than four times as much calcium, and babies fed cow's milk have larger and heavier skeletons. *Low-fat (2% milk fat) or skim milk should not be fed to infants because they will not gain weight and they need the fat content,* as described earlier (41, 44).

WATER

Infants have proportionally more body fluid than adults. About *70% of the infant's body weight is fluid.* More than 50% of the body fluid is extracellular, in contrast to 33% in the adult. Infants are more vulnerable to body fluid loss because extracellular fluid is more readily lost than cellular fluid. During the first 6 months, body fluid percentage changes rapidly; total body fluid percentage decreases (76).

The baby needs approximately 100 to 150 ml of water per kilogram of body weight daily to offset normal fluid losses. *Fruit juice is not a substitute for water. Water should be offered at least twice daily.* Some water is obtained through milk, but hot weather, fever, diarrhea, or vomiting quickly leads to dehydration. *Infants become dehydrated more quickly than adults because they have a smaller total fluid volume in the body compared with body size* (44). Parents should know the *signs of dehydration* (3, 76): (a) dry, loose, warm skin; (b) dry mucous membranes; (c) sunken eyeballs and fontanels; (d) slowed pulse; (e) lower blood pressure and increased body temperature; (f) concentrated, scanty urine; (g) constipation or mucoid diarrhea; (h) lethargy; and (i) a weak cry. Any combination of these symptoms implies the need for medical treatment (3, 76).

Water intoxication, *when the baby receives excess water and inadequate protein and other nutrients,* results in water retention, cerebral edema, and electrolyte imbalance. Convulsions ensue (76). The condition is a concern when babies are bottle-fed, especially in poor families when baby is given very diluted formula or only water to drink. The condition can be life-threatening. Thus, mothers in the lower socioeconomic levels are being encouraged to breastfeed (47).

NUTRIENT REQUIREMENTS

After the initial period of adjustment (7 to 10 days after birth), the baby needs a daily average of 2.2 g of *protein* and 110 to 120 *calories* per kilogram of body weight to grow and gain weight satisfactorily. Some *fats* are necessary because they contain essential fat-soluble vitamins, furnish more energy per unit than carbohydrates and protein, and promote development of the nervous system. Adequate intake of *vitamins and minerals* is essential. If the water supply is not fluoridated, *fluoride supplementation* should be given until 12 years of age to prevent dental caries. More information on nutrient recommendations can be found in a nutrition text (41, 44).

There is no rigid sequence in adding solid foods to the infant's diet. See **Table 9-5** for guidelines. The Case Situation also presents an effective approach. Whatever solid food is offered first or at what time is largely a matter of individual preference of the mother or of the pediatrician. Many physicians recommend later introduction of solid foods because fetal iron stores may last up to 6 months and because of an increasing incidence of allergies in infants introduced to a variety of solids before 3 months.

Infant nutritional status can be assessed by measuring head circumference, height, and weight. The fat baby, with a differential of two or more percentiles between weight and length, is more likely to become an overweight child or adult. However, weight at birth or weight gain in infancy is not a precise predictor of obesity. Small stature may indicate undernutrition unless there is a genetic influence from small-sized parents. Signs of nutritional deprivation include smaller-than-normal head size, pale skin color, poor skin turgor, and low hemoglobin and hematocrit levels (56).

Teach parents to avoid overfeeding—either milk or foods. Eating patterns are difficult to change, especially if food symbolizes love, attention, or approval. In addition to discussing the food quantities, quality, and nutrients needed by the baby, teach parents that food and mealtime are learning experiences. The baby gains motor control and coordination in self-feeding. He or she learns to recognize color, shape, and texture. Use of mouth muscles stimulates the ability to make movements necessary for speech development. The baby continues to develop trust with the consistent, loving atmosphere of mealtime. Food should not be used as reward or punishment (by withholding food). The child should learn moderation in feeding quantity. Between-feeding snacks should be avoided or, if used, should be healthful, small in quantity, and given because the child is hungry despite eating at mealtime.

Teach parents about nutritional value of foods and also about potential pollution of foods, depending upon where they are grown and how they are processed. For example, infants are very vulnerable to pesticide ingestion. Teach parents about the advantage of organically grown foods—to the infant and the rest of the family. More and more markets and stores sell organically grown foods, either fresh or processed, and cost is less prohibitive than in the past. Avoiding additives, preservatives, pesticides, and hormones used in meat production is increasingly viewed as health promotion and essential for the physically immature child. Refer also to Chapter 4 for more information about health effects of these substances. ∞

Case Situation

Breastfeeding and Weaning: The First Year

Sue has successfully breastfed her son for 9 months and she plans to continue for another 3 to 4 months because of the benefits to the mother and child. She believes that the attachment between mother and son is stronger because of breastfeeding.

Sue described how beneficial breastfeeding can be even for a short period of time. She explained that breastfeeding can continue if the mother is employed. Many work sites now have a specific room where the mother can use a breast pump in privacy and comfort.

For Sue, breastfeeding has been economical. A manual pump costs approximately $20 and an electric pump ranges from $75 to $250. This is a small cost, considering that formula will cost about $1,200 a year. (If the child has allergies and needs a special formula, such as soy, the cost will be about $2,000 the first year.)

Sue has followed the doctor's advice and introduced solids at 5.5 to 6 months, when the baby showed signs of reaching and pincer grasp, mouth movements, and teething.

She described the following routine, which should be a pleasant, untimed experience. Begin with a single grain cereal, such as rice, for the first few months after solid foods begin. Then add a single grain cereal each month, 1 tablespoon at a time, until the child is being given a serving of one-half cup a day. Use breast milk or formula to moisten the cereal. After 1 week of cereal, applesauce (1 to 2 teaspoons) can be mixed with the rice or given separately. When her son was first fed with a spoon, he expected to suck. She knew tongue protrusion was a result of immature muscle coordination and new items in the diet. The reflex disappeared between 7 and 8 months.

Sue explained that after the first week of feeding applesauce with cereal, strained, pureed, and blended prunes, peas, carrots, and other vegetables and fruits can be added each week to observe for any allergic reaction. Crackers, toast, teething biscuits, and zwieback toast can be started when the child starts teething and can sit up. A bagel that is frozen can be comforting for the child who is teething because it is hard to bite on and cool on the gums.

According to Sue, at about 6 to 8 months, an average serving size would be one-half cup of cereal, vegetable, and fruit each day. The routine for nursing and feeding can vary. For example, on waking, the mother can nurse and then give the solid food. At lunch that may be reversed. However, when introducing new food, give the solid food first before nursing, since a hungry baby is more likely to eat a new food.

Sue described that the breastfeeding mother may have the following feeding routine with her baby at 6 months.

6:00–6:30 a.m.	Breastfeed
8:30–9:00 a.m.	Rice cereal; breastfeed
12:00 noon	Vegetable/fruit; breastfeed
Mid-afternoon	Breastfeed
6:30 p.m.	Rice cereal with applesauce or breastfeed; a vegetable
8:30 p.m.	Breastfeed

Sue began to puree small chunks of meat at about 8 months; she started with white meat (by 8 months, chunky foods can be given). Unsweetened fruit juice was introduced at 8 months also. She diluted the juice with equal parts of water and gave 3 to 4 oz daily. If more than 4 oz of juice is given daily, the child may have dental problems from the sugar in the juice. Juice is given in a "sippy cup" to help the child learn to drink from a cup. Sue plans to follow the doctor's recommendation to add eggs at 1 year. Finely ground nuts or small amounts of peanut butter can also be given at 1 year. Sue will observe for possible allergy. No strawberries should be given until age 1 because of risk for allergy. Highly spiced, salty, and gas-forming foods should not be given until after 12 months of age, when the gastric secretions and motility are more developed. Solid foods should not have added sugar or salt. No honey should be given in any food because of possible infant botulism.

Sue plans to begin whole milk at 12 months. She will not use low-fat milk because the baby needs the fat and cholesterol in milk for normal brain development. Sue discussed that weaning should be initiated gradually. It is important not to wean during a crisis period, and it should not be done abruptly. She recommends dropping one feeding at a time and replacing that feeding with a bottle of whole milk and food (if baby is younger than 12 months).

At first, Sue nursed her son 8 times in 24 hours. By 10 months, she'll be nursing 4 times a day. She plans to allow 4 to 6 weeks to wean from the breast, since abrupt weaning can contribute to infection in the mother's breast caused by fullness from milk. The bedtime and awakening feedings will be the last to be stopped. She realizes that by 12 months the child will be able to eat solid foods; however, milk is still important in the diet.

The pediatrician continues to recommend later introduction of solid foods to avoid overfeeding and infant obesity (14% of 6-month-old infants are overweight) and risk of overweight adulthood.

When looking back upon the entire nursing experience, Sue is convinced her son is a healthier child emotionally and physically because of the months of nursing. That is why she plans to continue to nurse for the first year.

Contributed by Jill Burns, BS, RD.

FEEDING SCHEDULES AND WEANING

Weaning, *the gradual elimination of breastfeeding or bottle feeding in favor of cup and table feeding*, may be initiated about 6 months of age and is usually completed by the end of the first year. The baby shows signs of making this transition: muscle coordination increases, teeth erupt, appetite decreases, growth rate slows, and resistance to being held close while feeding is shown. The two methods should overlap and allow the baby to take some initiative and allow the mother to guide the new method. Her consistency in meeting the new feeding schedule is important to development of a sense of trust.

The most difficult feeding to give up is usually the bedtime feeding because the baby is tired and is more likely to want the "old method." After the maxillary central incisory teeth erupt, in order to reduce decay in the deciduous teeth, a night bottle should contain no carbohydrate. During periods of stress the baby will often regress. The baby is also learning to wait longer for food and may object vigorously to this new condition.

The need to suck varies with different children. Some children, even after weaning, will suck a thumb or use a pacifier (if provided). The baby should not be shamed for either of these habits because they are not likely to cause problems with the teeth or mouth during the first 2 years.

Teach parents the meaning of the baby's behavior and how to adapt to this new period of development. Assess for steady weight gain; normal developmental behavior; healthy-appearing hair, skin, teeth, and eyes; energy; ability to play and sleep; and infrequent colds or other infections.

CULTURAL INFLUENCES ON INFANT NUTRITION

Cultures vary in the extent to which they encourage breastfeeding. *Cultural values influence* (6): (a) women's perceptions about breastfeeding in terms of nutritional importance, (b) the father's beliefs and preferences, (c) acceptance of breast exposure, (d) sexuality issues, and (e) considerations related to convenience. For immigrant groups, bottle feeding may be viewed as more modern and prestigious.

In some cultures, for example Asian and Latino, breastfeeding is delayed for several days because colostrum is considered dirty and unacceptable. Some Latino women believe anger and stress in the mother produce "bad milk" and transmit illness and bad temper to her infant; thus, women with a bad temper may feel it is unwise to breastfeed (6). Some Asian-born immigrants have traditionally breastfed the baby for 1 to 3 years, after which the child is fed a plain diet of rice, lentils, some vegetables, occasionally eggs, fish, or fruit, and rarely meat. The Muslim parent, a vegetarian, cannot use, for religious purposes, commercially prepared baby food that has any meat product in it. They may occasionally eat animals slaughtered according to Muslim religious laws and rituals (meat is then classed as *halal*), but such meat is difficult to find in non-Islamic countries. Thus, eggs and milk are the primary sources of protein (6). Infant feeding and weaning patterns differ in many countries, including the dominant culture in the United States, United Kingdom, and Europe. The **Case Situation** gives an example of a Caucasian woman living in the United States; within one cultural group there can be considerable variations.

In some cultures, infants are given herbs to purge the intestines when they are a few days, weeks, or months of age to remove evil spirits from the body. Advise parents against the use of such purgatives because they cause fluid and electrolyte imbalance, and dehydration may occur rapidly.

In most cultures introduction of solid foods is associated with developmental markers, such as ability to hold up head, swallow, and sit with support; use of the tongue in motions besides sucking; reaching out for adult food; and tooth eruption. In some cultures, the mother is judged by when the baby is given adult food and by how much weight the baby gains (6, 99).

The use of *hot-cold* (**yin-yang**) *food practices* may be observed with Asian and Latino infants and children. See Chapter 5 for more information about hot-cold practices. ∞ Some parents refuse suggestions for certain foods or medicines because they violate hot-cold theory. Rather, the diet is to maintain or restore equilibrium or balance (6, 51, 53).

Discuss the infant's nutritional needs with the mother and other family members. Some culturally based practices can contribute to nutrient deficiencies. Careful developmental assessment and family teaching is necessary. When you or the physician suggests that the mother offer "table food" to the infant, ask what table food is in their home. Depending on the level of the household hygiene or the family food pattern, table food may or may not constitute an adequate or healthy diet. Family diet counseling may be necessary to ensure continued health of the family unit. Food supplies not only physical sustenance but also many personal and cultural needs. The introduction of foods characteristic of a culture provides the foundation for lifelong food habits and the basis for teaching a cultural pattern of eating.

Sleep Patterns

The baby should be placed on the back to sleep. Sleep patterns for baby vary with: (a) amount of active awake time, and later activity or exercise time; (b) feeding method and schedule (bottle-fed babies sleep for longer periods, especially at night, than do breastfed babies); (c) whether co-sleep is practiced; and (d) cultural or home practices related to fostering regular bedtime and consistent sleep rituals. Sleep patterns are unique to each infant, but some generalizations can be made.

The following is a typical sleep pattern (14, 99):

1. **Newborn** —Sleeps 16 to 20 hours daily. Rapid eye movement (REM) sleep starts the cycle and constitutes 50% of sleep.
2. **4 weeks** —Sleeps for longer period during night.
3. **6 weeks** —May sleep 6 hours at night without awakening. Not consistent.
4. **3 to 4 months** —Sleeps 14 to 15 hours daily and 9 to 11 hours through the night. More time in quiet sleep; 40% of sleep time is REM sleep. Morning and afternoon naps continue, but awake longer periods during day.
5. **8 months** —Sleeps about 8 hours at night without awakening. Daytime naps are shorter.

6. **12 months**—Sleeps through the night, about 12 to 14 hours. Naps once or twice daily for 1 to 4 hours. Morning naps are eliminated first (14, 87, 99).

The infant exhibits different levels of arousal (99):

1. **Regular or quiet sleep:** *Eyes are closed, breathing is regular, and the only movements are sudden, generalized startle motions. Baby makes little sound. This is the low point of arousal;* infant cannot be awakened with mild stimuli.

2. **Irregular, active rapid eye movement (REM) sleep:** *Eyes are closed. Breathing is irregular; rate of respirations is increased. Muscles twitch slightly from time to time. Facial responses of smiles or pouts in response to sounds or lights. Baby may groan, make faces, or cry briefly.*

3. **Quiet wakefulness:** *Eyes are open, the body is more active, breathing is irregular, and there is varying spontaneous response to external stimuli.*

4. **Active wakefulness:** *Eyes are open; there is visual following of interesting sights and sounds, body movements, and vocalizations that elicit attention.*

5. **Crying:** *Intensity of sounds ranges from sniffles to wailing.*

6. **Indeterminate state:** *Transition is made from one state of alertness to another.*

As the infant's nervous system develops, he or she will have longer periods of sleep and wakefulness that gradually become more regular. By *6 weeks*, biological rhythms usually coincide with daytime and nighttime hours. *Sleep is essential; growth hormone is released during sleep.* Some babies have chronic sleeplessness, which may result from an allergy to formula or cow's milk; if so, a suitable milk substitute should be used (44). Other conditions could be present. A pediatrician should be contacted.

Help parents understand that when a baby goes through the stage of separation anxiety at about 8 months of age, bedtime becomes more difficult because he or she does not want to leave mother or other people. Because the baby needs sleep, the parent should be firm about getting the child ready for bed. Prolonging bedtime adds to fatigue. A consistent routine and regular bedtime is important. Caressing or singing softly while holding the baby in a sleeping position in bed is calming. If the mother is available when the baby first awakes, he or she anticipates this pleasure, and sleep is associated with the return of mother. If the baby awakes and cries during the night, the parent should wait briefly. Many times the crying will subside. Persistent crying indicates unmet needs and should be attended.

Teach parents that the infant should have a consistent place for sleeping (be it box, drawer, or crib) and a clean area for supplies. A baby can sleep comfortably in an infant crib or bassinet during the first few weeks, but as soon as active arms and legs begin to hit the sides, he or she should be moved to a full-sized crib. The crib slats should be no more than 2.5 in. apart. No pillows should be used. The crib should have a crib border placed at the bottom of the slats to prevent catching the head between the bars. It should be fitted with a firm, waterproof, easy-to-clean mattress and with warm light covers loosely tucked in. The sides of the crib should fit closely to the mattress so that the infant will not get caught and crushed if he or she should roll to the edge. Thin plastic sheeting can cause suffocation and should never be used on or around the baby's crib. Advise parents that cribs made of composite wood and particle board contain high levels of formaldehyde, which can emit gas for years and is a source of air pollution. See Chapter 4 for description of formaldehyde as a pollutant. ∞ An older used crib may be preferable to a new one, since the older piece of furniture is more likely to be made from real wood and will not be toxic. However, check about width between slats.

Co-sleep, or **shared sleeping**, when *the baby sleeps in the bed with the parent(s),* is frowned on in the United States. However, this is considered normal in some cultures. Co-sleep can help the baby regulate respiration, heart rate, and body temperature in cold climates and is convenient for breastfeeding. Because of the baby's movements, it may be difficult for the parents to sleep, and the baby between the parents decreases their intimacy. It can be difficult to get the child to break this habit. There has been a higher risk of SIDS associated with co-sleep. Further, the baby can get wedged between the bed frame and mattress or be rolled on by the parent (56).

Rates of SIDS are lower because parents are following recommendations for positioning the infant during sleep. SIDS may have other causes; the occurrence is higher in infants whose mothers smoke tobacco or use addictive drugs (87, 99).

Play Activity

Play promotes health and holistic development. The infant engages in play with self: with the hands or feet, by rolling, by getting into various positions, and with the sounds he or she produces. The baby can remain satisfied playing with self for increasing amounts of time but prefers to have people around. He or she enjoys being held briefly in various positions, being rocked, swinging for short periods, and being taken for walks. The baby needs playful activity from both the mother and father to stimulate development in all spheres.

Certain toys are usually enjoyed at certain ages because of changing needs and developing skills. **Box 9-6**, Guide to Play Activities, lists age, characteristics that influence play interest, and suggested activities, toys, and equipment.

Because much of a baby's play involves putting objects into the mouth, a clean environment with lead-free paint is important. A small object that the baby swallows, such as a coin, is passed through the digestive tract; however, small batteries used in electronic toys may be hazardous if swallowed because they can rupture and release poisonous chemicals. Surgical removal may be necessary. Children gradually build an immunity to the germs encountered daily on various objects; however, health may be threatened by that which goes unnoticed. Sitting and playing in dirt or sand contaminated by dioxin, other pesticides or herbicides, or radiation is dangerous to the developing physiologic systems. Chapter 4 discusses such health threats in greater detail. ∞ Children's or parents' reading material, which can become play objects, may also be hazardous. The high lead content of the glossy color pages of magazines and newspaper inserts may account for some cases of lead poisoning in young children, who are eaters of the inedible. Although black-and-white newsprint, the comics, and black-and-white magazine stock are scarcely recommended for snacking, their lead content is dramatically lower than that of the shiny, colored pages. Ideally, the child does not eat paper; yet

BOX 9-6	Guide to Play Activities	

Age	Characteristics Development	Suggested Activities & Equipment
4 weeks	Tonic neck reflex position	Much tender loving care
	Rolls partway to side	Mobiles and other hanging objects that can be followed by
	Disregards ring in midplane	eyes but can't be grasped—bright in color
	Eyes follow ring in midplane	Musical mobiles
	Hand clutches on contact	
	Drops rattle immediately	
	Attends bell	
	Activity diminishes	
	Marked head lag when pulled to sitting position	
	Head sags forward; back evenly rounded	
	Head rotation; in prone position	
	Startles easily to sudden sounds or movements	
16 weeks	Head position in midplane	Enjoys cuddling and motion
	Plays with hands at midplane	Cradle gym for brief periods (20–30 minutes)
	Regards ring immediately, arms activate	Rattles
	Holds rattle in fist	Soft, stuffed, small toys to touch and squeeze
	Head fairly steady in sitting position	Soothing music (humming, singing, phonograph records)
	On verge of rolling	Rattles, bells, musical toys
	Laughs aloud; coos; carries on "conversation"	Crinkling paper, clap, or snap of fingers
	Spontaneous social smile	Large wooden or nonsplintering plastic toys, beads, spools
	Knows mother; stares at strangers	
	Smiles at strangers who are friendly	
28 weeks	Transfers small toys (blocks, bells, etc.) from one hand to the other	Small toys
		Soothing music
	Mouths objects	Cradle gym (30–40 minutes)
	Lifts head in supine position	Peek-a-boo
	Reaches with one hand	Pat-a-cake
	Sits momentarily by self leaning on hands	Noise makers (bells, squeak toys)
	Feet to mouth	Moderately active bouncing on lap
	Regards Image in mirror	Use of mirror to see self and others
	Polysyllabic vowel sounds	Outdoor excursions—walks
	Bounces actively	Reading to child, letting child touch and pat books
	Prompt grasp	Splashing in water, water toys
	Pivots in prone position	
	Plays contentedly alone	
40 weeks	Knocks blocks together in hands	Small one-square-inch blocks
	Approaches objects with index finger	Soft, small toys
	Prehends pellet with inferior pincer grasp	Assorted objects of varying color having interesting texture
	Grasps bell by handle and waves it	Peek-a-boo
	Sits with good control	Pat-a-cake
	Goes from sitting to prone position	Rides in buggy or stroller
	Creeps	Parallel play
	Pulls to standing position	Is fascinated with words and other sounds
	Waves bye-bye	Nesting, stack, or climbing boxes and blocks
	Increasing imitation	Kitchen utensils
	Adjusts to simple commands	Bath toys
		Cups and boxes to pour (water, sand) and fill

(continued)

BOX 9-6	Guide to Play Activities *(continued)*	

Age	Characteristics Development	Suggested Activities & Equipment
12 months	Walks with help	Open and close simple boxes
	Throws and rolls ball	Empty and fill toys
	Offers objects, but frequently does not release them	Push-pull toys
		Strongly strung large beads
	Vocabulary of 3–10 words	Small, brightly colored blocks
	Vigorous imitative scribble	Rag and oil cloth books
		Balls, bells, floating bath toys
		Cuddle toys
		Nursery rhymes
		Music and singing to child

most children have been observed sucking or chewing on corners of magazines or pieces of paper.

Toys need not be expensive, but they should be colorful (and without leaded paint), safe, sturdy, and easily handled and cleaned. They should be large enough to prevent aspiration or ingestion. They should be without rough or sharp edges or points, detachable parts, or loops to get around the neck. Some should make sounds and have moving parts. Some household items can be used for toys to provide fun and stimulate creativity, perhaps more so than some of the expensive toys on the market. The best educational toys are likely to be in household cupboards and closets.

A baby needs an unrestricted play area, such as the floor, that is clean and safe; use of a playpen may be necessary for short periods. Excess restriction or lack of stimulation inhibits curiosity, learning about self and the environment, and development of trust. Therefore, the baby should not wear clothing that is restraining and should not be kept constantly in a playpen or crib.

Stationary play stations, such as an exersaucer play gym that turns, rocks, and bounces, should be used no more than 20 minutes a day. If overused, the baby is likely to have poor posture and weak back and stomach muscles and delay walking. The child learns through activity. Babies need supervised "tummy time" and "scoot time" and a clean, safe floor to develop back, neck, abdominal, and buttock muscles. He or she needs play objects and loving parents who provide stimulating surroundings.

Teach parents how to touch, cuddle, talk to, and play with their baby. Parents should know the dangers of overstimulation and rough handling. Fatigue, inattention, and injury may result. The playful, vigorous activities that well-intentioned parents engage in, such as tossing the baby forcefully into the air or jerking the baby in a whiplash manner, may cause bone injuries or subdural hematomas and cerebrovascular lesions that later could cause physical or mental retardation. Compared to full-term female babies, premature infants and male babies are twice as vulnerable because of the relative immaturity of their brains.

Teach parents about the importance of avoiding plastic toys, especially those made outside of the United States, which contain polyvinyl chloride (PVC). Instead, select toys crafted from wood or cloth. Knowing the craftsman or manufacturing source ensures an environmentally safe product.

Health Promotion and Health Protection

At birth the neonate should have an antibiotic ointment instilled in the eyes to prevent gonococcal or chlamydial ophthalmia neonatorum. The possibility of blindness in the infant, along with the low cost and effectiveness of the treatment, makes this procedure mandatory (47, 56).

Injecting 1 mg of vitamin K is effective in preventing hemorrhagic disease, which is caused in 1 of 2,000 to 1 of 3,000 live births by a transient deficiency of factor VIII production. Sickle-cell screening can be obtained from in-cord blood (47, 56).

During the first week of life the infant should be screened for **phenylketonuria (PKU),** *an inborn metabolic disorder characterized by abnormal presence of phenylketone and other metabolites of phenylalanine in the urine.* Screening for thyroid function, hemoglobin abnormalities, sickle-cell anemia, galactosemia, congenital adrenal hyperplasia, and other disorders is recommended for all newborns (47, 56).

IMMUNIZATIONS

Immunizations, *promoting disease resistance through injection of attenuated, weakened organisms or products produced by organisms,* are essential to every infant as a disease prevention and health promotion measure. Before birth, the baby is protected from certain organisms by the placental barrier and the mother's physical defense mechanisms. Birth propels the baby into an environment filled with many microorganisms. The baby has protection against common pathogens for 4 to 6 months, but as he or she is gradually exposed to the outside world and the people in it, further protection is needed through routine immunizations, available from private physicians or public health clinics. Annually, millions of children in the developing world either are permanently disabled or die from childhood diseases that are preventable.

Immunization schedules change frequently as new knowledge is gained and new vaccines are developed. Recommendations for childhood immunizations are based on agreement of the Advisory Committee on Immunization Practices, the American Academy of Pediatrics, and the American Academy of Family Physicians. The recommended childhood and adolescent immunization schedules and catch-up schedules for children are available on the Websites of the three organizations:

American Academy of Pediatrics, www.aap.org

American Academy of Family Physicians, www.aafp.org

American Academy of Immunization Practice, www.cdc.gov.

Instruct parents about the importance of immunizations. Further, parents should be helped to get them, for example, through flexible clinic hours or low-cost mass immunizations in a community. *Parents should also keep a continuing record of the child's immunizations.* Your teaching, encouragement, community efforts, and follow-up are vital.

A mailed reminder about the date for immunization increases the chances that the infant will receive the scheduled immunization, especially in families that have a record of not keeping clinic appointments. A telephone reminder may help in getting mothers to return for well-baby immunizations.

DENTAL HEALTH

Dental health begins with maternal dental care and health and parental counseling during early infancy about dietary intake for promotion of optimal oral health. For example, the milk bottle should not be propped or given to the infant lying in bed, to avoid both aspiration and milk remaining in the mouth, which can contribute to dental caries. Fruit juices should not be given in the bottle before 6 months of age. Foods with concentrated sugar should be avoided. Cleaning of teeth should begin when primary teeth begin erupting. Teeth and gums should be initially cleaned by wiping with a damp cloth. A toothbrush should not be used because it could injure the tender gingiva. Stabilize the baby's head by cradling it with one arm and using the free hand to cleanse the teeth. Nearer 1 year of age, as more teeth erupt, a small, soft-bristled toothbrush dipped in water should be used to help the infant adjust to the routine of cleaning (56). An oral health examination by 6 months of age by pediatric health practitioners is recommended. Between 6 and 12 months infants at risk for dental caries should be seen by a dentist.

Fluoride is needed beginning at 6 months of age if the water is not fluoridated. Fluoride should not be given if the water supply is fluoridated to avoid **dental fluorosis,** *a discoloration of the teeth enamel.* Excess fluoride may also contribute to dental caries (56).

SAFETY PROMOTION AND INJURY CONTROL

Safety measures are discussed in the previous sections on sleep and play. Safety promotion and injury control are based on the understanding of infant behavior. Accidents and injuries are a major cause of death. *Risk factors that influence the occurrence of fatal childhood accidents include* (56, 65, 91): (a) host factors, such as age, gender, and developmental characteristics, such as increased mobility combined with insatiable curiosity; (b) environmental factors, such as hazardous play equipment, flammable clothing, and accessible poisons; (c) parental characteristics, such as socioeconomic status; and (d) developmental characteristics, such as increased mobility. Differences in infant mortality are noted in terms of socioeco-

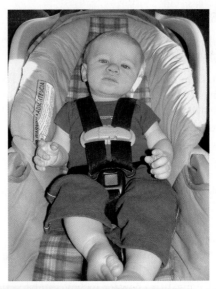

FIGURE ■ 9-5 Infants should be transported in an appropriate automobile infant seat or restraint.

nomic and educational variables. Substantial differences in infant mortality between the various ethnic and racial groups have been documented (6).

The main causes of death for the infant are drowning; suffocation by inhalation, by ingestion of food, or by mechanical means (in bed or cradle, by plastic bag, or by polystyrene-filled pillows); transport accidents; and falls. Contrary to common belief, the baby is not immobile. He or she will not necessarily stay where placed. A baby rolls, crawls, creeps, walks, reaches, and explores. The baby should never be left alone or with an irresponsible person while in water. A baby is helpless in water, unable to swim or lift the head above water level. The home and car have many often unnoticed hazards; thus, the baby should never be left alone at home or in a vehicle. Parents should use an approved car infant seat or restraint, as depicted in **Figure 9-5■**.

Prevent Falls

Falls can be avoided if the parents, nurse, or caregiver are responsible for doing the following:

1. Keep crib rails up at full height and securely fastened.
2. Maintain a firm grasp of the baby while carrying or caring for him or her and support the head during the first few months.
3. Use a sturdy high chair and federally approved car infant seat.
4. Strap the child securely in a high chair and grocery cart, if used.
5. Lock windows if the infant can climb onto windowsills.
6. Have a gate in front of windows or doors, especially those above the first story. Keep external doors locked, including the first floor.
7. Keep rooms free of loose rugs or trailing cables or cords.
8. Keep doors to stairways locked; have a gate at the top and bottom of stairs.
9. Keep furniture, lamps, and heavy or breakable objects secure so the child does not pull them on self.
10. Clean up spills immediately from the floor.

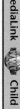

Prevent Suffocation

Suffocation at home and in the health care setting can be avoided through the following actions:

1. Remove any small objects from the floor or accessible surroundings that could be inhaled or ingested, such as safety pins, small beads, coins, toys, paper clips, parts of broken toys, balloons, string, and buttons.
2. Avoid access to food that may not be adequately chewed and may be aspirated, such as nuts, grapes, dried beans, peas, raisins, popcorn, chips, and pretzels.
3. Keep plastic bags, venetian blind cords, or other cords out of reach.
4. Avoid use of pillows or bumper pads in the crib or excessively tight clothing or bedcovers.
5. Choose stair gates with openings too small for the head; avoid accordion or expandable gates.
6. Avoid shaking baby powder or any similar product which would cause a cloud of dust.

Prevent Burns

Burns can be avoided through the following actions:

1. Test temperature of bath water and liquids or food to be consumed. Avoid use of microwave.
2. Use warm-air vaporizers with caution.
3. Disconnect unused appliances; cover electric outlets.
4. Avoid tablecloths that hang over the table's edge, especially when hot food is on the table.
5. Place crib, play materials, and high chair away from heaters, fans, radiators, or fireplaces.
6. Turn pot handles inward on the stove.
7. Avoid excessive sun exposure; use sunscreen.
8. Avoid smoking around the baby.
9. Use sturdy screens in front of the fireplace; keep child away from the stove.
10. Purchase flame-retardant sleepwear; discard after repeated laundering.

Prevent Motor Vehicle Injury

Motor vehicle safety must be enforced:

1. Use a proper-sized child restraint in the back seat of car; avoid seat placement where air bag deployment or impact may occur. **Figure 9-5** gives an example.
2. Avoid confinement in poorly ventilated vehicles, especially during hot weather.
3. Never leave the infant alone in the car.

Teaching parents about the child's normal developmental pattern will also enable them to foresee potential accidents and take precautions. For example, medicines, cleaning products, and all hazardous substances should be kept locked and out of reach, especially as the infant becomes more mobile. *Encourage parents to take a first aid course* (one directed toward cardiopulmonary resuscitation, preventing airway obstruction, and other home and family safety concerns) that enables them to recognize hazards and take appropriate measures to avoid injury to loved ones.

Parents must also consider another threat to the safety of the child and to the integrity of their family unit: stealing, kidnapping, or abduction of their infant. See Chapter 10 for more information about child abduction. ∞

Refer parents to the following Websites for safety information:

1. American Academy of Pediatrics, www.aap.org
2. American Association of Poison Control Centers, www. 1-800-222-1222.info
3. U.S. Consumer Product Safety Commission, www.cpsc.gov

COMMON HEALTH PROBLEMS: PREVENTION AND PROTECTION

Various conditions may occur in the infant. Refer also to Chapter 4 for illnesses that can result from various teratogens. ∞

Because of the contact with a variety of microorganisms, infants who are in day care centers or small group care have more respiratory infections than those who are reared entirely at home. However, when children raised entirely at home go to school, their illness rates are likely to be higher because of exposure to new germs (56).

Counsel parents about careful selection of day care services in relation to hygiene measures that are followed, the number of babies and children being served, and policies related to the ill child. Counsel parents against the harmful effects of smoking, both passive and active. The *incidence of acute respiratory disease, bronchitis, and pneumonia increases with the increasing number of cigarettes smoked by the mother or other family members, particularly in infants age 6 to 9 months.* Infants of smoking mothers have significantly more admissions for bronchitis or pneumonia and more injuries. In households in which the mother smokes, the infant's urine cotinine levels are higher, especially in breastfed babies during nonsummer months (35). However, infants in a family in which any member smokes will suffer the effects of passive smoking from absorption of environmental tobacco smoke.

Dental caries can be a problem beginning in late infancy. Fluoride concentration of the water supply must be determined by age 6 months, since tooth formation is occurring. If the water supply has less than 0.6 ppm, fluoride supplementation based on age should be explored.

Refer to the **Box** in Chapter 8 ∞ *Healthy People 2010:* Example of Objectives for Maternal and Infant Health Promotion, for a perspective on major health concerns and prevention strategies in the United States formulated by the U.S. Department of Health and Human Services (108).

Psychosocial Concepts

The *intellectual, emotional, and social components can be combined into what is often referred to as* **psychosocial development**. The separation of these facets of growth is artificial, for they are closely interrelated. Similarly, psychosocial, physical, and motor development greatly influence each other. Babies are born cognitively flexible rather than with preset instinctual behavior. A level of physiologic maturation of the nervous system must be present before environmental stimulation and learning opportunities can be effective in promoting emotional and cognitive development. In turn, *without responsive people, consistent love, and tactile, kinesthetic, verbal, and other environmental stimuli, some nervous system structures do not develop.* Babies adapt and react to the environment with which they are confronted. Low-birth-weight and premature infants have neurologic deficits that predispose to an increased risk for developmental delays, and they are apt to have behavioral styles that are more difficult to handle, which reduces maternal involvement and the stimulation needed for development (16, 47, 56, 110, 111).

COGNITIVE DEVELOPMENT

Intelligence is the *ability to learn or understand from experience, to acquire and retain knowledge, to respond to a new situation, and to solve problems.* It is a system of living and acting developed in a sequential pattern through relating to the environment. Each stage of operations serves as a foundation for the next life era (89). **Cognitive behavior** includes *thinking, perceiving, remembering, forming concepts, making judgments, generalizing,* and *abstracting.* Cognitive development depends on innate capacity, maturation, nutrition, gross and fine motor stimulation, touch, appropriate stimulation of all senses through various activities, language, and social interaction (15, 16, 109–111). *Thus, the home environment is crucial for intellectual development.*

Sequence in Intellectual Development

The infant is in the ***Sensorimotor Period of cognitive development*** (89, 90, 109). The sequence described by Piaget corresponds rather roughly in time span to those described for emotional development.

The infant arrives in the world as an active learner with great potential for intellectual development, but at birth intellectual capacities are undifferentiated. Piaget's theory laid a foundation for other research. More complex technology, such as electroencephalograms and magnetic resonance imagery, as well as audio and videotape recordings add to data collection and analysis of infant intelligence (77). Piaget's descriptions of general trends of cognitive development remain relevant, even though current research can give us detailed moment-by-moment or neuron-by-neuron descriptions (14, 16, 87, 99, 111).

STAGE 1: The Reflex Stage *This stage covers the neonatal period when behavior is entirely reflexive.* Yet all stimuli are being assimilated into beginning mental images through reflexive behavior and from human contact (89, 90). **Visible imitation,** *the ability to imitate facial movements that are observed,* such as sticking out the tongue, begins during this period (87). Refer also to **Table 9-3**, Assessment of Infant Reflexes.

STAGE 2: Primary Circular Reactions *Primary circular reactions are response patterns where a stimulus creates a response and gratifying behavior is repeated.* At 1 to 4 months, life is still a series of random events, but hand–mouth and ear–eye coordination is developing (89, 90). The infant's eyes follow moving objects; eyes and ears follow sounds and novel stimuli. The 1-month-old infant demonstrates habituation and dishabituation. The infant discriminates between stimuli, such as the sounds "*ba*" and "*pa*" or a circle with or without dots in the center. **Habituation** *is losing interest or becoming bored with repeated exposure to the same stimuli.* **Dishabituation,** *an increase in responsiveness after a change in stimulation,* is indicated by a longer or more focused gaze, change in heart rate, or change in tension of muscles around the mouth. The alert parent or caretaker responds to the infant's habituation to foster continued learning (87, 99). Responses to different objects vary. Baby begins to look for objects removed from sight, a beginning object permanence. Beginning intention of behavior is seen; he or she reproduces behavior previously done. For example, the 8-week-old infant can purposefully apply pressure to a pillow to make a mobile rotate, smile in response to familiar faces, and anticipate a routine such as diapering.

STAGE 3: Secondary Circular Reactions From 4 to 8 months, *a baby learns to initiate and recognize new experiences and repeat pleasurable ones. Intentional behavior is seen* (89, 90). Increasing mobility and hand control help him or her become more oriented to the environment. Reaching, grasping, listening, and laughing become better coordinated. Memory traces continue to be established. The baby anticipates familiar events or a moving object's position. After 6 months, **explicit memory,** *ability to consciously recall the immediate past,* is demonstrated (30, 77). **Categorization,** *ability to grasp at objects by basic function,* is beginning (87). The child repeats or prolongs interesting events. Activities that accidentally brought a new experience are repeated. Habits developed in previous stages are incorporated with new actions. The baby will imitate behavior if it is familiar and not too complex, as described in the Case Situation.

STAGE 4: Coordination of Secondary Schemata From 8 to 12 months, *the baby's behavior is showing clear acts of intelligence and experimentation. The baby uses certain activities to attain basic goals. He or she realizes that someone other than self can cause activity, and activity of self is separate from movement of objects* (89, 90). **Object permanence** *has developed; the infant realizes an object or person continues to exist even when out of sight.* He or she *intentionally* searches for and retrieves a toy that has disappeared from view. Shapes and sizes of familiar objects are recognized, regardless of the perspective from which they are viewed. Because of the baby's ability to differentiate objects and people from self and the increased sense of separateness, he or she experiences separation anxiety or seventh or eighth month anxiety when the mothering figure leaves. The baby is more mobile. Sitting, creeping, standing, or walking gives a new perception of the environment. The baby understands familiar words that are spoken. Thus coordination of schema involves using one idea or mental image to attain a goal and a second idea or image to deal with the end result. The baby systematically imitates another while observing another's behavior (56, 89, 90, 109, 111). **Deferred imitation,** *the ability to imitate actions seen a day earlier,* occurs by 9 months (77).

Reaffirm with parents that they can greatly influence the child's later intellectual abilities by the stimulation they provide, the loving attention they give, and the freedom they allow for their baby to explore and use his or her body in the environment. Many educational toys are on the market, but common household items can be made into educational toys. For example, a mobile of ribbons and colorful cutouts will attract as much attention as an expensive mobile from the store. Unbreakable salt and pepper shakers or small cardboard boxes partly filled with rice, sand, or pebbles and then taped securely shut make good rattles. Various sizes of pots, pans, lids, and unbreakable plastic wastebaskets or smooth blocks are effective play objects. Use **Box 9-7**, Examples of Educational Toys for the Infant, as a guide for teaching parents. Well-selected toys promote health and well-being.

COMMUNICATION, SPEECH, AND LANGUAGE DEVELOPMENT

Communication between people involves facial expressions, body movements, other nonverbal behavior, vocalizations, speech, and use of language. A newborn is ready to communicate if parents and caretakers know how to read the messages. The first communications are through eye contact, crying, and body movements. Emotions are the first language with which the parent and infant communicate (1).

Speech awareness *begins before birth. In utero the fetus hears a melody of language,* equivalent to overhearing two people talk through the walls of a motel room. *This creates a sensitivity that after birth provides the child with clues about sounds that accompany each other.* If babies have been read to *in utero,* after birth they appear to prefer the sound of the stories they had heard *in utero* (64, 87, 99).

Speech is the *ability to utter sounds.* **Language** refers to *the mother tongue of a group of people,* or the *combination of sounds into a meaningful whole to communicate thoughts and feelings.* Speech development begins with the cry at birth, and the cry remains the basic form of communication for the infant. The newborn cries an

Case Situation

Infant Development

Michael, 8 months old, is sitting on the lap of his babysitter, Aunt Jennifer, who is reading a story to him. Aunt Jennifer smiles and chuckles as she reads. Michael responds by mimicking her mouth movements. She says "Ooooohh" with a widened O-shaped mouth, and Michael imitates the O-shape of her mouth while she speaks. Michael makes a long, loud "Ooooohh" sound. Aunt Jennifer responds with smiles and exclamations of enthusiasm, recognizing his achievement. Michael smiles and continues to repeat "Ooooohh."

Michael then attempts to imitate Aunt Jennifer's actions in reading the book. He reaches toward the book and makes babbling sounds as he swats at the book. Michael's coordination of vision, hearing, and tactile senses as he repeatedly imitates his aunt's facial expressions, reaches for the book, and engages in prespeech babbling demonstrates a common behavior of children in this age group. These behaviors demonstrate Piaget's Stage 3, Secondary Circular Reactions of the Sensorimotor Stage, of cognitive development.

Contributed by Ruth Murray, EdD, MSN, N-NAP, FAAN.

BOX 9-7	Examples of Educational Toys for the Infant

1–3 Months—Mobiles, unbreakable mirrors, and large colorful rings attached over crib; rattles of various sizes and geometric shapes; stuffed animals with black and white patterns; music boxes or tapes of music—need to change the tune and words from time to time.

4–6 Months—Plastic or paper streamers attached over crib, so child sees but cannot chew or choke on them; squeaky toys; colorful stuffed animals that are not too large; small beach ball or soft plastic ball; chunky bracelets; books made of cloth or vinyl; small barriers that encourage playing peek-a-boo.

7–9 Months—Larger stuffed animals, without buttons or small parts that can be detached and cause choking; nesting cylinders of various size, unbreakable cartons; pop-up toys; cloth blocks; large dolls and puppets; bath toys; mirror available so child can see self during adult play of "so big" and pat-a-cake.

10–12 Months—Push-pull toys; household objects like empty egg cartons or large spoons; stacked rings on a spindle; balls—soft, of various sizes and colors.

Note: Toys or items like a music box or audiotape that were enjoyed in the prior months continue to be enjoyed throughout infancy, especially if they are not continuously available.

average of 1 to 4 hours a day. *A baby's cry is initially undifferentiated.* Parents learn to distinguish the meanings of different cries and grunts the baby makes. At first the baby responds to both soothing and distressing stimuli with similar sounds. Then *other prespeech sounds are as follows* (64, 99):

1. **Cooing**, *the soft murmur or hum of contentment,* beginning at 2 to 3 months.
2. **Babbling**, *incoherent sounds made by playing with sounds,* beginning before 6 months. The number of sounds produced by babbling gradually increases, reaches a peak at 8 months, and gives way for true speech and language development.
3. *Squealing* and *grunting.*
4. **Lalling**, *the movement of the tongue with crying and vocalization,* such as "m-m-m."
5. *Sucking sounds.*

Smiles, frowns, and other facial expressions often accompany the baby's vocalizations, as do gestures of reaching or withdrawing to convey feelings.

The brain's linguistic processes arise from a genetic coordination of a variety of brain structures that produce speech and language development. These processes are heavily dependent on environment and experience. A sensitive critical period exists for initial learning of language. If there is insufficient stimuli and interaction directed to the infant during the period when the brain is most ready, the infant, and later the child, may be impaired in speech and language development. Yet, when there is brain injury, the plasticity of the brain appears to allow these functions to be transferred from damaged to other regions of the brain (87, 99).

At first vocalizations are reflexive: No difference exists between the vocalizations of hearing babies and deaf babies before 6 months of age. Later, vocalizations are self-reinforcing; that is, the baby finds pleasure and reinforcement in making and hearing his or her own sounds, and responses from others provide further reinforcement. Reinforcement when desired sounds are made and when certain sounds are omitted is necessary for the infant to progress to language development. The child must also hear others speak to reinforce further the use of the sounds and language of the culture. Effective mothers speak to their children frequently, even while they are doing their housework (87). *Infants do not learn language by just listening to an audiotape or watching television* (111).

The *deaf baby of deaf parents* imitates their sign language and engages in **hand babbling,** *repeating motions over and over that are at random.* Parents reinforce appropriate gestures. The deaf baby may make up his or her own sign language. Inborn language capacity may underlay signed as well as spoken language (67, 74, 87, 88, 99). Parents are now teaching hearing babies to sign before they speak. The 4- to 6-month-old baby can learn to sign and convey needs that cannot yet be spoken.

From *birth to 7 months*, the baby is a **universal linguist** *capable of distinguishing 150 sounds that make up human speech* (14, 87, 111). By *9 months* the baby will have made every sound basic to any human language. The sounds made in infancy are universal, but when he or she learns a language, the potential to say all universal sounds is lost (87, 99).

At every age the child comprehends the meaning of what others say more readily than he or she can put thoughts and feelings into words. In speech comprehension, the child first associates certain words with visual, tactile, and other sensations aroused by objects in the environment. Between *9 and 12 months*, a baby learns to recognize his or her name and the names of several familiar objects, responds to "no," echoes and imitates sounds, repeats syllables, and may occasionally obey the parent's command (87).

The baby tries to articulate words from sounds heard. Words are invented, such as "didi" to mean a toy or food. By trial and error, by imitation, and as a result of reinforcement from others, the baby makes the first recognizable words, such as "mama," "dada," "no," and "bye-bye" between *10 and 18 months*. If the correct sound is directed to the appropriate parent, the sound is reinforced, and the baby continues speech. The parent is using operant conditioning, described in Chapter 1. ∞ Words such as "mama" and "nana" are universal to babies in every culture because they result from the sounds the infant normally makes in babbling (6, 53). By *12 months*, babies have a vocabulary of at least six words. Nouns typically are learned first. Meaning is associated with an object, such as its name, size, shape, use, and sound. Then a word becomes a symbol or label for the object. Learning to speak involves pronouncing words, building a vocabulary, distinguishing between sounds such as "p*e*t" and "p*a*t" or "*h*ear" and "*n*ear" and then making a sentence. The baby's first sentence usually consists of one word and a gesture (14, 87, 99).

Teach parents that many factors influence speech and language development: (a) innate intelligence, (b) ability to hear, (c) modification of the anatomic structures of the mouth and throat, (d) sense of curiosity, (e) parental verbal stimulation and interest, and

(f) encouragement to imitate others. Communication with others is essential for health throughout life.

EMOTIONAL DEVELOPMENT

In addition to the core problem or crisis at each level of development, the infant has other tasks to accomplish that relate to the psychosocial crisis, such as learning to walk and talk. Emotional or personality development is a continuous process. Emotional and social development occur together.

Babies differ from each other in several characteristics, which are demonstrated over the year and affect others' responsiveness. *These characteristics are* (21, 31):

1. Activity level or movement.
2. Rhythmicity; consistency in schedule (regular or irregular in routine—easy versus difficult to care for).
3. Approach to or withdrawal from something new (easy or difficult child to care for).
4. Adaptability, adjust quickly to new experiences (easy child to care for).
5. Intensity of reaction when crying, smiling, or laughing.
6. Threshold of responsiveness, reaction to sensory stimuli (positive, irregular, or low mood response).
7. Quality of mood (happy and positive, cry frequently, or slow to warm up).
8. Attention span and distractibility.

DEVELOPMENTAL CRISIS: TRUST VERSUS MISTRUST

According to Erikson (46), the psychosexual crisis for infancy is trust versus mistrust. **Basic trust** involves *confidence, optimism, acceptance of and reliance on self and others, faith that others can satisfy needs, and a sense of hope or a belief in the attainability of wishes in spite of problems and without overestimation of results.* A sense of trust forms the basis for a sense of hope and for later identity formation, social responsiveness to others, and ability to care about and love others. Over time, the person accepts self, develops reachable goals, assumes life will be manageable, and expects people and situations to be positive. *A sense of trust may be demonstrated in the newborn and infant by* (a) ease of feeding, (b) depth of sleep, (c) relaxation of the bowels, and (d) overall appearance of contentment. **Mistrust** is a *sense of not feeling satisfied emotionally or physically, an inability to believe in or rely on others or self.* See **Box 9-8**, Consequences of Mistrust in the infant, and later in the child and adult.

Teach parents that security and trust are fostered by the prompt, loving, and consistent response to the infant's distress and needs and by the positive response to happy, contented behavior. *Teach parents that they do not "spoil" a baby by promptly answering the distress signal—his or her cry. Rather, they are teaching trust* by relieving tension (1, 99). Parents should understand the meaning they convey through such care as changing diapers. Even if the techniques are not the best, the baby will sense the positive attitude if it exists. If the parents repeatedly fail to meet primary needs, fear, anger, insecurity, and eventual mistrust result. If the most important people fail him or her, there is little foundation on which to build faith in others or self. The world cannot be

<table>
<tr><td colspan="2">**BOX 9-8**   **Consequences of Mistrust**</td></tr>
</table>

INFANT

1. Is lethargic
2. Fails to gain weight
3. Eats poorly
4. Sleeps poorly
5. Experiences excessive, persistent colic
6. Fails to thrive

CHILD AND ADULT

1. Is pessimistic, hopeless
2. Lacks self-confidence
3. Is gullible, easily hurt
4. Is suspicious, unsure of self or others
5. Is dependent on others, clings to others
6. Is antagonistic toward others
7. Is bitter to others
8. Is withdrawn, asocial
9. Avoids new relationships or new experiences, *or*
10. Bullies others; is aggressive, sarcastic, controlling
11. Is pathologically optimistic (takes risks, gambles on everything, sure nothing can go wrong)
12. Is unable to delay gratification

trusted. If the **baby is abused, neglected, or deprived, he or she may suffer irreversible effects,** as discussed in this chapter and in Chapter 8. ∞

The infant who is in a nurturing, loving environment and who has developed trust is a happy baby most of the time. He or she is sociable and responsive to others, beginning at about 3 months. At 6 months, the baby reflects the mood of others and smiles and looks happy when seeing favorite people. By 1 year, a baby follows the gaze of others and tries to understand others and the environment. Gazing and listening lay the foundation for language development (102, 110, 111). **Stranger anxiety,** *fear or avoidance of strangers, occurs about 6 months, intensifies at 9 months, and lessens by 12 months.* Less stranger anxiety is seen if the baby is held by the mother when a stranger appears (99). **Separation anxiety or protest** *is distress when the baby is separated from the mother or caregiver and begins at about 7 to 8 months.* Extent of response varies with timing, family rituals, and the culture (99). After a time the infant will again respond to strangers and adapt to separation. Sociable babies have sociable mothers, and sociable, friendly babies score higher on cognitive tests than less sociable or mistrusting infants (1, 16, 99).

Many mothers work outside of the home. Emotional development of the infant is not compromised by the working mother if she has time and energy to maintain consistent, loving, and stimulating responses when she is with her baby. Often both parents work and share child care. The father's nurturance is important (68, 69).

Early emotional development may depend on the infant's experience. If the mother is severely depressed and cannot be responsive, studies show there is less activity in the left frontal lobe of the infant, the part of the brain involved in positive emotions, happiness, and joy. More activity occurs in the right front lobe, which is associated with negative emotions (87, 111). Sometimes corrective experiences can make up for past deprivation because of brain plasticity (87).

Discuss child care arrangements. Each parent has different ideas about how often, if at all, to leave the baby with a sitter. Discuss characteristics to consider in a sitter. Point out that parents will probably be most satisfied with a sitter whose childrearing philosophy and guidance techniques coincide with theirs and who has had some child care training or experience. The health of the child is maintained through the mother surrogate—the babysitter or nanny.

The *sitter* or *nanny should:* (a) be physically and emotionally healthy, (b) be acquainted with the baby and the home, and (c) like the baby. If possible, parents should keep the baby with the same person consistently, especially around 7 or 8 months when the baby recognizes the mother and familiar people and is experiencing separation anxiety. The *sitter or nanny should have exact instructions about:* (a) where the parents can be reached, (b) special aspects of care, (c) telephone numbers of the doctor and the police and fire departments, (d) name and telephone number of another family member, and (e) telephone number of a poison control center. Some mothers work and have no sitter available. Single-parent families may need an infant day care center. Factors to consider in choosing day care services for the young child are discussed in Chapter 11. ∞

During early infant care, the mother frequently feels low in mood. She may experience "postpartum blues" or sometimes depressive symptoms. A 10-week telephone/telecare support group for 20 mothers of infants who had been diagnosed with depression was found to be effective (107). Mothers were relieved to learn they were not alone in their depression and they felt a sense of growth and strength as a result of the supportive therapy. Further, scores on the Beck Depression Inventory were lower after the use of cognitive-behavioral therapy, relaxation techniques, and problem-solving strategies. Psychoeducation was viewed as a great help (107). You may utilize such an intervention method. The mother's health is a critical factor in promotion and stabilization of the infant's health.

DEVELOPMENT OF SELF-AWARENESS AND BODY IMAGE

At birth, the infant has diffuse feelings of hunger, pain, rage, and comfort but no image of the body. For the first month, the main goal is fulfillment of needs for survival and comfort. Pleasurable sensations come mainly from the lower face, the mouth and nose area, which has considerable innervation. At first all the baby knows is self. Gradually, the baby distinguishes his or her body from other animate and inanimate objects in the environment as he or she bites a hand, bangs the head, grasps and mouths a toy, and experiences visceral, visual, auditory, kinesthetic, and motor sensations (16, 100).

A primitive self-awareness begins at about 3 months. Later, weaning, having contact from others, and more exploration of the environment also heighten self-awareness. As the child approaches the first birthday, there is some coordination of these sensory experiences that are being internalized into the motor body image. There is increased locomotor function and ability to explore the environment, and a sense of separateness of self. He or she is aware that some body parts give greater pleasure than other parts and that there are differences in sensation when his or her body or another object is touched (16, 100).

Body image, the *mental picture of one's body, includes the external, internal, and postural picture of the body, although the mental image is not necessarily consistent with the actual body structure. Included also are attitudes, emotions, and personality reactions of the individual in relation to his or her body as an object in space,* with a distinct boundary and apart from all others and the environment. The body image, gradually formulated over a period of years, is included in the **self-concept** (*awareness of self or me*) and *derives from* (100): (a) *reactions of others to his or her body,* (b) *perceptions of how others react,* (c) *experiences with his or her own and other bodies,* (d) *constitutional factors, and* (e) *physiologic and sensory stimuli.*

Without adequate somatosensory stimulation, body image and ego development are impaired, as shown by studies of premature incubator infants who lacked rocking, stroking, and cuddling (63). The infant's initial experiences with his or her body, determined largely by maternal care and attitudes, are the basis for a developing body image and how he or she later likes and handles the body and reacts to others.

ADAPTIVE MECHANISMS

Adaptive mechanisms are *learned behavioral responses that aid adjustment and emotional development.* Research indicates that babies have initially two identifiable emotions: contentment when they are comfortable, and distress (99). At first the baby cries spontaneously. Soon the baby learns that crying brings attention; therefore, he or she cries when uncomfortable, hungry, or bored. Other tools besides crying used in adaptation are a social smile, beginning about 2 or 3 months. Laughter and curiosity become evident (14). Adaptation is gained through experimentation, exploration, and manipulation. The baby uses the body in various ways to gain stimulation. He or she grabs and plays with whatever is within reach, whether it is the father's nose or a toy. Between 8 and 12 months, emotions of anger, fear, delight, and affection are expressed through vocalization, facial expression, and gestures.

The young infant does not understand waiting and delayed gratification. But as the baby feels security and a sense of tenderness from caretakers, he or she begins to wait a short time between feeling hunger pains and demanding food. Instead of immediately screaming when a toy cannot be reached, the baby will persist in repeating the action that will get him or her to the object. The baby is beginning to respond to the expectations of others and adapt to the family's cultural patterns.

Emotional regulation is *effectively managing arousal responses, such as alertness or activity, to adapt and reach a goal.* The infant learns to inhibit or maximize the intensity and duration of emotional responses (45, 103). If, however, care does not foster trust, the infant constantly feels threatened. At first he or she cries and shows increased motor activity, perhaps expressing rage, but may eventually feel powerless and become apathetic.

Adaptive behavior is developed through structuring of the baby's potential. He or she needs freedom to explore and exercise and also consistent, pleasant restraints for personal safety, which together enable learning of self-restraint. Constantly saying "no" or confining the child to a walker or playpen does not help the learning of adaptive behavior. Research indicates that education of the mother about infant behaviors, emotional states, and communication cues facilitates mother-infant interaction, which has a positive effect on attachment, nurturing, and the child's development, health, and adaptation (70).

The infant may be temporarily deflected off course by premature birth, prolonged hospitalization, and illness around the time of birth, but once he or she is exposed to an even minimally appropriate environment, natural self-righting mechanisms have the potential to bring him or her back into the maturational trajectory characteristic of the species. The quality of the home environment and the passage of time significantly affect the outcome (12, 14, 71, 99).

DEVELOPMENTAL TASKS

The following developmental tasks are to be accomplished in infancy (43):

1. Achieve equilibrium of physiologic organ systems after birth and during the first year.
2. Begin to manage the changing body and learn new motor skills, develop equilibrium, begin eye–hand coordination, and establish rest–activity rhythm.
3. Establish self as a dependent person but separate from others.
4. Become aware of the alive versus inanimate and familiar versus unfamiliar and develop rudimentary social interaction.
5. Develop a feeling of and desire for affection and response from others.
6. Adjust somewhat to the expectations of others.
7. Begin to understand and master the immediate environment through exploration.
8. Develop a beginning symbol or language system, conceptual abilities, and preverbal communication.
9. Direct emotional expression to indicate needs and wishes.

Explore these tasks with parents. Help them realize specific ways in which they can enable their baby to achieve these tasks which contribute to the health and development of the child.

Health Promotion and Nursing Applications

ASSESSMENT: A HOLISTIC PERSPECTIVE

Utilize information throughout the chapter for assessment of family relationships in infancy, infant development, and concerns for the family. Tools to aid assessment are mentioned in several sections.

NURSING DIAGNOSES

Refer to the **Box** Nursing Diagnoses Related to the Infant, to summarize assessments and guide interventions (85). You may also formulate other diagnoses.

INTERVENTION TO PROMOTE HEALTH

Your intervention must reflect the concepts presented in **Box 9-9**, Considerations for the Infant and Family in Health Promotion. In addition, *your role with the infant and family has been discussed within each section throughout this chapter.* You can also be instrumental in establishing or working with community agencies that assist parents and infants. You may be called on to work with families who have adopted a child or with the single parent or with the stepfamily that then has their own child. Chapter 6 presents relevant information. ∞ You may work with a family whose child is not healthy or is born prematurely, or you may work with a family who experiences death of the infant.

As a nurse in a hospital or physician's office, you may provide postpartum home care services, especially for mothers and babies who are discharged from the hospital 24 to 48 hours after delivery. Early discharge has the advantages of treating the mother and baby as well rather than ill, reducing family separation time, and more directly involving the father in care. *Not every woman or family,*

Nursing Diagnoses Related to the Infant

Risk for Impaired Parent/Infant/Child **A**ttachment
Effective **B**reastfeeding
Ineffective **B**reastfeeding
Ineffective **B**reathing Pattern
Risk for Sudden Infant **D**eath Syndrome
Risk for **D**elayed Development

Delayed Growth and Development
Risk for **D**isproportionate Growth
Disorganized **I**nfant Behavior
Ineffective **I**nfant Feeding Pattern
Impaired **P**arenting

Source: Reference 85.

BOX 9-9	Considerations for the Infant and Family in Health Promotion

1. Cultural background and experiences of the family of the infant
2. Reaction of the mother and father to the crisis resulting from the baby's birth
3. Attachment behaviors and the binding-in process of the mother, attachment of father and other family members
4. Parental behaviors that indicate difficulty in establishing attachment or potential/actual abuse of the infant
5. Physical characteristics and patterns, such as eating, sleeping, elimination, and activity in the neonate/infant, that indicate health and are within the age norms for growth
6. Cognitive characteristics and behavioral patterns in the neonate/infant that indicate age-appropriate norms for intellectual development
7. Communication characteristics and behavioral patterns in the neonate/infant that indicate intact neurologic and

sensory status, speech awareness, and ability to respond with age-appropriate sounds (prespeech)
8. Overall appearance and behavioral and play patterns in the neonate/infant that indicate development of trust, rather than mistrust, and continuing age-appropriate emotional development
9. Behavioral patterns and characteristics that indicate the infant has achieved developmental tasks
10. Parental behaviors that indicate knowledge about how to care physically and emotionally for the neonate/infant
11. Parental behaviors that indicate they are promoting positive self-concept and sexuality development in the infant
12. Evidence that the parents provide a safe and healthful environment and the necessary resources for the neonate/infant
13. Parental behaviors that indicate they are achieving their developmental tasks for this era

however, is a candidate for early discharge, even though many insurance plans cover only 2 days or less. The mother and baby may not show complications until the third or fourth day after delivery. Medical backup care must be quickly available. Further, at times the mother may get more rest and emotional support in the hospital than at home, depending on home and family conditions. Even home visits by a nurse one hour daily for 2 or 3 days may *not* provide sufficient care.

Whenever visits are made in the home, one assessment tool that can be used is the *Denver II—Revision and Restandardization of the Denver Developmental Screening Test (DDST)*. See Figure 11-2 for a general scale that measures skills and gross and fine motor abilities ∞ (49). Another tool that can be used is the Home Observation for Measurement of the Environment (HOME), in which the home-rearing situation is assessed (29, 87). These tools can help guide intervention.

Special intervention challenges occur with the birth of a **premature baby** or child with congenital anomalies. The **family who is experiencing adoption or infant death also** has special care needs.

Use of Community Resources for Continuity of Care

Parents often lack awareness of available resources. Your referral to social support services, *especially informal support systems*, is impor-

tant (79). Some sources of help are summarized in the **Box** Client Education: Community Resources for Parents.

EVALUATION

Evaluation of your interventions and holistic care can be done by observing the infant's response and achievement of developmental tasks and the effectiveness of parental nurturing (59). Tools to determine attachment and developmental status and information in this chapter can be utilized for evaluation purposes or to formulate evaluation criteria. Determine also parental response to your client education, counseling, and advocacy through observation of parental behavior, asking questions to determine their retention of your teaching, or asking the parents to demonstrate how they respond to or handle the child in specific situations. When the mother brings the infant for routine well-baby checkups and immunizations, as well as when she returns for her postpartum checkup, are times to determine not only the status of the infant and mother but also to evaluate the effectiveness of prior professional care. These are also times to review prior education, initiate or continue counseling, or refer the mother for additional services for either baby, herself, or the family.

MediaLink ● Care of the Premature Baby and the Child with Congenital Anomalies

Client Education

Community Resources for Parents

CLASSES ON PARENTING, PRENATAL OR POSTNATAL CARE, LAMAZE OR PSYCHOPROPHYLAXIS METHOD OF CHILDBIRTH

- Junior or senior college presenting nonacademic courses
- Hospital clinics
- Individual childbirth educators who are members of local and international Childbirth Education Association
- Community health nursing services
- Local Red Cross chapter: www.redcross.org

BREASTFEEDING INFORMATION

- La Leche League: www.lalecheleague.org

PARENT SUPPORT

- Voluntary self-help agencies such as International Cesarean Awareness Network (ICAN): www.ICAN-online.org
- National Association of Mothers' Centers (NAMC): www.motherscenter.org

- Aiding Mothers and Fathers Experiencing Neonatal Death: www.amendgroup.com/
- The Arc of the United States (Association for Retarded Citizens): www.thearc.org
- National Association of Mothers of Twins Clubs: www.nomotc.org
- National SIDS/Infant Death Resource Center: www.sidscenter.org
- National Center on Shaken Baby Syndrome: www.dontshake.com
- Compassionate Friends: www.compassionatefriends.org

CRISIS ATTENDANCE OR COUNSELING

- Childhelp USA: www.childhelpUSA.org/
- National Child Abuse Hotline: 1-800-252-2783, 1-800-25A-BUSE

Summary

1. Childbirth is a crisis to the parents; life is changed with birth of a baby.
2. Culture influences all areas of the child's growth and development.
3. Development of infant and parent attachment is essential for the child's total development and health promotion.
4. Infant and parent behaviors are reciprocal; they affect each other's responses.
5. Maltreatment, abuse, and neglect of the infant by parents or others must be reported; intervention is essential to restore health and well-being.
6. The neonatal period, the first 30 days of life, and infancy, the first year of life, constitute an era that is a critical period for childhood and thereafter.
7. Physiologic adaptations are necessary to survive after birth.
8. The first year is a period of rapid physical growth and cognitive development.

9. Adequate nutrition, play, safety, health promotion measures, and illness prevention and protection are essential for the infant's growth and development.
10. The first year is also critical emotionally, in that the infant must be consistently loved and cared for as a whole person to thrive, learn to trust, and achieve developmental tasks.
11. **Box 9-9,** Considerations for the Infant and Family in Health Promotion, summarizes what you should consider in assessment and intervention with the infant and the infant's family.
12. Parents should be encouraged to use family, community, and other support systems.
13. Parents and the neonate/infant need special care if development does not follow a normal or healthy pattern.
14. Evaluate parental effectiveness in nurturing and your holistic care of the infant by observing the infant's progress toward meeting developmental tasks.

Review Questions

1. The mother of an infant tells the nurse she initially thought that being a parent would be "fun." However, now that the baby has arrived she is very stressed by this new role of a parent. The best response for the nurse to make to this woman is:
   1. "New parents have unrealistic ideas."
   2. "Didn't your mother tell you how hard being a parent can be?"
   3. "It will get easier."
   4. "Tell me about what you expected from parenthood."

2. Immediately after birth a healthy infant is handed to the new father. This interaction between the baby and father is best described by which of the following terms?
   1. Attachment
   2. Engrossment
   3. Bonding
   4. Parenting

3. On initial assessment at birth the newborn has a pulse of 110, is crying vigorously with regular respirations, and is moving all of the extremities. The infant's body is pink with cyanosis of the hands and feet. What Apgar score should the nurse assign to this child?
   1. 10
   2. 9
   3. 8
   4. 7

4. A woman who is pregnant with her first child tells the nurse that she would like to have a cesarean section rather than a vaginal delivery so the baby's head will "look normal" after birth. How should the nurse respond to this client's request?
   1. "The doctor will discuss your options for delivery with you."
   2. "Unnecessary surgery may harm the baby."
   3. "I will make a note of your request."
   4. "The infant's head will usually take on a round shape shortly after birth."

References

1. Ainsworth, M., Blehar, M., Waters, E., & Wall, S. (1978). *Patterns of attachment.* Hillsdale, NJ: Erlbaum.

2. American Academy of Pediatrics (AAP) Committee on Drugs. (1994). The transfer of drugs and other chemicals into human milk. *Pediatrics, 93,* 137–150.

3. American Academy of Pediatrics (AAP) Work Group in Breastfeeding. (1997). *Pediatrics, 100,* 1035–1039.

4. American Academy of Pediatrics and American College of Obstetricians and Gynecologists. (2002). *Guidelines for care* (5th ed.). Elk Grove, IL: American Academy of Pediatrics.

5. American Psychiatric Association. (1994). *Diagnostic and statistical manual of mental disorders* (4th ed.). Washington, DC: Author.

6. Andrews, M., & Boyle, J. (2003). *Transcultural concepts in nursing care* (4th ed.). Philadelphia: Lippincott.

7. Apgar, V. (1953). A proposal for a new method of evaluation in the newborn infant. *Current Research in Anesthesia and Analgesia, 32,* 260.

8. Aquilera, D. C. (1998). *Crisis intervention: Theory and methodology* (8th ed.). St. Louis, MO: Mosby.

9. Ballard, J., Novak, K., and Driver, N. (1979). A simplified score for assessment of fetal maturation in newly born infants. *Journal of Pediatrics, 95,* 769–774.

10. Battaglia, F. C., & Lubchenco, L. O. (1969). A practical classification of newborn infants by weight and gestational age. *Journal of Pediatrics, 71,* 159–163.

11. Beck, C. (1995). The effects of postpartum depression on maternal-infant interaction: A meta analysis. *Nursing Research, 44,* 296–302.

12. Becker, P., Grunwald, P., Moorman, J. and Stohr, S. (1991). Outcomes of developmentally supportive nursing care for very low birth weight infants. *Nursing Research, 40*(3), 150–155.

13. Behrman, R. E., Kliegman, R. M., & Jenson, H. B. (2004). *Nelson's textbook of pediatrics* (17th ed.). Philadelphia: Saunders.

14. Berger, K. (2005). *The developing person through the lifespan* (6th ed.). New York: Worth.

15. Berk, L. E. (2004). *Development through the lifespan* (3rd ed.). Boston: Pearson Allyn & Bacon.

16. Bettelheim, B., & Freedgood, A. (1988). *A good enough parent: A book on child-rearing.* New York: Random.

17. Bickley, L.S. (2003). *Bates' guide to physical examination and history taking* (8th ed.). Philadelphia: Lippincott.

18. Bowlby, J. (1969, January–February). Disruption of affectional bonds and its effects on behavior. *Canada's Mental Health Supplement,* No. 59, 2–12.

19. Bowlby, J. (1982). *Attachment and loss* (Vol. 1). New York: Basic Books.

20. Bowlby, J. (1988). *A secure base: Clinical applications of Attachment Theory.* London: Routledge.

21. Bowlby, J. (1989). *Secure and insecure attachment.* New York: Basic Books.

22. Bozett, F., & Hanson, S. (Eds.). (1991). *Fatherhood and families in cultural context.* New York: Springer.

23. Brazelton, T. B. (1992). *Touchpoints: Birth to 3.* New York: Perseus.

24. Brazelton, T. B., & Cramer, B. (1990). *The earliest relationship.* Reading, MA: Addison-Wesley.

25. Brazelton, T. B., & Nugent, J. (1996). *Neonatal Behavioral Assessment Scale.* London: MacKeith Press.

26. Bronfenbrenner, U. (1978). *The ecology of human development.* Cambridge, MA: Harvard University Press.

27. Bronfenbrenner, U., & Morris, P. (1998). The ecology of developmental processes. In W. Damon (Series Ed.) & R. Lerner (Vol. Ed.), *Handbook of child psychology: Vol. I. Theoretical models of human development* (5th ed., pp. 993–1028). New York: Wiley.

28. Brown, M. (1986). Social support, stress, and health: A comparison of expectant mothers and fathers. *Nursing Research, 36*(2), 74–76.

29. Caldwell, B. (1998). *Home Inventory for Infants.* Fayetteville, AK: Fayetteville Center for Development and Education, University of Arkansas.

30. Carver, L. J., Bauer, P. J., & Nelson, C.A. (2000). Associations between infant brain activity and recall memory. *Developmental Science, 3,* 234–246.

31. Cheffern, N. D., & Rannalli, D. A. (2004). Newborn biologic/behavioral characteristics and psychosocial adaptation. In S. Mattson & J. Smith (Eds.), *Core curriculum for maternal-newborn nursing* (3rd ed., pp. 433–464). Philadelphia: Elsevier-Saunders.

32. Chess, S., & Thomas, A. (1982). Infant bonding: Mystique and reality. *American Journal of Orthopsychiatry, 52,* 421–425.

33. Colyar, M. R. (2003). *Well-child assessment for primary care providers.* Philadelphia: F. A. Davis.

34. Crain, W. (2005). *Theories of development: Concepts and applications* (5th ed.). Upper Saddle River, NJ: Pearson Prentice Hall.

35. Cunningham, F. C., Leveno, K. J., Bloom, S. U., Hauth, J. C., Gilstrap, L. C., III, & Wenstrom, K.I. (2005). *William's obstetrics* (22nd ed.). Boston: McGraw-Hill.

36. D'Avanzo, C., & Geissler, E. (2003). *Cultural health assessment* (3rd ed.). St. Louis, MO: Mosby.

37. Davis, M., & Emory, E. (1995). Sex differences in neonatal stress reactivity. *Child Development, 66,* 14–27.

38. Deacon, J. J., & O'Neill, P. (Eds.). *Core curriculum for neonatal intensive care nursing* (2nd ed.). Philadelphia: Saunders.

39. DeHart, G. B., Sroufe, L. A., & Cooper, R. G. (2004). *Child development: Its nature and course* (5th ed.). Boston: McGraw-Hill.

40. Dubowitz, L., & Dubowitz, V. (1977). *A clinical manual: Gestational age of the newborn.* New York: Addison-Wesley.

41. Dudek, S. (2007). *Nutrition essentials for nursing practice* (5th ed.). Philadelphia: Lippincott Williams & Wilkins.

42. Duderstadt, K. G. (2006). *Pediatric physical examination: An illustrated handbook.* St. Louis, MO: Mosby/Elsevier.

43. Duvall, E., & Miller, B. (1984). *Marriage and family development* (6th ed.). New York: Harper & Row.

44. Duyff, R. (2006). *The American Dietetic Association's complete food & nutrition guide* (Revised and updated 3rd ed.). Hoboken, NJ: Wiley.

45. Eisenberg, N., Fobes, R., & Guthrie, I. (2002). The role of emotionality and regulation in children's social competence and adjustment. In I. Pulkkinen & A. Caspi (Eds.), *Paths to successful development.* New York: Cambridge University Press.

46. Erikson, E. (1963). *Childhood and society* (2nd ed.). New York: W.W. Norton.

47. Fenstermacker, K., & Hudson, B. T. (2004). *Practice guidelines for family practitioners* (3rd ed.). Philadelphia: Saunders.

48. Ferketich, S., & Mercer, R. (1995). Predictors of role competence for experienced and inexperienced fathers. *Nursing Research, 44,* 89–95.

49. Frankenburg, W. K., & Dodd, J. B. (1967). The Denver Development Screening Test. *Journal of Pediatrics, 71,* 181–191.

50. Garbarino, J., Guttmann, E., & Seeley, J. (1987). *The psychologically battered child: Strategies for identification, assessment, and intervention.* San Francisco: Jossey-Bass.

51. Geissler, E. (1998). *Pocket guide to cultural assessment* (2nd ed.). St. Louis, MO: Mosby.

52. Gesell, A., Irg, F. (1940). *The first five years of life.* New York: Harper Brothers.

53. Giger, J., & Davidhizar, R. (2004). *Transcultural nursing: Assessment and intervention* (4th ed.). St. Louis, MO: Mosby.

54. Greenburg, M., & Morris, N. (1974). Engrossment: The newborn's impact upon the father. *American Journal of Orthopsychiatry, 44,* 520–531.

55. Guyton, A., & Hall, J. (2006). *Textbook of medical physiology* (11th ed.). Philadelphia: Elsevier Saunders.

56. Hockenberry, M., & Wilson, D. (2007). *Wong's nursing care of infants and children* (8th ed.). St. Louis, MO: Mosby.

57. Hoff, L. (2001). *People in crisis: Clinical and public health perspectives* (5th ed.). Stanford, CT: Appleton-Lange.

58. Horowitz, J., Logsdon, M., & Anderson, J. (2005). Measurement of maternal-infant interaction. *Journal of the American Psychiatric Nurses Association, 11*(3), 164–172.

59. Johnson, M., Bulechek, G., Butcher, H., Dochterman, J., Maas, M., Moorhead, S., & Swanson, E. (2006). *NANDA, NOC, and MC linkages: Nursing diagnoses, outcomes, and interventions* (2nd ed.). St. Louis, MO: Mosby, Elsevier.

60. Kenner, C., Amlung, S. R., & Flandermeyer, A. A. (1998). *Protocols in neonatal nursing.* Philadelphia: Saunders.

61. Klaus, M., & Kennell, J. (1982). *Parent-infant bonding* (2nd ed.). St. Louis, MO: C.V. Mosby.

62. Koniak-Griffin, D. (1993). Maternal role attainment. *IMAGE: Journal of Nursing Scholarship, 25*(3), 257–262.

63. Kramer, M., Chamorro, I., Green, D., Knuttson, F., (1975). Extra tactile stimulation of the premature infant. *Nursing Research, 24*(5), 324–334.

64. Kuhl, P. (2000). A new view of language acquisition. *Proceedings of the Neonatal Academy of Sciences, 97*(22), 11850–11857.

65. Ladewig, P. A., London, M. L., & Davidson, M.R. (2006). *Contemporary maternal-newborn nursing care* (6th ed.). Upper Saddle River, NJ: Prentice Hall.

66. Lagona, K. (2003). *Come Bien, Camina y No Se Preocupe*—Eat right, walk, and do not worry: Selective biculturalism during pregnancy in a Mexican-American community. *Journal of Transcultural Nursing, 14*(2), 117–124.

67. Lai, C., Fisher, S., Hurst, J., Vaugh-Khaden, F., & Monaco, A. (2001). A forkhead-domain gene is mutated in a severe speech and language disorder. *Nature, 413,* 519–523.

68. Lamb, M. (1987). The emergent American father. In M. Lamb (Ed.), *The father's role: Cross cultural perspectives.* Hillsdale, NJ: Erlbaum.

69. LaRossa, R. (1988). Fatherhood and social change. *Family Relations, 37,* 451–457.

70. Letch, D. (1999). Mother-infant interaction: Achieving synchrony. *Nursing Research, 48*(1), 55–57.

71. Low-birth-weight infants catch up in adolescence. (1998). *American Journal of Nursing, 98*(10), 9.

72. Main, M., & Solomon, J. (1990). Procedures for identifying infants as disorganized/disoriented during the Ainsworth Strange Situation. In M.T. Greenberg, D. Cicchetti, & E.M. Cummings (Eds.), *Attachment in the preschool years* (pp. 121–126). Chicago: University of Chicago Press.

73. Maloni, J., & Ponder, M. (1997). Fathers' experience of their partners' antepartum bed rest. *IMAGE: Journal of Nursing Scholarship, 29*(2), 183–187.

74. Masataka, N. (1998). Perception of motherese in a signed language by 6-month-old deaf infants. *Developmental Psychology, 34*(2), 241–246.

75. Mercer, R. T., & Ferketich, S. L. (1990). Predictors of prenatal attachment during early parenthood. *Journal of Advanced Nursing, 15,* 268–280.

76. Metheny, N. (2000). *Fluid & electrolyte balance: Nursing considerations* (4th ed.). Philadelphia: Lippincott.

77. Metzoff, A. N. (2000). Learning and cognitive development. In A. Kazdin (Ed.), *Encyclopedia of psychology.* Washington, DC, and New York: American Psychological Association and Oxford University Press.

78. Mew, A., Holditch-Davis, D., Belzer, M., Miles, M., & Fischel, A. (2003). Correlates of depressive symptoms in mothers of preterm infants. *Neonatal Network, 22*(5), 51–59.

79. Molinari, D., & Freeborn, D. (2006). Social support needs of families adopting special needs children. *Journal of Psychosocial Nursing, 44*(4), 28–34.

80. Montagu, A. (1986). *Touching: The human significance of the skin* (3rd ed.). New York: Columbia University Press.

81. Monteleone, J. A. (1998). *Child maltreatment: A comprehensive photographic reference identifying potential child abuse* (2nd ed.). St. Louis, MO: G.W. Medical.

82. Monteleone, J. A., & Brodeur, A. E. (1998). *Child maltreatment: A clinical guide and reference* (2nd ed.). St. Louis, MO: G.W. Medical.

83. Murray, S., Baker, A., & Lewin, L. (2000). Screening families with young children for child maltreatment potential. *Pediatric Nursing, 26*(1), 47–65.

84. Murray, S. S., & McKinney, E. S. (2002). *Foundations of maternal-newborn nursing* (4th ed.). St. Louis, MO: Saunders/Elsevier.

85. NANDA International. (2007). *NANDA-I nursing diagnoses: Definitions and classifications 2007–2008.* Philadelphia: Author.

86. Palkovitz, R. (2002). *Involved fathering and men's adult development: Provisional balances.* Mahwah, NJ: Lawrence Erlbaum.

87. Papalia, D., Olds, S., & Feldman, R. (2004). *Human development* (9th ed.). Boston: McGraw-Hill.

88. Petitto, L. A., & Masentelte, P. F. (1991). Babbling in the manual mode: Evidence of the ontogeny of language. *Science, 251,* 1493–1495.

89. Piaget, J. (1952). *The origins of intelligence in children.* New York: International University Press.

90. Piaget, J. (1954). *The construction of reality in the child* (M. Cook, Trans.). New York: Basic Books.

91. Potts, N. L., & Mandleco, B. L. (2007). *Pediatric nursing: Caring for children and their families* (2nd ed.). New York: Thomson/Delmar Learning.

92. Robson, K. (1976). The role of eye-to-eye contact in maternal-infant attachment. *Journal of Child Psychology and Psychiatry, 8,* 13–25.

93. Rubin, M. (1964). The family-child relationship and nursing care. *Nursing Outlooks, 8,* 16–30.

94. Rubin, M. (1967). Attainment of the maternal role—Part I. *Nursing Research, 16,* 237–245.

95. Rubin, M. (1967). Attainment of the maternal role—Part II. *Nursing Research, 16,* 342–346.

96. Rubin, M. (1970). Cognitive style in pregnancy. *American Journal of Nursing, 70*(3), 502–508.

97. Rubin, M. (1977). Binding-in in the postpartum period. *Maternal-Child Nursing Journal, 6,* 67–75.

98. Rubin, M. (1984). *Maternal identity and the maternal experience.* New York: Springer.

99. Santrock, J. (2004). *Life-span development* (9th ed.). Boston: McGraw-Hill.

100. Schilder, P. (1951). *The image and appearance of the human body.* New York: International University Press.

101. Spector, R. (2003). *Cultural diversity in health and illness* (6th ed.). Upper Saddle River, NJ: Prentice Hall Health.

102. Spence, M., & DeCasper, A. (1987). Prenatal experience with low-frequency voice sounds influences neonatal perception of maternal voice samples. *Infant Behavior and Development, 10,* 133–142.

103. Thomas, A., & Chess, S. (1977). *Temperament and development.* New York: Brunner/Mazel.

104. Tiedje, L. B., & Darling-Fisher, C. (2003). Promoting father-friendly health care. *Maternal Child Nursing, 28,* 350–357.

105. Toney, L. (1983). The effects of holding the newborn at delivery on paternal bonding. *Nursing Research, 32*(1), 16–19.

106. Tulman, L. (1985). Mothers and unrelated persons' handling of newborn infants. *Nursing Research, 34*(4), 205–210.

107. Ugarizzo, R., & Schmidt, C. (2006). Telecare for women with postpartum depression. *Journal of Psychosocial Nursing, 44*(1), 38–45.

108. United States Department of Health and Human Services. (2000). *Healthy People 2010. With understanding and improving health and objectives for improving health* (2nd ed.) 2 vols. Washington: DC: U.S. Government Printing Office.

109. Wadsworth, B. (2004). *Piaget's Theory of Cognitive and Affective Development: Foundations of constructivism* (5th ed.). Boston: Pearson.

110. Walker, L., & Montgomery, E. (1998). Maternal identity and role attainment's long-term relations to children's development. *Nursing Research, 43*(2), 105–110.

111. Wingert, P., & Brant, M. (2005, August 15). Reading your baby's mood. *Newsweek,* 33–39.

112. Zitelli, B. J., & Davis, H. W. (2002). *Atlas of pediatric physical diagnosis* (4th ed.). St. Louis, MO: Mosby.

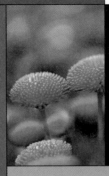

CHAPTER 10

The Toddler: Basic Assessment and Health Promotion

OBJECTIVES

Study of this chapter will enable you to:

1. Examine the effects of the family and the toddler on each other, the significance of attachment behavior and separation anxiety, and the family developmental tasks to be achieved.

2. Explore with parents ways to adapt to the toddler while they simultaneously socialize the child and meet their developmental tasks.

3. Assess a toddler's physical and motor characteristics; general cognitive, language, emotional, and self-concept development; and related needs.

4. Describe specific guidance and discipline methods for the toddler and the significance of the family's philosophy about guidance and discipline.

5. Discuss the toddler's developmental tasks and ways to help him or her achieve them.

6. Work effectively with a toddler and the family in the health care situation.

MediaLink **www.prenhall.com/murray**

Go to the Companion Website for interactive resources that accompany this chapter.

Glossary	Critical Thinking
Review Questions	Tools
Challenge Your Knowledge	Media Link Applications
Learning Activities	Media Links

Development of the toddler and family relationships are the basis for assessment and health promotion of the toddler and family in any setting. Nursing, health promotion, and health care responsibilities for the child and family are discussed throughout the chapter.

Within the first year of life, children make remarkable adaptations internally and externally to their environment. They sit, walk, remember, recognize others, begin to socialize, communicate more purposefully, and show more specific emotional responses.

The **toddler stage** *begins when the child takes the first steps alone at 12 to 15 months and continues until approximately 3 years of age.* The child makes a key transition from creeping to a pedestrian way of life. The family is very important as the child improves physical coordination, acquires language skills, increases cognitive achievement, and achieves control over bladder and bowel sphincters. These factors lead to new and different perceptions of self and the environment, new incentives, and new ways of dealing with problems.

Family Development and Relationships

Behaviorally, the toddler changes considerably between 12 months and 3 years, changes that in turn affect family relationships. Because of new skills, the child begins to develop a sense of independence, establishes physical boundaries between self and mother, and gains the sense of a separate, self-controlled, increasingly autonomous being who can do things on his or her own. The child attempts self-education through mastery and engaging parents and others to help when necessary. Without the myriad attempts to do things for self, the child would obtain no degree of autonomy in skills. The periods of practice that ensure reliable performance and skills are often periods of independent action; however, dependence on others and gratification of dependency needs are essential for optimum self-development. Dependency does not mean passivity, for the child is quite active in obtaining help by crying, screaming, taking an adult by the hand and pulling him or her to another area, or asking how to solve a problem. *The toddler should be neither kept too dependent nor forced too quickly into independence.*

The family of a toddler can be quiet and serene one minute and in total upheaval the next, resulting from the imbalance between the child's motor skills, lack of experience, and mental capacities. One quick look away from the toddler can result in a broken object, a spilled glass of milk, or an overturned dish. The toddler's quickly changing moods from tears to laughter or anger to calm, combined with energy, sense of "me do," and curiosity, also account for parents' labeling their toddler a "terrible two." The child could more appropriately be labeled a "terrific two."

Having a new sibling arrive in the toddler's world is a crisis. The child should be prepared for the arrival of a new baby with simple explanations about why the mother's shape is becoming larger or changing and that the toddler will sleep in a different bed if the crib is needed for the baby. Emphasis on the positive features of becoming a "big girl" or "big boy" is helpful. When baby arrives, the toddler will need more attention, especially while parents give the baby care.

The toddler is frequently jealous of younger siblings because of having to vie for the center of attention that was once his or her own; older siblings are resented because they are permitted to do things he or she cannot. Power struggles between parent and child often focus on feeding and toilet training. Family problems may also arise when the toddler's activities are limited because of parental anxieties concerning physical harm or because of their intolerance of the child's energetic behavior and unknowing infractions of societal rules.

Teach parents that this behavior is normal and necessary for maturation. Explain that expecting, planning for, and trying to handle patiently each situation will reduce parent and child frustration. Inform parents that their social teaching likely will center on consistency in life patterns, maintaining a healthy environment, guidance and even distraction to promote increasing social competency, and establishing reasonable controls over anger, impulsiveness, and unsafe exploration.

Influence of the Family

The chief molder of personality is the family unit, and home is the center of the toddler's world. Family life nurtures in the child a strong affectional bond, a social and biological identity, intellectual development, attitudes, goals, and ways of coping and responding to situations of daily life. The family life process also imparts tools such as language and an ethical system, in which the child learns to respect the needs and rights of others and which provide a testing ground before he or she emerges from home. A loving, attentive, healthy, responsible family is essential for maximum physical, mental, emotional, social, and spiritual development in childhood (7, 49).

The importance of the father's role with the child and with the mother is being affirmed (6, 17, 48, 49, 51, 66, 67). *Worldwide, the father or father figure is the one person whose role is increasingly recognized as significant to the young child* (48, 49). The mother has been, and usually still is, the main caregiver of the infant and toddler. A range of relatives, including father, grandparents, siblings, and other extended family members—and even neighbors, friends, and parents of peers—are also considered crucial to the child's development, especially in non-Caucasian cultures (3, 6, 15, 39, 66, 67). A father's frequent and positive involvement is increasingly seen among most groups in the United States. His role is directly related to the child's well-being and cognitive and social development (6, 15, 17, 51, 66, 67). In some cultures, the fathering role with the young child is intentionally shared or fulfilled by the mother's eldest brothers or a grandfather. The biological father becomes more involved when the child is older (3, 39). Some African and Caribbean countries report that at least 32% of families are headed by single mothers (67). In these families, a father's absence may affect the child in relation to financial loss, difficulty in meeting physical needs, and a sense of psychological distress (3, 43, 66).

Parents with high self-esteem provide the necessary conditions for the toddler to achieve trust, self-esteem, and **autonomy** (*self-control*) through allowing age-appropriate behavior. Parents with low self-esteem provoke feelings of shame, guilt, defensiveness, decreased self-worth, and "being bad" in the child. They tend to inappropriately or forcefully punish or restrain the child, deny necessities, and withdraw love (43, 73). If one or both parents are depressed and the condition is untreated, the toddler is likely to become depressed, which in turn affects attachment, self-esteem, language development, and biopsychosocial development (32, 55).

Changing parental attitudes are often evident. A parent who is delighted with a dependent baby and is a competent parent to an infant may feel threatened by the independence of the toddler and become less competent. Some parents have difficulty caring for the dependent infant but are creative and loving with the older child. But if the parent's development was smooth and successful, if the parent's inner child of the past is under control, and if the parent understands self, parental behavior can change to fit the maturing child (7). Some parents are more comfortable with either male or female offspring and may show **favoritism** *(more attention, positive reinforcement, or loving behavior)* to one gender in contrast to the other (14, 51, 56).

Educate and counsel parents to help them work out their feelings about self in relation to the child. Parents need validation and support for what they do effectively and reminders about normal development of the toddler. Discourage demonstration of favoritism behavior. Such intervention promotes mental health.

ATTACHMENT BEHAVIOR

Attachment behavior is very evident during the toddler years. The way adults recall early experiences with parents or caregivers affects the way they respond to their children. A mother who was securely attached to her mother, or who understands why she was insecurely attached, can more accurately respond with nurturing and foster secure attachment in her child. Negative childhood attachment experiences may negatively affect the parent's ability to remain nurturing and foster attachment (5, 23, 57, 66, 68). The mother-child relationship of infancy is slowly being replaced by more interaction with the father (48, 49) and the larger family unit, but the toddler still needs the mothering person close (41). Children need to be touched, cuddled, hugged, and rocked. All young mammals need physical contact for normal brain tissue development and for the brain to develop receptors that inhibit secretion of cortisol—the stress hormone (58). Thus, both the immune and neurologic systems are affected positively by touch and by emotional attachment (7, 8, 14, 43).

Although attachment is directed to several close people, such as father, siblings, babysitter, and grandparents, it is usually greatest toward one person, the mother or mothering person. The toddler shows attachment behavior by maintaining proximity to the parent. Even when out walking, the child frequently returns part or all the way to the parent for reassurance of the parent's presence: to receive a smile, to establish visual (and sometimes touch) contact, and to speak before again moving away (8). Securely attached toddlers, in contrast to insecurely attached toddlers, have more varied vocabularies, are more sociable, have more positive interactions with peers, and show more joy and positive emotions (23, 46, 47, 57, 66).

Effects of Day Care on Attachment

Attachment patterns do not differ significantly between children who stay home all day versus those who go to day care centers, because attachment is related to the consistency and intensity of emotional and social experience between child and adult rather than to physical care and more superficial contact. Attachment is as close if the mother or primary caretaker shows warm affection less frequently or if she (or he) is present all day but not affectionate (14). However, attending day care can lead to an increase in illness in the toddler, especially diarrhea, otitis media, respiratory tract infections (especially if the caregiver smokes), hepatitis A, meningitis, and cytomegalovirus (43). The strongest predictor of illness risk is the number of unrelated children in the room (43). Injuries can also occur, perhaps more so than if the child is at home (43).

Guide parents in selecting day care services, whether in the caregiver's home or in a day care center. *Advise parents to check* (a) accreditation and state licensure, which establishes minimum standards; (b) policies related to attendance and care of sick children; (c) infection control and injury prevention practices; and (d) control of environmental contamination with urine and feces, especially related to diapering and toilet training. Other criteria for day care selection are discussed in depth in Chapter 11. ∞ The Case Situation can be used to explain to parents about some activities and a typical environment of a day care center.

Explore with the parents feelings about the child's separation from home and regularly leaving the child in someone else's care. Explore ways to improve the quality of time they spend with the child, including reworking household routines as necessary to have more quality time with the toddler.

Effects of Longer-Term Separation

Separation anxiety, *the response to separation from the mother, intensifies at approximately 16 to 18 months and again at 24 and 30 months.* When separated, the child experiences feelings of anger, fear, and grief. Anxiety can be as intense for the toddler as for the infant if the child has had a continuous warm attachment to a mother figure (5, 14, 43, 54). The child who is more accustomed to strangers will suffer less from a brief separation. An apathetic, resigned reaction at this age is a sign of abnormal development. The *child who is separated from the parent for a period, as with hospitalization, goes through three phases of grief and mourning—protest, despair, and denial—as a result of separation anxiety* (8, 43, 71, 72).

During **protest,** *lasting a few hours or days and seen for short or long separations, the need for the mother is conscious, persistent, and grief laden.* The child cries continually, tries to find her, is terrified, fears he or she has been deserted, feels helpless and angry that mother left, and clings to her on her return. If he or she is also ill, additional uncomfortable body sensations assault the toddler. The child needs the mother at this time; strangers are rejected (8, 43, 71, 72).

Despair *is a quiet stage, characterized by hopelessness, moaning, sadness, less activity, and regression to earlier behavior.* The child does not cry continuously but is in deep mourning. The physical condition may worsen. He or she does not understand why mother

Case Situation

The setting is an urban day care center. The outdoor fenced, grassy area, with sandbox, a variety of active muscle play equipment, and wheeled toys, looks inviting. Inside, wide hallways, a cubicle for each child's personal items, and a large room for each specific age group indicate that this is a busy center. The large room has distinct play areas appropriate for the age group: a house corner, an area for large wooden blocks, a music area with a piano and other instruments for children, a reading corner with books, and an art area with plenty of paper and crayons, pencils, chalk, finger paints, and molding clay. Tables in the middle of the room have a variety of smaller toys that toddlers enjoy. Large windows face the playground. An aquarium and potted plants are on shelves, visible but posing no safety hazards. Two bathrooms with fixtures at toddler level adjoin the large room. Pictures of how to wash the hands are on the wall by the basin. Pictures of how to cover a cough are also posted.

Anna, 30 months old, is a typical toddler: 30 lb (13.6 kg) and 34 in. (86.4 cm) tall. She occasionally falls briefly while walking around the room but rises to her feet without help. She pulls a toy truck, then sits on a small tractor and pulls herself with her feet. In a few minutes, she sees a pink ball on a shelf. She runs to it, grasps it with her hands, and repeatedly places the ball off and on the shelf. Then it bounces out of her hands, and she goes to another shelf to get another toy.

While holding the toy, another toddler, Luis, approaches Anna to yank it out of her hands. Both toddlers yank back and forth. Anna is unable to share. Luis hits Anna, who starts to cry. The teacher approaches both children. She talks with both of them together and each child individually about the fun of sharing and playing together. She gives each child a hug on the shoulders and plays with the children briefly as they share the toy. In a few minutes, each child is distracted to engage in another activity in the room.

After an hour of active play, the teacher calls the group together for story time for 10 minutes to accommodate the toddler's short attention span. During this time, the toddlers repeat a nursery rhyme that was part of the short story. Then the toddlers move into music time. They sing the nursery rhyme as a group, demonstrating rote memory. After 10 minutes, the toddlers each select an instrument to play with as the teacher gives simple information about each one. Anna chooses a toy violin. Music time ends with the teacher turning on an audiotape of a march. Some children go through marching motions; others stand in place and stomp each foot. When the music and march ends, they all clap and laugh and shout.

The teacher reminds them it is bathroom time, to wash hands, and to sit at the table, which has been cleared for a morning snack of graham crackers and apple juice. The teacher and teacher aides assist the children as necessary, accommodating each child's developmental level. Anna manages toileting and hand washing. She is friendly to Luis as they sit together.

Contributed by Ruth Murray, EdD, MSN, N-NAP, FAAN.

has deserted him or her. The child neither makes any demands on the environment nor responds to overtures from others, including at times the mother. Yet the child clings to her when she is present. The mother may feel guilty and feel her visits are disturbing to the child, especially when the child does not respond to her (8, 32, 43, 71, 72). But if she does not visit, the child's reaction deepens.

Help parents to understand that the child's responses and their own reactions are normal and that the child desperately needs parental presence. If the mother, father, or other primary caregiver can be present, you can promote family-centered care through your explanations, not being rigid about visiting hours, attending to parental comfort and needs, encouraging the parent to stay overnight, and letting the parent help care for the child. Protests, in the form of the toddler's screams and crying, will thus be less intense. Be accepting if a parent cannot stay with the child. Parents may live great distances from the hospital or have occupational or family responsibilities that prevent them from visiting the child as often as desired. The parent may also be ill or injured. Be as nurturing to the toddler as possible while the parent is away. Tell the toddler how much Mommy and Daddy love him or her and want

to be present but cannot. If possible, have the parent leave an object with the child that is a familiar representation of the parent. Further, the same nurse should be assigned to care for the child each day if possible.

Denial, *which occurs after prolonged separation, defends against anxiety by repressing the image of and feelings for the mother and may be misinterpreted for recovery.* The child now begins to take more interest in the environment, eats, plays, and accepts other adults. Anger and disappointment at the mother or caregiver are so deep that the child acts as if he or she does not need her and shows anger by rejecting her, sometimes even rejecting gifts she brings. To prevent further estrangement, the mother should understand that the child's need for her is more intense than ever (8, 43, 71, 72). With prolonged hospitalization, the child may fail to discover a person to whom he or she can attach for any length of time.

Continue the interventions that promote family-centered care and family health. Give the parent and child time together undisturbed by nursing or medical care procedures. Provide toys that help the child to act out the fears, anxiety, anger, and mistrust experienced during the hospitalization and separation. Encourage the parent to talk about and work through feelings related to the child's illness and absence from the family.

Teach parents that immediate aftereffects of separation include changes in the child's behavior—regression (for example, in toilet training and eating and sleeping habits), clinging, and seeking out extra attention and reassurance. If extra affection is given to the child, trust is gradually restored. If the separation has been prolonged, the child's behavior can be very changed and disturbed for months after return to the parents. The parent needs support in accepting the child's expressions of hostility and in meeting his or her demands. Counteraggression or withdrawal from the child will cause further loss of trust and regression.

Attachment Disorder

Attachment disorder may occur when the child experiences (1, 47, 57):

1. Separation from the primary caregiver due to the child's or parent's illness; parental separation, death, or divorce; or parental maltreatment, abuse, or neglect.
2. Frequent changes in the primary caregiver, such as in foster care placement.
3. Maternal depression or addiction to alcohol or drugs.
4. A young or inexperienced mother with poor parenting skills and limited or no parenting role models.
5. Lack of connection between mother and child because of a congenital anomaly, developmental problems as a consequence of problems during pregnancy or delivery, or chronic or debilitating illness.

Attachment disorder is manifested by (1, 47, 57): (a) lack of eye contact with or resisting affection from parents or caregivers; (b) being difficult to handle, demanding, or aggressive; (c) relating poorly to peers, unable to engage in parallel play; (d) delays in speech, language, and cognitive development; (e) clinging or showing affection to anyone, even strangers; and (f) hypervigilant behavior. The Website for attachment disorder presents more information, www.attachmentdisorder.net.

CHILD MALTREATMENT, ABUSE, AND NEGLECT

Child maltreatment or abuse is contrary to health and may begin or continue at this age. Even when parents seem concerned and loving, a child is not immune from abuse. Further, children today are exposed to a variety of potential abusers—babysitters or day care workers; the parent's live-in companion, lover, or occasional friend; stepparents or extended family members; and neighbors. Be alert to signs and symptoms of child abuse, discussed in Chapters 8, 9, and 11. ∞ Chapter 11 presents in-depth information that is relevant to the toddler era.

You often must be very patient and observant to detect child maltreatment and abuse because the child does not have the language skills to tell you what has happened. The child's nonverbal behavior, play, and artwork may provide clues. Observation of the artwork takes time and patience as well as the parent's presence. Suspected abuse must be reported. Three boxes present relevant information to aid your assessment. **Box 10-1** summarizes parental behavior characteristic of psychological maltreatment of the toddler (36). **Box 10-2** summarizes signs of physical abuse to the child (43, 59–61). **Box 10-3** presents interaction behaviors that are typical between the child and parent if the child is being abused (43, 59–61). References 35 and 36 address psychological maltreatment in depth. References 59, 60, and 61 present information in pic-

---

BOX 10-1	**Parental Behavior Characteristic of Psychological Maltreatment of the Toddler**

REJECTING

1. Excludes actively from family activities
2. Refuses to take child on family outings
3. Refuses to hug or come close to child
4. Places the child away from the family

ISOLATING

1. Teaches the child to avoid social contact beyond the parent–child relationship
2. Punishes social overtures to children and adults
3. Rewards child for withdrawing from opportunities for social contact

TERRORIZING

1. Uses extreme gestures and verbal statements to threaten, intimidate, or punish the child

2. Threatens extreme or mysterious harm (from monsters or ghosts or bad people)
3. Gives alternately superficial warmth with ranting and raging at the child

IGNORING

1. Is cool and apathetic with child
2. Fails to engage child in daily activities or play
3. Refuses to talk to child at mealtimes or other times
4. Leaves child unsupervised for extended periods

CORRUPTING

1. Gives inappropriate reinforcement for aggressive or sexually precocious behavior
2. Rewards child for assaulting other children
3. Involves the child sexually with adolescents or adults

Source: From Garbarino, J. Guttmann, E., & Seeley, J. (1987). The psychologically battered child: Strategies for identification, assessment, and intervention. San Francisco: Jossey-Bass. Copyright 1986. Adapted by permission of Jossey-Bass, Inc., a subsidiary of John Wiley & Sons, Inc.

BOX 10-2	**Physical Signs of Abuse of a Child**

1. An injury for which there is no explanation or an implausible explanation is present.
2. Injury is not consistent with the type of accident described (e.g., child would not suffer both feet burned by stepping into hot tub of water, he or she would step in with one foot at a time, a child who tips a pot of hot coffee on his or her hand has a splash-effect burn, not a mitten appearance).
3. Inconsistencies exist in the parents' stories about the reason for child's injuries.
4. Parents quickly blame a babysitter or neighbor for an accidental injury.
5. Child does not have total appearance of an accident—dirty clothes, face smudged, hair tousled.
6. Large number of healed or partially healed injuries are observed.
7. Large bone fracture, multiple fractures, or tearing of periosteum caused by having limb forcibly twisted are evident.
8. Child flinches when your fingers move over an area not obviously injured, but it is tender due to abusive handling.
9. Human bite marks are evident.
10. Fingernail indentations or scratches are noted.
11. Old or new cigarette burns are evident.
12. Loop marks from belt beating are present.
13. Soft tissue swelling and hematomas are noted.
14. Clustered or multiple bruises are observed on trunk or buttocks, in body hollows, on back of neck, or resembling hand prints or pinch marks.
15. Bald spots are observed.
16. Retinal hemorrhage from being shaken or cuffed about the head is assessed.
17. History of unusual number of accidents exists.

Data from references 43, 59–61.

BOX 10-3	**Interaction Signs of Parental Abuse of a Child**

1. Child flinches or glances about nervously when you touch him or her.
2. Child seems afraid of parents or caregivers and is reluctant to return home.
3. Parent issues threat to crying child such as "Just wait till I get you home."
4. Parent remains indifferent to child's distress.
5. Parent blames child for his or her own injuries (e.g., "He's always getting hurt" or "He's always causing trouble").
6. Parental behavior suggests role reversal; parent solicits help or protection from child by acting helpless (when child cannot meet parent's needs, abuse results).
7. Parent repeatedly brings healthy child to emergency room and insists child is ill (parent feeling overwhelmed by parental responsibilities and may become abusive).
8. Child has had numerous admissions to an emergency room, often at hospitals some distance from the child's home.

Data from references 43, 59–61.

FAMILY DEVELOPMENTAL TASKS

Developmental tasks of the family with a toddler are to (25):

1. Meet the spiraling costs of family living that occur with the child's growth and changing needs.
2. Provide a home that is safe and comfortable, has adequate space, and provides needed resources for the toddler.
3. Maintain a sexual involvement that meets both partners' needs.
4. Develop a satisfactory division of labor for the couple related to care of the home and child.
5. Promote understanding of the toddler within the family related to behavior and needs.
6. Determine whether the couple will have any more children.
7. Rededicate themselves, among many dilemmas, to their decision to be a childbearing, nurturing family.

Help parents to be cognizant of these tasks. Encourage them to talk through concerns, feelings, and practical aspects related to fulfilling these tasks that promote health in the family and toddler. Encourage membership in a young parents' group, a play group for children and their parents, or a "mother's day out" child care situation. Give numbers for help lines, such as First Nurse, and remind them that being asked questions about the child's development is a positive response. Encourage them to seek support from family members, friends, or work colleagues. Refer them to a counselor or community agency if help is desired.

tures as well as in text that can help you more thoroughly assess the child.

One aspect of maltreatment is **child abduction**. There are 2,100 new *missing children* reports in the United States daily, including infants through adolescents. A significant number of young child abductions stem from **custody battles** between separated and divorced parents, *when one parent takes the child away from home base* (11). In an effort to thwart abductions, authorities use the AMBER (America's Missing Broadcast Emergency Response) alert system. Using television, radio, freeway signs, and other media outlets, governmental agencies pool resources to inform the public of the child abduction. The first few hours after the child is abducted are the most critical in recovering the child. More information is available at the National Center for Missing and Exploited Children Website, www.missingkids.com.

INTERVENTIONS FOR HEALTH PROMOTION

Teach parents the following safety information related to prevention of abduction or recovery of the abducted child:

1. Call **9-1-1** immediately if an abduction occurs.
2. Know the height, weight, and eye color of the child, and what the child was wearing—the most essential details. If possible, know where the child was at the time of abduction.
3. Keep easily retrievable: clear recent photographs of the child, a copy of the child's thumbprint, and an up-to-date list of physical data.
4. Accompany the young child consistently to any location; emphasize that the child should stay with the parent or caregiver.
5. Never leave the toddler alone in a car, public place, or grocery cart.
6. Avoid putting the child's name on his or her clothing, backpack, or tricycle to reduce the opportunity for someone to get familiar with the child's name.

7. Choose the babysitter or nanny carefully:
   a. Obtain references and do background checks (Child Protective Services and law enforcement checks for child maltreatment).
   b. Observe the person for general appearance, attitude, and approach to the child.
   c. Interview the person to determine experience with and knowledge about children.
   d. Determine the person's ability to do emergency measures for child safety.
   e. Observe the person's ability to play with and nurture the child, as well as manage a range of behavior.
   f. Determine the person's ability to do special care approaches and procedures if the child is a special-needs child, has a specific health impairment, or is visually or hearing challenged.
   g. Have the child and potential caregiver or nanny interact with the mother present. Observe the child's reaction.

Physiologic Concepts and Physical Characteristics

GENERAL APPEARANCE

The appearance of the toddler has matured from infancy. By 12 to 15 months, the child has lost the roly-poly look of infancy, with abdomen protruding, torso tilting forward, legs at stiff angles, and flat feet spaced apart. Limbs are growing faster than torso, giving a different proportion to the body. Chest circumference is larger than head circumference. By age 2 years, the child increasingly looks like a family member as face contours fill out with 16 deciduous teeth. Gradually the chubby appearance typical of the infant is lost; muscle tone becomes firmer as the fat-storing mechanisms change. Less weight is gained as fat; more weight is gained from muscle and bone (6, 18, 27, 33, 43, 66, 67). Review the principle of asynchronous growth described in Chapter 3. ∞

RATE OF GROWTH

During toddlerhood, *growth is slower than in infancy*, but it is even. Development follows the cephalocaudal, proximodistal, and differentiation (general-to-specific) principles discussed in Chapter 3. ∞ Although the rate of growth slows, bone growth continues rapidly with the development of approximately 25 new ossification centers during the second year (43).

Between the first and second years the average height increase is 4 to 5 in. (10 to 12 cm). Average height increase the next year is 2.5 to 3.5 in. (6 to 8 cm). Weight gain averages 5 to 6 pounds (2.27 to 2.72 kg) between the first and second years. Birth weight is quadrupled by age 2 years. The 2-year-old child stands 32 to 35 in. (81 to 87.5 cm) and weighs 26 to 28 pounds (11 to 13 kg). At *30 months average height* is 36 in. (91.5 cm), and *weight* is approximately 30 pounds (13.6 kg). *Generally, by age 2, the girl has grown to 50% of final adult height; by age 30 months, the boy has grown to 50% of adult height (6, 38, 43, 66, 67).* In the United States the African American child generally is taller and weighs more by age 2 than the Caucasian child (3, 39).

NEUROMUSCULAR MATURATION

The most dramatic change in the brain the first 2 years of life is **branching**, *the spreading connections of dendrites to each other*, and the myelination of axons (43, 67). **Pruning**, *elimination of redundant pathways, connections, and synapses* in each area of the brain, occurs from about 18 to 21 months. *The most used pathways are retained;* thus neuromuscular and cognitive stimulation are essential for retention and development of neurons (43, 67). Neuromuscular maturation and repetition of movements help the child further develop skills.

Myelination, *covering of the neurons with the fatty sheath called myelin, is almost complete by 2 years.* This enables the child to support most movement and increasing physical activity and to begin toilet training. Bowel control is accomplished before bladder control due to progressive development of the myelin sheath and muscular control and coordination (43). Additional growth also occurs as a greater number of connections form among neurons, and the complexity of these connections increases. **Lateralization or specialization of the two hemispheres of the brain** has been occurring; *evidence of signs of dominance of one hemisphere over the other can be seen.* The left hemisphere matures more rapidly in girls than in boys; the right hemisphere develops more rapidly in boys (43). These differences may account for language ability in girls and spatial ability in boys. Handedness is gradually demonstrated, and spatial perception is improving (38, 43, 66). (Spatial perceptual ability will be complete at approximately 10 years of age.) The limbic system is mature; sleep, wakefulness, and emotional responses become better regulated. The toddler responds to a wider range of stimuli, responds voluntarily to sounds, and has greater control over behavior. The brain reaches 80% of adult size by age 2 (43). The growth of the glial cells accounts for most of the change (43, 66).

The African American child is more advanced neurologically until 2 or 3 years of age, after which differences are not as noticeable (3, 39, 43). Children from other cultural backgrounds also may vary in age norms, but *sequence of skills is consistent across cultures* (3, 39).

MOTOR DEVELOPMENT AND COORDINATION

Size and strength of muscle fibers continue to develop due to muscle use and myelination of the corticospinal tract. Involuntary movement on one side is often accompanied by involuntary movement on the other side of the body (27, 38, 66). The toddler demonstrates use of either hand, although dominance may be established by age 2 years (66). Increasing gross motor coordination is shown by leg movement patterns and by hand-arm movements. **Table 10-1** summarizes the increasing motor coordination skills manifested during the toddler years in the United States (18, 27, 33, 43). **Figure 10-1** depicts an example.

Motor development follows an almost universal sequence (27), *but the timing of certain motor skills depends on* (a) physical health status, (b) opportunities provided by the family (27, 66), (c) child-rearing practices of the culture (37), and (d) possibly evolutionary or genetic foundations (3, 27). Children on the average walk and run by 10 months in Africa, 12 months in the United States, and 15 months in France. Asian children tend to develop motor skills more slowly, perhaps related to parenting practices and temperament (37, 66). However, at some point, children arrive at the same

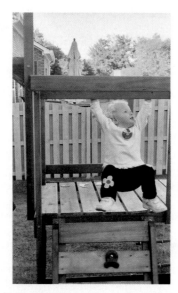

FIGURE ▪ 10-1 The toddler enjoys physical action and exploration.

destination and achieve the motor skills demanded by the culture (66). The chief difficulty with fine motor skills in the toddler years is that the child does not have necessary muscular control, patience, and judgment because of incomplete myelination and immaturity of the corpus callosum and prefrontal cortex (6, 27, 43).

VISION

Visual acuity and the ability to accommodate, to make adjustments to objects at varying distances from the eyes, are slowly developing. Vision is **hyperopic**, *farsighted*, testing approximately *20/40 at 3 years*. Depth perception is immature. Visual perceptions are frequently similar to an adult's, even though the child is too young to have acquired the richness of symbolic associations. The child's eye–hand coordination also improves. At *15 months* he or she reaches for attractive objects without superfluous movements. Between *12 and 18 months*, the toddler looks at pictures with interest and identifies forms (43, 66).

ENDOCRINE SYSTEM

Endocrine function is not fully known. Production of glucagon and insulin is labile and limited, causing variations in blood sugar. Adrenocortical secretions are limited, but they are greater than in infancy. Growth hormone, thyroxine, insulin, and corticoids remain important secretions for regulating growth (43).

RESPIRATORY SYSTEM

Respirations average 20 to 25 per minute. Lung volume continues to increase, and susceptibility to respiratory infections decreases as respiratory tract structures increase in size. The diameter of the upper respiratory tract is still comparatively small (43).

CARDIOVASCULAR SYSTEM

The *pulse decreases*, averaging 105 beats per minute (range 80 to 120 beats per minute). *Blood pressure increases*, averaging 80 to 100 systolic and 56 to 64 diastolic. The size of the vascular bed increases, thus reducing resistance to flow. The capillary bed has increased ability to respond to hot and cold environmental temperatures, thus aiding thermoregulation (43).

Juvenile hypertension has been defined as *sustained blood pressure levels above the 95th percentile on at least three measurements at different visits in circumstances where anxiety is minimized.* Another definition for children 3 to 12 years is a diastolic pressure greater than 90 mm Hg (33, 43). If hypertension is suspected, a complete investigation is warranted by a specialist interested in hypertension in children. Tell parents that many children will respond to an overall cardiovascular health program. Salt intake should be monitored to avoid excess ingestion, for example, from salty snacks. If at all possible, drug therapy should be avoided (33, 43).

GASTROINTESTINAL SYSTEM

By age 3 years, the child has a *complete set of 20 deciduous or primary teeth.* Swallowing patterns are not consistent or maturely developed. Foods move through the gastrointestinal tract less rapidly, and *digestive glands approach adult maturity.* Acidity of gastric secretion increases gradually. Liver and pancreatic secretions are functionally mature. *Stomach capacity is 500 ml* (24, 26, 43).

TABLE 10-1

Motor Coordination During the Toddler Years

Age (months)	Characteristics
12–15	Walks alone; legs appear bowed Climbs onto furniture Climbs steps with help; slides down stairs backward Stacks two blocks; scribbles spontaneously Grasps but rotates spoon; holds cup with both hands Takes off shoes and socks
15–18	Runs but still falls Walks backward and sideways (17 months) Climbs to get to objects Falls from riding toys or in bathtub Stoops and recovers Hammers on pegboard Grasps with both hands Picks up small items off floor; investigates electric outlets; grabs cords and table cloths (15 months) Clumsily throws ball; places ball in box Unzips large zipper Takes off easily removed garments Places three blocks in a row (15 months) Stacks three to four blocks (18 months) Climbs up stairs; bumps down (18 months)
18–24	Falls from outdoor play equipment Walks stairs with help (20 months) Can reach farther than expected, including for hazardous objects Fingers food Brushes paint; finger paints Takes apart toys; puts together large puzzle pieces Kicks ball forward (24 months)
24–30	Pushes a riding toy with both feet to operate (24 months) Runs quickly; falls less Walks upstairs and downstairs holding to rail; does not alternate feet Jumps off floor with both feet (28 months) Throws ball overhand Puts on simple garments Draws vertical scribbles Stacks six blocks; places "chimney" cube on house (row of cubes) Turns door handles Plays with utensils and dishes at mealtimes; pours and stacks Turns book pages correctly (24 months) Uses spoon with little spilling; feeds self Brushes teeth with help; chose own toothbrush
30–36	Walks with balance; runs well Balances on one foot; walks on tiptoes (30 months) Jumps from chair (32 months) Does broad jumps (30 months) Pedals tricycle (32 months) Jumps 10–12 in. off floor (36 months) Climbs and descends stairs, alternating feet (36 months) Sits in booster seat rather than high chair Stacks 8–10 blocks; builds with blocks Pours from pitcher Dresses self completely except tying shoes; does not know back from front Turns on faucet Assembles puzzles Draws; paints

Data from references 6, 38, 43, 67, 68.

Educate the parents about continuing dental health. Dental care is essential to preserve the temporary teeth and teach good dental health. A small, soft-bristled toothbrush should be used. Water is preferred to toothpaste, which the child may swallow. If toothpaste is fluoridated, the child may ingest excessive amounts of fluoride (43).

Pacifiers may occasionally be used when the child is teething or upset. The pacifier should not be honey- or sugar-coated to avoid allergies to honey and dental caries. Gum or hard candy should be avoided because of the danger of aspiration and excess sugar. A bottle in the bed by the child should be discouraged, as there is danger of aspiration, and holding milk in the mouth contributes to dental caries (43).

SKIN

The skin becomes more protective against outer invasion from microorganisms, and it becomes tougher, with more resilient epithelium and less water content. Less fluid is lost through the skin as a result. The skin remains dry because sebum secretion is limited. Eccrine sweat gland function remains limited. At this age eczema improves and the frequency of rashes declines (33, 43). Skin color depends on deposition of melanin, which varies between and within racial groups. For example, skin color of African Americans ranges from very light to very dark, even in the young child. Sunburn is less likely, but can occur in African American children who have light pigmentation. Latinos, Asians, and American Indians also vary in the hue of skin color and in risk for sunburn (39). Caucasians with less melanin are most likely to become sunburned with too much sun exposure, which over time increases the risk for skin cancer (39).

Assess for a baseline and uniform skin coloring. Areas of dark-skinned people not exposed to the sun, such as palms of hands, soles of feet, and buttocks, may be lighter in color and can be assessed for conditions that cause anemia. Lips and nail beds can also be assessed for color changes. **Birthmarks**, *pigmented, demarcated areas of the skin*, may persist beyond infancy.

URINARY SYSTEM

By age 3, the kidneys are differentiated in function. Renal function is mature; under stress, water is conserved, and urine is concentrated as in an adult level (43). The bladder has descended into the pelvis, assuming an adult position. Urine secretion daily for a 2-year-old is 500 to 600 ml, and it is 600 to 750 ml for the 3-year-old (33, 43).

IMMUNE SYSTEM

Specific antibodies have been established for most commonly encountered organisms, although the toddler is prone to gastrointestinal and respiratory infections when he or she encounters new microorganisms. Despite environmental exposure, antibody IgC increases, IgM reaches an adult level, and IgA gradually increases. Lymphatic tissues of adenoids, tonsils, and peripheral lymph nodes undergo enlargement, partly because of infections and partly from growth. By age 3 years, the adenoid tissue reaches maximum size and then declines, whereas tonsils reach peak size around 7 years (43, 69).

BLOOD CELL COMPONENTS

Blood cell counts are approaching adult levels, although the hemoglobin and erythrocyte (red blood cell) counts are lower. Sufficient iron intake is necessary to maintain an adequate erythrocyte level. Erythrocytes are formed in the bone marrow of the ribs, sternum, and vertebrae as in adulthood. During stress, the liver and spleen also form erythrocytes and granulocytes (43).

OVERALL DEVELOPMENT

Seasonal spurts in growth occur. Development does not proceed equally or simultaneously in body parts and maturational skills. Review the principles of development described in Chapter 3 ∞ for application to assessment of the child. For example, the anatomy of the ear, Eustachian tube, and nasal pharynx continues to resemble that of the infant, continuing the risk for otitis media (33, 43). The limbs grow faster than the torso. The head begins to rise above table height. The toddler develops greater stability and no longer needs arms for balance. Thus carrying and moving objects are favorite activities. Sometimes a child concentrates so intently on one aspect of development (e.g., motor skills) that other abilities (e.g., toilet training) falter or regress. Illness or malnutrition may slow growth, but a catch-up growth period occurs later so that the person reaches the developmental norms. The brain is more vulnerable to permanent injury because destroyed cells are not replaced, although some brain cells may take over some functions of missing cells (43).

There are also *cultural differences in growth and development.* Caucasian children, for example, show more height increase in spring and more weight increase in fall. The African American child develops motor skills at a greater pace than the Caucasian until age 3 years. The African American child may be walking alone at 7 or 9 months, in contrast to 12 or 15 months. If all variables are controlled, the African American child probably will be heavier and have more advanced skeletal development (3, 39, 66).

Teach parents about physical characteristics of the toddler to help them adjust to his or her changing competencies. Physical changes relate to health, safety promotion, and injury control.

PHYSICAL ASSESSMENT OF THE YOUNG CHILD

The approach to the physical examination depends on the specific age and developmental level of the toddler. Adequate time should be spent in becoming acquainted with the child and the accompanying parent. Get down to the child's level. Allow the child to examine equipment before testing. A friendly manner, quiet voice, and relaxed approach help make the examination more fruitful. Hands should always be warmed before giving an examination, but especially so in the case of the child. Before 6 months of age the infant usually tolerates the examining table. Between 6 months and 3 to 5 years, most of the examination can be done from the mother's or caretaker's lap. After age 4, much depends on the relationship established with the child.

No assessment is complete without knowing the antenatal, natal, and neonatal history. When the child is old enough, let him or her tell what conditions surround the visit even if the message is only "stomach hurt."

Many times you will be learning about the young child from the mother and will be learning about the mother's attitude. Observe and listen closely. If other siblings are present, observe the interaction among the family members. What are the mother's facial expressions? In what tone of voice does she talk? Does she look away or comfort the child if the child seems disturbed with a procedure? What are the other siblings' reactions toward the toddler, the mother, and the health care worker? What are the siblings' reactions in general?

Although the child may not talk much, general appearance can reveal much information. Does the child look ill or well? What is the activity level? Coordination? Gait, if walking? Reactions to parents, siblings, and examiner? Nature of cry, if present? Facial expressions?

The *sequence of the examination* with the young child should be from least discomfort to most discomfort. Undressing can be a gradual procedure as children are often shy about this process. Some examiners prefer to go from toe to head or at least to start with auscultation, which is painless and sometimes fascinating to the child. It is best to leave the ears, nose, and mouth to the end because examination of these areas often initiates a negative response.

Generally the *temperature* should be taken during the first years of life. Body temperature averages 99°F (37.2°C). Temperature may be taken by several methods: **axillary** *(under arm in axilla area, next to skin)*, **aural** *(probe inserted into ear)*, or by **temporal artery** *(infrared sensor probe scans forehead to detect heat from arterial blood flow)* (33). Through the age of 2, the *head circumference* is measured at its greatest width and plotted on a growth curve scale that is compared with the norm.

Blood pressure should be taken with the cuff that will snugly fit the arm. The first reading is recommended at age 3. The mean reading for the toddler is 100/58 (43). The inflatable bladder should completely encircle the arm but not overlap. Artificially high blood pressure results if the cuff is too narrow or too short. Because this procedure causes some discomfort and it is important to get readings in a low-anxiety state, sensitive timing is needed to get desired results. It sometimes helps to make a game out of the procedure by allowing the toddler to help pump up the bulb or read the numbers on the gauge.

The *skin* can be examined for turgor by feeling the skin over the chest or abdomen or feeling the calf of the leg; skin should be firm. **Spider nevi**, *pinhead-sized red dots from which blood vessels radiate*, are commonly found, as are **Mongolian spots**, *large, flat, black or blue-and-black spots.* **Café au lait spots**, *one or two patches of light brown, nonelevated stains*, are within normal findings, but more may be indicative of fibromas or neurofibromas. **Bruises** *(ecchymoses)* are not abnormal in healthy active children, but their location is important. Bruises not on the extremities or on areas easily hit when falling may indicate child abuse, or excessive bruising may indicate blood dyscrasias (33).

Lymph nodes are palpable in almost all healthy young children. Small, mobile, nontender nodes often point to previous infection. *When examining the head region, consider the following:*

1. The auricles of the ears should be pulled back and down in young children and back and up in older children to examine the ears.

2. A complete hearing test with an audiometer should be done before a child enters school. Before that, the whisper technique or the use of a tuning fork is adequate.

3. A Snellen E chart can be used for testing visual acuity before the child knows the alphabet. Visual acuity at 3 years is 20/40.

4. Other aspects of the visual examination depend on the child's age and the suspected problem (e.g., after surgery for congenital cataracts).

5. Teeth should be examined for their sequence of eruption, number, character, and position.

When examining the *thorax and lungs*, remember that breath sounds of young children are usually more intense and more bronchial and expiration is more pronounced than in adults. The heart should be examined with the child erect, recumbent, and turned to the left. Sinus arrhythmia and extrasystoles can be benign and are not uncommon.

When standing, a child's *abdomen* may be protuberant; when lying down, it should disappear. The skilled examiner should be able to palpate both the liver and the spleen.

Examination of the female *genitalia* is basically visual unless a specific problem in the area has developed. When examining the male genitalia, the testicles should be examined while the male is warm and in a sitting position, holding the knees and with the heels on the seat of the chair or examining table. Without warmth and abdominal pressure, the testes may not be in the scrotum.

When examining the *extremities*, the examiner may note bowlegs, which are common until 18 months. Knock-knees are common until approximately age 12 years. The toddler may appear flat-footed when first walking. All these characteristics are usually short term.

The *neurologic* examination is conducted throughout and is not much different from the sequence in the adult examination. However, the appropriate maturation level must be kept in mind (33, 43).

Nutritional Needs

No child under age 2 years should consume skim milk or eat only low-fat foods. Diets designed for adults wishing to lose weight or prevent heart disease, when eaten by toddlers, may retard growth and neurologic development (24, 26). See the Client Education MyPyramid for Kids: Recommended Daily Dietary Intake for Toddlers, for a summary of dietary needs (24, 26). More information is available from the United States Department of Agriculture (USDA) Food and Nutrition Service Website www.MyPyramid.gov.

Fat intake should be 30% to 35% of total calories daily. No more than 10% of total calories should be from saturated fats after 2 years of age. Two fatty acids not manufactured in the body, linoleic acid and alpha-linolenic acid, are essential for growth and brain development and must be supplied. Fat is also needed for absorption of the fat-soluble vitamins, A, D, E, and K, as well as for palatability and energy (26).

Toddlers like breads, sweets, mashed potatoes, sodas, milk, and snack foods. Such a diet, if served exclusively, would impair health. Too much milk without adequate amounts of other foods is also undesirable because omission of meats and vegetables could lead to iron deficiency anemia (26).

Client Education

MyPyramid for Kids: Recommended Daily Dietary Intake for Toddlers

1. Grains—Whole grain cereals (¼ cup serving), whole grain breads and crackers (6 servings).
2. Vegetable—A variety, including dark green and yellow/orange (3 servings, 2½ cups).
3. Fruits—A variety of fruit. Juice should be 100%, without added sugar or caloric sweetener (2 servings, 1½ cups).
4. Milk and milk products, such as yogurt, cottage cheese, and other cheeses (2 servings, 2 cups).
5. Meat, eggs, and beans—Lean meats, chicken, turkey, fish (baked, broiled, grilled), and beans (2 servings, 3 oz). Liver or other high-iron foods (2 servings weekly).
6. Fiber daily—At age 2 years, 7 g; at age 3 years, 8 g daily.

Source: References 24 and 26.

Because stomach capacity is comparatively small, more frequent, smaller meals are best. Each day offer the toddler three regular meals and three snacks; snacks may be fruits, vegetables, crackers, yogurt, a small sandwich, or juice. Avoid snacks that are high in sugar, fat, and salt; they may be permitted for special occasions. *Caloric needs* are not high and increase slowly throughout the toddler period. Artificially sweetened juices, all sodas, and sugary sweet foods should be limited for weight control, avoidance of dental caries, and overall health. Eating "empty calories" can interfere with eating healthy foods (24, 26, 43). The toddler's appetite typically declines at approximately 18 months. The child has finished a major growth spurt and needs fewer calories. Approximately 1,000 calories per day are needed at age 1, and only 1,300 to 1,500 calories are required by age 3 (100 cal/kg/d for each year above the basic 1,000 calories) because the child is growing less rapidly than during infancy. Body tissues are developing slowly; thus, *protein* needs are not high—between 1 g of protein/lb or 1.8 grams/kg of body weight daily. Vitamin supplements are rarely needed if food intake is balanced in nutrients. Fluoride supplements are helpful in areas without fluoridated water. From 6 months to 3 years of age, 0.25 mg fluoride daily is recommended if water fluoride content is less than 0.3 ppm. Parents should inquire about water fluoride content in their community (43). *Fluid* requirements are approximately 115 to 125 mL/kg per day (24,

26). Water should be offered throughout the day to allay thirst. It is recommended that juice be diluted with water (43). The rule for daily *fiber* intake is 5 grams plus years of age, for example 7 g for the 2-year-old (24).

Food intake, or its refusal, is one way for the toddler to show increasing independence. *Decreased food intake may result from:*

1. Slower growth rate; not hungry.
2. Short attention span and distracted by other stimuli.
3. Increased interest in the surroundings; curiosity about people's activities.
4. Need for attention.
5. Expression of independence, autonomy.
6. Sense of fatigue.

A hospitalized toddler frequently regresses; refusing to feed self is one manifestation. The child needs a lot of emotional support and to feel some kind of control over destiny, that he or she is not totally helpless and powerless. A way of assuring some area of control is by permitting the child to choose foods and encouraging him or her to feed self (43).

How well the child eats is determined to a great extent by how parents manage mealtime, parental behavior toward food, and the atmosphere surrounding the meal. Food preferences are established at an early age, depending on mealtime patterns, and

INTERVENTIONS FOR HEALTH PROMOTION

Teach parents the following suggestions to avoid having mealtime be a battleground:

1. Serve food in small portions. The average serving size can be calculated at about one tablespoon of food for each year of age.
2. Serve finger food or cut food so that it can be eaten with the fingers.
3. Let the child choose (it is not necessary for the toddler to sample every food served).
4. Avoid offering high-fat, high-salt, or carbohydrate foods such as soda, candy, and cake or empty nutrition snack foods.
5. Offer a food again if it has been rejected one time, without fussing about it.
6. Avoid insisting that the child eat everything on the plate.
7. Do not use food for reward or punishment, to bribe to get desired behavior, or as the main connection with love or nurturing.

predict later eating habits (24). The toddler is a great imitator and will eat what the parents eat. Parental pressure or reprimands when the child does not eat a particular food convey anxiety or anger and reinforce not eating, because of either the negative attention received or the stress response felt by the child. Toddlers can be fussy eaters or go on "food jags," preferring only a certain food. Parents can give the requested food for a few days until the child gets bored with it, while continuing to offer alternative foods. Or the toddler may overeat if parents overeat. If there is a high caloric intake, obesity may result. Excessive weight gain interferes with the physical mobility that is a part of being a normal toddler. In the United States, one in five children is overweight; 10 million children are obese (24).

Teach parents about the nutritional needs and eating patterns of the toddler. Avoid serving too large a portion, which can be the beginning of overeating or cause refusal to eat food, with resultant conflict between parent and toddler. Teach parents to maintain caloric balance by substituting fiber foods, which give a sense of fullness. Parents should also be aware of food insensitivities or allergies.

Play, Exercise, Rest, and Sleep

PLAY AND EXERCISE

Play is the business of the toddler. Play is essential to health. During play the child (a) exercises, (b) learns to manage the body, (c) improves muscular coordination and manual dexterity, (d) increases awareness and organizes the surrounding world by scrutinizing objects, (e) develops spatial and sensory perception, (f) learns to pay attention, (g) learns language, (h) releases emotional tensions and channels unacceptable urges, such as aggression, into acceptable activities, and (i) translates feelings, drives, and fantasies into action. The child learns about self as a person. Through play the toddler becomes socialized and begins to learn right from wrong. The child learns to have fun and to master. The cognitive skills discussed later are evident in play (6, 31, 43, 67).

Cultures vary in the way children are encouraged to play and in play activities or equipment that are utilized. Play provides practice for adult behavior (3). For example, Chinese toddlers often play with the caregiver rather than peers; the caregiver uses play to teach proper conduct, a major emphasis in Chinese culture (42, 66).

Different types of toddler play include (43, 66, 67):

1. **Solitary,** *playing alone.*
2. **Onlooker,** *observing others at play.*
3. **Unoccupied,** *standing in one spot and performing random movements.*
4. **Parallel,** *playing next to but not with other children with little overt exchange, but a satisfaction in being close to other children.*
5. **Functional,** *using repetitive muscular movements,* such as rolling or bouncing a ball.
6. **Constructive,** *using objects or materials to make something,* such as a house of blocks or a crayon drawing.
7. **Pretend/symbolic,** *beginning about 18 months, transforming an object or toy into another symbol, object, or toy,* such as the

box being a table, or under the table being a house, or pretending to be an animal or another person. By the end of 2 years, most children imitate adults in dramatic play by doing such things as setting the table and pretend cooking.

The toddler is unable to initiate sharing of toys and is distressed by demands of sharing, as he or she has a poorly defined sense of ownership. Toddlers will share and play cooperatively with guidance, however. Play time and positive relationships with the parents, siblings, and other family members help the toddler learn how to interact and to be sociable, and over time, how to make friends. A relation exists between the quality of attachment between mother and baby and the quality of play and problem-solving behavior at 2 years of age. Toddlers who are securely attached at 18 months of age are more enthusiastic, persistent, cooperative, and able to share than if secure attachment has not developed. There is also more frequent and sophisticated interaction with peers at 3 years when secure attachment has formed in infancy (47).

Gender influences play. Gender segregation in play seems universal across cultures. Boys and girls play differently beginning in the toddler years, even when they play with the same toys. Boys tend to be more boisterous and girls more sociable. This may be a result of genetics, hormones, and socialization (66).

The father continues the same kind of play pattern with the toddler as with the infant. Fathers tend to jostle the young child more and devote more time to play than do mothers. Fathers are more likely than mothers to use their own body as a portable, interactive monkey bar or rocking horse. From infancy on, the father helps the child to individuate by being willing to let the child move out of sight and will let a child crawl or move twice as far than the mother allows before retrieving the child. When a child confronts a novel situation, a new toy, a stranger, or a dog, mothers move closer to support the child and offer reassurance with their presence, whereas fathers stay back and let the child explore by self. The child needs to be exposed to both the comforting and the challenge (48, 49).

However, when the father is the primary caregiver, he interacts with the young child in much the same way as does the mother, by smiling frequently and imitating the child's facial expressions and vocalizations. The father still remains quite physical with the child in interaction (48, 49). As fathers assume greater responsibility for young child care due to changing social and cultural conditions and expectations, mothers and fathers are likely to interact more similarly with their young children.

Discuss play patterns and toys with the parents and remind them that talking to the child is a form of play. **Table 10-2** presents suggested play activities and equipment for the child 18 months or 2 years of age. **Box 10-4** lists examples of educational toys. *Teach parents the importance of play and safety.* Reinforce to parents, when selecting play materials for the toddler, to consider likes and dislikes and choose a variety of activities because the attention span is short. Refer to safety and durability aspects of toys, as discussed in Chapter 9. ∞

Help parents realize the importance of offering toys that can transform into any number of playthings, depending on the child's

TABLE 10-2

Suggested Play Activities and Equipment for Toddlers

Age (months)	Toy, Equipment, or Activity
18	Push-pull toys (cars, trucks, farm tools)
	Boxes and toys for climbing
	Empty and fill toys (plastic food containers, kitchen utensils, small boxes, and open-close toys)
	Big picture books—thick-paged, colorful, sturdy (child will turn two or three pages at a time, tear at thin pages, can identify one picture at a time)
	Stuffed animals with no detachable parts
	Baby dolls, large enough to hug, carry, cuddle, dress, feed
	Big pieces of plain paper or newspaper layers and crayons for scribbling
	Small blocks—builds a tower of two or three at a time
	Shape-sorting blocks or cubes
	Small chair; small furniture to play "house"
	Toy farm animals or equipment
	Rubber or soft ball; throws overhand
	Phonograph record, preferably sturdy plastic that child can manipulate by self; musical and sound toys; musical instruments simple to use
	Rocking horse; rocking chair
24	All of the above are enjoyed; child now turns book or magazine pages singly—still tears; builds tower of seven blocks and aligns cubes
	Makes circular strokes with crayon, enjoys finger paints
	Puppets
	Pedal toys; dumping toys (dump trucks)
	Sandbox toys
	Playdough and clay; mud
	Jungle gym for climbing; sandbox; small water pool for water play
	Pounding toys—hammer and pegs, drums, small boards
	Picture puzzles—two to four pieces (wooden or thick cardboard)
	Large, colored wooden beads to string
	Simple trains, cars, boats, planes to push–pull or sit on and pedal
	Kick ball
	Likes to run

mood and imagination at the time. The adult can be available or initially start a play activity with the child; however, the child should be encouraged to play independently, developing mastery, autonomy, and self-esteem in the process. *Recommend a variety of* (a) play interactions (alone, with children, with adults); (b) safe environments (own home, other children's home, outdoors); and (c) activities (active, quiet, organized, unstructured, fine and large muscular skills, reading, art, music, dress-up) (43). Explain that exercise helps the child learn a variety of physical, mental, and social skills. The child enjoys running, rolling, jumping, tumbling, walking and looking at nature, dancing, throwing and kicking, making objects move, swimming, or starting in a pre-ski program. Sedentary play, such as reading, should be balanced with plenty of active play. **Box 10-5**, Techniques for Using Play While Caring for the Child, summarizes how therapeutic play can be used effectively with the ill child.

REST AND SLEEP

Rest is as essential as exercise and play. Although a child may be tired after a day of exploration and exerting boundless energy, *bedtime is often a difficult experience.* Bedtime means loneliness and separation from fun, family, and, most important, the mother figure. Ritualistic behavior is normal and peaks at about 30 months. The toddler enjoys a bedtime ritual. The same ritual may last for several years; sometimes a favorite bedtime activity or ritual changes during this era. The toddler needs an average of 10 to 12 hours of sleep nightly plus a daytime nap of 1 to 2 hours. *Sleep is essential to physical growth, and healing if ill, because during sleep the growth hormone is produced in greater quantity.*

Cultures vary in child sleep practices. For example, among the Zuni people in New Mexico, the young child has no regular bedtime. Among the Canadian Hare people, 3-year-olds do not take a daytime nap but are put to sleep after the evening meal and are allowed to sleep as long as they wish in the morning (37). In mainstream U.S. culture, mothers who are employed outside the home and are the sole caregiver may take the sleeping toddler to a babysitter at an early morning hour or fully dressed to be placed in day care at 6 a.m.

The sleep schedule may be as follows:

15 months	Morning nap is shorter; needs afternoon nap.
17–24 months	Will have trouble falling asleep.
18 months	Brings stuffed toy or pillow.
19 months	Sleeps fairly well, tries to climb out of bed.
20 months	May awaken with nightmares.
21 months	May rest quietly and sleep well, may spend less time in afternoon naps.
24 months	Total sleep time reduced, tries to delay bedtime, continues to need afternoon nap or rest.
2–3 years	Can be changed from crib to bed; rails on side should be closely spaced so child does not tumble out or get caught between rails.

BOX 10-4   Examples of Educational Toys and Play for the Toddler

13–15 MONTHS

Toy telephone
Toy horse for rocking, rocking chair
Carriage or other toys for pushing and pulling
Household objects, such as pots or pans and unbreakable cups, or food cartons of various sizes for nesting and stacking
Pot lids for banging together
Wooden blocks of various sizes and shapes for stacking
Large plastic clothespins
Larger balls or stuffed animals
Toys that encourage acrobatic movement

16–18 MONTHS

Sandbox and toys that can be pushed through sand
Simple musical instruments, such as tambourine or drum
Large colored beads
Jack-in-the-box
Equipment for blowing bubbles, with adult help

19–21 MONTHS

Rocking horse
Kiddie cars
Toys to take apart and fit together
Small rubber balls
Digging toys
Large crayons, large sheets of paper
Easy puzzles with large and few pieces, colorful pictures of animals, foods, and other objects in the environment, made of sturdy material or wood

Dirt for making mud pies
Big cardboard boxes to play hide and seek (self and others)

22–24 MONTHS

Kiddie lawn mower
Kitchen sets for make-believe play, including toy utensils
Modeling clay
Construction blocks or sets
Actions toys, e.g., toy trains, dump trucks, cars, and fire engines
Old magazines that can be used to point out pictures and also torn up
Baskets, boxes, and tubes of various sizes for multiple uses in action and fantasy play
Containers (e.g., pots, pans) with lids

2–3 YEARS

Dolls, male *and* female, various ethnicity, with accessories like clothing, strollers, baby bottle, feeding utensils
Beginner tricycle
Kiddie swimming pool
Mini-trampoline
Age-appropriate roller skates
Swing set, mini-basketball hoop
Dress-up clothes (parents' and older siblings' clothing no longer used) for male *and* female
Crayons, markers, finger paints, large sheets of paper
Coloring books, not too detailed in design
Easel or chalkboard and chalk
Kiddie cassette player and tapes
Kiddie woodworking bench

Note: Toys played with at an earlier age continue to be enjoyed, especially if they can be used in different ways or with different actions. Puppets and age-appropriate musical tapes and cloth or vinyl books should be available throughout toddlerhood.

MediaLink   Centers for Disease Control and Prevention

Sleep problems may occur with co-sleeping, which can be stressful (44). During hospitalization, the child may experience restlessness, insomnia, and nightmares. Hospitals permit parents to spend the night in the child's room to lessen fears and separation anxiety. Cuddling is still important to a toddler, especially if hospitalized. If a parent cannot remain with a frightened child, you can hold and rock the child while he or she holds a favorite object.

Health Promotion and Health Protection

ROUTINE IMMUNIZATIONS

Immunizations remain a vital part of health care. *The toddler needs to continue the immunization process that was begun in infancy.* If the parent refuses to have the child immunized for religious reasons, emphasize the need to prevent exposure to these diseases, if possible, and the importance of continued good hygiene and nu-

trition. The *Healthy People 2010* Initiative addresses goals for effective vaccination of young children to prevent infectious diseases (75). The concern starts at birth and is global (19).

SAFETY PROMOTION AND INJURY CONTROL

The causes of accidental injury are motor vehicle accidents, burns, suffocation, drowning, poisoning, and falls. Accidents are the leading cause of death, and deaths from poisonings continue to increase. Areas outside the home—the playground at the child care center, the yard and street at home, the grocery cart—all pose hazards.

Motor vehicle accidents are a major cause of accidental death when car restraints are not used or are used improperly and when the child plays in areas of vehicle traffic. The toddler should be placed in a car seat or automobile restraint device appropriate for the size of the child, as shown in **Figure 10-2**. Many injuries occur in or near the home (6, 43, 66, 67). Thus, it is necessary to **childproof**

BOX 10-5 **Techniques for Using Play While Caring for the Child**

PHYSICAL ASSESSMENT

1. Talk soothingly and calmly. Explain what you are doing as you do it.
2. Blow on the stethoscope. Ask child to imitate.
3. Have child listen to own heartbeat with stethoscope.
4. Name body parts and touch them. "Foot. Here is my foot." "Where are your eyes?" "There are your eyes!" "Where is your nose?" Guide the child's hands to touch.
5. Use diversions—another toy, tickles (especially abdomen).
6. Play peek-a-boo: cover your eyes, then child's. Hide your head with blanket, then child's head. When child covers own head, say "Where's (name?)" Then delight in discovery.
7. Use body movement, exercising child's arms and legs rhythmically while doing assessment.
8. Sing a nonsense tune or talk animatedly.
9. Talk about sensations: warm or cold, soft or rough as sensations are presented.
10. Name body position: up or down, over.
11. Encourage child to do examination of doll, teddy bear, toy animal.

BATHING

1. Experiment with the properties of water in a small tub. Use items that float and sink—washcloth, plastic soap dish, paper cup, plastic lid, empty plastic cylinders, or toys at child's cribside. Talk about what happens.

2. Identify body parts as you wash them. Give simple directions: "Close your eyes." "Raise your arms." "Wash your hair." Be sure to praise all help.
3. Encourage child to "bathe" a doll, teddy bear, or toy animal.

FEEDING

1. Place the child in high chair or walker when he or she can sit unsupported. Tie toy or utensil to high chair to facilitate retrieval.
2. Discuss the food: hot or cold, colors, textures, which utensils to use.
3. Use an extra spoon and cup: one for you, one for baby.
4. Experiment with food: finger paint with food on tray, make lines.

DIAGNOSTIC PROCEDURES

1. Explain to the child what you plan to do and are doing. Be honest but gentle.
2. Tell the child it is all right to cry; comfort if child cries.
3. Set up situation so child can do procedure on doll or toy animal. While child is imitating, talk about how much it hurts. Cuddle and comfort the child, cooing, singing softly, rocking after the procedure.
4. Distract the child with empty dressing packages, encouraging crushing and listening to sounds.
5. Make the sounds and touch different parts of child's body.
6. Vocalize sounds related to procedure. Have child imitate you.

INTERVENTIONS FOR HEALTH PROMOTION

Teach the following guidelines to parents for establishing a bedtime routine for the toddler.

1. Set a *definite bedtime routine and adhere to it*. If the child is overly tired, he or she becomes agitated and difficult to put to sleep. *Bedtime routines become a precedent for other separations* and help the child strengthen a sense of trust and build autonomy.
2. Establish a *bedtime ritual*, including bath, reading a story, soft music (some young children prefer classical), having a favorite soft toy or blanket to hold when falling asleep, quiet talking and holding, and a tucking-in routine. Reduce noise and stimuli in the house. Avoid television, movies, or videos that show aggressive scenes and are too loud. Begin approximately 30 minutes before bedtime. The tucking-in should be caring and brief.
3. If the *child cries*, which most children do briefly, go back in a few minutes to provide reassurance. Do not pick up the child or stay more than 30 seconds. If the crying continues, return in 5 minutes and repeat the procedure. Thus the parent can determine whether there is any real problem, and the child feels secure.
4. If extended *crying continues, lengthen the time to return* to the child to 10 minutes. Eventually fatigue will occur, the cry will turn to whimpers, and the child will fall asleep.
5. The child *should remain in his or her bed* rather than co-sleep for all or part of the night with parents. Co-sleepers should plan to have the child in his or her own crib all night by no later than 3 years of age. However, if the parents make an occasional exception, such as during a family crisis of major loss, trauma, or transition or if the child is ill, neither the marriage relationship nor the child's development will be hindered. It is important that the exception not become the routine.
6. *As the child grows older, limit the number of times the child can get up*, for any reason, after going to the bathroom and to bed.

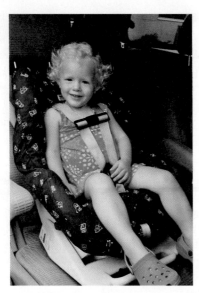

FIGURE ◻ 10-2 Toddler growth requires a change in the automobile restraint device.

the home, *to make it as safe as possible.* Some of the injury prevention suggestions presented in Chapter 9 are applicable. ∞

Explore thoroughly safety promotion and safety surveillance with the parents, and the following *normal developmental characteristics that make the toddler prone to accidents. The toddler:*

1. Moves quickly and is impulsive.
2. Likes to climb, stretch, and reach, but has limited physical coordination.
3. Is inquisitive, curious, and assertive.
4. Enjoys learning by touch, taste, and sight.
5. Enjoys playing with small objects.
6. Likes to attract attention.
7. Imitates the actions of others.
8. Has a short attention span and unreliable memory.
9. Lacks judgment and experience.
10. Has incomplete self-awareness.
11. Has rudimentary problem-solving skills.

Teach parents they can prevent falls by (a) avoiding hazardous waxing, (b) removing throw rugs, (c) keeping traffic lanes clear,
(d) placing locked gates at the tops and bottoms of stairways, (e) locking screens on the windows, (f) placing toys and favorite objects on a low shelf, and (g) using appropriate child safety seats in the car and grocery cart.

Burns are prevented by various measures. Teach parents to block access to electric outlets, heating equipment, candles, matches, lighters, hot water or hot food, stoves, ovens, fireplaces, and any appliances that heat. Handles of pans should be turned to the back of the stove. Electric cords attached to appliances that heat should not drape over the top edge of a work or counter surface. Fireworks should never be used when a young child is nearby.

Drowning may occur in various places. Teach parents that the child may drown within minutes in the bathtub, a bucket, the toilet, the backyard swimming pool, ditches, or larger bodies of water. The child is helpless in water and unaware of the danger (43). Water is fun to play in. Educate parents to *teach the toddler to swim,* but that will *not* prevent drowning in unsafe conditions. A responsible person should *always stay with the child when he or she is near water.* Emphasize to parents to *not* allow boisterous play or sharp objects near a swimming pool. Four-sided fencing should surround the pool and have a childproof latch.

Poisoning is common during childhood, especially in the 2-year-old group (43). Toddlers explore everything by mouth. Almost every nonfood substance, including vitamin supplements, are potentially harmful. Child-resistant closures on containers are essential. Storing hygiene, household, and gardening supplies out of reach and locked is important, yet difficult. Toddlers like to climb heights and unlatch doors; only a locked door or drawer is safe.

Teach parents to have two doses of ipecac syrup for each child in the house and know its proper use and administration in case of poisoning (43). Parents should have a poison treatment chart available. They should have the phone number and location of the nearest poison control center. Calls are routed to local centers. Refer to the **Box**, Client Education: Parent Teaching to Prevent Poisoning, for more suggestions to share with parents.

Teach parents the **Heimlich maneuver**, *a series of subdiaphragmatic abdominal thrusts, which is a first aid measure for choking* or to force out an aspirated object or piece of food. The procedure creates an artificial cough that forces air and the foreign object out of the child's airway. The procedure can be done while the child is standing, sitting, or lying down. In the conscious, choking child,

INTERVENTIONS FOR HEALTH PROMOTION

Teach parents they can reduce harm or prevent injury in the home by:

1. Selecting safe toys.
2. Avoiding tablecloths that extend over the edge when objects are on the table.
3. Selecting furniture with rounded corners and a sturdy base.
4. Packing away breakable objects.

5. Covering any sharp object, knife, or tool, or placing it out of the child's reach or in a locked cabinet.
6. Not allowing children to run, jump, wrestle, or throw objects in the house; parents should not initiate or encourage this kind of activity.
7. Putting safety catches on doors to prevent the child from opening furniture doors or pulling furniture onto self.
8. Disconnecting unused appliances, wrapping cords, and securing cords in use.

Client Education

Parent Teaching to Prevent Poisoning

1. Teach the child that medication and vitamins are not candy; keep them locked. Discard old medicine.
2. Keep medicines, polishes, insecticides, drain cleaners, bleaches, household chemicals, garage products, and other potentially toxic substances in a locked cabinet out of the child's reach. Do not store them in containers previously used for food.
3. Store nonfood substances in original containers with labels attached, not in food or beverage containers.
4. If you are interrupted while pouring or using a product that is potentially harmful, take it with you. The toddler is curious and impulsive and moves quickly.
5. Keep telephone numbers of the physician, poison control center, local hospital, and police and fire departments by the telephone.
6. Teach the child not to eat berries, flowers, or plants; some are poisonous.

INTERVENTIONS FOR HEALTH PROMOTION

Teach parents to *reduce risk of the toddler aspirating and choking through the following measures* (26, 43):

1. Supervise or be present when meals and snacks are served; watch what older siblings feed the child.
2. Prepare food in forms that are easy to eat and can be eaten as finger foods. For example, cut food such as bananas, strips of cheese, graham crackers, and bagels into small pieces.
3. Avoid foods that are difficult to chew or swallow, for example:
   a. Small, hard foods that can block the airway and cut off oxygen, such as nuts, seeds, popcorn, snack chips or puffs, pretzels, raw carrots, or raisins.
   b. Slippery foods, such as whole grapes, large pieces of meat, poultry, or frankfurters. Chop or cut these foods into small pieces.
   c. Sticky foods like peanut butter, unless spread as a thin layer on bread.
   d. Candy, cough drops, and chewing gum. These should not be given to the toddler.
4. Insist the child sit to eat or drink; encourage the child to chew thoroughly.
5. Do not allow the child to eat or drink while in a car seat, lying down, or physically active or running.

upward thrusts to the upper abdomen are delivered with a fisted hand below the rib cage and the xiphoid process of the sternum. Up to five thrusts should be repeated in rapid succession until the foreign body is expelled. After breathing is restored, the child should be allowed to rest in a side-lying position and should receive medical attention to check for complications (43).

Parents may call you to help when their child has been injured or is ill. Encourage parents to learn emergency care. The Red Cross is a source of first aid information.

COMMON HEALTH PROBLEMS: PREVENTION AND PROTECTION

Common health threats in the United States at this age are respiratory infections and home accidents. Communicable diseases are less a health threat than parasitic diseases (33, 43). Because respiratory conditions are common, teach parents and the child to "cover the cough" and "wash hands." *Demonstrate the following 1-2-3 steps to the toddler, and have the toddler imitate you in the procedure:*

1. Cover mouth and nose with a tissue during a cough or sneeze or cover the mouth with the upper sleeve. *Do not use bare hands.*
2. Put tissue in the wastebasket.
3. Then wash hands with soap and water after coughing or sneezing (to the count of 20, or 20 seconds, or teach the child a fun saying that takes 20 seconds to complete). Or clean with an alcohol-based hand cleaner.

Reinforce to parents that they follow through each time the toddler coughs or sneezes, and to use the same procedure themselves.

The child must be carefully assessed for infections and other disease conditions because he or she lacks the cognitive, verbal, and self-awareness capacities to describe specific discomforts. The child's pain level must be assessed when ill or injured. Pain documentation is inadequate in the pediatric population, especially in toddlers. In turn, he or she is unlikely to receive adequate treatment, analgesia, and subsequent relief and rest (22). Consult pediatric nursing texts for additional information on childhood illnesses and their assessment, care, and prevention.

MediaLink Common Toddler Health Problems and Health Promotion

Healthy People 2010

Example of Objectives for Toddler Health Promotion

1. Reduce toddler deaths or risk of death.
2. Increase percentage of healthy children who sleep in their own beds.
3. Ensure appropriate screening, follow-up, and referral to services for health problems.
4. Increase proportion of territories and states that have service delivery systems for children with special health care needs.

5. Increase the proportion of persons who have a specific source of ongoing care.
6. Prevent disease, disability, and death from infectious diseases, including vaccine preventable diseases.
7. Achieve and maintain effective vaccination coverage levels for universally recommended vaccines among young children.
8. Increase the proportion of preschool children age 5 years and under who receive vision screening.

Adapted from reference 75.

Health problems vary with the family and social culture. In the United States, respiratory infections, asthma, and otitis media are common health problems in toddlers (33, 43). Asthma has complex symptomatology and treatment; refer to a pediatric nursing text for in-depth information on care of the child. *The environment also contributes to health problems.* An estimated 3 to 4 million children in the United States live within one mile of at least one hazardous waste site. Children who live near waste sites, such as those described in Chapter 4, ∞ have greater exposure to and potential for associated health problems. The Agency for Toxic Substances and Disease Registry (ATSDC) presents a Website with additional information about child health issues, www.atrdr.cdc.gov.

Food allergic reactions occur in 6% to 8% of children younger than 3 years. Sensitivity to food additives also occurs as explained in Chapter 4. ∞ The most common allergens are cow's milk, eggs, peanuts, tree nuts, fish, shellfish, soybeans, and wheat. Some children outgrow reactivity by age 10; shellfish, peanut, and tree nut allergies are lifelong. The immune system identifies mistakenly a specific food or food component as harmful. B lymphocytes produce immunoglobulin E (IgE) antibodies to antagonize the food allergies. Ingestion of the food causes IgE antibodies to signal the immune system to activate mast cells and basophils. Inflammatory substances, histamine, and prostaglandins are produced that result in systemic symptoms. The skin, mucous membranes, and respiratory tract are affected. Itching, congestion, and oropharyngeal edema may progress to the life-threatening anaphylaxis and respiratory distress and must be treated immediately, with 4 to 6 hours of monitoring afterwards (43). *Preventive measures* include breastfeeding for 6 to 12 months, delayed introduction of solid foods in infancy, and total avoidance of peanuts and tree nuts. Some fruits may trigger cross-reactivity, such as bananas, pears, apples, cherries, and melon. Avoidance of contact with or ingestion of the allergens is the only safe strategy (24, 26, 33, 43). The Website by the Food Allergy and Anaphylaxis Network (FAAN) presents information about food allergies, www.foodallergy.org.

Malnutrition is a major global health problem, particularly in children under age 5 years. Causes include lack of food because of drought, famine, and inadequate food resources in the developing and underdeveloped countries of the world. Further, the trend to bottle feed in these countries deprives the infant of the nutrients in mother's milk and results in diarrhea from unsanitary preparation practices. Breastfed babies, weaned when a new sibling arrives, become malnourished in many countries where there is little or no food available. In the United States, poverty and parental feeding practices may contribute to less obvious malnutrition (24, 26, 33, 43). **Kwashiorkor**, *severe protein and other nutrient deficiency*, causes growth retardation; emaciation with the bloated abdomen typical of low serum albumin; dry, scaly, depigmented skin; hair loss; reduced immunity and increased rate of infections; dehydration with hypokalemia and hypernatremia; fatty infiltration of the liver; and eventual atrophy of muscles and vital organs. The child becomes more withdrawn, irritable, and apathetic. Death may ensue due to severe diarrhea, infection, or circulatory failure (24, 26, 43). **Marasmus**, *a syndrome of protein and calorie deficiency due to physical and emotional deprivation, is seen in failure-to-thrive children.* The condition may occur as early as 3 months of age if breastfeeding is not successful and there are no suitable alternatives (43). Refer to pediatric nursing texts for therapeutic management and nursing care. *Prevention is the critical community and global health issue.*

Teach parents to avoid smoking in order to reduce respiratory disease, asthma, and otitis media. Encourage parents to work with others to ensure a healthy community environment, as well as to monitor for health and safety in their own home. Be an advocate for environmental health. Review normal nutrition with parents and explain that there are degrees of malnutrition. Advocate for child nutrition and health globally through international organizations, including the International Council of Nurses, Doctors without Borders, and other agencies. Keep abreast of child health issues.

Refer to the **Box** *Healthy People 2010* Example of Objectives for Toddler Health Promotion for health concerns and prevention strategies in the United States, formulated by the U.S. Department of Health and Human Services (75). For more information, refer to the Website www.health.gov or call 1-800-367-4725.

Psychosocial Concepts

COGNITIVE DEVELOPMENT

The intellectual capacity of the toddler is limited according to adult capacities. However, the child has all the body equipment that allows for an assimilation of the environment and increasing intellectual maturity (34).

Learning occurs through several general modes, including (6, 38, 66, 67, 76):

1. Natural unfolding and maturation of the innate physical, sensory, and neuromuscular capacity.
2. **Guided participation**, *intellectual interaction with adults who structure opportunities and bridge the gaps between the child's and adult's understanding, which fosters imitation of others.*
3. Reinforcement from others as the child engages in acceptable behavior.
4. Insight, gaining understanding in increasing depth as he or she plays, experiments, or explores.
5. Imitation or primary identification, taking into self values and attitudes like those with whom he or she is closely associated.

The toddler experiences the world in a **parataxic mode**, *in that wholeness of experience and cause-and-effect relationships do not exist.* He or she experiences parts of things in the present; they are not necessarily events connected with past and future (73). It is necessary to repeat simple and honest explanations, for example, why a certain tool works or why he or she should not play in the street. Eventually this leads to understanding of cause and effect (34, 73).

The toddler's attention span lengthens. He or she likes songs, nursery rhymes, and stories, even if they are not fully understood. The child names pictures on repeated exposure, plays alone sometimes but prefers being near people, and is aware of self and others in a new way. *Part of the toddler's learning is through* (a) imitation of the parents and family members, (b) helping them with simple tasks such as bringing an object, (c) trying new activities on his or her own, (d) ritualistic repetition of activity, (e) experimenting with language, and (f) expressing self emotionally. According to Piaget, the toddler finishes the fifth and sixth stages of the Sensorimotor Period and begins the Preoperational Period at approximately 2 years (76).

In the **fifth stage of the Sensorimotor Period, Tertiary Circular Reactions** (12 to 18 months), *the child consolidates previous activities involving body actions into experiments to discover new properties of objects and events and to achieve new goals instead of applying habitual behavior.* He or she does not keep repeating the same behavior to achieve a goal, performs familiar acts without random maneuvers, and uses concepts to solve simple problems. The child differentiates self from objects in the environment. Understanding of object permanence, space perception, and time perception can be observed in new ways. The child is aware that objects continue to exist even though they cannot be seen; he or she accounts for sequential displacements and searches for objects where they were last seen or until they are found. The toddler manipulates objects in new and novel ways to learn what they will do.

The child is intrigued by the variety of properties that objects possess and by the many ways he or she can make something happen. For the first time, objects outside the self are understood as causes of action. Activities are now linked to internal representations, a developing memory, or symbolic meaning of events or objects (memories, ideas, feelings about past events) (76).

The **sixth stage of the Sensorimotor Period, Internal Representation of Action in the External World** (*making mental combinations*), extends from 18 to 24 months. *Now the child relies less on sensorimotor experiences for learning.* The toddler uses less trial-and-error thinking but uses memory of past experience and imitation to act *as if* he or she arrived at an answer. He or she imitates another who is out of sight. The toddler solves problems that combine motor and mental skills. The child can foresee maneuvers that will succeed or fail. The child thinks about an activity or situation without directly acting out the behavior. Increasing memory and symbolic thought allows the toddler to think about events and anticipate consequences without always resorting to actions—a beginning of insight (76).

In the **Preoperational Period** (2 to 7 years), *thought is more symbolic; memory continues to form; and the child internalizes mental pictures of people, the environment, and ideas about rules and relationships.* The child begins to arrive at answers mentally instead of through physical activity, exploration, and manipulation. *Symbolic representation is seen in* (38, 76): (a) use of language to describe objects, events, and feelings; (b) beginning of symbolic play (for example, crossing two sticks to represent a plane); and (c) **delayed imitation** (*repeating a parent's behavior hours or days later*).

In the early Preoperational Period, the toddler can understand simple concepts. Thinking is basically **concrete**, *related to tangible or observable events and literal in meaning.* The child is **egocentric**, *unable to take the viewpoint of another.* The ability to differentiate between subject and object, the real object and the word symbol, is not developed. He or she knows one word for an object and cannot understand how the one word, for example, *chair*, can refer to many different styles of chairs. If the flower is called *flower* and *plant*, the child will not understand that more than one word can refer to the same object. Concept of time is now, and concept of distance is whatever can be seen. The child imitates the thinking and behavior observed in another but lacks the past experience and broader knowledge that is essential for logical thought. This level of learning will continue through the preschool era (66, 67, 76).

The following behaviors in the home environment positively influence the child's cognitive performance (9, 66): (a) giving encouragement to explore the environment, (b) being involved with the child's daily events and play, (c) reinforcing the child's achievements, (d) providing books for the child and avoiding excessive use of television or computers, (e) guiding the child to practice and expand skills, (f) providing playthings that encourage concept formation, (g) stimulating language and social skills development, and (h) protecting the child from inappropriate disapproval or punishment for mistakes when trying skills. Poverty curbs cognitive growth by limiting parental ability to provide educational resources and exerts a negative psychological effect on the parents and parenting (9).

However, *pushing children to read and write or perform certain tasks at an early age has not been shown to produce long-lasting positive effects.* It may cause the child to lose initiative, curiosity, desire to use ingenuity, and ability to cope. Before parents put the child in a preschool that emphasizes formal academics, they should consider what the child is not learning from missed playtime. Play that is parallel to and cooperative with peers helps the child develop language, motor, cognitive, nonverbal, and social skills; positive self-esteem, a sense of worth as an individual; and unique problem-solving skills in the face of stress (6, 66).

Teach parents about cognitive development and the importance of opportunities without pressure on the child to achieve or succeed. Play is a natural medium for learning. This period can be trying and should be tempered by *supportive parental guidance and discipline:* (a) saying what is meant, (b) providing environmental stimulation, (c) showing interest in the child's activities and talking and working with the child, (d) reinforcing intellectual attempts, and (e) showing a willingness to teach with simple explanations. Explain that the amount and quality of parent–child interaction helps the child learn to enjoy learning, which forms the basis for later school achievement. Share information from **Box 10-4**, Examples of Educational Toys and Play for the Toddler (6, 20, 21, 38, 43, 66, 67).

LANGUAGE DEVELOPMENT

The toddler is still more focused on motor than verbal skills. *Learning to communicate in an understandable manner begins during this era.* The child understands words before they are used with meaning. Through speech the toddler will gradually learn to control unacceptable behavior, exchange physical activity for words, and share the view of reality held by society. The child cannot store a memory until he or she is able to talk about the event. The child is capable of considerable learning, including more than one language and words of simple songs and prayers (6, 7, 26, 40, 66, 67).

Various theories explain language acquisition. Although **Behavioral or Learning Theory** *explains some language learning through receiving reinforcement* for imitation of language sounds, the number of specific stimulus-response connections that would be necessary to speak even one language could not be acquired in a lifetime. Nor do behaviorists explain the sequence of language development, regardless of culture. However, learning principles can be used to modify acquired language deficits (6, 66).

Interactionist Theory is used by most theorists to explain language development. *Language develops through interaction between heredity, maturation, encounters with people and environmental stimuli, and life experiences.* Humans are biologically prepared for language learning, but experience with the spoken word and with loving people who facilitate language acquisition is equally essential. Further, the child has an active role in learning language rather than a passive one. The adult modifies their speech when talking to a child, and the child is more attentive to simplified speech. Mothers and fathers use different conversational techniques to talk with the child, which teaches children language in a broader way (6, 66).

The **Nativism Theory** *emphasizes the active role of the learner.* Language is universal among humans. There may be an inborn **language acquisition device (LAD)** *that programs children's brains to analyze language and figure out the rules as people speak to them.* There may be a simple set of universal principles that underlie all languages and a single multipurpose mechanism that connects sound to meaning, particularly as the child moves from infancy to toddlerhood. The mechanism may be located in the larger hemisphere, the left hemisphere for most people (12, 28, 66, 67).

Speech and language are major adaptive behaviors being developed during the second year. Speech enables the child to become more independent and to better make needs known. The greater the comprehension and vocabulary, the further a child can go in cognitive processes. As the child and parents respond verbally and nonverbally to each other, the child learns attitudes, values, behaviors, and ideas (28). The child first responds to patterns of sounds rather than to specific word sounds; if others speak indistinctly to the child, he or she will also speak indistinctly. The typical child will begin to speak by 14 months, although some children may make little effort to speak until after 2 years. By age 3, he or she may still mispronounce more than half the sounds (6, 7, 66, 67).

The toddler speaks in the present tense initially, using **syncretic speech**, in which *one word stands for a certain object, and represents an entire sentence.* For example, "go" means "I want to go." By *18 to 20 months* he or she uses **telegraphic speech**, *two- to four-word expressions that contain a noun and verb and maintain word order,* such as "go play" and "go night-night." Variety of intonation also increases. A *2-year-old* will introduce additional words and say "I go play" or "I go night-night." Conversation with parents involves contraction and expansion. *The child shortens into fewer words what the parent says but states the main message* (**contraction**). *The parent elaborates on, uses a full sentence, and interprets what the child says* (**expansion**). Expansion helps the child's language development (66). The toddler frequently says "no," perhaps in imitation of the parents and their discipline techniques, but may often do what is asked even while saying "no." Stuttering is common because ideas come faster than the ability to use vocabulary; attention should not be focused on stuttering. Gesturing is an important part of communication. Simple gestures and gesturing games begin in infancy. At *13 months,* the child understands and uses more elaborate gesturing. By *20 months,* the toddler uses fewer gestures and more words and labels for objects (66).

Recognizable language develops sequentially. See **Table 10-3** for a summary of language and speech development (6, 29, 38, 43, 66, 67). Apparently the child learns to speak in a highly methodical way, breaking down language into its simplest parts and developing rules to put the parts together. Children proceed from babbling to one-word and two-word sentences, use of word order and plurals, and negative sentences. Phonetics as a sound system is important. To communicate effectively, the child must learn not only the language and its rules, but also the use of social speech, which takes into account the knowledge and perspective of another person (29). This begins in toddlerhood and continues to develop through childhood as the child gains interpersonal and social experiences.

Learning at least a second language is essential in today's world. The best time to learn more than one language is during the language/auditory-sensitive years of early childhood when dendrites and axons adjust to the languages a child hears. Beginning

TABLE 10-3

Assessment of Language and Speech Development

Characteristics	Age			
	1 Year	1½ Years	2 Years	2½–3 Years
Language understanding and basic communication	Understands "no-no" inhibition; knows "bye-bye" and pat-a-cake; says "mama," "dada," or some similar term for caretakers	Understands very simple verbal instructions accompanied by gesture and intonation; identifies 3 body parts; points to 5 simple pictures; points for wants	Identifies 5 body parts; finds 10 pictures; obeys simple commands	Points to 15 pictures; obeys 2 or 3 simple commands
Appearance of individual sounds	10 vowels, 9 consonants in babbling and echoing	p, b, m, h, w in babbling		t, d, n, k, g, ng in words
Auditory memory imitation and repetition	Lalls; imitates sound; echoes or repeats syllables or some words (may not have meaning)		Meanings increasingly becoming associated with words	Repeats 2 digits; remembers 1 or 2 objects
Numerical size of vocabulary	1 or 2 words	50 words Adds 10–20 words a week	50–400 words if consistently spoken to	400–500 words 400 words by 3 years
Word type	Nouns	Nouns, action verbs, some adjectives	Nouns, verbs, adjectives, adverbs	Pronouns, "I"
Sentence length	Single word	Single words expanding to 3 or 4 words, noun and verb	2–5 words; elemental sentence	Basic sentence
Description of vocalization and communication	Babbling, lalling, echolalia (repeating sounds)	Leading, pointing, jargon, some words, intonations, gestures	Words, phrases, simple sentences	Developmental language problems first seen
Purpose of vocalization and communication	Pleasure	Attention getting	Meaningful social control; wish requesting	Interaction; express needs; convey yearnings
Speech content and style			Possessive "mine"; pronouns last grammar form learned; grammar depends on what is heard	
Percent intelligibility		20–25% for person unfamiliar with child	60–75%; poor articulation of some words	Vowel production—90%

Data from references 6, 38, 43, 67, 68.

in toddlerhood, the child can learn distinct grammars, gestures, pauses, and pronunciations. Bilingualism may slow down vocabulary development in one or both languages. However, young children can become fluent in two languages, especially if parents speak the two languages and expose the child consistently to both languages (4, 6, 40).

Teach parents that language and speech development is facilitated when they teach social language strategies to the child as they introduce him or her to life experiences. Through conversation,

mealtime experiences, and play with a variety of objects and stimuli, the toddler's vocabulary is enlarged, family expressions that aid socialization are learned, and positive reinforcement can be given. Language development requires a sense of security and verbal and nonverbal stimulation. For a child to speak, he or she must have a loving, consistent relationship with a parent or caretaker. Unless the toddler feels that this person will respond to his or her words, the toddler will not be motivated to speak. Emphasize to parents that using adult words rather than baby talk, being read to, and having an opportunity to explore the environment increase the child's comprehension of words and rules of grammar, organization and size of vocabulary, and use of word inflections.

Prepare the parents and health care providers to realize the toddler may not talk when separated from the parents, such as during hospitalization or the first day at day care. When being prepared for hospital procedures, the toddler needs simple and succinct explanations, familiar words with gestures pointing to the areas of the body being cared for, and verbal and physical displays of affection. *If a child is delayed in speech, carefully assess the child and family. Causes may include* (33, 43, 50, 53, 64, 70): (a) deafness or the inability to listen, (b) mental retardation, (c) emotional disturbance, (d) maternal deprivation or separation from the parents, (e) lack of verbal communication within the family and to the child, (f) inconsistent or tangential responses to the child's speech, (g) presence of multiple siblings, or (h) parents anticipating the needs of the child before he or she has a chance to communicate them. Direct your intervention to the cause, involving the child and family. A multidisciplinary team approach may be necessary.

EMOTIONAL DEVELOPMENT

The toddler demonstrates a range of emotions. The toddler is a self-loving, uninhibited, dominating, energetic little person absorbed in self-importance, always seeking attention, approval, and personal goals. Sometimes the toddler is cuddly and loving. At other times, he or she bites or pinches and looks almost happy, feeling no sense of guilt or shame. There is little self-control over exploratory or sadistic impulses. The toddler only slowly realizes that he or she cannot have everything desired and that some behavior annoys others. He or she experiments with abandon in the quest for independence, yet becomes easily frightened and runs to the parent for protection, security, reassurance, and approval. Sadness, joy, contentment, distress, and anger are shown by facial expressions, crying, and body movements.

Because the toddler still relies so much on the parents and wants their approval, he or she learns to curb the negativism without losing independent drives, to cooperate more frequently, and to develop socially approved behavior. *Need for attention and approval is one of the main motivating forces in ego development and socialization.* The toddler often repeats performances and behavior that are given attention and laughed at; he or she likes to perform for adults and pleases self as much as the audience. He or she has a primitive sense of humor; laughs frequently, especially at surprise sounds and startling incongruities; laughs with others who are laughing; and laughs at his or her own antics.

Teach parents to give sufficient attention but not make the child show off for an audience, verbally or physically. They should not overstimulate with laughter or games. Further, adults must realize the child fears separation, strangers, darkness, sudden or loud noises, large objects and machines, and hurtful events such as traumatic procedures.

The *effects of emotional, social, and physical deprivation* were demonstrated by infants and young children in Romanian orphanages in the late 1980s and 1990s, abandoned because of political dictatorship and upheaval. They were starving and had minimal contact with adult caregivers or each other. When they were found and humanitarian efforts were directed toward adoption (most by

Canada, some by the United States), the world learned of 2- and 3-year-olds who could not walk or talk. Radiological positron emission tomography (PET) scans of the brain showed extreme inactivity in the temporal lobes, which regulate emotions and receive sensory inputs. At the times of adoption, 80% of the children demonstrated delayed motor, language, and psychosocial development (13). Three years later, when these children were compared with those left behind in Romanian institutions, many of the adopted children showed significant progress. About 33% had no serious problems and were doing well. About 33%, those who had been in institutions the longest, had serious developmental problems. The other children were moving toward average performance and behavior (2). Those who had been adopted by 2 years of age had average IQs and verbal comprehension at age 5 years. But the orphanage group, as a whole, were not at the same performance level as Canadian-born nonadopted children nor with a group of Romanian children adopted by 4 months of age who had not been in an orphanage (2, 62, 63). At age 8 years, PET scans found persistent underactivity in portions of the children's brains (13, 74). Similar effects of deprivation had been described by Spitz following World War II and thereafter (71, 72).

Refer to the Abstract for Evidence-Based Practice for effects of very preterm birth on the emotional and behavioral development of the toddler. Maternal factors are also analyzed.

DEVELOPMENTAL CRISIS
Autonomy Versus Shame and Doubt

According to Erikson, the psychosexual crisis for the toddler is autonomy versus shame and doubt (30). **Autonomy** *is characterized by the oft-heard statement, "Me do it," the ability to gain self-control.*

Box 10-6, Characteristic Behaviors of Autonomy, presents what has been achieved gradually during the toddler years and manifested by the child who is about 3 years of age (30).

BOX 10-6	Characteristic Behaviors of Autonomy

1. Demonstrate increasing self-control over motor abilities and sphincters.
2. Maintain sense of security and control through:
   a. Using negativism; saying "no" although he or she may do as asked.
   b. Displaying temper, grabbing or pushing.
   c. Dawdling or being impatient, depending on situation.
   d. Using rituals, resisting change, insisting on the familiar.
   e. Exploring even when parents object.
3. Make and carry out discussions.
4. Cope with problems or get help; develop language skills.
5. Distinguish between possessions or wishes of self and others, hold on or share as indicated.
6. Demonstrate increasing patience, willingness to wait.
7. Manifest pride and increasing control over their body or situation.

Abstract for Evidence-Based Practice

Comparison of Behavioral Problems Between Very Preterm Children and Term Children

Delobel-Ayoub, M., Kaminski, A., Marrst, S., Burqult, A., Marchant, L., N'Guyon, S., et al. (2006). Behavioral outcome at 3 years of life in very preterm infants: The EPIPAGE Study. *Pediatrics, 117*(5), 1996–2005.

KEYWORDS

Very preterm child behavior, preschool age.

Purpose ➤ To compare prevalence of behavioral problems between very preterm children and term children when they were 3 years old and to examine factors associated with behavioral problems in preterm children. This study was part of the EPIPAGE Study (Etude Epidemiologique Sur les Petits Ages Gestational Study).

Conceptual Framework ➤ Studies on preterm children and behavior.

Sample/Setting ➤ This prospective, population-based cohort study included all infants born between 27 and 32 weeks of gestation and all infants born at term in nine regions of France in 1997. At age 3 years, 1,228 very preterm children without major neurodevelopmental disorders and 447 children born at term constituted the sample.

Method ➤ Data were collected at birth on neonatal status and sociodemographic status. Follow-up of neonates and parents at discharge from the hospital resulted in a prospective number of 2,382 parents of preterm infants and 666 parents of term infants. When the children were 3 years old, the parents were contacted; 2,276 (96%) of parents of preterm and 557 (84%) of parents of term infants responded. The responding parents were sent the Behavioral Strengths and Difficulties Questionnaire. Completed questionnaires were returned by parents of 1,880 (79%) preterm and 453 (68%) term babies. Parents were excluded from the study if the child was deaf, blind, or had major disabilities.

Findings ➤ Significant differences were found between the two groups. Higher difficulty scores were reported by parents of singleton preterm than term babies, for male than female children, and for children who had been hospitalized in the past year or who were diagnosed as having neurodevelopmental delay. Higher difficulty scores were also reported by mothers who were younger in age or reported lower socioeconomic status. Very preterm newborns with birth weight less than the 10th percentile for gender and gestational age were more likely at age 3 years to have behavioral problems than were term newborns (the controls). Preterm children were more likely to have hyperactivity, conduct disorders, emotional problems such as anxiety and depression, and difficulty relating to peers. Several medical conditions were associated with high total difficulty scores: major neonatal cerebral lesions diagnosed by cranial ultrasonic studies for children hospitalized in the past year, overall poor health, and psychomotor delay. Risk factors for preterm babies were high birth order for the child, young maternal age, and low educational level in the mother.

Implications ➤ Prevention and management of high-risk pregnancies are essential for the child's later developmental progress and health. Special long-term care should be directed to infants born very preterm and to their parents to reduce as much as possible complications and difficult behaviors in the child and to assist parents with the child's care. The study results in France parallel research findings in the United States. Implications for public health in the United States and globally are evident.

Although autonomy is developing, emotions are still contagious. The toddler reflects others' behavior and feelings. For example, if someone laughs or cries, the toddler will imitate for no apparent reason. Empathy is also evident. Empathy is related to ability to discern emotional expressions in people and a developing interest in others (6). By 13 to 15 months, the toddler attempts to comfort a crying child and will bring his or her own mother, if available, to help the crying child (6).

Shame and doubt are felt if autonomy and a positive self-concept are not achieved (30). **Shame** is the *feeling of being fooled, embarrassed, exposed, small, impotent, dirty, wanting to hide, and rage against self.* **Doubt** is *fear, uncertainty, mistrust, lack of self-confidence, and feeling that nothing done is any good and that one is controlled by others rather than being in control of self* (30). There is a limit to how exposed, dirty, mean, and vulnerable one can feel.

If the child is pushed past the limit or disciplined or toilet trained too harshly, or abused, he or she can no longer discriminate about self, what he or she should be and can do. If everything is planned and done for and to the child, he or she cannot develop autonomy. The toddler's self-concept and behavior will try to measure up to the expectations of parents and others, but there is no close attachment to an adult. **Box 10-7**, Consequences of Shame and Doubt, outlines traits and behaviors of a child who develops stronger feelings of shame and doubt than of autonomy. Too much shaming does not develop a sense of propriety but rather a secret determination to get away with things (6, 30).

Teach parents that reasonable limits help the toddler gain positive experiences and responses from others and build a sense of self and autonomy. Accepting the toddler's behaviors and allowing some self-expression and choice fosters autonomy.

BOX 10-7	Consequences of Shame and Doubt

1. Has difficulty with eating, digestion, elimination, sleep
2. Has low self-esteem
3. Has low frustration tolerance, gives up easily
4. Is apathetic, withdrawn
5. Is passive, too compliant, easily controlled or manipulated
6. Is excessively negative, defiant
7. Is impulsive
8. Is physically overactive, aggressive
9. Is angry about being controlled or manipulated by others
10. Is stubbornly assertive, obstinate
11. Has little sense of responsibility
12. Is sneaky, wanting to get away with things
13. Is compulsive
14. Hoards
15. Is overmeticulous or excessively messy

Discourage parents from creating an emotional climate of excessive expectations, criticism, blame, punishment, and over-restriction for the toddler, because within the child's consciousness a sense of shame and doubt may develop that will be extremely harmful to further development. The child should not be given too much autonomy or pushed unreasonably to achieve, or he or she will feel all-powerful. When a toddler fails to accomplish what he or she has been falsely led to believe could be achieved, the self-doubt and shame that result can be devastating. Aggressive behavior results if the child is severely punished or if parents are aggressive. With the proper balance of guidance and discipline, the toddler gains a sense of personal abilities and thus has the potential to deal with the next set of social adjustments.

While Erikson described the toddler achieving a sense of autonomy at the end of toddlerhood (30), this process was described in another way by Margaret Mahler (54). In her **Object Relations Theory**, Mahler explained the *process of separation-individualization from birth to 36 months, when a sense of separateness from the parenting figure is finally established. The six phases are as follows* (54):

1. **Phase 1 (birth to 1 month), Autistic Phase.** *The baby spends most of his or her time in a half-waking, half-sleeping state.* The main goal is fulfillment of needs for survival and comfort.
2. **Phase 2 (1 to 5 months), Symbiotic Phase.** *There is a type of psychic fusion of mother and child. The child views the self as an extension of the parenting figure, although there is a developing awareness of needs being fulfilled by external sources, especially the mothering one.*
3. **Phase 3 (5 to 10 months), Differentiation Phase.** *The child is beginning to recognize that there is a separateness between the self and the mothering one.*
4. **Phase 4 (10 to 16 months), Practicing Phase.** *Increased locomotor functioning and the ability to explore the environment independently are developing. A sense of separateness of the self is increased.*

5. **Phase 5 (16 to 24 months), Rapprochement Phase.** *Awareness of separateness of the self becomes acute.* This is frightening to the child, who wants to regain some lost closeness but not return to symbiosis. The child wants the mother there as needed for "emotional refueling" and to maintain feelings of security.
6. **Phase 6 (24 to 36 months), on the way to Object Constancy Phase.** *The child completes the individuation process and learns to relate to objects in an effective, constant manner. A sense of separateness is established. The child is able to internalize a sustained image of the loved object or person when out of sight.* Separation anxiety is resolved.

Development may not proceed as described above (50).

Toilet Training: Related to Development of Autonomy

Toilet training is a major developmental accomplishment and relates directly to the crisis of autonomy versus shame and doubt or to what Freudian theorists call the **Anal Stage**, described in Chapter 1 ∞ (7). *Independence and autonomy, not cleanliness, are the critical issues in teaching the child to use the toilet.* For the process to work, the parents must do little more than arrange for the child to use the toilet easily. The parent supports rather than acts as a trainer and is interested in the child, not just the act. The toddler is interested in the products he excretes. The toddler gradually learns to control bowel and bladder. *Neuromuscular maturity increases from 1 to 3 years. Bowel control occurs before bladder control because of neuromuscular maturation* (43).

Cultures vary in approaches to toilet training. In some cultures, the mother begins toilet training before the child is 1 year, and the child is expected to achieve dryness by 18 months. In other cultures, the child is not expected to be toilet trained until about 5 years of age (3). In the United States, there is more pressure to have toddlers trained by age 2 years. *Every well child can carry out this task by age 3, based on neuromuscular development.*

Many factors are involved besides biological readiness, since the toddler's fears, goals, and conflicting wishes also influence this learning experience. Psychologically, toilet training is complex. The mother gives approval not only for defecating properly but also for withholding feces. The sensations of expelling and withholding feces, imitation of parents and siblings, approval from family, and pride in the accomplishments hasten toilet training. Being forced may cause problems of negativism.

Teach parents that since elimination is a natural process, toilet training should be approached in a matter-of-fact and relaxed way. Some resistance can be expected. The information from this section can be shared with parents.

Bowel training *is a less complex task than bladder training and should be attempted first.* Some toddlers, after defecation, cry and indicate distress until they are changed. Others do not indicate discomfort and will play with and smear feces. They are curious, explore, and see nothing shameful about such behavior. They have not learned the aesthetic and cultural connotations of feces being "dirty" and "unsanitary" and not an object for play. *The toddler shows physical readiness for bowel training* when he or she (a) defecates regularly and (b) shows some signs of being aware of defecation, such as grunting, straining, and tugging at the diaper. It also helps if the child can speak, understand directions, and manipulate the clothing somewhat. *Mental readiness* includes the child (a) wanting to watch people use the toilet (which should be allowed), (b) wanting to flush the toilet, and (c) asking questions about it. *Emotional readiness* includes (a) feeling secure about using the toilet, (b) pretending to use it, and (c) asking to use it. Toilet training should not be started in turbulent periods, such as hospitalization of the toddler, homecoming of a new baby, absence of the main caretaker from home, or a family crisis. Even when started in a calm period, some regression is natural.

Teach parents about signs of readiness for toilet training. Teach them to have the child use a potty chair as it is mechanically easier than the family toilet, and the chair is his or her own. The potty chair should be in a place convenient for the child. Recommend that the child wear training pants and that training take place when disruptions in regular routine are at a minimum. The toddler should be praised for success. Parents should remain calm, reassuring, and supportive if the child has an accident.

Suggest to parents ways to prevent playing in feces: (a) changing diapers immediately after defecation, (b) having well-fitted training pants, (c) showing parental disapproval, and (d) encouraging opportunities for play and smearing with clay, sand, mud, paste, and finger paints. Play materials help the child develop natural potentials and divert instinctual urges into socially accepted behavior.

Bladder training is more complex because the reflexes appropriate for bladder training are less explicit, neurologic maturation comes later, and urination is a reflex response to bladder tensions and must be inhibited. Bladder control demands more self-awareness and self-discipline from the toddler and is usually achieved between the ages of 30 to 42 months, when physiologic development has progressed enough that the bladder can retain urine for approximately 2 hours. Waking hours and sleeping hours present two phases of control and differences in awareness of bladder function (33, 43).

The *series of events necessary for bladder training is that the toddler must* (a) first realize he or she is wet, (b) then know he or she is wetting, (c) next recognize impulses that tell that he or she is going to urinate, and (d) finally control urinating until he or she is at the toilet. A physiologically ready child is able to stay dry for 2 or more hours during the day, wakes up dry from naps, and may wake up dry in the morning.

Teach parents the process of urination. Make it clear that both boys and girls can sit down while urinating and that both may try to stand like daddy or the male in the household. Sleeping control will be effective when the child responds to bladder reflexes and not before. Cutting down on fluids before bedtime may reduce **enuresis**, or *bed-wetting*. After waking control has been well established, sleeping control usually follows.

SELF-CONCEPT AND BODY IMAGE DEVELOPMENT
Self-Concept

Self-concept *is made up of the feelings about self and body image, adaptive and defensive mechanisms, reactions from others, and one's perceptions of these reactions, attitudes, values, and many of life's ex-*periences. *The sense of self as a separate being* continues to develop; *the individuation process is complete between 24 and 36 months.* When the child is able to sustain a mental image of the loved person who is out of sight, separation anxiety is resolved (7, 10).

As the child incorporates approval and disapproval, praise and punishment, and gestures that are kind and forbidding, he or she forms an opinion about self as a person. How the person feels about self is determined to a great degree by the reactions of others and, in turn, later determines views of others. The young child is very aware of reactions that convey love, security, and approval as well as the gradient of anxiety: mild, moderate, or severe. He or she watches for signs of approval and disapproval from others in relation to self. Increasingly there is recall about what caused discomfort or anxiety. Experiences of discomfort are first with the child's mother and then are generalized to other people, and much behavior becomes organized to avoid or minimize discomfort around others (28, 73). Thus, he or she gradually evolves adaptive and defensive behaviors and learns what to do to get along with others (28, 73).

Self-awareness is demonstrated as the child says "mine" and "me" more often, beginning at about 18 to 24 months. The possessiveness with toys and inability to share that is typical of the 2-year-old may be a reflection of greater awareness of self, not just selfishness. The action may actually be an attempt to be sociable with another child (28, 73). By age 3 years, the child shows self-evaluative emotions of pride, shame, and guilt and can evaluate thoughts, plans, and behavior against what is socially acceptable (52). Building self-esteem involves more than praise. The toddler also needs to accomplish things and feel proud (46).

The various appraisals of others cause the child to form feelings of good-me or bad-me, as the self-concept (73). The toddler repeats words he or she has heard about self: "good boy," "bad girl," "stupid kid," "fat kid." A concept of **good-me** *forms in the presence of love and positive reactions. He or she likes self because others do, the basis of a* **positive self-concept**. *Reactions of disapproval or punishment from significant adults increase the child's anxiety,* and **bad-me, a negative self-concept**, results if the cycle continues. If the negative reaction is never-ending, the child may evolve defensive behaviors such as denial that prevent noticing the negative evaluations.

The child's major caretaker should have a positive self-concept and feel good about being a mother (or father). If the caretaker doubts personal worth and is depressive, these negative feelings will be conveyed nonverbally to the child and will have a direct bearing on his or her sense of security and self-worth. *This critical phase of development lies between 18 and 36 months* (7, 10, 28, 30).

Be mindful of self-concept formation as you care for toddlers, for it determines their reaction and promotes a healthy emotional development. Validate strengths that you observe in the parents, which fosters their ability to be positive with the child. Educate parents to reinforce the child's positive behavior and strengths. Emphasize to parents the importance of being consistently positive in their response. Fostering a positive self-image promotes emotional health. Emphasize that parents, especially during discipline, convey that they "do not like the behavior" but "love the child." Teach parents to provide an environment in which the child can successfully exercise skills and feel self-acceptance.

Body Image

Body image development gradually evolves as a component of self-concept. The toddler has a dim self-awareness, but with a developing sense of autonomy, he or she becomes more correctly aware of the body as a physical entity with emotional capabilities (7). The toddler is increasingly aware of pleasurable sensations in the genital area and on the skin and mouth and is learning control of the body through locomotion, toilet training, speech, and socialization. The toddler is not always aware of the whole body or the distal parts and might even consider distal parts such as the feet as something apart from self. Intrusive procedures are threatening because the child fears blood and thinks his or her insides will leak out (43).

By 18 months, if a colored sticker dot is placed on the toddler's nose, the toddler will be able to touch his or her own nose while looking in a mirror. *By age 2 years,* there is recognition of observable sexual differences. *By age 3,* the child can depict self in simple drawings or stick figures; however, assessment of body image must include the child's total behavior, language, and play, not just artwork (21). The toddler does not always know when he or she is sick, tired, too hot, or when his or her pants are wet. The child also has difficulty realizing that body productions such as feces are separate from self; therefore he or she may resist flushing the toilet. The toddler is not aware of the influences on his or her body but is aware of general feelings and thoughts and increasingly of others' reactions to his or her body and behavior. For example, when the toddler is in control of the environment, the body feels good, wonderful, and strong. When things are not going well, if he or she cannot succeed or is punished excessively, the child feels bad and shameful.

During your care of the child, show acceptance of and warmth to the child. Use a gentle touch. Use information from **Box 10-5** to incorporate playful activities into your holistic care. Use appropriate educational toys as a part of your care, as summarized in **Box 10-4**. Teach the child the correct names for body parts.

Teach parents about the importance of a positive body image and how to incorporate play to help the child better learn the names and functions of body parts. Encourage them to praise the child for functional skills. Help parents realize that their health practices are imitated; they teach health promotion and respect for the body by what they do for themselves and with the child. Emphasize that as the toddler develops, a more accurate mental picture of his or her body evolves, with parental guidance, which is essential for continuing skill development, autonomy, and ongoing physical and mental health. If the child has a physical disability or congenital anomaly, it should be spoken of realistically and approached with an accepting attitude. Encourage parents to help the child adapt or explore ways to overcome the disability when possible, thereby fostering a positive body image.

SEXUALITY DEVELOPMENT

Gender differences are based on (a) biology (hormones, brain structure, body size and musculature), and (b) environment (cultural and family patterns, explicit home teaching, parental response) (6, 51). Traditionally parents have handled sons and daughters differently during infancy, and the results became evident in toddlerhood. Because parents encourage independent behavior in males and more dependency in females, by *13 months* the son ventures farther from his mother, stays away longer, and looks at or talks to his mother less than does the daughter. The female at this age is encouraged to spend more time touching and staying near her mother than is the male. However, the separation process later seems less severe for the daughter. Perhaps sons should be touched and cuddled longer (6, 7, 51, 56, 66, 67).

Males play more vigorously with toys than do females, and they play more with nontoys such as doorknobs and light switches. Initially there is no sexual preference for toys, although parents may enforce a preference. Males show more exploratory and aggressive behavior than females, and this behavior is encouraged by the father. The female remains attentive to a wide variety of stimuli and complex visual and auditory stimuli. She demonstrates earlier language development and seems more aware of contextual relationships, perhaps because of the more constant stimulation from the mother (6, 7, 43, 51, 56, 66, 67).

Primary identification, imitation, and observation of the same-sexed parent contributes to sexual identity. The child by *15 months* is interested in his or her own and others' body parts (56). Both males and females achieve sexual pleasure through self-stimulation, although females masturbate less than males possibly because of anatomic differences (56). Demonstration of sensual activities include rocking, swinging, sliding, riding rocking horses, hugging people and toys, and posturing movements during the toddler period.

By *21 months* the child can refer to self by name, an important factor in the development of identity. By *2 years* of age, the child can categorize people into "boy" and "girl" and has some awareness of anatomic differences if he or she has had an opportunity to view them (7, 56, 65, 66). Gender preferences in play become apparent about 2 years of age, and toddlers play with their own gender (6).

By the *end of toddlerhood,* the child is more aware of his or her body, the body's excretions, and personal actions, and he or she can be more independent in the first steps of self-care.

Help parents to understand the developing sexuality of their child and to be comfortable with their own gender and sexuality so that they can cuddle the child and answer questions. Toddlers should be taught basic vocabulary associated with anatomy, elimination, and reproduction. Associations between words, functions, and behaviors can influence future sexual attitudes. Help parents understand that a wide variety of play experiences will prepare the child for adult behavior and competence. Help parents realize their son will not become a sissy if he plays with dolls or wears his mother's high heels in dramatic play, and a daughter playing with trucks does not mean she will become masculine.

ADAPTIVE MECHANISMS

Before the child is 2 years old, he or she is learning the basic response patterns appropriate for the family and culture. The child develops a degree of trust and confidence, or lack of it, in the parents; how to express annoyance, impatience, love, and joy; and how to communicate needs.

The toddler begins to adapt to the culture because of **primary identification**. He or she *imitates* the *parents and responds to their encouragement and discouragement*. With successful adaptation, the child moves toward independence. Other major adaptive mechanisms of this era include repression, suppression, denial, reaction formation, projection, and sublimation (7).

Repression *unconsciously removes from awareness the thoughts, impulses, fantasies, and memories of behavior that are unacceptable to the self.* The *bad-me* discussed earlier is an example and may result from child abuse. **Suppression** differs from repression in that it is a *conscious act*. For example, *the child forgets* that he or she has been told not to handle certain articles. **Denial** *is not admitting, even when warned, that certain factors exist,* for example, that the stove is hot and will cause a burn. **Reaction formation** *is replacing the original idea and behavior with the opposite behavior characteristics.* For example, the child flushes the toilet and describes feces as dirty instead of playing in them, thus becoming appropriately tidy. **Projection** *occurs when he or she attributes personal feelings or behaviors to someone else.* For example, if the babysitter disciplines a toddler, he or she projects dislike by saying, "You don't like me." **Sublimation** *is channeling impulses into socially acceptable behavior rather than expressing the original impulse.* For example, he or she plays with mud, finger paints, or shaving cream, which is socially acceptable, instead of playing with feces.

Teach parents that the child's adaptive behavior is strengthened when he or she is taught to do something for self and permitted to make a decision if that decision is truly his or hers to make. If the decision is one that must be carried out regardless of the toddler's wish, it can best be accomplished by giving direction rather than by asking the child if he or she wants to do something. Reinforce to parents that the child's use of denial, suppression, reaction formation, and projection is normal. The parents should not express anger at or punish the child for these adaptive behaviors. Urge parents to observe and listen closely to the child to determine the underlying needs. Encourage sublimation through artistic creations, singing, dancing, playing a musical toy, or playing in sand or with finger paints as a way to express anger or other uncomfortable feelings. Educate parents that depression may occur in the young child (16, 32, 43). Unusual or change in behavior, or lack of the usual emotional responsiveness, should be reported to a physician or graduate-prepared psychiatric clinical nurse specialist.

GUIDANCE AND DISCIPLINE

Discipline *is guidance that helps the child learn to understand and care for self and to get along with others.* It is *not* just punishing, correcting, or controlling behavior, as is commonly assumed.

From the toddler's point of view, everything is new and exciting and meant to be explored, touched, eaten, or sat on, including porcelain figurines from Spain or boiling water. In moving away from complete dependency, the toddler demonstrates energy and drive and requires sufficient restrictions to ensure physical and psychological protection and at the same time enough freedom to permit exploration and autonomy. Because the mother must now set limits, a new dimension is added to the relationship established between mother and toddler. Before, the mother met his or her basic needs immediately. With the toddler's increasing ability, freedom, and demands, the parent sometimes makes the child wait or denies a wish if it will cause harm. The transition should be made in a loving, consistent, yet flexible manner so that the child maintains trust and moves in the quest for independence. Excessive limitations, overwhelming steady pressure, or hostile bullying behavior might cause an overly rebellious, negativistic, or passive child. Complete lack of limitations can cause accidents, poor health, and insecurity.

The mother is usually the main disciplinarian at this age, and her approach is important. When the mother is under high, acute, or chronic stress, she needs support and help from others to avoid or reduce a negative discipline approach to the child, regardless of the mother's age, education, or marital status (7, 14).

Through guidance and the parent's reaction, the child is being socialized, learning what is right and wrong. Because the child cannot adequately reason, he or she must depend on and trust the parents as a guide for all activities. He or she can obey simple commands. Later, the child will be capable of internalizing rules and mores and will become self-disciplined as a result of having been patiently disciplined. Setting limits is not easy. Parents should not thwart the toddler's curiosity and enthusiasm, but they must protect from harm. Parents who oppose the toddler's desire of the moment are likely to meet with anything from a simple "no" to a temper tantrum.

Teach parents the importance of *constructive* and *consistent guidance and discipline*. Temper tantrums result because the toddler hates being thwarted and feeling helpless. Once the feelings are discharged, the child regains composure quickly and without revenge. If temper tantrums, a form of negativism, occur, the best advice is to ignore the outburst. It will soon disappear. The child needs the parent's reaction for the behavior to continue. Emphasize that belittling or whipping the child does not help temper tantrums. If he or she is given more frustration than can be handled, fear, hostility, and anger mount, and the lack of verbal ability inhibits adequate outlet. Hence he or she strikes out, bites, or hits physically. At this point, a toddler desperately needs the mother's support, firm control, and mediation. The parent's calm voice, expressing understanding of feelings, and introduction of a distracting, positive activity to restore self-esteem are important to teaching self-control. If a tantrum occurs in public and is annoying to others, the parent should remove the child from the area and leave, if possible.

MORAL-SPIRITUAL DEVELOPMENT

From birth through the toddler era might be termed the **prereligious stage**. The *toddler is absorbing basic intellectual, emotional, and moral patterns regardless of the religious conviction of the caretakers.* The toddler may repeat some phrases from prayers while imitating a certain voice tone or body posture that accompanies those prayers. The child only knows that when he or she

INTERVENTIONS FOR HEALTH PROMOTION

Because parents are sometimes confused about handling the toddler's behavior, you can assist them by teaching some *simple rules for guiding the toddler* (7, 14, 43, 66):

1. Provide an environment in which the child feels respected.
2. Decide what is important and what is not worth a battle of wills. For example, the child may not be wearing matched clothing but resists parental attempts to change. Avoid negativism and an angry scene by deciding that today it is all right for the child to wear an unmatched outfit.
3. Reconsider and pursue an alternative activity. To allow the child to have his or her way is not giving in, losing face, being a poor parent, or letting the child be manipulative. When limits are consistent, changing a direction of behavior can be a positive learning experience for the child. The child is becoming aware of being a separate person, able to assert self and influence others.
4. Remove or avoid temptations, such as breakable objects within reach or candy that should not be eaten, to avoid having to repeatedly say "no."
5. Do not ask open-ended questions for the child to decide about an activity when the decision is not really one the child can make.
6. Consider limits as more than restrictions but also as a distraction from one prohibited activity to another activity in which the child can freely participate. Distraction with alternatives or a substitute is effective with the toddler because attention span is short.
7. Reinforce appropriate behavior through approval and attention. The child will continue behavior that gains attention, even if the attention is punitive, because negative attention is better than none.
8. Set limits consistently so that the child can rely on the parent's judgment rather than testing the adult's endurance in each situation.
9. State limits clearly, concisely, simply, positively, and in a calm voice. For example, if the child cannot play with a treasured object, he or she should not be allowed to handle it. Say "Look with your hands behind your back" or "Look with your eyes, not your hands" rather than "Don't touch."
10. Set limits only when necessary. Some rules promote a sense of security, but too many confuse the child.
11. Provide a safe area where the child is free to do whatever he or she wants to do, as long as it is safe.
12. Do not overprotect the child, who should learn that some things have a price such as a bruise or a scratch.
13. Do not terminate the child's activity too quickly; tell him or her that the activity is ending.

Each situation will determine the extent of firmness or leniency needed. The toddler needs gradations of independence. The toddler also imitates how the parent disciplines, as described in the Case Situation.

imitates or conforms to certain rituals, affection and approval come that add to the sense of security. The "good" and "bad" are defined in terms of physical consequences to self.

Teach parents that the toddler can benefit from a nursery-school type of church program in which emphasis is on positive behavior and self-image and appropriate play and rest rather than on a specific lesson to learn. The toddler also needs to have others to imitate who follow the rules of society, and he or she needs rewards and reinforcement for good or desirable behavior. Refer to Chapter 1 ∞ for information about the use of behavioral therapy.

According to Kohlberg's Theory of Moral Development, *the toddler is in the Preconventional Stage.* Refer to Chapter 1 and Table 1-10 for an explanation. ∞

Case Situation

Imitation of Parental Discipline

Two-year-old Jill frequently displays anger through a temper tantrum of crying and hitting a toy on the floor when realistic limits are set. One day Jill's mother observed Jill sitting her doll on a stool in a corner of the central hallway. Jill was talking to the doll about her "bad behavior." When Jill looked satisfied that her point had been made, she removed the doll from the stool, gave the doll a hug, and said, "I love you." Then Jill continued to play with her doll and her toy kitchen appliances. Jill's mother recognized that Jill imitates parental behavior in her play and the importance of positive guidance.

Submitted by Carole Piles, PhD, MSN, RN.

DEVELOPMENTAL TASKS

Developmental tasks for the toddler may be summarized as follows (25):

1. Develop the physical skills and exercise patterns appropriate to the stage of motor development.
2. Master the basics of toilet training.
3. Master good eating and sleep habits.
4. Become more aware of being a family member, increase socialization skills.
5. Learn to communicate efficiently with an increasing number of other people.
6. Develop a sense of self-control and beginning independence in behavior.
7. Settle into healthy daily routines.

Help parents understand the sensitive situation of the toddler. At times, the child gains autonomy and independence. Sometimes the toddler overreaches and needs the mother's help. At other times, he or she needs freedom from too much protection. The child's future personality and health will depend partially on how these many opportunities are handled now. Your role in teaching and supporting parents and family members is critical.

Health Promotion and Nursing Applications

Your role in holistic assessment and health promotion intervention with the toddler and family has been discussed throughout this chapter. **Box 10-8**, Considerations for the Toddler and Family in Health Promotion, summarizes major points.

The **Box** Nursing Diagnoses Related to the Toddler lists some nursing diagnoses (65), based on *assessments* that would be made from knowledge presented in this chapter. Other nursing diagnoses would be applicable, depending upon the injury or illness situation.

Interventions are described throughout the chapter. They include your role-modeling of caring behavior and health promotion practices to the toddler and family; parent and family education, support, anticipatory guidance of parents, and counseling; or direct care to meet the toddler's physical, emotional, cognitive, and social needs. Refer to community resources as necessary for safety classes or family counseling. Parent groups may be helpful as members share their experiences with parenting a toddler. You may be instrumental in establishing parent discussion groups at a church, school, community agency, or health care site.

Criteria for **evaluation** of progression of toddler development and effectiveness of your health care measures can be generated from observation of the toddler, information presented in this chapter and various texts, and use of selected tools. Observation of and discussion with parents about toddler behavior and their use of health promotion practices also enhances your evaluation process (45). The goal is for the child to demonstrate age-appropriate milestones of physical, cognitive, emotional, and social development described in this chapter. Consideration for uniqueness of the individual and cultural background is essential. Influences described in Chapter 8 ∞ or challenges related to the child's progression during infancy, such as congenital anomalies, must be considered in evaluating the child's progress and parental behavior.

BOX 10-8	**Considerations for the Toddler and Family in Health Promotion**

1. Family cultural background and support systems for the family of the toddler
2. Attachment behaviors of the parents; separation reactions of the toddler
3. Parental behaviors that indicate difficulty with attachment or potential/actual abuse of the toddler
4. Physical characteristics and patterns, such as eating, toilet training, sleep/rest, and play, that indicate health and are within age norms for growth
5. Cognitive characteristics and behavioral or play patterns in the toddler that indicate age-appropriate norms for intellectual development
6. Communication patterns and language development that indicate age-appropriate norms for the toddler
7. Overall appearance and behavioral or play patterns in the toddler that indicate development of autonomy rather than shame and doubt, positive self-concept, sense of sexuality, and continuing age-appropriate emotional development
8. Behavioral patterns that indicate the toddler is beginning moral-spiritual development
9. Behavioral patterns and characteristics that indicate the toddler has achieved developmental tasks
10. Parental behaviors that indicate knowledge about how to physically and emotionally care for the toddler
11. Parental behaviors and communication approaches that indicate effective guidance of the toddler
12. Evidence that the parents provide a safe and healthful environment and the necessary resources for the toddler
13. Parental behaviors that indicate they are achieving their developmental tasks for this era

---

Nursing Diagnoses Related to the Toddler

Anxiety
Risk for Impaired Parent/Child **A**ttachment
Risk for Delayed **D**evelopment
Interrupted **F**amily Processes
Fear

Delayed **G**rowth and Development
Risk for **I**njury
Impaired **P**arenting
Risk for **P**oisoning

Source: Reference 65.

Summary

1. The toddler continues to develop parental attachment while developing the ability to relate to other adults and peers.
2. Parents may need help in meeting developmental tasks and avoiding maltreatment of the child.
3. The toddler grows at a slower pace physically than the infant, but physical growth is steady and there is considerable gain in neuromuscular skills.
4. Emotionally, socially, and behaviorally, the toddler makes great strides in development during these 2 years.
5. The child gains control over basic physiologic processes, for example, toileting, and a competency in physical behavior patterns.
6. Developmental or autonomy tasks are achieved in the child's unique way as parents and family members, and other significant people, provide consistent love, guidance, and adequate resources to foster physical, cognitive, emotional, social, and moral development.

7. The unique toddler characteristics of curiosity, impulsivity, advancement of motor skills beyond verbal and cognitive development, and assertion of will must be considered by parents and health care providers in relation to safety and health promotion measures.
8. Injury control or prevention can be achieved if appropriate social and environmental controls are in place.
9. **Box 10-8**, Considerations for the Toddler and Family in Health Promotion, presents some guidelines to consider in assessment and health promotion with the toddler. The family is included in considerations.
10. Holistic care includes your assessment, intervention, evaluation of parental nurturing as well as care of the toddler, and evaluation of your effectiveness with the toddler and family.

Review Questions

1. The nurse is working with the mother of a 2-year-old child who has started to have tantrums when being left at day care. The mother is concerned that she will lose her job as a result of tardiness associated with her child care situation. How should the nurse advise the mother?
   1. "Ask your boss if you can come in a little later."
   2. "The child may need to have a stay-at-home parent."
   3. "This is normal behavior for a child in this age group. It will likely pass with firm, consistent parenting."
   4. "Leave the child with a relative or neighbor until the behavior is outgrown."
2. The nurse is examining the ears of a 2-year-old child. How should the external ear best be positioned to insert the otoscope?
   1. Pull the earlobe up and back.
   2. Pull the earlobe down and back.
   3. Pull the earlobe straight down.
   4. Do not manipulate the earlobe.

3. Which toy should the nurse suggest that grandparents purchase as a gift for an 18-month-old grandchild?
   1. Tricycle
   2. Play kitchen
   3. Garden tools
   4. Tambourine
4. The nurse recommends to parents the use of bedtime rituals for their toddler because these activities:
   1. Promote a sense of security.
   2. Promote creativity.
   3. Encourage dependence.
   4. Offer options and choices.

References

1. American Psychiatric Association. (2000). *Diagnostic and statistical manual of mental disorders: Text revision* (4th ed.). Washington, DC: Author.
2. Ames, E. W. (1997). *The development of Romanian orphanage children adopted in Canada: Final report (National Welfare Grants, Programs, Human Resource Development, Canada)*. Burnaby, BC, Canada: Simon Fraser University Psychology Department.
3. Andrews, M., & Boyle, J. (2003). *Transcultural concepts in nursing care* (4th ed.). Philadelphia: Lippincott.
4. Bates, E., Devescovi, A., & Wulfeck, B. (2001). Psycholinguistics: A cross-language perspective. *Annual Review of Psychology, 52*, 369–396.
5. Bechwith, L., Cohen, S., & Hamilton, C. (1999). Maternal sensitivity during infancy and subsequent life events relate to attachment representation at early adulthood. *Developmental Psychology, 35*, 693–700.
6. Berger, K. (2005). *The developing person through the life span* (6th ed.). New York: Worth.
7. Bettelheim, B., & Freedgood, A. (1988). *A good enough parent: A book on child-rearing*. New York: Random.
8. Bowlby, J. (1969). *Attachment and loss, Vol. I: Attachment*. New York: Basic Books.
9. Bradley, R., Corwyn, R., Burchinal, M., McAdoo, H., & Coll, C. (2001). The home environment of children in the United States: Part II: Relations with behavioral development through age thirteen. *Child Development, 72*(61), 1868–1886.
10. Brazelton, T. (1997, Spring–Summer). Building a better self-image, *Newsweek* (special issue), 76–77.
11. Burgess, A., & Hartman, C. (2005). Sexually motivated child abductors: Forensic evaluation. *Journal of Psychosocial Nursing, 43*(9), 22–28.
12. Chomsky, N. (1995). *The minimalist program*. Cambridge, MA: MIT Press.
13. Chugam, H., Behen, M., Muezik, O., Juhasz, C., Nagy, F., & Chugani, D. (2001). Local brain functional activity following early deprivation: A study of postinstitutionalized Romanian orphans. *Neuroimage, 14*, 1290–1301.
14. Clark, A. M. (2003). *The ABC's of quality child care*. Clifton Park, NY: Thompson Delmar Learning.
15. Colby, R. (2001). Invisible men: Emerging research on low-income, unmarried, and minority fathers. *American Psychologist, 56*, 743–753.
16. Cole, P., Zahn-Waxler, C., Fox, N., Usher, B., & Welsh, J. (1996). Individual differences in emotional regulation and behavior problems in preschool children. *Journal of Abnormal Psychology, 105*, 518–529.
17. Coley, R. (1998). Children's socialization experiences and functioning in single-mother households. The importance of fathers and other men. *Child Development, 68*, 219–230.
18. Colson, E., & Dworkin, P. (1997). Toddler development. *Pediatric Review, 18*(8), 255–257.
19. Costello, A., & Manandhar, D. (2000). *Improving newborn infant health in developing countries*. London: Imperial College Press.
20. Cox, M. (1993). *Children's drawings of the human figure*. Hillsdale, NJ: Erlbaum.
21. DiLeo, J. (1973). *Children's drawings and diagnostic aids*. New York: Brunner/Mazel.
22. Drendel, A., Brousseau, A., & Goralick, M. (2006). Pain assessment for pediatric patients in the emergency department. *Pediatrics, 117*(5), 1511–1518.
23. Dozier, M., Stovall, K., Albus, K., & Bates, B. (2001). Attachment for infants in foster care: The role of caregiver state of mind. *Child Development, 72*, 1467–1477.
24. Dudek, S. (2006). *Nutrition essentials for nursing practice* (5th ed.). Philadelphia: Lippincott Williams & Wilkins.
25. Duvall, E., & Miller, B. (1986). *Marriage and family development* (6th ed.). New York: Harper & Row.
26. Duyff, R. (2006). *The American Dietetic Association complete food and nutrition guide* (Revised and updated 3rd ed.). Hoboken, NJ: Wiley.
27. Echrich, J., & Strohmeyer, S. (2006). Motor development. In K. Thies & J. Travers (Eds.), *Handbook of human development for health care professionals* (pp. 161–189). Sudbury, MA: James and Bartlett.
28. Eisenberg, N., Cumberland, A., Spinrad, T., Fabes, R., Shepard, S., Reiser, M., et al. (2001). The relations of regulation and emotionality to children's externalizing and internalizing problem behavior. *Child Development, 72*, 1112–1134.
29. Elmas, P. (1985). The perception of speech in early infancy. *Scientific American, 252*(1), 46–52.
30. Erikson, E. H. (1963). *Childhood and society* (2nd ed.). New York: W.W. Norton.
31. Erikson, E. H. (1977). *Toys and reason*. New York: W.W. Norton.
32. Fassler, D. (2003). *Help me, I'm sad: Recognizing, treating, and preventing childhood and adolescent depression*. New York: Little, Brown and Company.
33. Fenstermacker, K., & Hudson, B.T. (2004). *Practice guidelines for family practitioners* (3rd ed.). Philadelphia: Saunders.
34. Flavell, J. (1999). Cognitive development. Children's knowledge about the mind. In *Annual Review of Psychology* (Vol. 50). Palo Alto, CA: Annual Reviews.
35. Garbarino, J. (1992). *Children in danger*. New York: Jossey-Bass.
36. Garbarino, J., Guttmann, E., & Seeley, J. (1987). *The psychologically battered child: Strategies for identification, assessment, and intervention*. San Francisco: Jossey-Bass.
37. Gardiner, H., Mutter, W., & Kosmitzki, C. (1998). *Lives across cultures: Cross-cultural human development*. Boston: Allyn and Bacon.
38. Gesell, A., Ilg, F. C. (1946). *The first five years of life*. New York: Harper & Brothers.
39. Giger, J., & Davidhizar, R. (2004). *Transcultural nursing assessment and intervention* (4th ed.). St. Louis, MO: C.V. Mosby.
40. Gopnik, A. (2001). Theories, language, and culture—Whorf without wincing. In M. Bowerman & S. Levinson (Eds.), *Language acquisition and conceptual development* (pp. 45–69). Cambridge, England: Cambridge University Press.
41. Gottlieb, L., & Bailles, J. (1995). Firstborn's behaviors during a mother's second pregnancy. *Nursing Research, 44*, 356–362.
42. Haight, W., Wang, X., Fung, H. H., Williams, K., & Muntz, J. (1999). Universal, developmental, and variable aspects of young children's play: A cross-cultural comparison of pretending at home. *Child Development, 70*, 1477–1488.
43. Hockenberry, M., & Wilson, D. (2007). *Wong's nursing care of infants and children* (8th ed.). St. Louis, MO: Mosby.
44. Hunsley, M., & Thoman, E. B. (2002). The sleep of co-sleeping infants when they are not co-sleeping: Evidence that co-sleeping is stressful. *Developmental Psychology, 40*, 14–22.
45. Johnson, M., Bulechek, G., Butcher, H., Dochterman, J., Maas, M., Moorhead, S., & Swanson, E. (Eds.). (2006). *NANDA, NOC, and NIC linkages: Nursing diagnoses outcomes & interventions* (2nd ed.). St. Louis, MO: Mosby Elsevier.
46. Kelley, S., Brownwell, C., & Campbell, S. (2000). Mastery motivation and self-evaluative affect in toddlers: Longitudinal relations with maternal behavior. *Child Development, 71*, 1061–1071.
47. Kochansha, G. (2001). Emotional development in children with different attachment histories: The first three years. *Child Development, 72*, 474–496.
48. Lamb, M. (1987). The emergent father. In M. E. Lamb (Ed.), *The father's role: Cross-cultural perspectives* (pp. 1–26). Hillsdale: NJ: Lawrence Erlbaum.
49. LaRossa, R. (1988). Fatherhood and social change. *Family Relations, 37*, 451–457.
50. Larsson, H., Eaton, W., Madsen, K., Vestergaard, M., Oleson, A., Agerbu, E., et al. (2005). Risk factors for autism: Perinatal factors, history, and socioeconomic status. *American Journal of Epidemiology, 161*, 916–925.
51. Leaper, C. (2002). Parenting girls and boys. In M. Hornstein (Ed.), *Handbook of parenting. Vol. 2: Children and parenting* (2nd ed., pp. 189–220). Mahwah, NJ: Erlbaum.
52. Lewis, M. (1995). Self-conscious emotions. *American Scientist, 83*, 68–78.
53. MacNeil, J. (2005). Drugs make other autism interventions easier. *Clinical Psychiatry News, 33*(8), 51.
54. Mahler, M. (1979). *Separation–Individuation* (Vol. 2). London: Jason Aronson.
55. Mahoney, D. (2005). Children of depression: Breaking the cycle. *Clinical Psychiatry News, 33*(4), 54.

56. Margolis, D. (2006). Gender development. In K. Thies & J. Travers (Eds.), *Handbook of human development for health care professionals* (pp. 19–32). Sudbury, MA: James and Bartlett.

57. McCartney, K., & O'Connor, E. (2006). Psychosocial development: Attachment in young children. In K. Thies & J. Travers (Eds.), *Handbook of human development for health care professionals* (pp. 95–112). Sudbury, MA: James and Bartlett.

58. Montague, A. (1986). *Touching: The human significance of the skin* (3rd ed.). New York: Columbia University Press.

59. Monteleone, J. (1998). *A parent's & teacher's handbook on identifying and preventing child abuse.* St. Louis, MO: G.W. Medical.

60. Monteleone, J. (1998). *Child maltreatment: A comprehensive photographic reference identifying potential child abuse* (2nd ed.). St. Louis, MO: G.W. Medical.

61. Monteleone, J., & Brodeur, A. (1998). *Child maltreatment: A clinical guide and reference* (2nd ed.). St. Louis, MO: G.W. Medical.

62. Morison, S., Ames, E., & Chisholm, K. (1995). The development of children adopted from Romanian orphanages. *Merrill-Palmer Quarterly Journal of Developmental Psychology, 41,* 411–430.

63. Morison, S., & Ellwood, A. (2000). Resiliency in the aftermath of deprivation: A second look at the development of Romanian orphanage children. *Merrill-Palmer Quarterly, 46,* 717–737.

64. Multiple mutations may explain autism. (2005). *Neuropsychiatry Reviews, 6*(9), 15.

65. NANDA International. (2007). *NANDA-I nursing diagnoses: Definitions and classification 2007–2008.* Philadelphia: Author.

66. Papalia, D., Olds, S., & Feldman, R. (2004). *Human development* (9th ed.). Boston: McGraw-Hill.

67. Santrock, J. (2004). *Life-span development* (9th ed.). Boston: McGraw-Hill.

68. Slade, A., Belsky, J., Aber, J., & Phelps, J. (1999). Mothers' representation of their relationships with their toddlers: Links to adult attachment and observed mothering. *Developmental Psychology, 35,* 611–619.

69. Spittler, K. (2005). Unique immune response in children with autism. *Neuropsychiatry Reviews, 6*(6), 10–11.

70. Spittler, K. (2006). Autism may be identifiable in children as early as age 2. *Neuropsychiatry Review, 7*(7), 1, 18.

71. Spitz, R. (1945). Hospitalism. In *The psychoanalytic study of the child, Vol. I.* New York: International University Press.

72. Spitz, R. (1975). Hospitalism: The genesis of psychiatric conditions in early childhood. In W. Sze (Ed.), *Human life cycle* (pp. 29–43). New York: Jason Aronson.

73. Sullivan, H. S. (1953). *Interpersonal theory of psychiatry.* New York: W.W. Norton.

74. Thompson, S. (2001). The social skills of previously institutionalized children adopted from Romania. *Dissertation Abstracts International Section B: The Sciences & Engineering, 61*(7-B), 3906.

75. United States Department of Health and Human Services. (2000). *Healthy People 2010: With understanding and improving health and objectives for improving health* (2nd ed.) Vol. 2 Washington, DC: United States Government Printing Office.

76. Wadsworth, B. (2004). *Piaget's theory of cognitive and affective development: Foundations of constructivism* (5th ed.). Boston: Pearson.

CHAPTER 11

The Preschooler: Basic Assessment and Health Promotion

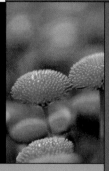

OBJECTIVES

Study of this chapter will enable you to:

1. Compare and contrast the family relationships between the preschool era and previous developmental eras and the influence of parents, siblings, and nonfamily members on the preschooler.

2. Explore with the family the expected developmental tasks and ways to meet them.

3. Assess and contrast physical, motor, mental, language, play, and emotional characteristics of a 3-, 4-, and 5-year-old.

4. Describe the health needs of the preschooler, including nutrition, exercise, rest, safety, and immunization, and measures to meet these needs.

5. Educate parents about their role in contributing to the preschooler's cognitive, language, self-concept, sexuality, emotional, and moral-spiritual development, and physical health.

6. Explore with parents effective ways for communication with and guidance and discipline of the preschooler to enhance the child's development.

7. Analyze the developmental tasks and crisis of initiative versus guilt, the adaptive mechanisms commonly used that promote a sense of initiative, and the implications of this crisis for later development.

MediaLink www.prenhall.com/murray

Go to the Companion Website for interactive resources that accompany this chapter.

Glossary	Critical Thinking
Review Questions	Tools
Challenge Your Knowledge	Media Link Applications
Learning Activities	Media Links

In this chapter, development of the preschool child and the family relationships are discussed. Nursing and health care responsibilities for health promotion for the child and family are presented throughout the chapter. The information regarding normal development and needs serves as a basis for assessment. Use information on assessment, health promotion, health education and counseling of families, and care of the preschooler.

The **preschool years**, *ages 3 through 5,* along with infancy and the toddler years, form a crucial part of the person's life. The preschool child is emerging as a social being: participating more fully as a family member, growing slowly out of the family, and spending more time in association with **peers,** who are *children of the same age.* Physical growth is slowing, but the body is well proportioned and control and coordination are increasing. Many body activities are becoming routine. Emotional and intellectual growth is progressively apparent in the ability to form mental images, express self in a range of emotions, and engage in a greater variety of behaviors. The child is becoming acquainted with the environment and has some perception of social relationships and the status of self as an individual compared with others. The child can identify with the play group and follow rules, control primitive (id) impulses, and begin to be self-critical with reference to a standard set by others (superego formation).

Explore with parents ways to separate themselves from their growing child and make decisions about how much free expression and initiative to permit the child while setting certain limits. The child's long step into the outside world is not always accomplished with ease for either the child or the parent. Thus, gradually promoting more independence during the preschool years allows both the child and parents to be more comfortable about the separation that occurs when he or she goes to school. Emphasize that parents need to spend time and exert energy to listen, talk with, and surround the child with educational opportunities. Preschoolers respond well to, and prefer, interaction and educational sessions that are fun. Watching television and videos decreases when parents provide other physical, cognitive, and social play opportunities (22).

Family Development and Relationships

The family unit, regardless of the specific form, is important to the preschooler. In turn, preschooler behavior affects family relationships. The baby's close relationship to the parents gradually expands to include other significant adults living in the home, siblings, and other relatives, who also affect the child's personality.

There are several dominant parenting styles (3–5, 7, 74, 75):

1. **Authoritarian:** *Parents are demanding, impose many rules, expect instant obedience, and do not give reasons for rules.* No consideration is given to the child's view. Physical punishment is used to gain compliance.
2. **Authoritative:** *Parents exert control and are demanding, but they are responsive to and accepting of the child.* They give reasons for rules, expect mature behavior, and encourage independence and the child meeting personal potential. Balance between control, socialization, and individualization is maintained.
3. **Permissive:** *Parents are accepting of and responsive to the child. They are indulgent. They rarely make demands or exert control.* The child is encouraged to express feelings and impulses.
4. **Neglectful:** *Parents are low in demand and control but also low in acceptance and responsiveness.* They are *uninvolved* in the child's upbringing and may be rejecting. They are involved in personal needs and problems, and there is little energy for the child.
5. **Intimidated:** *Parents lack the ability to be firm with the child or to direct the child's behavior.* Yet, they are frustrated or angry with themselves and the child's behavior.
6. **Secure:** *Parents are confident in their child rearing. They accept themselves and the child.* They realize they will make mistakes, are willing to change, and assume they and the child will cope successfully.

The effect of parenting styles on preschoolers and their parents can be divided into several categories of behavior, as depicted in **Box 11-1**, Effect of Parenting Style on Child's Behavior (3, 5, 69).

The important thing is the match between parenting behaviors and the child's temperament (4, 5, 74). Parenting behaviors also vary with the culture. Among some Asian Americans and American Indians, obedience and strictness are associated with caring, concern, involvement, and family harmony, not harshness and domination, as sometimes seen in North American culture. Traditional Chinese culture emphasizes respect for family and elders. Adults maintain social order by teaching socially proper behavior through firm control, even physical punishment. Strict parental control is combined with warm, supportive parenting (16). Some African American families have a **no-nonsense parenting style** *that falls between authoritarian and authoritative styles. Parents are warm and affectionate but maintain firm, stringent control,* **insisting on obedience to rules.** Children who grow up in dangerous neighborhoods see this as evidence of parental concern (9, 74). Refer to texts that describe family relationships in different cultures (1, 40).

RELATIONSHIPS WITH PARENTS

The preschooler's early emotional and physical closeness or attachment to the parents now leads to a different kind of relationship with them. The father may become more involved with care and guidance of the child at this age. The child needs interaction with the male (the father or father figure), which is different in approach than the interaction with the mother or female (60, 62). This is the *stage of the* **family triangle**, *or the* **Oedipus** *or* **Electra complex** *according to Psychoanalytic Theory explained in Chapter 1.* ∞

During this stage, *positive, possessive, or love feelings are directed mainly toward the parent of the opposite gender. The parent of the same gender may receive competitive, aggressive, or hostile feelings.* The daughter becomes "Daddy's girl" and imitates the mother's role; the father responds to her femininity. The son is "Mommy's boy" and imitates the father's role; the mother responds to his masculinity. The parent of the same gender may be told, "I hate you. Go away." The child may declare to the opposite-gender parent that he or she will marry the parent someday.

Help parents recognize these feelings as developmentally normal. During this phase the child is establishing a basis for an even-

BOX 11-1	Effect of Parenting Style on Child's Behavior	
Parent's Behavior	**Child's Behavior**
1. Controlling, detached, rather than loving and warm	1. Discontented, withdrawn, moody, unhappy, easily annoyed, aimless, lacks self-reliance, lacks confidence in own decision-making abilities
2. More overtly controlling, demanding, loving than most parents	2. Friendly, self-controlled, self-reliant, cheerful, socially responsible, cooperative with adults and peers
3. Highly permissive, warm and friendly	3. Low levels of self-reliance and self-control, rebellious, low levels of independence and achievement orientation
4. Relatively demanding, loving	4. Self-reliant, more independent, better adjusted
5. Warm, loving, expect a great deal of child at early age, demanding of child, show interest in child's activities	5. Highly creative, high need for achievement, independent, highly competent, works toward set goals

tual adult relationship. The parents' positive response is crucial. Help the parents feel comfortable with the sexuality of the child and with their own sexuality so that they are neither threatened by nor ignore or punish the child's remarks and behavior.

As the parents continue to show love to each other and the child, and as the parents desexualize the relationship with the child, the erotic aspects gradually disappear. The child can then get on with one of the major preschool tasks—identification. **Secondary identification** *occurs through internalization of attitudes, feelings, values, and actions about sexual, moral, social, and occupational roles and behavior. The child watches and listens to the parents and demonstrates what they do and say in his or her own unique way, depending on the child's perceptions.* Through this process of internalization and behaving, the child develops an inner parent, which is the core of the superego or conscience. Through identification, the child also gains sexual or gender identity.

Other theories previously discussed in Chapter 1 help explain parent-child relationships. ∞ **Behavioral Theory** *explains that the child learns patterns of behavior through parental reinforcement of their idea of appropriate behavior, including gender-appropriate behavior.* **Social Learning Theory** *explains that the child learns behavior patterns as the parents model the expected behavior and the child, in turn, observes and experiments with behavioral styles.* In reality, Psychoanalytic, Behavioral, and Social Learning Theories each explain some aspect of parent-child relationships and how the child achieves the behaviors that please the parents and strengthen their nurturing.

Attachment continues to develop in the preschool years. The attachment that began with parents in infancy is extended to other significant people in toddlerhood. Parallel and then cooperative play with other children is a continuation of the attachment learned in infancy and toddlerhood. From ages 3 to 5, *securely attached children,* in contrast to insecurely attached children, are more curious, competent, empathic, resilient, and self-confident. They get along better with parents and other adults, are more likely to form close peer friendships, and are better able to resolve conflicts (30). They tend to have a more positive self-concept (95). Some *adopted and foster children* experience insecure attachment and abuse, but when the child has a nurturing caregiver, the adopted and foster child develops secure attachment (47). The child adopted after 2 years of age is more likely to be insecurely attached to the adopted parents (47). *By age 3 years,* the child realizes that others may not think like him or her, but the child wants to interact. Thus the child learns to share or play, even when there are differences. The *4- or 5-year-old* has a best friend, likes to participate in many social activities, and plays with other peers because of the earlier experiences with attachment and parental guidance with socialization. In the process, a child learns to like and accept self, and then others. A nonresponsive, neglectful, or abusive environment produces angry, depressed, or hopeless children by age 2, 3, or 4 years (69, 71, 72, 85).

The importance of *parental nurturing* cannot be overemphasized. If the child has been neglected in infancy, brain scans show that the brain region responsible for emotional attachments has never fully developed (44). *Without early close relationships, there may be biological, as well as learned, reasons for the child to be unable later to form relationships and demonstrate social behavior* (69).

RELATIONSHIPS IN ONE-PARENT OR STEPPARENT FAMILIES

In the *one-parent* or *stepparent family* (or in the abusive home), achieving identification may be more difficult. In the *one-parent home,* the little girl raised by a male may not fit in with other girls at school or may not feel comfortable with and relate to females later in life. The boy raised by a female only may relate better to females than to males.

When *divorce* occurs, the child may live in a one-parent home, live with other family members in their home, or be placed in a stepfamily structure if the parent remarries (or lives with a partner). Review Chapter 6 ∞ for more information about the child's responses to the single-parent or stepparent family. The child believes divorce signifies rejection and that the missing parent no longer loves the child. The child may feel guilt about the separation or about the relief felt after the separation if much discord preceded the divorce. There are often practical problems, such as financial or lifestyle changes and emotional trauma. After the divorce the child may manifest insomnia, grief and depression, digestive and elimination problems, irritability, anger, aggression, regressive behavior, fear, anxiety, and withdrawal.

The child in a stepparent family needs (3, 5, 7, 24, 68, 69):

1. Help in expressing feelings (through art, play, music, and talking) and in adapting to the change.
2. Loving interactions with adult relatives or friends who are of the same and opposite gender. The mother or father should foster such a relationship.
3. An ongoing involvement with the divorced parent who is no longer in the home. The child loves and needs both parents in most cases.
4. Help to learn to live with and feel affection for and from the stepparent.
5. Help to develop a sense of history with the family of origin and the stepparent family, to maintain allegiance to the absent parent, and to develop new traditions.

Explore with parents the importance of identification with the same-gender parent or adult and ways to achieve this if the parent of the same gender as the child is not in the home. *These families benefit from* (a) your empathy and listening ear, (b) exploration of their own and the child's feelings, (c) suggestions of practical ways to help the child spend time with both biological parents, (d) discussion of ways to help the child mourn the loss and adjust to the changed life situation, and (e) counseling skills as the family works to resolve the crisis of separation, divorce, or remarriage.

Sometimes the one-parent family, usually a mother with a preschooler, is homeless. The child in this situation spends critical early years in an unstable, insecure, and often unsanitary environment. The parent and child, cut off from family ties and a supportive community, are at risk for injury, illness, malnutrition, and lack of immunizations and health care when they have to move from shelter to shelter. They are also at risk of being separated if the child is placed in foster care. The homeless child is likely to suffer neurologic and sensory deficits, anxiety, depression, developmental delays, and later learning and behavioral problems.

Be an advocate for community services for at-risk homeless mothers, children, and families. Advocate for low-income affordable housing, safe child care services, equitable wages, and accessible health care services. Become involved in community policy and development groups. Federal, state, local, foundation, and private funding is available for reclaiming neighborhoods and building low-income housing.

SEXUAL OR GENDER IDENTITY THROUGH PARENTAL RELATIONSHIPS

Gender Identity

This phase brings the development of sexuality to the foreground. By *2 to 3 years,* the child knows the personal gender and calls self a "boy" or "girl." By age *3 1/2 to 4 years,* the child has **gender constancy or stability,** *the realization that one will always be either a male or female.* At this point, the child *adopts gender-appropriate behavior through identification with the same-gender parent* (66, 85). The child is interested in the appearance and function of his or her own body, in variations of clothing and hairstyles (the child

at first assigns sex on this basis), and in the bodies of others, especially their sex organs (66). Children at this age feel a sense of excitement in seeing and feeling their own and others' nude bodies and of exposing themselves to other children or adults.

The gender of the child is a great determinant in personality development because each gender has different tasks and roles in every culture (1, 40). *However, you cannot predict the child's personality traits by knowing only the gender.* Some cultures have precise **gender roles,** *behaviors, interests, attitudes, skills, and personality traits considered appropriate for males or females.* The *process by which children learn the role* is called **gender typing.** However, children vary in the extent to which they follow the gender role. Many people, including in the United States, have **gender stereotypes,** *preconceived beliefs about male and female characteristics and behavior* (74, 85). Preschool boys and girls often describe boys as strong, fast, and cruel, and girls as fearful and helpless (84). They apparently learn stereotypes that surround them by observation, hearing, and interpretation about clothes, toys, and others' responses, even if they are not specifically taught. Achieving a firm identity as a male or female is basic to emotional stability and ego development, and cultural expectations and influences are important. These are expressed by the family socialization (7, 74, 85).

In the United States, most parents are less rigid about what clothing or colors are appropriate for boys and girls and make an effort to teach both daughters and sons to talk about feelings, to do the same household tasks, and to engage in the same play activities. In some homes, however, the daughter is reinforced for being cuddly, domestic, and emotional, and the son is reinforced for being physically aggressive or "tough." The 5-year-old son is not expected to set the table or help with dusting, and the daughter is not allowed to play with trucks.

Explore parental reactions to and expectations of the child. Help them clarify their feelings and behavior and convey their respect to the child, regardless of gender. The parents' feelings and needs strongly influence their reactions to the child so that gender assignment within the family can override biological factors. Parents can foster opposite-gender behavior by the way they name, handle, dress, play with, touch, or talk to the child.

Teach parents that sexual or gender identity is reinforced through name, décor of room, and behavior toward and expectations of the child. The innumerable contacts between the child and significant adults contribute to sexual and gender identification. Parents who have fixed ideas about sex role behavior may not be responsive to your suggestions about the importance of both daughters and sons having the same play, learning, or social experiences. Parental ideas frequently reflect their cultural values and norms.

Teaching Sexuality

Teaching sexuality to the child is enmeshed in the child's acquisition of gender identity and positive feelings about the self. The basis for sex education begins prenatally with the parents' attitudes about the coming child. Parents and other caretakers, including health care providers, continue daily thereafter to form attitudes in the child and impart factual knowledge in response to questions.

The child has many questions about conception and childbirth. The child usually develops or expands a personal theory: babies come from a seed placed in the mother's mouth, from eating foods with seeds, from kissing, or from animals; babies are manufactured like household items; prenatally the baby sits on the mother's stomach, ingesting food as she eats; and babies come out of the anus or the navel.

You can assist parents in acquiring information to answer the child's questions. Because of the child's consuming curiosity, he or she asks many questions: Will the man in the television come out? How do I tie my shoes? Why is that lady's tummy so big? What is lightning? These questions are originally asked with equal curiosity. The adult's response will determine into what special category the child places questions about gender and sexual behavior. Emphasize that if parent-child communication has been open—if the child feels free to ask questions about sex and other topics, and if the parent gives satisfactory and correct answers without embarrassment—the basis for a healthy sexual attitude exists.

Although sex education must be tailored to the individual child's needs and interests and to the cultural, religious, and family values, the following suggestions are applicable to all children and can be shared with parents:

1. Recognize that education about the self as a sexual person is best given by example in family life through parents' showing respect and love for the self, mate, and child.

2. Understand that the child who learns to trust others and to give and receive love has begun preparation for satisfactory adulthood, marriage, and parenthood.

3. Observe the child at play; listen carefully to statements of ideas, feelings, and questions related to sex. Ask questions to understand better the child's needs for education.

4. Respond to the child's questions by giving information honestly, in a relaxed, accepting manner, and on the child's level of understanding. Avoid isolated facts, myths, or animal analogies. The question, "Where does baby come from?" could be answered, "Mommy carried you inside her body in a special place." Religious beliefs can be worked into the explanation while acknowledging human realities.

5. Teach the child anatomic names rather than other words for body parts and processes. Parents may hesitate to do this because they do not want the child to blurt out the words *penis* or *vagina* in public. Parents can teach the child that certain topics such as sexual and financial matters are discussed in the home, just as certain activities such as urinating are done in private. Grabbing the genitals and some masturbation are normal in children as they explore their bodies, especially body parts not easily seen and that give pleasurable sensations when touched. Self-masturbation may be acceptable if it occurs in the home. The child should be taught that this is not normal behavior in public. Parents or other people should not engage in masturbation of the child.

6. Realize that playing doctor or examining each other's body parts is normal for preschool children. Parents should not overreact and should calmly affirm that they want the children to keep their clothes on while they play. Diversion from "playing doctor" is useful. If children seem to be using each other in a sexual way, they should be instructed that this is not acceptable and distracted to other play activity.

7. Realize that sex education continues throughout the early years. The child's changing self motivates the same or different questions repeatedly. Remain open to ongoing questions. An explanation about reproduction may begin with a simple statement, for example: "A man and a woman are required to be baby's father and mother. Baby is made from the sperm in the daddy's body and an egg in the mother's body." A simple explanation of sperm and egg would be needed. Later the child can be given more detail.

RELATIONSHIPS WITH SIBLINGS

Attachment that began with the parents extends to siblings in late infancy and continues to deepen during the toddler and preschool years. The discussion in Chapter 6 ∞ on the effect of the child's gender and ordinal position on family interaction is significant for understanding the preschooler.

Often the preschool child has **siblings,** *brothers or sisters,* either younger or older, so that family interaction is complex with many **dyads,** *groups of two people.* Siblings become increasingly important in directing the child's early development, partly because of their proximity but also because the parents change in their role with each additional child. In the following discussion, realize that the relationships described could occur at other developmental eras in childhood, but in the preschool years siblings begin to make a very definite impact (7, 74, 85).

The sibling may be part of a multiple birth: twins, triplets, or more. For the parents, raising twins or multiples creates a delicate balance.

You may give the following suggestions to parents:

1. Help the children realize they are individuals first and twins second. Parents do this by the way they talk to, dress, and handle twins (or other multiple-birth children).

2. Encourage each child to develop separate interests, pursue different hobbies and subjects, or go to different schools to reduce competition and rivalry.

3. Talk to the multiples about different kinds of relationships, their own special closeness, and the rewards of developing separate friendships.

Refer to Chapter 6 for more information on multiple births. ∞

Preschooler and New Baby

The arrival of a new baby changes life for the preschooler. He or she is no longer the center of attention but is expected by the parents to delight in the baby. It is important for parents to prepare the young child for a new arrival, as shown in **Figure 11-1** ■. Although a space of 3 to 4 years is ideal, such ideal spacing does not always occur. The firstborn, especially, has difficulty accepting family affection toward the newborn (85).

When pregnancy is apparent, counsel the parents about ways to prepare the older child:

1. Share the anticipation in discussions and planning, but not too far in advance. Let the child feel fetal movements. Show

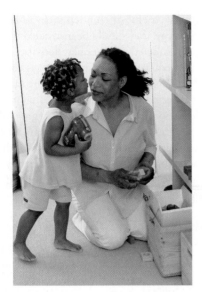

FIGURE ◼ 11-1 As birth approaches parents can prepare the preschooler. (Ruth Jenkinson © Dorling Kindersley)

the child a picture of when he or she was a newborn. Talk about what he or she needed as a baby and the necessary responsibilities. Read books that explain reproduction and birth on his or her level.

2. Include the child as much as possible in activities, such as shopping for furniture for the baby or decorating the baby's room. The preschool child likes to feel important, and being a helper enhances this feeling.
3. Accept that the child may act out, regress, or express dependency or separation anxiety during the pregnancy, as well as after the new baby arrives.
4. Prepare whether the child should be with the mother during birth, if permitted by the birthing center. The child may visit mother and baby at the hospital after delivery, if rules permit. Or the child can talk to the mother by phone.

Teach parents that the following behaviors may result from jealousy if more attention is focused on the baby than on the older child:

1. The preschooler may regress, overtly displaying a need to be babied. He or she may ask for the bottle, soil self, have enuresis, lie in the baby's crib, or demand extra attention.
2. The child may appear to love the baby excessively, more than is normal, and then harm the baby, directly or indirectly, through play or rough handling.
3. The child may show hostility toward the mother in different ways: direct physical or verbal attacks, ignoring or rejecting her, or displacing anger onto the teacher at day care, nursery school, or church.

Older Sibling and Preschooler

The older sibling in the family who is given much attention for accomplishments may cause feelings of *envy and frustration* as the preschooler tries to engage in activity beyond his or her ability and to seek attention also. If the preschooler can identify with the older sibling and take pride in the accomplishments while simultaneously getting recognition for his or her own self and abilities, the child will feel positive about self. If the younger child feels defeated and is not given realistic recognition, he or she may stop emulating the older sibling and regress instead. In turn, the older sibling can be helpful to the younger child if he or she does not feel deprived or is not reprimanded too much because of behavior toward the preschooler.

Often positive feelings exist between siblings. Quarrels are quickly forgotten if parents do not get overly involved. Because siblings have had a similar upbringing, they have considerable empathy for each other, similar values, similar superego development, and related perceptions about situations. Sibling values may be as important as the parents' values in the development of the child. *Often achievements of the older sibling are of such importance to the child that he or she may conceal ability rather than develop talents for which the sibling has gained recognition.* Children learn to develop roles

---

INTERVENTIONS FOR HEALTH PROMOTION

Teach the family ways to prevent or handle sibling jealousy:

1. Convey that the child is loved as much as before, provide a time for him or her only, and give as much attention as possible.
2. Do not leave the preschooler alone with the baby.
3. Give a pet or doll for the child to care for as mother cares for the baby.
4. Encourage the child to identify with the parents in helping to protect the baby because he or she is more grown up.
5. Avoid overemphasis that the child must show affection to the baby.
6. Involve the child in caring for the new baby. Although the preschooler may have to give up a crib, getting him or

her a new big bed can seem like a promotion rather than a loss.
7. Emphasize parental pleasure in having the child share in loving the new arrival. Give increasing responsibility and status without overburdening him or her.
8. Encourage the child to talk about the new situation or express feelings in play or through reading stories.
9. Encourage relatives and friends to bring a small surprise gift for the older child when they visit and bring a gift for the baby. Have them spend time with the older child also, rather than concentrating only on the baby.
10. Recognize that the child's outward behavior is linked to feelings. The child should not be punished.

and regulate space among themselves to avoid conflicts unless conflictual behavior is given undue attention.

To the preschooler, older siblings—the big guys—are important. The older sibling teaches the younger to swim, to ride a two-wheel bike, and to do school homework. The younger one may do anything to get attention, and at times, parents have to protect the older siblings. The preschooler must be taught that mean talk is not tolerated and that the older brother, sister, or anyone else must not be hit, kicked, or bitten. Older siblings remain loving and loyal, rather than angry, jealous, or rivalrous, when parents are fair in discipline of all concerned and when they explain normal developmental needs. Quality time, reassurance, and firm rules reduce sibling rivalry, squabbles, or avoidance. *A warm sibling relationship and playing together:* (a) promotes definition of self, (b) helps the child learn to consider others' perspectives, and (c) enhances the child's ability to form relationships later by learning to cooperate, compete, negotiate, and be sociable.

Explore sibling relationships with parents. Share the information presented in this chapter, and present suggestions for preventing conflicts.

Relationship with Grandparents

Attachment between grandparent and grandchild has emotional power and influence. Sometimes the relationship with the grandparent is deeper than with either parent, especially if the parents (58, 74): (a) are abusive or neglectful, (b) are busily employed professionals, (c) travel a great deal as part of a job, (d) have separated or divorced, or (e) suffer depression.

Grandparents are definitely more precious to, effective with, and necessary for a child than child development specialists or day care, Head Start, or after-school program staff. These elders, to the child, seem to have existed forever and play a number of valuable roles. An essential one is that of oral historian, whereby the child learns about "olden days," family history, the meaning of old pictures and objects, and the child's own roots. Grandparents are ideal mentors if they take the time and trouble; the child can learn to fix, build, and create. Grandparents provide spiritual sustenance to children and answer questions about God (58, 74).

Grandparents who live nearby are indispensable to *assist with babysitting or child care* while the single or divorced mother (and sometimes father) is employed outside the home. Often the grandparents play a key role when young unmarried daughters become pregnant. For example, African American grandmothers are likely to perceive themselves and to be perceived by the daughters as actively involved in child rearing (9, 40). The young African American couple may view the grandmother as the person to count on for child care assistance, advice, and emotional support. Often these grandmothers are themselves in late young adulthood or entering middle age. In the African American home, having a grandmother in the residence allows the mother to be more flexible and able to manage daily demands with less stress (40).

Yet, a growing number of grandparents are losing contact with their grandchildren as a result of parental divorce, conflict between parents, death of an adult child, or adoption of a grandchild after remarriage. After divorce, the grandparents may wish to be the child's legal custodians but may not be permitted by their own children or the courts. Increasingly, grandparents, in cases of divorce, are seeking legal means to ensure visitation rights and sometimes to gain custody (75).

INFLUENCE OF OTHER ADULTS AND NON-FAMILY MEMBERS

Significant Adults

Other significant adults may include relatives, especially aunts, uncles, and cousins who are peers; the teacher at the day care center or nursery school; the babysitter; or neighbors. Live-in help, the in-home caretaker, the babysitter, or the child's nurse-caretaker may be positive or negative identification figures and should be chosen with care, especially those who live in the home. Other relatives and friends also contribute to development of identity, if contact is frequent.

Guests introduce the child to new facets of family life and parents' behavior, to different people with unfamiliar behavior, and to different ideas, religions, or occupations. Visits to others' homes aid socialization through comparison of the households, ability to separate from home, and interaction with people in new places.

Even *domestic pets* can be useful in meeting certain needs: loving and being loved, companionship, learning a sense of responsibility, and learning about sex in a natural way.

Help parents realize that other people may be significant to the child, depending on frequency and duration of contact, warmth of the relationship, and how well the parents meet the child's needs. Explore the importance of pets and the child's involvement in pet care.

Day Care Services

Educate parents about the various types of agencies, the differences between them, their significance for the child, and the criteria for selection. You may also assist with primary prevention and health consultation to teachers, children, and parents in such an agency.

Day care is *a licensed, structured program that provides care daily for some portion of the day, for children away from home, throughout the year, for compensation. The age of the children can range from infancy to 13 years; most children will be of preschool age. Day care is child oriented in program and in the physical structure of the facilities. This program can be an important resource to many families when:* (a) the single parent works and is the sole support of the family, (b) both parents work, (c) one parent is ill or a full-time student and the other parent works, or (d) the mother needs relief from child care for health or other urgent personal reasons. Some day care programs are intergenerational, so that both preschoolers and elders come to the same site (61, 85). A positive relationship is fostered between preschoolers and grandparents, or surrogate grandparents (58, 61, 85). See the **Box** Client Education, Criteria for Selection of a Day Care Center.

Family day care is *the arrangement by a caregiver to provide care for a small group of mixed-age children in the home while their parents work.* In some states, if there are more than four children, the family day care must meet the requirements of a state license. Many caregivers choose to avoid undergoing the regulations, procedures, and remodeling that would be involved in licensing. Many providers formerly worked outside the home, but they want to remain at home with their own children while continuing to

Client Education

Criteria for Selection of Day Care Facility

1. **Operation by reputable person, agency, or industry.** Either profit or nonprofit programs can offer quality care.
2. **Licensed or certified by local and state regulatory bodies.** However, this only ensures meeting minimum standards, such as for space, safety, and staff-to-child ratio.
3. **Located convenient** to home or workplace, **open at the hours needed** by the parents.
4. Committed to a **philosophy** of and **beliefs about child rearing** and discipline that are similar to those of the parents.
5. **Staffed with certified teachers and other workers** in appropriate staff-to-child ratio. Teacher and staff have a low turnover rate in employment.
6. **Provision of an environment** in which children and staff are happy and interacting. Children are having fun and learning.
7. **Provision for grouping children** according to age and developmental level so that children are safe and can learn from each other.
8. **Provision of adequate space** that is safe and clean, with a well-controlled temperature and attractive decor. Psychomotor and sensory stimulation for age of child guided, supervised, or observed by staff.
9. **Provision of safe space and a variety of equipment, materials, and supplies** for different types of play, such as:
   - Creative: art, music, reading, water play
   - Quiet: games, puzzles
   - Active: pedal toys, blocks, balls
   - Outdoor: jungle gym, balls
   - Dramatic: playhouse, farm, fire station
10. **Provision of place for child to keep personal belongings.**
11. **Provision for snacks and mealtime. Kitchen facilities** meet health department standards. Tables and chairs are available for children and staff to sit and eat together. **Staff wash hands** before food is served. **Children wash hands** before eating.
12. **Provision for child to be alone for short period,** if desired, and for midday rest on floor mats.
13. **Provision of age-appropriate toilet facilities and sinks. Children wash hands** after toileting, play, touching animals, sneezing, and wiping nose.
14. **Provision of separate room supplied to give emergency health services** to an impaired or ill child until parents, or their designate, or emergency medical services can arrive.
15. **Provision for occasional extra event,** or short trip, such as a visit by a firefighter or a trip to the local fire station or park.
16. **Operated at a cost comparable to other similar facilities** or programs or on a sliding scale basis.
17. **Willingness by staff for anyone to visit unannounced. Security measures** at all entrances are implemented.
18. **Daily interaction of teachers with parents.** Talk with parents about child's behavior, progress, or health, as indicated.
19. **Discussion between teachers, administrators, and parents about the contract** for services, policies and procedures and their rationale, and explanation of planned changes well in advance.
20. **Satisfaction of parents, child, teachers, administrators, and staff with decision to have child attend program.**
21. **Discussion with administrators or teachers about suggestions for change** are openly received; appropriate suggestions are incorporated (e.g., posting menus, food preparation or selection).

contribute to family income. There is usually no structured program. The mixed ages of the children provide stimulation for each other, and the small number of children usually ensures that each child gets the needed attention.

Educate the parent that the criteria presented in the Client Education box also are *applicable to family or home day care,* although they would be *applied to one adult in a home setting. The following questions should be asked of the person in charge:*

1. Is there backup help available to the adult if needed (e.g., in case she is ill or if her child or another child was injured or became ill)?

2. Does the adult take the children for trips in a vehicle? If so, are there child safety seats or devices appropriate to the child's age? Is there insurance coverage? Does someone accompany the adult to help with the children?

3. Is care provided on weekends, on holidays, or in the evening?

Early School Experiences

At least 60% of U.S. children between ages 3 and 5 years have some type of early childhood education program. There is increasing emphasis on accountability and measurable outcomes to **evaluate** the effectiveness of early education efforts on child outcomes in school. It is difficult to link explicit performance to later school success. Some tools are being developed; they must be sensitive to child growth and development (76) and cultural variables (1, 40).

Montessori programs evolved from the Italian educator Maria Montessori. She developed preschool education in Europe, using the Piaget model (100). Activities are **child initiated.** *The child can discover and learn at his or her own pace, based on maturation. Programs emphasize* (100): (a) self-discipline of the child; (b) intellectual development through training of the senses; (c) freedom for the child within a structure and schedule; and (d) meaningful individual cognitive experiences that are provided in a quiet, pleasant, educational environment. Parents should explore the program and facilities. Criteria listed in the Client Education Box may be helpful.

Compensatory programs, which first began as Head Start and Follow Through Projects in the 1960s, *focus on making up for conditions in the child's life. They include* (7, 82, 85): (a) giving physical care (good nutrition, dental care, immunizations); (b) fostering curiosity, exploring creativity, and learning about the self and environment; (c) promoting emotional health through nurturing, positive self-concept, self-confidence, and self-discipline; and (d) teaching social skills and behaviors, how to interact with peers, teachers, and parents. Head Start is federally funded for children from low-income or minority experiences who need a "head start" on education because of their home environment (7). Children who participate in Head Start are less likely to be placed in special education or to repeat a grade, and they are more likely to finish high school than low-income children who did not attend compensatory preschool programs (7, 85). Outcomes are best when the child is enrolled at least 2 years (7, 75). Some programs extend from preschool through third grade; the added years of academic enrichment increase the child's achievements through high school and reduce behavior problems (7, 82, 83). The quality of the program is the key factor (7). Criteria listed in Client Education: Criteria for Selection of Day Care Facility are helpful for selection.

Nursery school or **prekindergarten** is usually a *half-day program that emphasizes an educational and socialization experience for the children to supplement home experiences.* The parents and child can also begin to deal with separation anxiety if the child has been with the mother at home until this time. Children may attend part-time or full-time. A midsession snack, but no lunch, is provided. Such a school is frequently sponsored by a church for their own and other children. The mother may consider it a morning that is "child-free" at home. Criteria listed in Client Education: Criteria for Selection of Day Care Facility may be helpful for selection.

Kindergarten *is a half- or whole-day educational program* for the 5-year-old child that may be either an extension of a nursery school or a part of the elementary school system. Cognitive learning that is begun is a foundation for the cognitive program of the first grade. The social behaviors that are learned also prepare the child to be better disciplined in the school setting and to interact appropriately with teachers and peers. The program also helps the child and parents to separate from each other, if that has not been done through nursery school or day care. As academic and emotional pressures increase in kindergarten, many parents are choosing to hold the child, especially the boy, back a year to start kindergarten at age 6 years (7, 85).

Discuss with parents that in **early child education**, *the child, under the guidance of qualified staff, will have many experiences and learn to:*

1. Follow rules.
2. Socialize with others and be cooperative in peer play.
3. Investigate the environment.
4. Do imaginative experimentation with a variety of toys.
5. Develop creative abilities.
6. Do basic problem solving.
7. Become more independent, secure, and self-confident in a variety of situations.
8. Handle emotions and broaden self-expression.
9. Follow basic hygiene patterns.
10. Become familiar with the surrounding community.

Emphasize to parents that pushing the child to develop reading and mathematics skills too early will create problems such as fatigue, stress-related illnesses, disciplinary problems, and cognitive burnout (7, 69, 74, 85). Advise parents to advocate for their children's holistic learning, not just academic or cognitive learning, even in kindergarten.

If parents use a day care center, family or home day care, nursery school, or early school program, reinforce that they remain the most important people to the child and that their love and involvement with the child are crucial for later learning and adjustment to life. The care or enrichment of a preschool center or program where children attend a few hours daily cannot undo family deprivation or abuse. Help the mother realize that her working outside the home does not necessarily deprive the child. Many career women tend to do better parenting than full-time homemakers. They allow the child to develop autonomy and initiative in creative ways because they have a sense of self-fulfillment in their own lives.

Help the parents and child prepare for the separation if the child will be enrolled in any program outside of the home. Help the parents realize, too, that the child's emotional and social adjustment and overall learning depend on many factors. Because each child interprets entrance into the agency on the basis of past experience, each differs in adjustment. Being with a number of children can be an upsetting experience. The child needs adequate preparation to avoid feeling abandoned or rejected. The mother must have confidence in the agency so that she can convey a feeling of pleasurable expectation to the child. The child should accompany the mother to see the building, observe the program, and meet the teachers and other children before enrollment. Ideally the child should begin attending when both mother and child feel secure about the ensuing separation. The mother should be encouraged to stay with the child the whole first day or for a shorter period for several days until he or she feels secure. If possible, the parent, rather than a neighbor or stranger, should take the child each day, assuring the child of the parent's return at the end of the day.

Share with parents that the National Institute of Child Health and Human Development studied 1,300 children over 10 years who were in day care for an average of 33 hours weekly. Findings indicated that preschool children placed in day care, compared to children who stay at home with their mothers, have a slightly weaker bond with their mothers at early ages and are slightly more aggressive and disobedient in the preschool years, regardless of gender or social class. Attachment is most affected in infancy, and only if the mother is insensitive to the child. *High-quality child care is associated with fewer behavior problems and better cognitive development* (81).

FAMILY DEVELOPMENTAL TASKS

While the preschool child and siblings are achieving their developmental tasks, the parents are struggling with child rearing and their own developmental tasks. *Parental developmental tasks while raising a preschooler include the following* (27):

1. Supply adequate housing, space, equipment, and other materials needed for life, comfort, health, and recreation.
2. Encourage and accept the child's evolving skills rather than elevating the parent's self-esteem by pushing the child beyond his or her capacity. Satisfaction is found through reducing assistance with physical care and giving more guidance in other respects.
3. Plan for predicted and unexpected costs of family life, such as medical care, insurance, education, babysitter fees, food, clothing, and recreation.
4. Maintain some personal privacy and an outlet for tension of family members, while including the child as a participant in the family.
5. Share household and child care responsibility with other family members, including the child.
6. Strengthen the partnership with the mate and express affection in ways that keep the relationship from becoming humdrum.
7. Learn to accept failures, mistakes, and blunders without piling up feelings of guilt, blame, and recrimination.
8. Nourish common interests and friendships to strengthen self-respect and self-confidence and to remain interesting to the spouse.
9. Maintain a mutually satisfactory sexual relationship and plan whether to have more children.
10. Create and maintain effective communication within the family.
11. Cultivate relationships with the extended family.
12. Tap resources and serve others outside the family to prevent preoccupation with self and family.
13. Face life's dilemmas and rework moral codes, spiritual values, and a philosophy of life.

Explore with parents the challenges and practical ways of meeting these tasks within the specific family unit. Refer also to Chapter 6. ∞

Physiologic Concepts and Physical Characteristics

GROWTH PATTERNS

Although development does not proceed at a uniform rate in all areas or for all children, *development follows a logical, precise pattern or sequence* (7, 39, 46, 74, 80). *Limb growth* is greater in proportion to trunk growth. See principle of asynchronous growth, Chapter 3. ∞ At *age 5,* leg length constitutes about 44% of body height, in contrast to age 2, when leg length is about 34% of body height. (In adulthood, leg length is about 44% of body height.) The *preschool child grows* approximately 2 1/2 to 3 inches (6 to 7.5 cm) and gains less than 5 pounds (2.2 kg) *per year.* The child appears taller and thinner because he or she grows proportionately more in height than in weight. The average *height* of the 3-year-old is 37 in. (94 cm); of the 4-year-old, 41 in. (104 cm) (*or double the birth length*); and of the 5-year-old, 43 to 52 in. (110 to 130 cm). At 3 years the child *weighs* approximately 30 to 33 pounds (15 kg); at 4 years, 38 pounds (17 kg); and at 5 years, approximately 40 to 50 pounds (18 to 23 kg).

Head circumference growth is slowing, and the preschooler looks more adult-like, in contrast to the top-heavy appearance of the infant and the bottom-heavy appearance of the toddler. Boys have a slight edge in height and weight, which continues until the growth spurt of puberty (7, 39, 46, 74, 80).

VITAL SIGNS

The *body temperature* ranges from 98 to 99°F (36.7 to 37.2°C). The *pulse rate* is normally 70 to 110 and the *respiratory rate* approximately 25 per minute. *Blood pressure* ranges from 101 to 115 mmHg systolic and 57 to 68 mmHg for diastolic between the ages of 3 and 5 years (46).

OTHER CHARACTERISTICS

Appearance changes as cartilage and bones develop further in the child's face. Fat pads in the cheeks decrease in size. Knees point forward, and legs are straight. Forelegs can be bent back along the thighs so that buttocks rest on or between the heels. The preschooler loses the toddler's ability to bend double, with legs straight, and rest the head on the ground.

Vision in the preschooler is farsighted; the 4- and 5-year-old has 20/30 vision and is visually discriminative. *Eye-hand coordination* improves (20). By age 4 1/2, the *motor nerves are fully myelinated* and the *cerebral cortex is fully connected to the cerebellum,* permitting better coordination and control of bowel and bladder. By *age 5,* hand, arm, and body all move together under better eye command and visual-body coordination. Precise fine muscle movements are demonstrated, such as tying shoelaces or building a church with steeple (74, 80, 85). *Internal organs* are larger. At *5 years,* the *brain* is at 90% of the weight of the adult brain. The child has 20 *teeth,* and by the end of the preschool period, the child begins to lose deciduous teeth (7, 46, 74, 80, 85).

Physical characteristics to assess in the preschool child are listed in **Table 11-1** (7, 20, 46, 74, 80, 85). Because each child is unique, the normative listings indicate only where most children of a given age are in the development of various characteristics. *Characteristics are listed by age for reasons of understanding sequence and giving comparison. Consideration of only the chronologic age is misleading as a basis for assessment and care.* The development of the whole and unique child and interrelations among various aspects must be considered. For example, opportunity for muscle movement and exercise and nutritional status, rather

TABLE 11-1

Assessment of Physical Characteristics: Motor Control

Age 3 Years	Age 4 Years	Age 5 Years
Occasional accident in toileting when busy at play; responds to routine times; tells when going to bathroom	Independent toilet habits; manages clothes without difficulty	Takes complete charge of self; does not tell when going to bathroom
Verbalizes difference between how male and female urinate	Insists on having door shut for self but wants to be in bathroom with others	Self-conscious about exposing self
Needs help with back buttons and drying self	Asks many questions about defecation function	Boys and girls to separate bathrooms
Nighttime control of bowel and bladder most of time		Voids four to six times during waking hours; occasional nighttime accident
Runs more smoothly than before, turns sharp corners, suddenly stops; trunk rotates with run, flops and tumbles, scoots and slides on knees	Runs easily with coordination	Runs with skill, speed, agility, and plays games simultaneously
	Skips clumsily	Starts and stops abruptly when running
	Hops on one leg 4 to 6 steps	Increases strength and coordination in limbs due to exercise
	Legs, trunk, shoulder, arms move in unison	
	Aggressive physical activity	
Walks backward	Heel-toe walk	May still be knock-kneed
Climbs stairs with alternate feet	Walks a plank	Jumps from 3 to 4 steps
Jumps from low step, about 12 inches	Hops on one foot	Hops on one foot for 16 feet
Jumps forward 15–24 inches	Climbs stairs without holding onto rail	Jumps 26–28 inches forward
Hops in irregular series of large jumps	Climbs and jumps without difficulty	Leaps, scrambles, swings through a turn
	Jumps 24–33 inches	
Tries to dance but has inadequate balance, although sense of balance improving	Enjoys motor stunts and gross gesturing	Balances self on toes on one foot briefly
Steps on footprint patterns		Dances with some rhythm
		Agile on rocky incline
		Swings self through a turn by holding on wall or furniture
Pedals tricycle	Enjoys new activities rather than repeating same ones	Rides bicycle with training wheels
Swings	Carries 12 to 16 objects	Jumps rope
Completes aided forward somersault	Pushes and pulls wagon or doll buggy	Roller skates
		Hops and skips on alternate feet
		Scales jungle gym and ladder
		Carries 16-pound object
		Kicks rolling ball
Sitting equilibrium maintained but combined awkwardly with reaching activity	Sitting balance well maintained; leans forward with greater mobility and ease	Maintains balance easily
	Exaggerated use of arm extension and trunk twisting; touches end of nose with forefinger on direction	Combines reaching and placing object in one continuous movement
		Arm extension and trunk twisting coordinated
		Tummy protrudes, but some adult curve to spine
Undresses self; helps dress self	Dresses and undresses self except tying bows, closing zipper, putting on boots and snowsuit	Dresses self without assistance; ties shoelaces
Undoes buttons on side or front of clothing	Does buttons	Requires less supervision of personal duties
Goes to toilet alone if clothes simple	Distinguishes front and back of self and clothes	Washes self without wetting clothes
Washes hands, feeds self	Strings and laces shoelace	
Can brush own teeth with supervision	Brushes teeth alone	

continued

TABLE 11-1

Assessment of Physical Characteristics: Motor Control—continued

Age 3 Years	Age 4 Years	Age 5 Years
Throws ball underhanded 4 feet	Greater flexion of elbow	Uses hands more than arms in catching
Catches large ball with arms fully extended one out of two to three times	Bounces ball	ball
	Catches ball thrown at 5 feet two to three times	Throws ball (boys 44 feet; girls 25 feet)
		Rolls ball to hit object
Hand movement becoming better coordinated	Throws ball overhand	Pours fluid from one container to another with few spills; bilateral coordination
Increasing coordination in vertical direction	Judges where a ball will land	Uses hammer to hit nail on head
	Helps dust objects	Interest and competence in dusting
Pours fluid from pitcher, occasional spills	Likes water play	
Hits large pegs on board with hammer		
Builds tower of 9 to 10 blocks	Builds complicated structure extending vertically and laterally; builds five-block gate from model	Builds complex things out of large boxes
Builds three-block gate from model		Builds complicated three-dimensional structure and may build several separate units
Imitates a bridge	Builds five-block bridge	
	Notices missing parts or broken objects; requests a parent to fix	Able to disassemble and reassemble small object
Copies circle or cross	Copies a square or simple figure	Copies triangle or diamond from model
Begins to use scissors	Uses scissors without difficulty, follows a line	Folds paper diagonally
Strings large beads		Definite hand preference
Shows hand preference	Strings 10 beads	Does simple puzzles quickly and smoothly
Pastes using pointer finger	Enjoys finer manipulation of play materials	Prints some letters correctly; prints first name; reproduces letters
Trial-and-error method with simple puzzle, force piece in hole or put it in vigorously	Surveys puzzle before placing pieces	Uses crayons appropriately
	Matches simple geometric forms	Makes clay objects with two small parts
	Prefers symmetry	
	Poor space perception	
Scribbles	Less scribbling	Draws clearly recognized lifelike representatives; differentiates parts of drawing
Tries to draw a picture and name it	Form and meaning in drawing apparent to adults	

Source: References 7, 35, 39, 46, 74, 80, 85.

than gender, influences strength. *By using the norms for the child at a given age, you can assess how far the child deviates from the norm. With more parental guidance, the child may reach norms ahead of age.* Certain situations, such as prenatal alcohol or drug exposure, may cause the child to be below the norms.

DEVELOPMENTAL ASSESSMENT

The Denver II—Revision and Restandardization of the Denver Developmental Screening Test (DDST) evaluates four major categories of development: gross motor, fine motor–adaptive, language, and personal–social. See **Figure 11-2■**. It is used to determine whether a child is within the normal range for various behaviors or is developmentally delayed. Like the original DDST, the Denver II is applicable to children from birth through 6 years of age. The age divisions are monthly until 24 months and then every 6 months until 6 years of age (15, 35).

Although it is not the purpose of this discussion to describe the administration and interpretation of the Denver II, the following points should be noted. First, to avoid errors in administration and interpretation, and hence invalid screening results, the examiner should carefully follow the protocol outlined by the test's authors. Second, before administering the test, explanations should be given to both the child and parents. Parents should be advised that the Denver II is not an intelligence test but rather a means of assessing what the child can do at a particular age (15, 35).

Because the Denver II is nonthreatening, requires no painful or unfamiliar procedures, and relies on the child's natural activity of play, it is an excellent way to begin the health assessment. It provides a general assessment tool that can help guide treatment and teaching. The Denver II form and instruction manual can be obtained from Denver Developmental Materials, Inc., P.O. Box 371075, Denver, CO 80237-5075; (303) 355–4729, 800-419-4729; or on the Denver II Website, www.denverii.com.

It is important to consider genetics, family factors, nutrition, and social environment when you assess and care for children, including those who are *developmentally delayed.* Occasionally a child

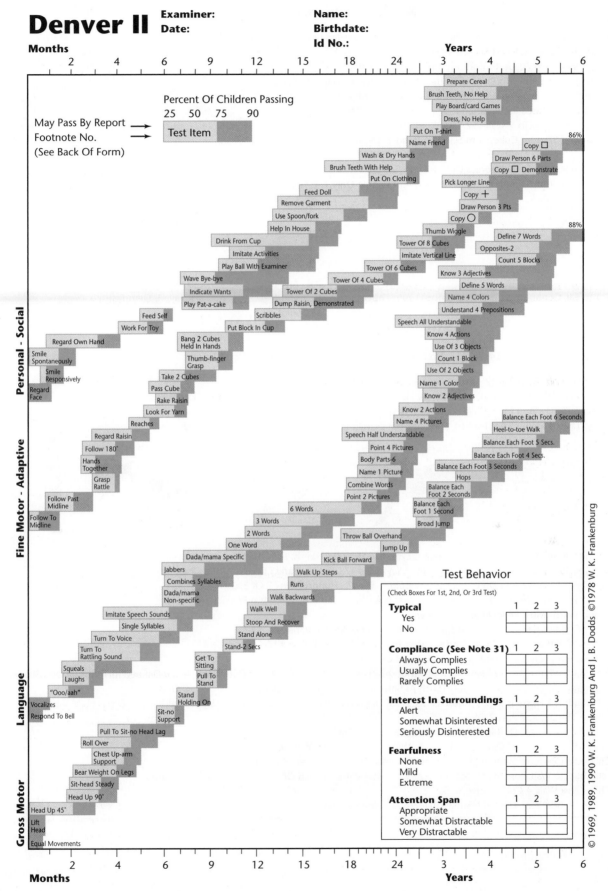

FIGURE ■ 11-2 Denver II—Revision and Restandardization of the Denver Development Screening Test

Source: From Frankenberg, W. K., & Dobbs, J. B. (1990) Denver II—Revision and Standardization of the Denver Developmental Screening Test. *Denver Developmental Materials. Used with permission.*

Directions For Administration

1. Try To Get Child To Smile By Smiling, Talking Or Waving. Do Not Touch Him/her.
2. Child Must Stare At Hand Several Seconds.
3. Parent May Help Guide Toothbrush And Put Toothpaste On Brush.
4. Child Does Not Have To Be Able To Tie Shoes Or Button/zip In The Back.
5. Move Yarn Slowly In An Arc From One Side To The Other, About 8" Above Child's Face.
6. Pass If Child Grasps Rattle When It Is Touched To The Backs Or Tips Of Fingers.
7. Pass If Child Tries To See Where Yarn Went. Yarn Should Be Dropped Quickly From Sight From Tester's Hand Without Arm Movement.
8. Child Must Transfer Cube From Hand To Hand Without Help Of Body, Mouth, Or Table.
9. Pass If Child Picks Up Raisin With Any Part Of Thumb And Finger.
10. Line Can Vary Only 30 Degrees Or Less From Tester's Line. ⃗
11. Make A Fist With Thumb Pointing Upward And Wiggle Only The Thumb. Pass If Child Imitates And Does Not Move Any Fingers Other Than The Thumb.

   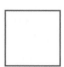

12. Pass Any Enclosed Form. Fail Continuous Round Motions.	13. Which Line Is Longer? (Not Bigger.) Turn Paper Upside Down And Repeat. (Pass 3 Of 3 Or 5 Of 6)	14. Pass Any Lines Crossing Near Midpoint.	15. Have Child Copy First. If Failed, Demonstrate.

When Giving Items 12, 14, And 15, Do Not Name The Forms. Do Not Demonstrate 12 And 14.

16. When Scoring, Each Pair (2 Arms, 2 Legs, Etc.) Counts As One Part.
17. Place One Cube In Cup And Shake Gently Near Childís Ear, But Out Of Sight. Repeat For Other Ear.
18. Point To Picture And Have Child Name It. (No Credit Is Given For Sounds Only.)
    If Less Than 4 Pictures Are Named Correctly, Have Child Point To Picture As Each Is Named By Tester.

 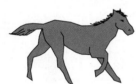 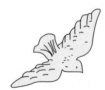 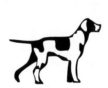 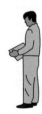

19. Using Doll, Tell Child: Show Me The Nose, Eyes, Ears, Mouth, Hands, Feet, Tummy, Hair. Pass 6 Of 8.
20. Using Pictures, Ask Child: Which One Flies?...Says Meow?...Talks?...Barks?...Gallops? Pass 2 Of 5, 4 Of 5.
21. Ask Child: What Do You Do When You Are Cold?...Tired?...Hungry? Pass 2 Of 3, 3 Of 3.
22. Ask Child: What Do You Do With A Cup? What Is A Chair Used For? What Is A Pencil Used For?
    Action Words Must Be Included In Answers.
23. Pass If Child Correctly Places *And* Says How Many Blocks Are On Paper. (1, 5).
24. Tell Child: Put Block **On** Table; **Under** Table; **In Front Of** Me, **Behind** Me. Pass 4 Of 4.
    (Do Not Help Child By Pointing, Moving Head Or Eyes.)
25. Ask Child: What Is A Ball?...Lake?...Desk?...House?...Banana?...Curtain?...Fence?...Ceiling? Pass If Defined In Terms Of Use, Shape, What It Is Made Of, Or General Category (Such As Banana <u>Is Fruit</u>, Not Just Yellow). Pass 5 Of 8, 7 Of 8.
26. Ask Child: If A Horse Is Big, A Mouse Is _____ ? If Fire Is Hot, Ice Is _____ ? If The Sun Shines During The Day, The Moon Shines During The _____ ? Pass 2 Of 3.
27. Child May Use Wall Or Rail Only, Not Person. May Not Crawl.
28. Child Must Throw Ball Overhand 3 Feet To Within Arm's Reach Of Tester.
29. Child Must Perform Standing Broad Jump Over Width Of Test Sheet (8 1/2 Inches).
30. Tell Child To Walk Forward ⬭⬭⬭⬭ → Heel Within 1 Inch Of Toe. Tester May Demonstrate. Child Must Walk 4 Consecutive Steps.
31. In The Second Year, Half Of Normal Children Are Non–compliant.

Observations:

FIGURE ■ 11-2 Continued

does not attain height within the norms for his or her age, although torso-to-leg proportions are normal, because the pituitary gland does not produce enough growth hormone (46). **Growth hormone deficiency,** *which causes dwarfism in a preschool child,* can be treated with a synthetic growth hormone. The person still remains short in stature but is within a normal height range (46). The treatment is important because children who lag behind peers in growth are often teased, are kept from participating in certain play activities, and may have difficulty finding clothes or play equipment that is of correct size. The child may be regarded by others as retarded intellectually. He or she may feel inferior, suffer a negative self-concept, lack initiative, and become withdrawn, depressed, or antisocial in later childhood or adult years (34, 46, 76).

Various endocrine conditions can affect growth and development. Early detection and treatment is essential. Refer to pediatric nursing texts for more information (46, 76).

Nutritional Needs

The child needs the same food groups as the adult each day, but in smaller quantities. **Box 11-2,** Recommended Daily Nutritional Intake for Preschoolers, summarizes basic nutritional needs, servings, and food examples. Information is based on the Food Pyramid (100) and revisions made for this age group (26, 28). The box presents the pyramid in reverse from the usual depiction: the grain group is first. Serving sizes are relevant for preschoolers: 1 tablespoon per year, or 3 tablespoons for the 3-year-old and 5 tablespoons for the 5-year-old. Other guides have been formulated. For example, MyPyramid is a symbol with vertical groups representing 12 patterns of food intake for caloric levels ranging from 1,000 to 3,200 calories (93). The MyPyramid Website gives data for age, gender, daily servings per group, and recommended activity level for estimated caloric needs. Information is also available at the Website for MyPyramid for Kids. The daily amounts are presented in ounces or cups, not number of servings. Stomach capacity is increasing and mouth muscles are stronger. The child eats a larger amount and greater variety of food.

The child needs a gradual increase in *caloric intake* (1,250 to 1,600 cal/day or 90 to 100 kcal/kg/day). A *guide is a daily baseline of 1,000 calories plus 100 calories for each year:* 1,300 calories for the 3-year-old, 1,500 calories for the 5-year-old. Calorie intake of 90 kcal/kg would give the larger-built child about 1,800 calories daily. Obesity is common in preschoolers related to excess calorie intake and insufficient exercise. Parental feeding practices, values related to food, preference for chubby children, and parental obesity may be related to the preschooler's being obese (26, 28). **Obesity,** *extreme overweight, is defined in childhood as having a* **body mass index** (**BMI,** *comparison of weight to height*) *at or above the 95th percentile for age and gender* (46, 74). More than 10% of 2- to 5-year-olds are obese (46, 74). As "junk food" of the United States spreads around the world, countries such as Egypt, Morocco, and Zambia report that 20% to 25% of their 4-year-olds are overweight or obese (74). Overweight or obese children set a pattern that continues into adulthood. Excess body mass is a health threat at all ages (46, 74, 85, 92).

Protein needs range from 13 g/day (3-year-old) to 19 g/day (5-year-old) (26). Saturated fatty acid consumption should be less than 10% of total caloric intake. *Total fat* should average no more than 30% and no less than 20% of total caloric intake. Some fat is necessary for taste and brain development and function (28, 46). *Calcium* (800 mg daily) is needed for growing bones and teeth and storage for ongoing growth (26). Equally important for bone and tooth building and muscle strength is *vitamin D* (at least 200 IU daily) (26); sunshine and vitamin-D-fortified milk and other foods are sources. *Iron* (10 mg daily)

BOX 11-2	**Recommended Daily Nutritional Intake for Preschoolers**
Grains 6 or more servings 6 oz	Breads (whole grain preferred), cereals, bagels, crackers, muffins, biscuits, tortilla, rice, grits, hominy, pasta, pretzels, popcorn.
Vegetable 3 or more servings	Any green, yellow, or white vegetable, legumes, plant oils.
Fruit 2 servings	Any fruit, including citrus and tropical.
Milk 2 cups or more; 2 servings	Milk, buttermilk, yogurt, milk puddings, any cheese. Ages 2–4 years—2 cups; 4 years and beyond—3 cups. Use soy milk, aged cheeses, cooked milk products if lactose deficiency/lactose intolerance.
Meat and Beans 2 servings 5 oz	Poultry, pork, red meats, organ meats, fish, shellfish, red beans, dried beans, pinto beans, black-eyed peas, nuts, peanut butter, eggs. Lean meat preferred. Ratio of white to red meat served should be 4:1.
Fats, Oils, Sugars *Use sparingly*	Oil from fish and nuts, liquid oils (corn, soybean, canola for cooking). Desserts—occasional.
Fruit Juice 4–6 oz 1/2–3/4 cup	Pure juices; no sugar or artificial sweeteners added. Juices with added vitamin C or calcium don't offer as much nutrition as pure fruit juice or milk.
Fiber Age +5	Whole grains, legumes, vegetables, fruits (e.g., slice of whole-grain bread, one serving broccoli, one serving carrot for a 3-year-old).
Water	Drink throughout the day. Avoid sense of thirst.

is needed for hemoglobin production and assists in the formation of muscle cells, proteins, and enzymes in the growing child (26, 28, 46). Iron deficiency anemia may occur because of fast growth and insufficient intake of iron; it can contribute to cognitive deficits (26). More information on nutrient requirements is available from the Food and Nutrition Board, Institute of Medicine Website, www.union.edu.

Without adequate fruits and vegetables, *vitamins A and C* usually are also lacking. Desserts should furnish protein, minerals, vitamins, and calories and should be a natural part of the meal, not used as a reward for finishing the meal or omitted as punishment.

A well-planned *vegetarian diet,* even a *vegan diet,* can supply the needed nutrients for growth and energy (28). If the family is **pure vegetarian,** *eating no meat, milk, or eggs,* the diet may be low in protein, iron, calcium, vitamins B_{12} and D, and zinc (30). The **lacto-ovo vegetarian diet** *excludes meat but includes milk, eggs, and rarely fish* and has fewer deficiencies. The diet may be low in protein since the major sources of all the essential amino acids are eliminated. Vegetarian diets require supplements for at least vitamins B_{12} and D, and zinc (28, 46). Careful monitoring is essential.

Slower growth rate and heightened interest in exploring the environment may lessen interest in eating. Midmorning, midafternoon, and evening snacks are necessary because of the child's high level of activity, but should be wisely chosen: milk, juice, fruit wedges, vegetable strips, cereals without added unrefined sugar and with fiber, cheese cubes, peanut butter with crackers or bread, or plain cookies. Sweets (candy, raisins, sodas, sugar-coated cereals) should be offered only occasionally, not as a reward for behavior and not before a meal. This pattern will help prevent health problems associated with overeating sweet foods, such as dental caries, malnutrition, and obesity, and associating only pleasure with food. Lifetime food habits are being formed (28, 46). Heart disease and cancer can occur at an early age. A diet high in saturated fat can cause, as early as age 3, fatty streaks in the vessel as a precursor to atherosclerosis (26, 28, 44, 46).

Eating assumes increasing social significance for the preschooler and is still an emotional and physiologic experience. The child needs the right foods physically and a warm, happy atmosphere in which he or she is included in mealtime conversation. The family mealtime promotes socialization in relation to meal preparation, behavior during mealtimes, language skills, and understanding of family rituals and situations. The training is positive or negative, depending on the parents' example. Such learning is missed if there are no family mealtimes. Table manners need not be rigidly emphasized; accidents will happen. Parental example is the best teacher.

The preschooler's eating habits are simple. There may be periods of overeating or not wanting to eat certain foods, but they do not persist. The overall eating pattern from month to month is more pertinent to assess. Preschoolers who follow their own appetite patterns are likely to maintain normal weight (26).

The sense of taste is keen; color, flavor, form, and texture are important. Foods should be attractively served, mildly flavored, whole, plain, separated, and distinctly identifiable in flavor and appearance rather than mixed (as in creamed foods, casseroles, and stews). An exception is spaghetti and pizza. Lukewarm, rather than too hot or too cold, including drinks, is preferred. The preschooler likes to eat one thing at a time. Of all food groups, vegetables are least liked, whereas fruits are a favorite. He or she prefers vegetables and fruits crisp, raw, and cut into finger-sized pieces. Strong-tasting vegetables, such as cabbage, onions, cauliflower, and broccoli, and those with tough strings, such as celery and green beans, are usually disliked. Meats should be easily chewed and cut into bite-sized pieces. New foods can be gradually introduced; if a food is refused once, offer it again after several days.

A child may be eating insufficiently for the following reasons:

1. Eats too much between meals
2. Experiences unhappy mealtime atmosphere
3. Seeks attention
4. Mimics parental eating habits
5. Responds to excessive parental expectations
6. Has inadequate variety and quantity
7. Suffers tooth decay, which may cause nausea or toothache with chewing
8. Feels sibling rivalry
9. Experiences overfatigue, physical illness, or emotional disturbance

Parents should consider, too, the difference in eating patterns of the 3-, 4-, and 5-year-old, which can influence food intake. The *3-year-old* either talks or eats, gets up from the table during meals but will return to eat more food, and rarely needs assistance to complete a meal. The *4-year-old* normally combines talking and eating, rarely gets up from the table, and likes to serve self. The *5-year-old* eats rapidly and is sociable during mealtime, so that family atmosphere is crucial.

Measures to increase food intake include letting the child help plan the menu, set the table, wash dishes, or prepare foods, such as stirring instant puddings or gelatin desserts, beating cake or cookie mix, or kneading dough. *Other measures are to:* (a) serve meals in courses in a quiet environment in which there are few distractions; (b) avoid coaxing, bribing, or threatening; (c) provide a premeal rest period; (d) give small, attractive servings; (e) provide a comfortable chair and table; (f) allow sufficient time for eating; and (g) avoid between-meal nibbling. Making food an issue and forcing the child to eat can create eating problems, and the child is likely to win the battle. The child's appetite will improve as the growth rate increases nearer school age.

Although vitamin-mineral supplements should not be a food substitute, many pediatricians recommend them as an adjunct, especially during these years when appetite fluctuates. Fluoride supplements should be continued if there is insufficient fluoride in the water (26).

Share information with parents about nutritional needs and eating patterns and the psychological aspects of food and mealtime. Refer them to Websites and other sources of information.

Exercise, Rest, and Sleep

EXERCISE NEEDS

The preschool child needs *at least 60 minutes of active exercise daily.* **Figure 11-3**◻ depicts an example. This is the period when the

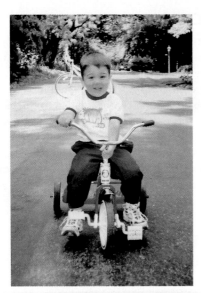

FIGURE ■ 11-3 The preschool child enjoys exercise on the tricycle.

child has a seeming surplus of energy and is on the move. The child needs time and space for physical exercise through play. Clothing and shoes should be comfortable and allow for movement. Shoes should provide flexibility, yet be stable, and conform to the plantar arch contours. The child may play to the point of fatigue. Thus the adult must initiate rest periods alternated with activity.

Share information with parents. Refer to the later sections about Play Patterns, Purposes, and Materials. Play is essential for physical development and exercise, as described in the Case Situation. Review types of play that can also promote rest.

REST AND SLEEP NEEDS

Sleep needs vary with age. The *3-year-old child* does not always sleep at naptime but will rest or play quietly for 1 or 2 hours if undisturbed. The *4-year-old child* resists naps but needs quiet periods. The *5-year-old child* is unlikely to nap if he or she gets adequate sleep at night.

The preschooler may still take a favorite toy to bed; he or she likes to postpone bedtime and is ritualistic about bedtime routines, such as prayers, a story, or music. *Sleeping time decreases from 10 to 12 hours for the younger preschooler to 9 to 11 hours for the older preschooler.* Dreams and nightmares may awaken the 3- or 4-year-old, causing fear and a move into bed with parents or older siblings. The 5-year-old sleeps quietly through the night without having to get up to urinate and has fewer nightmares. About 20% to 30% of children up to age 4 years have **bedtime struggles**, *difficulty falling asleep* because of co-sleeping, family stress or illness, or a mother who is depressed or who recently changed her schedule and is away most of the day (74).

Teach parents that co-sleep should not occur in this era on a regular basis. If the parent responds with special attention to the child who awakens during the night, the sleep disturbance becomes worse. Parents should not reinforce the waking behavior. Instead they should help the restless child develop sleep strategies, such as listening to soft age-related music or cuddling a teddy bear or blanket. Parents should provide reassurance and set and maintain limits.

Dreams, nightmares, and sleepwalking occur during the light sleep stages, most frequently in the 4-year-old. *Nightmares* occur more frequently when the child is overfatigued or overstimulated by frightening television, video, or video game scenes. They occur in the morning hours and can be recalled. Within an hour of falling asleep, during deep stages of sleep, the child may have night terrors. Often children do not awaken after they sleepwalk or have

Case Situation

Preschooler Development: The Fun of Exercise

Kalisha is an active, 38-month-old girl who weighs 34 pounds (15.45 kg) and is 38 in. (95 cm) tall. She is playing on the sidewalk in front of her parents' home with her brother, Mario, 4 years old, and her next-door neighbor, Lora, 5 years of age. Her parents are watching them play.

Kalisha is riding her small, two-wheeled bicycle that has training wheels. Mario and Lora are riding their small bicycles or scooters. Kalisha rides for a while, then stops to watch the others. Although involved in the same activity, she plays next to rather than with the older children. Several times she rides her tricycle toward her mother, calling to her, and when her mother answers, she rides away, showing typical preschooler attachment patterns.

When Mario and Lora ride down the street, leaving Kalisha, she asks her mother to go with her to join them. She pulls her mother's hand insistently, and her mother joins her for a walk down the street. When Kalisha hears the other two children, she runs to them, laughing, and gives each child a hug. Lora chases Kalisha; Kalisha turns to her mother, seeking protection and assurance.

As Mario and Lora ride their bicycles toward Kalisha, she laughs, waving her arms, and shouts, "I am the stop sign." Lora laughs and rides by her, saying, "You'll have to give me a ticket." As Lora rides by again, she stops. Kalisha and Lora repeat this pattern several times. Kalisha becomes more animated, demonstrating characteristics of autonomy and beginning initiative. Yet, her commands and wanting the other children to follow exactly her commands is typical egocentrism of this age.

Contributed by Ruth Murray, EdD, MSN, N-NAP, FAAN.

night terrors. In **night terrors** the *child screams or cries, may thrash and squirm, is confused, does not respond to parents, behaves abnormally, and has tachycardia and tachypnea, dilated pupils, and sometimes facial contortions and diaphoresis* (46, 74).

Help the parents understand that calm reassurance is needed with night terrors. Wait out the attack without trying either to comfort or to arouse the child. Further stimulation intensifies agitation. After 15 minutes or so, the child collapses back into sleep without memory of what happened. Sleep problems usually subside spontaneously. The child and parents may need therapy if the problem persists.

Health Promotion and Health Protection

IMMUNIZATION SCHEDULES

Before-school immunizations are recommended for the preschooler, between 4 and 6 years, prior to entry in Head Start or kindergarten (37, 51, 87). Refer to the Websites mentioned in the Immunizations section of Chapter 9 for more information. ∞

Counsel parents that the state law requiring immunizations before school entry is a beneficial one, because the organisms that cause childhood communicable diseases cannot be eliminated from the environment without broad immunizations. The decrease in these diseases and their harmful effects has resulted only because of mass *inoculations of a disease antigen* (**active immunity**) or *an antibody* (**passive immunity**). The minimum reaction is far better than acquiring the disease or, generally, the potential risks.

Before giving an immunization, ask yourself the following questions (34, 46, 80):

1. Has the parent given consent? Members of some religious groups, such as Church of Christ, Scientist (Christian Scientist), do not believe in immunizations. (The school district may allow these children to attend without immunization, based on parents' rights regarding their children.)
2. Is the vaccination (immunization) indicated based on the child's age and previous immunization record?
3. Are there any contraindications, such as allergy to any of the constituents of the vaccine; presence of another infectious disease (febrile condition, dermatitis) or immunodeficiency disease; presence of malignancy or immunosuppressive therapy; or administration of gamma globulin, plasma, or blood transfusion in the previous 6 to 8 weeks that would have given passive antibodies?
4. Has the parent been informed of the method (route of administration) and benefits and risks involved in inoculation?
5. Has the parent informed you of any reactions or difficulties that occurred with or after previous immunizations? If the child has a minor reaction, remaining doses may be cut in half or thirds to decrease the possibility of a systemic reaction. The child then returns an additional number of times to receive the full immunization series.
6. Has the vaccine been stored according to manufacturer's recommendations (usually refrigerated) and is there a date of expiration?

DENTAL CARE

Because caries frequently begin at this age and spread rapidly, dental care is important. Deciduous teeth guide in the permanent ones; they should be kept in good repair. Fluoride is important for preventing caries. If the child has teeth with deep grooves, a plastic coating can be applied to the teeth to prevent tooth decay and loss. If deciduous teeth are lost too early, permanent teeth grow in abnormally. Teeth should be brushed after eating, using a method recommended by the dentist, and intake of refined sugars limited to help prevent tooth decay. Before entering school the child is usually required to have a physical and a dental examination.

SAFETY PROMOTION AND INJURY CONTROL

The preschooler has more freedom, independence, initiative, and desire to imitate adults than the toddler but still has an immature understanding of danger and illness, and is reckless at times. Temperament may also be a factor (74, 89). This combination is likely to get him or her into hazardous situations.

Emphasize to parents that a major responsibility of caretaking adults is safety promotion and injury control. For example, the child needs to wear a seatbelt restraint in the car, appropriate for size and weight of the child, and wear a helmet when riding a tricycle or scooter or engaging in active play. The child needs watchfulness and a safe play area. The adult serves as a bodyguard while slowly teaching caution and keeping the environment as safe as possible. Begin safety teaching early. Teaching done in the toddler years, for example, pays off now. Other siblings can also take some, but not total, responsibility for the preschooler. Protecting the firstborn is simpler as the parent can put dangerous objects away and there is likely to be more time and energy for supervision. When there are a number of children in a family, the activities of the older children may provide objects or situations that are dangerous to the younger ones. As the child learns to protect self, he or she should be allowed to take added responsibility for personal safety and should be given appropriate verbal recognition and praise that reinforce safe behavior.

Discuss with parents how to be **effective in teaching safety to the child***:*

1. Avoid constant statements about need to be fearful, or natural curiosity and the will to learn will be dulled. The child may fear every new situation.
2. Avoid constant threats, frequent physical punishment, and incessant "don'ts" or the child will learn to ignore them, feel angry or resentful, and purposefully rebel or defy adults, thus failing to learn about real danger.
3. Use simple command words in a firm voice without anger to convey the impression that you expect the child to obey, for example, "Stop" or "No."
4. Phrase safety rules and their reasons calmly and in positive rather than negative terms when possible. For example, say: "Play in the yard, not the street, or you'll get hurt by cars" or "Put tiny things (coins, beads) that you find in here (jar, bowl, box)."

Teach **safety suggestions for parents to use when they teach the child** *about home and personal behavior:*

1. Teach the child his or her full name, address including zip code, and telephone number.
2. Teach the child how to access police or adults in service roles for help—for example, 9-1-1 (*not* nine-eleven), emergency services, police, or fire department.
3. Teach the child *not* to tell information about self or the family to another person on the phone.
4. Insist that the child *never* leave home alone or with a stranger.
5. Teach the child escape techniques, for example, how to unlock home doors or car doors, and when to use them.
6. Teach the child how to cross the street safely.
7. Teach the child to refuse gifts or rides from strangers, and to avoid walking or playing alone on a deserted street, road, or similar area.
8. Encourage the child to share any "secrets"; emphasize that he or she does not have to be afraid to say anything.

Teach parents **measures they can institute for the child's safety,** *including in the car, at home, or with supplies and equipment:*

1. *Never* leave the child alone in public or unattended in a car.
2. *Never* leave the child home alone. Make sure that the babysitter is reliable.
3. *Never* allow the child to play alone in or near a busy driveway, street, or garage. Teach children how to cross the street and to look carefully for cars. A fenced yard or playground is ideal, although not always available, especially for tricycles and similar toys.
4. Keep matches in containers and out of reach.
5. Dispose of or store out of reach and in a locked cabinet all of the poisons and caustic products you have in the house: rat and roach killer, insecticides, weed killer, kerosene, cleaning agents, furniture polish, and so on. The child should be taught their *correct* use. The child is less likely to pull them out of cabinets or swallow them than when he or she was a toddler, but brightly colored containers or pills, powders, or liquids stimulate curiosity and experimentation.
6. Keep medications, suntan lotion, shampoo, deodorants, nail polish, and cosmetics out of the child's reach. Brightly colored

pills can be mistaken for candy. Keep the Poison Control Center telephone number readily visible.

7. Store knives, saws, and other sharp objects or lawn or power tools out of reach.
8. Remove doors from abandoned appliances or cars. Dispose of them appropriately.
9. Discourage playing with or in the area of appliances or power tools while they are in operation.

Teach parents **measures to avoid falls** *and related injury:*

1. Keep stairways and nighttime play areas well lit.
2. Equip upstairs windows with sturdy screens and guards. Have hand rails for stairways.
3. Use safety glass in glass doors or shower stalls; place decals on sliding doors at child's eye level (and adult's eye level, too) to prevent walking or running through them.
4. Use adhesive strips on the bottom of the bathtub.
5. Avoid scatter rugs, debris, or toys cluttered on the floor in areas of traffic.

Explore with parents the possibility of **child abduction**, either from the home area, often by a person who knows the family, or while the family is in a large shopping area, with the child momentarily out of sight. Sometimes the abducted *child is enticed to follow the abductor or grabbed and forced into a vehicle* while en route to school or returning home or at play near the home. Some abductors are sexually motivated (14), or the child may be taken to the location of a cult (90). Refer to the section on cults in Chapter 7 ∞ for related information. Refer to information presented in Chapter 10 for immediate intervention. ∞ In addition, **teach parents to teach the child safety measures previously listed** that relate to the home and personal behavior. See Chapter 9 ∞ about education of parents in choosing an in-home caregiver or nanny.

Measures **for parents to teach the child related to the potential of abduction, running away from home, or getting lost** *include:*

1. Teach the preschooler about the neighborhood, how to get there from various locations (stores, church, day care center), and safe houses in the neighborhood. Introduce the child to the occupants of safe houses.

INTERVENTIONS FOR HEALTH PROMOTION

Explore the following with parents. If the child continually fails to listen and obey, ask the following questions:

1. Is the child able to hear?
2. Is he or she intellectually able to understand?
3. Are demands too many and expectations too great?
4. Are statements too lengthy or abstract?
5. Is anger expressed with teaching and discipline to the point that it interferes emotionally with the child's perception and judgment?

6. *Do the parents demonstrate safety-conscious behavior* with equipment, movements, or use of seatbelt or sun safety rules?
7. *Do parents understand that imitation is a major way to learn?*

2. Emphasize to avoid talking with or giving his or her name to strangers.
3. Review regularly the child's schedule, such as day care, nursery school, or special events, and set boundaries in relation to location and time when the parent will take the child and arrive later to get the child.
4. Encourage the child to discuss with the parent the events of the day, including any unusual happenings. Open communication gives the parent information that could prevent a future serious situation.

Parents often print the child's name on a backpack or clothing. The first and last initials or a special marker is sufficient for general identification and reduces the chance of a stranger/abductor learning the child's first name. It can be useful to place under the inner sole of the child's shoe a piece of paper with identification information that can be used by the child in an emergency.

Refer to the box *Healthy People 2010:* Example of Objectives for Preschool Health Promotion for a perspective on major health concerns and prevention strategies in the United States, formulated by the U.S. Department of Health and Human Services (94). The *Healthy People 2010* Initiative has established goals to reduce disease, disability, and death in young children through access to health screening, follow-up, and referral, and through accident prevention and immunization. For more information, refer to the Website www.health.gov or call 1-800-367-4725.

ACCIDENTS

Accidents are the most common cause of death (46, 74, 80, 85). Approximately 33% of accidental deaths are caused by motor vehicles; the next most common causes are drowning, burns from fire or hot water, falls, and poisonings. Running through sliding glass doors in homes, locking self in an abandoned refrigerator or freezer, and electric shocks from electrical equipment also frequently cause severe injury or death. Falls can cause minor bumps, bruises, lacerations, and even death. Animal bites are common.

Teach parents about prevention. See measures previously discussed. Encourage parents to seek information about emergency treatment.

Minor head injury *is any trauma to the head that does not alter normal cerebral functioning.* What appears to be a very minor head injury can result in a subdural or epidural hematoma—the preschooler bears very close monitoring.

Parents or caretakers should be taught to check the preschooler every 2 hours in the first 24 hours after injury for the following signs: (a) cannot be awakened; (b) is mentally confused; (c) is unusually restless, disturbed, or agitated; (d) starts vomiting; (e) has a severe headache; (f) has unequally sized pupils (unless previously that way); (g) has weakness of arms or legs; (h) has drainage from ears or nose; or (i) has some sort of fit or convulsion. Medical help must be sought (34, 46).

Minor lacerations, *cuts,* should be examined for dirt and foreign objects even after they have been cleaned with warm water and soap. The laceration may be covered with a loose bandage that will keep out dirt and protect the wound from additional trauma.

Have the parent or caretaker watch for signs of infection: redness, heat, swelling, and drainage. The child should have tetanus prophylaxis updated (34, 46).

Burns *are thermal injuries to the skin.* A **first-degree burn** *usually shows redness only.* A **second-degree burn** *causes blister formation,* sometimes with peeling and weeping. Scalds often produce this type of burn. A **third-degree burn** *chars the skin, causing a whitish appearance, and involves tissue under the skin.* It may cause anesthesia. Flame and hot metal often cause third-degree burns (46). Refer to pediatric nursing texts for information on emergency and long-term care of minor and major burns (34, 46). Care of these patients is complex.

Accidental ingestions and poisonings may occur in children under the age of 5, sometimes even when preventive measures as discussed in Chapter 10 ∞ are used. These ingestions can cause a great variety of symptoms and signs.

The following guidelines should be taught to parents:

1. Look for an empty container nearby if sudden unusual symptoms or abnormal odor of breath or clothes is observed.
2. Try to determine what and how much was ingested and when.
3. Call the Poison Control Center for help.
4. If there are no contraindications to vomiting (either from reading the container instructions or from directions of the

Poison Control Center), induce vomiting with syrup of ipecac. Mechanical stimulation of the posterior pharynx can be used to induce vomiting except with ingestion of corrosive agents, such as lye, gasoline, and kerosene.

5. Take the child to the nearest clinic that is set up to deal with these problems.

HEALTH RISKS

Respiratory problems, including asthma, are twice as common in children who are exposed to parental smoking, in contrast to children of nonsmoking parents (46, 49). Environmental tobacco smoke also lowers the blood level of vitamin C, a key nutrient for the immune system (28, 92).

The **bite of any animal** will probably have few symptoms other than pain at the site of puncture wounds or small lacerations. Dog bites are most common, although the child may have contact with other animals that bite or scratch. Bites from other children can also occur. The chief concern of animal bites is the possibility of rabies.

It is essential to establish the vaccination status of the biting animal, if possible. If the animal is properly vaccinated, there is little chance of acquiring and transmitting the disease to humans. Rabies prophylaxis will be determined by the physician. The wound should be washed with copious amounts of soap and water. Tetanus prophylaxis should be up to date (34, 46).

Lead poisoning, especially in preschoolers, will produce **encephalopathy,** or *brain dysfunction.* The onset is insidious, with weakness, irritability, weight loss, and vomiting, followed by personality changes and developmental regression. Convulsions and coma are late signs. The child puts fingers into the mouth, ingesting lead from cracking paint in old homes or lead-painted toys, old yellow and orange crayons, artist's paints, leaded gasoline, or fruit tree sprays. High blood lead levels contribute to lower intelligence and reduced achievement and to attention deficit/hyperactivity disorder (46).

Prevention lies in keeping the preschooler in a lead-free environment as much as possible. You may call the housing inspector, with the family's permission, to test paint for lead. In many cities landlords are required to repaint the house interior when lead paint is found. Treatment should be given as appropriate for the severity of the child's condition (34, 46).

COMMON HEALTH PROBLEMS: PREVENTION AND PROTECTION

Teach parents that scheduled health maintenance visits to the doctor or nurse practitioner are important for early detection of problems.

MALTREATMENT, ABUSE, AND NEGLECT

An all-too-common health problem for the young child is *maltreatment, abuse, or neglect* (10–14, 19, 37, 38, 52, 53, 60, 71, 72). See Chapters 9 and 10 for additional information. ∞

Be aware that when you encounter children with some of the previous accidental occurrences or health problems, the origin of the problems may be the beatings, burns, shakings, handling, sexual abuse or incest, or neglect received at the hands of a parent, stepparent, day care teacher, or other adult caretaker. Utilize the following information in assessment and intervention. *You are responsible for detecting, reporting, and treating the child and working with the parents.*

Role relationship of the child to the offender may be intrafamilial (family member) or extrafamilial (day care worker, teacher, babysitter, family acquaintance, or stranger). When the abuser is older, the age difference conveys that others will not believe the accusations by the child but rather the denial of the offender. Further, the role of the offender often involves one of caretaker so that trust would be the normal feeling for the child (10–14, 65, 71, 72, 79).

Abuse

The Federal Child Abuse Prevention and Treatment Act of 1996 defines **child abuse** as *any recent action, or failure to act, by a parent, caretaker, or agency staff who is responsible for the child's/youth's welfare, that results in risk of serious physical or emotional harm, sexual abuse, exploitation, or death of a person under age 18 years* (46). **Sexual abuse** *is defined by the Act as employment, persuasion, inducement, enticement, or coercion of any child to engage in, or assist any other person to engage in, any sexually explicit conduct, or stimulation of such conduct, such as for videotaping. Rape, statutory rape, molestation, prostitution or other forms of sexual exploitations, or incest with children are included in the definition* (46). The three types of abuse (physical, psychological, and sexual) may be present simultaneously, but frequently the child's symptoms and perceptions convey that one abuse experience is dominant (12).

Physically abusive acts *include being bitten, punched, kicked, beaten, burned, shaken, cut, physically restrained, and tied up.* It is also considered abuse if the child witnesses this behavior between an adult and a child or between adults (11, 46, 71, 72).

Psychological abuse *is characterized by behaviors, activities, and words that intimidate, threaten, humiliate, shame, or degrade the child; blaming the child for the abuse; and threatening the child with harm,* such as being locked in a box, removal of body parts, and death to self or family members, if he or she tells about the abuse (12, 38, 71, 72). A parent may belittle the child until her or she is convinced of being worthless, or physically abuse the child's pet or favorite toy to show power over the child.

Child sexual abuse *is defined as activities intended to sexually stimulate immature children and adolescents who do not fully comprehend the sexual act, who are unable to give informed consent, or who are forced to engage in activities that violate social taboos or family roles.* The child is victimized by the lack of choice involved (by force or trickery) because there is an unequal power relationship (abuser is older or a caretaker) (19, 72, 79). *Sexual abuse is defined as pressured or ritualistic* (10, 11, 37, 38, 79).

Pressured sexuality is an *adult's dominance used to ensure sexual control over the child so that there is no choice of consent and right to say "No" to the perpetrator; it often is accompanied by threats of violence to the child or family members* (10, 11, 52). Pressured sexuality may involve contact or noncontact with the child. See **Box 11-3**, Examples of Contact and Noncontact Sexual Abuse (10–14, 37, 38, 71, 72, 79).

Ritualistic abuse refers to the *systematic and repetitive sexual, physical, and psychological abuse of children by adults engaged in*

BOX 11-3 **Examples of Contact and Noncontact Sexual Abuse**

CONTACT

Touching, fondling, or kissing genital area of child's body

Making child touch, fondle, or kiss the person's genital area or breasts

Engaging in frottage, in which person rubs genital areas against child's clothing, genital area, or other body part

Masturbating the child

Making child masturbate the person

Performing fellatio, which is oral contact with male genitals (either by the child, male person, or both)

Performing cunnilingus, which is oral contact with female genitals (of child, female person, or both)

Performing digital or penile penetration of anus or vagina

Forcing child to perform sexual acts with others, either children or adults

NO DIRECT CONTACT

Voyeurism, which is sexual excitement from observing naked body of another or sexual acts of another, against the child's will or from a secret vantage point

Exhibitionism, which is exposing genital area or all of body to child

Making child disrobe or be nude, exposed to vision of offender or others

Photographing child's whole body or genitalia, when nude or partly nude, for pornographic purposes

Forcing child to observe sexual acts between others

Sexually harassing by verbally propositioning, belittling, intimidating, accusing, or emphasizing that this activity is the child's fault or the result of abnormal sexual interest

---

group secret activity or cult worship. The purpose of ritualistic abuse is to induce religious or mystical experiences for the adult participants. Ritualistic behavior is linked with symbols of overriding power, authority, and purpose, often pseudoreligious or satanic in nature ("It is God's will that you be punished in this way for your sins"). There is the determined intent by the offender to convert the abused person to a victim role (11, 37, 52, 79, 90).

Indications of satanic ritual abuse have been described by clients and researchers (37, 90):

1. Use of a special table or altar
2. Sexual behavior involving unusual practices
3. Imitations and reversals of the Catholic Mass
4. Ritual use of body fluids and excrement
5. Ritual use of a circle
6. Ritualized use of chants and songs, especially using names of demons
7. Use of animals and insects in ceremonies
8. Wearing of special masks and robes in ceremonies
9. Use of torches, candles, darkness, and body parts in ceremonies
10. Administration of drugs and potions
11. Dismemberment of infants and young children
12. Cannibalism of animals or humans; drinking of human or animal blood in ceremonies

The *autonomic response to abuse is of two types: numbing or hyperarousal (great anxiety). Affective states may include passivity, anxiety, depression, anger, hostility, defiance, and rebellion.* With **numbing,** *there may be acting out of aggressive and sexualized behaviors and a lack of empathy for others.* With **hyperarousal,** there may be *night terrors, stomachaches, startle reflexes, avoidance of people and places, crying, and enuresis.* Alcohol and drug use may be a way to avoid the emotional pain (11–14, 52, 53, 79). Of particularly harmful impact are acts demanding sexual activity with other children, pornographic photography, and forced participation in rituals. The children vacillate between great anxiety and

numbness, for when children reach a panic state, they go into a dissociative state (11, 12). More information about nursing assessment and intervention for the abused child is presented. See **Box 11-4**, Signs and Symptoms of Sexual Abuse in a Child (10–14, 46, 52, 71, 72).

Neglect

Not all abused children are battered. Some suffer just as cruelly from another type of abuse—parental neglect, either willful or unintentional. **Neglect** is defined by the Federal Child Abuse Prevention and Treatment Act as *failure by a parent or persons legally responsible for the child's welfare to provide for the child's physical, emotional, or educational needs* (46). *Neglect can take many forms.* The child is denied food, clothes, shelter, medical care, emotional love, nurturance, security, and necessary socialization opportunities. A parent may neglect a child by being uninvolved and not making an emotional connection, or by simply "forgetting" about him or her (e.g., leaving him or her behind at a bus terminal after rounding up the other children). Or a parent may sedate a rejected child to keep him or her quiet or not expressive of basic needs. Such action may be rooted in anger at the child, ignorance of the child's needs, and poor parenting skills (46). Lack of financial and social support system resources, the parent having been neglected as a child, and parental physical or mental illness also contribute to inability to nurture the child.

The neglected child demonstrates any of the following (12, 46, 71, 72):

1. Effects of malnutrition, including wasting of subcutaneous tissue, abdominal distention, thinness, pallor, dull eyes, sore gums
2. Wearing inadequate clothing in cold weather
3. Expression of apathy, resentfulness, or depression
4. Hyperexcitability, lack of self-control, unruliness
5. Frequent temper tantrums, increasing hostility, aggressiveness, antisocial behavior, often for many years

BOX 11-4   Signs and Symptoms of Sexual Abuse in a Child

DISCLOSURES OF CHILD

1. States that someone removed child's clothes or handled or had contact with the genital area in some way
2. Complains that an adult or older child touched or penetrated child's bottom, vagina, rectum, or mouth or that child touched an older child or adult's bottom, vagina, penis, or rectum
3. Refers to blood or "white stuff" in genital area
4. Describes detailed and age-inappropriate understanding of sexual behavior
5. Hints about engaging in sexual activity

PHYSICAL SYMPTOMS OF CHILD

1. Somatic complaints: stomachaches, nausea, vomiting, headaches, leg aches
2. Underwear excessively soiled resulting from reluctance to clean self or a relaxed anal sphincter
3. Semen or blood stains on child's underwear, skin, hair, or in mouth
4. Bruises or abrasions in the genital or rectal area
5. Vaginal or anal pain, burning when washed, pain when urinating or defecating
6. Chronic constipation or urinary infections
7. Constant fatigue, illness, flare-ups of allergies, vomiting
8. On examination, relaxed anal sphincter, anal or rectal lacerations, or scarring; child relaxes rather than tenses rectum when touched
9. On examination, enlargement of vaginal opening and vaginal lacerations in girls, sore penis in boys; blood or trauma around genital area
10. Presence of venereal disease, including infections, such as trichomoniasis, herpes, and moniliasis

BEHAVIOR OF CHILD

1. Uncontrolled, hyperactive, wild
2. Accident-prone or deliberately hurts self
3. Negativistic, resistant to authority; mistrusts adults

4. Overcompliant with authority; overly pleasing with adults
5. Withdrawn, does not play; plays in lethargic, unfocused way
6. Exhibits short attention span; has difficulty staying on task
7. Does not learn readily
8. Regressive, babyish, delayed, or disordered speech; significantly decreased speech production
9. Sleep disorders: nightmares or night terrors, bed-wetting, fear of going to bed
10. Does not clean himself or herself after going to the bathroom
11. Masturbates excessively; attempts to insert finger or other object in rectum or vagina
12. Pulls down pants, lifts dress, or takes off clothes inappropriately
13. Touches others sexually or asks for sexual activity
14. Is sexually provocative or seductive in behavior
15. Excessive bathing; preoccupation with cleanliness of self and surroundings
16. Unusual reluctance to remove clothes (e.g., during visit to pediatrician, insistence on wearing underwear to bed)

EMOTIONAL RESPONSES OF CHILD

1. Low self-esteem, feeling of being "bad"; feels deserving of punishment
2. Perceives self as dumb, ugly, unloved
3. Is fearful and clingy; regressed to "baby" behavior
4. Shows an unusual fear of people of a particular age group or sex, of policemen, or of doctors
5. Is angry, aggressive, acts out
6. Shows rapid mood changes inappropriate to the circumstances
7. Sudden onset of anxiety or anxiety-related behavior (e.g., nail biting, grinding teeth, rocking)
8. Is fearful of being touched; fears having genital area washed

6. Disturbed relationships with peers and adults, often for many years
7. Physical illness or infections
8. Parental role-playing among siblings (When all the children in a family are neglected, older children will sometimes "mother" the younger ones.)

For more information, refer to the following Websites:

The Kempe Center, www.childwelfare.gov
Prevent Child Abuse America, www.preventchildabuse.org
Health Resources and Services Administration (HRSA): Maternal and Child Health Bureau, wwwmchb.hrsa.gov

Health Promotion and Nursing Applications for the Maltreated Child

Because maltreatment, abuse, and neglect are so common in the United States, detail about the nurse's role is described. It is critical that the nurse and other health team members intervene to protect the child and work with the family to improve parenting. Neither the child who is being abused nor the abusive family can develop and mature normally. The same is true for the family in which the child has been abused by someone from outside the family.

ASSESSMENT

Be careful and patient in assessment. *The TRIADS Checklist assesses the dimensions of child abuse (12). This acronym represents the following assessment areas:*

Type of abuse (physical, psychological, sexual)

Role relationship of victim to offender (intrafamilial or extrafamilial)

Intensity of abuse (way abuse began and ended, number of times abuse occurred, and number of offenders involved)

Autonomic response of the child

Duration of abuse (length of time over which abuse occurred, ranging from days to years)

Style techniques or access of offender (spontaneous, explosive, without anticipation on the part of the child, cues that alert the child, if acts are repetitively patterned, ritualistic, or ceremonial)

If you suspect abuse, establish rapport and talk with the child alone; however, do not pry. If the child finds it difficult to talk, gently offer to draw some pictures or play with the child to *gain information as follows:*

1. *What* has happened to you?
   a. Has anyone ever told you to take off your clothes (e.g., panties)?
   b. Has anyone ever put his or her finger (or another object) between your legs? Into your mouth? Ears? Has anyone rubbed their body against yours? If so, how?
   c. Does anyone ever get in bed with you at night?
2. *Who* did this to you? Explain. Who saw this happen to you?
3. *How* did it happen? Tell me what happened just before that.
4. *Where* did this happen?
5. *When* did this happen?
6. *Who* else have you told? What did they say? What did they do?

The child may not answer because abuse is considered normal or deserved. The child may know the parents will be more abusive if they learn he or she told. Some children feel loyal to the parents and fear desertion.

When you talk with the parents about the subject of child maltreatment or abuse, do not give the impression that you are criticizing or judging them. Putting them on the defensive will not make them cooperate. It may keep them from accepting help from other health care professionals or cause them to leave the agency and the area. Do your best to be tolerant and understanding. Try to determine how realistically they perceive the child, how they cope with the stresses of parenting, and to whom they turn for support.

Attempt to get parental answers to the following questions as applicable for the child's age (10–14, 37, 38, 46, 71, 72, 79):

1. What do you do when he or she cries too much? If that does not work, what do you do?
2. Does the child sleep well? What do you do when he or she does not sleep?
3. How do you discipline the child?

4. How do you feel after you have disciplined the child?
5. Are you ever angry because the child takes so much of your time?
6. Does this child take up more time than your other children or require more disciplining? If yes, explain.
7. Do you think he or she misbehaves on purpose?
8. Whom do you usually talk to when your child upsets you? Is that person available now?
9. Does the child remind you of a relative or former spouse that is disliked? (Explore this possibility with gentle questions: "It must be really upsetting for you when he acts like his father. What goes through your mind then?" "In what ways is she like your mother? Do those characteristics irritate you?")

As you discuss, try to determine what the situation is at home. Does one or both of the parents seem unduly distressed or depressed? Perhaps they are facing other stresses with which they cannot cope, such as a job loss, loneliness, physical or mental illness, or substance abuse or addiction.

Consider cultural factors and definitions during assessment (1, 40, 69):

1. Cultural differences in childrearing practices may appear to be abuse to an outsider (for example, harsh discipline), but not be so defined by the culture.
2. Cultural beliefs about how children should behave may be considered maltreatment by an outsider. For example, demanding strict obedience through verbal belittling may be the norm.
3. Cultural beliefs about sexual practices may vary by culture. For example, it may be acceptable to fondle the genital area to quiet or comfort the child, although the culture would define fondling for the adult's pleasure as abuse.
4. Cultural living conditions, such as poverty, isolation, inadequate housing or health care, or lack of nutritional resources, may be considered maltreatment or neglect by outsiders but be considered normal by the cultural group.

If you suspect **sexual abuse,** *seek the following information:*

1. What words or names does the child use to describe various body parts?
2. What are the names of family members and frequent visitors?
3. Who babysits for the child?
4. What are the family's sleeping arrangements?
5. Does the child have behavioral problems, such as excessive masturbation?
6. Does the child demonstrate unusual behavior, such as withdrawal, sleeping or eating problems, or anger outbursts not previously noticed?
7. Does the child have any phobias or excessive fears of any person or place? Any nightmares?

Parents may not be involved in the sexual abuse and may be unaware of its occurrence. Work up gradually to the subject of their child's abuse. Inform them of your suspicions in private and without judgment. Do not bombard the parents with questions they will interpret as accusatory.

A pelvic examination is necessary if the child has been sexually abused; however, this procedure should be done carefully after explanation is given to the child, questions are answered, rapport is established, and the child feels some sense of security. A visual examination of the whole body, including the genital and rectal regions, should be done before a pelvic examination. Allow plenty of time for every step of the examination. The prepubescent vagina is extremely sensitive, and the doctor may want to sedate or anesthetize the child before the examination. A sterile plastic medicine dropper lubricated with sterile water should be used to obtain specimens. A nasal speculum or infant-sized vaginoscope, lubricated with water and warmed, can be used with the young child. Test the child for sexually transmitted disease (girls who are past menarche should be tested for pregnancy) (40, 46, 80).

INTERVENTION

You are a key factor in intervention; however, do not engage in rescue fantasies. You are limited in what you can do. **Reporting to the appropriate professionals and agencies is mandatory.** Tell parents of your concern for the child whether or not they are the abusers. Suggest counselors who would be helpful for the child and parents. Give them ideas on how to help the child work through feelings about the trauma. Advise parents not to punish or scold the child when he or she works through emotions through masturbation or by playing with dolls.

Interventions with the abused child include the following (10–14, 38, 46, 69, 71, 72, 80):

1. Supportive, gentle counseling techniques: listening, encouraging the child to speak, taking time in a calm atmosphere and approach, being careful in use of space and touch. Avoid judgmental statements toward the child or about the parents or other abusive adults.
2. Relaxation techniques to reduce hyperactivity, nightmares, enuresis, and startle responses.
3. Desensitization and play techniques to help the child overcome fearful involvement with others, to discriminate threatening exploitative behavior from safe behavior, and to develop coping techniques to reduce interpersonal disruption.

Play therapy can be used to help the child (a) express feelings; (b) reenact incidents of sexual trauma, such as through use of anatomic dolls to show abuse and vent anger, shame, humiliation, and tension from secrecy, fear, and guilt; (c) learn respect for the body and the right to have physical and psychological boundaries; and (d) reveal bad dreams and nightmares and be reassured of safety. Crayons, paints, chalkboards, punching bags, bean bags, and dolls may be used in treatment (24, 70). Simple teaching tools, basic vocabulary, and keen observation are essential. Repetition of stories, re-creation of telephone conversations with the perpetrator, and drawing and painting (25) are effective for beginning resolution.

Carefully document all evidence of abuse, your interview of and actions with parents and child, any agencies or persons contacted about the abuse, and any agencies to which the parents were referred. All 50 states and the District of Columbia provide immunity to professionals who report suspected or actual abuse. Failure to report abuse is a crime.

A **neglected child** needs help as much as one who has been abused. Careful assessment and interviewing of the child and parents are essential. Notify your community's Child Protection Service and document thoroughly your findings and interventions. Many of the guidelines described in this chapter are applicable.

REACTIONS TO ILLNESS

During the preschool stage, the child has heightened feelings of sexuality, fears of dependency and separation, various fantasies and feelings of self-importance, and rivalry with parents. He or she is particularly vulnerable to fears about body damage. The child perceives and fears dental, medical, and surgical procedures as mutilating, intrusive, punishing, or abandoning. The resulting conflicts, fears, guilt, anger, or excessive concern about the body can persist and influence personality development into adulthood.

Teach parents that many of these negative reactions can be averted by introducing the child to medical facilities and health workers when he or she is well. The best teaching is positive example. If the parent takes the child with him or her to the physician and dentist and if the child observes courteous professionals, a procedure that does not hurt (or an explanation of why it will hurt), and a positive response from the parent, a great deal of teaching is accomplished. These visits can be reinforced with honest answers to the many questions the preschooler will have.

Interventions for the child and family are presented.

Psychosocial Concepts

COGNITIVE DEVELOPMENT

Brain scans reveal that between ages 3 and 4 years, the child's brain undergoes rapid spurts developmentally. Overall brain size does not increase dramatically, but by *age 5 years* brain weight is 90% of the adult brain weight (59). Some neurons branch, others are pruned, and the brain reorganizes itself. The most rapid growth is in the frontal lobe of the cerebral cortex, the area involved in planning and organizing new actions, creating memories, and attending to tasks (44). Thus, cognitive abilities emerge. The child's ability to learn is also affected by sensory function—vision, hearing, and tactile and kinesthetic sensations (59, 85).

The child in this stage is **perceptually bound,** *unable to reason logically about concepts that are discrepant from visual cues.* The child learns by interacting with more knowledgeable people, being confronted with others' opinions, and being actively involved with objects and processes (97, 98). More important than the facts learned are the attitudes formed.

Help parents understand the cognitive development of their child, including concept formation. Help them stimulate intellectual growth realistically, without expecting too much. **Concepts** *come about by giving events, things, and experiences a meaningful label.* The name or label implies similarity to some other things having the same name, and difference from things having a different name. **Concept formation** *progresses from diffuse to increasingly differentiated awareness of stable and coordinated objects.* A word comes to designate a crudely defined area of experience. As the late toddler and early preschooler acquires a number of words, each presenting a loosely defined notion or thing, the global meaning becomes a simple concrete concept. Perceived characteristics of things and events become distinguished from each other. The child becomes aware of differences among words, objects, and experiences, such as dog and cat, baby and doll, man and Daddy, approval and disapproval. The preschooler cannot yet define attributes or make explicit comparisons of the objects. The attributes are an absolute part of the object, such as bark and dog; hence the child is said to *think concretely.* What he or she sees or hears can be named, which is different from conceptual or abstract thinking about the object (77, 78, 98).

The late preschooler can compare, combine, describe, and think and talk about various attributes. At this point the child can deal with differences between concepts, such as "dogs bark, people talk." Not until after age 6 or 7 will he or she be able to deal with opposites and similarities together. See **Box 11-5**, Categories of Concepts That Develop in the Preschool Years, for more information (39, 74, 77, 78, 98, 100).

Influences on cognitive development include:

1. Prenatal and birth history, gestational age at delivery, and consequent health status.
2. Physiologic factors, such as genetics, nervous system myelination, and brain maturation (weight increase, branching, and pruning).
3. Nurturing, physical and health care, and nutritional status during infant and toddler eras.
4. Parental emotional and intellectual status and ability to interact with the child.
5. Birth order and gender of the child and opportunities provided in the family accordingly.
6. Cultural, societal, and geographic variables, and related opportunities.
7. The child's perception of events and inability to distinguish obvious from essential features.
8. Emotional or contextual significance of an event or of the verbal and nonverbal language used to describe it.

The concreteness typical of a preschooler's concepts is found in the rambling, loosely jointed circumstantial descriptions. Everything is equally important and must be included. One must listen closely to get the central theme as young children learn things in bunches and not in a systematic, organized way. They can memorize and recite many things, but they cannot paraphrase or summarize their learning (98).

Concepts of Relationships

These *concepts involve time, space, number, and causation. They are more abstract than those based on the immediately observable properties of things. They are greatly determined by culture* (44). See **Table 11-2** for the pattern of mental development (7, 39, 74, 77, 85, 98, 100).

Time Concepts

For the preschooler, time is "now" but beginning to move. The past is measured in hours, perhaps, or several days; the future is vague. Clock time has nothing to do with personal time. Adults are seen as changeless, and the child believes that he or she can mature in a hurry. Thus the preschooler thinks he or she can grow up fast and marry the parent. Time concepts are further described in **Table 11-2** (7, 39, 74, 77, 85, 98, 100).

Spatial Concepts

These concepts differ markedly in children and adults. There are five major stages in the development of spatial concepts. First, **action space** *consists of the location or regions to which the child moves.* Second, **body space** *refers to the child's own awareness of directions and distances in relation to his or her own body.* Third, **object space** *refers to where objects are located relative to each other and without reference to the child's body.* The fourth and fifth stages, **map space** and **abstract space,** *are interrelated and depend on knowing directions of east, west, south, and north; allocating space in visual images to nations, regions, towns, and rooms; and the ability to deal with maps, geographic or astronomic ideas, and three-dimensional spaces* that use symbolic (verbal or mathematical) relationships (39, 77, 78, 98).

BOX 11-5   Categories of Concepts That Develop in the Preschool Years

1. *Life:* ascribes living qualities to inanimate objects
2. *Death:* associates death with separation, lack of movement; thinks dead people capable of doing what living people do
3. *Body functions:* has inaccurate ideas about body functions and birth process
4. *Space:* judges short distances accurately; aware of direction and distance in relation to body
5. *Weight:* estimates weight in terms of size; by age 5 can determine which of two objects feels heavier, notion of quantity—more than one, big, small
6. *Numbers:* understands up to 5
7. *Time:* has gradually increasing sense of time; present oriented; knows day of week, month, and year

8. *Self:* knows sex, full name, names of outer body parts by age 3; when begins to play with other children, self-concept begins to include facts about his or her abilities and race but not socioeconomic class
9. *Sex roles:* has general concept of sex, identity, and appropriate sex roles developed at age 5 or 6
10. *Social awareness:* is egocentric but forms definite opinions about others' behavior as "nice" or "mean"; intuitive, concept of causality is magical, illogical
11. *Beauty:* names major colors; prefers music with definite tune and rhythm
12. *Comedy:* considers as comic funny faces made by self or others, socially inappropriate behavior, and antics of pets

TABLE 11-2

Assessment of Mental Development

Age 3 Years	Age 4 Years	Age 5 Years
Knows he or she is a person separate from another	Senses self as one among many	Aware of cultural and other differences between people and the two sexes
Knows own sex and some sex differences		Mature enough to fit into simple type of culture
		Can tell full name and address
		Remains calm if lost away from home
Resists commands but distractible and responsive to suggestions	States alibis because more aware of attitude and opinions of others	Dependable
Can ask for help	Self-critical; appraises good and bad of self	Increasing independence
Desire to please	Does not like to admit inabilities; excuses own behavior	Can direct own behavior; but fatigue, excessive demands, fantasy, and guilt interfere with assuming self-responsibility
Friendly	Praises self; bosses or criticizes others	Admits when needs help
Sense of humor	Likes recognition for achievement	Moves from direct to internalized action, from counting what he or she can touch to counting in thought; uses more clues
	Heeds others' thoughts and feelings; expresses own	
Uses language rather than physical activity to communicate	Active use of language	Improves use of symbol system, concept formation
	Active learning	Repeats long sentences accurately
	Likes to make rhymes, to hear stories with exaggeration and humor, dramatic songs	Can carry plot in story
	Knows nursery rhymes	Defines objects in terms of use
	Tells action implied in picture books	States relationship between two events
Imaginative	Highly imaginative yet literal, concrete thinking	Less imaginative
Better able to organize thoughts		Asks details
Can be bargained with	Can organize his or her experience	Can be reasoned with logically
Sacrifices immediate pleasure for promise of future gain	Increasing reasoning power and critical thinking capacity	More accurate, relevant, practical, sensible than 4-year-old
	Makes crude comparisons	Asks to have words defined
		Seeks reality
Understands simple directions; follows normal routines of family life and does minor errands	Concept of 1, 2, 3; counts to 5; does some home chores	Begins to understand money
	Generalizes	Does more home chores with increasing competence
		Can determine which of two weights is heavier
		Idea in head precedes drawing on paper or physical activity
		Interested in meaning of relatives
Knows age	Realizes birthday is one in a series and that birthday is measure of growth	Understands week as a unit of time
Meager comprehension of past and future	Knows when next birthday is	Knows day of week
Knows mostly today	Knows age	Sense of time and duration increasing
	Birthday and holidays significant because aware of units of time	Knows how old will be on next birthday
	Loves parties related to holiday	Knows month and year
	Conception of time	Adults seen as changeless
	Knows day of week	Memory surprisingly accurate
Has attention span of 10–15 minutes	Has attention span of 20 minutes	Has attention span of 30 minutes

The preschool child has *action space* and moves along familiar locations and explores new terrain. He or she is beginning to orient self to *body space* and *object space* through play and exploration of body, up and down, front and back, sideways, next to, near and far, and later left and right. The child is not able until approximately age 6 to understand object space as a unified whole; he or she will first see a number of unrelated routes or spaces. *The child is generally aware of specific objects and habitual routes.* The child does not see self and objects as part of a larger integrated space with multiple possibilities for movement. *Map space and abstract space are not understood until later* (39, 74, 77, 78).

Quantitative Concepts

Notions of quantity, such as one and more than one, or bigger and smaller, are developed in the early preschool years. Understanding of the quantity or amount represented by a number is not related to the child's ability to count to 10, 20, or higher, nor can he or she transfer numbers to notions of value of money, although he or she may imitate adults and play store, passing money back and forth. Ordinal numbers, indicating successions rather than totals, develop crudely in "me first" or "me last." The concept of second or third develops later. The preschooler cannot simultaneously take account of different dimensions such as 1 quart equals 2 pints and equal volume in different-shaped containers. **Table 11-2** presents additional information (39, 98, 100).

Concepts of Causality

Perceiving cause and effect is marginal. Things simply are. The child may be pleased or displeased with events but does not understand what brought them about. He or she does **precausal thinking**, *confusing physical and mechanical causation or natural phenomena with psychological, moral, or sequential causes.* He or she frequently says "n' then," indicating *causal sequence.* When the child asks "Why?" he or she is probably looking for justification rather than causation. Most things are taken for granted. The child assumes that people, including self, or some motivated inanimate being is the cause of events. Perception of the environment is **animistic**, *endowing all things with the qualities of life that Westerners reserve for human beings.* There is little notion of accident or coincidence. It takes some time to learn that there are impersonal forces at work in the world. Thinking is also **egocentric**: *things and events are seen from a personal and narrow perspective and are happening because of self* (39, 77, 78, 98).

The late preschooler fluctuates between reality and fantasy and a materialistic and animistic view of the world (78, 98). Most adults never completely leave behind the magical thinking typical of the preschooler. The child plays with the idea of a tree growing out of the head, what holes feel like to the ground, and growing up starting as an adult. The adult finds no meaning in music, art, literature, love, and possibly even science and mathematics without a sense of fantasy or magic that is a normal part of preschooler thinking.

PREOPERATIONAL STAGE

According to Piaget, the preschooler is in the Preoperational Stage of cognitive development (77, 78). The **Preoperational Stage** *is divided into the Preconceptual and Intuitive phases* (77, 78, 98).

During the **Preconceptual Phase**, *from 2 to 4 years of age, the child gathers facts as they are encountered but can neither separate reality from fantasy nor classify or define events in a systematic manner.* Ability to define properties of an object or denote hierarchies or relationships among elements in a class is lacking. He or she is beginning to develop mental strategies from concept formation; concepts are constructed in a global way. The child is capable of perceiving overall outward appearances but sees only one aspect of an object or situation at a time. For example, if you say, "Take the yellow pill," he or she will focus on either *yellow* or *pill* but cannot focus on both aspects at once. The child is unable to use time, space, equivalence, and class inclusion in concept formation. During the **Intuitive Phase**, *lasting from approximately 4 to 7 years, the child gains increasing, but still limited, ability to develop concepts.* He or she defines one property at a time, has difficulty stating the definition, but knows how to use the object. The child uses **transductive logic**, *going from general to specific in explanation,* rather than deductive or inductive logic. He or she begins to label, classify in ascending or descending order, do seriation, and note cause–effect relationships, even though accurate cause–effect understanding does not occur (77, 78, 98, 100).

In addition to the previously described characteristics of concept development, *the Preoperational Stage is characterized by the following* (77, 78, 98, 100):

1. Literal thinking with absence of a reference system.
2. Intermingling of fantasy, intuition, and reality.
3. **Absolute thought,** *seeing all or nothing without shades of gray or any relativity.*
4. **Centering,** *focusing on a single aspect of an object,* causing distorted reasoning.
5. Difficulty remembering what he or she started talking about, so that when the sentence is finished he or she is talking about something else.
6. Inability to state cause–effect relationships, categories, or abstractions; believing that events that occur together belong together and sequence denotes causation. The preschooler lacks the concept of **reversibility**: *for every action, there is one that cancels it.*

In general, the preschooler has a consuming curiosity. Learning is vigorous, aggressive, and intrusive. The imagination creates many situations to be explored. Judgment is overshadowed by curiosity and excitement. *The preschooler has begun to develop such concepts as* (a) friend, aunt, and uncle; (b) accepting responsibility; (c) independence; (d) passage of time and spatial relationships; (e) use of abstract words, numbers, and colors; and (f) the meaning of cold, tired, and hungry. Attention span is lengthening. The child's ability to grasp reality varies with individual and potential intelligence, the social milieu, and opportunities to explore the world, solve problems independently, ask questions, and get answers.

SOCIOCULTURAL PERSPECTIVE

Another approach to understanding how people learn is **Vygotsky's Sociocultural Theory** (97). *Cognitive growth occurs in a sociocultural context and evolves out of the child's social interactions. Knowledge, thought, and language are shaped by the culture and historical time.* Each culture has certain "tools of the mind,"

TABLE 11-3

Comparison of Piaget's and Vygotsky's Theories of Cognitive Development

Piaget's Cognitive Theory	Vygotsky's Sociocultural Theory
1. Cognitive development is mostly the same universally.	1. Cognitive development differs from culture to culture and in different historical eras.
2. Cognitive development results from the child's independent exploration of the world.	2. Cognitive development results from guided participation or social interactions.
3. Each child constructs knowledge on his or her own.	3. Children and adults or more knowledgeable persons or peers co-construct knowledge.
4. Individual egocentric processes and language become more social.	4. Social processes or interactions with others become individual psychological processes.
5. Peers are important because children must learn to take peers' perspectives.	5. Adults are important because they know the culture's way and tools of thinking.
6. Development precedes learning; children cannot master certain things until they have the requisite cognitive structures.	6. Learning precedes development; tools learned with adult help are internalized.

knowledge, languages, problem-solving tactics, and memory strategies (97). Thereby cognitive development differs between cultures; some cultures do not demonstrate formal operational thinking as described by Piaget (1). However, the child, with an adult's help at a new task, expands the zone of cognitive development as the adult questions, demonstrates, explains, and encourages independent thinking or praises a decision or outcome (7). Refer to **Table 11-3** for a summary of Piaget's and Vygotsky's theories (7, 74, 77, 78, 85, 97, 98).

THE FAMILY'S ROLE IN TEACHING THE PRESCHOOLER

Emphasize to parents that they enhance the child's growth and health through the following approaches and their work with the child. *Consider the needs of the family with a challenged child, as well as the cultural background.* The Abstract for Evidence-Based Practice presents a cultural example.

Emphasize to parents that the single most critical factor in the child's learning is a loving caretaker, because that is who the child imitates. How the parenting person speaks to, touches, and plays with the child governs the potential for socialization and cognitive development. **Figure 11-4**■ shows an example of how the father is teaching about the physical, emotional, cognitive, and social dimensions to his two sons.

This is true even for the child who had a low birth weight and was at risk for developmental lag or disability (7, 8, 46). A child's problem-solving abilities are shaped by the parents' method for handling problems and by opportunities for problem solving. In families in which everyone gets a chance to speak out and jointly explore a problem, the child learns to express logically. *In the home, the child learns how to learn.* Teaching the child is more than telling him or her what to do. It involves demonstration, listening, and talking about the situation in direct and understandable terms and giving reasons. Cognitive development includes more than fluency with words, a good verbal memory, and information. It includes

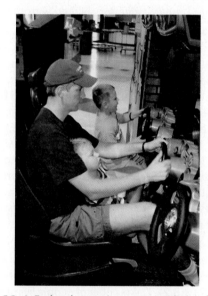

FIGURE ■ 11-4 Father has an important role in playing with the preschool child and infant sibling.

ability to use imagination, engage in fantasy appropriately, and enjoy and use art, music, and other creative activities. It includes expanding skills in logical thinking. Most important, it involves increasing integration of many kinds of brain functions and branching of dendrites, as described earlier. Much integrated learning comes from the child's engaging in motor activity, play, and language games; talking with adults and peers; and paying attention to both trivial and important aspects of the environment (7, 8, 32, 55, 59, 63, 66, 67, 70).

Television, videotapes, and video games are used extensively and are meant to captivate children. Children should watch no more than one hour daily of slow-paced TV before age 6 years, according to the American Academy of Pediatrics. Parents report an average of 3 1/2 hours daily of TV watching by age 4 years; video time may

Abstract for Evidence-Based Practice

Mothers' Adaptation to Children with Intellectual Disabilities

Azar, M., & Badr, L.K. (2006). The adaptation of mothers of children with intellectual disability in Lebanon. *Journal of Transcultural Nursing, 17*(4), 375–381.

KEYWORDS

intellectual disability, developmentally disabled, developmentally impaired, mental retardation, coping, adaptation.

Purpose ➤ To identify factors that influence mothers' adaptation to the care of their children who have intellectual impairments.

Conceptual Framework ➤ Stress, adaptation, and coping resources of families caring for children with disabilities and the Double ABC X Model.

Sample/Setting ➤ A convenience sample of 127 Lebanese mothers who resided in an urban area of Lebanon were recruited from centers caring for children with special needs.

Method ➤ Four standardized questionnaires were used to collect data. The Parenting Stress Index (PSI), to assess the mother's stress, had already been translated into Arabic and tested. The other three questionnaires were translated from English to Arabic using back-translation, verified by an expert panel for equivalency and cultural appropriateness, and pilot tested. The Family Inventory of Life Events (FILE) tested family stress. The Family Crisis Oriented Personal Evaluation Scale (FCOPES) tested family coping. The Center of Epidemiologic Studies Depression Scale (CES-D) measured depressive symptoms. Mothers were interviewed in their homes for 30 to 45 minutes by a research assistant to obtain questionnaire answers and descriptive data.

Findings ➤ Age range of the mothers was 25 to 56 years ($\times$ 40.3 years). Age range of their children was 2 to 18 years ($\times$ 10.2 years). The number of children in the home ranged from 1 to 9 ($\times$ 3.2). The number of people living in the home ranged from 2 to 10 ($\times$ 5.3). Intermediate level of education was most common in this sample (30%). Most women (85.8%) were not employed outside of the home. Boys were more likely to be the disabled child (59%), and most of the disabled children were moderately affected. Of the mothers, 46.5% had depressive symptoms, 60% reported high levels of personal stress, and most reported moderate family strain. Families with high income and medical insurance reported less strain than families with low incomes and no insurance. Mothers with large families and less education reported fewer coping resources. Family stress correlated positively with maternal stress and depressive symptoms. Family strain was the best predictor of maternal depressive symptoms.

Implications ➤ Study results concur with a large number of similar studies done in the United States and Europe, especially the high percentage of mothers with depressive symptoms. Family strain often arises from intrafamily and financial stressors that occur when caring for an intellectually disabled child. Mothers with higher education are more likely to seek and mobilize resources to manage the complexity of the situation. Demands of modern life may make people less available to offer support to each other, and Lebanese society is not well prepared to offer help to families who have children with developmental deficiencies. Rather, most mothers and families encounter stigma and criticism, and thereby may isolate themselves, adding to their burden. Strain and depressive symptoms may be heightened by the fact that mothers in Lebanon are the sole caretakers of the children, and by the unsettled political and economic situation. This study has implications for policy development internationally, considering cultural factors, since 30% of children internationally are estimated to be intellectually disabled.

be additional. Most programming and many videotapes are too fast-paced, aggressive or violent, and scary (22, 23). Preschoolers have difficulty distinguishing reality from fantasy in portrayals. They think monsters or scary creatures are in the box and will come out to get them. Children are disoriented by form, such as changes in angle, cuts in time, and zooming in and out. Exposure to hours of rapid image and scene changes makes regular life seem boring. Further, commercials are aimed at children as consumers who influence parents (54). *Children of all ages who watch violent TV or videotapes become more aggressive and violent in behavior* (7, 23, 48, 51, 91). Repeated visual experience of TV may slow or divert brain development and contribute to distractibility and hyperactivity, and a diagnosis of attention deficit/hyperactivity disorder (2). *Video games* can be more detrimental because children not only watch, but also behave with aggressiveness. *Early childhood is the most vulnerable period for the impact of video games because* (7, 23): (a) the amount of exposure time is likely to be excessive; (b) society, culture, and emotions are not clearly understood; (c) depiction of violent solutions for problems does not foster realistic problem solving or empathy; (d) sexist, racist, and ageist stereotypes are perpetuated; and (e) quick, reactive emotions are encouraged rather than thoughtful regulation. *Excess exposure to TV, videos, and video games reduces physical activity, social skills, and creativity* (7, 23, 48, 51, 91).

INTERVENTIONS FOR HEALTH PROMOTION

Parents can stimulate the intellectual development of their child by various practices:

1. Give daily individual attention to the child.
2. Create many and varied opportunities to learn about people and their environment.
3. Avoid doing too much for the child; share activities with the child.
4. Talk about situations the child is engaged in (shopping, cooking a meal, laundering).
5. Provide interesting in-home and out-of-home activities.
6. Give the child freedom to roam and follow natural curiosity within safe limits, and opportunity to handle objects, explore, and ask questions.
7. Obtain information about child development and rearing from books, films, and other parents.
8. Experiment with games and observe feedback from the child to determine which meet his or her needs.
9. Avoid the push to learn academic subjects too early, causing undue frustration and a negative attitude about learning and school later.

Creative methods of teaching for preschoolers are seen in educational programs such as *Sesame Street,* presented as a lively, fast-moving, colorful program that emphasizes the alphabet, number concepts, similarities and differences, and positive body image. *Veggie Tales,* videotapes in which vegetables depict Bible stories, are popular with parents who are interested in content and child-appropriate depiction related to religion, moral values, and prosocial behavior. It is difficult to assess the effect of these programs on the overall cognitive development of the child. *Parents should monitor what is watched, and watch with the child and explain the lessons to be learned.* Most important, *parents should encourage active play.*

Explore the use of television with parents. Children should be playing actively, creating their own "movie" world that they can control. Teach parents to see themselves as a parent educator rather than as "only a housewife" or "his pal, Dad."

COMMUNICATION PATTERNS

People use three types of communication: (a) somatic or physical symptoms such as flushed skin color and increased respirations; (b) action such as play or movement; and (c) verbal expression. The preschool child uses all of them. Preschool children learn words with remarkable speed, flexibility, and efficiency. Related to communication ability is myelination of hearing pathways, which is completed by about age *4 years* (44, 76). Maximum synapse density in the language area of the brain occurs around *3 years of age,* which fosters language production and comprehension. Later, the excess neurons are pruned (44, 76).

Learning to use verbal expression—language—to communicate is an ongoing developmental process that is affected directly by the child's interaction with others. Vygotsky's sociocultural approach to language development helps us understand the preschooler as he or she learns (7, 97). Two preschoolers together may be in a **collective monologue,** *each talking but not truly conversing with each other. Preschoolers often talk to themselves as they play or go about daily activities.* Instead of the egocentric speech of preoperational thought, such speech can be considered **private speech,** *speech that guides one's thoughts and behavior. It is a step toward mature thought and a forerunner of the silent thinking-in-words that*
adults use daily. Private speech is heavily used when the child is struggling to solve difficult problems. Private speech gets expanded by **social speech,** or *conversations with others.* Then the child develops **inner speech**, or *mutterings, lip movements, and silent verbal thoughts.* Use of private speech increases during preschool years and then decreases during early elementary school years. **Guided participation,** or *learning in collaboration with more knowledgeable adults or companions who are more knowledgeable,* helps the child incorporate the learned problem-solving strategies into thinking (7, 74, 76, 85, 97).

Children learn words quickly when information is offered in a novel way or when the word is unusual. *Children learn new words when* (76, 86): (a) they are used with familiar words or applied to familiar objects, (b) words and information are linked with experience (e.g., play), (c) the word or information is linked to them personally (e.g., "the butterfly has a thorax or chest"), and (d) information contains whole–part associations ("see the bird; the bird has a beak"). Thus, the preschooler learns differentiation or multiple levels of information.

The child uses language to: (a) maintain social rapport, (b) gain attention, (c) get information, (d) seek meaning about experience, (e) note how others' answers fit personal thoughts, (f) play with words, (g) gain relief from anxiety, and (h) learn how to think and solve problems. He or she asks why, what, when, where, and how, repeatedly.

Directing one's life depends on language and an understanding of the meaning of words and the logic with which they are used. When the child acquires language, he or she gradually internalizes visual symbols, develops memory and recalls the past, thinks about the future, and differentiates fantasy from reality (59, 86).

Share the following suggestions with parents. Books and stories foster language development. Choose books that are durable, have large print that does not fill the entire page, and are colorfully illustrated. The concepts should be expressed in simple sentences and should tell a tale that fits the child's fantasy conception of the world, such as a story with animals and objects that talk and think like people. Or the story should tell about the situations he or she ordinarily faces, such as problems

TABLE 11-4

Guidelines for Communication with a Preschooler

1. Be respectful as you talk with the child.
2. Do not discourage talking, questions, or the make-believe in the child's language; verbal explorations are essential to learn language. Answers to questions should meet needs and give him or her an awareness of adult attitudes and feelings about the topics discussed.
3. Tell the truth to the best of your ability and on the child's level of understanding. Do not say an injection "won't hurt." Say, "It's like a pin prick that will hurt a short time." Admit if the answer is unknown, and seek the answer with the child. A lie is eventually found out and causes a loss of trust in that adult and in others.
4. Do not make a promise unless you can keep it.
5. The child takes every word literally. Do not say, "She nearly died laughing," or "I laughed my head off." Do not describe surgery as "putting you to sleep."
6. Respond to the relationship or feelings in the child's experience rather than the actual object or event. Talk about the child's feelings instead of agreeing or disagreeing with what he or she says. Help the child understand what he or she feels rather than why he or she feels it.
7. Precede statements of advice and instruction with a statement of understanding of the child's feelings. When the child is feeling upset emotionally, he or she cannot listen to instructions, advice, consolation, or constructive criticism.
8. Do not give undue attention to slang or curse words, and do not punish the child for using them. The child is demonstrating initiative and uses these words for shock value, and attention or punishment emphasizes the importance of the words. Remain relaxed and give the child a more difficult or different word to say. If he or she persists in using the unacceptable word, the adult may say, "I'm tired of hearing that word, say _____"; ask him or her not to say the word again since it may hurt others, or use distraction. Children learn unacceptable words as they learn all others, and parents would be wise to listen to their own vocabulary.
9. Sit down if possible when participating or talking with children. You are more approachable when at their physical and eye level.
10. Seek to have a warm, friendly relationship without thrusting yourself on the child. How you feel about the child is more important than what you say or do.
11. Through attentive listening and interested facial expression, convey a tell-me-more-about-it attitude to encourage the child to communicate.
12. Regard some speech difficulties as normal. Ignore stuttering or broken fluency that does not persist. Do not correct each speech error and do not punish. Often the child thinks faster than he or she can articulate speech. Give the child time when he or she speaks.
13. Talk in a relaxed manner. Do not bombard the child with verbal information.

with playmates, discovery of the preschooler's world, nightmares, and the arrival of a new baby.

Use, and share with the parents and significant adults in the child's life, effective ways of talking with the preschooler, presented in **Table 11-4.** These guidelines will make life and learning more enjoyable for the preschooler and family and enhance your health care practice. Educate that if the child has speech problems, it may be related to hearing deficits, which should be evaluated and treated by experts in the field as early as possible. Cochlear implants are now available for the young child, if indicated; hearing aids are also an option. Cochlear implants better magnify high-frequency sounds, plurals, verb tenses, and endings. The ability to communicate and overcome any hearing or visual challenges is essential to health promotion.

Table 11-5 is a guide for assessing language skills of the preschooler. During assessment, keep in mind that how the child's parents and other family members speak, the language opportunities, and response to the child influence considerably the child's language skills. Realize that *language skills may be ahead of these norms due to factors discussed earlier.*

PLAY PATTERNS

Play is the work of the child (32) and promotes physical, mental, emotional, and social health. Play occupies most of the child's waking hours and *serves to consolidate and enlarge previous learning and promote creativity and adaptation.* Play has elements of reality, and there is an earnestness about it. Piaget described play as **assimilation**; *play behavior involves taking in, molding, and using objects for pleasure and learning* (78).

The *preschooler is intrusive in play,* bombarding others by purposeful or accidental physical attack. He or she is into people's ears and minds by loud, assertive talking; into space by vigorous motor activities; into objects through exploration; and into the unknown by consuming curiosity (31, 32).

Peer Relationships

The preschool years are the **pregang stage,** *in which the child progresses from solitary and parallel play to cooperating for a longer time in a larger group.* The child identifies somewhat with a play group, follows rules, is aware of the status of self compared with others,

TABLE 11-5

Assessment of Language Development

Age 3 Years	Age 4 Years	Age 5 Years
Appearance of individual sounds *y, f, v* in words	Appearance of individual sounds *sh, zh, th* in words	Appearance of individual sounds *s, z, th, r, ch, j* in words
Vocabulary of at least 900, up to 2,000, words	Vocabulary of at least 1,500, up to 3,000, words	Vocabulary of at least 2,100, up to 5,000, words
Uses language understandably; uses same sounds experimentally	Uses language confidently	Uses language efficiently, correctly
Understands simple reasons	Concrete speech	No difficulty understanding other's spoken words
Uses some adjectives and adverbs	Increasing attention span	Meaningful sentences; uses future tense
	Uses "I" and other pronouns	Increasing skill with grammar
	Imitates and plays with words	Knows common opposites
	Defines a few simple words	
	Talks in sentences; uses past tense	
	Uses plurals frequently	
	Comprehends prepositions	
Talks in simple sentences about things	Talks incessantly while doing other activities	Talks constantly
Repeats sentence of six syllables	Asks many questions	No infantile articulation
Uses plurals in speech	Demands detailed explanations with "why"	Repeats sentences of 12 or more syllables
Collective monologue; does not appear to care whether another is listening	Carries on long, involved conversation	Asks searching questions, meaning of words, how things work
Some random, inappropriate answers	Exaggerates; boasts; tattles; may use profanity for attention	Can tell a long story accurately, but may keep adding to reality to make story more fantastic
Intelligibility is 70–90%	Frequently uses "everything"	Intelligibility good; some distortion in articulation of *t, s*
Sings simple songs	Tells family faults outside of home without restraint	Sings relatively well
	Tells story combining reality and fantasy; appears to be lying	
	Intelligibility is 90%; articulation errors with *l, r, s, z, sh, ch, j, th*	
	Variation in volume from a yell to a whisper	
	Likes to sing	
Knows first and family name	Calls people names	Counts to 10 or further without help
Names figures in a picture	Names three objects he or she knows in succession	Repeats five digits
Repeats three digits	Counts to 5 without help	Names four colors, usually red, green, blue, yellow
Likes to name things	Repeats four digits	
	Knows which line is longer	
	Names one or more colors	
Talks to self or imaginary playmate	Talks with imaginary playmate of same sex and age	Sense of social standards and limits seen in language use
Expresses own desires and limits frequently	Seeks reassurance	
	Interested in things being funny	
	Likes puns	

develops perception of social relationships, begins the capacity for self-criticism, and states traits and characteristics of others that he or she likes or dislikes. At first the child spends brief, incidental periods of separation from the parents. The time away from them increases in length and frequency, and eventually the orientation shifts from family to peer group (70, 74).

A **peer** is a *person with approximately equal status, a companion, often of the same sex and age,* with whom one can share mutual concerns. The **peer group** is a *relatively informal association of equals who share common play experiences with emphasis on common rules and understanding the limits that the group places on the individual.* The preschool play group differs from later ones in that it is loosely organized. The activity of the group may be continuous; but membership changes as the child joins or leaves the group at will, and the choice of playmates is relatively restricted in kind and number. This is the first introduction to a group that assesses the preschooler as a child from a child's point of view. The preschooler is learning about entering a new, different, very powerful world when he or she joins the group. Although social play is enjoyed, the child feels a need for solitary play at times (74, 85).

The number and gender of siblings and the parent's handling of the child's play seem to influence behavior with the play group. If the family rejects the child, he or she may feel rejected by peers, even when the child is not rejected, causing self-isolation, inability to form close friendships, and ultimately real rejection.

Purposes of Play

The natural mode of expression for the child is play. *Purposes of play include the following:*

1. Develop and improve muscular strength, coordination, and balance; define body boundaries.
2. Release excess physical energy; provide exercise.
3. Communicate with others, establish friendships, learn about interpersonal relations, and develop concern for others.
4. Learn cooperation, sharing, and healthy competition.
5. Express imagination, creativity, and initiative.
6. Imitate and learn about social activity, adult roles, and cultural norms.
7. Test and deal with reality; gain mastery over unpleasant or overwhelming experiences.
8. Explore, investigate, and manipulate features of the adult world; sharpen the senses and concentration.
9. Learn about rules of chance and probability, rules of conduct, and that at times one loses, but it is all right.
10. Build self-esteem and self-confidence.
11. Feel a sense of power, make things happen, explore, and experiment.
12. Provide for intellectual, sensory, and language development.
13. Assemble novel aspects of the environment.
14. Organize life's discrepancies privately and with others.
15. Learn about self and how others see him or her.
16. Practice leader and follower roles.
17. Have fun, express joy, and feel the pleasure of mastery.
18. Act out and symbolically work through a painful physical or emotional state by repetition in play so that it is more bearable and assimilated into the child's self-concept.
19. Develop the capacity to gratify self and to delay gratification.
20. Formulate a bridge between concrete experiences and abstract thought.

Box 11-6, Types of Play Related to Social Characteristics (46, 63, 69, 70, 74, 80), and **Box 11-7**, Common Themes in Children's Play (7, 8, 24, 67, 74, 99), give more insight into children's play.

Play Materials

These materials should be simple, sturdy, durable, easily cleaned, and free from unnecessary hazards. They need not be expensive. Often creative, stimulating toys can be made from ordinary household articles such as string, beads, empty thread spools, a bell, yarn, or empty boxes covered with washable adhesive paper. The child may like the box more than the toy. The child should have adequate space and equipment that is unstructured enough to allow for cre-

BOX 11-6	**Types of Play Related to Social Characteristics**

1. *Unoccupied play:* Child stands by, aimlessly engaged in activity, such as pace, run, hit.
2. *Onlooker play:* Child watches others with no interactions or movement toward participation (e.g., use of television).
3. *Parallel play:* Child plays independently but next to other children; displays no group association.
4. *Associative play:* Children play together in similar or identical play without organization, division of labor, leadership, or mutual goals.
5. *Cooperative play:* Play is organized in group with others. Planning and cooperation begin before play starts to form goals, division of labor, and leadership.
6. *Solitary play:* Child, either by choice or because of lack of peers, entertains self in play. Play is often imaginative or studious in nature.
7. *Supplementary play:* Play shifts from large group activities or games to focus on smaller group or board games.

BOX 11-7	**Common Themes in Children's Play**

Various issues in the child's life will be repeated four to five times in each play session. These issues are shown in different styles of play, but the theme is the thread that ties all the different styles together, as the pieces of a quilt unite to form the pattern of the whole.

1. Power/control
2. Anger/sadness
3. Trust/relationships/abandonment
4. Nurturing/rejection/security
5. Boundaries/intrusion
6. Violation/protection
7. Self-esteem
8. Fears/anxiety (separation, monsters, ghosts, animals, the dark, noises, bad people, injury, death)
9. Confusion
10. Identity
11. Loyalty/betrayal
12. Loss/death
13. Loneliness
14. Adjustment/change

ativity and imagination to work unfettered. He or she will enjoy trips to parks and playgrounds. The parents should be sure the child is not playing at dumps or at contaminated landfills.

Increasing emphasis is being placed on high-technology, interactive, and weaponry toys. These toys actually stifle imagination and discovery, and weaponry toys may cause fears, heighten aggressive fantasies, and cause injury and sometimes death. **Refer to the earlier discus-**

sion about use of television, videos, and video games. Weaponry toys should be avoided as much as possible (98). Young children need to direct their games to be in control of their play and their fantasies, which is health promotive. Some toys from infancy and toddlerhood are still enjoyed.

The play materials that are available determine the play activities. *Play materials are enjoyed for different reasons* (8, 24, 46, 63, 67, 70, 74, 80, 85). For example, **physical activity,** *which facilitates development of motor skills,* is provided through play with musical instruments and records for marching and rhythm; balls; a shovel and broom; a ladder, swing, trapeze, slide, and climbing apparatus; blocks, boxes, and boards; a sled, wheelbarrow, and wagon; and a tricycle and bicycle with training wheels. Swimming, ice skating, roller skating, skiing, and dance are being learned. **Dramatic play,** *which is related to the ability to classify objects correctly, take another's perspective, and do problem solving,* is afforded through large building blocks, a sandbox and sand toys, dolls and housekeeping toys, nurse and doctor kits, farm or other occupational toys, cars and other vehicles, and worn-out adult clothes for dress-up. This is a predominant form of play in childhood and also can include aspects of physical play. **Creative playthings,** *which promote constructive, nonsocial, cognitive, and emotional development,* include blank sheets of paper; various art supplies, such as crayons, finger or water paints, chalk, beads or glitter, clay, plasticine, or other manipulative material; blunt scissors, paste, cartons, and scraps of cloth; water-play equipment; and musical toys. **Symbolic play,** *creating new images or symbols to represent objects, people, and events,* results from opportunities to do dramatic and creative play. **Quiet play,** *which promotes cognitive development and rest from physical exertion,* is achieved through books, puzzles, audiotapes, CDs or records, and table games. Children's songs, nursery rhymes, and fairy tales can absorb anxiety, entertain, soothe, reassure that life's problems can be solved, and support the child's superego.

The role of the adult in child's play is to provide opportunity, equipment, and safety and to avoid interference or structuring of play. Mothers and fathers tend to play differently with the child. How fathers play with their children appears to be determined not just by biology but also by cultural influences (1). Studies of fathers in Sweden, Germany, Africa (the Aka), and New Delhi showed that they do not play with children in a highly physical way, in contrast to the United States. Rather, they play more quietly; the Aka and New Delhi fathers were notably gentle (74).

Even when free time, space, and toys are limited, most children find a way to play. They use household objects such as pots, pans, and furniture. Outdoors they find trees, sticks, rocks, sand, empty cans, and discarded equipment for dramatic and fantasy play. In countries such as Kenya, India, Ecuador, and Brazil, as well as in Appalachia, American Indian reservations, farmlands, and poorer households of the United States, many children spend a large part of the day doing household chores and assisting their families in daily routines, or in getting food or money. Yet even these children find time and opportunity for play.

Table 11-6 summarizes play characteristics as a further aid in assessment and teaching (7, 8, 24, 32, 39, 46, 67, 70, 74, 80, 85).

Share this information with parents. Explore their feelings about child's play and their role with the child. Utilize play principles as you care for the child.

GUIDANCE AND DISCIPLINE

The child learns how to behave by imitating adults and by using the opportunities to develop self-control. If the adult tells the child, "Tell him I'm not home" when the child answers the door, the child may at first be astonished, then accept the lie, and eventually use this behavior too.

The *child needs consistent, fair, and kind limits to feel secure,* to know that the parents care and love the child enough to provide protection—a security he or she does not have when allowed to do anything, regardless of ability. Limits should be set in a way that preserves the child's and parent's self-respect. Limits and discipline should not be applied angrily, violently, arbitrarily, or capriciously, but rather with the intent to educate and build character. Only when the child can predict the behavior of others can he or she accept the need to inhibit or change personal behavior and work toward predictable and rational behavior. The parent should be an ally to the child as he or she struggles for control over inner impulses. The child often gets confused by the many expectations and commands, and often spontaneously follows the inner impulses. Parents must work daily to socialize and avoid unnecessary doubt or guilt.

Some children are more difficult to discipline even though the parents appear to be using the right strategies. Some people are born with a larger variety of dopamine-4 receptor genes and are biologically predisposed to be thrill seekers. The gene makes them less sensitive to pain and physical sensation (44). Such children are

INTERVENTIONS FOR HEALTH PROMOTION

Parents should be taught the following:

1. Encourage the child to try and enjoy a variety of activities, including self-designed activities.
2. Assist only if he or she is in need of help or help is requested. Let the child lead.
3. Avoid showing amusement or ridicule of play behavior or conversation. The child is not natural in play when he or she thinks adults are watching.
4. Allow playmates to work out their own differences.
5. Distract, redirect, or substitute a different activity if the children cannot share and work out their problems.
6. Avoid overstimulation, teasing, hurry, or talking about the child as if he or she were not present.
7. Try to enter the child's world. If he or she wants you to attend the teddy bear's 100th birthday party, go.

TABLE 11-6

Assessment of Play Characteristics

Age 3 Years	Age 4 Years	Age 5 Years
Enjoys active and sedentary play	Increasing physical and social play	More varied activity
		More graceful in play
Likes toys in orderly form	Puts away toys when reminded	Puts away toys by self
Puts away toys with supervision		
Fantasy not yielding too much to reality	Much imaginative and dramatic play	More realistic in play
Likes fairy tales, books	Has complex ideas but unable to carry out because of lack of skill and time	Less interested in fairy tales
		More serious and ready to know reality
		Restrained but creative
Likes solitary and parallel play with increasing social play in shifting groups of two or three	Plays in groups of two or three, often companions of own sex	Plays in groups of five or six
	Imaginary playmates	Friendships stronger and continue over longer time
	Projects feelings and deeds onto peers or imaginary playmates	Chooses friends of like interests
	May run away from home	Spurred on in activity by rivalry
Cooperates briefly	Suggests and accepts turns but often bossy in directing others	Generous with toys
Willing to wait turn and share with suggestion	Acts out feelings spontaneously, especially with music and arts	Sympathetic, cooperative, but quarrels and threatens by word or gesture
		Acts out feelings
		Wants rules to do things right; but beginning to realize peers cheat, so develops mild deceptions and fabrications
Some dramatic play—house or family games	Dramatic and creative play at a peak	Dramatic play about most life events, but more realistic
Frequently changes activity	Likes to dress up and help with household tasks; plays with dolls, trucks	Play continues from day to day
Likes to arrange, combine, transfer, sort, and spread objects and toys	Does not sustain role in dramatic play; moves from one role to another incongruous role	Interested in finishing what started, even if it takes several days
	No carryover in play from day to day	More awareness of yesterday and tomorrow
	Silly in play	
Able to listen longer to nursery rhymes	Concentration span longer	Perceptive to order, form, and detail
Dramatizes nursery rhymes and stories	Sometimes so busy at play forgets to go to toilet	Better eye-hand coordination
Can match simple forms		Rhythmic motion to music; enjoys musical instruments
Identifies primary colors	Reenacts stories and trips	Likes excursions
Enjoys cutting, pasting, block building	Enjoys simple puzzles and models with trial-and-error method	Interested in world outside immediate environment; enjoys books
	Poor space perception	Interested in the many hues and shades of colors
Enjoys simple puzzles, hand puppets, large ball	Uses constructive and manipulative play material increasingly	Enjoys cutting out pictures, pasting, working on special projects, puzzles
Enjoys sand and water play	Enjoys sand and water play; cups, containers, and buckets for carrying and pouring	Likes to run and jump, play with bicycle, wagon, and sled
Enjoys dumping and hauling toys	Identifies commonly seen colors	Enjoys sand and water play; dramatic and elaborative in play
Rides tricycle	Enjoys crayons and paints, books	Enjoys using tools and equipment of adults
	Enjoys swing, jungle gym, toy hammer or other tools, pegboards	

Data from references 7, 43, 51, 73, 81, 87, 92.

INTERVENTIONS FOR HEALTH PROMOTION

Techniques for guidance and limit setting should be shared with parents and utilized by you when indicated. The Case Situation, Positive Parental Guidance, gives an example.

1. Be positive, clear, and consistent; let the child know what is acceptable behavior.
2. Convey authority without anger or threat to avoid feelings of resentment, fear, or guilt.
3. Place specific limits on special actions when the occasion arises; maintain some flexibility in rules.
4. Recognize the child's wish, and put it into words: "You wish you could have that but . . . ." Point out ways the wish can be partially fulfilled when possible.
5. Help the child express resentment likely to arise when restrictions are imposed: "I realize you don't like the rules but . . . ."
6. Enforce discipline by adhering to the stated rules kindly but firmly. Do not argue about them or initiate a battle of wills.
7. State positive suggestions rather than commands and "don'ts." This helps the child to learn how to get what is desired and to form happy relationships with others.
8. State directions that convey what he or she has to do if the child has no choice about a situation. For example, "It is time now to . . . ."
9. Convey that adults are present to help the child solve problems that cannot be solved alone.
10. Control the situation if the child has temporarily lost self-control. Remove him or her from the stimulating event; stay with the child. Talk quietly.
11. Use an inductive approach. Explain to the child how an undesirable act or word hurt another, how the person may feel, and how the child would feel if someone acted to the child in this manner.
12. Encourage thinking through the problem and finding a fair solution after a discipline situation when the child has become calm.
13. Convey, in any discipline situation, that you love the child but the behavior is unacceptable.
14. End the discipline situation by affirming that the child can regain self-control and handle situations appropriately.
15. Encourage the child to rejoin the group or continue the former activity when he or she feels ready.

---

more likely to crash a tricycle into a wall, to jump from high places, to not listen to cautious directions, to pound fists on hard objects, to break objects, and to be a daredevil. They want to experience a feeling, and it takes more of the experience for them to feel anything (44). The child can be taught to modulate and channel overactive curiosity and aggressive action (99).

Explore with parents the child's behavior. "Bad behavior" springs from wanting to get attention, from the desire to exert independence or control, or from frustration and anger. Children learn to strike out or hit by imitating parents or others, including children. Stop immediately any behavior that hurts another by holding the child's arm gently and quietly saying, "No." Explain the reason. Spanking should be avoided; it only teaches the child it is all right to hit. It shows the child an undesirable way of handling frustration. Spanking may interfere with superego development by relieving guilt too easily; the child feels that he or she has paid for the misbehavior and is free to return to mischievous activity.

Effective guidance and limit setting fosters emotional and social health. A *behavior modification technique* that can be used to discipline an aggressively acting-out child is *time-out*. **Time-out** *involves immediately placing the child after an undesirable act in a quiet, uninteresting place (hall, small room, or corner of a room) for about 5 minutes to remove the child from positive reinforcement.* Time-out stops the misbehavior and is unpleasant enough to increase the possibility that the child will not repeat the undesirable act. The child learns accountability for behavior when time-out is linked to breaking rules and extreme behavior. The child as part of

the family unit should have input into formulating rules and limits. This method should not be viewed by the child as a way to get out of cleanup or other tasks. Time-out is a method to help parents avoid nagging, spanking, screaming, lecturing, or being abusive. The method helps parents feel in control and handle misbehavior so the child's behavior can improve. *The child should be helped to realize that time-out means the behavior, not he or she, is rejected. Thus, parents should use rewards to reinforce desired behavior in conjunction with this time-out method.*

Work with parents to implement effective time-out methods. Explore parental guidance and discipline measures and the effectiveness of their methods of discipline. Share information presented in this chapter. The method of guidance and discipline should be appropriate to the age and developmental level of the child.

EMOTIONAL DEVELOPMENT

If the child has developed reasonably well and if he or she has mastered earlier developmental tasks, the preschooler is a source of pleasure to adults, more a companion than someone to care for. The various behaviors discussed under development of physical, mental, language, play, body image, and moral-spiritual aspects contribute to emotional status and development. *The child appears more self-confident and relaxed because of:*

1. Increasing motor self-control.
2. Feeling a high-energy level.
3. Using language.

Case Situation

Every morning when he woke up, 3-year-old Steve called for his mother to get him out of bed even though he was capable of doing it himself. His mother decided that she would no longer respond to his call, so he continued to call for about 15 minutes as he waited for her to come. Finally, he hollered, "Hello, is anybody home!" Thinking it rather humorous, his mother explained calmly, firmly, and in a positive way what he should do and that he was able to help himself in lots of ways. Thereafter, he'd leap out of bed in the morning and run to her, saying, "I'm here." She would respond with smiles and positive statements. That ended his calling. She wondered why she had not done this sooner. She realized Steve's self-esteem and confidence had increased as a result.

Contributed by Carole Piles, PhD, MSN, RN.

4. Delaying somewhat immediate gratification.
5. Tolerating separation from the mother.
6. Experiencing curiosity, strong imagination, and desire to move.

These characteristics propel him or her to plan, attack problems, start tasks, consider alternatives, learn aggressively, and direct behavior with some thought, logic, and judgment. Tolerance of frustration is still limited, but flares of temper and frustrations over failure pass quickly. As the child is learning to master things and handle independence and dependence, so is he or she increasing mastery of self and learning to get along with more people, both children and adults. The preschooler attempts to behave like an adult in realistic activity and play and is beginning to learn social roles, moral responsibility, and cooperation. However, the child still grabs, hits, and quarrels for short bursts of time. **Table 11-7** summarizes common causes and emotional manifestations of various emotional states in preschoolers (7, 8, 33, 46, 69, 74, 80, 85).

If the child has the opportunity to establish a sense of gender and to identify with mature adults, the attitude about self is sound and positive. If he or she has learned to trust and have some self-control, the child is ready to learn about and move into the broader culture. The preschooler begins to decide what kind of person he or she is, and self-concept, ego strength, and superego will con-

TABLE 11-7

Common Emotional Patterns of Preschooler

Emotion	Cause	Manifestation
Anger	Conflicts over playthings, thwarting of needs or wishes, attacks from another child	Temper tantrums; cries, screams, stomps, kicks, jumps, hits
Fear	Conditioning, imitation, and memories of unpleasant experiences; stories; pictures; TV; movies; darkness; being locked in closed-in space or room	Panic reaction; runs away and hides, cries, avoids situation; withdraws from source of punishment
Jealousy	Attention from parent shifted to someone else in family, especially younger sibling	Open expression; regresses to infantile behavior; pretends to be ill; is naughty; seeks attention
Curiosity	Anything new; their own and others' bodies; replaces normal fears	Sensorimotor exploration, questions
Envy	Abilities or material possessions of another, e.g., older sibling	Complains about what he or she has, states wish for something else, steals object wanted
Joy	Physical well-being; incongruous situation; sudden or unexpected noises; slight calamities; playing pranks on others; accomplishment of difficult task; music; drama; art	Smiles, laughs, claps hands, jumps up and down, hugs object or person
Grief	Loss, separation from loved person, pet, or object	Cries, is apathetic about daily activities, appears sad
Affection	Pleasure-giving persons, objects, or situations	Expresses verbally or nonverbally through smile, laugh, shout, hug, or words

tinue to mature. Self is still very important, but the sense of omnipotence is gradually being overcome.

Thus, the child is ready to learn **prosocial behavior**, *voluntary activity intended to benefit another.* Helpful actions, sharing, self-denial, and offering comfort reflect increasing empathy and may reflect genetics, temperament, or role-modeling by parents, other adults, and children (29). *Cultures vary* in the way they teach prosocial, cooperative, and caring behavior versus aggressive or competitive behavior. Cultures in which people live in extended family groups and share work foster prosocial behavior more than cultures that emphasize individualism (29, 40). The child who is securely attached and has well-regulated emotional response demonstrates prosocial behavior (41, 55).

Educate parents about the range of emotional responses, patterns, causes, and manifestations. Emphasize to parents the importance of their being a role model for standards of behavior. Stories read, songs sung, games played, and television and videos chosen to foster prosocial behavior and avoid depiction of violence and aggression are effective methods. The preschooler needs the opportunity to demonstrate caring and helpfulness, including visits to the elderly and household chores. If the child disobeys, encourage parents to use the guidance methods previously discussed.

Developmental Crisis: Initiative Versus Guilt

The *psychosexual crisis for this era is initiative versus guilt,* and all the aforementioned behaviors are part of achieving initiative (31). **Initiative** is *enjoyment of energy displayed in action, assertiveness, learning, increasing dependability, and ability to plan.* Natural initiative is desirable; however, it is important for parents not to expect too much or to push the child excessively. If the child does not achieve the developmental task of initiative, there is an overriding sense of guilt from the tension between others' expectations, the demands of the superego, and actual performance.

Guilt is a *sense of defeatism, anger, feeling responsible for things that he or she is not really responsible for, feeling easily frightened from what he or she wants to do, and feeling bad, shameful, and deserving of punishment.* A sense of guilt can develop from sibling rivalry,

---

BOX 11-8	**Consequences of Excessive or Unrealistic Guilt**

Guilt is an expression of rigid superego. The child exercises strong self-control but displays evidence of resentment or bitterness to the restrictive adult.

1. Stammering speech
2. Poor motor coordination
3. Eating and elimination problems
4. Regressed or immature behavior
5. Inability to separate from mother without extreme anxiety
6. Fear of strangers
7. Temper tantrums
8. Lack of interest in childhood activities or peers
9. Anxiety, easily frightened, irritability
10. Nightmares
11. Disorganized in behavior, not demonstrating age-appropriate neuromuscular, mental, or social skills

---

lack of opportunity to try things, or restriction on or lack of guidance in response to fantasy. Parents stifle initiative by doing things for the child or by frequently asking, "Why didn't you do it better?" If the guilt feelings are too strong, the child is affected in a negative way. Excessive guilt does not enhance moral or superego development, although the child must experience realistic guilt for wrong behavior. See **Box 11-8**, Consequences of Excessive or Unrealistic Guilt for a summary of this topic (7, 8, 31, 69, 88).

Self-Concept and Body Image Development

Self-concept, body image, and gender role behavior are gradually developing in these years (46, 80, 84, 87, 95, 96). *Positive self-concept develops* from parental love, effective relations with peers and others, success in play and other activities, and gaining skills

---

INTERVENTIONS FOR HEALTH PROMOTION

Help parents understand that *if the child is to develop a sense of initiative and a healthy personality, they and other significant adults must:*

1. Encourage use of the child's imagination, creativity, activity, and planning.
2. Limit punishment to those acts that are truly dangerous, morally wrong, socially unacceptable, or have harmful or unfortunate consequence for self or others.
3. Encourage the child's efforts to cooperate and share in the decisions and responsibilities of family life.
4. Reinforce appropriate behavior so that it will continue. The child develops best when commended and recognized for accomplishments.

5. Affirm a child's emotional experience, which is as important as affirming physical development.
6. Set aside a time each day, perhaps near bedtime, for the child to review emotional experiences. If there has been joy, pride, or anger, it can be recounted to the parents. Talking integrates these feelings with the event.
7. Help the preschooler to learn what feelings of love, hate, joy, and antagonism are and how to cope with and express them in ways other than physically. This promotes more mature behavior.

INTERVENTIONS FOR HEALTH PROMOTION

Teach parents ways to increase the child's self-esteem and positive self-concept. These guidelines will also be useful as you work with the child and family.

1. Identify causes of low self-esteem, such as lack of competence (real or perceived) in cognitive or physical skills, or negative perceptions about attractiveness and social acceptance.
2. Provide opportunities for the child to achieve and gain competence. Achievement in even one area can improve self-esteem significantly.
3. Use puppets, art, dolls, dramatic play, and playing with the child, for example, games and sports, to increase achievement and work through feelings.
4. Provide emotional support and realistic approval or reinforcement for achievements, as well as personal appearance and other behavior.

5. Explore and role-play ways for the child who is achieving and competent to handle negative comments from other children who are jealous. Recalling positive statements made by significant others can be a strong inner resource.
6. Role-play ways for the child to handle negative experiences or comments that threaten self-esteem or self-concept, for example, comments about race, ethnicity, religion, appearance, or skill level.
7. Seek support outside the home, for example, day care staff, teachers, a coach, friends or extended family, church friends, or a Big Sister or Big Brother agency. (This is a difficult step in abusive families.)

and self-control in activities of daily living. *Body boundaries and sense of self become more definite because of:* (a) developing sexual curiosity, greater awareness of his or her own genital area, and awareness of how he or she differs from others; (b) increasing motor skills with precision of movement and maturing sense of balance; (c) improving spatial orientation and a sense of the body in space, for example, on a slide, swing, or jungle gym; (d) maturing cognitive and language abilities to understand and describe the body and its sensations; (e) ongoing play activities; and (f) identifying with his or her parents. When the child is asked, "Are you a boy or a girl?" the 3-year-old child is likely to give his or her name. The 4-year-old can state gender, thus showing a differentiation of self (66).

The pleasurable feelings associated with touching the body and genitals, with masturbation, and play involving rocking or riding toys heighten self-awareness but also anxiety and anticipation of punishment. If the child is threatened or punished because of sexual curiosity, he or she may repress feelings about and awareness of the genitals or other body parts and develop a distorted body image. Of course, he or she must be taught that society does not condone handling of genitals in public. The preschooler must be able to stroke the body with affection and needs adult caresses as well.

Learning about the body—where it begins and ends, what it looks like, and what it can do—is basic to the child's self-awareness and eventual identity formation. Included in the growing self-awareness is discovery of feelings and learning names for them. The child is beginning to learn how he or she affects others and the meaning of others' responses. Control over feelings and behavior is being learned. The concept of body is reflected in the way the child talks, draws pictures, and plays.

The artistic productions of the preschooler convey self-perceptions and feelings. The *3-year-old* draws a man consisting of one circle, sometimes with an appendage, a crude representation of the face, and no differentiation of parts. The *4-year-old* draws a

man consisting of a circle for a face and head, facial features of two eyes and perhaps a mouth, two appendages, and occasionally wisps of hair or feet. Often the 4-year-old has not really formulated a mental representation of the lower part of the body. The *5-year-old* draws an unmistakable person. There is a circle face with nose, mouth, eyes, and hair and a body with arms and legs. Articles of clothing, fingers, and feet may be added. The width of the person is usually approximately 50% the length (24). The happy child draws a smile and uses bright colors. The sad or angry child expresses feelings in the face drawn and colors used (25). The child may think of the body as a house (24, 45). For example, while eating, he or she may name the various bites as fantasy characters who will go down and play in his or her house. The child may create an elaborate play area for them. (You can take advantage of this fantasy if eating problems arise.)

The child feels greater self-esteem when a problem is faced and handled than when it is avoided. The results can lead to positive self-evaluation (6, 74, 85, 95, 96).

Discuss with parents ways to develop the child's concept of body image. The child needs opportunities to learn the correct names and basic functions of body parts and to discover his or her body with joy and pride. Mirrors, photographs of the child, drawings of self and others such as parents and siblings, weighing, and measuring height enhance the formation of the mental picture. The child needs physical and mental activity to learn body mastery, self-protection, and the difference between self and machines, equipment, or tools. The child needs help to express and understand feelings of helplessness, doubt, or pain when the body does not accomplish what is desired or during illness and to "listen" to the body—the aches of stretched muscles, tummy rumblings, and stubbed toes. To deny, misinterpret, misname, or push aside physical or emotional feelings promotes an unrealistic self-understanding and eventually a negative self-concept, an unwhole body image, and health risks.

Specific nursing, physical therapy, or occupational therapy measures after illness or injury help the child reintegrate body image. Utilize play principles discussed in Chapter 10 ∞ and in this chapter.

Adaptive Mechanisms

Development proceeds toward increasing differentiation, articulation, and integration. **Differentiation** involves a *progressive separation of feeling, thinking, and acting and an increased polarity between self and others.* Differentiation is seen in the child's ability to **articulate** or *talk about the perceived experience of the world and the experience of self as a being.* **Integration** is seen in the *development of structured controls and adaptive or defensive mechanisms* (8).

Fears are common during the preschool years (17). With increasing differentiation, articulation of language, description of perceptions, and integration of experience and adaptive mechanisms into self, the child is better able to talk about fears and other feelings. The *infant demonstrates behaviorally and through crying the fears* of sudden movements, loud noises, loss of support, flashing lights, pain, separation from familiar people, and strange people, objects, or situations. The *toddler expresses vocally and behaviorally the fears* of being alone, the draining bathtub, the vacuum cleaner, the dark, dogs or other animals, high places, insecure footing, and separation from familiar people. There are times the *preschooler will regress* to infantile or toddler behaviors when fearful situations are encountered. However, the *preschooler has gained both language and conceptual ability, greater experience, and a greater imagination.* Now he or she *can talk about and play out* feelings. *Fears commonly expressed by the preschooler* include being alone; ghosts, masks, the dark, strange noises, and strangers; dogs, tigers, spiders, bears, and snakes; closed or unfamiliar places; thunderstorms; monsters, robbers, kidnappers, and other fantasized characters; and separation from loved ones. These fears decline by age 5 but may persist until age 7 or 8, especially if parents do not talk about them and help the child differentiate between reality and imagination (17, 18, 69).

What the preschool child sees through the media or hears in stories (including traditional fairy tales) may produce great fear. The child has no way of knowing, unless explanations are given, that the big bad wolf will not eat him or her, or that the Indians attacking wagon trains will not attack the home.

Help parents realize that to instill realistic fear is adaptive. Viewing and reading experiences that do not emphasize violence, bad people, or fearsome objects or animals, but rather gentle and calm experiences, are helpful for the child to gain a sense of self-control over fears.

Frustration arises in the child in response to self- and other's expectations as new activities and experiences are encountered. *Aggressive behavior may result. A variety of factors may be involved* (25, 36, 42, 74):

1. Lack of maternal warmth and social support; presence of maternal depression
2. Stressful home environment, lack of learning stimulation, low levels of parent-child interaction
3. Overcrowding in the home, severe housing problems
4. Single motherhood, lack of social support for the mother
5. Harsh discipline consistently
6. Transient peer groups, lack of stable friendships
7. Exposure to aggressive adults and neighborhood violence
8. Surroundings that foster antisocial behavior and attitudes despite parental effort to socialize the child positively

These variables may or may not all exist together (39).

Affirm to parents the importance of listening to the child and showing concern about his or her feelings. Emphasize not to make excessive demands on the child. Explore ways to overcome factors that contribute to the child's frustration and aggressivity. Art, music, and play activities may help both the child and adult express frustration and aggression. Examine other coping and problem-solving strategies for use with the child and for the parents.

The parents need your listening, validation, and suggestions to cope with fears, frustrations, and problems. Parental behavior is a role model to the child. Refer parents to community resources. Help them find social support linkages. The problem is often bigger than the family. Your advocacy efforts may extend to local, state, or national agencies for greater resources to families. Policy development and legislation may also be needed, especially in relation to affordable and livable housing and mental health services.

Emotional regulation is a task for the preschooler (7). Children do not develop this ability at the same age because of genetic and experiential differences. In fact, a range of expressive or inhibited behavior is found from infancy through adulthood. Brain scans show that people who are more fearful and inhibited demonstrate greater right prefrontal cortex activity. In contrast, people who are more expressive or exuberant show more left prefrontal cortex activity (18). Emotional regulation seems to be attained more easily for females than males, possibly related to the XX chromosomes (7, 18, 44).

Repeated exposure to extreme stress interferes with emotional and physical regulation. Early stressors can change electrical activity, dendritic growth, and production of various hormones in the brain (7, 21, 43, 44). With extreme stress, some neurons are killed; others do not develop. The brain becomes unable to respond normally to ordinary stressors, and excess cortisol is released with many experiences. Thus, the preschooler may not be able to tolerate an unexpected loud noise or even a critical remark and may demonstrate hyperactivity. One preschooler may express fury or terror whereas another, not having experienced extreme stress, would have a mildly upsetting experience to the same stimuli (7, 21, 43, 44). Sometimes children have experienced so much stress (for example, abused children) that they have a blunted stress response because the body is responding to stress with lower cortisol levels. Emotions are dampened and diluted, instead of regulated; the child may demonstrate depression (7, 21, 43, 64).

Specific adaptive mechanisms are at a peak during the preschool years. They include introjection, secondary identification, fantasy, repression, and suppression. These mechanisms may be used in other developmental eras to aid or hinder adjustment. Mechanisms discussed in Chapter 10 are also used in response to situations. ∞

Introjection, *integrating attitudes, information, and actions into the self through empathy, learning, and imitation,* is essential for secondary identification to occur. Through **secondary identification** the *child internalizes standards, moral codes, attitudes, and role behavior, including gender, as his or her own, in a personally unique way.*

Through **fantasy,** or *imagination,* the child handles tension and anxiety related to the problems of becoming socialized into the family, culture, and peer group. As the child mentally restructures reality to meet personal needs, he or she is gradually learning how to master the environment realistically. Because the child has difficulty distinguishing between wish and reality, parents must be gently realistic when necessary without shattering fantasies when they are needed or cause no problem. Parents must realize that an active imagination is normal at this age, provides tension release, and is the basis for creativity.

Repression, *unconscious submersion of prior experiences,* and **suppression,** *forgetting or inability to recall,* occur as the parents and culture continue to insist firmly on reality and following the rules. Excessive *repression* is related to guilt feelings, harsh punishment, or perceived strong disapproval and will later interfere with memories of this period and result in constricted creativity and restricted behavior. Some repression, such as that related to the Oedipal conflict, is necessary to free the child's energies for new tasks to be learned (42). *Suppression* is overcome with realistic consistent reminders.

You can help parents understand the processes of differentiation, articulation, and integration as related to emotional development, the adaptive mechanisms commonly used, and ways to help the child learn coping skills. Affirm the normality and importance of these health-promoting adaptive mechanisms.

MORAL-SPIRITUAL DEVELOPMENT

The child is in the preconventional stage of moral development (56). Influences on the child during these early years are the parents' attitude toward moral codes (the human as creative being, spirituality, religion, nature, love of country, the economic system, education) and their behavior in the presence of the child. They convey to the child what is considered good and bad, worthy of respect or unworthy. With the developing superego, imitation of and identification with adults, and development of prosocial behavior, the child is absorbing a great deal of others' attitudes and will retain many of them throughout life. The preschooler begins to consider how personal actions affect others (42).

Moral and Religious Education

There are some general considerations pertaining to moral and religious education. *The child cannot be kept spiritually neutral. He or she hears about morals and religion from other people and will raise detailed questions about the basic issues of life:* Where did I come from? Why am I here? Why did the bird (or Grandpa) die? Why is it wrong to do . . .? Why can't I play with Joey? How come Billy goes to church on Saturday and we go to church on Sunday? What is God? What is heaven? Mommy, who do you like best: Santa Claus, the Easter Bunny, the tooth fairy, God, or Jesus? These questions, often considered inappropriate from the adult viewpoint, should not be lightly brushed aside, for how they are answered is more important than the information given.

Example is the chief teacher for the child. If adult actions do not match the words, the child quickly notices and learns the action. For the child, the parent is like God—omnipotent. Parents would be wise to remember this and try to live up to the high ideals of the child while at the same time introducing the reality of the world,

for example, that parents do make mistakes. Talking with the child about such a mistake and asking forgiveness (if the child was wronged) will foster understanding of the redeeming power of a moral code, religion, or an ideal philosophy.

There are *two major methods of religious education: (a) indoctrination, or (b) letting the child follow the religion of choice. Neither meets the real issues.* The preschooler does not follow a religion because he or she understands it but because it encompasses daily life, offers concomitant pleasure, and is expected. The preschooler accepts the religion of the parents, if a religion is practiced, because to the child they are all-powerful. He or she is trusting and literal in the interpretation of religion. The first religious responses are social in nature; bowing the head and saying a simple prayer is imitated like brushing the teeth. The child likes prayers before meals and bedtime, and the *3-year-old* may repeat them like nursery rhymes. The *4-year-old* elaborates on prayer forms, and the *5-year-old* makes up prayers.

Interpretation of religious forms and practices is marked by mental processes normal for the age: (a) egocentrism, (b) **anthropomorphism***, in which the child relates God to human beings who are known,* (c) fantasy rather than causal or logical thinking, and (d) animism. The child thinks either God or human beings are responsible for all events. God pushes clouds when they move; wind is God blowing; thunder is God hammering; the sun is God lighting a match in the sky.

The child needs consistent, simple explanations matched with the daily practices and religious ceremonies, rituals, or pictures. The preschool child is old enough to go to Sunday school, vacation Bible school, or classes in religious education that are on an appropriate cognitive level. Religious holidays raise questions, and the spirit of the holiday and ceremonies surrounding it should be explained. In the United States, where Christmas and Easter have become secularized and surrounded with the myths of Santa Claus and Easter Bunny, the child's fantasy and love of parties may minimize the religious significance of the days. There is no harm in telling the child about these myths but convey the religious spirit of the days rather than as an end in themselves. The child thinks concretely, and embodiments of ideas such as the material objects used in any religion convey abstract meanings that words alone do not. When he or she expresses doubt about the myths, a more sophisticated explanation may be presented.

Conscience or Superego Development

This development is related to moral-spiritual training, discipline, conditioning of behavior (smiles, loving words), modeling of parents and others for correct behavior, being given reasons for behavior, and other areas of learning. The **superego,** *that part of the psyche that is critical to the self and enforces moral standards,* forms as a result of identification with parents and an introjection of their standards and values, which at first are questioned (8, 31, 42). The child is in the Preconventional Period, Stage 2 of moral development, which is described in Chapter 1, Table 1-10 ∞ (57, 58).

The preschooler usually behaves even if there is no parent or external authority nearby, to avoid disapproval, although he or she will slip at times. The child continues use of social referencing, or *turning to the mother or father for guidance in unfamiliar situations to seek tacit permission, or to determine disapproval.* Just as children imitate language, gestures, and other behaviors, they imitate moral principles, from saying, "thank you" to not torturing the family pet. Thus, the child learns to feel proud or a realistic guilt about what is done.

The superego can be cruel, primitive, and uncompromising. The child can be overobedient or resentful because parents do not live up to what the child's superego demands. The child is likely to overreact to punishment. This all-or-nothing quality of the superego is normally tempered later. A strict superego does not necessarily mean that the child has strict parents, but rather that he or she perceives them as strict. It is the result of the child's interpretation of events, teaching, admonitions, demands of the environment, discipline, punishment, fears, and guilt and anxiety about fantasized and real deeds. Superego development will continue through contact with teachers and other significant adults through the years.

If the superego does not develop and if no or few social values are internalized, the child will be increasingly regarded as mischievous or bad. Eventually the child may have no guilt feelings and no qualms about not following the rules. The child is then on the way to truancy or delinquency (69, 88).

The child continues the moral development previously begun, learning a greater sense of responsibility, empathy, mercy, compassion, and fairness. The parents are the major teachers as they relate to the child fairly, courteously, with compassion and gentleness, and are reliable and responsive. They teach when they point out the consequences of behavior upon others. If the child hurts another child physically or emotionally, the child needs to know that. Then the child learns an appropriate sense of guilt. That does *not* mean that the parent abuses the child or uses brute force to teach pain. Rather, discussion and reasoning, along with asserting authority (restraining and calming an angry, aggressive child) when necessary, are ways to influence positively the child's moral outlook. Withdrawal of love and physical punishment are not effective ways to teach moral behavior. In response to physical punishment, the child acts out even more physically or verbally because of consequent anger. Withdrawal of love results in a terrified, withdrawn, passive child who cannot respond to messages to be caring to others (88). If the child feels valued and values self, he or she will in turn treat other people, animals, the environment, and things as valuable.

Encourage parents to discuss religion and related practices with the child. Discuss with parents the importance of superego development and beginning moral development during this period.

DEVELOPMENTAL TASKS

In summary, the *developmental tasks for the preschooler are to* (27):

1. Settle into a healthful daily routine of adequately eating, exercising, and resting, and follow health promotion behavior of the family.
2. Master physical skills of large- and small-muscle coordination and movement.
3. Become a participating member in the life and activities of the family.
4. Identify with the parent of the same gender.
5. Conform to others' expectations that are appropriate for this era.

6. Express emotions healthfully and for a wide variety of experiences.
7. Become more realistic; relinquish some fantasies.
8. Learn to communicate effectively with an increasing number of others.
9. Learn to use initiative tempered by a conscience.
10. Develop ability to handle potentially dangerous situations.
11. Lay foundations for understanding the meaning of life, self, the world, and ethical, religious, and philosophic ideas.

Discuss with parents how these tasks may be achieved, and encourage them to talk about their concerns or problems as they help the child mature in these skills. If delays in cognitive or language development, destructiveness, or excessive bed-wetting persist, the parents and child need special guidance. Obtain information on causes, associated behavior, and care for these and other special problems from a pediatric nursing book (46, 80).

Health Promotion and Nursing Applications

ASSESSMENT

Your role with the preschooler and family has been discussed in each section throughout this chapter. Use the information in your assessment while you also recognize the uniqueness of the child and family situation. Be aware of variations related to cultural background (1, 40).

NURSING DIAGNOSES

The **Box**, Nursing Diagnoses Related to the Preschooler, lists some nursing diagnoses that may apply to the preschooler (73). Assessments that result from information presented in this chapter may help you formulate other nursing diagnoses to guide your care.

INTERVENTION

Interventions have been interwoven throughout the chapter as they apply to the topic being discussed. Your therapeutic relationship and role-modeling of caring behavior to the preschooler and family are basic. Educate, support, and counsel the preschooler and family, based on their needs. Give direct care to meet the preschooler's physical care as you simultaneously meet emotional and cognitive needs. At times, intervention will be directed to socialization needs. Your caring behavior will contribute toward moral development. As you implement the preschooler's care, you will also contribute toward meeting the parental needs, often emotionally and cognitively, if not in direct physical care. Your moral integrity may strengthen theirs.

You will find opportunity in many settings—the neighborhood, day care center, compensatory program, church group, clinic, doctor's office, school, industrial setting, or hospital—to correct parents' misconceptions and validate their sound thinking about their child's development and the importance of the family's behavior for the child's emotional, physical, and social health. Principles of communication, health teaching, and crisis counseling also apply. Become active as a citizen to educate the public

Nursing Diagnoses Related to the Preschooler

Ineffective **A**irway Clearance
Impaired Verbal **C**ommunication
Readiness for Enhanced **C**ommunication
Ineffective **C**oping
Risk for Delayed **D**evelopment
Diarrhea
Risk for **F**alls
Fear
Delayed **G**rowth and Development
Risk for Disproportionate **G**rowth

Risk for **I**nfection
Risk for **I**njury
Imbalanced **N**utrition: Less than Body Requirements
Imbalanced **N**utrition: More than Body Requirements
Risk for **P**oisoning
Bathing/Hygiene **S**elf-Care Deficit
Dressing/Grooming **S**elf-Care Deficit
Risk for Situational Low **S**elf-Esteem
Disturbed **S**leep Patterns
Risk for **T**rauma

Source: Reference 73.

about needs of children. Promote needed legislation. Directly advocate about problems that affect children's health, such as child abuse and lead poisoning. Promote quality day care or preschool programs. The range of possible effective intervention is wide and will depend on your work setting and interest.

You have a critical role as advocate in the local or broader community for the maltreated child, family in distress, and cultural group suffering poverty and its consequences. Interventions have to extend beyond the individual client to the broader society, through community and societal awareness, public policy, legislation, and overcoming of negative forces. Citizens, schools, churches, health care and social agencies, and political parties all have responsibility for healthy children and families.

EVALUATION

Sometimes care can be **evaluated** by the verbal and nonverbal responses of the preschooler and family at the time of care. Sometimes you receive a later report. Evaluation is not just a measurement. It is an approach of self-review of actions and thoughtfulness about the agency or system response. At times, it involves advocacy on behalf of the preschooler and continuing work with the family, for example, in cases of child maltreatment. The statements in **Box 11-9**, Considerations for the Preschool Child and Family in Health Promotion, may also be used in **evaluation.** Reference 50 is also a resource for determining outcomes in practice.

BOX 11-9 Considerations for the Preschool Child and Family in Health Promotion

1. Family, cultural background and values, support systems, and community resources for the family
2. Parents as identification figures for the child, secondary identification of the preschool child with the parents
3. Behaviors that indicate gender identity and sense of sexuality in the preschool child
4. Behaviors that indicate ability of the preschool child to relate to siblings, adults in the extended family, and other adults and authority figures in the environment
5. Parental behaviors that indicate difficulty with parenting or potential of actual abuse of the preschool child
6. Physical characteristics and patterns, such as neuromuscular development, nutrition, exercise, and rest or sleep, that indicate health and are within age norms for growth for the preschool child
7. Cognitive characteristics and behavioral patterns in the preschool child that demonstrate curiosity, increasingly realistic thought, expanding concept formation, and continuing mental development
8. Communication patterns—verbal, nonverbal, and action—and language development that demonstrate con-

tinuing learning and age-appropriate norms for the preschool child
9. Behaviors that indicate that the child can participate in and enjoys early childhood education experiences
10. Overall appearance and behavior and play patterns in the preschool child that indicate development of initiative rather than excessive guilt, positive self-concept, body image formation, and sense of sexuality
11. Use of adaptive mechanisms by the preschool child that promote a sense of security, control of anxiety, and age-appropriate emotional responses
12. Behavioral patterns that indicate the preschool child is forming a superego or conscience and continuing moral and spiritual development
13. Behavioral patterns and characteristics that indicate that the preschool child has achieved developmental tasks
14. Parental behaviors that indicate knowledge about how to guide and discipline the child and assist the child in becoming more independent
15. Parental behaviors that indicate the child is achieving the developmental tasks for this era

Summary

1. Family relationships and nurturing are important to the child's development in all areas.
2. The child begins to participate within the family, and to communicate and relate more effectively with adults who are either extended family, friends, or authority figures in the community.
3. Parents' provision of consistent love, guidance, and new experiences is essential for holistic, healthy development.
4. The preschooler grows at a steady pace; coordination is increasing.
5. The preschooler gains considerable neuromuscular, cognitive, emotional, social, and moral and spiritual competencies.
6. The child develops the ability to carry out basic hygiene and routine activities.
7. The child slowly grows out of the family, establishes beginning peer relationships, and learns to follow rules of the play group.
8. Health promotion is important and lays the foundation for future health status.
9. Health problems, including maltreatment and injuries, must be addressed.
10. **Box 11-9**, Considerations for the Preschool Child and Family in Health Promotion, summarizes what you should consider in assessment and health promotion with the preschooler. The family is included in considerations.

Review Questions

1. A nurse in the pediatric clinic observes that a 4-year-old female child is being consoled by her father but rejects her mother's attempts to calm her. The nurse concludes that this behavior is:
   1. A definitive indication of physical abuse by the mother.
   2. A sign of sexual abuse by the father.
   3. Symptomatic of developmental delay.
   4. Normal for a child of this age group.
2. The parent of a 5-year-old is concerned that the child is obese. The child's weight is 22 kg. The nurse should explain to the parent that the child is:
   1. Underweight for age.
   2. Overweight, but not obese.
   3. Normal weight for age.
   4. Obese.
3. Nutrition education for parents of preschool children should emphasize:
   1. Limiting between-meal snacks.
   2. Providing desserts only as a reward for finishing a meal.
   3. Recognizing that times of not wanting to eat are normal behavior for preschoolers.
   4. Offering large portions to provide adequate calories.
4. A parent is concerned that a 3-year-old child refuses to play with others, preferring to play alongside other children. The nurse should base the response to the parent's concern with one of the following facts:
   1. Children of this age group usually enjoy games and activities involving groups.
   2. Parallel play is a characteristic of this age group.
   3. This play behavior may reflect a developmental delay.
   4. The child is too young to play with other children.

References

1. Andrews, M., & Boyle, J. (2003). *Transcultural concepts in nursing care* (4th ed.). Philadelphia: Lippincott Williams & Wilkins.
2. Attention deficit disorder: Old questions, new answers. (2006). *Harvard Mental Health Letter, 22*(8), 3–5.
3. Baumrind, D. (1967). Child care practices anteceding three patterns of preschool behavior. *Genetic Psychology Monographs, 75,* 43–88.
4. Baumrind, D. (1971). Harmonious parents and their preschool children. *Developmental Psychology, 41,* 92–102.
5. Baumrind, D. (1989). Rearing competent children. In W. Damon (Ed.), *Child development today and tomorrow* (pp. 349–378). San Francisco: Jossey-Bass.
6. Bednar, R., Wells, M., & Peterson, J. (1995). *Self-esteem* (2nd ed.). Washington, DC: American Psychological Association.
7. Berger, K. (2005). *The developing person through the lifespan* (6th ed.). New York: Worth.
8. Bettelheim, B. (1987). *A good enough parent: A book on child-rearing.* New York: Alfred A. Knopf.
9. Brody, G., & Flor, D. (1998). Maternal resources, parenting practices, and child competence in rural, single-parent, African-American families. *Child Development, 69,* 805–816.
10. Burgess, A. (1984). Intra-familial sexual abuse. In J. Campbell & I. Humphreys (Eds.), *Nursing care of victims of family violence.* Reston, VA: Reston.
11. Burgess, A., Hartman, C., & Baker, T. (1995). Memory presentations of childhood sexual abuse. *Journal of Psychosocial Nursing and Mental Health Services, 33*(9), 9–16.
12. Burgess, A., Hartman, C., & Kelley, S. (1990). Assessing child abuse: The TRIADS Checklist. *Journal of Psychosocial Nursing and Mental Health Services, 28*(4), 6–14.
13. Burgess, A., McCausland, M., & Wolbert, W. (1981). Children's drawings as indicators of sexual trauma. *Perspectives in Psychiatric Care, 19*(2), 50–58.
14. Burgess, A., et al. (1987). Child molestation: Assessing impact in multiple victims (Part I). *Archives of Psychiatric Nursing, 1*(1), 33–39.

15. Cadman, D., et al. (1984). The usefulness of the Denver Developmental Screening Test to predict kindergarten problems in a general community population. *American Journal of Public Health, 74*(110), 1093–1097.

16. Chao, R. (2001). Extending research on the consequences of parenting style for Chinese Americans and European Americans. *Child Development, 72,* 1832–1843.

17. Children's fears and anxieties. (2004). *Harvard Mental Health Letter, 21*(6), 1–3.

18. Codder, C., Mott, J., & Berman, A. (2002). The interactive effects of infant activity level and fear on greater trajectories of early childhood behavior problems. *Development and Psychopathology, 14,* 1–23.

19. Cook, L. (2005). The ultimate deception: Childhood sexual abuse in the church. *Journal of Psychosocial Nursing and Mental Health Services, 45*(10), 19–24.

20. Crowley, A., Bams, P., & Pellici, L. (2005). A model preschool vision and hearing screening program. *American Journal of Nursing, 105,* 52–56.

21. DeBallis, M. (2001). Developmental traumatology: The psychological development of maltreated children and its implications for research, treatment, and policy. *Development and Psychopathology, 13,* 539–564.

22. Dennison, B., Russo, T., Burdick, P., & Jenkins, P. (2004). An intervention to reduce television viewing by preschool children. *Archives of Pediatric and Adolescent Medicine, 158,* 170–176.

23. Dietz, T. (1996). An examination of violence and gender role portrayals in video games: Implications for gender socialization and aggressive behavior. *Sex Roles, 38,* 425–442.

24. DiLeo, J. H. (1971). *Young children and their drawings.* Springfield, IL: Springer.

25. Dodge, K., Pettit, G., & Bates, J. (1994). Socialization mediators of the relation between socioeconomic status and child conduct problems. *Child Development, 65,* 649–665.

26. Dudek, S. (2007). *Nutrition essentials for nursing practice* (5th ed.). Philadelphia: Lippincott Williams & Wilkins.

27. Duvall, W., & Miller, B. (1984). *Marriage and family development* (6th ed.). New York: Harper & Row.

28. Duyff, R. (1998). *The American Dietetic Association's complete food and nutrition guide.* Hoboken, NJ: John Wiley & Sons.

29. Eisenberg, N., & Fabes, R. (1998). Prosocial development. In W. Damon (Series Ed.) & N. Eisenberg (Vol. Ed.), *Handbook of child psychology: Vol. 3, Social, emotional, and personality development* (5th ed., pp. 701–778). New York: Wiley.

30. Elicker, J., Englund, M., & Stronfe, L. (1992). Predicting peer competence and peer relationships in childhood from early parent-child relationships. In R. Parke & G. Ladd (Eds.), *Family-peer relationships: Modes of linkage* (pp. 77–106). Hillsdale, NY: Erlbaum.

31. Erikson, E. H. (1963). *Childhood and society* (2nd ed.). New York: W.W. Norton.

32. Erikson, E. (1977). *Toys and reasons.* New York: W.W. Norton.

33. Fassler, D. (2003). *Help me, I'm sad: Recognizing, treating, and preventing childhood and adolescent depression.* New York: Little, Brown and Company.

34. Fenstermacker, K., & Hudson, B.T. (2004). *Practice guidelines for family practitioners* (3rd ed.). Philadelphia: Saunders.

35. Frankenburg, W., & Dobbs, J. B. (1990). *Denver II—Revision and Restandardization of the Denver Developmental Screening Test.* Denver, CO: Denver Developmental Materials.

36. Galboda-Liyanage, K. C., Prince, M. J., & Scott, S. (2003). Mother-child joint activity and behavior problems of preschool children. *Journal of Child Psychology and Psychiatry, 44*(7), 1037–1048.

37. Garbarino, J. (1992). *Children in danger.* New York: Jossey-Bass.

38. Garbarino, J., Guttmann, E., & Seeley, J. (1987). *The psychologically battered child: Strategies for identification, assessment, and intervention.* San Francisco: Jossey-Bass.

39. Gesell, A. Ilg, F. (1990). *The first five years of life.* New York: Harper & Brothers.

40. Giger, J., & Davidhizar, R. (2004). *Transcultural nursing: Assessment and intervention* (4th ed.). St. Louis, MO: Mosby.

41. Gilliam, M., Shaw, D., Beck, J., Schoenberg, M., & Lukon, J. (2002). Anger regulation in disadvantaged preschool boys: Strategies, antecedents, and the development of self-control. *Developmental Psychology, 38,* 222–235.

42. Grusec, J., Goodnow, J., & Kuczynski, L. (2000). New directions in analysis of parenting contributions to childhood acquisition of values. *Child Development, 71,* 205–211.

43. Gunner, M., & Vasquez, D. (2001). Low cortisol and a flattening of expected daytime rhythm. Potential indices of risk in human development. *Development and Psychopathology, 13,* 515–538.

44. Guyton, A., & Hall, J. (2006). *Textbook of medical physiology* (11th ed.). Philadelphia: Elsevier Saunders.

45. Harter, S. (1998). *The conservation of the self.* New York: Guilford.

46. Hockenberry, M., & Wilson, D. (2007). *Wong's nursing care of infants and children* (8th ed.). St. Louis, MO: Mosby.

47. Howe, D. (2001). Age at placement, adoption experience and adult adopted people's contact with their adoptive and birth mothers: An attachment perspective. *Attachment & Human Development, 3,* 222–237.

48. Huesemann, I., Moise-Titus, J., Podolski, C. L., & Eron, L. (2003). Longitudinal relations between children's exposure to TV violence and their aggressive and violent behavior in young adulthood 1977–1992. *Developmental Psychology, 39,* 201–221.

49. Jaakkola, J., Nafstad, P., & Magnus, P. (2001). Environmental tobacco smoke, parental atopy, and childhood asthma. *Environmental Health Perspectives, 109,* 579–582.

50. Johnson, M., Bulecheck, G., Butcher, H., Dochterman, J., Maas, M., Moorhead, S., & Swanson, E. (2006). *NANDA, NOC, and NIC Linkages: Nursing diagnoses, outcomes, & intervention* (2nd ed.). St. Louis, MO: Mosby Elsevier.

51. Johnson, J., Cohne, P., Smarles, E., Kasen, S., & Brock, J. (2002). Television viewing and aggressive behavior during adolescence and adulthood. *Science, 295,* 2468–2471.

52. Kelley, S. (1990). Parental stress response to sexual abuse and ritualistic abuse of children in day care centers. *Nursing Research, 39*(1), 25–29.

53. Kelley, M., Howe, T., Dodge, K., Bates, J., & Pettit, S. (2001). The timing of child physical maltreatment: A cross-domain growth analysis of impact on adolescent internalizing and externalizing problems. *Development and Psychopathology, 13,* 89–92.

54. Kelly, K., & Kulman, L. (2004, September 13). Kid power. *U.S. News and World Report,* 47–51.

55. Kochanska, G., Coy, K., & Murray, K. (2001). The development of self-regulation in the first four years of life. *Child Development, 72,* 1091–1111.

56. Kohlberg, L. (1977). *Recent research in moral development.* New York: Holt, Rinehart, Winston.

57. Kohlberg, L. (1981). *Essays on moral development.* San Francisco: Harper & Row.

58. Kornhaber, A., & Woodward, K. (1995). *Grandparent power.* New York: Random House.

59. Krimer, L., & Goldman-Rakic, P. (2001). Prefrontal microcircuits. *Journal of Neuroscience, 21,* 3788–3796.

60. Lamb, M. (1987). The emergent father. In M. B. Lamb (Ed.), *The father's role: Cross-cultural perspectives* (pp. 1–26). Hillsdale, NJ: Lawrence Erlbaum.

61. Latimer, D. (1994). Involving grandparents and other older adults in the preschool classroom. *Dimensions of Early Childhood, 22*(2), 26–30.

62. LaRossa, R. (1988). Fatherhood and social change. *Family Relations, 37,* 451–457.

63. LeVieux-Anglin, L., & Sawyer, E. (1990). Incorporating play interventions into nursing care. *Pediatric Nursing, 19,* 456–462.

64. Mahoney, D. (2005). Children of depression: Breaking the cycle. *Clinical Psychiatry News, 33*(4), 54.

65. Manlyn, J., Todd, K., Jungmeen, E., Rogosch, F., & Cicohetti, D. (2001). Dimensions of child maltreatment and children's adjustment. Contributions of developing timing and subtype. *Development and Psychopathology, 13,* 759–782.

66. Margolis, D. (2006). Gender development. In K. Thies & J. Travers (Eds.), *Handbook of human development for health care professionals* (pp. 19–32). Boston: Jones and Bartlett.

67. Marzolla, J., & Lloyd, J. (1972). *Learning through play.* New York: Harper & Row.

68. McCartney, K., & O'Connor, E. (2006). Psychosocial development: Attachment in young children. In K. Thies & J. Travers (Eds.), *Handbook of human development for health care professionals.* Boston, MA: Jones and Bartlett.

69. McGoldrick, M., Geordano, J., & Garcia-Presto, N. (2005). *Ethnicity and family therapy* (3rd ed.). New York: Guilford.

70. Millar, S. (1974). *The psychology of play.* Harmonds-Worth, England: Penguin Books.

71. Monteleone, J. A. (1998). *A parent's & teacher's handbook on identifying and preventing child abuse.* St. Louis, MO: G.W. Medical Publishing.

72. Monteleone, J. A., & Brodeur, A. E. (1998). *Child maltreatment: A clinical guide and references* (2nd ed.). St. Louis, MO: G.W. Medical.

73. NANDA International. (2007). *NANDA-I nursing diagnoses: Definitions and classification 2007–2008.* Philadelphia: Author.

74. Papalia, D., Olds, S., & Feldman, P. (2004). *Human development* (9th ed.). Boston: McGraw-Hill.

75. Pettit, G., Bates, J., & Dodge, K. (1997). Supportive parenting, ecological context, and children's adjustment: A seven-year longitudinal study. *Child Development, 68,* 908–923.

76. Phaneuf, R., & Silberglitt, B. (2003). Tracking preschooler's language and preliminary development using a general outcome measurement system. *Topics in Early Childhood Special Education, 23*(3), 114–124.

77. Piaget, J. (1953). *Origins of intelligence in childhood* (2nd ed.). New York: International Universities Press.

78. Piaget, J. (1989). *The equilibration of cognitive structures: The central problem of intellectual development* (T. Brown & K. J. Thampy, Trans.). Chicago: University of Chicago Press.

79. Polk-Walker, G. (1990). What really happened? Incidence and factor assessment of abused children and adolescents. *Journal of Psychosocial Nursing and Mental Health Services, 28,* 17–22.

80. Potts, N.L., & Mandleco, B.L. (2007). *Pediatric nursing: Caring for children and their families* (2nd ed.). New York: Thomson/Delmar Learning.

81. Questioning child care. (2002). *Harvard Mental Health Letter, 19*(6), 1–3.

82. Ramey, S. (1999). Head Start and preschool education. Toward continued improvement. *American Psychologist, 54,* 344–346.

83. Reynolds, A., Temple, J., Robertson, D., & Mann, E. (2001). Long-term effects of an early childhood intervention on educational achievements and juvenile arrest. *Journal of the American Medical Association, 285,* 2339–2346.

84. Ruble, D. N., & Martin, C. L. (1998). Gender development. In W. Damon (Series Ed.) & N. Eisenberg (Vol. Ed.), *Handbook of child psychology: Vol. 3, Social, emotional, and personality development* (3rd ed., pp. 993–1016). New York: Wiley.

85. Santrock, J. (2004). *Life-span development* (9th ed.). Boston: McGraw-Hill.

86. Saylor, M., & Sabbagh, M. (2004). Different kinds of information affect and learning in the preschool years: The case of part-term learning. *Child Development, 75*(2), 395–408.

87. Schilder, P. (1951). *The image and appearance of the human body.* New York: International Universities Press.

88. Schulman, M. (1985). *Moral development training: Strategies for parents, teachers, and clinicians.* Menlo Park: CA: Addison-Wesley.

89. Schwebel, D., & Plumert, J. (1999). Longitudinal and concurrent relations among temperament, ability estimation, and injury proneness. *Child Development, 70,* 700–712.

90. Singer, M. (1995). *Cults in our midst.* San Francisco: Jossey Bass.

91. Singer, M., Slovak, K., Frierson, T., & York, P. (1996). Viewing preferences, symptoms of psychological trauma, and violent behaviors among children who watch television. *Journal of the American Academy of Child and Adolescent Psychiatry, 37,* 1041–1048.

92. Strauss, R. S. (2001). Environmental tobacco smoke and serum vitamin C levels in children. *Pediatrics, 107,* 540–542.

93. United States Department of Agriculture, Center for Nutrition Policy and Promotion. (2005, April). *My Pyramid.* Washington, DC: Author.

94. United States Department of Health and Human Services. (2000). *Healthy People 2010: With understanding and improving health and objectives for improving health, Vol. 2* (2nd ed.). Washington, DC: United States Government Printing Office.

95. Verschueren, K., Buyck, P., & Marcoen, A. (2001). Self-representations and socioemotional competence in young children: A 3-year longitudinal study. *Developmental Psychology, 37,* 126–134.

96. Verschueren, K., Marcoen, A., & Schoefs, V. (1996). The internal working model of the self, attachment, and competence in five-year-olds. *Child Development, 67,* 2493–2511.

97. Vygotsky, L. (1978). *Mind in society. The development of higher psychological processes* (M. Cole, V. Johnsteiner, S. Scribner, & E. Souberman, Eds.). Cambridge, MA: Harvard University Press.

98. Wadsworth, B. (2004). *Piaget's Theory of Cognitive and Affective Development: Foundation of constructivism* (5th ed.). Boston: Pearson Education.

99. Warren, S., Oppenheim, D., & Emde, R. (1996). Can emotions and themes in child's play predict behavior problems? *Journal of the American Academy of Child and Adolescent Psychiatry, 35*(10), 1331–1337.

100. Webb, P. (1980). Piaget: Implications for teaching. *Theory into practice, 19*(2), 93–97.

CHAPTER 12

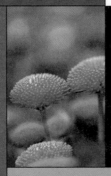

The Schoolchild: Basic Assessment and Health Promotion

OBJECTIVES

Study of this chapter will enable you to:

1. Discuss family relationships of the school-age child and the influence of peers and other adults.

2. Explore with the family members their developmental tasks and ways to achieve them.

3. Examine effects of the types of child maltreatment upon the health and development of the child.

4. Compare and assess the physical changes and needs, including nutrition, rest, exercise, safety, and health promotion.

5. Assess intellectual, communication, play, emotional, self-concept, sexuality, and moral-spiritual development in the juvenile and preadolescent phases and influences on these areas of development.

6. Describe the crisis of school entry and ways to help the child adapt to the experience of formal education, including latchkey care.

7. Relate the physical and emotional adaptive mechanisms of the schoolchild and how they contribute to healthy development, including to meet the developmental crisis of industry versus inferiority.

8. Evaluate the significance of peers and the chum relationship to the psychosocial development and health of the child.

9. Explore with parents their role in communication with and guidance of the child to foster healthy development in all spheres of personality.

10. Discuss the influence of media on health, development, and behavior of the child.

11. Describe the developmental tasks of the schoolchild and relate your role in helping him or her to achieve them.

MediaLink www.prenhall.com/murray

Go to the Companion Website for interactive resources that accompany this chapter.

Glossary	Critical Thinking
Review Questions	Tools
Challenge Your Knowledge	Media Link Applications
Learning Activities	Media Links

As growth and development continue and the child leaves the confines of the home, he or she emerges into a world of new experiences and responsibilities. If previous developmental tasks have been met and the child has developed a healthy personality, new knowledge and skills are acquired steadily. If previous developmental tasks have not been met and the child's personality development is immature, the child may experience difficulties mastering developmental tasks. Peers, parents, and other adults can have a positive, maturing influence if the child is adequately prepared for experiences outside the home, if individual needs are considered, and if he or she has some successful experiences.

The **school-age** years can be divided into **middle childhood** (*6 to 8 years of age*) and **late childhood** (*8 to 12 years of age*). The school-age years can also be divided into the juvenile and preadolescent periods. The **juvenile period** *begins at approximately age 6, marked by a need for peer associations.* **Preadolescence** *usually begins at 9 or 10 years of age and is marked by a new capacity to be loving, when the satisfaction and security of another person of the same sex (a chum) is as important to the child as personal satisfaction and security* (137). *Preadolescence ends at approximately 11 to 12 years with the onset of puberty. Preadolescence is also called* **prepubescence** *and is characterized by an increase in hormone production in both sexes, which is preparatory to eventual physiologic maturity.* Psychological and social changes also occur as the child slowly moves away from the family. This chapter discusses characteristics to assess and intervention measures for you to use in relation to health promotion for the child and family.

In many societies of the Western world, children are considered precious, valued, and vulnerable; they are protected and often are the first to be saved in an emergency. In less developed societies, many children do not live to adulthood. Thus, a child's life may be viewed as less valued. But each child is precious to his or her parents and loved ones. Illness or death of the child causes grief in the family in every country (7).

Some of the characteristics described in this chapter are not applicable to every child in the United States or children in underdeveloped, war-torn, or famine-stricken countries. Children in rural Appalachia and the Horn of Africa may grow up stunted in physical and intellectual potential from the malnutrition they suffer. The children in every war-torn country grow up with the haunted eyes of battle fatigue (90). Children in city slums worldwide may die early from communicable diseases and violence. Both the diary of Zlato Filipovic, age 10, a Bosnian girl of mixed heritage (46), and the diary of Anne Frank, a Dutch Jewish girl in World War II (49), as well as the daily newscasts, reveal the horrors of war and represent the uncertainty that many school-age children face.

Millions of children in the world are homeless street children living on garbage. Many of them are outcasts sold for prostitution, and they die young unless some humanitarian or religious agency takes them in for care and education. In some parts of the world, children are exploited and constantly exposed to danger. In 2000, 1.2 million children were victims in trafficking (144). Children between the ages of 6 and 12 are sold or given away by poor families to become bonded servants; the World Health Organization estimates 5.7 million children in 2000 (144). The children may be lured away or kidnapped from their impoverished homes to end up in slave labor, beaten, degraded, and often sexually abused. An estimated 1.8 million children were forced into prostitution and pornography in 2000 (144). Some are forced into being child soldiers (89, 90), or to toil as domestic servants or bonded laborers in factories or mines, or on farms or construction projects. In the United States, many urban children have learned to drop to the floor when there is a sound like a gunshot. For many children, violence is routine. Our media continues to have frequent reports of community, school, and family violence.

In the United States, the number of families with children who are homeless, or at risk for homelessness, is increasing because of societal, economic, employment, and housing trends. Homeless school-age children constitute a large percentage of homeless youth. They are more likely to have physical illness such as asthma, and emotional health problems such as anxiety, depression, or aggressive behavior. An estimated 25% of these children have witnessed family violence (66). Families who are homeless, often the working poor, can no longer live with relatives. Some shelters take the mother and school-age children, but the homeless family is forced to move from shelter to shelter because of residency time limits (2 weeks to 2 months).

Family income strongly correlates with optimal child development. Household wealth makes it easier for families to fulfill their developmental tasks (13, 57, 156). For example, children of teenage mothers encounter more risks to optimal development related to the mother's socioeconomic status than to her age (13, 140, 156). Children in single-mother households achieve more in school if their father regularly pays adequate child support (13, 62, 159). Yet, affluent families who satisfy the schoolchild's every material desire, allow the child to have a lifestyle appropriate for a teen or young adult, give little structure or limits on activities or peer group associations, and reinforce the child's "fast forward" behavior (growing up too fast) are not letting the child be a child. Overindulgence does not foster optimal development or health (40, 68, 141, 143).

Collaborate with other health care professionals to combat poverty and homelessness and their effects on children and families. Advocate that money, effort, and time be directed to:

1. Provide affordable housing to families who have low income or are in poverty, and provide wraparound services of health care, parent education, and employment opportunities.
2. Help children who are at risk of dropping out of school for physical, emotional, or social reasons with special tutoring so that academic performance and self-esteem can be strengthened.
3. Counsel parents and children in homes where abuse and violence are present; provide avenues for child safety.
4. Assist parents with child care; support efforts of parents who are trying to improve their incomes and life patterns.
5. Provide after-school services for children when parents cannot be in the home because of job demands.
6. Work at the community level to reduce violence in the neighborhoods, community, and school.
7. Support families in their efforts to protect their children from violence through church, community, and school programs.

8. Establish governmental policies and programs that will assist children, such as healthy school lunches, as well as eliminate causes of poverty, such as employment conditions, for families.

Family Development and Relationships

RELATIONSHIPS WITH PARENTS

Although parents remain a vital part of the schoolchild's life, the child's position within the family is altered with entry into school. *Both mother and father play a major role in socializing the child to the adult world as they* (15, 82, 83, 107):

1. Assume the role of love providers and caretakers.
2. Serve as identification figures and socialization agents.
3. Determine the sort of experiences the child will have.
4. Participate in the development of the child's self-concept.

The schoolchild channels energy into intellectual pursuits, widens social horizons, and becomes familiar with the adult world. He or she has identified with the parent of the same sex and, through imitation and education, continues to learn social roles and the tasks and routines expected by the culture or social group. The family atmosphere has much impact on the child's emotional development and future response within the family when he or she becomes an adolescent. Research indicates that children can become positive in their behavior whether they are reared in authoritarian or permissive homes, if parents are consistent in their approach and promote harmony and stability in the home (13, 124). In Asian American, African American, and Mexican American families that are authoritarian but convey encouragement and warmth, children perceive parents positively—as caring (7, 60). Rejecting and neglectful families foster harmful effects (7).

Although parental support is needed, the schoolchild pulls away from overt signs of parental affection. Yet during illness or when threatened by his or her new status, the child turns to parents for affection and protection. Parents get frustrated with behavioral changes, antics, and infractions of household rules.

The child changes ideas about and behavior toward parents and adults as he or she grows. See **Box 12-1**, The Schoolchild's View of Parents and Adults (107).

There is no "typical family" for school-age children. The nuclear family in the traditional roles does exist. Yet, *in the United States, millions of children experience* (13, 107):

1. Both parents (or parent and stepparent) working outside of the home; 75% of mothers with school-age children are employed. Many children have never known a time when their mother was not working for pay outside of the home.
2. One parent in the home; 25% of all children under age 18 live with a single parent, and this type of family is more likely to be poor.
3. A sibling or parent with a physical or mental disability or an emotional or behavioral disorder. Some children grow up while their parents are hospitalized or in prison or jail.

> ### BOX 12-1   The Schoolchild's View of Parents and Adults
>
> **AGES 6–8**
> 1. Is still primarily family oriented
> 2. Sees parents as good, powerful, and wise
> 3. Seeks parental approval
> 4. Becomes emotionally steadier and freer from parents
>
> **AGES 9–12**
> 1. Begins to question parental authority
> 2. Tends to feel smarter than parents, teachers, and adults in general
> 3. Sees same-sex parent as more harsh disciplinarian

4. No home of their own; they live doubled up with relatives or in shelters.
5. The grind of poverty on a daily basis. In the United States, 33% of all children live in poverty at some time. Most American Indian children living on reservations live in poverty. The number of children of families who recently emigrated from another country to the United States who live in poverty is unknown; however, the percentage is believed to be high.

Proportionately more children in the United States live in poverty than in any other industrialized country. Being poor affects all dimensions of development (13, 14, 107, 124). Refer to Chapter 6 ∞ for more information about trends in family life.

Children growing up in homes without fathers more often have lowered academic performances, more cognitive and intellectual deficits, increased adjustment problems, and higher risks for psychosexual development problems (107). However, another nurturing man or a grandfather can serve as a "social father," or a grandmother may provide guidance, warmth, and practical help (for example, in some African American homes). Children in these homes are effectively nurtured and achieve well in school. The children try to stay out of trouble and make the family and community proud of them (13). Children who experience parental divorce, compared with children in continuously intact two-parent families, exhibit more symptoms of psychological maladjustment and social problems, lower academic achievement, and lower self-concept. *Variations in reactions to divorce exist, however, depending on* (107):

1. Amount and quality of contact with the nonresidential parent.
2. Custodial parent's psychological adjustment and parenting skills.
3. Level of interparental conflict preceding and following divorce.
4. Degree of economic hardship.
5. Number of stressful life experiences that accompany and follow divorce.

In families with many disruptive or transitional relationships, repeated cohabitation, and divorce, the children are more likely to quit school, leave home, use drugs, become delinquent, and become a parent before age 20 (13, 124).

Review with families the **tasks that must be resolved by children after divorce** (13, 93, 107, 124). Refer to **Table 12-1** for specific information. Encourage schools to have counselors to conduct group sessions for students who are experiencing separation or divorce of parents. These sessions can help students toward resolution of the tasks listed in Table 12-1, which in turn should enhance their scholastic ability.

Because of one-parent homes or homes with both parents employed, the child may face another kind of experience. The **latchkey child**, *the child who is given the door key to let self into the home after school because the parents are still at work, may not see the parents from early morning until late afternoon or evening.* The child is unsupervised from 2 to 4 hours daily after school and probably for the whole day during the summer months when school is not in session (124, 143). Children voice different feelings about the working mother and having no one at home to meet them after school. Some like it. They enjoy the solitude, privacy, responsibility, and closeness of each other at day's end. Some hate it for the same reasons. Some tolerate it out of necessity, disliking the separation and lack of time together. Some are afraid for themselves and their mothers. Some are proud of their mother and how they are managing together (143). Some become discipline problems. Without limits and parental supervision, they may get themselves into trouble, especially using the computer and e-mail, playing video games, or calling peers. They are more likely than supervised children to abuse a sibling, have academic or social problems at school, steal or vandalize, or engage in juvenile delinquent behavior (74). All understand the financial reasons and sometimes the career and emotional reasons that are usually the basis for their mother working. Some girls say they want to work as a result, and some want to be homemakers when they grow up (124). Programs such as YWCA Latch Key Programs and day care centers that provide longer hours of care accommodate the child after school. Safety measures are critical.

Educate parents, as needed. Not only poor, single-parent, or stepparent families need help. Many middle-class or upper-class families need education and counseling because they do not feel confident about raising their children. Explore stressors in the family. Explore feelings of family members. Although the poor child frequently shares the helplessness of an unemployed parent, the higher-income child often feels the relentless pressure on the parent who is a high-powered corporate executive, lawyer, professor, or government official preoccupied with his or her own survival. Too often the demands of the workplace encroach on the needs and happiness of the family. Educate about and validate use of stress management measures.

Educate parents that the child must be given time—physically, emotionally, mentally, and socially—to be a child and to learn about the world at an individual pace. Too often parents want to hurry the child into adulthood (13, 40, 141, 142). Television, films, advertisements, peers, and neighbors all exert pressure on the child to wear adult clothes and cosmetics; to be sexually precocious; to manipulate parents into fewer limits and less guidance; to take technology, materialism, and money for granted; and often to

TABLE 12-1

Psychological Tasks for Children After Divorce

Task I: Understanding the Divorce

Schoolchildren

1. Understand the immediate changes.
2. Differentiate fantasy from reality.
3. Manage concerns regardng abandonment, placement in foster care, not seeing departed parent again.

Adolescents and Young Adults

1. Understand what led to marital failure.
2. Evaluate parents' actions.
3. Draw useful conclusions for their own lives.

Task II: Strategic Withdrawal

1. Acknowledge concern and provide appropriate help to parents and siblings.
2. Avoid divorce as the total focus and get back to their own interests, pleasures, activities, peer relationships.
3. Children allowed to remain children.

Task III: Dealing with Loss

1. Deal with loss of intact family and loss of presence of one parent, usually the father.
2. Deal with feelings of rejection and blame for making one parent leave.
3. Task is easier if child has good relationship with both parents; this may be most difficult task.

Task IV: Dealing with Anger

1. Manage anger at parents for deciding to divorce.
2. Be aware of parents' needs, anxiety, and loneliness.
3. Diminish anger and forgive.

Task V: Working Out Guilt

1. Deal with sense of guilt for causing marital difficulties and driving wedge between parents.
2. Separate guilty ties and get on with their lives.

Task VI: Accepting Permanence of Divorce

1. Overcome early denial and fantasies of parents getting back together.
2. Task may not be completed until parent remarries or child mourns loss.

Task VII: Taking a Chance on Love

1. Remain open to love, commitment, marriage, fidelity.
2. Able to turn away from parents' model.
3. Most important task for growing children, adolescents, and young adults.

INTERVENTIONS FOR HEALTH PROMOTION

If the child is to return home before the parent arrives, advise parents to teach the following measures to the child:

1. Do not display keys and always lock doors. Keep a spare key at a neighbor's house.
2. Do not go into the house after school if the door is ajar, a window is open, or anything looks unusual. Families who will be at home and available for help with emergencies should be known by the child.
3. Do not open the door to anyone unless the person has been approved by the parent.
4. Do not get in cars with strangers.
5. Use first aid procedures; know where the safety kit is located.
6. Use safety rules if expected to cook. Microwave ovens are the safest. Parents should not expect too much from the child.
7. Use fire safety rules, such as leaving the house and not returning to it if a fire starts. Practice fire drills and evacuation at home, including a safe place to meet outside the home.
8. Use weather-related safety rules: (a) stay in the house in an electric storm and (b) stay in the basement or in the safest part of the house during a tornado warning. Practice tornado drills with children and keep a flashlight handy in case of power failures.
9. Use water safety rules, such as not playing in the backyard pool when alone and no swimming without adult supervision. If the older child is expected to care for an infant or toddler, teach safe bathing methods.
10. Do not handle firearms that are in the home. Firearms should be locked in storage.
11. Tell people who call on the telephone that the parents are busy rather than saying, "They're not here."
12. Keep police, fire department, and other important telephone numbers by the phone. Know how to report emergencies.
13. Follow rules about what may or may not be done until the parent gets home. Offer a choice of activities other than television.
14. Report anything of concern that happened before the parent arrived home.

If parents provide a cell phone for the child to foster safety, the child should be thoroughly taught about the reasons for having it, safe usage, and cost factors.

---

participate in a multitude of after- (or before-) school activities. Parents believe their child must be the "early maturer" (40, 141, 142). The pressures and hurry, especially in the middle-class and lower-upper-class urban family, are contributing to a growing number of troubled children who are emotionally distressed or ill or who are antisocial (13, 141, 142). If the child must be hurried through childhood and if the child cannot be accepted for who he or she is, feelings of being unloved, rejected, and inferior grow ever deeper and bigger.

As a health care professional, you care for the family and the individual child. Help parents clarify and act on their values. As a school nurse, your assessment may be the key to a child receiving necessary care; many children do not have a family doctor. Conduct many of the health promotion activities that are described throughout this chapter. Counsel and teach both parents and children in any health care setting. Be aware of cultural beliefs and practices as you work with children and families. A family who has lived in this country for several generations may follow the same cultural patterns as the new immigrant family. Finally, as a citizen, your vote to pass health-related legislation is important and may be as crucial to health promotion as immunizations.

RELATIONSHIPS WITH SIBLINGS

Although parental influence is of primary importance, the child's relationship with siblings affects personality formation. The influence of siblings on the development of the school-age child depends on a number of factors, including age and sex of the siblings,

number of children in the family, proximity of their ages, and type of parent-child interaction.

Relationships between the school-age child and siblings vary from jealousy, rivalry, and competition to protectiveness and deep affection. Siblings tend to get along more harmoniously when they are the same gender, but boys usually are more physically aggressive at all ages. School-age children need privacy and personal space. Quarrels and conflicts erupt when this need is violated. Although sibling jealousy is less acute in school-age children than in preschool children, it still exists. An older child may be jealous of the attention given to younger siblings and may resent having to help with their care. The younger school-age child may feel jealous of the freedom given to older siblings. School-age children may feel the need to compete for parental attention and academic excellence. Parental comparisons of siblings' scholastic and artistic abilities or behavior should be avoided as they add to jealousy and resentment.

Adjustment outside the home is generally regarded as easier for the child with siblings than for the only child, who may develop a very close, intense relationship with the parents. The only child may cling to the notion of being the center of the family and may expect to be the center of attention in other groups as well. As a result, he or she may find the give and take of social living difficult. The differences in socialization between small and large families and for the only child are discussed in Chapter 6. ∞

Sibling relationships are likely to influence social interactions in later life. Siblings teach each other how to negotiate, cooperate, compete, support, and reward one another and how to work and play with others. One child's illness or disability will have an effect on a healthy sibling, either positive or negative. Siblings of chronically ill children may work hard at being helpful to parents and the ill child, or even be overprotective, to receive attention and approval as well as to convey love. The siblings may also become depressed, withdraw, or act out in various ways to receive attention. They may have more school problems, or they may excel at school if that is the reinforcer. In part, *how the siblings react depends on the psychological health of parents and their marital adjustment, and on the parents' ability to allow siblings to express their feelings:* (a) anger, guilt, exclusion, deprivation, and jealousy; (b) fears of family breakup; and (c) feelings related to how their life differs from the life patterns of their friends (e.g., fewer outings, increased chores, less money for desired items).

Explore with the family the strategies used to handle sibling conflicts and maintain positive, healthy relationships. Discuss with the children their feelings about each other's behavior and how they resolve issues. If one of the children is chronically ill—physically, mentally, or emotionally—discuss how the other children cope with the stressors involved, the caregiving role, and their feelings about the situation.

FAMILY DEVELOPMENTAL TASKS

Family activities with the school-age child revolve around expanding the child's world. Tasks include the following (37, 156):

1. Take on parenting roles; provide food, clothing, shelter, and basic necessities that the child cannot provide for self.
2. Adjust the family system and lifestyle to allow physical, emotional, and social space for the child.
3. Keep lines of communication open among family members.
4. Form a cooperative parental alliance that supports each other.
5. Work together to achieve common goals.
6. Plan a lifestyle within economic means.
7. Find creative ways to continue a mutually satisfactory married life or satisfactory single parenthood.
8. Maintain close ties with extended family or supportive friends.
9. Realign relationships with the extended family to include their nurturing or grandparenting roles.
10. Expand family life into the community through various activities and through peers.
11. Validate the family philosophy of life. The philosophy is tested when the child brings home new ideas and talks about different lifestyles, forcing the family to reexamine patterns of living.
12. Encourage learning: Ensure that the child receives the necessary education, motivate and guide the child to master academic skills, and foster an understanding of the family history.
13. Love and nurture the child to foster a sense of being loved and accepted, positive self-esteem, and competence.
14. Provide predictable family routines, safety, security, harmony, and stability.

These tasks are manifested differently by families from various cultural backgrounds, such as those who are homeless, live in poverty, work as migrants, or live in war-torn or Third World countries.

As you care for families and assist them to achieve their developmental tasks and foster a healthy family, consider the uniqueness of the family situation and system. Prepare families for their changing functions. Educating parents about their roles and the developmental needs and abilities of children and discussing the parents' personal belief systems may be a better way to help them accomplish parenting tasks than to dwell on their parenting behaviors (15).

Adoptive families have the same developmental tasks as other families. An issue for adoptive parents, however, is how to help their adopted child feel part of the family, especially if adoption occurs at an age when the child remembers the process. Refer to Chapter 6 ∞ for more information about adoptive families. **Table 12-2** describes the adopted child's perception of adoption during the school years and how adoptive parents may respond.

The adopted child especially struggles with identity issues because of uncertainties about the past, especially if the child is of different racial or ethnic origin than the parents. The child may become rebellious, saying, for example, "I don't have to obey you—you're not my real mom." Parents must remain open to the youth's questions, sustain an accepting and open atmosphere, expect challenges, and help him or her find other supportive adults. Parents should not smother with concern, give in to unreasonable demands, or hold a grudge against the child who is acting ungratefully. (Most children do.) Adoption is not a constant issue, but parents cannot ever completely retreat from it (13, 94).

Counsel with the parents and adopted child about the issues and related feelings that arise at home, at school, or in community activities. *Explore with the family how to work with the child's teacher in relation to class assignments about:* (a) genetic diseases in the family (which may be unknown); (b) a genogram or family tree (ambivalent feelings in the older child about who to include—biological, foster, or adoptive family); (c) a child or family picture (potential embarrassment in transracial families); or (d) a story about the family history, which can trigger strong feelings of loss and grief, embarrassment, anger, or guilt in the case of past abuse or multiple foster families because of behavioral problems. Discuss with elementary teachers how these assignments can be approached in a culturally sensitive way and that these assignments can be equally difficult for children from other family structures: single-parent, stepparent, foster, lesbian/gay, multiethnic, or transracial. Family diversity must be a consideration in the classroom when discussing family issues or tasks and types of families. Teachers and school administrators need to understand that certain lessons can affect children very differently. Encourage parents to collaborate with the child's teacher. Explore ways that the parent, teacher, and child can handle negative statements about adoption in the media or peer conversations. Such discussions of feelings, coping strategies, and the circles of caring people will set the foundation for the child to face his or her own later identity issues. Prepare adoptive families for when the adopted child may initiate search for the birth parent.

RELATIONSHIPS OUTSIDE THE FAMILY

As the child's social environment widens, other individuals begin to function as role models and to influence the child. The child strives for independence and establishes meaningful relationships

TABLE 12-2

Adopted Child's Perceptions and Suggested Parental Responses

Age	Child's Perception	Suggested Parental Response
5–7	Begins to grasp full notion of adoption, that parents are not blood relatives, and that most children live with biological parent(s) Feels sense of loss	Emphasize that child is important to them and was chosen. Answer questions comfortably and naturally. Explain it is normal for child to have mixed emotions about adoption.
8–11	Fantasizes and wonders about birth parents Realizes he or she is different from nonadopted children Wants to question parents about adoption but fears appearing disloyal or ungrateful Feels grief and goes through mourning process Frequently asks questions about why birth parents relinquished him or her, parent's appearance, and whether there are siblings	Discuss the adoption openly, when appropriate, to help the child vent curiosity and feelings. Help child accept fact that he or she is different and emphasize other differences as well. Answer questions truthfully. Do not criticize or overpraise birth parents. Adjust depth of answer to age of child. Realize children who are not adopted also fantasize that they are.

with peers, teachers, and other significant adults. These relationships provide the child with new ideas, attitudes, perspectives, and modes of behavior. Although the parents remain role models, the influence of the family and the time spent with family diminish. Parents may feel a loss of control and may actually experience ambivalent feelings toward the child's peers and new adult role models. Influences outside the family may cause the child to verbalize less love and respect for parents, to resent limits imposed by the family, and to question ideas, attitudes, and beliefs held by the family. Through contacts with the peer group, the child acquires a basis for judging the parents as individuals and learns that parents can make mistakes.

The schoolchild has a growing sense of community that changes with increased mobility and independence and added responsibility. His or her understanding broadens to include a sense of boundaries, distance, location, and spatial relationships of resources and organizations, demographic characteristics, and group identity.

You are in a key position to listen to and explore with families their concerns about being parents and adjusting to the growing and changing child. Discuss ways to handle problems between siblings, and with relatives, peers, and other adults outside the home. At times you may validate their approach to a given situation. At other times you may help them clarify their values so they can, in turn, better guide the child. Such practical suggestions as how to plan nutritious meals more economically or how to handle sibling rivalry can help a distraught parent feel and become more effective. Validate parental behavior that promotes holistic health. Instill confidence. Give information. Help the family use community resources effectively to meet basic needs and promote physical and emotional health.

MALTREATMENT, ABUSE, AND NEGLECT

Refer to information presented in Chapters 8, 9, 10, and 11 ∞ as a base for understanding the health risk that may begin in this life era or continue from prior eras. Maltreatment, abuse, and neglect destroy health—physically, emotionally, cognitively, socially, and spiritually. Health care professionals and systems must address this epidemic for individual, family, and societal health promotion.

Abuse

A history of a perceived negative relationship with parents in childhood and abuse or neglect during childhood are significant risk factors for engaging in child abuse (3, 13, 43, 50, 68, 98, 107, 112, 124). If the parent received severe punishment as a child or recalls the punishment as unfair, severe, and persistent, the person is more likely to have difficulty controlling aggressive impulses and to freely express violence. Abusive families tend to be more isolated, have fewer supportive relationships, and have low self-esteem (68, 98). *Maltreatment frequently involves physical, verbal, and emotional dimensions;* it is difficult to separate effects of each of these upon the child. In addition, sexual abuse may also be present. *Maltreatment includes* (a) discrimination; (b) humiliating punishment at school; (c) neglect and use of physical restraint in the child's home; (d) brutality by law enforcement officers; (e) witnessing violence in the home against a parent, siblings, other family members such as grandparents, or pets; and (f) witnessing gang activities, gunshots, or physical assaults in the home or residential area. Infanticide and "honor killings," which are a part of some cultures, are considered as maltreatment outside of that culture (144).

A thorough *assessment* is necessary to differentiate organically caused physical disease states from conditions caused by maltreatment, abuse, or neglect. The disease state may be the same; the etiology has to be differentiated. In addition to overt injury, *exposure to the violence of maltreatment and abuse contributes to* (a) symptoms of the Alarm Stage of the General Adaptation Syndrome described in Chapter 2 ∞, (b) acute stress disorder at the peak of the incident, (c) symptoms of chronic stress because of persistence of maltreatment, and (d) various physical injuries or illnesses. Assessment may involve a multidisciplinary team approach and a variety of diagnostic measures. *Treatment should be directed to the presenting condition. The holistic approach and health promotion focus will assess and care for the individual and the family system.* Consider dynamics of behavior; execute necessary documentation and reporting; and conduct intervention, follow-up, and referral in an approach relevant for the schoolchild and family.

Educate parents and adults who work with children about attitudes and behaviors that will help the child protect self. Refer to Chapter 11 ∞; some of the guidelines for personal safety of the child are applicable. Also refer to **Table 12-3**, Personal Safety Skills to Be Taught to the Child. Teach parents and caregivers in the home about appropriate and inappropriate touch of the child, how to detect symptoms or behaviors in the child that indicate any form of maltreatment, and how to handle the situation when sexual abuse or other maltreatment has occurred.

Educate parents about their responsibility to keep their children safe from maltreatment and abuse from others. *That may mean speaking alone to the mother* about potential or actual abusive behavior from the child's father, her live-in partner, other family members or friends who spend time alone with the child, or the babysitter or caretaker. *Your approach must be gentle and unhurried, and convey caring, not a judgmental approach.* Clarify and summarize what her nonverbal and verbal behavior implies, especially if she has "hunches" about sexual abuse or conveys guilt about verbal, emotional, or physical "punishment," which may in reality be abuse. Encourage the parent (usually the mother) to tell the child about personal safety skills, to carefully listen to the child, and to monitor the child's behavior and responses around people. Teach information presented in **Table 12-3**, Personal Safety Skills to Be Taught to the Child, and **Table 12-4**, How Parents Can Prevent or Intervene in Child Abuse, which is pertinent to physical, verbal, or emotional abuse, as well as sexual abuse.

Refer the parents to community resources, including professionals/agencies where the child and parent can receive counseling. Emphasize that the parent will be fostering health of the child, the self, and the family when seeking help.

Psychological and sexual abuse may be especially difficult to assess. Therefore, it is difficult to implement intervention measures. More secrecy surrounds these forms of abuse. Refer to **Box 12-2**, Parental Behavior Characteristic of Psychological Maltreatment of the Schoolchild, for assessment information (51, 52). Risks for sexual abuse occurrence and common family characteristics are presented in **Table 12-5**, Sexual Abuse of the Schoolchild (13, 17–20, 44, 98, 130, 144).

Sexual maltreatment or abuse can be assessed and categorized as (2, 3, 44, 98):

1. **Incest**—*Any physical-sexual activity between family members other than legally sanctioned spouses; blood relationship is not required.* Thus, stepparent sexual activity with the child is considered incest.
2. **Molestation**—*Indecent behavior, such as unwanted, inappropriate, or forced touching, fondling, kissing, forced individual or mutual masturbation, or genital contact or penetration.*
3. **Cunnilingus**—*Oral contact with female genitals.*
4. **Fellatio**—*Oral contact with male genitalia.*
5. **Exhibitionism**—*Indecent exposure of the genitals, usually with the desire to shock or surprise the observer.*
6. **Child pornography**—*Arranging and photographing (in any media) sexual acts with or involving children, either alone or*

TABLE 12-3

Personal Safety Skills to Be Taught to the Child

1. **Walk and behave in a confident manner,** *especially if a peer is a bully or an adult is overwhelming;* **trust his or her own judgment** if "things don't seem right."
2. **Believe that his or her body belongs to the self;** that the child has a right to love, be proud of, and protect his or her body.
3. **Avoid playing in deserted or dark places.**
4. **Avoid talking with strangers,** or replying, even if they seem friendly.
5. **Break rules to protect self in a potentially dangerous situation.**
6. **Talk with a parent or a trusted adult, such as a teacher, about situations that are threatening to the child,** including being bullied at school.
7. **Realize that hugs and kisses are nice but are never to be kept secret.**
8. **Say "No" and get away from anyone who is touching the child's "private places," the genital area, or any area of the body that feels uncomfortable.**
9. **Refuse to keep "secrets,"** even if an adult says to keep a hug, kiss, touch, or activity a secret.
10. **Refuse invitations to go to a "special" or "secret" place,** even if the person is known to the child.
11. **Realize that there is the responsibility of each person to treat the body respectfully** through personal behavior, careful use of gestures, manner of dress, and nonseductive use of nonverbal behavior.
12. **Believe that if someone is abusive in any way, it is not the child's fault. The child cannot consent to sexual abuse.**

TABLE 12-4

How Parents Can Prevent or Intervene in Child Abuse

1. **Build the child's self-esteem** with praise, love, and appropriate attention; maintain a positive relationship.
2. **Choose appropriate caregivers;** avoid leaving the child alone at home if at all possible.
3. **Discuss all types of personal safety behavior** in a matter-of-fact way, using words the child can understand.
4. **Maintain supervision or awareness of the child's activities** throughout the day/week.
5. **Avoid overnight visits in other homes,** whether with relatives or friends.
6. **Maintain open communication** at any time of the day or night, between the parent and child; **be available** as much as possible.
7. **Encourage the child to share fears, concerns, or secrets** about being with another adult, including the other parent, or a child, including siblings and peers.
8. **Believe what the child says; children seldom lie about abuse.**
9. **Listen to the child's verbal and nonverbal behavior,** especially when with specific people (any relative, the other parent, a caregiver), or changes in the child's behavior toward these individuals.
10. **Observe for inconsistencies between verbal statements and overall behavior** when the child is in the presence of others, for example, saying "I love you," but avoiding a hug or kiss that had been part of the behavior pattern.
11. **Repeat regularly to the child the list of personal safety skills** in order to empower the child.
12. **Seek professional help** (individual or community agency) to explore personal feelings, observations, and "intuitions" or "hunches" about the child's behavior or changing patterns.

with peers, adults, or animals, regardless of consent of the child or by the child's legal guardian. Distribution of such material, with or without profit, that occurs publicly in various forms is considered pornography.

7. **Child prostitution**–Involving children in sex acts for profit and usually with changing partners.

8. **Pedophilia**–Preferring children, often of a specific age, gender, or ethnicity, as a means of achieving sexual excitement; sexual activity with a prepubescent child, generally 13 years or younger. The pedophile is at least 16 years of age and at least 5 years older than the child and has been involved with the child for at least 6 months (2, 3, 93).

BOX 12-2 — Parental Behavior Characteristic of Psychological Maltreatment of the Schoolchild

REJECTING

1. Communicates negative definitions of self to the child
2. Creates a sense of "bad-me" or negative self-concept by consistently calling child negative names such as stupid, dummy, monster
3. Belittles child's accomplishments regularly
4. Scapegoats child in the family system
5. Criticizes constantly so that child has no prospect of meeting expectations

ISOLATING

1. Removes child from normal social relations with peers
2. Prohibits child from playing with or inviting children into the home
3. Withdraws child from school

TERRORIZING

1. Places child in double bind
2. Demands opposite or conflicting behavior or emotions simultaneously from the child
3. Forces child to choose one of the two parents
4. Changes rules of the house or of relationships with parents frequently

IGNORING

1. Fails to protect child from threats or intervene on behalf of the child
2. Does not protect child from assault from siblings or other family members
3. Does not respond to child's request for help or feedback

CORRUPTING

1. Rewards child for stealing, substance abuse, assaulting other children, and sexual precocity
2. Goads child into attacking other children
3. Exposes child to pornography
4. Encourages drug use
5. Reinforces sexually aggressive behavior
6. Involves child sexually with adolescents or adults

Source: From Garbarino, J., Guttmann, E., & Seeley, J. (1987). The psychologically battered child: Strategies for identification, assessment and intervention. San Francisco: Jossey-Bass. Adapted by permission of Jossey-Bass, Inc., a subsidiary of John Wiley & Sons, Inc.

TABLE 12-5

Sexual Abuse of the Schoolchild*

Risk Factors

1. Having a stepfather
2. Poor relationship between child and parent
3. Mothers who work outside the home or are emotionally distant
4. Having a parent who does not live with the child
5. Sex: 25% of all females and 10% of all males by age 18

Family Characteristics

1. An emotionally dependent adult male in the home
2. Sexual estrangement between the parents or parental figures
3. Mother deserted the family (literally or figuratively)
4. Sexual offender suffers a crisis, i.e., loss of job
5. Daughter begins to mature sexually
6. Parent has poor impulse control
7. Problems such as substance abuse, personality disorders, psychoses, and mental retardation in parent(s)

*The legal definition differs from state to state.

Pedophiles may limit activity to their own children, stepchildren, or relatives (incest) or may victimize children outside their family. Access to children may occur through the Internet, child abduction in the community, or taking in foster children, especially from other countries. The pedophile may threaten the child to prevent disclosure. Or, the pedophile may be attentive to the child's needs in order to gain the child's affection, interest, and loyalty, and to prevent disclosure (2, 3, 98). Often behavior to the child is inconsistent, which adds to the child's fear and confusion.

Mandatory reporting is the first step, but assessment and intervention takes time and a careful approach. Use of art or play therapy principles may initially be more effective in assessment or counseling than verbal interview. (Refer to References 17–20, 34, 68, 93, 98, 158, 159.) The child may be unable to explain the sexual activity verbally, either because of lack of knowledge of words to use, or because of fear, anxiety, or anger. The child will need time to vent feelings, resolve unrealistic guilt, reintegrate self-concept and body image, and resolve relationship issues, especially if the perpetrator remains visible and active in the child's life. How state agencies and authorities handle the situation will affect the approach of you or another professional with the perpetrator.

Neglect

Neglect, *deprivation of necessities,* is easier to identify when manifested physically. However, emotional neglect, which has less obvious signs, may take months or years to be manifested in behavior (107, 124). Emotional neglect or abuse is also more difficult to substantiate. Any persistent or unexplained change in the child's behavior may be caused by **emotional abuse,** *threats to self-concept and personhood,* or **neglect of emotional needs,** *lack of attention, love, or security.* Refer to Chapter 11 ∞ for information about neglect, which is also relevant to the schoolchild.

Abduction

Abduction of the schoolchild is as much a concern as earlier, as the child is more likely to be away from parents—walking to school or going places with peers. The child who is abducted is likely to be abused and neglected or even killed. Information presented in Chapters 10 and 11 is also relevant. ∞

Educate parents to have the child fingerprinted and to have other identifiers, such as dental imprints, available. Educate parents about risks of abduction; potential reasons for the kidnapping, such as pedophile behavior; preventive measures; and ways to cope with unplanned situations. Explain also the Amber Alert System and how law enforcement officers can be helpful. Explore with parents how to teach the child safety behavior described in this and previous chapters and to reinforce that they will always be the parents, will always love the child, and will always want the child to be in the family and in the home. Parents should build the child's confidence so that he or she would not believe anyone who speaks otherwise. Reinforce the importance of the child seeking help from a police officer if ever in a scary or dangerous situation. Discuss ways to warn the child without creating unnecessary fear about everything and everyone. The parent has to choose the timing and what to say based on the child's development.

Educate professionals and volunteers who work with children how to (a) effectively communicate with and observe children for signs and symptoms of maltreatment, abuse, or neglect; (b) teach children how to protect themselves and seek help; (c) identify and intervene with these children; and (d) detect people who may be or are molesting children. *Work with child-serving institutions and programs* (churches, day care centers, schools, Boy/Girl Scouts, other children's clubs, and competitive sports teams) to develop policies and procedures for screening, training, and monitoring all staff and volunteers about health-promoting and effective ways to work with children. *Consult with institutions* to design the physical environment to provide openness and visibility within the facility to prevent any staff or volunteer from having the opportunity to be unseen or unsupervised with a child.

Educate the public about the hidden prevalence and detrimental effects of maltreatment, abuse, or neglect. Work with community agencies and professionals in creating safe environments and prevention programs, and in de-emphasizing aggression, violence, and sexuality in media programming.

Physiologic Concepts and Physical Characteristics

GENERAL APPEARANCE

The *principles of growth or growth patterns* are comparable across cultures, generally. For example, progression of maturation of body organ systems is similar in all cultural groups (7, 60). The child between 6 and 12 years old exhibits considerable change in physical appearance (13, 58, 59, 68, 107, 112, 126). Growth during this stage of development is **hypertrophic** (*cells increase in size*) instead of **hyperplastic** (*cells increase in number*). The growth rate is usually slower than infancy or puberty/adolescence but steady, characterized by periods of accelerations in the spring and fall and by rapid growth during preadolescence. Children are generally taller and mostly wiry.

WEIGHT, HEIGHT, AND GIRTH

These measurements vary considerably among children and depend on genetic, environmental, nutritional, gender, and cultural influences. It is essential to look at the individual child and compare growth patterns to his or her own norms and history. Females have more adipose tissue than males (58, 59, 68, 107).

Children from high socioeconomic levels are taller in all cultures. Generally, African American and Caucasian children are tallest, followed by American Indians and Asian Americans (7). African American children and Caucasian children from lower socioeconomic groups usually are smaller in weight and height. Growth retardation is more reflective of socioeconomic than ethnic and genetic factors (7, 60, 68, 107).

African American children may be taller than Caucasian children during the school years. At age 6 years, the African American female has more bone and muscle mass than the European American or Mexican American female (7, 107, 112). Around puberty, the growth rate of African Americans slows and Caucasian children catch up, so the two races achieve similar heights in adulthood. Most Asian children born and raised in the United States or Canada are larger and taller than those children born and raised in Asian countries because of differences in diet, climate, and social milieu (7). The Latino child has a higher percentage of body adipose tissue than the Caucasian child of the same age (107).

The *average schoolchild grows* 2 to 2.5 in. (5 to 6 cm) per year to gain 1 to 2 ft (30 to 60 cm) in height by age 12. A *weight gain* of 4 to 7 pounds (2 to 3.5 kg) occurs per year. The average weight for a 6-year-old boy is 48 pounds (21.5 kg), and the average height is 46 in. (117 cm). By 8 years, the child weighs about 55 pounds (25 kg). At age 10 years, the child weighs about 70 pounds (32 kg) and is 54 in. (1.37 meters) tall (13, 124). At age 11, the female is taller than the male. By age 12, the average child weighs approximately 88 to 90 pounds (40 kg) and is more than 59 in. tall (150 cm). By age 12, the child has usually attained 90% of adult height (13, 68, 107, 112, 124).

During the *juvenile or middle childhood period*, females and males may differ little in size. Their bodies are usually lean, with narrow hips and shoulders. There is a gradual decrease in the amount of baby fat with an increase in muscle mass and strength. Although the amount of muscle mass and adipose tissue is influenced by muscle use, diet, and activity, males usually have more muscle cells, which accounts for heavier weight and greater strength, compared to females. Females have more adipose tissue. Muscle growth is occurring at a rapid rate. The muscles are changing in composition and are becoming more firmly attached to the bones. Muscles may be immature in regard to function, resulting in vulnerability to injury stemming from overuse, awkwardness, and inefficient movement. Muscle aches may accompany skeletal growth spurts as developing muscles attempt to keep pace with the enlarging skeletal structure. As the skeletal bones lengthen, they become harder. **Ossification,** *the formation of bone,* continues at a

steady pace. The schoolchild loses the potbellied, swayback appearance of early childhood. Abdominal muscles become stronger, the pelvis tips backward, and posture becomes straighter (13, 68, 112, 124, 126).

NEUROLOGIC SYSTEM

The *brain* of the child is very active. Brain development is affected by genetics, culture, and practice. Functional brain imaging reveals that different brain regions are activated when the individual engages in different cognitive activities, for example, reading and arithmetic (35). Throughout the school years *myelination is completed and dendritic branching continues* in the sensory and motor cortices. *Hemispheric specialization* makes the brain more efficient. The areas of the brain governing use of language, logic, memory, and spatial knowledge become more complex in function. *Prefrontal cortex development* allows the child to better control emotional outbursts and inattention, analyze consequences of behavior before an emotional outburst, and respond to routines (35). **Selective attention** improves: *The child can select, attend to, and coordinate impulses from all neurologic regions simultaneously through use of both active and inactive processes,* heeding the most important elements, analyzing simultaneous stimuli, and responding to the most appropriate stimuli (35). Studies reveal that from age 4 to puberty, glucose metabolism by brain cells is twice that of the adult brain (63). Thus the child is capable of processing new information readily (68).

By age 7 the brain has reached 90% of adult size. The growth rate of the brain is slowed after age 7, but by age 12 the brain has virtually reached adult size. Memory has improved. The child can listen better and make associations between incoming stimuli (68). However, the child does not have the mental maturity of an adult. A national database on the range of normal brain development in healthy children is being developed through the MRI Study of Normal Brain Development conducted by the National Institutes of Health (75).

Refer to **Table 12-6** for a summary of neuromuscular development from 6 to 12 years of age (13, 68, 107, 124, 126).

MUSCULOSKELETAL SYSTEM

Neuromuscular changes are occurring, related to completed *myelination,* along with skeletal development. Myelination improves fine motor skills. *Ossification* continues; bones harden (13, 68). Neuromuscular coordination is sufficient to permit the schoolchild to learn most skills he or she wishes. Reaction time in performance shortens. By *10 to 12 years of age, hand manipulative skills* are similar to that of adults; females outperform males. The child can master almost any basic skill with grace and precision as long as the task does not require strength or split-second judgment of speed and distance (13). *Improved coordination* of each side of the body and performance of complex tasks occur because of neuronal connections formed in the brain. The *corpus callosum* continues to mature between hemispheres. Practice and play help the brain process faster and more efficiently (13). Play advances brain development. Rough-and-tumble play appears to help regulate and coordinate the *frontal lobes of the brain,* in turn reducing attention

TABLE 12-6

Neuromuscular Development in the Schoolchild

Age (Yr)	Characteristic
6	High activity level but clumsy
	Moves constantly: skips, hops, runs, roller skates
	Can do manipulative skills: hammer, cut, paste, tie shoes, fasten clothes
	Grasps pencil or crayon, makes large letters or figures
	Can throw with proper weight shift and step
	Walks chalk mark with balance
	Tandem gait
	Girls are superior in movement accuracy
	Boys are superior in forceful, less complex activity
7	Lower activity level; enjoys being quiet or active
	Pedals a bicycle
	Prints sentences, reverses letters less frequently
	Spreads with a knife
	Can balance on one foot without looking
	Can walk 2-inch-wide balance beam
	Can hop and jump accurately into small squares
	Can do accurate jumping jack exercise
8	Moves energetically but with grace and balance
	Enjoys vigorous activity
	Improved coordination
	Can engage in alternate rhythmic hopping in 2-2, 2-3, or 3-3 pattern
	Faster reaction time
	More skillful at throwing because of longer arm, girls can throw small ball 40 feet
	Better grasp of objects
	Begins cursive writing rather than printing, better small muscle coordination
	Has 12-pound pressure in grip strength
9	Less restless
	Bathes self
	Refined eye-hand coordination, skilled in manual activities
	Draws a 3-dimensional geometric figure
	Enjoys models
	Uses both hands independently
	Spaces words and slants letters when writing
	Strives to improve coordination and perfect physical skills, strength, and endurance
	Boys can run 16½ feet per second
	Boys can throw a small ball 70 feet
10	More energetic, active, restless movements
	Finger drumming or foot tapping
	Balances on one foot for 15 seconds
	Can judge and intercept pathway of small ball thrown from a distance
	Girls can run 17 feet per second
11–12	Standing broad jump of 5 ft is possible for boys, 6 in. less for girls
	Standing high jump of 3 ft possible by age 12
	Can catch a fly ball
	Skillful manipulative movements nearly equal to those of adult
	Physical changes preceding puberty begin to appear

deficit/hyperactivity disorder and learning disabilities (13). Refer to **Table 12-6** for more information on muscular development (13, 68, 107, 112, 126).

CARDIOVASCULAR SYSTEM

The *heart* grows slowly during this age period; the left ventricle of the heart enlarges. After 7 years of age, the apex of the heart lies at the interspace of the fifth rib at the midclavicle line. Before this age, the apex is palpated at the fourth interspace just to the left of the midclavicle line. By age 9, the heart weighs 6 times its birth weight. By puberty, it weighs 10 times its birth weight. Even though cardiac growth does occur, the heart remains small in relation to the rest of the body (63). Because the heart is smaller proportionately to body size, the child may tire easily. Sustained physical activity is not desirable. The schoolchild should not be pushed to run, jog, or engage in excessively competitive sports, such as football, hockey, and racquetball (58, 68, 112).

Hemoglobin levels are higher for Caucasian than African American 10- to 15-year-olds. Racial differences are consistent with those for infants, preschool children, teenagers, pregnant women, and athletes, unrelated to nutritional variables (7, 60).

VITAL SIGNS

Vital signs of the schoolchild are affected by size, gender, and activity. Temperature, pulse, and respiration gradually approach adult norms, with an average *temperature* of 98 to 98.6°F (36.7 to 37°C), *pulse rate* of 70 to 80 per minute, resting pulse rate of 60 to 76 per minute, and *respiratory rate* of 18 to 21 per minute. The average *systolic blood pressure* is 107 to 120, and average *diastolic blood pressure* is 70 to 76 mmHg. As respiratory tissues achieve adult maturity, *lung capacity* becomes proportional to body size. Between the ages of 5 and 10, the respiratory rate slows as the amount of air exchanged with each breath doubles. Breathing becomes deeper and slower. By the end of middle childhood, the lung weight will have increased almost 10 times. The ribs shift from a horizontal position to a more oblique one. The chest broadens and flattens to allow for this increased lung size and capacity (63, 68, 112).

HEAD DEVELOPMENT

The *growth of the head* is nearly complete. Head circumference measures approximately 21 in. (53 cm) and attains 95% of its adult size by the age of 8 or 9. The sinuses strengthen the structured formation of the face, reduce the weight of the head, and add resonance to the voice. The child loses the childish look as the face takes on features that will characterize him or her as an adult. Jaw bones grow longer and more prominent as the mandible extends forward, providing more chin and a place into which *permanent teeth* can erupt. *Loss of the first baby tooth is considered the beginning of the middle school years. This period ends about the time the permanent teeth* (except wisdom teeth, third molars) *finish erupting.* Females lose teeth earlier than males; deciduous or baby teeth are lost and replaced at a rate of four teeth per year until approximately age 11 or 12. The "toothless" appearance, beginning with the lower front teeth and moving symmetrically back, may produce embarrassment for the child. The first permanent

teeth are 6-year molars that erupt by age 7 and are the key teeth for forming the permanent dental arch. Evaluation for braces should not be completed until all four 6-year molars have appeared. The second permanent molars erupt by age 14, and the third molars (wisdom teeth) come in as late as age 30. Some persons' wisdom teeth never erupt. **Figure 12-1** depicts the normal developmental sequence of primary and permanent teeth. When the first permanent central incisors emerge, they appear too large for the mouth and face. Generally the teeth of males are larger than those of females (68).

Myelination is complete and also enables signals from one part of the brain to travel more rapidly to another part of the brain. Thoughts and actions repeated in sequence at first require careful, slow, focused concentration. After many repetitions, the neurons fuse together in a particular sequence; behavior becomes more habitual and requires less effort. **Automatization**, whereby *thoughts and actions repeated in sequence become automatic or routine*, occurs, and less neuron effort is required (13). This would account for the skills seen in children who excel in gymnastics, dance, competitive sports, or other complex activities.

Children who live in areas with high fluoride content in the drinking water may demonstrate **fluorosis** or **fluoride mottling,** *yellowish or brownish permanent discoloration of the tooth enamel* (23). Because of better dental care and widespread use of fluoride in toothpaste and water, about 50% of children between the ages of 5 and 17 have no dental decay (68, 107).

VISION

Overall, vision is keener than during the preschool years. The shape of the eye changes during growth, and the normal farsightedness of the preschool child is gradually converted to 20/20 vision by age 8 (68, 112). By age 10 the eyes have acquired adult size and shape. Binocular vision is well developed in most children at 6 years of age, and peripheral vision is fully developed. Females tend to have poorer visual acuity than males, but their color discrimination is superior. Large print is recommended for reading matter. Regular vision testing should be part of the school health program (68, 107). About 13% of children are visually impaired or blind (107).

GASTROINTESTINAL SYSTEM

Secretion, digestion, absorption, and excretion become more efficient. The stomach shape changes and its capacity increases. Stomach capacity at age 10 is 750 to 900 ml. Maturity of the gastrointestinal system is reflected in fewer stomach upsets and better maintenance of blood sugar levels (68, 112).

URINARY SYSTEM

The urinary system becomes functionally mature during the school years. Between the ages of 5 and 10, the *kidneys* double in size to accommodate increased metabolic functions. Fluid and electrolyte balance becomes stabilized, and *bladder capacity* is increased, especially in females. *Urinary constituents* and specific gravity become similar to those of an adult; however, 5% to 20% of school-age children have small amounts of albuminuria (68, 112).

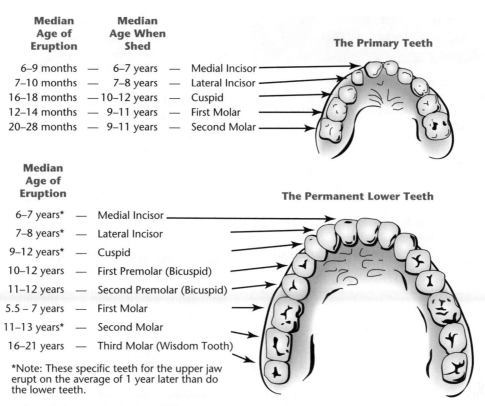

Median Age of Eruption	Median Age When Shed	
6–9 months	6–7 years	Medial Incisor
7–10 months	7–8 years	Lateral Incisor
16–18 months	10–12 years	Cuspid
12–14 months	9–11 years	First Molar
20–28 months	9–11 years	Second Molar

The Primary Teeth

Median Age of Eruption	
6–7 years*	Medial Incisor
7–8 years*	Lateral Incisor
9–12 years*	Cuspid
10–12 years	First Premolar (Bicuspid)
11–12 years	Second Premolar (Bicuspid)
5.5 – 7 years	First Molar
11–13 years*	Second Molar
16–21 years	Third Molar (Wisdom Tooth)

The Permanent Lower Teeth

*Note: These specific teeth for the upper jaw erupt on the average of 1 year later than do the lower teeth.

FIGURE ▪ 12-1 Normal tooth formation in the child.

IMMUNE SYSTEM

Lymphoid tissues reach the height of development by age 7, exceeding the amount found in adults. The body's ability to localize infection improves. Enlargement of adenoidal and tonsillar lymphoid tissue is normal, as are sore throats, upper respiratory infections, and ear infections, which are caused by the excessive tissue growth and increased vulnerability of the mucous membranes to congestion and inflammation. The *frontal sinuses* are developed near age 6. Thereafter, all sinuses are potential sites for infection. Immunoglobulins G (IgC) and A (IgA) reach adult levels by age 9, and the child's immunologic system becomes functionally mature by 12 years of age (68, 112).

PREPUBERTAL SEXUAL DEVELOPMENT

During the *preadolescent* or *prepuberty period*, both males and females develop preliminary characteristics of sexual maturity. In females, pubertal timing is correlated with percent of body fat. The female who has a higher percent of body fat at 5 years of age or a larger waist circumference at 7 years of age is more likely to demonstrate earlier pubertal development, for example at 9 years (33). This period is characterized by the growth of body hair, a spurt of physical growth (peak weight before peak height), changes in body proportion, and the beginning of primary and secondary sex characteristics. The child demonstrates physical changes such as increased weight and height, vasomotor instability, increased perspiration, and active sebaceous glands. There is an increase in fat deposition approximately 1 year before the height spurt. These fat deposits last approximately 2 years or until skeletal growth and muscle mass increase. Females have more subcutaneous fat de-

posits, and the fat is lost at a slower rate, accounting for the fuller appearance of the female figure (13, 33, 68, 112, 124, 126).

The female's growth spurt begins as early as 8 years. The average is 10 or 11 years, and maximum height velocity is reached around 12 years. The male's growth spurt begins about 12 to 13 years, and maximum height velocity is reached by approximately 14 years. The male grows approximately 4 in. (10 cm) per year for 2½ years and then begins a slower rate of growth. The female grows an average of 3 in. (7.5 cm) per year until menarche begins. For both males and females, the growth spurt begins in the hands and feet and progresses to the calves, forearms, hips, chest, and shoulders. The trunk is the last to grow appreciably (13, 68, 107, 124, 126).

As sebaceous glands of the face, back, and chest become active, acne (pimples) may develop. These skin blemishes are caused by the trapping of collected sebaceous material under the skin in small pores. The preadolescent and later the adolescent is concerned with appearance; these blemishes cause considerable embarrassment. The young person and the family may resort to numerous remedies, such as visits to skin specialists or use of sun lamps, diets, makeup, lotions, and creams. Basically, the skin should be kept clean. If the problem persists, a dermatologist should be seen. To prevent the youth's withdrawal from social contact, the parents and youth should be encouraged to seek medical attention as early as possible after acne occurs (68). Acne is further discussed in Chapter 13. ∞

Vasomotor instability with rapid vasodilation causes excessive and uncontrollable blushing. This condition usually disappears when physical growth is completed.

BOX 12-3	**Physical Changes in Girls During Prepuberty**

1. Increase in transverse diameter of the pelvis
2. Broadening of hips
3. Tenderness in developing breast tissue and enlargement of areolar diameter
4. Axillary and body sweating
5. Change in vaginal secretions from alkaline to acid pH
6. Change in vaginal layer to thick, gray, mucoid lining
7. Change in vaginal secretion flora from mixed to Döderlein's lactic-acid-producing bacilli
8. Appearance of pubic hair from 8 to 14 years (hair first appears on labia and then spreads to mons, adult triangular distribution does not occur for approximately 2 years after initial appearance of pubic hair)

These physical changes for females are listed in the approximate sequence of their occurrence.
Assembled from references 13, 53, 63, 112, 124, 126.

For a summary of physical changes, refer to **Box 12-3**, Physical Changes in Girls During Prepuberty, and **Box 12-4**, Physical Changes in Boys During Prepuberty (13, 58, 68, 107, 124, 126).

Teach parents about the physical and growth characteristics of the school-age child and the importance of nutrition, rest, immunizations, healthful activity, and regular medical and dental care. Health promotion practices in this era lay the foundation for later health.

Educate parents about the changing physical characteristics of the schoolchild. Discuss implications for the child's needs and resources, whether it is space, food, clothing, changing interests and activities, or changing health status. Counsel parents, also, about how they will need to change in their approach and expectations as the child grows and matures physically. Emphasize that the changing physical status will influence the psychosocial and spiritual dimensions of the child and, therefore, parenting strategies.

Reinforce that parents should maintain contact with a pediatrician or pediatric nurse practitioner so that concerns or questions related to the child's health can be addressed. Educate parents

BOX 12-4	**Physical Changes in Boys During Prepuberty**

1. Axillary and body sweating
2. Increased testicular sensitivity to pressure
3. Increase in size of testes
4. Changes in color of scrotum
5. Temporary enlargement of breasts
6. Increase in height and shoulder breadth
7. Appearance of lightly pigmented hair at base of penis
8. Increase in length and width of penis

The physical changes for males are listed in the approximate sequence of their occurrence.
Assembled from references 13, 53, 63, 112, 124, 126.

about what they can teach their child in relation to normal physical growth changes. Also educate the child about these changes, and validate normality.

Teach parents and the child dental health promotion measures. Emphasize the importance of regular dental examinations, cleaning, removal of plaque, and carrying out the dentist's recommendations about brushing and flossing. Parents should check the child's efforts until he or she is old enough to have the fine motor skills to brush teeth properly (usually *7 or 8* years) and to floss (*8 or 9* years). Teeth should be brushed after meals, after snacks, and at bedtime. If a sweet snack has been eaten, advise parents to have the child follow with eating an apple if flossing and brushing is not practical. While the child has a mix of permanent and deciduous teeth, a toothbrush with soft nylon bristles should be used.

PHYSICAL ASSESSMENT OF THE SCHOOL-AGE CHILD

Information will be gained from the child, the parents or caretakers, or both when assessing the child. Initial identifying information should include the informant (parent or another person) accompanying the child and any special circumstances, such as use of an interpreter or conflicting answers given by more than one person (45). The health status and developmental history should be obtained by asking open-ended, neutral questions. Listen carefully. Ask related questions to obtain a full perspective.

A child may be better at drawing than at explaining what is wrong. For example, when asked to draw a big circle where it hurts, the child can normally identify the part if given a simple outline drawing of a child.

The child over age 10 may wish to talk to the health care provider without the parent present. Being alert to the child's chronologic and developmental stage and his or her relationship with parents or caretakers will guide you in interviewing. Remember that the child is not there in isolation. *In the health assessment consider the following:*

1. Where the child lives (house or apartment, rural or urban area).
2. How much personal space he or she has (own room, own bed).
3. Parents' marital situation or family system, presence or absence of siblings.
4. What is usually eaten, the amounts of exercise and rest in 24 hours.
5. Who cares for the child after school if parents are working. How the child spends free time.

When doing a review of systems, remember to use words the child understands. For example, instead of asking if the child has ever experienced any otitis problems, simply ask as follows: "Do your ears ever ache?" "Can you always hear when people talk to you?"

In assessing skin, remember that the school-age child is subject to allergic contact dermatitis, warts, herpes type 1, ringworm, and pediculosis (lice). When any rash is present, a thorough history is necessary to determine the diagnosis and treatment (45).

Understand that visual function is more than reading the 20/20 line on a Snellen chart. Suggest a more comprehensive visual examination when a child is experiencing difficulty with schoolwork.

Children and their parents do not always react predictably when there is a need for corrective lenses. Some children may feel self-conscious with their peers when wearing glasses. Parents may react as if the child's visual problem is a flaw and deny it, stating that they are sure the child will outgrow the problem. Or they may ignore the information, or even go from doctor to doctor in search of re-assurance. If you are able to provide accurate information, using the principles of therapeutic communication, it will be valuable to a child and family who are having difficulty adjusting to the need for therapy for a visual impairment. (This also holds true when therapy or a corrective device is needed on another body area.)

When assessing a child's hearing and ears, remember that hearing should be fully developed by age 5. By age 7, most children should speak clearly enough to be understood by adults. If either of these factors seems deficient, a thorough investigation into congenital or inherited disorders and how this deficiency affects daily activities and communication is in order (45).

In the young child, the ear canal slants up. Therefore, you should pull the auricle down, but not back as you would in an adult, when using the otoscope. Also, the ear canal is short in the young child, so take care not to insert the ear tip too far. The otoscope should be controlled so that if the young child moves suddenly, you can protect against the otoscope's hitting the eardrum. The cone of light is more indistinct in a child than in an adult (45, 68).

Keep in mind the following as you continue assessment of the child's body systems (45, 68): (a) if you think you hear fluid in the lungs, check the child's nose because sounds caused by nasal fluid can be transmitted to the lungs; (b) an S_3 sound and sinus arrhythmia are fairly common in children's heart sounds; (c) a child's liver and spleen usually enlarge more quickly than an adult's in response to disease; (d) the bladder is normally found much higher in a child than in an adult, and the kidneys can more often be palpated; (e) the genitalia should be inspected for congenital abnormalities that may have been overlooked and for irritation, inflammation, or swelling; and (f) developmental guidelines must be used to assess the nervous system, specifically language development, motor and sensory functions, and cerebral function.

Musculoskeletal and posture problems, especially scoliosis detection, should be assessed. **Scoliosis,** *lateral curvature of the spine,* is more common in females than in males and is of two types, functional and structural. Ask the child to bend over and touch the toes without bending the knees and keeping the palms of the hands together. If the child has **functional scoliosis,** the *external curve will disappear with this exercise;* if it is **structural,** *the curve will remain and sometimes become more pronounced.* Early diagnosis is extremely important to arrest this problem (45). Refer the child and family to an orthopedic specialist. If scoliosis is not corrected early in life, it can result in mobility problems, obstructive pulmonary disease, and problems with body image.

Nutritional Needs

NUTRIENT NEEDS

Although *caloric requirements* per unit of body weight continue to decrease for the schoolchild, nutritional requirements remain relatively greater than for the adult. The young schoolchild requires approximately 80 calories per kilogram daily or 35 calories per pound. By age 10 there is a decrease in the calories needed per kilogram for both boys (45 calories/kg) and girls (38 calories/kg). An individual child may require more or fewer calories, depending on size, activity, and growth rate. Therefore the total caloric range is approximately 1,600 to 2,200 daily. *Daily caloric needs can be approximated for the child by the following formula:* 1,000 calories the first year plus 100 calories for each additional year (36, 38).

Protein requirements for growth are 0.5 to 1 g per pound or 36 to 40 g of protein daily. *Vitamin and mineral requirements* are slightly higher from 4 to 8 years than in the toddler years, and they increase for children 9 to 13 years. Vitamin requirements for males and females are the same during these years. Because of enlargement of ossification centers in the bone and to prevent rickets, *vitamin D* (400 IU) and a large intake of *calcium* (800 mg to age 8 years; 1,300 mg from ages 9 to 13) are needed daily. *Vitamin C* needs are 25 mg to 8 years of age, and 45 mg from ages 9 to 13 years. Fruit-flavored juices may supply some ascorbic acid but are often high in sugar content and should be limited. Regular fruit juice should be consumed. Vitamin A, iodine, iron, and major micronutrients are often not supplied adequately; these deficiencies can threaten school and work output and health (36, 38). Vitamin and mineral supplements are not necessary. Eating a variety of food supplies what is needed. *A variety of foods includes* (a) 5 to 6 oz of lean meats, fish, nuts, and beans; (b) 3 cups of 2% or 1% milk, or yogurt or other milk products; (c) 2.5 cups of vegetables, including green and yellow; (d) 1.5 cups of fruit (a variety, include citrus); (e) 6 oz minimum of bread and bread products, including whole grain, to equal about 30% of daily calories; and (f) limited unsaturated fats and carbohydrates.

Water intake may be overlooked. The schoolchild needs 1.5 to 3 quarts daily, depending on size and activity. *In children, four signs are predictive of dehydration or fluid volume deficit:* decreased tearing, prolonged capillary refill, dry mucous membranes, and a generally ill expression (97).

The MyPyramid for Kids depicts the balance between nutritional and exercise requirements. More information is available at the Website www.mypyramid.gov. Because the prepubertal growth spurt begins later in the male than in the female, nutritional needs increase later for males than females.

Solid fats and foods that supply them should be limited. Sugars, sweeteners, and salty snacks should be eaten sparingly. Overall, children in the United States eat too much salt, sugar, fat, and high-cholesterol foods (36, 38). *More fiber (age +5 = g)* is recommended. For example, the 6-year-old needs 11 g daily. Fiber establishes normal gastrointestinal muscle tone and reduces constipation. Because fiber is filling, especially when accompanied with adequate fluid intake, the child is less likely to consume foods with high fat or empty calories (36, 38).

Lunch for schoolchildren is often made up of snacks. The school lunch program offers some children the best chance for a daily nutritious meal. However, the lunch may be high in fat. Foods in this program should be baked, not fried. Students may not eat the school lunch because they do not like the menu. Food sent from the home may not be nutritious. Further, in many homes, eating at restaurants, especially those serving fast food, is commonplace. Such a dietary intake is unlikely to be nutritious.

Nutritional assessment is determined by obtaining a history of the child's food intake. Observe the general appearance and skin color and turgor. Correlate height and weight. Measure subcutaneous tissue. Check for dental caries, allergies, and chronic illness. Test hemoglobin and hematocrit levels. Determine physical, cognitive, emotional, and social well-being. Utilize information from **Box 12-5**, Subjective Global Assessment for Nutritional Status, for a comparison of normal and malnourished characteristics (36, 38).

Discuss with parents the importance of a balanced diet and foods that supply specific nutrients. Refer to **Appendix A**, Major Sources and Functions of Primary Nutrients.

EATING PATTERNS

Culture determines the type of foods eaten, when certain foods are to be eaten, and the manner in which they are consumed. The many dietary variations must be assessed for nutritional adequacy (7). By *age 8*, children have increased appetites. By *age 10*, their ap-petites are similar to those of adults. Despite increasing appetites, children seldom voluntarily interrupt activities for meals. Television, e-mails, sports, and other activities compete with mealtimes. A consistent schedule for meals should be established. The school-child is capable of learning about healthful eating and helping to plan and prepare meals. Such activities develop a healthy sense of industry and independence in the child if they are not overdone. Having healthy snacks, such as vegetables and fruit wedges, easily accessible teaches healthy eating habits.

Mealtime continues to cause dissension within many families. Parents are often upset by their child's table manners. The time the family spends together eating can be much more pleasant if manners are not overemphasized. If discipline during meals is necessary, it should be kept to a minimum. When mealtime becomes a time of stress, digestive problems, poor eating habits, or a temporary aversion to food may occur. Making a fuss over eating certain foods may cause the child to reject them more strongly. Experience and time will improve eating patterns, as

---

BOX 12-5 Subjective Global Assessment for Nutritional Status

Normal

Hair: Shiny, firm in the scalp

Eyes: Bright, clear pink membranes; adjust easily to darkness

Teeth and gums: No pain or cavities, gums firm, teeth bright

Face: Good complexion

Glands: No lumps

Tongue: Red, bumpy, rough

Skin: Smooth, firm, good color

Nails: Firm, pink

Behavior: Alert, attentive, cheerful

Internal systems: Heart rate, heart rhythm, and blood pressure normal; normal digestive function; reflexes, psychological development normal

Muscles and bones: Good muscle tone, posture; long bones straight

Malnourished

Hair: Dull, brittle, dry, loose; falls out

Eyes: Pale membranes; spots; redness; adjust slowly to darkness

Teeth and gums: Missing, discolored, decayed teeth; gums bleed easily and are swollen and spongy

Face: Off-color, scaly, flaky, cracked skin

Glands: Swollen at front of neck, cheeks

Tongue: Sore, smooth, purplish, swollen

Skin: Dry, rough, spotty; "sandpaper" feel or sores; lack of fat under skin

Nails: Spoon-shaped, brittle, ridged

Behavior: Irritable, apathetic, inattentive, hyperactive

Internal systems: Heart rate, heart rhythm, or blood pressure abnormal; liver, spleen enlarged; abnormal digestion; mental irritability, confusion; burning; tingling of hands, feet; loss of balance, coordination

Muscles and bones: "Wasted" appearance of muscles; swollen bumps on skull or ends of bones; small bumps on ribs; bowed legs or knock-knees

TABLE 12-7

Summary of Eating Patterns of Schoolchildren

6 Years	7 Years	8 Years	9 Years	10 Years	11 Years	12 Years
Has large appetite	Has extremes of appetite	Has large appetite	Has controlled appetite	Goes on eating sprees	Has controlled appetite	Has large appetite
Likes between-meal and bedtime snacks	Improves table manners	Enjoys trying new foods	Eats approximately an adult meal	Likes sweet foods	Improves table manners when eating in a restaurant	Enjoys most foods
Is awkward at table	Is quieter at table	Handles eating utensils skillfully	Acts more adultlike	Criticizes parents' table manners	Enjoys cooking	Has adultlike table manners
Likes to eat with fingers	Is interested in table conversation	Has better table manners away from home	Becomes absorbed in listening or talking	Has lapses in control of table manners at times		Participates in table discussions in adult manner
Swings legs under table, often kicking people and things	Leaves table with distraction			Enjoys cooking		
Dawdles						
Criticizes family members						
Eats with better manners away from family						

shown in **Table 12-7**, Summary of Eating Patterns of Schoolchildren (36, 38, 58, 59, 68).

Food preferences and dislikes become strongly established during the school years. By age 8, the child will try new or previously disliked foods. Food likes and dislikes are often carried over from the eating experiences of the toddler and preschooler. In addition, it is easy for the schoolchild, influenced by peers, television commercials and other forms of advertisement, and the availability of "junk" (nonnutritious) food, to avoid nutritious foods and to fill up on empty calories.

The child mimics family attitudes toward food and eating. In many families, food is equated with love and affection, an attitude that may result in the child's becoming overweight. Companionship and conversation at the child's level are essential during mealtime, for the child wants to talk and participate in a group. Mealtime conversation should be enjoyable, provide for learning conversational skills, and allow for participation by all. The give-and-take of good family discussion stimulates learning, confidence, and digestion. The child especially likes picnics and eating with peers. Because food and eating are such vital social and cultural concerns, the source of a nutritional problem may be as much a psychosocial problem as a physiologic one.

Diet is also influenced by a child's activities. If the child has been active all day, he or she will be hungry and ready to eat. On the other hand, if the child has had limited activity or emotional frustrations during the day, he or she may have no appetite. The schoolchild has more freedom to move without parental supervision and often has small amounts of money to spend on candy, soft drinks, and other treats. In addition, the schoolchild is eating on his or her own for the first time. Peer influence will frequently determine the child's lunch. Total and saturated fat, sugar, and sodium content should be reduced in both school lunches and home meals. Schools are a critical setting for prevention of overweight or obesity and for health promotion. Schools can foster physical activity and provide healthy foods at mealtime and healthy snacks in the vending machines (48).

NUTRITIONAL DEFICITS

Undernutrition and *malnutrition* in children can be manifested in retarded growth, underweight, fatigue, behavioral changes, and poor school performance and work output. Anorexia and digestive disturbances, such as diarrhea and constipation, signal improper use of nutrients. Poor muscular development may be evidenced by a child's posture—rounded shoulders, flat chest, and protuberant abdomen. Prolonged undernutrition may cause irregularities in dentition and may delay epiphyseal development and puberty. See **Box 12-5**, Subjective Global Assessment for Nutritional Status (36, 38, 68).

Undernutrition and *malnutrition* are problems throughout the world and are present in 20% of U.S. children (36, 107). Many immigrants and refugees, migrants, and poor families of any ethnic group living in cities and rural areas may not be able to provide

INTERVENTIONS FOR HEALTH PROMOTION

Share the following suggestions with parents to improve nutrition and mealtime (36, 38):

1. Create an environment of respect, love, acceptance, and calm. Parents are the role models.
2. Make food attractive and manageable; the intake is likely to be adequate for the child.
3. Establish basic rules regarding table etiquette and table language, topics of conversation, and behavior. Provide a rest period before meals.
4. Have a firm understanding with the child that play and television do not take precedence over eating. Turn the television off and avoid telephone calls during mealtime.

5. Between-meal snacks are necessary and enjoyed and do not interfere with food intake at meals if eaten an hour or longer before mealtime. Milk, cheese, fresh fruits and vegetables, peanut butter, and fruit juices are desirable snacks for both general nutritional needs and dental health.
6. Breakfast is crucial for providing the child with sufficient calories to start the day. The child who attends school without breakfast frequently exhibits fatigue and poor attention.

their children with adequate food intake. However, many middle- and upper-socioeconomic-level children, including some obese children, are also inadequately nourished (7, 68, 124).

There are currently many more overweight children than in the past decades. **Overweight** *is defined as up to 20% above ideal weight for height and growth patterns; body mass index is 25 to 29.9* (68). **Obesity** is *20% or more above ideal weight for age and height; body mass index is 30 or higher* (68, 124). Obesity is the most frequent nutritional disorder of children in developed countries (36, 38, 48). Childhood obesity can have serious social, emotional, and physical effects that may carry into adulthood (36, 38). Obese children have a higher risk for childhood hypertension. They also have an increased risk for adulthood obesity, diabetes, cardiac and pulmonary disease, and stroke (68). The obese child may suffer peer ridicule or isolation, exclusion from sports and other play activities, lower self-esteem, negative self-image, and depression (36, 38, 124). Diet and a sedentary lifestyle, such as increased time watching television or sitting at the computer, less physical exercise and outdoor play, and family eating patterns, contribute to overweight or obesity (36, 38). Exercise helps to control weight (107, 124).

Undernutrition and overnutrition may have the same causative factors: (a) the child may be reflecting food habits of other family members, (b) the parents and child may displace unrelated anxieties on food and mealtime, or (c) eating may serve as a reward or punishment for both parents and child. In some cultures, being overweight is considered a sign of health and family affluence. In other cultures, obesity is considered unsightly and unhealthy (7).

Eating disorders may begin during this era, either as anorexia nervosa or picky eating and difficulty with swallowing (16, 65). Body image disturbance and anxiety may be apparent. It is important to begin treatment early for food refusal or eating problems (16). More information is presented in Chapter 13. ∞

Encourage parents to promote food to their children as nourishment for their bodies, not as a reward or punishment. A healthy child's appetite corresponds to physiologic needs and should be a valuable index in determining intake. Tell parents not to expect young children to eat as much as adults do. The child should be neither forced to eat everything on the plate nor made to feel guilty if second portions of mother's special dish are not eaten. Help parents learn about adequate nutrition for their child as well as what behavior to expect at each age. Aid teachers as they plan lessons on nutrition. In addition to nutrition education, emphasize the importance of established exercise patterns, which can help prevent obesity.

Rest and Exercise

Information about the new guidelines on physical activity for children and adolescents can be obtained from MyPyramid for Kids (145).

REST AND SLEEP

Hours of sleep needed depend on such variables as age, health status, and the day's activities. Schoolchildren usually do not need a nap. They are not using up as much energy in growth as they were earlier. A *6-year-old* usually requires approximately 11 hours of sleep nightly. The *11-year-old* needs 9 to 9.5 hours (68). The schoolchild does not consciously fight sleep but may need firm discipline to go to bed at the prescribed hour. Lack of sleep can lead to excess weight gain (snacking to overcome daytime sleepiness), contribute to behavior that mimics symptoms of attention deficit disorder, and contribute to depression. Children who get insufficient sleep achieve lower grades in school and have more emotional problems (68). Sleep may be disturbed with dreams and nightmares, especially if the child has considerable emotional stimulation before bedtime. Fewer bedtime problems occur during this era (13, 68, 107).

EXERCISE

Exercise is essential for developing muscles and bone, refining coordination and balance, gaining strength and endurance, controlling weight, decreasing anxiety, and enhancing other body functions such as metabolism, circulation, aeration, and waste elimination. Children need to be active. They become more fatigued by long periods of sitting or passive activity than by running, jumping, or bicycling (13). Males of all ages are more physically active than females (124).

Children need 60 minutes of physical activity daily, including active play and games involving large muscles of the body: climbing, tumbling, and activities that require lifting the body or relocating the body in space. Walking, involvement in household chores, and activities done for longer than an hour without stopping are suggested. Recreational swimming, family walking, riding a bike, other short-term (30 minutes or less) aerobic activities, sports, games of longer duration, and more continuous activity are effective. An accumulation of several hours daily is encouraged. Some of the child's activities each day should be of moderate to vigorous exercise that lasts 10 to 15 minutes or more (95). This is a time for the child to learn fundamental motor skills; develop fitness in a practical, safe, and gradual manner; and enjoy being active. Coordination, timing, and concentration needed to participate in adultlike activities are being acquired, although the child has not yet achieved the strength, stamina, and muscular control of the adolescent and adult (68, 107). During middle childhood, both genders have the same basic body structure, strength, and response to systematic exercise training (13, 68, 107, 124).

The schoolchild should have a safe place to play and simple pieces of equipment. Because there are times when bad weather will keep a child from going outdoors, supplies should be available that will facilitate exercise indoors. Parents should play actively with their children sometimes. Children benefit from their parents' knowledge of various activities and are encouraged by the attention. Exercise then becomes fun, not work. *In the United States, where the child can be constantly entertained by television, the computer, or video games, parents must encourage exercise* (95).

Organized athletics, the trend to earlier participation in competitive sports, and the amount and type of competitive sports that are appropriate for children in the elementary grades are widely debated topics. Coaches must be carefully chosen. Children, if participating, should be matched to their interests, abilities, and physical and emotional constitutions. Most children of this age enjoy competition. *Goals of organized athletics should focus on* (68, 107, 124):

1. Enjoyment of sports and physical fitness that can be sustained through adulthood.
2. Inclusion of as many children as want to participate, rather than concentrating on a few athletic stars.
3. Basic motor skills, physical fitness, and a variety of activity or games.
4. Positive self concept, self-esteem, and body image; increased self-confidence.
5. Balanced perspective on sports in relation to other activities in the home, school, and community.
6. Commitment to the values of teamwork, fair play, and sportsmanship, rather than focus on winning.

Review the child's rest and exercise needs with parents. At the same time, discuss with parents how they are meeting their own needs for rest and exercise and how the parents and child can engage in activities that are mutually interesting and healthful, such as walking, bicycling, or swimming. Some families enroll the schoolchild with a personal trainer in a health club to encourage nonathletic children to be more active. Emphasize the importance of having a trainer who understands and knows how to motivate children, and who will not demand perfect achievement, expect skills beyond the child's capabilities, or insist the child engage in activity that could cause injury and even long-term negative neuromuscular effects. Affirm that although exercise is important to holistic health and development, participation in organized or competitive sports is *not* essential. *Refer the family to the following Websites for more information*:

1. *MyPyramid*, which integrates physical activity and nutrition. www.mypyramid.gov
2. Kids Activity Pyramid from the Pennsylvania State College of Agricultural Sciences, Cooperative Extension.

Children who are physically fit have lower cholesterol, low-density lipoprotein cholesterol, and triglyceride levels and higher high-density lipoprotein cholesterol levels than physically unfit children (36, 38). Regular physical activity at this age, and thereafter, helps to prevent coronary artery disease, hypertension, obesity, and type 2 diabetes in the years ahead (36, 38, 68, 102).

Health Promotion and Health Protection

IMMUNIZATIONS

Emphasize to parents the importance of immunizations and record keeping. Supply parents with information about an appropriate immunization schedule, free immunization programs, and school requirements for immunization. Before a child receives an immunization, he or she should be told why and where it will be given.

Immunizations reduce deaths from infectious diseases. Measles, tetanus, and whooping cough are still leading causes of childhood death around the world, although the death rate is decreasing because of expanding global immunization (68).

In the United States, the Advisory Committee on Immunization Practices (ACIP) of the Centers for Disease Control and Prevention, the Committee on Infectious Diseases of the American Academy of Pediatrics, and the American Academy of Family Physicians recommend policies and procedures. In Canada, the National Advisory Committee on Immunization, under authority of the Minister of Health and Public Health Agency of Canada, governs immunization recommendations. Recommendations change as the field of immunology advances. Keep informed of the changes (68, 112).

SAFETY PROMOTION AND INJURY CONTROL

Accidents are the leading cause of severe injury and death for children. Motor vehicle accidents, either as pedestrian or passenger, are the most common cause, accounting for about half of the accidental deaths of schoolchildren (68, 124). Other accidents that threaten children are fires, falls, drownings, poisonings, bicycling, and using skateboards, roller skates, and sports equipment (112, 124). Though school-age children have developed more refined muscular coordination and control, their activities and desire for independence increase their risk for injury. They are susceptible to cuts, abrasions, fractures, strains, sprains, and bruises. The incidence of injury and death is significantly higher in school-age males than females (69). Some of the injuries sustained during sporting activities may cause permanent disability because of damage to the epiphyseal cartilage or the neuromuscular system (68).

Some children apparently are **high risk takers** or *accident-prone; they suffer more accidental injuries than the overall childhood population.* Although the causative factors have not been completely determined, children who are overreactive, restless, impulsive, hostile, and immature are frequently found in this group (68, 112).

Encourage parents to provide supervision and attention and to repeat, even to children who are not accident-prone, cautions as necessary. The child forgets when involved in play. Conceptual thinking and judgment are not well developed so that the child does not foresee dangers.

Accident prevention should be taught and enforced in school and at home. Promote safety by helping parents and children identify and avoid hazards. The school-age child has increasing cognitive maturity, including improved ability to remember past experiences and anticipate probable outcomes of his or her actions. This makes the child a good candidate for safety instructions.

Safety education should include information about the hazards of (a) risk taking, (b) improper use of equipment, and (c) the variety of toys that can cause injuries, including slingshots, water balloons, lawn darts, and chemistry sets. *Injury prevention* should address motor vehicle injuries, equipment used in play, and risk of drownings, burns, poisonings, falls, and sports-related injuries. The child should be taught the proper use of seat belts in motor vehicles. Safe pedestrian behavior should be emphasized. Stress the safety and maintenance of two-wheeled vehicles (such as bicycles) and the use of safety apparel. Water safety and survival skills should be taught with basic swimming skills at an early age. Families who go boating must teach related safety measures to their children and insist the children wear flotation devices.

Emphasize that the schoolchild may not have sufficient coordination, strength, judgment, or maturity to operate motorized vehicles or use motorized equipment, such as power mowers, all-terrain vehicles (ATVs), snowmobiles, motorized skateboards, or farm equipment. Confirm that parents should not push the child into risky situations or acquiesce when the child is demanding. The skill level of the child should be evaluated on an ongoing basis.

Teach parents about ways to prevent accidental injury. (Refer to Chapter 11 for safety measures that remain relevant.) ∞ Advise parents of hazards associated with organized contact or competitive sports. Emphasize that the *child must wear protective head, elbow, and knee gear* when engaged in the following play activities: bicycling, baseball, softball, football, hockey, roller skating, in-line skating, skateboarding, scooter riding, horseback riding, or speed sledding or tobogganing. *Protective eye gear and mouth guards* must be worn to decrease head and facial injuries. *"Heading" the ball should not be allowed because of danger of brain injury.* If necessary, *role-play with parents how to explain the latter measure, as well as other safety rules,* such as care in crossing the street, riding the bicycle with the traffic and not against it, and using and reading traffic signals. Recommend that parents do *not* buy a trampoline or allow the child to use one at playgrounds or at school. Supervision is necessary at public playgrounds and amusement parks (especially water slides), as well as around the home. Explain that *the parent needs to follow the same rules.* The parent is a role model; the child follows the behavior observed.

INTERVENTIONS FOR HEALTH PROMOTION

Children who live on a farm or who work in agriculture are at risk for accidental injury or death when they accompany or assist parents or other adults with farm work. Teach these parents or adults the following rules to reduce hazards:

1. Do not allow children as extra riders on equipment.
2. Do not allow children to play with machinery that is parked in "idle."
3. Leave any equipment that might fall, such as front-end loaders, in the down position.
4. When self-propelled machinery is parked, brakes should be locked and keys removed from the ignition.
5. Always leave a tractor power-takeoff unit in neutral.
6. When starting machinery—and especially when reversing it—know where the children are to avoid contact and possible injury or death.
7. Maintain machinery in good repair, particularly protective shields and seat belts.
8. Do not permit children to operate machinery until they have completed safety training.
9. Fence farm ponds and manure pits.
10. Place fixed ladders out of reach, or fit them with a special barrier; store portable ladders away from danger areas.
11. Shield dangerous machinery components, electric boxes, and wiring; place out of easy reach or fit with locking devices.
12. Place warning decals on all grain bins, wagons, and trucks.
13. Maintain lights and reflectors for all equipment used on roads.
14. Do not expect children to work with farm animals or with machinery that is beyond their maturity physically or mentally.

Explore with parents that *meal preparation* can be fun for the school-age child, but the *hazards* of sharp knives, hot stoves, microwave ovens, and hot liquids must be kept in mind. Supervise the use of matches or flammable chemicals, and teach the child the proper behavior if clothing becomes ignited. A family-designed fire escape plan should be initiated and practiced monthly.

Advise parents to teach all children how to climb in the safest possible way. Explain the dangers involved in climbing trees, electric poles, water towers, silos, and other structures. Instruct the child in the proper use of playground equipment and in the need to pick up toys from the floor to prevent falls.

Instruct parents to keep potentially dangerous products in properly labeled receptacles. Educate the child about the dangers of ingesting nonprescription drugs and chemicals. Emphasize that firearms, including air guns and air rifles, should not be accessible to the schoolchild. Gun accidents are common during the school-age period. *Parents who have a gun should keep it under lock and place the key in a childproof location.* Children of this age should be taught safety rules concerning guns. Gunshot wounds and homicides are an increasing risk because of firearms in the home. Share with parents that the incidence of *homicides* in the United States for children under age 15 years is nearly 16 times higher than the incidence found in 25 other industrialized countries (13, 124).

Reinforce any teaching with books, films, and creation of mock situations to supplement verbal instruction. You and the parents will repeat the same cautions endlessly. Reinforce to parents the necessity of shifting responsibility to the child with increasing age.

Emphasize to parents the importance of regular examinations at a clinic or from a family physician or nurse practitioner and dentist. Every child should have a thorough preschool examination, including visual and auditory screening and posture and general health examination. Correction of health problems is essential, as they may be a cause for injuries, ongoing illness, or difficulties with schoolwork or peers (78). Millions of children receive basically no health care. Advocate to eliminate such health care disparities.

As a nurse you have a responsibility to strengthen the school health program in your community through direct services. Teach the board of education, teachers, parents, and students about the value and use of such a program despite costs. Work for legislation to finance and implement programs that do more than first aid care. A school health program should supervise not only the child's physical health, but also emotional, mental, and social health. Instruction in personal hygiene, disease prevention, nutrition, safety, family life, and group living is of interest to the schoolchild and should be under the direction of the school nurse.

If there are students who have chronic illnesses or disabilities in school, special preparation should be given to the teachers, students, and parents. Promote understanding of the child and the condition, of the child's need to reach individual potential, and of a total rehabilitation program (4, 9, 10, 25, 27, 72, 77, 78, 110, 153, 154).

COMMON HEALTH PROBLEMS: PREVENTION AND PROTECTION

Although the child should remain basically healthy, health problems that limit school performance and function exist in 12% of all schoolchildren. School-age children get sick about one half as often as preschoolers and about twice as much as their parents (68). *Inform parents* about health problems and both acute and chronic conditions.

A considerable number of schoolchildren have *risk factors that are predictive of adulthood coronary heart disease:* hypertension, increased serum cholesterol and triglycerides, and obesity. The elementary school population may also be the main reservoir of *infectious hepatitis A*, because schoolchildren often have a mild undiagnosed disease that is spread person to person (45, 68, 112).

Because of the short urethra, females are prone to *urinary infection.* This may be diagnosed by reddened genitals, a feeling of burning on urination, and abnormal appearance and chemical analysis of the urine. Normal urinary output from 6 to 12 years ranges from 500 ml to 1,000 ml (adult output is 1,500 ml daily). Bladder capacity is greater in females than in males. Output depends on amount of fluid ingested, environmental temperature and humidity, time of day and emotional state (68). Pinworms accompany urinary tract infections in approximately 50% of the cases (45).

The *7-year-old* has fewer illnesses but may complain of fatigue or muscular pain. Tension, overactivity or exertion, bruising, or injury may cause leg pains. Pain in the knees with no exertional signs are also common in school-age children. Such pain usually occurs late in the day or night and disappears in the morning. Children with persistent leg pain should be referred to a physician.

The *8- or 9-year-old* is generally healthy but may complain of minor aches to get out of disagreeable tasks. Such behavior should not be reinforced by undue attention.

Visual impairments that occur in the younger child may be undetected and untreated until the child attends school. Visual acuity may not develop normally. For more information, see **Box 12-6**, Signs and Symptoms Indicating Defective Vision in Schoolchildren (45, 68, 112). It is essential that visual problems be corrected.

Refer to **the Box** *Healthy People 2010:* Example of Objectives for Schoolchild Health Promotion, for health concerns and prevention strategies in the United States, formulated by the U.S. Department of Health and Human Services. The health status of school-age children is a major focus of this initiative, since their health lays the foundation for the health of our future adult population (146). For more information, refer to the Website www.health.gov or call 1-800-367-4725.

Increasingly, the ill effects of *smoking and drug and alcohol abuse* are emerging as a regular health problem. These habits are influenced by the habits of parents, siblings, and peers. *The child may not enjoy these experiences* but will smoke, take drugs, and drink to show off and follow peer influence. *Knowledge of the negative effects is not necessarily a deterrent; health teaching must consider this situation.*

Interventions to teach health promotion to children must consider family assessment and the child's self-esteem and motivational levels, and foster a positive personal responsibility in the child for healthful practices, such as exercise, healthy snacks, and avoiding risky behaviors. It is essential to consider cultural differences in definitions of disease prevention and health promotion practices.

MediaLink Common Health Problems and Health Promotion Measures

MediaLink Healthy People 2010

BOX 12-6 **Signs and Symptoms Indicating Defective Vision in Schoolchildren**

BEHAVIOR

1. Attempts to brush away blur; rubs eyes frequently; frowns, squints
2. Stumbles frequently or trips over small objects
3. Blinks more than usual; cries often or is irritable when doing close work
4. Holds books or small playthings close to eyes
5. Shuts or covers one eye, tilting or thrusting head forward when looking at objects
6. Has difficulty in reading or in other schoolwork requiring close use of the eyes; omits words or confuses similar words
7. Exhibits poor performance in activities requiring visual concentration within arm's length (e.g., reading, coloring, drawing); unusually short attention span; persistent word reversals after second grade
8. Disinterested in distant objects or fails to participate in games such as playing ball
9. Engages in outdoor activity mostly (e.g., running bicycling), avoiding activities requiring visual concentration within arm's length

10. Sensitive to light
11. Unable to distinguish colors
12. Steps carefully over sidewalk cracks or around light or dark sections of block linoleum floors
13. Trips at curbs or stairs
14. Poor eye–hand coordination for age, excessively hard-to-read handwriting, difficulty with tying shoelaces or buttoning and unbuttoning

APPEARANCE

1. Crossed eyes (iris of one eye turned in or out and not symmetric with other eye)
2. Red-rimmed, encrusted, or swollen eyelids
3. Repeated styes
4. Watery or red eyes

COMPLAINTS

1. Cannot see blackboard from back of room
2. Blurred or double vision after close eye work
3. Dizziness, headaches, or nausea after close eye work
4. Itching or burning eyes

Data from References 45, 68, 112.

The school nurse and teacher can do considerable health teaching, introducing students to positive health habits. Some programs emphasize that the body is a beautiful system, that no one should abuse the system by doing or using anything damaging, and that children should "just say no." Education should emphasize that people can be happy and active when they avoid the use of alcohol, drugs, or cigarettes. This can help to offset the preponderance of advertising that links youth, beauty, and excitement with these activities.

Emphasize to adults that *more effective than organized educational attempts is the influence of significant adults, those who take a personal interest in the child and who set an example.* These include (a) parents who neither smoke, drink, or use drugs nor give cigarettes, alcohol, or drugs to their children; (b) the teacher who not only teaches content but also lives the teaching; (c) parents and health care providers who have quit smoking; (d) the athletic coach who is committed to no smoking, drinking, or drugging; and (e) the health care professional who role-models healthy behaviors. *Equally important, or more so, is the peer group. Leaders of the peer group who have positive health habits should be used as models.* You may have a role in working with the peer group.

Health diaries can be used to note assessment of problems and disease, monitoring of medication, teaching about health behaviors, and evaluation of effectiveness. Advise parents and children about the importance of keeping health records.

Promote healthy behavior and design and implement health promotion interventions in various sites. Traditional sites (schools, clinics) and nontraditional sites (shelters, social service programs, correctional institutions, shopping malls, religious institutions, and work and recreational settings) in rural and urban areas are places to implement health promotion programs and teaching. Information can also be given to parents in their occupational settings, and health screening and immunizations for children can be set up at the work site. Advocate with employees for such health programs.

Psychosocial Concepts

COGNITIVE DEVELOPMENT

The schoolchild has a strong curiosity to learn, especially when motivation is strengthened by interested parents and opportunities for varied experiences in the home and school. Learning, behavior, and personality are complex and are not easily explained by one theory. This section uses information from a number of theorists. Refer to Chapter 1 for a review of the major theorists. ∞

Bandura's research demonstrated the importance of adult role-modeling behavior (11). The child pays attention to the adult's behavior and remembers what has been demonstrated. Actions impress the child, affect motivation and behavior, and give a reason to perform. Vygotsky also emphasized that the child learns a great deal by being with adults and peers—observing and imitating (148).

Concrete Operations Stage: Pattern of Intellectual Development

Children manifest a **cognitive style**, *the characteristic way in which information is organized and problems are solved.* The style varies from child to child, but there are *four major cognitive styles* (126, 139):

1. **Analytic.** Examine minute details of objects or events.
2. **Superordinate.** Observe for shared attributes of objects or similarities of events.
3. **Functional-relational.** Link objects or events because they have interactional value.
4. **Functional-locational.** Recognize that objects or events have a shared location.

Older children are more likely to use analytic and superordinate cognitive styles.

In addition to cognitive style, children differ in their **conceptual tempo**, *the manner in which they evaluate and act on a problem.* Tempo may be either **impulsive**, *where the first idea is accepted and hurriedly reported without consideration for accuracy or thoughtfulness*, or **reflective**, *where a longer period is used to consider various aspects of a situation.* Reflective children are more likely to be analytic than are impulsive children (126).

Teach parents that certain kinds of questions or statements help the child learn to think more analytically and reflectively, which promotes cognitive health and maturity:

1. Why? Give an explanation.
2. If that is so, what follows? What is the cause of _____?
3. Aren't you assuming that _____?
4. How do you know that?
5. Is the point you were making that _____?
6. Can I summarize your point as _____?
7. Is this what you mean to say?
8. What is your reason for saying that?
9. What does that word mean?
10. Is there another way of looking at _____?
11. Is it possible that _____?
12. How else can we view this? How else can we approach this situation?

The pattern of intellectual development can be traced through the school years (115–119, 149).

In American culture, the 6-year-old is supposed to be ready for formal education. The child in first grade is frequently still in the Preoperational Stage. See **Table 12-8** for a summary of cognitive abilities of the child from ages 6 to 12 (13, 58, 59, 107, 115–119, 124, 149).

At approximately *age 7* the child enters the **Concrete Operations Stage**, *which involves systematic reasoning about tangible or familiar situations and the ability to use logical thought to analyze relationships and structure the environment into meaningful categories.* The child must have interactions with the environment, equipment, and materials and with tangible, visible references to build understanding that is basic for the next stage (115–117, 119, 149).

The following mental operations are characteristic of this stage (115, 120, 149):

1. **Classification.** *Sorting objects in groups according to specific and multiple attributes,* such as length, size, shape, color, class

401

TABLE 12-8

Cognitive Characteristics of the School-Age Child

Age (Yr)	Cognitive Ability
6	Thinking is concrete and animistic
	Beginning to understand semiabstract concepts and symbols
	Defines objects in relation to their use and effect on self
	May not be able to consider parts and wholes in words at the same time
	Likes to hear about his or her past
	Knows numbers
	Can read
	Learning occurs frequently through imitation and incidental suggestion and also depends on opportunities
	May not be able to sound out words; may confuse words when reading, such as *was* and *saw*
	High correlation between ability to converse and beginning reading achievement; may have vocabulary of 8,000 to 14,000 words when reading, if assisted with language
7	Learns best from interaction with actual materials or visible props
	Learning broad concepts and subconcepts, e.g., car identified as Ford or Chevrolet, based on memory, instruction, or experience
	A number of mental strategies or operations are learned
	Becoming less egocentric, less animistic
	Better able to do cause–effect and logical thinking
	More reflective; has deeper understanding of meanings and feelings
	Interested in conclusions and logical endings
	Attention span lengthened; may work several hours on activity of interest
	More aware of environment and people in it; also interested in magic and fantasy
	Understands length, area or mass
	Sense of time practical, detailed; present focus; plans the day
	Knows months, seasons, years
	Serious in inventing, enjoys chemistry sets
8	Less animistic
	More aware of people and impersonal forces of nature
	Improvises simple activities
	Likes to learn about history, own and other cultures, geography, science, and social science
	Intellectually expansive; inquires about past and future
	Tolerant and accepting of others
	Understands logical reasoning and implications
	Learns from own experience
	Extremely punctual
	Improvises simple rules
	Can read a compass
9	Realistic in self-appraisal and tasks
	Reasonable, self-motivated, curious
	Needs minimal direction
	Competes with self
	Likes to be involved with activities and complex tasks
	May concentrate on project for 2 or 3 hours
	Plans in advance; wants successive steps explained and wants to perfect skills
	Focuses on details and believes in rules and laws (they can be flexible), as much as luck or chance
	Enjoys history
	Tells time without difficulty
	Likes to know length of time for task
	Likes to classify, identify, list, make collections
	Understands weight

TABLE 12-8

Cognitive Characteristics of the School-Age Child—continued

Age (Yr)	Cognitive Ability
10	Is matter-of-fact
	Likes to participate in discussions about social problems and cause and effect
	Likes a challenge
	Likes to memorize and identify facts
	Locates sites on a map
	Makes lists
	Easily distracted; many interests and concentrates on each for a short time
	Greater interest in present than past
11	Curious but not reflective
	Concrete, specific thinking
	Likes action or experimentation in learning
	Likes to move around in the classroom
	Concentrates well when competing with one group against another
	Prefers routine
	Better at rote memorization than generalization
	Defines time as distance from one event to another
	Understands relationships of weight and size
12	Likes to consider all sides of a situation
	Enters self-chosen task with initiative
	Likes group work but more inner motivated than competitive
	Able to classify, arrange, and generalize
	Likes to discuss and debate
	Beginning formal operations stage, or abstract thinking
	Verbal formal reasoning possible
	Understands moral of a story
	Defines time as duration, a measurement
	Plans ahead, so feels life is under own control
	Interested in present and future
	Understands abstractness of space
	Understands conservation of volume

of animals, and trademark. Schoolchildren can identify which kind of Ford car is approaching on the highway. Usually one characteristic is focused on first; then more characteristics are considered. Simpler relationships between classes of objects are understood.

2. **Seriation.** *Ordering objects according to decreasing or increasing measure* such as height, weight, and strength. The child knows A is longer than B, B is longer than C, and A is longer than C.

3. **Nesting.** *Understanding how a subconcept fits into a larger concept.* For example, a German shepherd is one kind of dog; a reclining chair and a dining room chair are both chairs.

4. **Multiplication.** *Simultaneously classifying and seriating,* using two numbers together to come out with a greater amount.

5. **Reversibility.** *Returning to the starting point or performing opposite operations or actions with the same problem or situation.* The child can add and subtract and multiply and divide the same problems. A longer row of clips can be squeezed together

to form a shorter row and vice versa; the child realizes the number of clips has not changed.

6. **Transformation.** *Being able to see the shift from a dynamic to static or constant state, to understand the process of change, and to focus on the continuity and sequence, on the original and final states.* For example, the child realizes or anticipates how a shorter row of pennies was shifted to become a longer row, or the shift in level of fluid in a container as it is poured from one container into a second container of a different size.

7. **Conservation.** *Understanding transformation conceptually and that a situation has not changed, to see the sameness of a situation or object despite a change in some aspect and that mass or quantity is the same even if it changes shape or position.* There is an order to conservation: mass and number first, weight and volume last. *Three concepts contribute to conservation:*

   a. *Identity, or remaining essentially the same.* A lump of clay rolled into different shapes is the same clay; six paper clips moved from a 6-inch line to an 8-inch line remain six paper clips.

   b. *Reversibility, operations can be reversed and their effects can be nullified.* Water in boiled form is vapor, which can return to water and freeze. It is still the same amount of water; nothing is lost in the process.

   c. *Reciprocity, changing from one form to another but remaining the same.* A change of a mass of clay in one direction is compensated for by a change in another direction, but the total mass remains the same. A small, thick ball of clay can be flattened to be large and thin; but no clay material was added or taken away.

8. **Decentering.** *Coordinating two or more dimensions, or the ability to focus on several characteristics simultaneously.* For example, space and length dimensions can be considered; the younger child would consider only one or the other. When 12 paper clips are spread from 6 to 12 inches, the child realizes the clips are spread and there are not more clips.

9. **Combination.** *Being able to combine several tasks or operations at once, to see the regularities of the physical world and the principles that govern relationships among objects. The original or essential idea is retained when conflicting or unorganized information is presented. Perceptions alone become less convincing* than a logical understanding of how the world operates. For example, a sunset on the ocean looks like the sun is sinking into the water; science teaches that what we see is a result of the earth's rotation on its axis. The child recognizes number, length, volume, area, and weight as the same even when a view or perception of an object changes.

The Case Situation gives an example of some of the child's thought processes in the Stage of Concrete Operations.

The cognitive operations increase in complexity as the child matures from an empirical to logical orientation. The child can look at a situation, analyze it, and come up with an answer without purposefully going through each step. **Cause-and-effect versus sequence of events** is increasingly understood; *causation is not necessarily what preceded an event.* The child learns and can recall associations between sequences and groupings of events. At first he or she makes associations within a certain context or environment; later memory is used to transfer these associations to different contexts or environments. **Accommodation** is utilized; *the child is less egocentric due to social relationships and understands that others can form a different conclusion.* The child **rehearses,** *going over mentally what has been learned* in the time between a learning experience and a memory test or application of learning (149).

Educate parents about the child's changing cognitive abilities and ways they can contribute to the cognitive achievement. If parents do not understand that certain cognitive behavior is age-appropriate, their interactions with and guidance of the child may be less effective. Emphasize that nurturing parental responsiveness throughout the early years, even for children of very low birth weight, positively influences the schoolchild's cognitive development (131).

Fears held by the child change with an increasing understanding of implications and consequences of cause-and-effect relations. *By age 7 or 8, most fears that are typical of preschoolers (darkness, spooks) have been resolved.* New fears arise. **Table 12-9** presents a comparison of fears of the young and older school-age child. Some of the fears presented in Table 12-9 (e.g., fear of vehicles or dangerous people) are realistic as the child increasingly moves out into the community alone (26, 58, 59, 132). Children from different cultures or in other countries may state or order fears differently (7, 60). Adults also express some of these same fears.

Case Situation

Sarah, age 10, and Joshua, her 6-year-old brother, are visiting their grandmother, aunt, uncle, and cousins for the day. Sarah is thin, with narrow shoulders and hips and little adipose tissue, although she has considerable muscle mass.

A luncheon is being held for her grandmother's birthday, and Sarah is eager to help her aunt and cousins prepare the food, set the table, and make party favors. Sarah and Megan, her 9-year-old cousin, divide the nuts and candies into party cups to set at each person's plate. They do this systematically and logically, using the concepts of seriation and classification, so that each person receives an identical number of candies and nuts. This is typical of the Concrete Operations stage of cognitive development.

Sarah and Megan go to play school in Megan's room where there are a toy chest, dolls, bookshelves, and a chalkboard.

Sarah plays the teacher, writing multiplication tables on the board and talking to Megan and to pretend students. She demonstrates concrete *transformations* as she solves multiplication problems. Sarah pretends the class is being bad and reprimands them as a teacher would. In this behavior she demonstrates understanding of *relationships between various steps in a situation.* It is apparent that Sarah's teacher is a role model for her; this is common among school-age children.

Sarah asks Megan for advice on solving the problems and on reprimanding the pretend class. This exchange of information is typical of the syntaxic mode of communication and consensual validation that is observed in the schoolchild. By incorporating Megan's ideas and answers, she shows that she cares about Megan's thoughts.

Contributed by Ruth Murray, EdD, MSN, N-NAP, FAAN.

TABLE 12-9

Fears of the Schoolchild

Young Schoolchild	Older Schoolchild
Loss of or separation from family	Separation from or death of loved ones
Unsafe conditions, natural environmental hazards	Natural environmental hazards
Body injury or disease, death	Disease, personal death
School problems, bullying peers, teachers, not achieving	Dangerous people and animals, machines, or vehicles, weapons
Breaking the moral code, punishment	Breaking the moral code, punishment
War, when the country is involved in war	War, the Atom Bomb, terrorists
Hell (depending on how this concept is taught)	Hell (depending on how this concept is taught)

Adapt your care and approach, as the child is likely to be fearful in the health care setting. Coming for screening, immunization, diagnosis, or treatment can heighten fear of damage to the body and punishment. (Most procedures seem like punishment.) Give appropriate explanations. Fears of separation from loved ones or death can be diminished by having the parent remain with the child. Affirm the child is doing all right during a procedure to avoid fear that the crying, screaming, or thrashing about is considered "being bad." Use the newly developed cognitive operations to help the child cope with the health care visit, such as classification or seriation of equipment, decentering, combination, or imitating your behavior (role-modeling).

CONCEPT OF TIME The concept of time evolves during the early school period. See **Table 12-10** for a summary of how the schoolchild develops a concept of time (58, 59, 107, 119, 124).

Help parents understand that school-age children do not have adult concepts of time. Teach the mother who is distraught because her *6- or 7-year-old* constantly dawdles in getting ready for school that this is normal behavior. The mother must still be firm in direction but not expect the impossible. She can look forward to *improvement in the 8-year-old*. Understanding maturing time concepts will also help you explain the sequence of a procedure to the schoolchild in a health care setting.

SPATIAL CONCEPTS Spatial concepts also change with more experience. The *6-year-old* is interested in specific places and in relationships between home, neighborhood, and an expanding community. He or she knows some streets and major points of interest. By *age 7* the sense of space is becoming more realistic. The child wants some space of his or her own, such as a room or portion of it. The heavens and various objects in space and in the earth are of keen interest (28, 58, 59, 118, 126).

For the *8-year-old*, *personal space* is expanding as the child goes more places alone. He or she knows the neighborhood well and likes maps, geography, and trips. He or she understands the compass points and can distinguish right and left on others as well as self (28, 58).

Space for the *9-year-old* includes the whole earth (global space). He or she enjoys pen pals from different lands, geography, and

TABLE 12-10

School-Age Child's Concepts of Time

Age (Yr)	Conceptualization of Time
6	Time counted by hours; minutes disregarded
	Enjoys past as much as present; likes to hear about his or her babyhood
	Future important in relation to holidays
	Duration of episode has little meaning
7	Interested in present; enjoys a watch
	Sense of time practical, sequential, detailed
	Knows sequence of months, seasons, years
	Plans days; understands passage of time
8	Extremely aware of punctuality, especially in relation to others
	More responsible about time
9	Tells time without difficulty
	Plans days with excess activities; driven by time
	Wants to know how long a task will take to complete
	Interested in ancient times
10	Less driven by time than the 9-year-old
	Interested primarily in present
	Able to get to places in time on own initiative
11	Feels time is relentlessly passing by or dragging
	More adept at handling time
	Defines time as distance from one event to another
12	Defines time as duration, a measurement
	Plans ahead to feel in control
	Interested in future as well as present

BOX 12-7	**Categories of Concepts Developed During the School Years**

- ***Life:*** Is aware that movement is not sole criterion of life.
- ***Death:*** Accepts death as final and not like life. Thinks of death as an angel or bogeyman. Thinks personal death can be avoided if one hides, runs fast, or is good. Traumatic situations arouse fear of death. By age 10 or 11, realizes death is final, inevitable, and results from internal processes. Belief in life after death depends on religious teachings.
- ***Body functions:*** Has many inaccurate ideas about body functions until taught health class. Needs repetitive sex education. Becomes more modest for self but interested in seeing bodies of adults. Performs complete self-care by 9 years.
- ***Money:*** Begins to understand value of coins and bills.

- ***Self:*** Clarifies ideas of self when sees self through eyes of teachers and peers and compares self with peers. By 11 or 12 years, considers self to be in brain, head, face, heart, and then total body.
- ***Sex roles:*** Has clear concept of culturally defined sex role and that male role is considered more prestigious.
- ***Social roles:*** Is aware of peers' social, religious, and socioeconomic status. Accepts cultural stereotypes and adult attitudes toward status. Group conscious.
- ***Beauty:*** Judges beauty according to group standards rather than own aesthetic sensibilities.
- ***Comedy:*** Has concept of comedy or what is funny influenced by perception of what others think is funny.

history. For the *10-year-old*, space is rather specific, such as the location of a building. The *11-year-old* perceives *space as nothingness* that goes on forever, a distance between things. He or she is in good control of getting around in the *personal space* (28, 59). The *12-year-old* understands that *space is abstract* and has difficulty defining it. Space is nothing, air. He or she can travel alone to more distant areas and understands how specific points relate to each other (28, 59). The child has difficulty understanding **velocity,** *the relationship between time and space,* which has safety implications. This concept is useful in safely using motor-driven tools or engaging in certain activities or sports, such as skateboarding.

Encourage the parents to discuss spatial concepts with the child to facilitate abstract reasoning. Piaget's concepts in care and teaching of children are a basis for practical suggestions. **Box 12-7,** Categories of Concepts Developed During the School Years, summarizes other concepts formulated at this time.

Multiple Intelligences

More than one kind of intellectual competence, **multiple intelligences,** rather than one intelligence, exist. The **Triarchic Theory of Intelligence** proposed by Robert Sternberg *incorporates three realms of cognition* (133, 134). *These realms are* (13, 133, 134): (a) how thinking occurs and the main components of thinking based on the information-processing model, including skills at coding, representing, combining information, planning, and self-evaluation in problem solving; (b) how individuals cope with experiences, how they respond to novelty in solving new problems, or how quickly they adjust to a new form of the task; and (c) the context of thinking—the extent to which children adapt to, alter, or select environments supportive of their abilities.

The **Theory of Multiple Intelligences** proposed by Howard Gardner *presents factors that reflect the influence of culture and society on intellectual ability* (53, 54). *Multiple intelligences take the following forms* (13, 53, 54, 107, 124, 126):

1. **Language skills.** *Thinks in words. Speaks fluently to express meaning, learns new words easily. Memorizes easily.*

2. **Mathematical skills.** *Carries out and performs well with mathematical operations.*
3. **Spatial skills.** *Thinks in three dimensions; finds the way around easily without getting lost, more so than other children of the same age.*
4. **Body-kinesthetic skills.** *Manipulates objects, is physically skilled. Sensitive to the internal sensations created by body movements, and easily learns dancing and gymnastics.*
5. **Musical skills.** *Plays one or more musical instruments, sings, discerns subtle musical effects, and has a sense of timing, rhythm, melody, and pitch.*
6. **Interpersonal skills.** *Understands and effectively handles social encounters, interacts with others, and relates easily to others.*
7. **Intrapersonal skills.** *Has an understanding of self that is accurate and promotes empathy; directs own life effectively.*
8. **Naturalistic skills.** *Observes patterns in nature; understands natural and human-made systems; understands ecology, botany, and nature.*

Information Processing and Metacognition

The schoolchild can increasingly receive and use information more rapidly. Various mental processes to remember and apply information are used (35). The working or present memory is more effective in speed and capacity. Long-term memory utilizes knowledge and experience, which allows more learning, analysis, and evaluation. The more the child learns, the more he or she can learn (35). The child increasingly uses **selective attention,** the ability *to concentrate on what is important* (13, 28).

Metacognition, *thinking about thinking* and a higher form of thinking, develops in the older schoolchild. The child becomes increasingly accurate and efficient in cognition, and more focused on the relevant. Evaluation is used to determine how to best accomplish a task or achieve a goal (28, 107, 124). **Mnemonic devices,** *memory aids or strategies,* are increasingly used for storage and retrieval of information and for analytic thinking (28, 107, 124).

ENTERING SCHOOL AND THE EDUCATIONAL EXPERIENCE

School entry is a developmental crisis for the child and family, even with preparation of early child education, for behavior must be adapted to meet new situations. Regular attendance at school starts early for some children, perhaps at 2½ to 3 years in nursery school. But *not all children are emotionally or cognitively ready for school, even at age 6 or 7.* If the child is unprepared for school, separation anxiety may be intense. The demands of a strange adult and the peer group may be overwhelming (126, 141). The school experience has considerable influence on the child and is formative. School systems vary throughout the United States and from country to country (107, 138).

School is society's institution to help the child (a) develop the fullest intellectual potential and a sense of industry, (b) learn to think critically and make judgments based on reason, (c) accept criticism and different viewpoints, (d) develop social skills and a sense of accomplishment, (e) cooperate with others from various backgrounds, (f) accept adult authority other than from parents, and (g) be a leader and follower among the peer group.

Teaching the child personal identifying information, independence in self-care, and basic safety rules prepares the child for school. The preentry physical and dental examination and an orientation to the school and teacher promote a sense of anticipation and readiness. Parents should examine their own attitudes about the child entering school. Some parents seem eager to rid themselves of a portion of responsibility. Others are worried about the new influences and fear loss of control. Because the parents' attitudes so strongly affect the child, they should verbalize the positive aspects.

The parent or classroom teacher (and the nurse in the health care setting) can stimulate the child's learning through a variety of learning experiences that consider the child's individual abilities and interest, as well as the demands of the educational system and society. A child can quickly learn a specific and advanced task but often with limited retention and transfer. Success at learning tasks of increasing complexity depends on levels and interactions of subskills already possessed by the learner (149, 150).

Second Language Education

Certain skills are learned more easily at an early age, such as language, art, and music. The United States is one of the few countries where most students learn only one language. In most other countries, children begin learning several languages in the early school years.

Second language education has become important in the United States because of the rising number of immigrant children. An estimated 10 million U.S. children speak a language other than English in the home (107, 124). The federal Equal Education Opportunity Act aims to help non-English-speaking students learn English well enough to compete academically with native English speakers. Schools may have **bilingual education programs,** *where students are taught first in their native language and then in English.* Thus students are bilingual and can feel pride in their cultural identity. Some schools use an **English-immersion approach,** *where non-English-speaking students are immersed in English in*

special classes from the beginning. The bilingual approach appears more effective (107). Another approach is the **dual-language approach,** *in which English-speaking and non-English-speaking students learn together in their own and each other's languages.* This avoids separate classrooms, values both languages, helps build self-esteem, and improves school performances. English speakers learn a foreign language at an early age, when they can acquire it most easily (107). Bilingually proficient students have higher cognitive and linguistic achievement as long as bilingualism is valued and the second language addition is not at the sacrifice of the first (13, 107, 124).

The Diverse School Population

Most schools today have a *culturally diverse student body.* The child who attends a school with children from various ethnic or racial backgrounds or with children who have immigrated will also learn about cultures, and possibly several languages. However, mainstream culture perspectives usually prevail. The cultural orientations of American Indians, African Americans, Asian Americans, and Hispanic Americans may be misunderstood. Students benefit when educators understand their unique culture. However, *there are many intracultural, socioeconomic, geographic, generational, religious, and individual differences among families and children.*

Encourage teachers to foster understanding of cultural differences and social health in the classroom through the following measures:

1. Listen to the behavior as well as the words of the child.
2. Emphasize that each person is unique and worthy of respectful behavior, regardless of perceived differences.
3. Read stories, books, and articles about the history, life patterns, and achievements of people from various cultures and religions to the class.
4. Have bulletin board displays that commemorate the special days or historical leaders for each cultural group represented in the classroom.
5. Encourage parents from various cultural groups to come to the classroom, bring artifacts that are important or representative, and discuss commonly held beliefs or practices.
6. Encourage children to find similarities as well as differences among the cultural and religious groups represented in the classroom.

Problems of the family and concerns for the child's health are brought into sharp focus when the child enters school. *The teacher sees many difficulties:* (a) the loneliness of an only child, a foreign-born child, or a child who is from a minority culture; (b) the pain of the child with divorce or death in the family; (c) the negative self-image of the child who is not as physically attractive or coordinated or intellectually sharp as his or her peers; and (d) the child with learning difficulties. The child may demonstrate separation anxiety or **school phobia,** *fear of or refusal to attend school* (3, 93). School phobia or separation anxiety can be an indicator of a larger medical problem, the consequence of peer behavior and being bullied at school (108), or nothing more than a normal child with a temporary conflict (13, 68, 107, 124, 127).

Educate parents that school experiences are vivid in the child's memory. The child needs someone to listen to and talk about these experiences when he or she arrives home. This strengthens

MediaLink Cultural Difference in the Classroom

language skills, self-concept, and self-respect. If the child is put off or no one is there to listen, he or she may increasingly turn inward and refuse to talk when the adult is ready. The parents' taking a few minutes from supper preparation can be very important to the child. Collaborate with health care providers, parents, and educators to create a school environment that promotes health.

Influences on Ability to Learn

The *child's ability to learn and achieve in school is affected by factors other than intellectual ability.* Adult role models and other children influence the child in and out of school (141, 148). The educational level and vocalization patterns of the parents are strong predictors of a child's academic performance and measured intelligence (150). Failure to achieve may be the child's reaction to a hostile home environment, poor nutrition, physical illness, a troubled classroom, or a teacher's personal problem. Even the design of the school or physical attributes and appearance of the classroom may affect achievement. If the child cannot see or hear well, is uncomfortable or bothered by distractions and noise, feels unsafe, or has insufficient space, his or her attention, interest, and learning are reduced. Parents may project their inferiority feelings onto the child, and he or she believes that it is useless to try. He or she may have been placed in the wrong learning group, either above or below personal abilities. Occasionally negative factors cause a child to try harder, to sublimate and compensate, and to achieve well if ability is present.

Too much pushing by parents for the child to be a success, perfect in physical skills, the most intellectual, or a hard worker can backfire. The pressure that is generated may be so intense that the child eventually does not succeed. The child may become a perfectionist from parental example and behavior. *The perfectionistic child manifests* (14, 40, 107, 124, 126, 141):

1. Extreme concern about appearance.
2. Avoidance of tasks, play, or school because of fear of failure.
3. Dawdling or procrastinating on easy tasks to avoid harder ones or working so slowly on projects that creativity is lost.
4. Jealousy and envy of the apparent success and perfection of others.
5. Wanting to do something for which the child has no ability or talent.
6. Low tolerance for mistakes (e.g., the child who wins the race may feel unsuccessful because no records were set).

If these behaviors are present, teach the parents to work on relaxing themselves and the child and developing a sense of tolerance and humor. They can join the child in new activities—done for fun and without competition. They and the child can set realistic goals. They can praise the child's efforts, not focus on the outcome.

School difficulty may arise from the misuse of intelligence quotient (IQ) testing. IQ scores are not the same as intelligence. IQ scores can predict academic success generally, but they say nothing about a child's curiosity, motivation, inner thoughts, creativity, ability to get along with people, or ability to be a productive citizen (113, 134, 137). *A number of factors may negatively affect the IQ score* (13, 68, 107, 124, 126): (a) hunger and poor nutrition, (b) homelessness, (c) health problems, (d) sensory impairments, (e) lack of concentration, and (f) family stress. IQ test scores are also affected by very low birth weight; ethnic, racial, cultural, and language biases; the testing environment; and gender (68, 107, 126). Vocabulary use by the young schoolchild, based on parent-child interaction, is the best prediction of school achievement and overall intelligence (150). Minimal conversation between the parent and child, for example at meals or chore times, limits learning. Poverty places the child at risk for low achievement, but if the mother or caregiver talks frequently and expansively with the child, the child enters school with a larger vocabulary and greater capacity to learn (13, 150). Early childhood enrichment programs for disadvantaged children improve performance in the school years (107, 126).

Studies by the American Association of University Women revealed sexism in elementary school education in the United States. Teachers and the educational system historically favored males over females. Some females experience decreasing self-esteem and academic achievement from the time they begin elementary school to the time they enter high school (96, 99–101). Yet females are as capable as males in all avenues of educational attainment if society allows, expects, or demands it (99, 107, 124). There is, however, growing concern about school-age males having difficulty in school and not achieving because of lack of attention to their needs, emphasis on early testing, lack of a father figure for many boys, and gender differences physiologically. By the seventh grade, a high correlation exists between personality characteristics and IQ scores (56, 99, 101, 107, 124, 150).

Education for Children with Special Needs

Past legislation regarding special education in the United States included (13, 68, 107, 124):

1. Children with Specific Learning Disabilities Act; 1969 (PL [Public Law] 91-230), which recognized learning disabilities as a category within special education.
2. Education of All Handicapped Children, 1975 (PL 96-142), which mandated education of all schoolchildren, no matter what the disability, in the least restrictive environment, which meant with other children in a regular classroom, mainstreaming, if possible (68).
3. Individuals with Disabilities Education Act (IDEA), 1990, and updated 1997 (PL 105-17), required all states to provide education for all children, preschool and thereafter. Parents could agree or refuse referral, testing, placement, and the IEP (Individual Educational Plan) and appeal the decision. School districts within the United States interpret these laws in various ways (68).
4. The Americans with Disabilities Act (ADA) broadened educational integration opportunities for all Americans with disabilities, in both private and public schools (124).
5. The Elementary and Secondary Education Act (ESEA) was enacted in 1995 to eliminate sex bias in schools and promote equity for females in schools (107, 124).

A *classroom with diversity* in the children's intellectual abilities, skills, and personalities is helpful to the child; he or she learns about the real world. Putting the exceptional child in a regular classroom, however, may not make him or her feel normal; he or she may still be perceived, and perceive self, as different. The exceptional child may need special classes to get the help needed. Most students benefit from **mainstreaming** or **inclusion,** *placing the child with special needs and abilities in the regular classroom to participate in academic skills and play* (13).

The Gifted Child

The **gifted child** is *above average intellectually (IQ 130 or higher) and has superior talent for or aptitude in a specific area.* The child is *characterized by superior consumption of information and by outstanding ability to produce information, concepts, and new forms and is* **precocious,** *able to perform consistently at a higher level than most children of the same age.* The gifted child *demonstrates to a greater extent than other children the many types of intelligence:* mathematical, linguistic, musical, spatial, body-kinesthetic, interpersonal, and intrapersonal. The child is *adept at problem solving and problem finding and has a passion to learn.* The gifted child is considered *educationally exceptional. The child's full intellectual, creative, and leadership potential may be neglected if* (1, 68, 107, 124, 126):

1. Parents are not attuned to the child's abilities and needs.
2. Parents or teachers are threatened by the gifted child who grasps concepts more quickly than they do.
3. Parents do not value cognitive, creative, or leadership abilities.
4. The child is not given freedom to explore and be different.
5. The school system does not have a program suited for his or her abilities.

Often the gifted child is misunderstood. Research indicates, however, that gifted students have higher self-esteem than others and are popular with their peers (107, 124, 126). Yet, the gifted child may not excel or be ahead of the norm in all dimensions. The child may be intellectually ahead of chronologic age but may be behind in physical growth and coordination, emotional development, or social skills. The inconsistency inherent in lack of developmental synchrony may be difficult for parents, teachers, and peers to accept.

Encourage parents to respect the individual interests and talents of their child. Help parents not to be intimidated by the child's unusual interests and behavior and to avoid crushing budding interests or creativity. *Emphasize that the essence of raising a gifted child is to facilitate and provide opportunity,* not hold back or insist that something be done a certain way. Validate that it takes courage and patience to let a child develop at his or her pace. Support parents as they let their child assert his or her own initiative in a situation, even if the child is not at first successful. Foster empathy for the child and an individualized educational program to enhance cognitive health and development and competency. Reinforce that the impulse toward growth and development must first come from the child's budding inclinations, not from a desire to conform to another's expectations.

Home Schooling

Home schooling, *teaching the child at home according to a curricular plan,* is conducted by some parents who believe the present public school system is inadequate to teach their children the needed skills. There are established lesson plans for the grade level and academic year with subject content, suggestions for teaching, and evaluation methods. The parents have a choice, depending on cost factors and perceived needs and interests of the child. Often all the parents and children in a locale who are enrolled in home schooling gather periodically for social events to foster social skills and friendships among the children. Parents, or groups of parents, may also plan field trips to enhance the child's education, for example to museums, parks, and historical sites (107, 121, 124).

Work with these parents to help them realize the importance of curricular integrity, that if the child graduates from a home school program, he or she is expected to have achieved a certain standard. Further, emphasize the child's need for friendships and interaction with people from diverse backgrounds. Explore whether the child will have opportunities such as regular physical education activities, playing a musical instrument, choral singing, and art classes. Explore whether the parents will be able to consistently engage the child in learning activities and monitor the necessary testing or evaluation. Home schooling should not be an excuse to keep the child home and sheltered from the world. *Some parents do not have the persistence or skill to implement home schooling. Some children need to be away from the home and with other people a few hours each day,* just as parents need to interact with other parents. In certain situations, if the child is geographically isolated or in an adverse school environment, home schooling may be an answer.

Educate parents about the importance of being alert to the feelings and emotional status of the child, which may be less obvious than physical symptoms and diseases. Educate parents that the child having emotional or behavioral problems is not a disgrace; help them work through feelings of embarrassment or stigma. Emphasize the importance of seeking treatment as early as possible, learning ways to overcome the disorder, and preventing more serious consequences or chronicity. Encourage careful observation. For example, there *is* a difference between attention deficit disorder and attention deficit/hyperactivity disorder, depression and grief related to crises and losses, and the various disorders that make up the autism spectrum disorders. Affirm that parents are the child's advocates. Refer parents to professional counselors and agencies that work with the individual child and also include the family in assessment and management. Educate parents about the local and national organizations that present information.

Box 12-8 presents a list of resources that give information about various diseases and their prevention, support groups, treatment, and the importance of avoiding overmedication. Educate parents that overmedication of mentally or emotionally ill children is increasingly a problem and must be avoided (94, 109, 153). Often school-age children (and younger) are given medications that have not been tested for use in children and are recommended only for adults (94, 153).

Counsel parents that behavior that is challenging to them may not be a sign of illness but may actually be a sign of the child's giftedness or creativity. Recommend a holistic family counselor and discussion with the teacher, as well as appropriate screening, in order to determine the child's IQ and behavioral and emotional status. Refer to **Box 12-8** for resources that give information to clarify parental concerns.

Educate parents about negative effects of much of what is presented on television—certainly the aggressive, violent, sexually suggestive, and pornographic content. Refer to the section later in this chapter on the effects of media on the child. The American

BOX 12-8	**Resources for Information About Emotional and Behavioral Disorders**

Autism Society of America (toll-free phone 800-328-8476)— *www.autism-society.org*

Asperger Syndrome Coalition of the United States— *www.asperger.org*

Online Asperger Syndrome Information and Support (OASIS)—*www.udel.edu/bkerby/asperger*

Depression and Bipolar Support Alliance (toll-free phone 800-826-3632)—*www.dbsalliance.org*

Depression Awareness, Recognition, and Treatment Program of the National Institute of Mental Health— *www.nimh.nih.gov/publicat/index.cfm*

MacArthur Foundation Initiative on Depression and Primary Care—*www.depression-primarycare.org*

Children and Adults with Attention Deficit Hyperactivity Disorder (toll-free phone 800-233-4050)— *www.chaad.org*

Attention-Deficit Hyperactivity Disorder (ADHD) /Children & Adults with Attention Deficit Disorders (CHADD)— *www.chadd.org*

Comorbidity—*www.depression-guide.com/adhd-disorders.htm*

National Alliance for the Mentally Ill (toll-free phone 800-969-6642)—*www.nmha.org*

American Academy of Child and Adolescent Psychiatry (202-966-7300)—*www.ascap.org*

American Academy of Pediatrics—*www.aap.org/policy/ s0120.html*

Attention Deficit Disorder Facts, Prevention and Treatment Strategies—*www.healingwithnutrition.com/*

National Resource Center—*www.help4adhd.org/*

Behavior Problems National Institute of Mental Health (NIMH)—*www.nimh.nih.gov/anxiety*

Academy of Pediatrics recommends that children watch no more than one hour daily of *slow-paced programming, preferably educational* (2). This would be critical for children with cognitive, emotional, and behavioral challenges or disorders.

You, the teachers, and administrators must work together for the *health and safety of all children.* Guns and other weapons do not belong in school, and the school must be kept safe from gunmen and snipers. All adults must know how to protect the children and themselves. Work with the child, parents, teachers, and administrators as a consultant or counselor. Treating difficulties early is likely to prevent major problems (32, 47, 107, 109).

Increasingly schools are inviting parents to participate in the **Parents As Teachers Program,** *whereby the parent attends school with the child, learning with and assisting the child.* Teachers are developing partnerships with families to foster student development. Parents, who are trained to be school volunteers, learn parenting and communication skills. The parent can better assist the child with homework and becomes more active in school governance and decisions as well as in the broader community (5, 106, 107, 124). Special efforts should be made to involve parents from diverse cultural groups. A helpful organization is the Parents As Teachers National Center. Information is available from their Website, www.parentsasteachers.org.

Reaffirm to parents that they are ultimately responsible for their child's behavior and learning. The **Box** Client Education: Suggestions for Parents' Participation in the Child's Education suggests how parents can assist the child. Educate parents about growth and development, the teacher's role, and the importance of attending parent–teacher association meetings and working with the child's teacher.

COMMUNICATION PATTERNS

Many factors influence the child's communication pattern, vocabulary, and diction. Some of these factors have been referred to in previous chapters. *Influences include:*

1. Speech and verbal and nonverbal communication patterns of parents, siblings, and other adults such as teachers and peers.
2. Attitudes of others toward the child's effort to speak and communicate.
3. General environmental stimulation.
4. Opportunity to communicate with a variety of people in a variety of situations.
5. Intellectual development.
6. Ability to hear and articulate.
7. Vocabulary skills.
8. Contact with television or other technology such as computers, the Internet, and video games.

The *6-year-old* has command of nearly every form of sentence structure and can understand from 8,000 to 14,000 words, depending on home and environmental experiences and innate ability. The child experiments less with language, using it more as a tool and less for the mere pleasure of talking than during the preschool period. Now language is used to share in others' experiences. He or she also swears and uses slang to test others' reactions. The child enjoys printing words in large letters (58, 59, 107).

Eye–hand coordination continues to improve. *At age 7* the child can print several sentences, and at *age 8* he or she can write instead of print. By *9 years* the child participates in family discussions, showing interest in family activities and indicating an individuality. Verbal fluency has improved, and common objects are described in detail. Writing skill has improved; he or she can write with small, even letters. *By age 10* the child can write or type for a relatively long time with speed. Increasingly, schoolchildren use computers to type rather than write. The preadolescent may seem less talkative, withdrawing when frustrated instead of voicing anger. Sharing feelings with a best friend is a healthy outlet (58, 59, 107, 126).

As the child shares ideas and feelings, he or she learns how someone else thinks and feels about similar matters. The child expresses self in a way that has meaning to others, at first to a chum and then to others. Thus he or she is validating and expanding vocabulary,

Client Education

Suggestions for Parents' Participation in the Child's Education

DO	DO not
1. Let your children know you believe they can do well. Encourage self-evaluation.	1. Dwell on the negative by criticizing.
2. Minimize time spent watching television.	2. Allow the television to be your babysitter.
3. Help your children organize. Encourage them to do the most difficult task first.	3. Do homework for the children.
4. Talk and read to your children.	4. Leave them to their own devices.
5. Go to your children's school and volunteer.	5. Forget to encourage verbal exchange.
6. Encourage outside activities and having friends at home.	6. Push them to have every minute scheduled or send them off to play.
7. Work with your children's teachers and let the teacher know you understand and are supportive.	7. Criticize and interfere with everything you do not understand.
8. Insist on good eating habits.	8. Allow constant eating.
9. Plan activities with your children.	9. Send them off without you to family functions (e.g., school plays, potluck dinners).
10. Be a good example.	10. Say, "Do as I say and not as I do."

ideas, and feelings. The child learns that a friend's family has similar life patterns, demands of the child, and frustrations. He or she learns about self in the process of learning more about another. The child recalls what has happened in the past, realizes how this has affected the present, and considers what effect present acts will have on future events. The child uses **syntaxic, or consensual, communication** *when he or she sees these cause-and-effect relationships in an objective, logical way and can validate them with others* (137). *By sixth grade,* the child who has had opportunity to learn may have a vocabulary 10 to 20 times that of the 6-year-old (13, 124, 126).

Convey love and caring, not rejection, when you talk with children. Love is communicated through nonverbal behavior, such as getting down to the child's eye level, and through words that value feelings and indicate respect. Children understand language directed at their feelings better than at their intellect and the overt action. Do not overreact to normal behavior. Avoid talking about touchy areas, if possible, or the child's babyhood. He or she is struggling to be grown up; any reminder of younger behavior creates anxiety about potential regression. The principles of communicating with the preschooler discussed in Chapter 11 are also applicable to the schoolchild. ∞

EFFECTS OF MEDIA ON THE CHILD'S DEVELOPMENT AND HEALTH

This section is presented in detail because of the continuing pervasiveness of the problem and the short- and long-term health effects on the child, cognitively, emotionally, socially, and even physically and spiritually, and ultimately on society. *Electronic media* such as television and movies, video and computer games, the Internet, and text messaging *exert a powerful influence on a child's health, communication, and behavior patterns.* The effects of televi-

sion, related media, and the Internet, and the portrayal of violence and pornography in the media, will be discussed in this section.

Children watch an average of 25 to 29 hours of television weekly—more time than is spent on school homework or any activity except sleeping (2, 28, 68, 76). Generally females, in contrast to males, begin in the preschool years to view more television that is educational and read more books, if available. Positive characteristics continuing into adolescence have been demonstrated in these females: higher grades during the school years, a higher value on achievement, and more creative behavior. However, preschool females who watch more aggressive, violent television shows have lower grades in the school years (6, 124, 128). Males watch more TV than females, and they are more likely to watch violent and action-packed programs. Saturday morning cartoons may be the worst for viewing, with 20 to 25 violent actions shown per hour, in contrast to 5 or 6 times per hour in prime-time programs. The highest rates of violence are in programs broadcast when children are most likely to be viewing: 6:00 to 9:00 a.m. and 2:00 to 5:00 p.m. (2, 124, 128).

Effects of Television Viewing

If watching television is controlled by responsible parents and caregivers, cognitive and social learning can be enhanced. Educational programs for children are presented about 3 hours weekly by the commercial channels as a result of the Children's Television Act, passed in 1990, which requires stations to meet the educational and informational needs of children in order to renew their license.

Increasingly, research indicates short- and long-term negative effects on children when they watch violent (2, 6, 12, 21, 22, 29, 35, 43, 69, 71, 85, 86, 114, 128, 129, 135), sexually seductive (29, 67, 111, 135, 159), or pornographic (29, 116, 135, 157) material on television, in films, or in other media. Heavy television viewing is

INTERVENTIONS FOR HEALTH PROMOTION

Parents must help children select educational programming in order to (31, 68, 86, 135, 157):

1. Gain information about specific topics that add to understanding of the world in general and beyond the immediate environment.
2. Observe positive images of people from various ethnic groups or people who have disabilities.
3. Observe positive or prosocial behavior and cultural values such as work, sacrifice, and goal setting.

4. Convey positive ethical messages about the value of family life, friendship, and commitment to relationships.
5. Feature females and males in positions of authority or performing heroic acts.
6. Present and reinforce techniques associated with various sports or exercise routines.
7. Stimulate creativity and problem solving.

associated with lower school achievement. Schoolteachers report that more children are entering school with decreased imaginative play and creativity and increased aimless movement, low frustration level, poor persistence and concentration span, and confusion about reality and fantasy. Rapid speech and constantly changing visuals on television prevent reflection. The child does not learn correct sentence structure, use of tenses, or the ability to express thoughts or feelings effectively. The result may be a child who is unable to enunciate or use correct grammar and who is vague in the sense of time, history, and cause-and-effect relationships (21, 39, 43, 86).

Most studies emphasize that children are more likely to be violent after watching violence on television if they see violence in their own home, receive harsh discipline, or have no nurturing father in the home, and if there is excessive television viewing without parental supervision or discussion (13, 29, 68, 86, 111, 135, 147). Children from dysfunctional homes lack the supervision or guidance to help them handle and sort through what they see and hear. Children who have grown up in stable families, who feel secure and loved, and who have a variety of interests and relationships are less adversely affected by the aggression and violence presented on tele-

vision. They learn to separate fantasy from fact, and all of their fantasy is not based on television (13, 29, 111, 135).

Understanding television can involve active mental work for the young child, but often the child does not understand content, motives, or feelings; integrate events shown; or infer conditions not shown. Those are the mental processes that are stimulated by adult and peer interactions and reading of literature (148, 149). Excess television viewing is associated with lower school achievement (39). Often television is used in the home to the extent that it stifles family interaction and bombards with noise, excitement, speed, and misdirected humor or aggression.

Discuss with parents the need *to limit the amount of television viewing (less than 2 hours a day)*, limit time spent playing video games, do alternative activities with their children, and screen what their children are viewing. This is a significant area of life that affects the child and the family in all aspects. Review with parents the information presented in the **Box**, Client Education, Guidelines for Parents: Healthy use of Media in the Home.

Review with parents the negative effects of excess media viewing. Refer to **Table 12-11**. Encourage parents to be vigilant about

Client Education

Guidelines for Parents: Healthy Use of Media in the Home

1. Keep televisions and computers in public places in the home, such as the kitchen, family or living room, office, or large hallway, so that when children are viewing media, they are in full view of others.
2. Avoid having a computer or television in the child's bedroom or the playroom, which interferes with supervision and can interfere with sleep.
3. Screen the programs that are available via television, films, video games, and Internet. Be direct about wanting to know what the child is viewing. Explain that this is a family activity and give logical reasons.
4. Stay in touch with the child's viewing habits, video games acquired, and online activities. Do not let their desire for

privacy override their need for parental supervision. Give positive feedback for the child's open communication.
5. View questionable movies and television serial programs before allowing children to view them.
6. View and discuss programs with the child. Get the child's feedback about reasons for his or her interest in various programs.
7. Establish boundaries. A television with adults-only channels or computer with access to adult sites should not be available to the child or placed in the child's room.

TABLE 12-11

Negative Effects of Excessive Media Viewing

Physical

1. Arouse aggressive impulses and actions in response to environment, others.
2. Promote sedentary lifestyle and snacking rather than participating in play, sports, physical exercise, community events, discussions, or interaction with others.
3. Foster increased ingestion of carbonated beverages, fried foods, and high-fat, high-sugar snacks.
4. Decrease imaginative play, increase aimless movements.
5. Foster difficulty falling asleep, nightmares related to fears aroused by scary, violent, or fictional content.
6. Create a desire through the advertisements for unhealthy products, such as high-sugar or high-fat content foods, cigarettes, alcoholic beverages.

Cognitive

1. Promote passive rather than active learning.
2. Increase passivity from continual information overload.
3. Reduce creative thinking and creativity of the child.
4. Encourage short attention span and hyperactive thought because of fast-paced presentation verbally and visually.
5. Reduce concentration ability and persistence at problem-solving tasks.
6. Interfere with correct enunciation of words, grammar, vocabulary use, sentence structure, reading comprehension, and spelling achievement.
7. Interfere with ability to express thoughts and feelings effectively.
8. Contribute to confusion or uncertainty about what is real and what is fantasy.
9. Contribute to vague understanding of historical events, cause-and-effect relationships.
10. Contribute to lack of understanding about what is seen and consequences of the behavior because of content or fast pace of programming.
11. Create a desire for superficial rather than depth of information; media teaches simplified, superficial solutions.
12. De-emphasize complexity of life with simplistic plots and fast action; no lasting consequences to behavior, no visual or cognitive depth.
13. Teach unrealistic, stereotyped view of men and women and gender roles; women depicted as sexual objects and with limited problem-solving skills.
14. Heighten aggressive tendencies, thoughts, feelings, and memories in consciousness, causing overt aggression.
15. Stimulate consumerism; become highly focused on buying things related to advertisements, value on materialism to which parents have difficulty saying "no."

Behavioral/Social

1. Promote aggressive or violent behavior as a way to resolve problems or conflicts, to protect self.
2. Increase incidence of aggressive and violent behavior because of program pace and content; loud music or intense, rapid rhythm; camera tricks.
3. Keep the child occupied, use in lieu of a babysitter, avoid interfering with parental activities.
4. Reduce social interaction; foster loneliness, shyness, inability to interact with peers.
5. Compete with parents, school, and peers as a socializing agent.
6. Promote passivity and withdrawal from direct involvement in real life.
7. Arouse aggressive sexual tendencies through depiction of overt sexual behavior, perversions, pornographic content.

Emotional/Motivational

1. Contribute to poor control of impulses and frustrations.
2. Reduce interest in less exciting but necessary classroom and home activities.
3. Promote passive acceptance of aggressive or violent behavior.
4. Formulate unrealistic or negative attitude about authority figures.
5. Increase anxiety, fears, suspicion of others.
6. Increase emotional problems, including conduct disorders, post-traumatic stress disorder (nightmares, flashbacks, suspicions, poor concentration, impaired relationships with others).

Moral

1. Contribute to confusion about values and value systems, especially related to gender, race, and age.
2. Model lack of commitment in relationships, emphasize sexuality and immediate gratification, without showing consequences of such behavior.
3. Foster attitude of domination of others, inequality of people; most frequent victims are women, children, and elders.
4. Become desensitized to violence in general.

programs their children watch. Explore ways they can work with children to avoid being enticed by product advertisements (76, 142, 157). Encourage parents to be active advocates for healthy media programming. They can write letters to television stations, newspapers, legislators, and program advertisers. Parents can refuse to buy the products advertised during negative programming. They can join advocacy groups that are concerned about unhealthy media and effects on children and families.

Effects of Internet Use

The **Internet**, which began as a defense project in the 1960s, is a *huge network of computers electronically linked via phone, cable lines, and satellites, which enables users to communicate and access information while "online."* It is a major tool to obtain information, an education, or access to various resources; to conduct ministries; to do shopping; and to conduct conversations. It is also a major tool for negative programming, including violence and pornography. Many X-rated Websites disguise their programming so that they are accessed in innocent Internet searches, including searches used by children for homework (2, 13, 68, 92, 98, 124). As with all technologic advances, parents must guide, monitor, and protect their children and look for creative, commonsense solutions. Parents can "surf the net"—sit at the computer—with the child. Or the child, often very knowledgeable, can teach the parent about computer and Internet use, online sites, and available services. Such collaboration can open lines of communication and raise the child's self-esteem.

Educate parents how they can protect the child and reduce risks of Internet use. Review with them the information in the **Box**, Client Education, Guidelines for Parents: Healthy Use of the Internet.

Portrayal of Violence and Pornography in the Media

The stereotype about people living in the United States is that everyone engages in violent and pornographic behavior because of the messages on mass media. In fact, most of what the mass media depict, whether newscasts, sitcoms, cartoons, movies, or negative Internet programming or online messages, do not reflect behavior of the majority of people in the United States. They do not reflect the entire real world, here or abroad. For example, many people in the United States may see homicides in the media; few people, *comparatively*, see or experience murder in real life. If as much murder occurred in real life as on the screen, the U.S. population would be rapidly decreasing. For every harmful or negative act depicted in newscasts, for example, there are hundreds or thousands of positive, helpful acts daily between people that go unreported.

However, research studies over the past three decades indicate increased portrayal of violence in the media (television, including cable; video games, movies, and the Internet). There is a correlation between overall national maltreatment or abuse of children and adults and more incidences of aggressive behavior by people of all ages (2, 6, 22, 39, 43, 85, 92, 98, 111, 135, 136). Even children's cartoons shown on Saturday mornings depict as many as 25 aggressive or violent scenes in an hour (124), and 80% of prime-time television programs depict violent acts (124).

Some media programming is planned to be pornographic. The child who has unsupervised television watching cannot avoid programs that teach unhealthy family and life values; stereotyped views of males and females; the apparent normality of uncommitted, brief, unloving relationships; and the female as a sex object. Consequences of such behavior are rarely shown (2, 67, 92, 98, 111, 135, 136). Some groups also object to frequent depiction of stepparent or same-sex partners.

Children of all ages (and adults) who watch violence on television, movies, videos, or the computer screen become more aggressive and violent. Such programming is graphic, explicit, realistic, and intensively involving. Children are especially affected short and long term, because they have less ego control or less maturely developed coping mechanisms. They act out more directly what they see. *Video games are even worse*, because the child is not a passive observer but has to be an active participant in the violence to play the game and score points (6, 12, 31, 43, 47, 68, 98). Males may be vulnerable to the effects because they play these games more frequently and for longer periods (12). Further, video games tend to be more violent, racist, and sexist than other programming, although considerable media programming is actually X-rated (12, 43, 47). Many programs directly or indirectly teach the viewer how to carry out violent acts. It is not unusual when arson, rape, hostage taking, suicide, or homicide is described on newscasts that, either locally or nationally, such incidents are repeated within a few days. The live, explicit portrayals suggest such action is normal, justified, courageous, rewarded (media attention), and even socially acceptable.

Alternatives to violence are seldom shown, and violence is glorified (107). The school-age child seeks heroes. In violent programming, perpetrators go unpunished (107). Since victims appear unharmed, the child is likely to imitate the filmed model, especially when there is lack of parental supervision. The influence is stronger if the child believes the violence on the screen, identifies with the violent character, and watches without parental supervision (29). The more television and active violent programming watched daily, the greater the incidence of trauma symptoms (anxiety, stress responses, anger, depression) reported by the child, as well as aggressive or violent behavior that is observable (68, 129, 130). Children with psychological and behavioral problems report more trauma symptoms (130).

Educate parents by reviewing information previously discussed. Emphasize that viewing aggressive, violent, sexually seductive programs or pornographic scenes on television, movies, videos, and computer screens has negative short- and long-term effects on behavior. Video games, often used outside the home, are worse than television. Review **Table 12-11**, Negative Effects of Excessive Media Viewing, and the **Box**, Client Education: Guidelines for Parents: Healthy Use of the Internet. Discuss the information in relation to the parent's and child's individual needs and situation.

Reducing Risks and Protecting the Child

Discuss with parents how they handle media viewing in the home. Explore ways to make better choices (31, 98). Empower parents to intentionally turn off objectionable television programs, the video game, or computer, and give reasons. ("We don't allow violence in this house.") ("Watching such programs [playing this kind of video game] interferes with your health [well-being, learning, creativity].") Effective parental behavior fosters holistic health in the

Client Education

Guidelines for Parents: Healthy Use of the Internet

1. Become familiar with sites and services that are available on the Internet. Emphasize to the child that online exploration is an activity for the whole family, just as families watch television together.

2. Share information and concerns about Internet use with other parents and teachers.

3. Set up and post guidelines for online usage. Specify the sites they can visit and the amount of time online for fun and for school activities. Curb late-night usage, especially of chatrooms and bulletin boards.

4. Use options for blocking programs that are objectionable or unwanted, and ensure that the children or babysitters cannot override the block.

5. Use Internet filters that can be purchased and downloaded directly from the Internet to block objectionable Websites. One especially effective filter was created by a Christian company—Integrity Online.

6. Reinforce that parents review behavior related to strangers (presented in Chapter 11) ∞ ; avoidance behaviors are as applicable to the computer as to the street or play area.

7. Forbid the child to reveal the password, send a picture, or reveal personal identifying information about the self or family online, via e-mail, no matter how friendly the person is, even if the person acts like the child's friend or poses as another child. Give the child reasons for the limits.

8. Be present with the child to meet another child or adult if an online relationship has progressed to that point. Explain reasons to the child; meet in a public place, and advise that if the person is a child, he or she should bring along a parent. If this is to be a solid friendship, having a chaperone should not be a problem.

9. Emphasize that the child never accept offers of delivery of merchandise or information without first getting parental permission.

10. Tell the child to never continue an uncomfortable conversation or one that is demanding of personal information, but rather to "hang up" by going to another site or area. Affirm that the child should report the event to the parents. Reinforce such positive behavior.

11. Validate that the child should never answer e-mail or bulletin board items that are suggestive, rude, uncomfortable, or obscene, but to tell the parents so that the message can be forwarded to the service provider. Emphasize that such a message is not the child's fault and that the child does not deserve such a message. Reinforce the child's decision to share the event.

12. Explain, on a level the child can understand, about activities of a pedophile, "a person who hurts children." Explain gently and over time, often with other health or sex education, how the pedophile uses the computer. Online conversations escalate from giving attention and showing interest, to gaining trust, to lowering the child's sexual inhibitions, to descriptions of sexual experiences. The pedophile will emphasize the need for secrecy, ask the child to delete the messages, and eventually, ask for a secret meeting. Emphasize that the parents love the child and always want to protect the child.

13. Engage the child in a variety of activities that are fun and involve the family such as (a) playing table games, working on puzzles in the home, pursuing a hobby; (b) visiting parks or museums; (c) going on day trips, as a mini-vacation; (d) visiting with family friends or relatives; or (e) volunteering in a community activity, such as helping at a food pantry or an agency for elders. Such activities reduce the child's need to entertain self on the Internet, keep the parent or another adult as an active, positive role model, and provide a range of educational and fun-filled experiences. Encourage the child to invite a friend to the home or on the outing.

child. Encourage parents to spend time watching television, movies, and the Internet with their children. After viewing they can plan to discuss the themes and values portrayed. This allows exploring perceptions, fosters open communication, presents a time for teaching family values, and strengthens the relationship.

Explore negative behaviors presented in **Table 12-11** that the parents may have observed in the child. Explore ways to prevent short- and long-term effects. School, church, or community resources can help the child and family overcome negative effects.

Educate parents about organizations that are engaged in advocacy against programming that contains violent and sexual excesses. These organizations include the American Academy of Child and Adolescent Psychiatry, the American Academy of Family Physicians, the American Academy of Pediatrics, the American Medical Association, the American Psychiatric Association, the American Psychological Association, and the National Education Association. Many parents, schools, and community, health care, and religious leaders are joining efforts to gain more educational and less destructive programming.

One national organization, the Parents Television Council (PTC), has consistently for years educated the public about the increasing obscenities and pornography depicted in movies and national television shows and in the electronic media (video games, the Internet, computer programming). Their monitoring reveals this trend even in prime-time, family-oriented television programs. Executives and board members of PTC have testified before congressional hearings in an effort to obtain better federal regulation. Although progress is slow, some states, such as Illinois, are passing laws to protect children from violent programming. PTC explains that inadvertently we all support such programming, often unaware, by the company stocks we own or the products we buy that are advertised during such programming. More information about the work of PTC and how to be involved as an advocate for less violent or pornographic media programming can be obtained through their Website, www.parentstv.org.

Another organization dedicated to protecting family values and reducing violent and pornographic programming in television, movies, and electronic media is Focus on the Family. This *spiritually based organization* focuses its efforts both nationally and worldwide. More information, including extensive references, books, and CD-ROM sets related to healthy living, and listings of video games and computer games that present lessons about Christian values rather than violence or pornography is available through their Website, www.family.org. The materials offered may also be helpful to families of the Jewish or Muslim faiths.

Actions for preventing and responding to violence against all children, across all settings in which violence occurs, have been recommended. Promoting nonviolent values and transforming attitudes that condone or normalize violence are basic. Public information campaigns should be used to sensitize the public about harmful effects on children. Policies, programs, and budget allocations should address various risks, such as family breakdown, abuse of alcohol or drugs, and access to guns and other weapons. Social and cultural attitudes and actions must be confronted because of attachment to traditions. Continuing education of professionals and all who work with and for children about elimination of violence must be developed and disseminated. Codes of conduct and ethical standards of practice should be formulated and enforced. Recommendations that address national strategies and practices in all systems, data collection, and accountability, as well as international involvement, are presented in detail in the Medical News Today Website, www.medicalnewstoday.com.

PLAY PATTERNS
Peer Groups

The healthy child plays with peers, not just electronic media. Peer groups, including the group or gang and the close chum, provide companionship, shared time, conversation, and activity with a widening circle of persons outside the home. They are extremely important to the school-age child. Between the *ages of 7 and 9*, children usually form close friendships with peers of the same sex and age. Later in this age group, peers are not necessarily of the same age. Functions of the peer group are listed in **Table 12-12.**

Children must earn their membership in the peer group, and being accepted by one's peers and belonging to a peer group are major concerns for this age group. Many factors determine a child's acceptance, including attractiveness and friendliness. Most children find acceptance with at least one or two peers; rejection and loneliness are always a risk. Children may be rejected because they are either too aggressive or too passive. Being an outsider carries all the risks that are implied if the peer group functions cannot be attained. Effects of not being a peer group member can be cor-

TABLE 12-12

Functions of the School-Age Peer Group

1. Reinforces gender role behavior
2. Accepts those who conform to social roles
3. Provides an audience for developing self-concept, self-esteem, and unique personality characteristics
4. Provides information about the world of school and neighborhood, games, dress, and manners; decreases egocentrism
5. Provides opportunity to compete and compare self to others of same age
6. Develops a personal set of values and goals; conformity is expected
7. Teaches rules and logical consequences; punishes members who disobey rules
8. Provides opportunity to test mastery in a world parallel to adult society, with rules, organization, and purposes
9. Provides emotional support during stressful or crisis points in a member's life
10. Protects against other peers who may threaten, bully, or intimidate, or actually harm if the member were alone

rected through having a chum, as explained in the following section, or may set the foundation for either a shy, withdrawn personality or an overtly assertive or aggressive personality that tries to maneuver into groups. These effects may still be evident in adulthood. **Figure 12-2■** depicts the peer group.

Chum Stage

The chum stage occurs around *9 or 10 years of age* and sometimes later when affection moves from the peer group and gang to a **chum**, a *special friend of the same sex and age*. This is an important relationship because it is the *child's first love attachment outside the family, when someone becomes as important to him or her as self* (137). Initially, a person of the same sex and age is easier than someone of the opposite sex to feel concern for and to understand. The friend becomes an extension of the child's own self. As he or she shares ideas and feelings, the child learns a great deal about both self and the chum. The child discovers that he or she is more similar to than different from others and learns to accept self for what he or she is. Self-acceptance of uniqueness increases acceptance of others so that the child of this age is very sociable, generous, and sympathetic; enjoys differences in people; and is liberal in ideas about the welfare of others. He or she learns that others can do things differently but that they are still all right as people. It is also through the chum relationship that the child learns the **syntaxic mode of communication** *to validate word meanings in talking with the chum and others*. Thus ideas about the world become more realistic. Loyalty to the chum at this age may be greater than loyalty to the family (137). **Altruism,** a *concern for others in various situations*, and an ability to respond to others' happiness and distress, to develop intimate associations, including with individuals of the opposite sex, and a sensitivity and concern for all humanity result from high-level chumship (137).

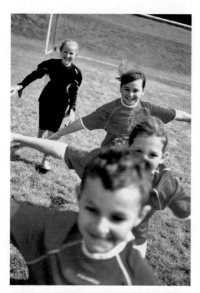

FIGURE ■ 12-2 Exposure to a variety of peers and learning to work and play cooperatively are important for the school age child. (Russell Sadur © Dorling Kindersley)

The chum stage provides the foundation for later intimacy with an individual of the opposite sex and close friends of both sexes. If the child does not have a chum relationship, he or she has more difficulty with adolescent heterosexuality or adult intimacy.

Help parents understand the importance of the chum stage. The chum stage fosters emotional health. Parents should monitor who is chosen as the chum; prior social opportunities foster choosing a close friend who can be trusted. Parents need to be receptive to the chum and include the chum in some family activities.

Play Activities

Play activities change with the child's development. From *age 6 to 8*, he or she is interested chiefly in the present and in the immediate surroundings. Because he or she knows more about family life than any other kind of living, the child takes the role of parents or various occupational groups with which there is contact: mail carrier, firefighter, carpenter, nurse, occupational therapist, teacher, and clergy. Although the child is more interested in playing with peers than parents, the *6- or 7-year-old* will sometimes enjoy having the parent participate in their play or games.

Both sexes enjoy some activities in common, such as painting, music, cutting and pasting, reading, collecting items such as baseball cards or stamps, simple table games, television, digging, riding a bicycle, construction sets or models, puzzles, kites, running games, team sports, rough-and-tumble play, skating, and swimming. The parent can enjoy these activities with the child, especially if the parent has a special talent the child wishes to learn. The child often imitates the roles of his or her own gender and becomes increasingly realistic in play.

By *age 8*, collections, more advanced models, radio, television, computers, art materials, "how to" books, farm activities, and train sets are favorite pastimes. Loosely formed, short-lived clubs with fluctuating rules are formed.

Computerized and electronic games give a sense of control and power; of being a peer with, or even superior to, the adult;

and of challenge and inventiveness. They foster an enjoyment of complexity and expandability. Computer and video toys can help the schoolchild understand the nature of systems and control of information—skills needed in the adult world. Let the child take the lead in when to move into computer games. There is no need to rush the child. Further, some schoolchildren will prefer reading, painting, playing an instrument, doing crafts, camping, or playing sports. These skills and what these activities teach are as essential to the workplace as the ability to operate a computer.

At approximately *age 10*, gender differences in play become pronounced. Each gender is developing through play the skills it will later need in society; this is manifested through the dramatizing of real-life situations. The child's interest in faraway places is enhanced through a foreign pen pal and through travel.

From *age 9 to 12*, the child becomes more interested in active sports but continues to enjoy quieter activity. He or she wants to improve motor skills. The child may enjoy carpentry or mechanics' tools, advanced models or puzzles, arts and crafts, science projects, music, dance, cameras and film, and camping. Adult-organized games of softball, football, or soccer lose their fun when parents place excessive emphasis on winning. The hug from a teammate after hitting a home run means more than just winning. Further, adults' taking over the games robs the child of independence, autonomy, and industry.

Throughout childhood, females compare favorably with males in strength, endurance, and motor skills, and in late childhood, females are physically more mature than males (69). At about *age 12*, females begin to perform less well than males on tests of physical skills; they run more slowly, jump less far, and lift less weight *if* they are given no physical training. *The traditional poorer performance is probably the result of gender expectations about behavior.* Athletic activity is attractive to both genders and is becoming more accessible to females than in the past (13, 68, 124, 126).

Discuss peer relationships and play activities with the parents. Refer to the section that describes safety and health promotion measures and the effects of media on the child.

Group or Gang Behavior

In preadolescence, the group, gang, or clique becomes important. The **gang** is a *group whose membership is earned on the basis of skilled performance of some activity, frequently physical in nature. Its stability is expressed through formal symbols, such as passwords or uniforms.* Groups or gang codes take precedence over almost everything. They may range from agreement to protect a member who smoked in the boys' restroom at school to boycotting a school event. Generally, gang codes are characterized by collective action against the mores of the adult world. In the gang, children discharge hostility and aggression against peers rather than adults and begin to work out their own social patterns without adult interference. Unfortunately, some gangs do turn their hostility or sexual harassment against other youths or adults. When this occurs, the pattern is laid for delinquent behaviors. However, these groups are not necessarily offenders against the law. Group or gang formation is loosely structured at first, with a transient membership that cuts across all social classes. Early gangs may consist of both genders in the same groups. Later, gangs separate by gender.

Help parents understand the importance of the group. You can work with the group to promote health and positive behavior. Become familiar with the community in which you live. Is there gang formation that is different from the usual school-age cliques? Are there groups of children in the schools that belong to an antisocial gang in the community? Explore with school administrators and teachers. Convey to parents the importance of their knowing with whom the child interacts and to be familiar with the broader community.

Peer aggression or **bullying** is *aggressive behavior meant to harm that is deliberately, persistently directed against a particular target, a victim who is weak, vulnerable, and defenseless.* Male bullies use physical force. Female bullies may also use physical force and also use teasing, ridicule, rejection, or other verbal psychological/relational aggression to bully other children. These highly aggressive children typically have a history of extensive watching of violent media. Children who are lonely, have low self-esteem, are physically weak, are without family support, or are highly sensitive to relational or other aggression are likely to be bullied and taunted

repeatedly (13, 50, 104, 107, 124). Children from cultures that value gentle or submissive behavior, who come from punitive homes, or who do poorly in school are also more likely to be victimized (7, 60). Being victimized contributes to fear, loneliness, low self-esteem, and being sensitive to teasing, being isolated, or being attacked. Having friends in school offers some protection against bullying (13, 32, 50, 64, 107, 108, 122, 124). A child's self-concept can be traumatized by peer behavior that is aggressive and bullies the child. Victims of bullying behavior may develop emotional disorders or hyperactive behavior, and may at some point themselves become aggressive or violent at school or in the community (13, 64, 109, 132). The Abstract for Evidence-Based Practice presents research about bullying behavior in diverse cultures of school-age children.

This kind of school violence can be prevented, reduced, or stopped, as indicated by the review of literature in the Cochrane Collaboration Review. A variety of school-based violence programs have been implemented in the past 25 years, and they do appear to reduce aggressive behavior and improve general behavior (102). An

Abstract for Evidence-Based Practice

Predictors of Bullying Among School Children

Zimmerman, F., Glow, G., Christakis, D., & Katon, W. (2005). Early cognitive stimulation, emotional support, and television watching as predictors of subsequent bullying among grade-school children. *Archives of Pediatric and Adolescent Medicine, 159,* 384–388.

KEYWORDS

cognitive stimulation, emotional support, grade-school children, bullying behavior, Social Learning Theory.

Purpose ➤ Examine links between early home environment (cognitive stimulation, emotional support, and television viewing) and the child's subsequent bullying behavior.

Conceptual Framework ➤ Cognitive deficits, poor inhibition control, and lack of academic self-efficacy decrease social competence with peers and can contribute to the child's bullying behavior. Parental maltreatment of the young child is associated with the child's later bullying behavior. Evidence clearly links increased viewing of television violence to aggressive behavior (Social Learning Theory).

Sample ➤ A national survey of mothers of 1,266 children ages 6 to 11 years. Participants included Caucasians, African Americans, and Latinos.

Methods ➤ Data were collected through interview of the mothers and the mothers' completion of a Likert-type scale designed to measure the child's characteristics, including bullying behavior (e.g., cruel or mean to others). A multivariate logistic regression model was used to determine which variable constituted an independent risk factor for subsequent bullying. Analysis controlled for socioeconomic status as a confounding factor.

Findings ➤ Children ages 6 to 11 years characterized as bullies had a higher mean score for antisocial, oppositional, hyperactive, and other problem behaviors than children characterized as nonbullies (p < .001). Children who were not bullies had a higher mean score for parental cognitive stimulation and emotional support at age 4 years than did children who were characterized as bullies. Children who were bullies had watched television at least 5 hours daily in contrast to 3.5 hours daily for nonbullying children. More hours of television viewing at 4 years of age was a predictor of subsequent bullying behavior at 6 to 11 years of age (p < .001). Early emotional support was protective against bullying behavior (p < .05). Cognitive stimulation was not statistically significant as a predictor.

Implications ➤ Since 60% of television programming demonstrates disrespectful, aggressive, or violent behavior, the child who spends more hours watching television is more likely to learn such behavior, which can become a habit. Early parental emotional support and cognitive stimulation may increase the child's comfort level with peers and confidence about academic matters and may endorse parental views about prosocial behavior and the importance of school. Parents should control the number of hours the young child spends viewing television and the type of programming. Parents should be educated that the early childhood period is formative; their nurturing behavior is important to the child's development.

INTERVENTIONS FOR HEALTH PROMOTION

Educate school administrators, teachers, and parents about strategies to reduce bullying (102, 124):

1. Have older peers to serve as monitors for bullying and give permission to intervene when they see bullying behavior.
2. Develop schoolwide rules and sanctions against bullying, educate personnel and students, and post them throughout the school.
3. Encourage students to develop friendships.
4. Incorporate the message of the antibullying program into church, school, and other community agencies where schoolchildren are involved.

5. Encourage school administrators, teachers, other personnel, parents, students, and the broader community to embrace diversity and people who demonstrate characteristics that appear or are perceived as "different" in any way.
6. Educate the school, community, and parents about factors that contribute to bullying: physical appearance, personal behavior, family and environmental factors, and school relations.
7. Educate parents and students about ways to minimize factors that contribute to the child being bullied.
8. Explore feelings of victimization in students who have been bullied to reduce long-term negative consequences.

---

intervention program in Norway for grades 4 through 7 reduced bullying by 50% and also reduced other antisocial behavior. This was accomplished by creating an authoritative atmosphere—warmth, interest, and involvement—combined with firm limits and consistent, nonphysical punishment. More adult supervision at recess and lunch time, class rules against aggressive or bullying behaviors, and serious discussions with bullies, victims, and parents were interventions (64). A growing number of schools in the United States are adopting similar programs (102). There are long-term effects on the victim who is bullied (64).

Tools of Socialization

The child becomes socialized through having opportunities for cooperation, competition, compromise, and collaboration. The child is typically taught sharing and cooperation from an early age.

Cooperation, an *exchange between equals by adjusting to the wishes of others*, results from the chum relationship with its syntaxic mode of communication (137). Through the **morality of cooperation** the *child begins to understand the social implications of acts*. He or she learns judgment through helping make and carry out rules (114, 149).

Competition *comprises all activities that are involved in getting to a goal first, of seeking affection or status above others*. When the child is competing, he or she has rigid standards about many situations, including praise and punishment. For example, regardless of the circumstance, the child believes that the same punishment should be given for the same wrongdoing. He or she cannot understand why a 3-year-old sibling should not be punished in the same way for spilling milk on the kitchen floor. Similarly, the child thinks he or she should be praised for dressing self as much as the 3-year-old is. *The child accepts adult rules as compulsory and rigid; he or she experiences a* **morality of constraint** (114, 149).

Compromise, a *give-and-take agreement*, is gradually learned from peers, teachers, and family. The child becomes less rigid in standards of behavior (137).

Collaboration, *deriving satisfaction from group accomplishment rather than personal success*, is a step forward from coopera-

tion. It enables experimentation with tasks and exploration of situations (137).

Teach parents that competition, compromise, cooperation, and beginning collaboration are progressive tools that the schoolchild uses in accomplishing satisfying peer relationships (137). If a child is not relating well with peers, you may conduct a group assertiveness training program to effectively increase social and assertive behavior through reinforcement procedures, relaxation techniques, guided imagery, and behavior contracts.

GUIDANCE AND DISCIPLINE

In guidance, parents should invite confidence of the child as a parent, not as a buddy or pal. The child will find pals among peers. The parents should see the child as he or she is, not as an idealized extension of themselves. Middle childhood is a transitional period of **coregulation**, *whereby parents and the child share power. Parents monitor and guide; the child exercises moment-to-moment self-regulation* (13, 14, 124). Parents do more discussion, rather than direct management, related to school, family, and peer issues. The child is more likely to follow parental wishes or advice when parents are fair and express concern about the child's welfare. Parents who defer to the child's maturing judgment and take a strong stand only on important matters are more effective in guidance.

The schoolchild has a rather strict superego and also uses many rituals to maintain self-control. He or she prefers to initiate self-control rather than be given commands or overt discipline. Stability and routine in his or her life provide this opportunity (14).

During preadolescence, the child strives for more autonomy and independence. The child becomes more argumentative; family problem solving and negotiation may deteriorate (113). The way parents resolve conflicts may be more important than the specific outcome. Constructive family conflict can help the child realize the need for rules and standards of behavior, what issues are worth an argument, and effective strategies for coping (107). Effects of various parenting styles are discussed at the beginning of the chapter.

Discuss with parents about methods of guidance and the importance of not interfering with behavior too forcefully or too often. The child needs some alternatives from which to choose in order to learn different ways of behaving and coping and to be better able to express self later. If development has been normal during the preschool years, the child is now well on the way to absorbing and accepting the standards, codes, and attitudes of society. He or she needs ongoing guidance rather than an emphasis on disciplinary measures.

Help parents learn the value of positive guidance techniques. Teach the following guidelines. When expressing anger to children, describe what you see, feel, and expect. Do not lower the child's self-esteem by humiliating him or her, especially in front of others. The child's dignity can be protected by using "I" messages: "I am angry. I am frustrated." Such statements are honest and are safer than "What's your problem? You are stupid!" If repeated frequently, the child may believe that he or she is stupid and carry that self-image for years. Although shouting is not recommended, the parent who occasionally *only* shouts displeasure at danger or inconvenience is probably harming the child much less than the parent who quietly and continually verbalizes personal assaults against the child. Ideally, the limit should be set with firm conviction and should deal with only one incident at a time. More than one message can confuse the child.

Explore with parents the value of using inductive techniques and reasoning to guide and discipline. Parents may appeal to the child's self-esteem, use a gentle sense of humor, integrate moral values, and state consequences of behavior. It is essential to convey recognition and appreciation of appropriate and mature behavior when it occurs. Too often parents think of guidance or discipline as focusing only on the negative or what has not been done.

Our grandparents are reputed to have disciplined their children with authority and certainty. By contrast, some of today's parents seem afraid of their children. The child needs an understanding authority and a good example. He or she needs to know what constitutes unacceptable behavior and what substitute will be accepted (142). For instance, say, "Food is not for throwing; your baseball is." He or she will not obey rules if parents do not. Inconsistent discipline, or the "Do as I say, not as I do" approach, will lead to maladjustment, conflict, and aggression. Suggestions about guidance listed in Chapter 11 are applicable to the schoolchild as well. ∞

Guidance at this age takes many other and less dramatic forms. A mother can turn the often harried "getting back-to-school clothes" experience into a pleasant lesson in guidance. She can accompany the child on a special shopping trip in which he or she examines different textures of material, learns about color coordination, understands what constitutes a good fit, and appreciates how much money must be spent for certain items. This principle can be carried into any parent-schoolchild guidance relationship, such as learning responsibility for some household task or earning, handling, and saving money.

EMOTIONAL DEVELOPMENT

The schoolchild consolidates earlier psychosocial development and simultaneously reaches out to a number of identification figures, expands interests, and associates with more people. *Behavioral char-*

acteristics change from year to year. **Table 12-13** summarizes and compares basic behavior patterns, although individual children will show a considerable range of behavior (13, 42, 58, 59, 107, 124, 126). *Cultural, health, and social conditions may also influence behavior* (7, 60).

Developmental Crisis: Industry versus Inferiority

The psychosexual crisis for this period is industry versus inferiority. **Industry** is *an interest in doing the work of the world, the child's feeling that he or she can learn and solve problems, the formation of responsible work habits and attitudes, and the mastery of age-appropriate tasks* (42). The child has greater body competence and applies self to skills and tasks that go beyond playful expression. The child gets tired of play, wants to participate in the real world, and seeks attention and recognition for effort and concentration on a task. He or she feels pride in doing something well, whether a physical or cognitive task. A sense of industry involves self-confidence, perseverance, diligence, self-control, cooperation, and compromise rather than only competition. There is a sense of loyalty, relating self to something positive beyond the moment and outside the self. Parents, teachers, and nurses may see this industry at times as restlessness, irritability, rebellion toward authority, and lack of obedience.

The danger of this period is that the child may develop a sense of **inferiority**, *feeling inadequate, defeated, unable to learn or do tasks, and unable to compete, compromise, or cooperate*, regardless of his or her actual competence (42). See **Box 12-9**, Consequences of Inferiority Feelings, for a summary of behaviors and traits of the child (42), and later the adult, if this stage is not resolved. If the child feels excessively ashamed, self-doubting, guilty, and inferior from not having achieved the developmental tasks all along, physical, emotional, and behavioral problems may occur. Sometimes opposite behavior may occur as the person tries to cope with feelings of being no good, inferior, or inadequate. The person might immerse self in tasks. If work is all the child can do at home and school, he or she will miss out on a lot of friendships and opportunities in life, now and later, and eventually become the adult who cannot stop working.

Educate parents to talk to children about feelings, including fears. Children often do not disclose openly because they do not want to be labeled a "baby," "sissy," or "chicken." Children need to know that parents and teachers are concerned about their feelings, including sadness, fears, and loneliness. Parents should avoid being overprotective while teaching personal safety and coping skills.

Stress Response

Stress is experienced by the school-age child. Often stress response occurs from the demands placed on the child in relation to school achievement or for extracurricular performance, being overprogrammed in activities, or the fear of violence at home, during transportation, or at school. One study indicated *three major areas of stress* (70):

1. Actual or anticipated loss of loved ones, pets, or space, such as home, school, and neighborhood.
2. Threats to self; situations of anger, fear, aggression, or violence against self or personal belongings; threats to personal safety such as being bullied.

TABLE 12-13

Assessment of Changing Behavioral Characteristics in the Schoolchild

6 Years	7 Years	8 Years
Self-centered	Self-care managed	Expansive personality but fluctuating behavior
Body movement, temper outbursts release tension	Quiet, less impulsive, but assertive	Curious, robust, energetic
Behavioral extremes; impulsive or dawdles, loving or antagonistic	Fewer mood swings	Rapid movements and response; impatient
Difficulty making decisions; needs reminders	Self-absorbed without excluding others; may appear shy, sad, brooding	Affectionate to parents
Verbally aggressive but easily insulted	Attentive, sensitive listener	Hero worship of adult
Intense concentration for short time, then abruptly stops activity	Companionable; likes to do tasks for others	Suggestions followed better than commands
Security of routines and rituals essential; periodic separation anxiety	Good and bad behavior in self and others noted	Adult responsibilities and characteristics imitated; wants to be considered important by adults
Series of three commands followed, but response depends on mood	High standards for self but minor infractions of rules: tattles, alibis, takes small objects from others	Approval and reconciliation sought, feelings easily hurt
Self-control and initiative in activity encouraged when adult uses counting to give child time ("I'll give you until the count of 10 to pick up those papers")	Concern about own behavior, tries to win over others' approval	Sense of property; enjoys collections
Praise and recognition needed	Angry over others' failure to follow rules	Beginning sense of justice but makes alibis for own transgressions
		Demanding and critical of others
		Gradually accepts inhibitions and limits

9 Years	10 Years
More independent and self-controlled	More adultlike and poised, especially girls
Dependable, responsible	More self-directive, independent
Adult trust and more freedom without adult supervision sought	Organized and rapid in work; budgets time and energy
Loyal to home and parents; seeks their help at times	Suggestions followed better than requests, but obedient
More self rather than environmentally motivated; not dependent on but benefits from praise	Family activities and care of younger siblings, especially below school age, enjoyed
More involved with peers	Aware of individual differences among people, but does not like to be singled out in a group
Own interests subordinated to group demands and adult authority	Hero worship of adult
Critical of own and others' behavior	Some idea of own assets and limits
Loyal to group; chum important	Preoccupied with right and wrong
Concerned about fairness and willing to take own share of blame	Better able to live by rules
More aware of society	Critical sense of justice; accepts immediate punishment for wrongdoing
	Liberal ideas of social justice and welfare
	Strong desire to help animals and people
	Future career choices match parents' careers because of identification with parents
	Sense of leadership

continued

TABLE 12-13

Assessment of Changing Behavioral Characteristics in the Schoolchild—continued

11 Years	12 Years
Spontaneous, self-assertive, restless, curious, sociable	Considerable personality integration; self-contained, self-competent, tactful, kind, reasonable, less self-centered
Short outbursts of anger and arguing	Outgoing, eager to please, enthusiastic
Mood swings	Sense of humor; improved communication skills
Challenges enjoyed	More companionable than at 11; mutual understanding between parents and child
On best behavior away from home	Increasingly sensitive to feelings of others; wish good things for family and friends; caught between the two
Quarrelsome with siblings; rebellious to parents	Others' approval sought
Critical of parents, although affectionate with them	Childish lapses, but wishes to be treated like adult
Chum and same-sex peers important; warm reconciliation follows quarrels	Aware of assets and shortcomings
Secrets freely shared with chum; secret language with peers	Tolerant of self and others
Unaware of effect of self on others	Peer group and chum important in shaping attitudes and interests
Strict superego; zeal for fairness	Ethical sense more realistic than idealistic
Future career choices fantasized on basis of possible fame	Decisions about ethical questions based on consequences
Modest with parents	Less tempted to do wrong; basically truthful
	Self-disciplined, accepts just discipline
	Enthusiastic about community projects

BOX 12-9 Consequences of Inferiority Feelings

1. Does not want to try new activities, skills
2. Is passive, excessively meek, too eager to please others
3. Seeks attention; may be "teacher's pet"
4. Is anxious, moody, depressed
5. Does not persevere in tasks
6. Is very fearful of body injury or illness
7. Does not volunteer to do tasks alone, always works with another on tasks
8. Isolates self from others, withdraws from peers
9. Tries to prove personal worth, a "good worker" with directives or assistance
10. Lacks self-esteem unless praised considerably
11. Is overcompetitive, bossy
12. Insists on own way, experiences difficulty with cooperation or compromise
13. May immerse self in tasks to prove self, gain attention
14. Acts out to prove self; lying, stealing, fire setting
15. Displays extreme antisocial behavior, destructive or aggressive acts
16. Manifests illnesses associated with emotional state: enuresis, complaints of fatigue
17. In adulthood, is unable to pursue steady work or become involved in life tasks as expected
18. May become "workaholic"; in adulthood, is unable to engage in leisure

3. Feelings of being hassled, extra responsibility or restrictions, sibling relations, peer relations, violence in the home, maltreatment, abuse and neglect, or divorce.

These areas of stress may be magnified because of societal changes and problems presented in Chapters 5 and 6. ∞ Abuse and violence in the home and demonstrations of aggression and violence socially are major stressors (68, 112). Excess stress may cause fatalistic orientation to the future, anxiety, and depression (84). **Table 12-14** lists signs of stress that can be observed in the classroom and school.

There are differences in how children bear up under stress. Some children are **vulnerable** to stressors: *They are sensitive to or drawn in by the events around them. They become nervous and withdrawn, and feel inferior. Some are illness-prone and slow to develop.* Other children are **resilient**: *They shrug off the stressors, thrive, and go on to be industrious, have high self-esteem, and lead highly productive lives as adults.* True, some children are born with an innately easygoing temperament and handle stressors better than do children with a nervous, overreactive disposition. Children who have robust, sunny personalities are lovable and readily win affection, which further builds self-esteem and an identity. **Resilient children** are likely to have a number of protective factors, but the *key is a basic, consistent, lasting, trusting relationship with an adult who is supportive and who is a beacon presence from infancy on* (8, 13, 40, 41, 91, 107, 151, 152).

Vulnerable children, if placed in the right environment, become productive and competent adults. They need help to find a solid relationship—neighbor, teacher, relative—until they find at least one such adult. Then they distance self from the conflictual

TABLE 12-14

Signs of Stress Observed at School

Physical Signs

1. Morning stomachaches, leg cramps
2. Frowning, squinting, clenched jaw, facial expressions reflecting misery
3. Mixes cursive and manuscript, lower- and upper-case letters when writing
4. May invert, omit, or substitute letters and words
5. Laborious writing, tiring easily when writing
6. Frequent erasures, hates writing activities
7. Negotiates to minimize writing assignments
8. Alert and attentive to noises and distractions not associated with learning task
9. Misses teacher instruction, directions
10. Needs directions repeated, instruction repeated
11. Reading is difficult
12. Falls asleep during the school day
13. Nail-biting, throat-clearing, coughing, eye-blinking, incontinent of urine at school, bed-wetting at home
14. Exhaustion from performing school tasks
15. Low resistance to illness
16. Absenteeism
17. Relieves tension through constant physical activity

Emotional Signs

1. Seeks adult approval and reassurance
2. Needs a lot of praise
3. Needs immediate feedback and response from teacher
4. Fear of making a mistake, does not volunteer
5. Lacks confidence
6. Fears getting hurt
7. Withdraws from touch
8. Does not seek to try new things, does not take risks
9. Cannot readily change activities
10. Loses place in lessons

11. Daydreams
12. Often gives the right answer to the wrong question
13. Fears getting hurt
14. Cries easily
15. Picked on by classmates
16. Behavior at school is acceptable, but parents report bad behavior at home

Intellectual Signs

1. Inconsistent performance
2. Trouble keeping up the pace
3. Trouble completing assignments within the time limit
4. Has potential, but does not apply self
5. Loses the "low-grade" papers
6. Parents blame teacher for not challenging the child

Social Signs

1. Favorite at-home activity is watching television
2. Passive, apathetic, no initiative at school
3. Does not fit in with peer group
4. Avoids other children, tries to remain anonymous
5. Tries to annoy other children
6. Has few friends, feels uncomfortable in social situations
7. Does not take responsibility for not having assignments, makes excuses
8. Feels hurt and left out, may become angry or jealous of classmates
9. Can be a class bully
10. May show off in one area
11. Seeks out younger children to play with
12. Afraid to take risks
13. Avoids competition
14. Prefers to play alone

or abusive home, at least emotionally (8, 13, 40, 41, 107, 151). The Case Situation about resilient children presents an example.

As children get older, they are more able to accurately appraise a stressful situation and their control over it. They use more coping strategies and intentionally shift their thoughts to less stressful situations or reframe perceptions. If families are not supportive, children may be more overwhelmed by stress (24, 41, 124).

Teach the child to identify signs of stress within the self and their source. Ways to cope with and reduce stress levels can be explored. Physical exercise is useful to reduce tension. Relaxation methods and stress management can be taught through individual and group counseling, play therapy, and use of art and music (34, 68, 84, 158, 159). Alternative coping methods, steps in problem solving, and potential support systems can be explored. Encouraging expression of feelings is important. Help the child identify a role model for effectively handling similar situations. Repeated rehearsal of how to handle stressors can also be useful so that effec-

tive responses become more automatic. Information about the stress response and stress management presented in Chapter 2 can be applied to education of the schoolchild and the parents. ∞ Engel describes the use of cognitive behavioral therapy within the American Indian cultural context as a way to help the child identify inner strengths, build self-esteem, gain a sense of the Creator as healer, and achieve stability that continues beyond the school years (41).

Basic health and social and educational programs must be provided to assist the child to adapt to the extent possible (8, 68, 112). When the child's environment is overwhelmingly stressful, extra support and love are especially important. If the child is facing multiple stressors, it is more difficult for outside intervention to help the child. The more the risk factors, the worse is the outcome for the child, regardless of the intervention.

Teach parents that they can contribute to a sense of industry and avoid inferiority feelings by not having unrealistic expectations of

Case Situation

Resilient Children: The Importance of School Relationships

"What do the children think as they ride by here on the way to school?" I wondered as I stood by the ditch on a desolate stretch of highway, twenty miles from Red Cloud Indian School, that was full of beer bottles glistening in the sun. Several people had asked me how so much could have been dumped in such a short time. Going to see for myself, I realized what others had missed: The bottles had been accumulating for a long time, but one of the recent prairie fires had burned off the grass and revealed their ugly presence. The burned-out ditch stretched for miles. Before the fire, most people driving by would only notice an occasional sparkle as the sunlight reflected off the bottles covered by the long grasses. Only if they stopped and took time to investigate could they begin to see the evidence that is a sad part of the Pine Ridge Indian Reservation tragedy.

I couldn't help but think of all the factors that lie "just beneath the surface" in so many of the children's lives. What overwhelming challenges so many of the children face every day. To come to school, to work hard, to dream, to graduate, and to pursue those dreams takes every ounce of courage and strength that they have—every day.

Many of the challenges that surround these children on a daily basis can easily destroy the hopes and dreams of a young American Indian child. Too many of the children live with the effects of alcohol abuse. Only 5 miles from Red Cloud Indian School, 4 million cans of beer are sold each year in a Nebraska border town that has a population of 35 people. This is the yearly equivalent of 133 cans of beer for every man, woman, and child living on the reservation. Drug abuse is rampant and continues to rip families apart. In today's newspaper there is a report of an organized cocaine drug ring that operated just a few miles away. The incidence of diabetes is epidemic here on the Pine Ridge, and many young children know what it means to have a family member needing a ride to get to dialysis. More young people are turning to violent gangs as a way to express themselves and extort money to support their alcohol and drug needs. Children are being raised by grandparents in record numbers because their parents are unable to care for them.

Knowing the challenges that so many of the children face, one would not expect them to dream, let alone thrive. Yet, with outside help they are! What we are doing here at Red Cloud is so important. Every day the children hear "Of course you can!" when so much in their lives tells them not to even try. I have seen children arrive at Red Cloud hungry and cold, but with a smile that warms your heart. They are happy to be here because they know that they can focus on learning. They will be warm, they will be fed, and they will have a teacher who cares about them.

More than one visitor has told me, "Red Cloud is a ray of hope." HOPE! That is what Red Cloud is all about. Hope that takes root in the lives of the children. Hope that helps them to break through the rock of despair and to succeed when so many would say that their future is hopeless. At Red Cloud we know that we are doing something right. Our graduates are thriving, not merely surviving, at colleges and universities across the country. We know that what we can provide is often all the learning tools that a child has. Few have any resources at home. A caring teacher who takes the children's learning seriously is so important for their future.

Daily, we say to each other here at Red Cloud Indian School, "May the Great Spirit bless you with all good—*Wakan Tanka niya Wastepi!*"

Contributed by Fr. Peter Klink, SJ, President, Red Cloud Indian School, Pine Ridge, SD.

---

the child and by using the suggested guidance and discipline approaches. They can encourage peer activities and home responsibilities, help the child meet developmental crises, and give recognition to his or her accomplishments and unique talents.

SELF-CONCEPT, BODY IMAGE, AND SEXUALITY DEVELOPMENT

Self-Concept and Body Image Development

Self-concept, body image, and sexuality development are interrelated. They are affected by cultural, ethnic, or racial background; gender; grade level of the child; parents' education; history of illness; and health status. Until the child goes to school, self-perception is derived primarily from the parents' attitudes and reactions toward him or her. The child who is loved for what he or she is learns to love and accept self.

The child with a **positive self-concept** *likes self; accepts his or her physical characteristics, abilities, values, and self-ideals; has an idea of self in relation to others; and accepts others.* The child believes that what he or she thinks, says, and does makes a difference; believes he or she can be successful and can solve problems; and expresses feelings of happiness.

In studies of children in grades 1 through 3, females develop an accurate self-perception earlier than males, although males become more accurate in their self-perceptions between 7 and 10 years of age. Children reflect social stereotypes in their self-evaluations. For example, males evaluate highly their mathematic skills and physical abilities, and females evaluate highly their social competence, "being a good student," academic skills such as language arts, and "learning quickly." Children's self-perceptions do not consistently correlate with teachers' evaluations of how children perceive themselves (87).

Body image refers to *the mental image of one's body, as a person in relation to others, and as a person who interacts with the environment. The child is aware of how he or she differs from others* in appearance, body, muscular function, and physical ability, including physical disabilities in other children. The child will conceal physical characteristics that are perceived by self or others as undesirable. The child may feel excluded by the group if he or she is physically disabled or different in any way.

Younger children use mostly surface or visible characteristics to describe themselves (87). At about *age 8* the child describes the self with less focus on external characteristics and more on enduring internal qualities and is more realistic. Because of concern with appearance or body image, children may try to lose weight, influenced by the ultrathin models in the media. At about *age 9 or 10*, Caucasian girls are more likely to be dissatisfied with their bodies and to try to lose weight, although they are on average thinner than African American girls. African American girls are more likely to try to gain weight. Mothers exert a strong influence over their daughters' weight-control efforts (107).

If parental reactions have been rejecting, or if he or she has been made to feel ugly, ashamed, or guilty about self or personal behavior, the child enters school feeling bad, inadequate, or inferior. A negative self-image causes the child to feel defensive toward others and hinders adjustment to school and academic progress. Children with a low self-concept show more social withdrawal, academic difficulties, and inappropriate attention seeking than children with a high self-concept (42, 96).

At school, the child compares self and is compared with peers in appearance and motor, cognitive, language, and social skills. If he or she cannot perform as well as other children, peers will perceive the child negatively. Eventually he or she will perceive self as incompetent or inferior because self-image is more dependent on peers than earlier in childhood. Schoolchildren are frequently cruel in their honesty when they make derogatory remarks about peers with limitations or disabilities.

Unattractive children may receive discriminatory treatment from parents, teachers, and babysitters because adults have learned the social value of beauty. Attractive children are better liked by peers and adults and are judged to be more intelligent. Because people tend to act as others expect them to, the prophecy may be self-fulfilling, likely to become true (96). It is important to overcome this kind of reaction.

Biracial children have a special status related to racial identification and self-concept. They may deal with overt racism affecting children of color, cope with outsiders who may view their families as abnormal, and sometimes cope with the loyalty issues and negative feelings from the extended family of each parent. Positive parental feelings about racial identification and positive extended family relationships are critical to sound emotional adjustment of the child and a positive self-concept. The child may have difficulty identifying with either parent because of racism, and these feelings and issues must be worked through (95).

The *child's body image* is still developing. Schoolchildren are more aware of the internal body and external differences. They can label major organs with increasing accuracy. Heart, brain, and bones are most frequently mentioned, along with cardiovascular, gastrointestinal, and musculoskeletal systems. The younger child thinks that organs change position, and organ function, size, and position are poorly understood. Organs such as the stomach are frequently drawn at the wrong place (this may reflect the influence of television ads). Children generally believe that they must have all body parts to remain alive and that the skin holds in body contents (34, 87, 107, 124). Consider the effect of injury or surgery on the child. This is an excellent age to teach about basic anatomy and physiology. **Table 12-15** shows how aspects of the child's view of self change through the school years (13, 14, 34, 55, 58, 59, 87, 96, 107, 124).

Assist parents in promoting a positive self-concept and body image. During prepuberty, males and females are similar in many ways, but differences are taught. Females reportedly are less physically active, but they have greater verbal, perceptual, and cognitive skills than males. Females supposedly respond to stimuli—interpersonal and physical, including pain—more quickly and accurately than males. They seem better at analyzing and anticipating environmental demands; thus their behavior conforms more to adult expectations, and they are better at staying out of trouble. Females are encouraged to depend and rely on others' appraisals for self-esteem more than males. Females are not usually forced to develop internal controls and a sense of independent self in the way that males are because of the difference in adult reactions to each gender. Innate physiologic differences become magnified as they are reinforced by cultural norms and specific parental behaviors. However, females can be aggressive and competitive, and cope in each situation similarly to males (14, 61, 68, 95, 113).

Sexuality Development and Education

Sexuality education, *learning about the self as a person who is a sexual being*, has begun by the school years. **Sex education,** *factual information about anatomy, physiology, and birth control methods*, should begin now for both genders. By *7 or 8,* children usually know that both sexes are required for childbirth to occur, but they are not sure how.

The child can learn that both genders have similar feelings and behavior potential, which can instill attitudes about maleness and femaleness for adulthood. *At this age both sexes are dependent and independent, active and passive, emotional and controlled, gentle and aggressive.* Keeping such a range of behavior will contribute to a more flexible adult who can be expressive, spontaneous, and accepting of self and others.

Explore and clarify the attitudes of parents and teachers during the early planning phases for presentation of sexual education. Assist as needed in choosing content. *Guidelines for parents, teachers, or yourself when handling this subject include:*

1. Know the facts; do not lecture or preach.
2. Do not skip anything because the youngster says, "I already know." Chances are the child has received some inaccurate information.
3. Answer all questions as honestly as possible.
4. Do not force too much at one sitting. Aim the information at the child's immediate interest. Do not pry into the child's feelings and fantasies. Try to make the conversation as relaxed as possible.

TABLE 12-15

Assessment of Changing Body Image Development in the Schoolchild

6 Years	7 Years	8 Years
Is self-centered	Is more modest and aware of self	Redefines sense of status with others
Likes to be in control of self, situations, and possessions	Wants own place at table, in car, and own room or part of room	Subtle changes in physical proportion; movements smoother
Gains physical and motor skills	Has lower-level physical activity than earlier	Assumes many roles consecutively
Knows right from left hand	Does not like to be touched	Is ready for physical contact in play and to be taught self-defense mechanisms
Regresses occasionally to baby talk or earlier behavior	Protects self by withdrawing from unpleasant situation	Is more aware of differences between the sexes
Plays at being someone else to clarify sense of self and others	Dislikes physical combat	Is curious about another's body
Is interested in marriage and reproduction	Engages less in sex play	Asks questions about marriage and reproduction; strong interest in babies, especially for girls
Distinguishes organs of each sex but wonders about them	Understands pregnancy generally; excited about new body in family	Plays more with own sex
May indulge in sex play	Concerned he or she does not really belong to parents	
Draws a man with hands, neck, clothing, and six identifiable parts	Tells parts missing from picture of incomplete man	
Distinguishes between attractive and ugly pictures of faces		

9 Years	10 Years
Has well-developed eye–hand coordination	Is relatively content with and confident of self
Enjoys displaying motor skills and strength	Has perfected most basic small motor movements
Cares completely for body needs	Wants privacy for self but peeks at other sex
Has more interest in own body and its functions than in other sexual matters	Asks some questions about sexual matters again
Asks fewer questions about sexual matters if earlier questions answered satisfactorily	Investigates own sexual organs
Is self-conscious about exposing body, including to younger siblings and opposite-sex parent	Shows beginning prepubertal changes physically, especially girls

11 Years	12 Years
States self is in heart, head, face, or body part most actively expressing him or her	Growth spurt; changes in appearance
Feels more self-conscious with physical changes occurring	Muscular control almost equal to that of adult
Mimics adults; deepening self-understanding	Identifies self as being in total body or brain
Masturbates sometimes; erection occurs in boys	May feel like no part of body is his or hers alone but like someone else's because of close identity with group
Discusses sexual matters with parents with reticence	Begins to accept and find self as unique person
Likes movies on reproduction	
Feels joy of life with more mature understanding	

ADAPTIVE MECHANISMS

The schoolchild is losing the protective mantle of home and early childhood and needs order and consistency in life to help cope with doubts, fears, unacceptable impulses, and unfamiliar experiences. *Commonly used adaptive mechanisms are presented in the following paragraphs. Assess for these behaviors.*

Ritualistic behavior, *consistently repeating an act in a situation,* wards off imagined harm and anxiety and provides a feeling of control. Examples include avoiding stepping on cracks in the sidewalk while chanting certain words (so as not to break mother's back), always putting the left leg through trousers before the right, having a certain place for an object, or doing homework at a specific time. Reaction formation, undoing, and isolation are related to ritualistic behavior.

Reaction formation, *demonstrating behavior opposite to the actual feelings,* is used frequently in dealing with feelings of hostility. The child may unconsciously dislike a younger brother because he infringes on the schoolchild's freedom, but such impulses are unacceptable to the strict superego. To counter such unwanted feelings, the child may become the classic example of a caring, loving sibling.

Undoing is *unconsciously removing an idea, feeling, or act by performing certain ritualistic behavior.* For example, the gang has certain chants and movements to follow before a member who broke a secret code can return. The child is taught to apologize after engaging in rude or unacceptable behavior.

Isolation is a *mechanism of unconsciously separating emotion from an idea because the emotion would be unacceptable to the self.* The idea remains in the conscious, but its component feeling remains in the unconscious. A child uses isolation when he or she seems to talk very objectively about the puppy who has just been run over by a truck.

Fantasy *compensates for feelings of inadequacy, inferiority, and lack of success* encountered in school, the peer group, or home. Fantasy is necessary for eventual creativity and should not be discouraged if it is not used excessively to prevent realistic participation in the world. Fantasy saves the ego temporarily, but it also provides another way for the child to view self, thus helping him or her aspire to new heights of behavior.

Identification *is seen in the hero worship* of a teacher, scoutmaster, neighbor, or family friend, someone whom the child respects and who has the qualities the child fantasizes as his or her own. The child continues to identify with the parent or caregiver of the same sex while *incorporating other models of behaviors.*

Regression, *returning to a less sophisticated pattern of behavior,* is a defense against anxiety and helps the child avoid potentially painful situations. For example, he or she may revert to using the language or behavior of a younger sibling if the child feels that the sibling is getting undue attention.

Malingering, *feigning illness to avoid unpleasant tasks,* is seen when the child stays home from school for a day or says he or she is unable to do a home task because he or she does not feel well.

Rationalization, *giving excuses when the child is unable to achieve wishes,* is frequently seen in relation to schoolwork. For example, after a low test grade, the response is, "Oh well, grades don't make any difference anyway."

Projection is seen as the child says about a teacher, "She doesn't like me," when really the teacher is disliked for having reprimanded him or her.

Sublimation is a major mechanism used during the school years. The child increasingly *channels sexual and aggressive impulses into socially acceptable tasks* at school and home. In the process, if all goes well, he or she develops the sense of industry.

Help parents understand the adaptive mechanisms used by the child and how to help the child use healthy coping mechanisms. Counsel that use of any and all of these mechanisms in various situations is normal, but overuse of any one can result in a constricted, immature personality. If constricted, the child will be unable to develop relationships outside the home, to succeed at home or school, or to balance work and play. Achieving a sense of identity and adult developmental tasks will be impaired.

Encourage parents to foster certain adaptive mechanisms because they contribute to stress management and to a healthy personality: (a) identification with mature adults, as well as with the parents and other adult family members; (b) sublimation of aggressive or sexual impulses through crafts, games and play, reading materials, music, art, sports or other exercise, and creative individual or group projects; and (c) a healthy or creative expression of fantasy. Validate with parents that excess attention should not be given to regressive behavior or malingering.

Parents need to discuss with the child feelings that underlie the excessive use of rituals, reaction formation, undoing behaviors, rationalization, and projection. If the child demonstrates emotional isolation, refer parents to a counselor in order to detect early the manifestations of grief, depression, maltreatment, or school or peer difficulties. The child and family can benefit from counseling. Suggest that parents explore the option of a pet with the child. Pets, especially a dog, can be a companion to whom the child can divulge secrets and work through problems.

CHILD IN TRANSITION

American families are on the move. Moving from one part of the country to another, or even from one community and school system to another, brings a special set of tasks that should be acknowledged and worked through. Some families, because of the military or other career or as part of an exchange program, may live in another country for a number of years or move from country to country. This poses another kind of adjustment and set of tasks. Children who were born in a foreign country and then return with their parents to the United States undergo culture shock. They feel like citizens of another country and visitors in the land of which they are citizens. They know more than one language and accept various lifestyles. They may behave as if they were still in another land. Family and employment dynamics, education, and peer relationships and adjustment to school must be considered.

The school-age child is especially affected by a geographic move if he or she is just entering or is well settled into the chum stage. The child cannot understand why he or she cannot fit into the new group right away. Because routines are so important to the schoolchild, he or she is sometimes confused by the new and different ways of doing things. The parents will need to consult with the new school leaders about their child's adjustment.

Foster adjustment in the school setting through noticing a new child, watching his or her behavior, working with the teacher and peers, and contacting parents if necessary. Foster a welcoming attitude in the school and community.

MORAL-SPIRITUAL DEVELOPMENT

Assist parents in understanding the importance of their role and that of peers, school, and even literature and the media in moral and spiritual development. If you care for a child over a period, you will also contribute to this development (30).

INTERVENTIONS FOR HEALTH PROMOTION

Share the following ideas with parents when there is a geographical move:

1. If a family can include the schoolchild in the decision about where to move, the transition will be easier.
2. Ideally, the whole family should make at least one advance trip to the new community. If possible, the new home and town should be explored, and the child should visit the new school so that he or she can establish mentally where he or she is going.
3. Contacting one of the new classmates before the actual move can enhance a feeling of friendship and belonging.
4. If the child has a special interest such as gymnastics or dancing, a contact with a new program can form another transitional step.
5. When parents are packing, they are tempted to dispose of as many of the child's belongings as possible, especially if they seem babyish or worn. They should *not do this*. These items are part of the child, and they will help him or her feel comfortable and at home during adjustment to a new home and community.

6. Sometimes parents in the new community are reticent about letting their children go to another child's house. The new parents should make every attempt to introduce themselves to the new playmates' parents and ensure that the environment will be safe for play. Parents can have a get-acquainted party for a few children who are especially desired as playmates or chums.
7. Just as the family initiated some ties before they moved, so should they keep some ties from the previous neighborhood. If possible, let the child play with old friends at times. If the move has been too far for frequent visits, allow the child to call old friends occasionally.
8. If possible, plan a trip back so that some old traditions can be revived and friends can be visited. The trip to the old neighborhood will cement in the child's mind that "home" is no longer there but in the new location.
9. The parents must accept as natural some grieving for what is gone. Let the child express his or her feelings. Accept these feelings, and continue to work with the above suggestions to foster the adjustment.

Moral Development

The schoolchild is in the Conventional Stage of moral development, according to Kohlberg (82–84). See Chapter 1, Table 1-10 ∞, for a summary of Kohlberg's Theory and explanation of the Conventional Stage (79–81). Beliefs about right and wrong have less to do with the child's actual behavior than with the likelihood of getting caught for a transgression and the gains to derive from the transgression. Other factors that influence moral development include the child's intelligence, ability to delay gratification, and sense of self-esteem. The child with high self-esteem and a favorable self-concept is less likely to engage in immoral behavior, possibly because he or she will feel more guilty with wrongdoing. Thus, moral behavior may be more a matter of strength of will or ego than of strength of conscience or superego. Morality is not a fixed behavioral trait but rather a decision-making capacity. The child progresses from an initial premoral stage, in which he or she responds primarily to reward and punishment and believes rules can be broken to meet personal needs, through a rule-based highly conventional morality, and finally to the stage of self-accepted principles (79–81, 107, 124).

Part of moral development is the ability to follow rules. Unlike the preschooler who initiates rules without understanding them, the *7- or 8-year-old* begins to play in a genuinely social manner. Rules are mutually accepted by all players and are rigidly followed. Rules come from some external force such as God and are believed timeless. Not until the *age of 11 or 12*, when the formal operations level of cognition is reached, does the child understand the true nature of rules—that they exist to make the game possible and can be altered by mutual agreement (68, 107, 114, 124, 149).

Piaget identified *stages of moral development based on the child's pattern of reasoning to think about moral issues* (114):

1. **Premoral.** *The child has no regard for rules.*
2. **Heteronomous.** *The child obeys rules because of fear of authority or powerful figures.*
3. **Autonomous.** *The child follows rules freely, expressing mutual rights and obligations.* The person is increasingly able to distinguish between principles and rules. At more advanced stages the person applies principles to guide behavior in specific situations instead of automatically following established rules.

Moral development is related to self-discipline and empathy, and how this is taught varies with the culture (7, 60). Educate parents that this era is a crucial time for learning moral views and to obey rules. Almost all children in all cultures realize that laws and rules are norms that guide behavior and require obedience from all, and they realize that chaos would result without them (107, 124, 125). Parental and adult use of affiliative nurturant strategies rather than punitive ones is most effective in inducing compliance and ensuring the stability of systems (125).

Spiritual Development

In the school years, the child usually moves from the fairy tale stage of God being like a giant to a more realistic or concrete view of God. For the Christian child, Jesus may be an angelic boy growing into a perfect man.

The child is learning many particulars about his or her religion, such as Allah, God, Jesus, prayer, rites, ancestor worship, life after death, reincarnation, heaven, and hell, all of which are developed into a religious philosophy and used in interpretation of the world. These ideas are taught by family, friends, teachers, church, books, radio, and television (30).

The child of *6 years* can understand God as Creator, expects prayers to be answered, and feels the forces of good and evil with the connotation of reward and punishment. The 6-year-old believes in a creative being, a father figure who is responsible for many things, including thunder and lightning. The adult usually introjects the natural or scientific explanation. Somehow the child seems to hold a dual thinking without contradiction. The adult's ability to weave the supernatural with the natural will affect the child's later ability to do so. Most children, even those from an atheistic background, develop a concept of God and are likely to believe in God. Children may not discuss their views if they fear ridicule or rejection from adults or peers who follow a secular society (30).

The developing schoolchild has a great capacity for reverence and awe, continues to ask more appropriate questions about religious teaching and God, and can be taught through stories that emphasize moral traits. The child operates from a simple framework of ideas and will earnestly pray for recovery and protection from danger for self and others (30). The child believes that a supreme being loves him or her, gives the earth and a house, and is always near. He or she may ask, "How does God take care of me when I can't see him?" "Allah's here, but where?" "I don't know how to love God like I love you, Mommy, because I've never touched him."

In *prepuberty* the child begins to comprehend disappointments more fully and realize that his or her answers to problems or desires to change the world quickly are not always possible (136). He or she realizes that self-centered prayers are not always answered and that no magic is involved. The child can now accept totally the scientific explanation for thunder and lightning. He or she may drop religion at this point; or because of strong dependence on parents, the child may continue to accept the family preference. An active program for this age group at the family's house of worship can be instrumental in deepening knowledge about the belief system and development of personal faith. Spiritual leaders and educators are important role models for the child and a support system to parents.

DEVELOPMENTAL TASKS

Although the schoolchild continues working on past developmental tasks, he or she is *engaged in achieving new developmental tasks* (37):

1. Decrease dependence on family and gain some satisfaction from peers and other adults.
2. Increase neuromuscular skills so that he or she can participate in games and work with others.
3. Learn basic adult concepts and knowledge to be able to reason and engage in tasks of everyday living.
4. Learn ways to communicate with others realistically.
5. Become a more active and cooperative family participant and more aware of his or her culture.
6. Engage in safe and health-promoting behavior, integrating the guidance of parents, teachers, and others.

7. Give and receive affection among family and friends without immediately seeking something in return.
8. Learn socially acceptable ways of getting money and save it for later satisfactions.
9. Learn how to handle strong feelings and impulses appropriately.
10. Adjust the changing body image and self-concept to come to terms with the cultural expectations of the masculine or feminine social role.
11. Discover healthy ways of becoming acceptable as a person to self and others.
12. Develop a positive attitude toward his or her own and other social, racial, economic, and religious groups.
13. Begin to formulate a set of beliefs that contribute to a sense of well-being.

The accomplishment of these tasks gives the schoolchild a foundation for entering adolescence, an era filled with dramatic growth and changing attitudes. Support, teaching, and guidance from family, other adults at church or in the community, and health professionals can assist the child in this progression.

Health Promotion and Nursing Applications

ASSESSMENT

Your role with the schoolchild and family has been discussed in each section throughout this chapter. Use the information from this chapter and other sources in your assessment while you also recognize the uniqueness of the child and the family situation. Be aware of variations related to the community, school, or cultural background.

NURSING DIAGNOSES

The **Box** Nursing Diagnoses Related to the Schoolchild, lists some nursing diagnoses that may be applicable (103). Assessments that result from information presented in this chapter may help you formulate other nursing diagnoses to guide your care.

INTERVENTION

Interventions have been interwoven throughout the chapter as they apply to the topic being discussed. Your therapeutic relationship and role-modeling of caring behavior to the child and family continue to be essential for health promotion and teaching. Continue the interventions described in Chapter 11 that are relevant. ∞ Refer also to **Box 12-10** for a summary of intervention points.

Interventions may occur in many settings and involve measures that promote health (e.g., immunization or control of hazards); teaching, support, counseling, or spiritual care with the child or family; or direct care measures to the ill child. Establish parent support groups and education programs, and involve parents in planning and implementation (15). Their shared knowledge can be instrumental in more effective parenting in family units, in development of resources in the community, and in legislative advocacy

Nursing Diagnoses Related to the Schoolchild

Disturbed **B**ody Image
Readiness for Enhanced **C**ommunication
Ineffective **C**oping
Impaired **D**entition
Risk for Delayed **D**evelopment
Risk for **F**alls
Fear
Delayed **G**rowth and Development

Risk for Disproportionate **G**rowth
Risk for **I**njury
Imbalanced **N**utrition: Less Than Body Requirements
Imbalanced **N**utrition: More Than Body Requirements
Acute **P**ain
Situational Low **S**elf-Esteem
Impaired **S**ocial Interaction
Social Isolation

Source: Reference 103.

Practice Point

Your understanding of the child developmentally will enable you to give holistic care—care that includes physiologic, emotional, cognitive, social, and spiritual aspects of the person. Your approach will differ, depending on age and maturity of the child, as well as the specific needs or condition to be treated. The other family members are always your clients as you care for the child.

and policy development for the health and welfare of children—our future leaders.

Become active as a citizen to educate the public about needs of schoolchildren and issues related to education and the school system. Promote needed legislation. Directly advocate about problems that affect children's health and education.

EVALUATION

Evaluation criteria of progression of the schoolchild in achieving developmental tasks and the effectiveness of your health care can be generated from observation of the schoolchild and family, from information and related references presented in this chapter and various sources, and from use of selected tools (73). Several references mention tools that have been used to evaluate intervention effectiveness. Discussion with the child's parents, teachers, and other health care professionals about their use of health promotion practices with the child also enhances your evaluation process. Keeping abreast of findings from the National Institutes of Health MRI Study of Normal Brain Development will help to develop relevant assessment, education, and evaluation tools (75). Self-evaluation and team review is an important part of analysis for evaluation. Each statement in **Box 12-10**, Considerations for the Schoolchild and Family in Health Promotion, may also be used in the evaluation process.

BOX 12-10   **Considerations for the Schoolchild and Family in Health Promotion**

1. Family and cultural background and values, the school, the support systems available, community resources
2. Parents' ability to guide the child, to help the child develop coping skills and gain necessary competencies
3. Relationships between family members
4. Behaviors that indicate a parent(s) or another significant adult, such as a relative or teacher, is perpetuating abuse, neglect, or maltreatment
5. Relationships between the family, school, and other community organizations (church, clubs) and resources
6. Physical growth patterns, characteristics and competencies, nutritional status, and rest/sleep and exercise patterns that indicate health and are within age norms for the school-age child
7. Growth spurt and secondary sex changes in prepubescence that indicate normal development in the boy or girl; self-concept and body image development related to physical growth
8. Nutritional requirements greater than those for the adult
9. Immunizations, safety education, and other health promotion measures
10. Cognitive characteristics and behavioral patterns in the preschool child that demonstrate curiosity and concrete

operations (concept formation, realistic thinking, and beginning social and moral value formation)
11. Educational/school programs, demonstration of development of cooperation, compromise, and collaboration as well as competition
12. Communication patterns; effect of television, computer, or the other media on communication, learning, and behavior
13. Overall appearance and behavioral patterns at home, in school, and in the community that indicate development of industry, rather than inferiority
14. Use of adaptive mechanisms that promote a sense of security, assist the child with relationships, promote realistic control of anxiety and age-appropriate emotional responses in the face of stressors
15. Behavioral patterns that indicate ongoing superego development and continuing moral–spiritual development
16. Behavioral patterns and characteristics that indicate the child has achieved developmental tasks
17. Parental behaviors that indicate they are achieving their developmental tasks

---

Summary

1. The schoolchild grows at a steady pace and continues physical growth and cognitive, emotional, social, and moral-spiritual development.
2. The growth spurt at prepuberty or preadolescence accelerates and influences development in all dimensions. Sexual identity is strengthened.
3. Relationships with parents, siblings, peers, and other adults change and influence development in all dimensions.
4. The child is learning to get along with a variety of people and in diverse situations.
5. Family is important as a base as peer relations become more important.
6. The chum of the same gender is a major support and is vital in psychological, self-concept, and social development.
7. The child meets many challenges, faces and overcomes insecurities, and develops competence that indicates a sense of emotional and social industry and cognitive development of Concrete Operations.
8. School, home, and community provide the avenues for development in all dimensions.
9. The parents are responsible for the child's health and safety; the professional reinforces monitoring to prevent maltreatment of the child.
10. **Box 12-10**, Considerations for the Schoolchild and Family in Health Promotion, summarizes what you should consider in assessment and health promotion with the schoolchild and evaluation of care. The family is included.

Review Questions

1. The school nurse overhears two 11-year-olds discussing their families. One child states, "My parents are so stupid. They don't know anything!" What is the best action for the nurse to take?
   1. Notify the parent.
   2. Ask the child about the statement.
   3. Ignore the comment.
   4. Notify the child's counselor.

2. A 9-year-old girl complains of breast tenderness. On physical assessment, the nurse notes increased diameter of the areola. The nurse concludes that the child:
   1. Is experiencing changes associated with prepuberty.
   2. Is experiencing precocious puberty.
   3. Should be scheduled for a mammogram.
   4. Should be counseled regarding birth control.

3. A 6-year-old child frequently is fatigued during the school day and is not doing well academically. How much sleep should the nurse suggest to the parents is needed by a child in this age group?
   1. 8 hours
   2. 9 hours
   3. 11 hours
   4. 17 hours

4. A 12-year-old child responds to the death of a grandparent by playing with younger siblings' toys and displaying behaviors consistent with an earlier age group. The nurse is aware that the child is using the adaptive mechanism of:
   1. Fantasy.
   2. Undoing.
   3. Regression.
   4. Projection.

References

1. Agne, K. (2001). Gifted: The lost minority. *Kappa Delta Pi Record, 37*(2), 168–172.
2. American Academy of Pediatrics, Committee on Public Education. (2001). Media violence. *Pediatrics, 108*(5), 1222–1226.
3. American Psychiatric Association. (2000). *Diagnostic criteria from DSM-IV-TR.* Washington, DC: Author.
4. An update on attention deficit disorder. (2004). *Harvard Mental Health Letter, 20*(11), 4–7.
5. Anderson, A., & Smith, A. (1999). Community building with parents. *Kappa Delta Pi Record, 35*(4), 158–161.
6. Anderson, C., & Bushman, B. (2002). Human aggression. In *Annual review of psychology* (Vol. 53). Palo Alto, CA: Annual Reviews.
7. Andrews, M., & Boyle, J. (2003). *Transcultural concepts in nursing care* (4th ed.). Philadelphia: Lippincott Williams & Wilkins.
8. Anthony, E. J., & Cohler, B. (1987). *The invulnerable child.* New York: Guilford.
9. Asperger's syndrome. (2005). *Harvard Mental Health Letter, 21*(8), 4–6.
10. Attention deficit disorder: Old questions, new answers. (2006). *Harvard Mental Health Letter, 22*(8), 3–5.
11. Bandura, A. (1991). Social Cognitive Theory of Self-Regulation. *Organizational Behavior and Human Decision Processes, 50,* 248–287.
12. Begany, T. (2005). Violent video games heighten aggression, literature review confirms. *Neuropsychiatry Reviews, 6*(9), 10–11.
13. Berger, K. (2005). *The developing person through the life span* (6th ed.). New York: Worth.
14. Bettelheim, B., & Freedgood, A. (1988). *A good enough parent: A look on child-rearing.* New York: Random.
15. Bond, L., & Burns, C. (2006). Mothers' beliefs about knowledge, child development, and parenting strategies: Expanding the goals of parenting programs. *Journal of Primary Prevention, 27*(6), 555–571.
16. Brunt, D. (2005). Two subtypes of food refusal in preteens found. *Clinical Psychiatry News, 33*(12), 34.
17. Burgess, A. (1988). Sexually abused children and their drawings. *Archives of Psychiatric Nursing, 2*(2), 65–73.
18. Burgess, A., Hartman, C., & Kelley, S. (1990). Assessing child abuse: The TRIADS Checklist. *Journal of Psychosocial Nursing and Mental Health Services, 28*(4), 6–14.
19. Burgess, A., McCausland, M., & Wolbert, W. (1981). Children's drawings as indicators of sexual trauma. *Perspectives in Psychiatric Care, 19*(2), 50–58.
20. Burgess, A., Hartman, C., Wolbert, W., and Grant, C. (1997). Child molestation: Assessing impact in multiple victims (Part I). *Archives of Psychiatric Nursing, 1*(1), 33–39.
21. Bushman, B., & Anderson, C. (2001). Media violence and the American public. *American Psychologist, 56,* 477–489.
22. Bushman, B., & Huesmann, L. (2001). Effects of televised violence on aggression. In D. Singer & J. Singer (Eds.), *Handbook of children and the media.* Thousand Oaks, CA: Sage.
23. Butler, W., Segreto, J., & Collins, E. (1985). Prevalence of dental mottling in school-aged lifetime residents of 16 Texas communities. *American Journal of Public Health, 75,* 1408–1412.
24. Campa, B., Connor-Smith, J., Saltzman, H., Thomsen, A., & Wadsworth, M. (2001). Coping with stress during childhood and adolescence: Problems, progress, and potential in theory and research. *Psychological Bulletin, 127,* 87–127.
25. Cashin, A. (2005). Autism: Understanding conceptual processing deficits. *Journal of Psychosocial Nursing, 43*(4), 22–30.
26. Chaiyawat, W., & Jezewski, M. (2006). Thai school-age children's perception of fear. *Journal of Transcultural Nursing, 17*(1), 74–81.
27. Characterizing the bipolar spectrum in pediatrics. (2006). *NeuroPsychiatry Reviews, 7*(11), 10.
28. Chenz, Z., & Siegler, R. (2001). Intellectual development in childhood. In B. J. Sternberg (Ed.), *Handbook of intelligence.* New York: Cambridge University Press.
29. Cole, J., & Dodge, K. (1998). Aggression and antisocial behavior. In W. Damon (Series Ed.) & N. Eisenberg (Vol. Ed.), *Handbook of child psychology: Vol. 3. Social, emotional, and personality development* (5th ed., pp. 781–862). New York: Wiley.
30. Coles, R. (1990). *The spiritual life of children.* Boston: Houghton Mifflin.
31. Cooke, P. (2004). Making the right media choices. *Enjoying Everyday Life, 18*(12), 22–23.
32. Crick, N., Casas, J., & Nelson, D. (2002). Toward a more comprehensive understanding of peer maltreatment. Studies of relational victimization. *Current Directions in Psychological Science, 11*(3), 98–101.
33. Davison, K., Susman, E., & Birch, L. (2003). Percent body fat at age 5 predicts earlier pubertal development among girls at age 9. *Pediatrics, 111,* 815–821.
34. DiLeo, J. (1971). *Young children and their drawings.* Springfield, IL: Springer.
35. Dowker, A. (2006). What can functional brain imaging studies tell us about typical and atypical cognitive development in children? *Journal of Physiology-Paris, 9,* 333–341.
36. Dudek, S. (2007). *Nutrition essentials for nursing practice* (5th ed.). Philadelphia: Lippincott Williams & Wilkins.

37. Duvall, E., & Miller, B. (1984). *Marriage and family development* (6th ed.). New York: Harper & Row.

38. Duyff, R. (2006). *American Dietetic Association complete food and nutrition guide* (Revised and updated 3rd ed.). Hoboken, NJ: John Wiley & Sons.

39. Effects of violence on children's ability to learn highlighted in new report from NHEC (1995). *The National's Health 25*(10), 23.

40. Elkind, D. (1981). *The hurried child: Growing up too fast, too soon.* Reading, MA: Addison-Wesley.

41. Engel, B. (2007). Eagle soaring: The power of the resilient self. *Journal of Psychosocial Nursing, 45*(2), 44–49.

42. Erikson, E. (1963). *Childhood and society* (2nd ed.). New York: W. W. Norton.

43. Exposure to violence adversely affects children. (1993). *Journal of Psychosocial Nursing, 31*(8), 45.

44. Fauman, M. (2002). *Study guide to DSM-IV-R.* Washington, DC: American Psychiatric Association.

45. Fenstermacher, K., & Hudson, B.T. (2004). *Practice guidelines for family practitioner* (3rd ed.). Philadelphia: W.B. Saunders.

46. Filipovic, Z. (1994). *Zlata's diary: A child's life in Sarajevo.* New York: Viking Penguin/Penguin Books.

47. Fink, P. (2005). Why do kids kill? *Clinical Psychiatry News, 33*(6), 12.

48. Flynn, M., McNeil, D., Maloff, B., Mutasingwa, D., Wu, M., Ford, C., & Tough, S. (2006). Reducing obesity and related chronic disease risk in children and youth. A synthesis of evidence with "best practices" recommendations. *Obesity Review, 7* (Suppl. 1), 7–66.

49. Frank, A. (1967). *The diary of a young girl.* New York: Doubleday.

50. Frazier, C. (2004, Fall). Unwelcome advances. *Teaching Tolerance,* Issue 26, 45–47.

51. Garbarino, J. (1992). *Children in danger.* New York: Jossey-Bass.

52. Garbarino, J., Guttmann, F., & Seeley, J. (1987). *The psychologically battered child: Strategies for identification, assessment and intervention.* San Francisco: Jossey-Bass.

53. Gardner, H. (1993). *Frames of mind: The theory of multiple intelligences* (2nd ed.). New York: Basic Books.

54. Gardner, H. (1993). *Multiple intelligence: Theory in practice.* New York: Basic Books.

55. Gelbert, E. (1962). Children's conceptions of the content and functions of the human body. *Genetic-Psychologic Monographs, 65,* 293–411.

56. Gender equation. (1995). *American Association of University Women Outlook, 88*(3), 28–29.

57. Gennetian, L., & Miller, C. (2002). Children and welfare reform: A view from an experimental welfare program in Minnesota. *Child Development, 73,* 601–620.

58. Gesell, A., & Ilg, F. (1977). *The child from five to ten* (Rev. ed.). New York: Harper Collins.

59. Gesell, A., Ilg, F., & Ames, L. (1956). *Youth: The years from ten to sixteen.* New York: Harper & Brothers.

60. Giger, J., & Davidhizar, R. (2004). *Transcultural nursing: Assessment and intervention* (4th ed.). St. Louis, MO: Mosby.

61. Gilligan, C. (1982). *In a different voice: Psychological theory and women's development.* Cambridge, MA: Harvard University Press.

62. Graham, J., & Beller, A. (2002). Nonresident fathers and their children: Child support and visitation from an economic perspective. In C. Tamis-LeMenda & N. Cabrera (Eds.), *Handbook of father involvement: Multidisciplinary perspectives* (pp. 431–453). Mahwah, NJ: Erlbaum.

63. Guyton, A., & Hall, J. (2006). *Textbook of medical physiology* (11th ed.). Philadelphia: Elsevier.

64. Hanish, L., & Guerra, N. (2002). A longitudinal analysis of patterns of adjustment following peer victimization. *Development & Psychopathology, 14*(1), 69–89.

65. Harris, M., & Cumella, E. (2006). Eating disorders across the life span. *Journal of Psychosocial Nursing, 44*(4), 21–26.

66. Haynie, L., Lofton, S., Ragland, G., & Norwood, A. (2007). Homesickness: No place to call home. *Journal of Christian Nursing, 24*(3), 153–155.

67. Henley, J. (2002, May 25). Pornography forms children's views on sex. *The Guardian,* 16.

68. Hockenberry, M., & Wilson, D. (2007). *Wong's nursing care of infants and children* (8th ed.). St. Louis, MO: Mosby.

69. Huesmann, R., Moise-Titis, J., Podolski, C.L., & Eron, L. (2003). Longitudinal relations between children's exposure to TV violence and their aggressive and violent behavior in young adulthood: 1977–1992. *Developmental Psychology, 39,* 201–221.

70. Jacobson, G. (1994). The meaning of stressful life experiences in nine-to-eleven-year-old children: A phenomenological study. *Nursing Research, 43,* 95–99.

71. Johnson, J., Cohen, P., Smailes, E., Kasen, S., & Brook, J. (2002). Television viewing and aggressive behavior during adolescence and adulthood. *Science, 295,* 2468–2471.

72. Johnson, L., Safranek, S., & Friemoth, J. (2005). What is the most effective treatment of ADHD in children. *Public Health, 94*(9), 1580–1586.

73. Johnson, M., Bulechek, G., Butcher, H., Bochterman, J., Maas, M., Moorhead, S., & Swanson, E. (2006). *NANDA, NOC, and NIC linkage: Nursing diagnoses, outcomes, & interventions* (2nd ed.). St. Louis, MO: Mosby Elsevier.

74. Kantrowitz, R., & Wingert, P. (1999, October 18). The truth about tweens. *Newsweek,* 60–72.

75. Kelly, J. (2007). Massini NIH Database tracks normal brain development in health children. *Neuro Psychiatry Review, 8*(7), 10.

76. Kelly, K., & Kulman, L. (2004, September 13). Kid power. *U.S. News & World Report,* 47–51.

77. Khonzam, H., El-Gabajawi, F., Pirwani, N., and Priest, F. (2004). Asperger's disorder: A review of the diagnosis and treatment. *Comprehensive Psychiatry, 45*(3), 184–191.

78. Klinnert, M., Nelson, H., Price, M., Odenoff, A., Leung, D., & Mrazek, D. (2001). Onset and persistence of childhood asthma: Predictors from infancy. *Pediatrics, 108*(4), e69.

79. Kohlberg, L. (1964). Development of moral character and moral ideology. In M.L. Hofman (Ed.), *Review of child development research,* Vol. 1 (pp. 383–432). New York: Russell Sage.

80. Kohlberg, L. (1977). *Recent research in moral development.* New York: Holt, Rinehart & Winston.

81. Kohlberg, L. (1972). Stages of moral development as a basis for moral education. In C.M. Beck, B.S. Crittenden, & E.V. Sullivan, *Moral education: Interdisciplinary approaches* (pp. 23ff). New York: Paulist Press.

82. Lamb, M. (1987). The emergent father. In M.E. Lamb (Ed.), *The father role: Cross-cultural perspectives* (pp. 1–26). Hillsdale, NJ: Lawrence Erlbaum.

83. LaRossa, R. (1988). Fatherhood and social change. *Family Relations, 37,* 451–457.

84. Law, B. (2002). Stress in children: Can nurses help? *Pediatric Nursing, 28*(1), 13–19.

85. Lego, S. (1998). Children killing children. *Perspectives in Psychiatric Care, 34*(3), 3–4.

86. Liebert, R., & Spraskin, J. (1989). *The early window: Effects of television on children and youths* (3rd ed.). New York: Pergamon Press.

87. Mantzicopoulos, P. (2006). Younger children's changing self-concepts: Boys and girls from preschool through second grades. *Journal of Genetic Psychology, 167*(3), 289–309.

88. Martin, S. (2002). Children exposed to domestic violence: Psychological considerations for health care practitioners. *Holistic Nursing Practice, 16*(3), 7–15.

89. Masland, T. (2002, May 13). Voices of the children: We beat and killed people. *Newsweek,* 24–27.

90. Masland, T. (2003, July 14). Wars without end. *Newsweek,* 28–31.

91. Masten, A. (2001). Ordinary magic: Resilience processes in development. *American Psychologist, 56,* 227–238.

92. McColgan, M., & Giardino, A. (2005). Internet poses multiple risks to children and adolescents. *Pediatric Annals, 34*(5), 405–414.

93. McGoldrick, M., Giordano, J., & Garcio-Preto, N. (2005). *Ethnicity and family therapy* (3rd ed.). New York: Guilford.

94. McGuinness, T. (2007). How young is too young for psychotropic medication? *Journal of Psychosocial Nursing, 45*(6), 20–23.

95. McGuinness, T. (2006). Active living for healthy youth. *Journal of Psychosocial Nursing, 44*(6), 13–16.

96. McKee, A. (1992). *The AAUW Report: How schools short-change girls.* New York: American Association of University Women.

97. Metheny, N. (2000). *Fluid and electrolyte balance: Nursing considerations* (4th ed.). Philadelphia: Lippincott.

98. Monteleone, J. (1998). *A parent's & teacher's handbook on identifying and preventing child abuse*. St. Louis, MO: G.W. Medical Publishing.

99. Morse, S. (1995). Growing smart. *American Association of University Women Outlook, 88*(3), 17–19.

100. Morse, S. (1995). Why girls don't like computer games. *Association of University Women Outlook, 88*(4), 16–19.

101. Morse, S. (1996). Girls in the middle. *American Association of University Women Outlook, 90*(3), 33–36.

102. Mytton, J., DiGuiseppi, C., Gough, D., Taylor, R., & Logan, S. (2007). *School based secondary prevention programs for preventing violence (Review). The Cochrane Collaboration*. New York: John Wiley.

103. NANDA International. (2007). *NANDA-I nursing diagnoses: Definitions and classification 2007–2008*. Philadelphia: Author.

104. Nansch, T., Overpeck, M., Pilla, R., Ruan, W., Simone-Morton, B., & Scheidt, A. (2001). Bullying behavior among U.S. youth: Prevalence and association with psychosocial adjustment. *Journal of the American Medical Association, 285*, 2094–2100.

105. Owens, D. (1995). Bullying or peer abuse at school. Facts and intervention. *Current Directions in Psychological Science, 4*, 196–200.

106. Parent training. (2006). *Harvard Mental Health Letter, 22*(10), 1–3.

107. Papalia, D., Olds, S., & Feldman, P. (2004). *Human development* (9th ed.). Boston: McGraw-Hill.

108. Pellegrin, A. (2002). Bullying, victimization, and sexual harassment during the transition to middle school. *Educational Psychologist, 37*, 151–164.

109. Perrin, M. (2005). *Psychiatric medications for children: Medication and treatment for children & youth with emotional and behavioral challenges*. New York: Stillwater Press.

110. Perry, C., Hatton, D., & Kendall, J. (2005). Latino parents' account of attention deficit hyperactive disorder. *Journal of Transcultural Nursing, 16*(4), 312–321.

111. Perse, E. (2001). *Media effects and society*. Mahwah, NJ: Erlbaum.

112. Potts, N., & Mandleco, B. (2007). *Pediatric nursing: Caring for children and their families* (2nd ed.). New York: Thomson/Delmar Learning.

113. Phelps, P. (1999). The power of partnership. *Kappa Delta Phi Record, 35*(4), 154–157.

114. Piaget, J. (1965). *The moral judgment of the child*. New York: Free Press.

115. Piaget, J. (1963). *The origins of intelligence in children*. New York: W. W. Norton.

116. Piaget, J. (1965). *The child's conception of numbers*. New York: W.W. Norton.

117. Piaget, J. (1985). *The equilibration of cognitive structures: The central problem of intellectual development* (T. Brown & K.J. Thampy, Trans.). Chicago: University of Chicago Press.

118. Piaget, J., & Inhelder, B. (1969). *The psychology of the child*. New York: Basic Books.

119. Piaget, J., & Inhelder, B. (1973). *Memory and intelligence*. New York: Basic Books.

120. Pontious, S. (1982). Practical Piaget: Helping children understand. *American Journal of Nursing, 82*(1), 115–117.

121. Rakestraw, J., & Rakestraw, D. (1990). Home schooling: A question of quality, an issue of rights. *Educational Forum, 55*(1), 67–77.

122. Rigby, K. (2002). Bullying in childhood. In P. Smith & C. Hart (Eds.), *Blackwell handbook of childhood social development*. Malden, MA: Blackwell.

123. Sadock, B., & Sadock, V. (2004). *Kaplan & Sadock's concise textbook of clinical psychiatry* (2nd ed.). Philadelphia: Lippincott Williams & Wilkins.

124. Santrock, J. (2004). *Life-span development* (9th ed.). Boston: McGraw-Hill.

125. Schulman, M. (1985). *Moral development training: Strategies for parents, teachers, and clinicians*. Menlo Park, CA: Addison-Wesley.

126. Seifert, K., Hoffnung, R., & Hoffnung, M. (2000). *Lifespan development* (2nd ed.). Boston: Houghton Mifflin.

127. Separation anxiety. (2007). *Harvard Mental Health Letter, 23*(7), 1–3

128. Singer, J., & Singer, D. (1998). *Television imagination and aggression: A study of preschoolers*. Hillsdale, NJ: Erlbaum.

129. Singer, M., Slovak, K., Friersen, T., & York, P. (1998). Viewing preferences, symptoms of psychological training and violent behaviors among children who watch television. *Journal of the American Academy of Child and Adolescent Psychiatry, 37*(10), 1041–1048.

130. Skybo, T. (2005). Witnessing violence: Biopsychosocial impact on children. *Pediatric Nursing, 31*(4), 263–270.

131. Smith, K., Landry, S., & Swank, P. (2006). The role of early maternal responsiveness in supporting school-aged cognitive development for children who vary in birth status. *Pediatrics, 117*(5), 1608–1617.

132. Smith, S., & Reynolds, C. (2002). Innocence lost: The impact of 9-1-1 on the development of children. *Annals of the American Psychotherapy Association, 5*(5), 12–13.

133. Sternberg, R. (1994). *Thinking and problems solving*. San Diego: Academic Press.

134. Sternberg, R., & Wagner, R. (Eds.). (1994). *Mind in context: Interactionist perspectives in human intelligence*. New York: Cambridge University Press.

135. Strasburger, V., & Donnerstein, E. (1999). Children, adolescents, and the media: Issues and solutions. *Pediatrics, 103*, 129–139.

136. Study links online porn to sex crimes in children. (2003, December 27). *Calgary Herald*, 0511.

137. Sullivan, H.S. (1953). *The interpersonal theory of psychiatry*. New York: W.W. Norton.

138. Tichenor, M., Tichenor, J., Hannah, T., Paterniti, N., & Wilson, S. (2003). Education in Germany. *Kappa Delta Pi Record, 39*(2), 94–95.

139. Tobias, C. (1996). *Every child can be successful: Making the most of your child's learning style*. New York: Tyndale.

140. Turley, R. (2003). Are children of young mothers disadvantaged because of their mother's age or family background? *Child Development, 74*, 465–474.

141. Tyre, P. (2006, September 11). The new first grade: Too much too soon? *Newsweek*, 34–44.

142. Tyre, P., Scelfo, J., & Kantrowitz, B. (2004, September 13). The power of "No." *Newsweek*, 42–51.

143. Ulrich, B. (2005, September). Switchin' roles. *Focus on the Family*, 22–23.

144. UN Secretary-General's study reveals full range and scale of violence against children. (2006, October 12). Retrieved January 11, 2007.

145. United States Department of Agriculture, Food and Nutrition Service. (2005). *MyPyramid for Kids*. www.mypyramid.gov/kids

146. United States Department of Health and Human Services. (2000). *Healthy People 2010. With understanding and improving health and objectives for improving health* (2nd ed.). 2 vols. Washington, DC: U.S. Government Printing Office.

147. Violent crimes linked to early childhood factors. (1995). *Menninger Letter, 3*(7), 7.

148. Vygtosky, L. (1978). Mind in society. In M. Cole, V. Johnsteiner, S. Scribner, & E. Scriberman (Eds.), *The development of higher psychological processes*. Cambridge, MA: Harvard University Press.

149. Wadsworth, B. (2004). *Piaget's theory of cognitive and affective development* (5th ed.). Boston: Pearson Education.

150. Weizman, Z., & Snow, C. (2001). Lexical input as related to children's vocabulary acquisition: Effects of sophisticated exposure and support for meaning. *Developmental Psychology, 37*, 265–279.

151. Werner, E. (1989). *Vulnerable but invincible*. New York: Adams-Bannister-Cox.

152. Werner, E., & Smith, R. (1992). *Overcoming the odds: High-risk children from birth to adulthood*. Ithaca, NY: Cornell University Press.

153. Wilens, T. (2004). *Straight talk about psychiatric medications for kids* (Rev. ed.). New York: Guilford Press.

154. Willey, L.H., et al. (1999). *Pretending to be normal: My life with Asperger's syndrome*. New York: Jessica Kingsley Publishers.

155. Wolfe, J. (2006). How the tobacco industry targets children. *American Journal of Nursing, 106*(11), 13.

156. Yeung, W.J., Linver, M., & Brooks-Gunn, J. (2002). How money matters for young children's development: Parental investment and family processes. *Child Development, 73*, 1861–1879.

157. York, F., & Larue, J. (2002). *Protecting your children in an X-rated world*. New York: Tyndale.

158. Zimmerman, M., Wolbert, W., Burgess, A., & Hartman, C. (1987). Art and group work: Interventions for multiple victims of child molestation (Part I). *Archives of Psychiatric Nursing, 1*, 33–39.

159. Zimmerman, M., Wolbert, W., Burgess, A., & Hartman, C. (1987). Art and group work: Interventions for multiple victims of child molestation (Part II). *Archives of Psychiatric Nursing, 1*, 40–46.

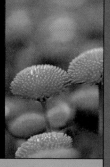

CHAPTER 13

The Adolescent: Basic Assessment and Health Promotion

OBJECTIVES

Study of this chapter will enable you to:

1. Examine the impact of the crisis of adolescence on family life and the influence of the family on the adolescent.

2. Explore with the family its developmental tasks and ways to achieve them while giving positive guidance to the adolescent.

3. Contrast the physiologic changes and needs of early, middle, and late adolescence and compare to changes in preadolescence.

4. Discuss with parents the cognitive, self-concept, sexual, emotional, and moral-spiritual aspects of development of the adolescent and ways in which the family can foster their healthy progress.

5. Identify examples of adolescent peer group dialect and use of leisure time in your region, and discuss how knowledge of them can be used in your health promotion activities and teaching.

6. Explore the developmental crisis of identity formation with the adolescent and the parents and the significance of attaining identity formation for ongoing maturity.

7. Examine ways to counteract influences that interfere with identity formation.

8. Evaluate the developmental tasks of adolescence and how the adaptive mechanisms commonly used assist the adolescent in achieving them.

MediaLink www.prenhall.com/murray

Go to the Companion Website for interactive resources that accompany this chapter.

Glossary	Critical Thinking
Review Questions	Tools
Challenge Your Knowledge	Media Link Applications
Learning Activities	Media Links

Historical and Cultural Perspectives

Adolescence is a developmental stage that differs cross-culturally. Before the 20th century, children in the United States entered the adult world when they matured physically. That is still true in many countries. The female may begin childbearing. The male enters the adult work world. In the United States, children are physiologically maturing at an earlier age than previously. *The increase in height and earlier age at which puberty and physical maturation occur is called a* **secular growth trend**. This trend is attributed to improved nutrition and health practices. The developmental era is also being extended because of social, economic, employment, industrial, and family changes. For some people adolescence ends in the teens, but for most the period ends in the middle 20s (46, 62). However, adolescence is not so prolonged in all countries or cultures. In some cultures when puberty occurs, **rites of passage**, *specific age-related ceremonies or community responsibility,* such as completing the spiritual development markers for the bar mitzvah, signal adulthood. Some cultures practice female circumcision, which mutilates the external genitalia and carries a number of health risks. (Female circumcision is described in Chapter 14.) ∞ Some encourage the male to perform acts of bravery. Some cultures expect certain types of behavior at a specific age (6, 58).

Definitions

In the past many people equated puberty and adolescence; they are now considered separate components. Puberty is preceded by **prepuberty**. **Preadolescence**, the *stage of prepuberty*, is discussed in Chapter 12. ∞ *These children are a part of the school-age population in the United States.*

Puberty is the *state of physical development between 10 and 14 years for females and 12 and 16 years for males, when sexual reproduction first becomes possible with the onset of* **menstruation** (*onset of menses*) or **spermatogenesis** (*production of spermatozoa*) (73, 140).

Adolescence is the *period that begins with puberty and extends for about 8 to 10 years or longer, until the person is physically and psychologically mature, ready to assume adult responsibilities and be self-sufficient* (140). Exceptions occur; some people never become psychologically mature. This definition does not reflect the individuality or culture of the adolescent.

For the purpose of this chapter, the adolescent period is divided into the subperiods of preadolescence, and early, middle, and late adolescence. Although age ranges are assigned to each subperiod, they are approximate. Each adolescent may vary as to when and how he or she proceeds through the various stages.

Early adolescence *begins with puberty and lasts for several years.* Growth is rapid and reaches peak velocity. Secondary sexual characteristics are evident (16, 140, 155). Age ranges vary considerably: 8–10 up to 12–14 years for females, and 9–12 up to 14–16 years for males (73, 140).

Middle adolescence *begins when physical growth is completed and usually extends from age 13–14 to 16 for females and 14–16 to 18–20 for males* (73).

| BOX 13-1 | The Adolescent's View of Parents |

EARLY ADOLESCENCE

1. Views parents as less powerful.
2. Feels loved but misunderstood by parents.
3. Feels dependent on parents, seeks their support.
4. Perceives parents as less ideal than selected adults, begins to emotionally distance from parents.

MIDDLE ADOLESCENCE

1. Feels constrained by parents, yet continues to want parental support while exerting sense of power and importance.
2. Believes parents are old-fashioned and lack good judgment; seeks affirmation from peers.
3. Feels parents do not understand or care, needs to demonstrate uniqueness by rebelling against selected aspects of parental values and behaviors.
4. Values parental restraints, despite protests, if restraints are reasonable.

LATE ADOLESCENCE

1. Feels renewed respect and affection for parents.
2. Perceives parental feedback as important in self-evaluation.
3. Desires to integrate parental values, attitudes, and behavior into own identity.
4. Realizes autonomy and identity incorporate cooperation and collaboration rather than rebellion and egocentrism.
5. Realizes continued economic and physical dependence on parents if unable to support self economically.

Late adolescence *may occur from approximately 18 to 22, or as late as 25 years of age.* The male may continue to grow in height until 22 to 25 years of age. The person is physically mature and is transitioning into young adulthood (73, 140). Emotionally, some individuals remain immature or adolescent-like—they do not "grow up"—until they are nearly 30 years of age. These **"adultolescents"** *do not desire to engage in the traditional benchmarks of independence—* moving out of the parents' home to establish their own home, financial autonomy, marriage, and children (177). After high school, they may be employed but live at home. After college graduation, they move back home. Parents may encourage this extension of adolescence and demand little of the offspring. Refer to **Box 13-1**, The Adolescent's View of Parents (16, 140, 155). Some teens are expected to move into the tasks of young adulthood at this point.

Family Development and Relationships

THE MOSAIC OF THE FAMILY

The family and home are expected to be a stable environment, the base for meeting needs and feeling security and acceptance. The importance of the family discussed in previous chapters continues throughout this era. For some teens, there is too much family conflict, unstable behavior or illness in the parents, or divorce. For some teens, there is little family life, not even discord. Some teens go to work part-time to help support the one-parent family. In many U.S. homes, both parents work, so the adolescent helps to care for younger siblings and juggles school and home responsibilities. Some parents want the child to be active and succeed. Extracurricular activities, especially team sports, are juggled with the school schedule and fewer home responsibilities. Sometimes parents in these families complain about the time spent in chauffeuring until the teen can drive the automobile. In contrast to the materialism seen in some families, about 20% of children, including teens, live in poverty, which negatively affects all spheres of the family and individual environment (16).

CHANGING BEHAVIORS IN THE ADOLESCENT AND FAMILY

Adolescence is a developmental stage spanning a number of years. Family relationships change during that time.

In **early adolescence,** *the child begins to separate emotionally from the parents,* especially the early-maturing female (16). The dependency-independency struggle is shown by less involvement in family activities, arguing or bickering about daily routines and chores, and expressing criticism or embarrassment about parental behavior. Rebellion against parental discipline and authority may begin (73, 140, 155). See **Box 13-1**, The Adolescent's View of Parents, for other characteristics.

In **middle adolescence,** *the independency and emancipation behaviors become stronger.* Bickering about and testing parental limits occur in relation to any parental limits, especially when parents confront the teen with behavior they do not like. This is often the low point in parent-child relationships as the teen does the opposite of what parents suggest; risk-taking behavior is common. There is greater detachment from parents and more dependence on peers (73, 140). Each generation has its own **generational stake**, *the tendency to interpret interactions from the view of the respective generation* (16, 184). It is not easy for parents to show love, caring, and involvement without appearing to interfere, and to communicate without appearing intrusive. It is difficult to confront the adolescent about behavior without feelings of guilt and anger rising in each generation. Even suggestions by the parent stated calmly and objectively may trigger the teen's denial of behavior or rebellion (16).

Parents want to show love and protect; the teen views this as domination, outmoded values, or lack of trust. Parents want to believe their teen is loyal to the family despite overt rebellion. Adolescents want to believe their parents are limited, old-fashioned, and out-of-touch. This helps the teen to **emancipate,** *to break free to establish a personal identity* and eventually a family (16, 184). See **Box 13-1**, The Adolescent's View of Parents, for other characteristics.

In **late adolescence,** *the emotional separation is being completed. More autonomy is granted by the parents, and the adolescent demonstrates more stability. These behavioral changes may be due to* (16, 140, 155): (a) increasing hormonal equilibrium; (b) parental consistency; (c) earlier stabilizing influences of adults outside of the family, such as teachers and friends; (d) participation in organizations or a church that provides support to parents and the teens; and (e) healthy peer group relationships. There is less conflict with parents. Emancipation is nearly secured (73). At this point, the adolescent and parent generations have similar values, attitudes, and aspirations (16, 41, 155). There has been an ongoing adjustment in both generations. Mutual appreciation, respect, and friendship between parent and adolescent develop. The late adolescent becomes less dependent on parents for help in meeting physical needs. There is greater financial independence as the individual becomes employed part- or full-time even if continuing in the student role. The youth may take the final step of establishing independence from parents by moving out of the home, being employed, and supporting self. See **Box 13-1**, The Adolescent's View of Parents, for other characteristics.

Adultolescence is a *stage that follows late adolescence for some individuals in their 20s. The youth, often Caucasian, stays at home during college or returns after college to live with the parents to be financially and physically supported.* Parents often demand little. This lifestyle is an extension of their philosophy to make the child feel secure, with the idea the youth will eventually become adult-like (177). The offspring is not likely to establish a home or partnership until the late 20s. The female may have a child in her mid-30s, having enjoyed the traditional freedom of opportunities of the adolescent to age 30 or beyond. There is a kind of drift between traditional late adolescence and young adulthood, which has become socially acceptable (177). Beyond the economic realities, there are complicated psychological bonds that keep able-bodied college graduates on their parents' payroll. The youth may not build an adult identity in reaction to the parents' way of life—the "Me Generation." Apparently most of the youth (the "Mini-Me Generation") do like and respect their parents (177).

Families high in conflict and low in support impair normal adolescent development. The adolescent does not benefit from parents that are too permissive or too strict. The adolescent's mother who was a teen when her child was born often has a difficult time with establishing boundaries or limits; she may be reliving adolescence through her child (16).

In addition to other conflicts, the teen must also work through feelings for the parent of the opposite gender and unravel the ambivalence toward the parent of the same gender. He or she reworks some of the gender identity and family triangle problems that remain from the preschool era. In an attempt to resolve this ambivalence, the adolescent may strive to be as different as possible from the parent of the same gender. Frequently affection is turned to an adult outside the family. "Crushes" or "idol worship" of this nature are very common; they are usually brief and may occur once, twice, or on numerous occasions. Idolizing another adult person causes the adolescent to want to please that person; therefore, the adolescent's actions and language may change when the idolized person is present. Frequently the adolescent identifies so completely with this person that he or she absorbs some of the person's adult characteristics into the personality. These relationships are not harmful to the adolescent unless the idolized person still feels confused and rebellious toward society and fosters immaturity. The "idol" who is a public or media figure is likely to be an unstable identification figure. However, a stable adult outside the family usually will be more objective than the parent and can help the adolescent grow toward psychological maturity. Parents are experiencing sexuality changes at the same time as they face middle age.

Listen to parents as they try to resolve feelings of rejection and anger about the adolescent's critical, argumentative, defiant, and remote behavior. Affirm that the mood changes will level off. As the offspring matures, a previously close relationship will be restored if parents are patient. Validate that even now, at times, the relationship can be close and positive. The adolescent may actually support the parents in the presence of peers.

STRESSORS FOR PARENTS

In addition to dealing with a loss of authority, parents are faced with other stresses. They are forced to redefine past child-parent relations and rethink their own values. Parents may also be forced to evaluate their own career choices as their adolescent begins vocational pursuits. Competition between parents and the teen may exist. They may be anxious to relinquish financial, physical, and emotional childrearing responsibilities to increase their own freedom.

Teens use the computer to send instant messages or e-mail, visit chat rooms, download songs, or do homework. Increasingly, some teens are in their own secret world. The computer and Internet, video games, and no-holds-barred music are creating new worlds unknown to adults. New technologies and the entertainment industry, combined with changes in family structure, have isolated parents and other adults from teens. Many teens have a reality that excludes parents and adults. Teens are often unsupervised with the technology, looking at what they please. They often do not get an adult perspective on stimulation to which they are exposed. Teens have less access to parents and more access to potentially damaging information and more opportunity for damaging behavior. The anonymity of the Internet protects teens online but also engages them in potentially dangerous behavior. Refer to Chapter 12 for information on the effects of media. ∞ The teen may become addicted to the computer, neglecting family and school tasks and even self, for peer e-mails, chat rooms, and Internet sites (24, 137, 159). See also the information on Internet use in Chapter 12. ∞

Stresses that frequently produce family discord in the United States grow out of conflicting value systems. Today's adolescents are a generation born with technology (and less emphasis on people skills) that has brought remote corners of the world into their homes and minds and has fostered questioning of instead of reliance on authority. Parents need help to see that the adolescent is a product of his or her time and is reflecting what is happening socially. Further, teens may be confused by their parents' behavior. Some grow up with little parental supervision. Some are in single-parent or stepparent families. In some families, a parent may announce that he or she is bisexual or homosexual, or the teen may turn to alternate sexual orientation (16, 34, 62).

Parental and adolescent response to the ambivalence and conflicts of this period varies. In the United States, parents often say "boys will be boys," believing males get into more trouble than females. Some parents also believe that females, but not males,

should be hugged and are thereby less likely to keep close relationships with adolescent sons (91). Parents may adhere to rules and the status quo to bolster their own security or cultural traditions rather than change for the offspring's benefit. Parents may overprotect. Others may be reluctant to admit that their child is establishing an independent lifestyle. *If the adolescent has come from a family that has provided past opportunities to learn responsibility, self-reliance, skills, and self-respect, he or she will make a smoother transition from childhood dependency to adulthood independence.* If parents have been too liberal, overly permissive, or uninterested, the adolescent will have more difficulty adjusting because the past lacked structure and a system of standards or values. He or she has no point of reference other than peers to determine if the behavior is suitable and decisions are appropriate (16).

Fortunately some parents trust their offspring to live the basic values they taught, although at times behavior may appear differently. Effective parents work at being communicative and flexible, yet supportive, following suggestions such as those in the **Box**, Client Education: Communicating with Your Teen (33, 63, 73, 148). They accept that the adolescent may be as large as an adult but still behave childishly at times. The parents' adultlike behavior is a model for their offspring. They feel enough self-confidence that they do not have to belittle the adolescent. They are not threatened by the offspring's sexuality, so that the adolescent can rework sex identity. If the parent-child relationship has been close in the past, it can remain close now in spite of problems and responses.

A factor that may affect parent-adolescent communication and relationships is the *stepfamily, adoptive family,* or *foster family structure.* Often, adolescents struggle with whether they really belong to the family. Refer to Chapter 6 ∞ for discussion about these family structures. The adopted and foster child may search for the birth parents. Adoptive parents should cooperate rather than feel threatened. The search should not be interpreted as rebellion.

Encourage adoptive or foster parents to work with the adolescent, utilizing community resources as needed. They may join a group to assist with legal issues as well as resolve feelings. Encourage parents to *continue* to learn about the adolescent's native culture in the case of an international adoption. When possible, the adolescent can join a group to be with others and share commonalities of heritage, ethnicity, and appearance. Thus, identity and self-esteem can be strengthened.

FOREIGN-BORN PARENTS AND THEIR CHILDREN IN THE UNITED STATES

In your practice, you will increasingly have contact with children and adolescents with one or both parents who were born abroad. In the United States, 20% of children and adolescents are of foreign-born parentage and the number is increasing. *There are emotional, social, educational, and clinical issues to be aware of when addressing the needs of children and of their immigrant parents* (5, 10, 58, 175, 191):

1. **Language issues:** The offspring live in linguistically isolated households, which require them to be translators for the parents. The adolescent could be exposed to inappropriate or untimely information. Translators should be provided. Refer parents to classes in English as a second language and support

Client Education

Communicating with Your Teen

1. Make time for listening and talking.
2. Create a beginning and an ending to the day.
3. Respect the teen's privacy; do not insist on his or her disclosure.
4. Do not judge or shame; state facts and recognition of differences.
5. Say "thank you" and "please" as appropriate.
6. Be generous with honest praise.
7. Apologize when it is appropriate.
8. Let the teen make choices and the inevitable mistakes.
9. Talk about ways to cope with the consequences of unwise decisions.
10. Avoid lectures, preaching, talking down, or sarcasm.
11. Use open-ended questions, such as "How was your day?"
12. Speak to feelings, "you look frustrated," or reflect back feelings that are disclosed.
13. Nurture mealtime conversation; turn off the television, radio, computer, and stereo.
14. Plan family times that emphasize casual talk.
15. Take advantage of driving time, especially when you are alone with the teen, to talk. The need for the parent who is driving to keep "eyes on the road," avoiding eye contact, often helps exploration of sensitive issues.
16. Welcome their friends; engage them in conversation, often through activity.
17. Use "I" statements. If you have a plan, be open about it (e.g., a shopping trip).
18. Keep the teen and self in perspective.
19. Criticize the behavior, not the person.
20. Talk about one issue at a time; do not bring in past events or behavior unrelated to the current topic.
21. Make requests in a neutral, kind tone of voice, assertively but not commandingly.

their attendance. The youth may also wish to continue classes in English.

2. **Parental guidance:** During resettlement in the United States, parents are coping with many demands on their time and emotional energy and often are working long hours in low-paying jobs. Thus, they can give less time and attention to their children.

3. **Coping with stresses related to immigration:** Children and parents have to deal with a new life pattern, resolve losses, face discrimination, and adjust to the fast pace of the United States. Some immigrant families have to work through their memories of past traumatic experiences. Family stress is associated with depression, aggression, anxiety, low self-esteem, and delinquency in the offspring.

4. **Parental overmonitoring:** Because of the experiences prior to immigration, and the scenes portrayed in the U.S. media, parents are hypervigilant about the offspring's safety. They have difficulty permitting independent behavior.

5. **Cultural and religious conflicts related to differing norms and expectations:** Conflicts between the parents and adolescents arise in relation to social and gender differences in behavior between the United States and the country of origin. The adolescent may transgress and shame the family in relation to dress, modesty, association with the opposite gender, or experimentation with alcohol, drugs, or sexual activity.

6. **Parental concerns about Americanization of the offspring and loss of cultural heritage:** Youth in immigrant families are more likely to manifest adjustment and emotional problems. They experience the conflicts between parental expectations of conformity and obedience and demands at school or from peers or society.

Do not miss critical cues or discredit parental concerns. Listen to both nonverbal and verbal expressions of parents and youth. Encouraging discussion can be difficult because in many cultures feelings and family conflicts are not discussed with nonfamily members. Focus first on the physical complaints that brought them to the health care setting. Then speak to the "possible feelings." Refer to Chapter 2, Table 2-2, ∞ to review therapeutic principles of communication. A calm, objective but empathic statement, such as "How are you managing with everything?" can open the door to a response. State concerns about their dilemma in promoting well-being of their offspring.

CULTURAL VARIATIONS IN PARENT-CHILD RELATIONSHIPS

In some cultures, the conflict typical of U.S. adolescents with the parents may not exist. For example, in Asian American, African American, Mexican American, American Indian, Hispanic and African cultures, a basic value is respect for older individuals (5, 58). Further, the family is considered more important than the individual. Thus, families in many cultural groups are dismayed by the emphasis in the United States on adolescent "rights" and acceptance of their behavior, regardless of family or social consequences (5, 58). In some cultural groups, for example, Asian and Mexican, conflict with parents may not be apparent because parents encourage the child to remain close to the family—physically and emotionally (5, 16, 156). In many cultures, including some European countries, behavior norms and role expectations provide a basis for a smoother transition to adolescence than is expected in the United States. Less technologic societies have less parent-child conflict because there is less choice in occupations and lifestyles and less generational variances (5, 10, 156). In Asian cultures, the youth is expected to consider expectations of the extended family. There are different expectations of male and female behavior and achievement in many cultures that extend to adolescents. The adolescent may behave differently at home than with peers at school or in the community (5, 10, 156).

Adolescents belong not only to their own cultural group but to other groups that form the basis for the person's values, attitudes, and beliefs. In Westernized societies, they also belong to the **subculture of adolescence**, *a system of socially transmitted values, attitudes, and behaviors that may or may not be in harmony with the larger culture.* Status symbols, material goods, clothing, hair styles, equipment, music, and art also vary with each generation of adolescents. Laws or codes for this subculture may be unwritten, but they are powerfully enforced through peer pressure. Communication patterns of the adolescent subculture often differ from that of the adult population (10, 16, 58, 140, 155).

Culturally competent care of adolescents *requires sensitivity to the* (a) sociocultural background of the adolescent and the family, (b) family structure and organization (who is the major decision maker), (c) religious values and beliefs, and (d) role assignment related to age and gender within the family and cultural group. The adolescent's family should be approached as a client. The family environment must be assessed; it is a major factor in the adolescent's health promotion practices and illness prevention. Further, other family members, in addition to the adolescent, may need assessment and intervention. Consider the family's support system and network of relatives, friends, and neighbors who are important for the adolescent's well-being, recovery, and continuing health. Diet, exercise, use of leisure, stress management, and control of disease states, such as hypertension or diabetes, depend upon family support (5, 10, 58).

FAMILY DEVELOPMENTAL TASKS

The overall family goal at this time is to allow the adolescent increasing freedom and responsibility to prepare him or her for young adulthood. Although each family member has personal developmental tasks, *the family unit as a whole also has developmental tasks.* The family members (37, 70):

1. Provide facilities for individual differences and needs of family members.
2. Work out a system of financial responsibility.
3. Establish a sharing of responsibilities.
4. Reestablish a mutually satisfying marriage relationship.
5. Strengthen communication with the members.
6. Rework relationships with relatives, friends, and associates.
7. Broaden horizons of the adolescent and parents.
8. Formulate a workable philosophy of life.

Discuss the developmental tasks and how to achieve them with the family. Discuss information about developmental markers and the points in the **Box**, Client Education: Communicating with Your Teen. Explore the interaction between parents and offspring. Validate that the parental behavior and the home situation affect the teen's adjustment.

Emphasize that this era usually creates family turmoil, conflict, and ambivalence as both parents and adolescents learn new roles.

Explore how parents can gradually increase the teenager's responsibilities and allow privileges formerly denied, yet resist granting instant adult status when the child reaches teen years. Reinforce that the adolescent feels more self-confident in exploring the environment if reasonable limits are imposed. Encourage parents to listen to their adolescent's viewpoints concerning restrictions, which may offer hints about the readiness for more independence and freedom.

Explore how teenagers may fight for grown-up privileges that they never use—the actual battle is more important than the privilege. Discuss or role-play ways to handle disagreements and conflicts about sexual behavior, dress, drugs, school performance, homework, friendship, family car, telephone privileges, manners, chores and duties, money, and disrespectful behavior that frequently disrupt family harmony.

MALTREATMENT, ABUSE, AND INCEST

Careful screening and *astute communication skills are essential when maltreatment is suspected.* Establish a relationship and interview the adolescent alone. Then you are more likely to learn of physical, sexual, and psychological abuse (maltreatment) or neglect and to pick up the cues. Utilize information from **Box 13-2**, Parental Behavior Characteristics of Psychological Maltreatment of the Adolescent for your assessment (54, 55).

The adolescent who is physically abused may be present in the emergency room with some of the same kinds of injuries that are seen in the younger child. Review Chapters 9, 10, 11, and 12 ∞ for a description of possible injuries. Sometimes bruises and lacerations are concealed from peers, teachers, and health care providers by cosmetics and clothes.

Adolescent girls who were sexually abused as children are likely to demonstrate the following behaviors (67, 113, 147):

1. Engage in voluntary intercourse at a young age.
2. Use drugs and alcohol, even when most of the peers do not.
3. Have older sexual partners who use drugs and alcohol.
4. Avoid use of contraceptives; get an abortion if pregnant.
5. Remain in an abusive or violent relationship during the teen years.
6. Report experiencing emotional and physical abuse in childhood.

Discuss signs of all types of abuse with the adolescent in a matter-of-fact way, which may encourage the teen to confide about being abused. Discuss with the parent the importance of listening if the teen discloses having been abused as a child or implies a current abusive situation. Interventions suggested in previous chapters are applicable but must be modified for the adolescent era. Personal safety rules should be emphasized. Advise the parent to discuss with the teen how to evaluate and get out of various unsafe situations. Assure the parent that the teen rarely lies about sexual assault if there is a close and trusting relationship. Validate that an important warning sign is the "gut feeling," the intuitive feeling held by a mother or father that something is wrong in the relationship between the teen and another person, including the other parent, a close relative, or friend.

Incest is sexual intercourse between persons in the family too closely related to marry legally. The adolescent, either male or female, is at

---

BOX 13-2   Parental Behavior Characteristics of Psychological Maltreatment of the Adolescent

REJECTING

1. Refuses to acknowledge changing social roles and to move to autonomy and independence
2. Treats adolescent like a young child
3. Subjects adolescent to verbal humiliation and excess criticism
4. Expels youth from family

ISOLATING

1. Tries to prevent youth from participating in organized and informal activities outside the home
2. Prohibits adolescent from joining clubs or after-school activities
3. Withdraws youth from school to work or perform household tasks
4. Punishes youth for engaging in normal social activity such as dating

TERRORIZING

1. Threatens to expose youth to public humiliation such as undressing youth, forcing encounter with police or stay in jail

2. Threatens to reveal intensely embarrassing characteristics (real or fantasized) to peers or adults
3. Ridicules youth in public regularly

IGNORING

1. Abdicates parental role
2. Shows no interest in youth as person or in activities; refuses to discuss adolescent's activities, plans, interests
3. Concentrates on activities or relationships that displace adolescent from affections

CORRUPTING

1. Involves youth in more intense or socially unacceptable forms of sexual, aggressive, or substance abuse behavior; forces youth into prostitution
2. Rewards aggressive or scapegoating behavior toward siblings, peers, or adults
3. Encourages trafficking in illicit drug use or alcohol use or in sex rings

Source: From Garbarino, J., Guttmann, E., & Seeley, J. (1987). Psychologically battered child: Strategies for identification, assessment, and intervention. San Francisco: Jossey-Bass. Adapted by permission of Jossey-Bass, Inc., a subsidiary of John Wiley & Sons, Inc.

---

risk for incest or for youth prostitution (20, 113). Either the mother or the father may be the abuser. Incestuous relations usually begin when the child is young and continue through adolescence (20, 73, 113, 140). The behavior and consequent signs and symptoms that occur are like those of the sexually abused child, described in Chapter 12. ∞ Incest may involve stepparents or stepsiblings, grandparents, or uncles or cousins.

In incestuous families, the man is often the sole economic support. The female partner or mother is often isolated. The daughter singled out for the sexual relationship is usually spared the beatings or other abuse given other family members, but she clearly understands what happens if she incurs the displeasure of the male. Incestuous males are described as family tyrants, but when confronted with the behavior, or in the presence of health care professionals, will appear pathetic, meek, bewildered, and ingratiating (20).

Typically the mother is working outside of the home, is ill or disabled, and cannot effectively care for herself or her children. Incestuous males do not assume maternal caretaking roles when the female partner is disabled. Rather they expect the eldest daughter to assume the "little mother" role for housework and child care responsibilities. The daughter's sexual relationship with the male often evolves as an extension of her other duties. When the oldest daughter becomes resistant, the male often turns his attention to the next daughter, or nieces, stepchildren, or granddaughters (20, 62, 77).

Incest should be suspected between daughter and father, stepfather, or mother's boyfriend in any family that includes (a) a violent or domineering and suspicious male; (b) a battered, chronically ill, or disabled mother; and (c) a daughter who appears to have assumed major adult responsibilities. If incest has been reported with one daughter, it should be suspected with all of the other daughters. Incest should be suspected as a precipitant in the runaway, delinquent, drug abusing, sexually acting-out, pregnant, or suicidal adolescent female. False accusations of sexual abuse or incest are rare; however, the female commonly retracts a true allegation because of family pressure (20, 77).

Discovery of incest is a family crisis. **Immediate reporting to authorities and crisis intervention are essential.** Typically the behavior has been going on for many years, and the family's defenses are organized around preservation of the incest secret. Disclosure interrupts patterns of functioning. The male faces loss of sexual activity and possible criminal sanctions. The mother faces possible loss of a husband or partner, social stigmatization, and the prospect of raising her family alone. The male denies his behavior. The wife is torn between husband and daughter. Unless she is given rapid support, her initial belief of the daughter gives way to rallying to the husband's side in 1 or 2 weeks. The daughter then finds herself discredited, shamed, punished for bringing trouble on the family, and still unprotected from sexual abuse. Suicide and runaway behavior are likely at this time as the offspring is being segregated and driven out of the family (20, 62, 77).

An active, directive, even coercive approach is necessary. Treatment requires ongoing cooperation between the therapist and agencies of the state—both law enforcement and child protective services. It may be necessary to remove the offspring from the home to ensure safety. This intervention, however, reinforces the couple's bonding against the offspring. It is preferable to have the male leave during this period. He may be imprisoned for a time (20, 62).

Crisis support for the offspring involves the following (20, 77, 113):

1. Reassure the adolescent (or child) that there are protective adults outside of the family that believe the story.
2. Praise the adolescent (or child) for the courage to reveal the incest secret.
3. Assure the offspring that he or she is *not* to blame for the incest.
4. Tell the offspring explicitly that many children retract their initial complaint because of pressure or fear. Encourage him or her not to do so.

Crisis support for the mother involves encouragement and assistance to (20, 77, 106, 113):

1. Continue to believe the offspring, even if this is painful.
2. Resist the tendency to bond with the husband against the offspring.
3. Talk about her feelings of shame, guilt, anger, fear, and inadequacy.
4. Explore ways she can handle the issues of survival and seek needed help.
5. Obtain treatment for health problems.

Group treatment for the mother, father, and offspring is more effective than family or individual therapy alone. Individual therapy can be combined with group therapy. Family therapy may be used in the late stages of treatment. The best motivator for the offender to remain in therapy is the court mandate.

Restoration of the incestuous family centers on the mother-daughter relationship. Safety for the daughter comes first. The mother may give up the marital partner relationship. Help the mother feel strong enough to protect herself and her children. Ensure that the daughter feels and is safe.

Destructive effects of incest continue into adult life related to self-esteem, intimate relationships, sexual functioning, and a higher-than-normal risk for repeated victimization (battering and rape). Incest occurs between siblings and may have consequences similar to those described (20).

Rape and *other sexual abuse* may be part of the adolescent's experience as a victim. *Several types of sex rings exist* (20): (a) child sex initiation rings, (b) youth prostitution rings, and (c) syndicated pornography and prostitution rings. The adolescent may be lured into these experiences through the Internet. Be aware that sex rings may exist in your area.

As you work with sexual assault victims, be aware of various types of assault and entanglements that exist so that you can better detect verbal and nonverbal cues and give immediate assistance (143). Refer the youth (and parents) to receive the necessary medical and legal assistance. Work with law enforcement agents as needed for the assaulted person's safety.

Physiologic Concepts and Physical Characteristics

NEUROENDOCRINE INFLUENCES ON PHYSICAL GROWTH

The hypothalamus-pituitary-gonadal system is dormant in childhood. *Events of puberty* begin with the hypothalamus, which is related to brain maturation. The hypothalamus initiates secretion of neurohumoral-releasing factors. These neurohumors stimulate the anterior pituitary gland to release gonadotrophic hormones, somatotropic hormone (STH) or growth hormone (GH), thyroid-stimulating hormone (TSH), and adrenocorticotropic hormone (ACTH). The amygdala in the limbic system also apparently changes function and promotes hormonal production (65, 73).

Gonadotropin-releasing hormone (GnRH), via the anterior pituitary, causes the follicle-stimulating hormone (FSH) and luteinizing hormone (LH) to stimulate the gonads to mature and produce sex hormones. FSH stimulates the ovaries in females to produce estrogen and the development of seminiferous tubules in males; LH stimulates the Leydig cells in the testes to produce testosterone. FSH and LH act together to stimulate sperm production. Growth and development of the adrenal cortex and stimulation of the secretion of androgens are promoted by ACTH. These androgens are responsible for producing secondary sex characteristics. Deoxyribonucleic acid (DNA) synthesis and hyperplastic cell growth, particularly of the bones and cartilage, are stimulated by STH. Under the influence of TSH, thyroxine secretion is increased during the pubertal period to meet body metabolic needs (65, 73). The **sex steroids or hormones**, *estrogen, progesterone, and testosterone, and other androgens*, are released from the gonads. Serum levels of these hormones increase, and the rise provides a feedback to the hypothalamus to decrease GnRH secretion, and to the anterior pituitary gland to decrease stimulation of FSH, LH, and androgen production. When the serum sex hormones decrease to a certain level, the feedback system causes the hypothalamus to increase GnRH secretion. The cycle is repeated (65, 73).

Both male and female hormones are produced in varying amounts in both genders throughout life. During the prepubescent years, the adrenal cortex secretes a small amount of sex hormones. The sex hormone production that accompanies maturation of the ovaries and testes is responsible for the physiologic changes observed in puberty. Both forms of gonadal hormones stimulate epiphyseal fusion by repressing the growth hormone, which slows physical growth at the end of puberty (65, 73, 140). Hormone levels also affect emotional status after puberty begins (65, 73).

Discuss the hormonal changes that are occurring with the adolescent and family. Factual knowledge enhances adjustment and health.

PHYSICAL CHARACTERISTICS

Teach the adolescent, and help parents understand what they should teach their children, about the physical changes of this era, in structure, size, shape, and function. They both need realistic information about these subjects and an opportunity for discussion.

This knowledge can help the adolescent understand his or her *normal* development. If the parents are knowledgeable about growth changes, they can predict coming physical changes based on how the teen presently looks, which can be reassuring to the child whose onset of puberty is delayed.

Growth

Adolescence is the second major period of accelerated growth (infancy was the first). The adolescent growth spurt occurs approximately 2 years earlier in the female than in the male.

By the beginning of adolescence, females tend to be as tall as or taller than males of their age. By the end of early adolescence or the end of the middle school years, most males have caught up or even surpassed the females in height. The *secular growth trend* is apparent, including in Japan, Western European countries, and the United States.

Changes in appearance occur, and growth is likely to be asymmetrical. See Chapter 3 for information on the Asynchronous Principle of Development. ∞ The nose, lips, and ears often grow larger before the head increases in size. *The typical growth progression is manifested in the following order:* (a) hands and feet become larger and hand strength increases, (b) arms and legs are longer and gangly, and (c) the chest and trunk lengthen and the shoulders broaden. Large muscles grow and develop faster than small muscles. Weight is likely to be gained before height increases occur. The female is likely to gain in cumulative volume of fat; the male tends to drop fat tissue. In early adolescence, females outweigh males. By age 14 years, males begin to surpass females (73, 155). There is a steady increase in strength. Late-maturing individuals tend to be taller than their peers in late adolescence (140).

The growth spurt begins as early as 9 years of age in females and about 11 years in males. The peak for pubertal changes is 11.5 years in females and 13.5 years in males (73, 155). During each year of the growth spurt, females grow 2.5 to 5 in. (6 to 12.5 cm) and gain 8 to 10 pounds (3.5 to 4.5 kg); males average 3 to 6 in. (7.5 to 15 cm) and gain 12 to 14 pounds (5.5 to 6.5 kg). In the initial phase of the growth spurt, the increase in height is due to lengthening of the legs. Later, most of the increase is in the trunk length. The total process of change takes approximately 3 years in females and 4 years in males (73, 140). Between age 15 and 18, females (and most males) are approaching full adult size and appearance. During adolescence, the person gains 15% to 20% of adult height and 50% of adult weight (36). By late adolescence, the person is more physically stable; body equilibrium is being reestablished. The person is less awkward and handles his or her body more efficiently (140).

Every system of the body is growing rapidly, but physiologic changes occur unevenly within the person. Variation exists in age of onset of puberty and rapidity of growth between different groups of people as well. For example, Chinese adolescents show an earlier height spurt and menarche and more advanced skeletal maturity than Europeans (5, 58). In the United States, low-birth-weight babies catch up in adolescence to expected height and weight, according to parental size (73).

Sexual Development

Physical characteristics define puberty. The sequence is almost always the same (16, 62, 73, 140, 148, 155).

Females evidence:

1. Initial breast development, enlargement, and tenderness: 8 to 13 years, peak at 11 years.
2. Initial pubic hair growth: 8 to 14 years.
3. Growth spurt: 9 to 12 years, usually peak at 10 to 11.5 years, cease at 16 to 17 years.
4. Menarche: 9 to 15 years, average 11 to 12 years.
5. Change in vaginal secretions, increase acidity or lower pH.
6. Widening of hips, pelvis wider than shoulders: 9 to 10 years.
7. Completion of growth of pubic and underarm hair: 2 years after appearance of pubic hair.
8. Final breast development: 18 years.
9. Increased output of oil and sweat-producing glands: about same time as appearance of underarm hair.

Males evidence:

1. Growth of testes and increased sensitivity to pressure, growth of scrotal sac and change in color and skin texture: 10 to 13.5 years.
2. Initial pubic hair growth: 12 to 16 years.
3. Growth spurt: 10.5 to 16 years, peak at about 12 to 13.5 years, usually cease about 21 years.
4. Growth of penis, prostate gland, seminal vesicles: 11 to 14.5 years.
5. Deepening voice, temporary enlargement of breasts, complexion changes: about same time as penis growth.
6. First ejaculation of seminal fluid: about one year after beginning of penis growth.
7. Nocturnal emission.
8. Facial and underarm hair: about 1 to 2 years after appearance of pubic hair.
9. Increased output of oil and sweat-producing glands, change in body odor: about same time as appearance of underarm hair.

Menarche, *the first menstrual period, is the indicator of puberty and sexual maturity in the female.* Ovulation usually occurs 12 to 24 months after menarche. The onset of menarche varies among population groups and countries and is influenced by heredity, nutrition, percent of body fat, health care, and other environmental factors (73). The onset of puberty correlates with weight in both genders; it is more obvious in females. Stocky or overweight individuals experience puberty earlier than do those with thinner, taller build. Menarche does not usually occur until a female weighs about 100 pounds (45 to 48 kg). Females who are severely malnourished or who are serious athletes have little body fat menstruate later than the average female (73). In many nations, puberty begins earlier than in the past because of better nutrition (16). Secondary sex characteristics in the female begin to develop in prepuberty, as described in Chapter 12, ∞ and may take 2 to 8 years for completion (73).

Spermatogenesis (*sperm production*) and *seminal emissions mark puberty and sexual maturity in the male.* The first ejaculate of seminal fluid occurs approximately 1 year after the penis has begun its adolescent growth, and **nocturnal emissions,** *loss of seminal fluid during sleep,* occur at approximately age 14 (73). Production of viable sperm follows the first ejaculation. Secondary sex characteristics in the male begin in prepuberty, as described in Chapter 12, ∞ and may take 2 to 5 years for completion. Changes in body shape, growth of body hair, muscle development, changes in voice and complexion, and stronger body odor may continue to develop until 19 or 20 or even until the late 20s. North American males usually complete growth in stature by 18 or 19 years, with an additional 0.5 to 1 in. (1 to 2 cm) in height occurring during the 20s because of continued vertebral column growth (62, 73, 140).

Sex hormones are *biochemical agents that primarily influence the structure and function of the sex organs and appearance of specific sexual characteristics.* **Androgens** are *hormones that produce male-type physical characteristics and behaviors.* The main androgen is testosterone. Testosterone stimulates descent of the testes and development of sexual characteristics, such as male distribution of hair and the deeper voice due to larynx hypertrophy. Testosterone causes a thicker skin texture, increases musculature and bone thickness, and unites the epiphyses of the long bones. In both males and females, androgens promote growth of pubic, axillary, facial, and body hair. Androgens are also associated with acne, body odor, voice deepening, height, and increased red blood cell production (65, 73). **Estrogens** are *hormones that produce feminine characteristics.* Estrogen stimulates growth by increasing total body protein and the subcutaneous adipose deposits. It is responsible for female hair distribution, soft skin texture, and retention of sodium, water, calcium, and phosphates. **Progesterone** is a *female hormone that promotes development of breast alveoli and breast development during pregnancy, inhibits ovulation during pregnancy, and enhances sodium, chloride, and water reabsorption to prepare the uterus to accept a fetus and maintain the pregnancy.* All three sex hormones are in both genders. Androgens are in greater amounts in males; the other two hormones are in greater amounts in females (65, 73). More information about the function of sex hormones can be obtained in any physiology text.

The **menstrual or reproductive cycle** (usually 28 days), *is controlled by an intricate feedback system involving* (65, 73, 140): (a) the hypothalamus, which audits the level of the hormones in the bloodstream; (b) the anterior lobe of the pituitary and its hormones, follicle stimulating hormone (FSH) and luteinizing hormone (LH); (c) the ovaries and their hormones, estrogen and progesterone; and (d) the interplay between the ovarian hormones and FSH and LH.

In *early puberty,* FSH stimulates the female's ovaries to begin producing estrogen. By *midpuberty,* a larger estrogen production causes formation of the endometrial lining of the uterus. *Menarche* begins. As puberty progresses, an ovarian follicle becomes dominant each menstrual cycle, producing a larger amount of estrogen during the *follicular phase* (65, 73, 155). The hypothalamus stimulates the pituitary gland to release FSH, which causes maturation of one of the ovum-containing ovarian or Graafian follicles and increased production of estrogen (65, 73, 140).

In response to the high level of estrogen, the anterior pituitary releases LH. The sudden increase in LH triggers **ovulation**, *release of the mature ovum,* from the follicle, which happens approximately 14 days after the onset of the cycle. The LH moves to the ruptured follicle, which causes development of the glandular corpus luteum. This produces both estrogen and progesterone, which,

when acting together, cause the glands of the endometrium to form the endometrial lining of the uterus and prepare further for the nourishment of a possible zygote (65, 73, 140).

If fertilization of the ovum by a sperm cell does not occur, the ovum deteriorates. The pituitary stops production of both FSH and LH, and the corpus luteum becomes dormant and atrophies. The resulting drop in estrogen and progesterone levels stimulates shedding of the endometrial lining, which consists of blood, mucus, and tissues, or the menstrual discharge. Menstruation lasts 3 to 5 days. The cycle then begins anew. As serum estrogen and progesterone decrease, the feedback mechanism arises that involves the pituitary gland to produce more FSH. A new menstrual cycle begins (65, 73).

Primary dysmenorrhea, *painful menstruation occurring without any evidence of abnormality in the pelvic organs,* may occur. The cause is unknown, but endocrine factors, natural pain processes, and psychological factors have all been considered. Various analgesics have been used for this condition through the years. More recently the nonsteroidal anti-inflammatory agents have been used with some success. Some females find that adherence to a certain diet, such as one with decreased caffeine and sugar and increased protein intake, and exercise habits may decrease symptoms. Heat to the painful area may be palliative (65).

In the **male hormonal and reproductive system** *no cyclic pattern occurs.* The **male gonads**, *the testes, produce sperm continuously and secrete androgens.* The major androgen is testosterone (73). Just as FSH promotes the development of the ovum in the female, FSH acts on testicular cells, which stimulates sperm production. FSH and LH are responsible for acting on a different group of testicular cells to produce sperm. A continuous level of sperm production takes place in the seminiferous tubules inside the testes. The secretion of LH (also called interstitial cell-stimulating hormone [ISCH]) stimulates the Leydig cells lying between these tubules to secrete androgen (65).

Neurologic System

Beginning at puberty, the *brain is reshaped* (62, 117). Neurons, the gray matter, and synapses, the junctions between neurons, proliferate in the cerebral cortex and then are gradually pruned in adolescence. Cerebral white matter volume increases through ages 4 to 21 years, and there is increasing density, organization, and integrity of white matter pathways through the teen years (117). Meanwhile, the *myelin coat,* or white matter, on the axons that carry signals between nerve cells continues to accumulate, which improves the precision and efficiency of neuronal communication. This process is completed in the early 20s; thus, a greater capacity for more complex physical and cognitive skills is possible. The *corpus callosum,* which connects the right and left brain hemispheres, consists mostly of this white matter and continues to mature (65). The *parietal and temporal lobes,* which are important in spatial and language skills, continue to develop through puberty (16, 65, 173).

Also under construction is a circuit that links the prefrontal cortex to the *midbrain reward system* where romantic love and addictive drugs exert their powers (65). There is evidence that adolescent and adult brains react differently to drugs; most addictions begin in adolescence (73). Teens and adults process reward stimuli differently; teens are hypersensitive to novel experiences (16, 140, 155, 173).

Adrenal stress hormones, sex hormones, and the growth hormone also influence brain development. Sex hormones act on the limbic system and the raphe nucleus, a source of serotonin, a neurotransmitter that regulates mood and arousal. Stress retards hippocampus growth, which consolidates memory (173).

Biological rhythms also differ from those of the adult. The 24-hour circadian rhythms get reset in adolescence. The timing of melatonin secretion takes place later at night. The day-night cycle almost reverses. The teen stays awake late in the night and has difficulty with early morning awakening (173).

The *reaction time* shortens each year until about age 16, then stabilizes. A gradual slowing begins at about age 20 and continues into old age (65, 140, 173).

Musculoskeletal System

Structural changes—growth in skeletal size (45% is added), muscle mass, adipose tissue, and skin—are significant in adolescence. The skeletal system grows faster than the supporting muscles; hands and feet grow out of proportion to the body, and large muscles develop faster than small muscles. Poor posture, disrupted balance, and decreased coordination result. Performance in motor tasks decreases during maximum or rapid growth stages because of the inability of the neurologic system to rapidly adapt during the growth spurt. Males demonstrate more difficulty with balance and coordination than females in early adolescence. Male performance in motor skills improves through adolescence.

Males and females differ in skeletal growth patterns. Females have less bone growth than males (36). Males have greater length in arms and legs relative to trunk size, in part because of a prolonged prepubertal growth period in boys. Males have a greater shoulder width, a difference that begins in prepuberty. Thus, males have greater leverage and rotational torque for throwing and striking tasks. Ossification of the skeletal system occurs later for males than females. In females, estrogen influences ossification and early unity of epiphyses with shafts of the long bones, resulting in shorter stature (40).

Muscle growth continues in males during late adolescence because of androgen production. Muscle growth in females is proportionate to growth of other tissue. Differences in muscle movement and walking patterns are more a function of social and cultural factors than gender differences, physically (46). Adipose tissue distribution over thighs, buttocks, and breasts occurs predominantly in females and is related to estrogen production (36, 62, 140). Males have less body adipose tissue and proportionately more muscle. Thus, oxygen transportation is more efficient in males (40).

Skin

Skin texture becomes coarser. Sebaceous glands become extremely active and increase in size. Eccrine sweat glands are fully developed, are especially responsive to emotional stimuli, and are more active in males. Apocrine sweat glands also begin to secrete in response to emotional stimuli (140). Because facial glands are more active, **acne** (*pimples*) emerges, especially in males, related to testosterone level.

Cardiovascular System

The *heart* grows slowly at first compared with the rest of the body, resulting in inadequate oxygenation and fatigue. The heart continues to enlarge and blood volume to increase until age 17 or 18. Systolic *blood pressure* and *pulse pressure* increase; blood pressure averages 100 to 120/50 to 70. *Pulse rate* averages 60 to 68 beats per minute. Females have a slightly higher pulse rate and basal body temperature and lower systolic pressure than males (16, 73, 140).

Hypertension is increasing in adolescents, both Caucasian and African American, in males, in obese persons, and in those with a family history of hypertension. Higher systolic pressure occurs in urban dwellers; higher diastolic pressure has been seen in those who smoke and lack regular exercise (73). Higher systolic and diastolic blood pressure is associated with stressed or negative mood states, such as feeling anger, anxiety, work stress, rushed, or depressed, and in association with lack of exercise (108). Cardiac control, mediated by the autonomic nervous system, buffers blood pressure fluctuations, especially in response to challenge or stress. Lower systolic and diastolic blood pressure is associated with a relaxed, happy, or bored mood or a sense of engagement or accomplishment, especially in females. These findings are the same as in adulthood (108).

Routine hypertension screening should be done. The upper limit for normal blood pressure in individuals from 11 to 17 years old is 130/90 (73, 140). Because puberty may bring a transition in selective frequency of specific moods, referral to a counselor may be effective in stabilizing moods. Psychosocial intervention, including cognitive behavioral therapy and stress management, is recommended as a part of therapy for hypertension.

Respiratory System

The respiratory system also grows slowly relative to the rest of the body, contributing to inadequate oxygenation. Respiratory rate averages 16 to 18 per minute. Males have a greater shoulder width and chest size, resulting in greater respiratory volume, greater vital capacity, and increased respiration. The male's lung capacity matures later than that of the female, which is mature at 17 or 18 years (73, 148).

Respiratory system changes, and the relative slowness to mature, have implications for the teen who participates in competitive sports. Parents and coaches should be aware that the teen may not be able to meet expectations for physical skill and muscular performance.

Blood Components

Red blood cell mass and hemoglobin concentration increase in both genders because of increased hormone production. Hematocrit levels are higher in males, platelet count and sedimentation rate are increased in females, and white blood cell count is decreased in both genders. Blood volume increases more rapidly in males. By late adolescence, males average 5,000 ml and females 4,200 ml of blood (73, 148).

Monitoring for signs of anemia and susceptibility to infection is important. Educate about healthful habits to reduce these risks.

Gastrointestinal System

The gastrointestinal system matures rapidly from 10 to 20 years. By age 21 all 32 *teeth* have usually appeared. The third molars may not erupt until later; extraction may be necessary. If the person resides in an area with inadequate fluoride supply (less than 0.6 ppm), fluoride supplementation may be necessary to prevent dental cavities. Toothpaste with added fluoride should be used unless there is high fluoride content in the water supply. Dental health is maintained with visits to a dental care provider every 6 months, daily flossing, and brushing at least twice daily. *Stomach capacity* increases to approximately 1 quart (more than 900 ml), up to 1,500 ml, which correlates with increased appetite as the stomach becomes longer and less tubular. Increased gastric acidity occurs to facilitate digestion of the increased food intake. *Intestines* grow in length and circumference. Muscles in the stomach and intestinal wall become thicker and stronger. Elimination patterns are well established and are related to food and fluid intake. The *liver* attains adult size, location, and function (73, 148).

Fluid and electrolyte balance changes reflect changes in body composition in terms of bones, muscle, and adipose tissue. Percentage of body water decreases, reaching adult levels (40% cellular and 20% extracellular) at puberty (112). Approximately 60% of the male's total body weight is fluid, compared with 50% in the female. The difference is caused by the greater percentage of muscle mass in the male. Electrolyte composition approaches adult norms. Exchangeable sodium and chloride decline; intracellular fluid and body potassium levels rise with the onset of puberty. Because of their greater muscle mass, males have a 15% higher potassium concentration (112).

Urinary System

Urinary bladder capacity increases. The adolescent voids up to 1,500 ml daily. Renal function is like that of the adult (49, 73).

Educate about the need for adequate fluid intake, especially water, especially related to activity level and environmental conditions. Explore with the teen what fluids are regularly consumed in order to encourage healthful liquids.

Special Sense Organs

The eyeball lengthens, increasing the incidence of myopia in early adolescence. Depth perception and tracking are improved. Auditory acuity peaks at 13, and from that age on, hearing acuity gradually decreases. Sensitivity to odors develops at puberty. The female's increased sensitivity to musklike fragrances may be related to estrogen levels (49, 73).

Unique Differences

Racial differences in physical development exist, although adult statures are approximately the same. For example, African American males and females attain a greater proportion of their adult stature earlier. Skeletal mass is greater in the African American person; using Caucasian norms means that bone loss could go undetected. The normal value for hemoglobin concentration is 1 g less for African Americans. Thus, a lower hemoglobin reading for African Americans has a different nutritional implication; the person may not be iron deficient (5, 58, 73).

PHYSICAL ASSESSMENT OF THE ADOLESCENT

Regular physical examinations should be encouraged. The examination is conducted much as for the adult. However, it is crucial that the examiner knows and understands the special emotional needs, developmental changes, age and maturation level of the person, and physiologic differences specific to adolescence. Adolescents often have intense feelings, may perceive health care workers in extreme terms, and have trouble trusting adults. If the teen feels misunderstood, he or she may withdraw or become hostile. A straightforward and listening approach is useful to establish rapport. Neutral phrasing, voice tone, and body language is effective to elicit the adolescent's participation (49). The adolescent, and parents if present, should have an opportunity to talk privately with you, as well as in a shared session, if appropriate. The Home, Education, Employment, Activities, Drugs, Sexuality, Suicide/Depression (HEADSS) assessment tool is an objective, routine way to assess the person and begin discussion (140). (Review therapeutic communication principles in Chapter 2.) ∞

Honest and genuine interest in the adolescent and not "speaking down" as though the young person is a child are essential. Confidentiality and trust are key issues. Be sure to express honestly to the teen what part of the interview and examination can be kept in strict confidence and what may need to be shared. Specific age of the person and the nature of the findings determine these factors. Above all, do not say, "This is completely confidential," only to say later, "I believe we better share that."

Physical complaints and emotional symptoms may relate to underlying problems of drug abuse, alcoholism, sexual uncertainties and stress, date rape, pregnancy or fear of pregnancy, fear of or actual sexually transmitted disease, depression, family or peer adjustment problems, school problems, or concerns about future plans.

Because the adolescent may be extremely shy about his or her body, every effort must be made to protect privacy within the confines of the situation. With the advent of the female nurse practitioner and physician's assistant conducting examinations on male patients, the traditional "embarrassment roles" are switched. Much has been written on the conduct of the male examiner with the female patient but not on the reverse. The younger the adolescent male in terms of sexuality development, the more concern he has about a female examiner seeing and touching his body parts that are considered private. The female examiner must provide proper draping and touch as little as possible. She may make the preliminary statement, "It is important that I palpate your scrotum to detect. . . . I know this is a tender area and I will proceed as quickly as possible while being thorough in my exam."

The blood pressure should be at adult levels. The athlete may have a slower pulse rate than peers. Pallor, especially in girls, is a clue to check hemoglobin levels (49).

The teen needs frequent dental visits because most have caries. Many young adolescents whose parents have insurance for the service or have sufficient funds have orthodontic work in progress.

Because myopia seems to increase during these years, increased reading, studying, and viewing computer screens encourage eye strain.

Although breast neoplasms are not common to this age group, females should be taught breast self-examination and that some asymmetric development may occur. Some increase in breast tissue can also be expected in adolescent males. Excessive growth should be referred for evaluation. Both male and female breasts should be examined. The male should be taught testicular self-examination.

The heart is located at the fifth left intercostal space as in the adult; most functional murmurs should be outgrown. Obtain serum cholesterol and triglyceride levels if there is a family history of cardiovascular disease (49). Discuss preventive dietary and exercise regimens.

Striae may be found on the abdomen of females because of the rapid weight gain and loss experienced by fad diets followed by a return to overeating.

Be acutely aware not only of the pattern of sexual development of both males and females, but of the concerns and questions that may be voiced. The presence of the testes in the scrotum is of primary importance because undescended testicles at this age can mean sterility.

Papanicolaou (Pap) smears and pelvic examinations are done when the adolescent becomes sexually active. These procedures, done the first time with explanation and as much gentleness as possible, can set a positive tone for future examinations (49, 114).

Some have suggested that urine cultures be taken periodically on females between the ages of 15 and 18 because of the number of asymptomatic urinary infections.

Scoliosis is common in teenagers, so a close look for asymmetry of the musculoskeletal system is essential. Any severe, persistent pain in the long bone area should also be referred.

Nutritional Needs

RECOMMENDATIONS FOR ADOLESCENTS

During this time of accelerated physical and emotional development the body's metabolic rate increases; accordingly, nutritional needs increase. Requirements peak in the year of maximum growth, between 10 and 12 years in females and approximately 2 years later in males. *Calorie* and *protein* requirements during this year are higher than at almost any other time of life. The adolescent female's requirements are equaled or surpassed only during pregnancy and lactation. An inactive 15-year-old female may need fewer than 2,000 calories daily to avoid weight gain (36, 38). An active 15-year-old male may need 4,000 calories daily to maintain weight. Even after the obvious period of accelerated growth has ended, nutritional intake must be adequate for muscle development and bone mineralization, which continue (36, 38). The adolescent's nutritional status encompasses the life span; it begins with the nutritional experience of childhood and determines the nutritional potential of adulthood.

Both males and females have an increased appetite; they are constantly hungry. A fast-growing male may never feel full. His stomach capacity may be too small to accommodate the amount of food required to meet growth needs unless he eats at frequent intervals. Adolescent females between 11 and 14 years of age may need 2,200 kcal per day. Males of the same age need 2,500 to 2,700 kcal. Females between 15 and 18 years of age need 2,400 kcal and males need 2,800 to 3,000 kcal (36, 38). However, stage of sexual maturation, rate of physical growth, and amount of physical and social activity should be considered before determining exact caloric needs. In addition, the nutritional needs differ for the pregnant and nonpregnant adolescent.

Protein helps to maintain a positive nitrogen balance within the body during the metabolic process (36). Protein needs increase. Approximately 15% to 30% of the total caloric intake daily (34 g for 9- to 13-year-olds, to 46 g for females and 52 to 56 g for males) should be derived from protein consumed in adequate quantities. Protein may be obtained from milk, cheese, eggs, meat, legumes, nuts, and whole grains. Today's teens often emphasize vegetarian diets rather than meat as a protein source.

Fats should be limited to 30% or less of total calories. Adolescents consume high-fat diets. Saturated fat intake should be less than 10% of total calories. Dietary cholesterol intake should be less than 300 mg daily (193).

Fiber from fruits, vegetables, whole-grain bread and cereals, and psyllium is necessary. Youth need more fiber as they grow to meet changing needs and reduce risk for cardiovascular disease and constipation.

Calcium and phosphorus are needed for bone growth and continued teeth formation. Calcium intake should be increased to 1,300 mg daily. If the adolescent drinks a quart of milk daily, this dietary requirement can be easily met (36).

Phosphorus intake should be increased to 1,250 mg daily (42). Calcium intake tends to decline because of substitution of soft drinks for milk. The phosphoric acid in soft drinks works against calcification and may lead to bone resorption (36).

Iron needs increase because of expanding blood volume, increased hemoglobin concentration, and muscle mass growth. Iron daily requirements for females almost double between the 9- to 13-year-old age group (8 mg) and the 14- to 18-year-old age group (15 mg). In males, iron requirements decrease after the growth spurt (36). Females are more likely to develop iron deficiency because of poor eating habits or fad dieting and menstrual losses (36, 148). Iron deficiency is prevalent in both genders and all races and socioeconomic levels. Females are especially susceptible to iron deficiency at menarche (36).

Vitamin requirements for males and females, unless the female is pregnant, generally decrease a small amount from requirements for the school-age child (36).

Snacking is part of the social pattern of teens. The real issue is what is eaten for snacks. High-calorie snacks replace nutrition-rich snacks and meals. Emotional snacking adds excess calories. Supersize portions, often with added fat and sugars, and excess soft drinks add calories.

Underweight and overweight are probably the two most common but overlooked symptoms of malnutrition. **Malnutrition** *refers to excess imbalance, or deficient nutrient availability in relation to tissue needs* (36, 38). **Protein energy malnutrition (PEM)** *refers to undernutrition and is usually diagnosed when the adolescent is below normal in weight and height.* Psychomotor and cognitive development are negatively affected (111). Assess the adolescent for physical, cognitive, and emotional indicators of poor nutritional status.

Abstract for Evidence-Based Practice

Use of Technology to Promote Healthy Eating

Long, J., & Stevens, K. (2004). Using technology to promote self-efficacy for healthy eating in adolescents. *Journal of Nursing Scholarship, 36*(2), 134–139.

KEYWORDS

Self-efficacy, nutrition education, technology, healthy eating, adolescent.

Purpose ➤ To compare the effectiveness of classroom and technology, using the World Wide Web (WWW) and educational interventions on self-efficacy and healthy eating patterns, and to examine the relationships of theoretical concepts in a hypothetical model of adolescent eating behaviors.

Conceptual Framework ➤ Social cognitive theory and theory on developmental characteristics of adolescents guided the research design.

Sample/Setting ➤ A random sample of 121 adolescents, 12 to 16 years old, from the 7th, 8th, and 9th grades in two schools, who did not have eating disorders or learning difficulties, volunteered to participate. The sample was comprised of Caucasian, African American, and Latino students; 52.1% were females and 47.9% were males. Approvals from the Institutional Review Board, parental consents, and adolescent assents were obtained prior to the study.

Methods ➤ The design was a pretest-posttest quasi-experimental study. Volunteers were assigned by the researcher to either a comparison or intervention group. The intervention students had computers with WWW access; the comparison students did not. The variables self-efficacy (SE), healthy eating (HE), usual food choices, dietary knowledge, and fruit, vegetable, and fat intake were measured at baseline and one month later in both groups. The questionnaires measuring eating habits were administered in the same sequence for the pre- and posttests to minimize socially acceptable or prearranged answers. The intervention consisted of 5 hours of WWW-based nutrition education through three modules using a gaming approach or 10 hours of classroom activity-oriented curriculum developed and tested by the American Cancer Society and the National Cancer Institute. The content was consistent with the WWW modules. Six instruments were used to measure study variables.

Findings ➤ Students in the intervention group had significantly higher scores for self-efficacy (SE) for healthy eating (HE), dietary knowledge, and healthier food choice than did those in the comparison group. There were no significant changes in eating behaviors in the intervention group. No significant difference was found between the groups in food intake.

Implications ➤ The use of dietary measurements sensitive to subtle changes in eating behavior is important for future research. The time needed for WWW intervention may need to be lengthened to create a change in eating behavior. A longitudinal design is suggested. The self-efficacy model is useful for future research. Adolescents need sufficient SE for HE to make healthy choices and change eating behavior. Innovative methods of delivering nutrition education might help adolescents to lead healthier, longer lives.

Intervention with undernourished youth must focus not only on providing nutritional food but also on the environment—parenting skills, socioeconomic status, and accessibility of nutritious food at school. Public education and advocacy are essential to correct environmental factors that contribute to poor nutrition.

Educate parents and teens about normal nutrition. Validate with parents the need to make time for family meals. If the teen has a heavy extracurricular schedule, *write the family meal dates and times on an easily seen calendar.* Discuss that family meals are linked to consuming more fruits and vegetables, and fewer soft drinks and foods high in fat and sugar. Suggest that parents involve the teen in nutrient-dense meal planning and preparation. Discuss options and portion sizes at fast-food restaurants. Emphasize that *parents are the main role model for a healthy lifestyle: eating habits, sensible portions, regular exercise patterns, not smoking, and no excess drinking.* Encourage parents to help the teen deal with peer pressure. Even when the teen disregards what the parents say, he or she is likely to hear their concerns about the teen growing normally,

looking and feeling good, and doing well in school and other interests (such as sports, dance, art, music, and drama). You may also use electronic media for nutrition education. The Abstract for Evidence-Based Practice describes research comparing effectiveness of classroom and electronic presentations about nutrition and eating habits to adolescents. For more information, refer to the MyPyramid Website to teach recommended nutrients for the adolescent (178).

THE VEGETARIAN EATING PATTERNS

The person who is a *vegetarian or vegan has to knowledgeably manage the diet.* Protein, calcium, vitamin B_{12}, vitamin D, calcium, iron, and zinc have to be monitored so that the recommended nutrients are eaten. The vegan has more challenges, especially with adequate vitamin B_{12} intake, because the best food sources for some nutrients are of animal origin. Vitamin D can be obtained with 20 to 30 minutes of sunlight twice weekly to the hands and face, not covered by sunscreen. If the person lives in a northern cli-

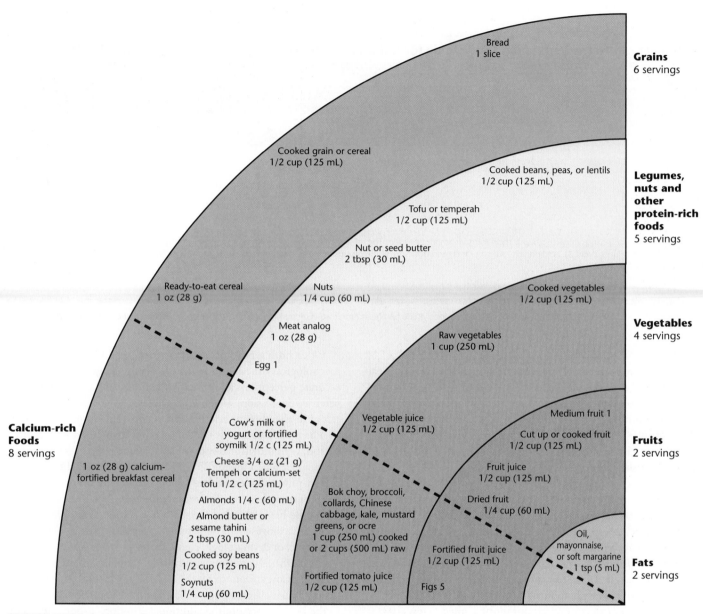

FIGURE ■ 13-1 Vegetarian food guide rainbow.

Source: Messina, V., Melina, V., & Mangels, R. (2003). A new food guide for North American vegetarians. *Journal of the American Dietetic Association, 103*(6), 771–775.

mate or has a darker skin, a vitamin D supplement is needed (36, 38, 87, 110). For a summary of information, refer to **Appendix A**, Major Sources and Functions of Primary Nutrients.

Refer to **Figure 13-1■**, The vegetarian food guide rainbow, for information on calcium and protein-rich foods, as well as other recommended foods and servings (110). Refer to **Table 13-1** for comparisons related to needs for vegetarian adolescents, pregnant women, and lactating women (110). Information from both the table and figure is relevant to health teaching.

If the teen is a *vegetarian*, help him or her make food choices that promote growth and health. Suggest to parents that the teen's choice may be a way of reflecting independence. The vegetarian eating pattern, when followed knowledgeably, can supply the needed nutrients and energy. A strict vegetarian diet with no animal foods may not. Explore, also, what "vegetarian" means to

the teen. It may mean "no meat," but no limits on soft drinks, cheese pizza, french fries, and ice cream. Such a diet has implications for not only malnutrition, but also later chronic illness. The teen needs this information, even if there is no immediate response. Explore also if "being a vegetarian" is a way to hide an eating disorder.

If the teen is a *vegan*, cover all of the above points. In addition, teach the teen about the importance of a vitamin B_{12} supplement (not seaweed, algae, spirulina, tempeh, or miso, in which the B_{12} is in an inactive form for humans). The label on the supplement should say "cyanocobalamine," the bioavailable form the human can use (36, 38, 110). Calcium sources, in addition to supplements, should be explored. Encourage the family and teen to choose a variety of foods. Teach about limiting saturated fat content if the person is eating a dairy-rich diet.

TABLE 13-1

Modifications to the Vegetarian Food Guide for Children, Adolescents, and Pregnant and Lactating Women

Life Cycle	Food Group[a]		
	B-12-Rich Foods (servings)	Beans/Nuts/Seeds/ Egg (servings)	Calcium-Rich Foods (servings)
Child[b]	2	5	6
Adolescent[c]	2	6	10
Adolescent[d]	3	5	10
Pregnancy	4	7	8
Lactation	4	8	8

[a]The number of servings in each group is the minimum amount needed. The minimum number of servings from other groups is not different from the vegetarian food guide (Figures 2 and 3). Additional foods can be chosen from any of the groups in the vegetarian food guide to meet energy needs.
[b]4 to 8 years.
[c]9 to 13 years.
[d]14 to 18 years.

Source: Messina, V., Melina, V., & Mangels, R. (2003). A new food guide for North American vegetarians. *Journal of the American Dietetic Association, 103*(6), 771–775.

UNDERWEIGHT

Weight loss may negatively affect adult height. Underweight can be caused by an inadequate intake of calories or poor use of the energy. The adolescent's preoccupation with weight and appearance triggers monitoring of food intake, dieting, and sometimes eating disorders (107). *Inadequate food intake is often accompanied by* (a) fatigue and irritability, (b) anorexia and digestive disturbances such as constipation or diarrhea, (c) poor muscular development evidenced by posture, and (d) hypochromic anemia. Growth and development may be delayed. Permanent arrest of growth and development and serious health problems, such as osteoporosis in the teen, may occur (73, 107). Even with the recommended dietary intakes, malabsorption of protein, fat, or carbohydrate can result in undernutrition. Underweight may be a symptom of an undiagnosed disease (73, 148). The most severe form of underweight is seen in individuals with anorexia nervosa and bulimia, which affects people from all cultural groups in the United States (107).

Anorexia nervosa is a *syndrome*, occurring usually in females between the ages of 12 and 18, although onset may occur in the 20s and 30s, *in which the person refuses to eat, presumably because of lack of hunger but related also to distorted body image and conflictual relationships. The person refuses to maintain body weight at or above 85% of what is expected for age and height.* Refer to **Box 13-3**, Signs and Symptoms of Anorexia Nervosa (2, 16, 36, 73, 107, 140, 148). Males (10% to 30%) also suffer from this disease but may be even more reticent than women to reveal symptoms or seek treatment (36, 73, 107, 140, 148).

Bulimia nervosa is a *syndrome characterized by recurring self-restriction of food intake followed by extreme overeating and self-induced purging, such as vomiting, laxative abuse, excess exercise, fasting, or diuretic abuse. These behaviors are associated with a sense of loss of control over eating during the episode, followed by recurrent, compensatory behaviors to prevent weight gain.* Refer to **Box 13-4**, Signs and Symptoms of Bulimia, to assist your assessment (36, 73, 107, 140, 148).

Often both syndromes exist together. Impaired physiologic and psychological functioning, disturbed body image, confused or inaccurate perceptions about body functions, and a sense of incompetence, depression, anger, and helplessness are present to some extent in all anorectic and bulimic clients (36, 38, 43, 73, 98).

The person usually is treated on an outpatient basis. Hospitalization, with nutritional support and intense psychotherapy, is recommended when loss of 25% or more of body weight leaves the person physically, emotionally, and socially compromised to the point of being in a life-threatening situation. The anorectic person should be hospitalized if there is a low serum electrolyte or fluid level or cardiovascular, hematologic, gastrointestinal, neurologic, endocrine, or dermatologic complications—all of which can be severe (73, 98). Depression with suicidal thoughts or attempts, substantial disorganization of the family, or failure of outpatient treatment are other reasons to hospitalize. These criteria also apply to the bulimic person; the additional criterion is spontaneous induced purging after binges. Hospitalization may also be helpful in diffusing parent-adolescent tensions and the resultant power struggle and in preventing suicide (73, 107, 140, 148).

The following Websites give information about eating disorders and treatment.

1. National Association of Anorexia Nervosa and Associated Disorders, www.anad.org
2. National Eating Disorders Association, www.edap.org
3. Remuda Ranch Programs for Eating Disorders, www. remudaranch.com

The intervention approach is holistic. *Treatment involves any of the following methods:* behavior modification, and insight-oriented, supportive, individual, group, and family therapy. *The teen should be warned against relying on Internet sites that give inaccurate or dangerous information, for example, "Pro-ana" and "Pro-mia" Websites. Such Websites treat eating disorders as a choice, not an illness.* Parents should be warned also.

BOX 13-3	Signs and Symptoms of Anorexia Nervosa

1. Refusal to eat or eating only small amounts yet feeling guilt about eating; excuses about not eating; inability to tolerate sight or smell of food
2. Denial of hunger (hunger becomes a battle of wills) but preoccupation with food (plays with food when eating; collects recipes)
3. Intense fear of becoming obese, even when underweight; refusal to maintain body weight; compulsive exercise and weighing
4. Large (at least 20% to 25%) weight loss with no physical illness evident
5. Abuse of laxatives or diuretics; frequent trips to bathroom, especially after meals
6. Distorted body image; perception of self as fat even when below normal weight
7. Vital sign changes: bradycardia, hypotension, hypothermia
8. Interruption of normal reproductive system processes in females: at least three consecutive menses missed when otherwise expected to occur
9. Malnutrition adversely affecting (1) the skeleton, causing decalcification, decreased bone mass, and osteoporosis; (2) muscular development; (3) cardiac and liver function, arrhythmia; and (4) body metabolic functions, which may decrease as a result of liver involvement
10. Skin dry, pale, yellow-tinged; presence of lanugo; hair loss
11. Enlargement of brain ventricles, with shrinkage of brain tissue surrounding them
12. Apathy, depression, irritability, low motivation, poor concentration
13. Regular use of loose-fitting clothing

BOX 13-4	Signs and Symptoms of Bulimia

1. Binge eating—consumption of excessively large amount of food—followed by self-induced vomiting or laxative and/or diuretic abuse (at least twice weekly); secretive eating; frequent trips to bathroom, especially after eating
2. Fear of inability to stop eating voluntarily
3. Feeling of lack of control over the eating behavior during eating binges
4. Preoccupation with food and guilt about eating
5. Weight fluctuations and fluid and electrolyte imbalances due to binges, fasts, and vomiting/laxatives
6. Use of crash diets to control weight
7. Weakness, headaches, fatigue, depression, dizziness
8. Orthostatic hypotension due to fluid depletion
9. Scars on dorsum of hand from induced vomiting
10. Loss of tooth enamel and esophageal and gastric bleeding in vomiters
11. Chest pain from esophageal reflux or spasm
12. Parotid gland enlargement in vomiters; swollen or infected salivary glands
13. Increased peristalsis, rectal bleeding, constipation if laxative abuser
14. Menstrual irregularities
15. Bursting blood vessels in eyes
16. Red knuckles from forced vomiting
17. More time alone or engaged in cooking

Teaching adolescents only about the dangers of eating disorders is ineffective. *More effective interventions include to increase the teen's resilience and enhance self-esteem and coping.* Explore the teen's feelings about self, underlying conflicts, and family dynamics. Convey caring with explanations of treatment measures and rationale. Do not focus on weight or food intake, although monitoring is necessary to prevent physiologic complications. Explore parental feelings and concerns; avoid being judgmental. Strengthen parental coping and reinforce their consistent caring behavior when it is not controlling of the teen. Reinforce the parents and teen working together to cope with problems underlying the illness and to pursue the necessary treatment, which can be long term. Emphasize to the teen and parents that some of the Internet sites on eating disorders give inaccurate information and should be avoided. Information should be obtained from their health care providers.

OVERWEIGHT AND OBESITY

Excess body weight is a national epidemic for all ages in the United States. Overweight is rarely the result of an endocrine, metabolic, or neurologic disturbance (36, 38, 39, 68). Genetic predisposition to obesity may exist, but genes do not change as quickly as the U.S. incidence has. *Often weight status is a result of lifelong food and activity habits.* Children grow up associating food with much more than nourishment for their bodies. Food means celebration, consolation, reward, or punishment. People give and receive food as symbols of their love. Food and drink are chief forms of entertainment (36, 38, 39). Portion sizes are larger. The misuse of food, accompanied by a decrease in physical activity levels, has led to a steady increase in the prevalence of obesity. Energy input is greater than energy output. One pound of body fat equals 3,500 calories; eating an extra 500 calories daily for 7 days will cause a 1-pound weight gain (36, 38). Research about causative factors continues (36, 38, 74). Cultures also vary in their attitude toward body size, weight, and obesity. The overweight person in some cultures has special status or is considered the ideal beauty (5, 58). In those cultures, even in the United States, education about losing weight is likely to go unheeded. *Education has to focus on what is to be gained by losing weight, not on what is being lost.*

Various theories are proposed regarding the deposition of fat in the body, including physical, emotional, and sociocultural. There are many environmental and societal contributing factors (36, 38, 65, 73). In some people, the body compensates for variations in caloric intake by adjusting the rate at which it burns calories during inactivity. The **set-point theory of weight control** *proposes that when weight falls below the innate body "ideal," metabolic rate*

INTERVENTIONS FOR HEALTH PROMOTION

Teach the teen the following strategies to help with weight loss:

1. Consciously ask self before eating, "Am I really hungry?"
2. Eat only at mealtimes and at the table; avoid snacks. To lose 1 pound weekly, dietary intake must be reduced by 500 calories daily.
3. Cut food into small pieces and eat slowly to eat less.

4. Keep a food diary, with the goal of reinforcing the adherence to the traditional food groups and avoiding empty calories.
5. Engage in planned, regular exercise such as bicycle riding, walking, calisthenics, or various sports.
6. Maintain proper posture and an overall attractive appearance.

---

is adjusted downward to conserve fat stores. When caloric intake increases, some people are able to burn the extra calories. Others do not, depending on the compensatory increase in nonexercise energy expenditure (36, 155).

Overweight is defined as *being up to 20% above ideal weight for age and height (body mass index or BMI between 25 and 29).* **Obesity** *is defined as being 20% or more above ideal weight or a BMI of 30 or above (16, 36). Body fat is in excess of age and gender standards (193).* Normal values of adipose tissue are 12% to 18% for males and 18% to 24% for females (36, 193).

Major health problems that can result are (a) coronary heart disease and hypertension; (b) certain cancers; (c) glucose metabolic abnormalities, insulin resistance, and type 2 diabetes; (d) osteoarthritis; (e) dyslipidemia and fatty liver; (f) pulmonary complications; and (g) reduced life span. Obese children and teens are at increased risk for becoming obese adults. *Emotional problems that can result are* (a) negative body image, (b) depression, (c) low self-esteem, (d) peer rejection and social isolation, and (e) conflicts with parents, siblings, and peers (73, 98, 148, 171, 185, 193). Just a 5% reduction in body weight will begin to decrease insulin resistance and lower blood pressure (98, 103).

Therapeutic management includes (a) diet modification, (b) exercise programs (60 to 90 minutes daily), (c) behavior modification programs to change lifestyle and eating habits, (d) medications, (e) individual or group support or counseling, (f) use of community resources such as Weight Watchers, and (g) surgical techniques. Medications must be carefully prescribed and monitored. Surgical treatment is a drastic option that needs careful exploration by the

parents and teen, as well as a multidisciplinary team (73). Nutritional counseling, behavior therapy, a group approach designed for the teen, and family involvement are effective (73).

Assess all dimensions of the teen and family. Compare the teen's weight and size to that of the parents. Assess food intake and activity habits and prior efforts at weight loss or control.

Teach the teen, and parents if available, about physiologic processes involved in obesity. Teach about lifestyle modification to promote health and gain the desired appearance. Motivational interviewing can direct discussion toward emotional and physical challenges. Give information about BMI. Explore the teen's and family's schedules. Overscheduled days may lead to fast-food meals, which are high in calories and often limited in nutrients. Explore physical activity interests; set up a routine. Even walking stairs instead of taking the elevator, or parking to allow for walking to the destination, can build in activity.

Encourage the teen and parents to join you in action at the policy level, such as expansion of school physical education programs and nutrition education, removal of "junk food" vending machines from schools, options for portion sizes in restaurants, and media regulation about marketing of calorie-dense food to children.

Reinforce the permanence of new food habits and achievement of weight loss through your continued guidance and realistic praise. The key to successful treatment may be in improving the adolescent's self-image. If emotional problems exist, counsel the adolescent or refer him or her to an appropriate source. Regardless of the methods of treatment used, parental understanding and co-

---

INTERVENTIONS FOR HEALTH PROMOTION

Teach families the following strategies to help the adolescent achieve weight loss:

1. Limit purchases and cooking and baking of carbohydrate foods or snacks.
2. Remove tempting snacks such as candy and cookies from the home.
3. Ban eating in front of the television or reading while eating.

4. Make dining at the table a pleasant time.
5. Avoid using food as reward or punishment.
6. Serve food in individual portions on the plate rather than in bowls on the table to avoid second helpings, and serve food on smaller plates.
7. Praise even a small weight loss; avoid nagging.
8. Participate in physical activity with the adolescent when possible.

operation are needed. You are a member of the health team with whom both parents and the adolescent can discuss their concerns. Your listening, discussing, teaching, and referral, when necessary, can help the adolescent prevent or overcome the health hazard of obesity.

In addition, work with the school system to establish daily physical exercise programs that stimulate the teen to remain physically active, give dietary instructions, check weight, and provide low-calorie refreshments. Explore community programs to foster ways to behavioral changes for health. Focus on preventing adolescent obesity through education of the teen and the parents and treating it when it occurs in order to eliminate future health problems.

ADOLESCENT PREGNANCY

Adolescent pregnancy, discussed later in the chapter, presents another health problem related to nutrition as well as to medical, physical, social, and emotional factors. Clearly, many teenagers lack the physiologic maturity needed to withstand the stresses of pregnancy. The adolescent's nutritional intake may be only barely sufficient to support her own development, not adequate to satisfy two nutritional requirements (36, 38). Risks depend on biological maturity, ethnic background, economic status, prenatal care, and lifestyle (36, 37, 73, 103, 155). Educate the female adolescent about the importance of healthful eating during the teen years, as the foundation is being laid for her health during adulthood and the prenatal period, if she chooses pregnancy, and for her baby's health. To begin eating healthful when she knows she is pregnant is insufficient for her or the baby's health.

Exercise, Play, and Rest

EXERCISE AND PLAY ACTIVITIES

Three types of play predominate in this age group: cooperative play, exemplified in games; team play, exemplified in sports; and construction play, exemplified in hobbies, crafts, or the arts. All of these types of play promote growth and brain development in the adolescent (62, 73). Rough-and-tumble play helps regulate and coordinate the frontal lobes of the brain and reduces attention deficit/hyperactivity disorder and learning disabilities (2, 16).

Benefits of exercise include to (36, 38, 140, 193):

1. Increase calorie expenditure, which can prevent or reduce weight gain and obesity, and promote and maintain weight loss.
2. Suppress the appetite.
3. Offset decline in basal metabolism created by dieting.
4. Reduce body fat and prevent loss of lean body mass during weight loss.
5. Produce positive effects on plasma insulin levels, blood pressure, and coronary efficiency.
6. Reduce risk of cardiovascular disease, cancer, and diabetes.
7. Foster a realistic body image and increase confidence.
8. Promote peer acceptance and social skills.

Good exercise patterns begun in childhood carry over into adulthood (36, 140).

Refer to the MyPyramid Website for information about physical activity related to nutritional needs, gender, and age. *Other sources of information on exercise are:*

1. Kids' Activity Pyramid by the Pennsylvania State College of Agricultural Sciences, Cooperative Extension, www.pubs.cas.psu.edu.
2. Activity Pyramid from Well Span Health, www.wellspan.org.

Outdoor play space that is welcoming and recreational areas in or near residential communities encourage participation in physical activity. Adolescent females who live closer to recreational centers are more likely to be active physically and participate in sports (103). Unfortunately, neighborhoods with low socioeconomic status face the barrier of reduced access to parks, trails, and recreational facilities compared to more affluent neighborhoods. Neighborhood design is integral to children and adolescent activity levels (88, 103).

Teenage males are concerned with activities that require physical abilities and demonstrate their manliness, such as practicing and participating in sport-related activities. Some males work on cars, machines, or electronic equipment. There is growing acceptance, however, of the male who wants to cook, garden, or do other activities that traditionally were not so popular or acceptable.

Some cultures still expect females to develop the traditional interests in social functions and domestic skills such as cooking, cleaning, and serving. In the United States, adolescent females are involved in a variety of physical activities and competitive sport teams. Those who try out for and succeed on "boys' teams" are challenging long-accepted ideas about feminine and masculine roles, strength and endurance of each gender, and competition. However, excess athletic participation may have negative health effects (4, 51). The **female athlete triad** is *a syndrome involving three interrelated conditions: disordered eating, menstrual irregularity, and low bone mass.* This syndrome has been observed in female Olympic elite athletes since the early 1990s. About 20% of high school females who participate in sports also manifest the condition. Disordered eating is often the first condition to appear, which increases risk of menstrual irregularity, and poor nutrition and low estrogen levels are risk factors for osteoporosis. Suboptimal bone growth during adolescence may not be fully reversible (4, 51).

Male adolescents are more likely than female adolescents to engage in vigorous physical activity. High levels of physical activity and fitness may reduce risk for cardiovascular disease, obesity, high blood pressure, and hyperlipidemia, as well as depression and emotional distress. A positive relationship exists between level of physical activity and fitness during adolescence (73).

Help parents and teens realize that competitive activities are one way to prepare young people to develop a process of self-appraisal that will last them throughout their lives. Learning to win and to lose can also be important in developing self-respect and concern for others. Physical activities provide a way for adolescents to enjoy the stimulation of conflict in a socially acceptable manner. Participation in sports training programs in junior and senior high schools can also help decrease the gap between biological and psychosocial maturation while providing exercise. Some form of physical activity should be encouraged to promote physical development. Being

MediaLink Physical Activity and Exercise

an observer on the sidelines or engaging in sedentary activities will not promote health.

Discuss with the adolescent the need for and types of physical exercise, as well as the frequency and intensity of his or her participation. Review positive physical, emotional, and social effects. Encourage the adolescent to engage in safe exercise daily on a regular basis (60 minutes a day is recommended), as a part of play, games, sports, work, transportation, and school physical education. Advocate for community and neighborhood environments that foster physical activity and areas and facilities for planned and spontaneous exercise. Also work with sports team coaches and parents to reduce team sports-related injuries through use of safety rules and proper equipment. Emphasize the grouping of players by size, developmental skill, and maturational level. Interests of the individual adolescent must always be considered. Some prefer the arts or music to sports; physical activity can be planned into the routine. Emphasize also the need for rest, quiet time, and sleep.

REST AND SLEEP

During adolescence bedtime becomes variable; the adolescent is busy with an active social life. The teen is expending large amounts of energy and functioning with an inadequate oxygen supply because the heart and lungs do not enlarge rapidly enough at the time of growth spurt. Both contribute to fatigue and need for additional rest. In addition, protein synthesis and growth hormone production occur more readily during sleep. Because of the growth spurt during adolescence, protein synthesis needs are increased (38, 65, 73). Increased rest also is needed to prevent illness. Lack of sleep in adolescents can contribute to depression and suicidal thoughts or attempts. Adolescents need at least 8 hours of sleep nightly for good mental health; 9 hours daily are needed by early adolescents (140). "Sleeping in" on weekends does not make up for sleep deprivation. The change in circadian rhythms and changing sleep cycle may also affect daily mood cycles. Teens tend to be least alert and most stressed early in the morning (140).

Educate parents about limit setting to ensure adequate opportunities for rest. Rest is not necessarily sleep. A period spent with some quiet activity is also beneficial. Every afternoon should not be filled with extracurricular activities or home responsibilities. When there is school the next morning, the adolescent should be in bed at a reasonable hour.

Psychosocial Concepts

Adolescence is a time of self-evaluation, decision making, commitment, and carving out a place in the world. It is a time of transition; physical changes affect the cognitive, social, and moral-spiritual development. The person is getting ready to be self-sufficient because of changes in intellect, attitudes, and interests and is moving to a stable sense of self. Parents sometimes underestimate the cognitive abilities of the adolescent.

Help parents work with the adolescent from an intellectual and creative perspective. Discuss with parents how they can learn from adolescents, just as adolescents learn from parents. Discuss with the adolescent how to use cognitive skills in a way that will not antagonize parents.

COGNITIVE DEVELOPMENT
Formal Operations Stage

Changes in cognitive functioning may first be evident in that *the person moves to more abstract thinking*, but returns to more concrete operations during stressful times (62, 70, 168). This is the **Formal Operations Stage**, according to Piaget's theory (144, 145). Tests of mental ability indicate that adolescence is the time when the mind has great ability to acquire and use knowledge. One of the adolescent's developmental tasks is to develop a workable philosophy of life, a task requiring time-consuming abstract and analytic thinking and **inductive** (*specific to general*) and **deductive** (*general to specific*) reasoning. Yet, according to media reports, some teens read at a fourth-grade level or are functionally illiterate.

The adolescent uses available information to combine ideas into concepts and concepts into constructs, develop theories and look for supporting facts, consider alternative solutions to problems, project thinking into the future, and try to categorize thoughts into usable forms. He or she is capable of highly imaginative thinking, which, if not stifled, can evolve into significant contributions in many fields—science, art, or music. The adolescent's theories at this point may be oversimplified and lack originality, but he or she is setting up the structure for adult thinking patterns. The adolescent can solve hypothetical, mental, and verbally complex problems; use scientific reasoning; deal with the past, present, and future; appreciate a wide range of meanings and complex issues; and understand causality and contrasting features. Formal operations differs from concrete operations in that a larger range of symbolic processes and imagination, along with memory and logic, are used (144, 145, 168, 180).

Cognitive development of youth or late adolescence proceeds through a complex transition of dualism such as a simple understanding of right and wrong and "either-or" of an issue to an awareness of multiplicity, a realization of relativism, and a more existential sense of truth. An aspect of this stage of cognitive development is to think about thinking: the ability to achieve a new level of consciousness, an awareness of consciousness, and a decrease in self-consciousness. Thus, the teen enjoys intellectual tricks, experiential games, and a higher level of creativity. This stage involves being very aware of inner processes, focusing on states of consciousness as something to control and alter, and thinking about the ideal self and society (16, 140, 144, 145, 155, 180).

Even though there are no overall differences between female and male adolescents' intelligence, females have shown greater verbal skills, whereas males have shown more facility with quantitative and spatial problems. These differences are apparently the result of interest, social expectations, training, and neurologic differences.

The School Experience

In the United States, the emphasis in education and the work world is on logical, analytical, critical, and convergent thinking. The goals of these linear thinking processes are precision, exactness, consistency, sequence, and correctness of response. The source of such thinking is the left hemisphere of the brain. Yet original concepts do not necessarily arise from logical thinking. Thinking that is creative or novel is marked by exploration, intentional ambiguity, problem solving, and originality. Creativity is a multivariate mental process that is divergent, intuitive, and holistic in nature; its source is the right hemisphere of the brain. It is an intellectual skill in which the person creates new ideas rather than imitating existing knowledge.

Creativity, problem-solving ability, and cognitive competence can be encouraged when the educational process requires the following (5, 140):

1. Opportunity to gain skills in all facets of sciences and technology.
2. Written assignments that necessitate original work, independent learning, self-initiation, and experimentation.
3. Reading assignments that emphasize questions of inquiry, synthesis, and evaluation rather than factual recall.
4. Questions that are divergent or ask for viewpoints.
5. Group work to encourage brainstorming or exposure to creative ideas of others.
6. Tests that include both divergent and convergent questions that engage the student in reflective, exploratory thought (questions should become increasingly complex in nature).
7. A creative atmosphere, whereby the learner is autonomous, self-reliant, internally controlled, and self-evaluated. The teacher provides a supportive atmosphere and recognizes creativity.

In addition, students cannot learn unless they are ensured of an environment that feels safe and supportive and that is as free as possible from the threats of bullies or the fear of system violence.

The adolescent does not always develop intellectual potential by staying in school. Students drop out of school for a variety of reasons, not just because of socioeconomic disadvantage (140). Dropping out has many negative consequences, including unemployment and legal problems. Providing special classrooms for the teen during pregnancy and after delivery so that she can bring the baby for day care while she attends class is one way to prevent school dropouts in that population.

A study of immigrant male and female adolescents from a number of countries, including Latino, Chinese, and Haitian immigrants, revealed differences in their school experiences in the United States (169). Adolescent males who came to the United States faced more debilitating prejudice. They faced more peer pressure to adopt the ways of the adolescent culture —the dress, slang, and disdain for education. They were disciplined more often in school and thus developed negative relationships with teachers. For example, Latino males were perceived as "macho" even before they were known as individuals; teachers perceived all of their behavior as aggressive. They carried these negative attitudes and experiences into the broader community. In contrast, immigrant females were perceived positively. Female peers wanted to "get to know them" and showed empathy. Teachers perceived females as "pure sweetness." Females were kept closer to home, having greater domestic responsibility, in contrast to the adolescent males who were more likely to spend their time at home playing computer games. Females were often the translators for the parent generation and mediated between parents and the outside world. Thus, females were thrust into a responsible role more often than males and lived up to the expectations (the self-fulfilling prophecy) (169, 170).

PEER GROUP INFLUENCES AND RELATIONSHIPS
Influences and Purposes

The **peer group**, or *friends of the same age*, influences the adolescent to a great extent. Because peer groups are so important, the adolescent has intense loyalty to them, more so than to parents, teachers, religious leaders, or other adults. Yet, the family's values, beliefs, lifestyles, socioeconomic level, and patterns of interaction, as well as other adults, influence peer selection and relationships. Refer to **Figure 13-2**.

Purposes of the peer group include promotion of (16, 62, 140, 155):

1. Opportunities for friendships, to counteract feelings of emptiness, isolation, and loneliness.
2. A sense of acceptance, prestige, belonging, and approval.
3. A sense of stability, based on the rules set by the group.
4. A sense of immediacy, concentrating on the here-and-now, what happened last night, and who is doing what today.
5. A reason for *being* today, a sense of *importance right now*, and not just dreams or fears about what he or she might become in some vague future time.
6. Role models and relationships to help define personal identity as he or she adapts to a changing body image, more mature relationships with others, and heightened sexual feelings.
7. Experiences to integrate accepted masculine or feminine behavior although adults may not recognize the distinctions.
8. Opportunities to try a variety of acceptable behaviors within the safety of the group.
9. Opportunities to learn behavior related to later adult roles.
10. Incorporation of new ideas into the body image and self-concept. The adolescent who is rejected by peers may be adversely affected, as he or she does not learn the high degree of social skill and ability to form relationships that are necessary for the adult culture.

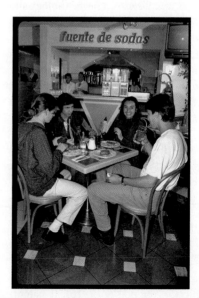

FIGURE ■ **13-2** Peer relations are strong during adolescence.

Relationship Changes

In *early adolescence*, peers are important to counter the instability felt from rapid growth changes. The person seeks close, idealized friendships with the same gender and group standards in a struggle for mastery within the peer group. Peer group activities are popular; there is beginning interest in the opposite gender, especially for females (62, 73, 140).

In *middle adolescence*, group allegiance is strong and manifested in choice of food, clothing, music, leisure activities, and other fads. Pressure to conform is greater during periods of uncertainty (16). Friends of the same ethnicity, for example, African American, Latino, or Asian, are more likely to maintain close contact, "to stick together" (140). Fear of rejection is so great the person follows the group, even against his or her better judgment (16, 73). The teen explores ways to attract attention of the opposite gender. Relationships become less superficial; for some, sexual experimentation begins now, if not earlier (62, 73). Females are more likely to describe romance in terms of interpersonal qualities, males in terms of physical attraction (155). The most common trigger for the first episode of depression is a romantic breakup (62, 73, 140, 155). The intensity and importance of friendships and time spent with friends are greater now than at any other life era (140).

In *late adolescence*, the peer group recedes in importance. The person maintains contact with a number of people of the same gender and with older individuals who have similar interests (155). Several individual friendships are formed and strengthened. Individual dating is more frequent; romantic relationships are considered in terms of a longer or permanent partnership. There is more giving and sharing, cooperation, compromise, and collaboration in a relationship (62, 140).

The *Internet* is often used to initiate and strengthen peer relationships. It provides a way to present a mask. Teens think they are untouchable; some deliberately engage people online whom they call "creeps" or "perverts." Pushing discussions into inappropriate areas and even setting up meetings are part of risk-taking behavior (17, 60, 148). In turn, the teen may experience harassment, by *phone, including cell phone,* or **cyberbullying,** *harassment via e-mail, text messages, and Websites.* The technology allows adolescents (and children) to engage in bullying not only at school but also at home, at all hours of the day and night (17, 60, 61, 150, 167).

Same-gender (gay, lesbian) relationships and couples may be slower to connect based on later awareness of sexual orientation or hesitancy to acknowledge orientation. There are variations, but acceptance in school, churches, teen organizations, and communities of same-gender relationships is increasingly evident (18, 25).

Cultural groups vary in the extent to which peer relationships are emphasized, related to (5, 16, 155): (a) age of initiation; (b) amount of time allowed away from home with peers; (c) contacts with same-gender and opposite-gender peers or mixed groups; (d) when dating begins, freedom allowed, and use of chaperones; and (e) formation of heterosexual couples with private intimacies. African Americans are likely to maintain close contact, to "stick together" in peer groups (140). Latino and Asian cultures are conservative in standards related to dating behavior, which can be a cause for generational conflicts in the family (5, 16). If parents are too strict, "sneak" dating may occur. The mainstream societal and media influences are difficult for parents to contradict (6, 16, 25, 155).

In schools and in teen organizations, there are females who are the "queen bees" and males who are "macho"—these teens are popular but often mean to peers and will not allow their omnipotence to be threatened. Some teens do whatever it takes to be recognized by the leader of the group. There are other youth who are studious, participate in school and church activities, volunteer in the community, work part-time, and pursue their own hobbies and interests. Today, in the United States, the adolescent has many choices. Parents are likely to attend their youth's activities, provide encouragement, and sincerely put effort into "raising good kids." Family activities may involve the parents and all the children, or it may be "dinner with Dad" or "lunch with Mom." Church attendance is another layer of protection; teens may participate in youth group discussions or work together on a Habitat for Humanity house-building project. The social life at school, church, or various social clubs or organizations allows "goof-off" time, being with reliable peers, having adult support, and decreasing the likelihood of substance abuse or other risky behaviors.

Peer group relations can also direct the adolescent into antisocial behavior because of pressure to conform and the teen's need to gain approval. The adolescent may participate in drug and alcohol abuse, sexual intercourse, or various delinquent acts not because he or she wants to or enjoys them, but rather to prove self, to vent aggression, or to gain superiority over younger or fringe members of the group. He or she may even gain pleasure from sadistic activities toward others.

Validate with parents that they have reason to be concerned about their adolescent's peers. It is their role to guide the teen into wholesome activities and groups that will reinforce the values they have taught. Help parents and teachers understand peer group relationships and work through crises related to peer relations. Reinforce with parents that if the teen is engaging in risk-taking behavior, parents must emphasize safety issues and how important it is that the teen stop and become involved in healthy behavior. Parents can also discuss with the teen information that was presented in Chapter 12 on the effects of media. ∞

Peer Group Dialect

Slang is one of the trademarks of adolescence and may be considered a **peer group dialect**. *It is a language that consists of coined terminology and of new or extended interpretations attached to traditional terms.*

Slang is used for various reasons:

1. To provide a sense of belonging to the peer group.
2. To use a small, compact vocabulary to avoid wasting energy on words.
3. To exclude authority figures and other outsiders.
4. To permit expression of hostility, anger, and rebellion.

Unknowing adults do not understand the insults given with well-timed pieces of slang. Other adults sense the flippancy of underlying feelings but to their chagrin can do little other than try to understand. By the time they learn the meanings of the current terms, new meanings have evolved.

Help parents understand the purposes of teenage dialect and the importance of not trying to imitate or retaliate verbally. In addition, encourage parents to enter into discussion with their teenager to understand more fully him or her and the teenage dialect.

Use of Leisure Time

Leisure time with both the family and peer group is important for normal social development and adjustment. The adolescent spends an increasing amount of time away from home, either in school, in other activities, or with peers, as he or she successfully achieves greater independence. School is a social center, even though abstract learning is a burden to some students. In school, students seek recognition from others and determine their status within the group, depending on success in scholastic, athletic, or other organizations and activities.

For some teenagers there is little leisure time. They may have considerable home responsibility, such as occurs in rural communities, or work to earn money to help support the family. Other youths are active in volunteer work. Ideally, the adolescent has some time free for personal pursuits, to stand around with friends, and to sit and daydream.

In the United States, the teen can pursue a variety of individual interests or group or community activities. Political activism draws some youth. "Everybody's doing it" is seemingly a strong influence on the adolescent's interests and activities, as are personal talents or interests.

Socioeconomic and educational levels determine to some extent how teens use free time. Upper-economic-level teens may travel extensively and attend cultural events or debutante parties. Middle-class teens emphasize participation in activities. During adolescence these teens are involved in church- or school-related functions, such as sports, theater, and musical events. Lower-economic-level teens may spend more time in unstructured ways, such as talking to peers, or finding ways to earn extra money. In many homes, however, the absence of money does not mean the absence of healthy leisure activity. Smoking and using alcohol and drugs cannot be attributed primarily to lower-economic-level teens, for a great deal of money is required to supply some of these habits. However, shoplifting or burglary may be done for "kicks" or to obtain money for desired items; the teen does not think ahead to the possibility or consequences of "getting caught."

Many parents consider a party in the home for a group of teenagers a safe use of leisure time. This is undoubtedly true if parents and other adults are on the premises and can give guidance as needed and if the parents are not themselves supplying the teens with alcohol and drugs. The latter sometimes happens; however, parents rationalize by saying that they prefer their youngster to be at home (or at a friend's home) if they are using alcohol and drugs. They may even drive home teens who are unsafe to drive. Drug and alcohol parties are also hosted by teens when parents are not in the home or are out of town. Teenagers chip in for beer for an "open" party (any number of people may attend). When behavior becomes boisterous, police are often called by the neighbors, but police find the situation difficult to handle if there is no responsible authority figure on the premises.

Police in various communities give guidelines to help parents and teens host and attend parties. Share suggestions from law enforcement agents with parents:

1. Set the ground rules *before* the party.
2. Notify parents of the guest teens who will attend, whether adults will be present, and address and phone number of the host.
3. Notify neighbors about the party, and if the host parents will be out of town.
4. Notify the police when planning a large party and plans for guest parking.
5. Plan to have plenty of food and a variety of beverages on hand.
6. Plan activities with the teen before the party so the party can end before guests become bored.
7. Limit party attendance and time (3 to 4 hours is suggested as sufficient party time). Discourage crashers; ask them to leave. Open-house parties are difficult for parents and teenagers to control.
8. Plan transportation home for each teen who attends.
9. Remain at home during the entire time of the party. The parent's presence helps keep the party running smoothly. It also gives the parent an opportunity to meet the teenager's friends. Invite other adults to help chaperone.
10. Decide what part of the house (not bedrooms) will be used for the party. Choose where guests will be most comfortable and the parent can maintain adequate supervision.
11. Do not offer alcohol or drugs to guests under the age of 21 or allow minors to use drugs in your home. In some states, parents face criminal charges or have to pay monetary damages in a civil lawsuit if they furnish alcohol or drugs to minors.
12. Do not allow a guest who leaves the party to return in order to discourage teenagers from leaving to drink or to use drugs elsewhere and then return to the party.
13. Ask guests who refuse to cooperate with parental expectations to leave. Notify the parents of any teenager who arrives at the party drunk or under the influence of any drug to ensure his or her safe transportation home. Do not let anyone drive under the influence of alcohol or drugs.
14. Notify parents and teens before the party that these guidelines are in effect at all parties. If, despite precautions, things get out of hand, do not hesitate to call the local police department for help.

Educate parents about state laws related to their responsibility in the home, such as endangering the welfare of a child under 17 years of age, failure to exercise reasonable diligence in the care or control of a minor, and unlawful transactions with a child if they knowingly permit a minor child to enter or remain in a place where illegal activities are conducted. Parents have responsibility (possibly in all states) if a minor is killed or injured after leaving their home in which an illegal substance was consumed.

The teenager may also feel more secure when the parent is actively interested in knowing where he or she will be, and what he or she will be doing even though rebellion may ensue. Parents should be awake or have the teen awaken them when arriving home from a party. This is a good sharing time. Peers are important, but if peer activity and values are in opposition to what has been learned as acceptable, the adolescent feels conflict. Parental limits can reduce feelings of conflict and give an excuse to avoid an activity in which he or she does not want to engage. Parental limits appropriate to the situation without undue constraints develop ego strength within the adolescent.

Explore with parents the adolescent's need for constructive use of leisure time and the importance of participation in peer activities. You may be involved in implementing constructive leisure activities. Reinforce to parents that they are role models for the youth in relation to use of leisure time.

Dating Patterns

Dating is one use of leisure time and is influenced greatly by the peer group but also varies according to the culture and social class and religious and family beliefs. Dating prepares the adolescent for intimate bonds with others, marriage, and family life. The adolescent learns social skills in dealing with the opposite gender.

Cyberdating, *dating over the Internet*, is popular, starting in early adolescence. By the time the teen can drive, dating has evolved into more traditional patterns (17, 27, 60, 155). Adolescents assume various dating patterns (25). Some begin early to date one person and continue that pattern until marriage. Some may date a number of people with no intent of moving into a serious relationship. Dating may begin with shared group activities, move to groups of couples, double dating, and finally single dating (25, 184).

Some teens prefer homosexual relationships; isolated homosexual encounters are not unusual (16). Because the person is usually a young adult when homosexuality is declared the preferred sexual pattern, the topic is discussed in greater detail in Chapter 14. ∞ However, the adolescent may have always felt more comfortable with or more cared for by the same-gender person (25).

As you work with adolescents, assess the stage of peer group development and dating patterns. *Build your teaching on current interests and attitudes.* Adolescents from another culture may sharply contrast in pattern with American adolescents. For example, in Egypt the male is not supposed to have any intimate physical contact with the female until marriage. In the United States, certain physical contact is expected.

Dating Violence

Dating violence, *a traumatic event that may include intimate partner rape, physical assault, and stalking*, is a major health care problem, involving extensive physical and psychological morbidity and great financial costs. Violence from a known person is more likely than from a stranger, and the consequences are devastating (1, 16, 44, 75, 150).

Adolescents, including those in early adolescence (ages 11 or 12 to 14 years), may be involved in serious sexual and dating relationships; there may be negative consequences. Sexual dating behaviors beginning in teen years for the female may be coerced. Acquaintance rape is more frequent than suspected. Pregnancy or sexually transmitted diseases may result from casual or romantic relationships. Adolescent relationships emulate the violence found in other segments of U.S. society. Sustained verbal

aggression and pushing and shoving may occur between dating partners.

Risk factors for dating violence include (1, 44, 75) (a) jealousy, (b) need for power or control, (c) disagreements about sex and sexual activity, (d) riding in a car with someone consuming alcohol or illegal drugs, (e) use of marijuana, alcohol, or injection of illegal drugs, (f) inhalant use, (g) frequent unwanted sexual experience, and (h) a number of sexual partners. Exposure to violence in one context, such as in the home or community, tends to have a crossover effect related to being a victim or a perpetrator in another situation, such as dating violence (1, 16, 44, 75).

The female who has experienced dating violence feels great emotional distress, including (a) distrust in potential dating partners, (b) a sense of distance or disengagement from relationships, (c) negative judgment of self, (d) disenfranchisement or being abandoned by previously supportive groups, and (e) disruption in life patterns. Some females may deny or disown the experience and its harmful effects (1, 75). The perpetrator may also feel negative about self and the behavior.

Prevention must be addressed before dating begins. Prevention programs sponsored by schools, churches, or social service agencies can address health, sexual education, maltreatment and abuse, and avoidance of drug and alcohol abuse. Various programs that have been instituted and policy issues are discussed by Ely (44).

Every female, during every health care visit, should be asked about experiences with violent behavior. Explore physical, emotional, sexual, and stalking violence and effects on personal feelings and behaviors. Discuss ways to reduce risks. Counseling and education are essential. Support the female's attempts at sublimation or channeling negative feelings into constructive outlets and efforts to try new coping strategies.

Refer the teen to the following toll-free hotlines:

1. National Domestic Violence Hotline: 800-799-SAFE or 800-787-3224 (TDD). Offers crisis intervention and exploration about relationships.
2. National Runaway Switchboard: 800-621-4000. Offers crisis intervention, message relay, conference calling to parents, and referrals to shelters and other services in the person's geographic area.
3. Rape, Abuse, and Incest National Network (RAINN): 800-656-HOPE. Provides counseling on how to help a survivor of sexual abuse or assault.
4. Child Help USA—National Child Abuse Hotline: 800-422-4453. Offers crisis intervention and referrals.

Sexual Harassment in School and with Peers

Sexual harassment has occurred in the schools and workplace for decades but has only recently been defined as an illegal activity. **Sexual harassment**, or *troubling behavior toward the self as a sexual object from another*, has been endured from peers and adults in school because children did not know what to call it or do about it. *Sexual harassment behavior has traditionally included* (16):

1. Uninvited touching from other students, teachers, or other adults at school.
2. Sexually provocative statements or sexual innuendos in conversation.

3. Rumors about sexual behavior of the person.
4. Rude, degrading, and wounding remarks toward a student who participates in classes not frequently enrolled in by others of the same gender.
5. Activities called teasing, horseplay, or flirting. These include blocking the passage; grabbing, touching, pinching, or brushing against the person; spying on another; forcing a kiss or any unwanted sexual behaviors; calling another names or words with a sexual connotation; commenting about body parts, clothing, or looks; or whistling, howling, or lip smacking.

Schools no longer dismiss these behaviors because sexual harassment is a form of discrimination. It undermines self-confidence and denies the victim full educational opportunities.

Sexual harassment exists on a continuum of unwanted behaviors ranging from spoken or written comments and stares, to electronic messages, to actual physical assault and attempted rape. Sexual harassment is defined by the victim. If the individual finds the comments or physical contact to be unwelcome, it is sexual harassment. The most common area of complaints has been harassment of students by other students, often on the school bus as well as on the school grounds. Children as young as 6 years of age can understand language and conduct that expresses hostility based on sex. Certainly education, emotional and social development, and health are compromised in the process.

Students of both genders report the same debilitating impact from either same- or opposite-gender harassment. The effect on girls appears more profound and longer lasting. *Effects of harassment include* (16): (a) not wanting to go to school; (b) talking less in class; (c) difficulty with attention; (d) feeling embarrassed; (e) having difficulty with sleeping, eating, and daily activities; (f) losing self-confidence, self-esteem, and trust in others; (g) changing behavior, classes, routes home, and friends; and (h) anxiety, depression, and suicidal thoughts or attempts.

Students consistently state that when they report harassment to adults, they often encounter disbelief, find themselves blamed for the behaviors, and suffer much agony because of the lack of responsiveness of teacher and administrators. The lack of support for the students and their parents is demoralizing. Unfortunately, students who have been harassed often turn around and harass others. The behavior spirals (16).

Teachers may harass students. There often appears to be a conspiracy of silence about student-teacher sex in high school reports of harassment. Any student's report should be listened to seriously and investigated. False allegations can be detected when interrogated students back down or there are inconsistencies in the reports. Females who are abused by male members of the family may report a male teacher because it is too scary to report the real abuser. Some districts suspend students who falsely accuse teachers. Accused teachers who have been found innocent report a sense of betrayal, self-doubt, stigma, and rejection by colleagues and the wider community, and may never again feel competent as teachers or acceptable as people. Yet, people who investigate these charges say that students are more likely to avoid reporting actual incidents than to fabricate incidents.

EMOTIONAL DEVELOPMENT
Emotional Characteristics

Emotional characteristics of the personality cannot be separated from family, physical, intellectual, and social development. Emotionally, the adolescent is characterized by mood swings and extremes of behavior, as summarized in **Table 13-2** (45–47). Coping with psychological problems can be done through internalizing or externalizing. **Internalizing** *refers to turning emotional problems inwardly, so that the individual harms the self.* Examples are eating disorders, self-mutilation, overuse of prescription (antidepressant or sedative) medications or use of illicit street drugs, clinical depression, and suicide. **Externalizing** *refers to manifesting emotional problems outwardly*, so that the acting out injures others, destroys property, or defies authority. Aggressive behavior, violent deaths, provoked homicides, or deliberate accidents may be an externalizing outgrowth of depression, an attempt to establish an identity. There are *gender differences:* internalizing is more common in girls; externalizing is more common in boys (16). Emotional development requires an interweaving and organization of opposing tendencies into a sense of unity and continuity. This process occurs during adolescence in a complex and truly

TABLE 13-2

Contrasting Emotional Responses of Adolescents

Independent Behaviors	Dependent Behaviors
Happy, easygoing, loving, gregarious, self-confident, sense of humor	Sad, irritable, angry, unloving, withdrawn, fearful, worried
Energetic, self-assertive, independent	Apathetic, passive, dependent
Questioning, critical or cynical of others	Strong allegiance to or idolization of others
Exhibitionistic or at ease with self	Excessively modest or self-conscious
Interested in logical or intellectual pursuits	Daydreaming, fantasizing
Cooperative, seeking responsibility, impatient to be involved or finish project	Rebellious, evading work, dawdling, ritualistic behavior, dropout from society
Suggestible to outside influences, including ideologies	Unaccepting of new ideas
Desirous for adult privileges	Apprehensive about adult responsibilities

impressive way to move the person toward psychological maturity (16, 168, 188).

Media and best-selling books in the United States do not adequately explain the U.S. adolescent. There are many variations, not just based on ethnic or racial lines. Some teens are apparently very popular—either well known by many peers or very selective with whom they associate. Some appear insecure and immature, having adjustment difficulties. Some are obviously emotionally healthy and socially secure with peers and adults at the school and in selected community or team sports activities. They are confident, accepting of themselves and others, and attractive but not necessarily fashionably beautiful or handsome. Youth demonstrate healthy behavior when they have supportive parental and other adult relationships, values bolstered by attendance at a house of worship, and participation in character-building activities, such as Boy or Girl Scouts, 4-H clubs, local sports teams, or other activities at the school. These youths still constitute the norm in the United States. Many can delay gratification, behave as adults, and have positive relationships with family and authority figures. These youth are a model for other teens.

Counsel parents to reinforce the positive characteristics and strengths of their teen. Parental mature behavior is a role model to help the teen stabilize emotional responses, achieve a sense of ego identity, and demonstrate an appropriate sense of independence.

Developmental Crisis: Identity Formation Versus Identity Diffusion

The psychosexual crisis of adolescence is identity formation versus identity diffusion: "Who am I?" "How do I feel?" "Where am I going?" "What meaning is there in life?" Identity means that an *individual believes he or she is a specific unique person;* he or she has emerged as an adult. **Identity formation** *results through synthesis of biopsychosocial characteristics from a number of sources: parents, friends, social class, ethnicity, religion, membership in other groups, and personal experiences* (45–47).

A number of influences can interfere with identity formation (45–47):

1. Telescoping of generations, with many adult privileges granted early so that the differences between adult and child are obscured and there is no ideal to which to aspire.
2. Contradictory American value system of individualism versus conformity in which both are highly valued and youth believe that adults advocate individualism but then conform.
3. Emphasis on sexual matters and other risk-taking behaviors, and encouragement to experiment without frank talking with parents.
4. Diminishing hold of Judeo-Christian traditions and ethics throughout society so that the adolescent sees that failure to live by the rules is not necessarily followed by unpleasant consequences.
5. Increasing emphasis on education for socioeconomic gain, which prolongs dependency on parents when the youth is physically mature.
6. Lack of specific sex-defined responsibilities. Blurring of the traditional male-female tasks has its positive and negative counterparts; although eventually allowing more individual freedom, it can be very confusing to the adolescent who must decide how to act as a male or female.
7. Rapid changes in the adolescent subculture and all of society, with emphasis on conforming to peers.
8. Diverse definitions of adulthood, for example, driving and voting age.

Identity formation implies an *internal stability, sameness, or continuity, which resists extreme change and preserves itself from oblivion in the face of stress or contradictions.* It implies emerging from this era with a sense of wholeness, knowing the self as a unique person, and feeling responsibility, loyalty, and commitment to a value system. *There are three types of identity, which are closely interwoven* (45–47): (a) **personal,** or **real identity**—*what the person believes self to be;* (b) **ideal identity**—*what he or she would like to be;* and (c) **claimed identity**—*what he or she wants others to think he or she is.*

Identity formation is enhanced by having support not only from parents but also from another adult who has a stable identity and who upholds sociocultural and moral standards of behavior (45). If the adolescent has successfully coped with the previous developmental crisis and feels comfortable with personal identity, he or she will be able to appreciate the parents and others on a fairly realistic basis, seeing and accepting both their strengths and shortcomings. The values, beliefs, and guidelines they have given are internalized. The adolescent needs parents less for direction and support. He or she must now decide what is acceptable and unacceptable behavior.

Students from different ethnic and racial backgrounds have unique needs and ways of adapting to stressors and unique aspects of the developmental crisis of identity formation. Some may feel isolated and alienated in relation to mainstream culture values (5, 58). Parents, schoolteachers, and health care professionals can help these teens work through values and cognitive and emotional conflicts.

Identity diffusion *results if the adolescent fails to achieve a sense of identity* (45, 47). The youth feels self-conscious and has doubts and confusion about self as a human being and his or her roles in life. With identity diffusion, he or she feels impotent, insecure, disillusioned, and alienated. Some researchers believe females enter puberty and adolescence feeling self-confidence and high self-esteem and, because of classroom and socialization processes, are more likely than males to enter their 20s feeling low self-esteem and insecure (97). Yet, females report less ego diffusion in all age groups than males (97). Erikson (45, 46) believes such feelings exist in both males and females until identity formation occurs.

Identity diffusion is manifested in other ways as well, as listed in **Box 13-5**, Negative Consequences of Identity Diffusion (45–47, 135). The real danger of identity diffusion looms when a youth finds a negative solution to the quest for identity. He or she gives up, feels defeated, and pursues antisocial behavior because "it's better to be bad than nobody at all." Aggressive or delinquent behavior may result; such behavior is a risk factor for a variety of social and health problems (22, 48, 53, 83, 116). Identity diffusion is more likely to occur if the teenager has close contact with an adult who is still confused about personal identity, who is in rebellion against society, and who is engaged in aggressive or violent behavior (45–47, 71, 135, 181).

BOX 13-5	Negative Consequences of Identity Diffusion

1. Feels he or she is losing grip on reality
2. Feels fragmented; lacks unity, consistency, or predictability with self
3. Feels impatient but is unable to initiate action
4. Gives up easily on a task; feels defeated
5. Vacillates in decision making; is unable to act on decisions
6. Is unable to delay gratification
7. Appears brazen or arrogant, sarcastic
8. Is disorganized and inconsistent in behavior; avoids tasks
9. Fears losing uniqueness in entering adulthood; displays regressive behavior; acts out behavioral extremes to attract attention
10. Has low self-esteem, negative self-concept, low aspirations
11. Is unable to pursue academic or career plans; may drop out of school
12. Isolates self from peers; is unable to relate to former friends or significant adults
13. Feels cynical, disillusioned, excessively angry or suspicious
14. Engages in antisocial or illegal behavior; acts out sexually
15. Seeks association with gang, cult, or negative community or media leader

The identity-seeking processes are even more diffused or abnormal if the child has encountered repeated stresses, such as abuse, neglect, or terror. Such experiences cause physical changes in the brain. The steady flood of stress chemicals keeps the person in a fight-or-flight pattern of behavior, as described under Stress and Adaptation Theory in Chapter 2, ∞ which results in the impulsive aggression that is seen in some teens (22, 48, 57, 90, 181). The outcast and bullied and the one who bullies have similar reactions at some point. Any stimulus can increase the level of stress hormones and reaction, because the nervous system is highly reactive to anything perceived as a stressor. If parents and other adults are not available, supportive, or empathic, the youth may decide to "take things" into his or her own hands (48). Sometimes the youth does not act out against others but instead harms self through risk-taking behaviors, such as substance abuse or self-harm in other ways, for example, cutting self (57, 71, 79).

Parents who are withdrawn, remote, neglectful, self-centered, or passive are at risk of shaping a child who shuts down emotionally, who feels no remorse for any violent plan or action. This lack of parental love and compassion impairs development of the brain cortex, which controls feelings of belonging and attachment. Such early life experiences result in an underdeveloped capacity to form relationships. Thus, cults or the pop culture may offer attention and inclusion, offsetting feelings of shame, humiliation, ostracism, inferiority, and diffusion. But in the process, the group (whether nearby persons or on the Internet) may create further diffusion, antisocial behaviors, and emotional and behavioral problems (48, 83).

In the process of achieving identity and committing to goals in life, the person may have experienced **identity moratorium**, a *time of making no decisions but a rethinking of values and goals*, a step beyond *identity diffusion*, when *the person has not begun to examine his or her own life's meaning and goals*. In some cultures, identity formation is not a task for the individual. Rather, **identity foreclosure** exists: *The goals, values, and life tasks have been established by the parents and the group, and the individual is not allowed to question or examine them but is expected to follow the pattern set by elders*. Usually roles are related to gender and socioeconomic or caste status (47).

Assist parents to work with the adolescent who feels and demonstrates identity diffusion. Emphasize that parents must never give up trying to form a loving bond with offspring, showing attention and empathy, and stimulating participation and emotional feelings in the teen, whether they are a nuclear, stepparent, or single-parent family (69, 106, 161). Refer parents to counseling services when needed to overcome the teen's neurologic and behavioral vulnerability, just as you would refer patients to an allergist for asthma.

Collaborate with other professionals to develop a program within the school system to counter aggressive behavior. School-based prevention programs aimed at reducing aggressive behavior in adolescents appear to produce behavioral improvement. For example, use of behavioral therapy principles, as described in Chapter 1, ∞ combined with positive role models, supportive groups, and education designed to improve relationship and social skills, are effective (116). *Individual and group education and counseling should focus on* (a) listening skills, (b) behavior that is a positive response to self and others, (c) understanding of personal behavior and how it affects other people's response, (d) how to work cooperatively with others, and (e) use of assertive rather than aggressive behavioral responses. These interventions can be initiated in mixed-gender or same-gender groups. Schoolwide activities can also be implemented that focus on youth and adults being considerate of others (116).

Your education and counseling of youth and families can incorporate these points of intervention whenever you have contact with any adolescent. A consistent approach is effective.

Self-Concept and Body Image Development

Development of self-concept and body image is closely akin to cognitive organization of experiences and identity formation. The adolescent cannot be viewed only in the context of the present; earlier experiences have an impact that continues to affect him or her. The earlier experiences that were helpful enabled the adolescent to feel good about the body and self. If the youngster enters adolescence feeling negative about self, the body, or appearance, this will be a difficult period. Self-esteem drops in females and rises in males as they move through adolescence (62). Parents and teachers need to support assertive, autonomous, outgoing, and nonconforming behavior in females, just as they support males.

Various factors influence the adolescent's self-concept, including (5, 16, 58, 60, 78, 133, 140, 155): (a) age of maturation, (b) degree of attractiveness, (c) name or nickname, (d) size and physique appropriate to sex, (e) degree of identification with the same-sex parent,

(f) level of aspiration and ability to reach ideals, (g) residence, (h) peer relationships, and (i) culture and family background.

The rapid growth of the adolescent period is an important factor in *body image* revision. *Physical changes in height, weight, and body build cause a change in self-perception and in how the adolescent uses the body.* Females and males are sometimes described as "all legs." They are often clumsy and awkward. Because the growth changes cannot be denied, the adolescent is forced to alter the mental picture of self to function. More important than the growth changes is the meaning given to them. The mother who says, "That's all right, Tom, we all have our clumsy moments," is providing understanding that a comment such as, "Can't you ever walk through the room without knocking something down?" denies. The adolescent needs understanding because he or she fears rejection and is oversensitive to the opinions of others. To some male adolescents, the last chance to get taller is very significant.

Most teenage females are not satisfied with the body or its appearance. The Caucasian female is likely to think she is "too fat," which can lead to nutritional deprivation or eating disorders (16, 36, 134). Some females engage in self-mutilation, for example, cutting (57, 134). The male is likely to perceive self as "too weak," which can be a factor in acting aggressive (compensation) or drug use (16).

The body is part of one's inner and outer world. Many of the experiences of the inner world are based on stimuli from the external world, especially from the body surface. Therefore the adolescent focuses attention on the body surface. He or she spends a great deal of time in front of mirrors and with body hygiene rituals, grooming, and clothing styles. These are normal ways for the early adolescent to integrate a changing body image. Growth and physical changes draw the adolescent's attention to the body part that is changing, and he or she becomes more sensitive about it. This can cause a distorted self-view.

Considerable time can be spent in training to build muscles. Adolescent males are especially aware of body size, strength, muscle mass, and function. The temptation to use anabolic-androgenic steroids has been great, perhaps due to the practices of some professional athletes who may serve as role models. Some males are influenced by pictures of the ideal male model with minimal body fat and developed lean muscles. Female athletes have also used performance-enhancing drugs, including growth hormone, amphetamines, or thyroid preparations (1, 43, 73, 140).

Anabolic-androgenic steroids are *medications available by prescription, chemically similar to male sex hormones, used to slow loss of muscle mass in wasting diseases* (e.g., AIDS). The term **anabolic** *refers to muscle-building properties;* **androgenic** *refers to the ability to increase male secondary sex characteristics* (131). Those who use steroids illegally take them at much higher doses than given by prescription and with the intent of improving body appearance and athletic performance and thereby the body image. Unlike other illicit drugs, their initial use is not prompted by seeking a "high." They are taken orally or injected, typically in cycles of weeks or months rather than continuously. This "cycling" of use promotes muscular development. Different types of steroids are combined (called "stacking") to maximize effectiveness and decrease side effects (131).

Steroids obtained through various means are initially taken related to body image issues. *Major physical side effects may occur, including* (131): (a) fluid retention, (b) trembling, (c) severe acne, (d) high blood pressure, (e) jaundice, (f) increases in low-density lipoprotein (LDL) and decreases in high-density lipoprotein (HDL) cholesterol, and (g) liver and kidney tumors and cancer. *Feminine characteristics may occur in males:* (a) shrinking of the testicles, (b) reduced sperm count, (c) infertility, and (d) breast development. Baldness and increased risk for prostate cancer also occur. *Masculine characteristics may occur in females:* (a) growth of facial hair, (b) male-pattern baldness, (c) menstrual cycle irregularities, and (d) deepened voice.

Psychological side effects may also occur. The **euphoria,** *heightened mood,* may progress to irritability, suspicion, hypersexuality, aggression, insomnia, and impaired judgment. When the steroids are stopped, depression may result, which contributes to dependence.

Adolescents who use steroids are prone to accelerated puberty changes and possible growth halt due to premature maturation of the joints and bones, which have negative effects on body image (73, 131). Since teens often share needles to administer the drugs, they risk contracting HIV or hepatitis through contamination. In addition, users may turn to other drugs, primarily opiates, to relieve the insomnia and irritability brought on by steroids.

By late adolescence, self-image is complete, self-esteem should be high, and self-concept should have stabilized. The person feels autonomous but no longer believes he or she is so unique that no one has ever experienced what he or she is currently experiencing. The older adolescent no longer believes everyone is watching or being critical of his or her physical or personality characteristics. Egocentricity has declined. Interactions with the opposite gender are more comfortable, although awareness of sexuality is keen.

Your understanding of the importance of the value the adolescent places on self can help you work with the adolescent, parents, teachers, and community leaders. Your goal is to avoid building a false self-image in the adolescent. Rather, help him or her evaluate strengths and limits, accept the limits, and build on the strengths. Listen and respond carefully to the adolescent's statements about self and the sense of future. You will have to sense when you might effectively speak and counsel, and when silence is best. Share an understanding of influencing factors on body image and self-concept development with parents, teachers, and other adults so that they can positively influence adolescents.

You may implement a therapeutic group to help adolescents think more positively about themselves and reduce anxiety. Small group sessions outside the regular classroom have been found effective in enhancing self-concepts of junior high students. Group sessions can focus on personal and social awareness and how to cope with age-related problems.

Body Art, Self-Image, and Health Promotion

Body art *refers to tattoos, piercings, branding, and pocketing.* These are increasingly perceived as an aesthetic addition to the self-concept and body image in females and males of all ages and economic levels (9, 73, 76, 102, 158). A **tattoo** *is an indelible mark made by pigments and multiple punctures or cuts under the skin (1/16 to 1/64 inch depth) to produce a decorative design. Metallic elements may be present in the pigments* (9, 158). **Piercing** *entails threading a stud, hoop, or other object through a section of skin* (158). **Branding**

involves burning a design onto a person's flesh. The branding artist often also works with cattle and horses (158). **Pocketing** *is placing three-dimensional objects, such as wood, plastic, and acrylic, into areas of the body. A portion of the jewelry is buried; the exposed area creates designs in the skin* (76). **Splitting the tongue** *in lizard-like fashion* has become popular but is being banned in some states as a form of mutilation that would require a medical procedure (158). *Use of body art may not be healthy.*

Body art is acquired for a variety of reasons, including to:

1. Express individuality, uniqueness, self-confidence, personal progressiveness, rebellion, and a personal philosophy (9, 76, 158).
2. Identify with others (peers, celebrities) who display body art (9, 76, 158).
3. Respond to support of friends who have body art (9, 76, 158).
4. Mark significant life events or new relationships (73).
5. Apply a permanent cosmetic effect, such as eye makeup, or as an adjunct to reconstructive surgery (face, breasts) (158).
6. Engage in a rite of passage (102).
7. Manifest sign of group membership (158).
8. Experience an erotic act (158).

Body art or modification, including scarification, may be a way for high-risk adolescents to reduce suicidality (a substitute activity) or to convey risk prior to a suicide attempt (80).

Because these procedures are unregulated and people who do these procedures have no standardized education, there are health and safety risks. In 2006, Switzerland passed a regulatory federal law, the first country reflecting an international concern (190). Physical and psychosocial risks, even physical pain, have been minimized; however, they exist.

Physical health risks related to invasive body art procedures include:

1. Bloodborne diseases such as HIV and hepatitis B and C, due to the small to moderate amount of serosanguineous fluid released (9, 73).
2. Allergic reactions to the pigment, especially red, or to metallic pigments (9, 73).
3. Infection of the skin, the nipples, or soft tissue with vesicles and drainage, and swelling, due to unsterile equipment and techniques, and unsanitary conditions of the physical environment (9, 73, 76, 104).
4. Cyst or **keloid** (*scar*) formation at the site (73).
5. Unattractive lesions on the nose and ears, which are primarily cartilage, as there is a poor blood supply. Thus the area heals slowly (3 to 6 months) and scars easily (73). *Pseudomonas aeruginosa* and staphylococcal infections may occur (73).
6. Bleeding, bruising, and disfigurement of the body site, which may last many weeks (76).
7. Systemic disease, such as impetigo, cellulitis, bacteremia, lymphadenopathy, endocarditis, glomerulonephritis, Ludwig's angina, and toxic shock syndrome, especially with piercing and pocketing (76, 104).
8. Gingivitis, contact lesions, chipped and broken teeth, edema, and bleeding of the lips, tongue, and mouth tissue with tongue piercing. Excessive bleeding may occur if the blood vessels of the tongue are inadvertently pierced (76, 104).
9. Speech impediments, choking, and tooth damage due to oral (lip or mouth) jewelry. Inhalation of jewelry can occur (76).
10. Allergic reactions, infections, and scarring with genital piercings (104).
11. Spread of the scar to 2 to 3 times the size of the original brand (158). Branding done on curved body areas may cause severe third-degree burns (or at least uneven designs) and be very painful (158).
12. Delayed healing. Branding may take 1 to 2 months to heal; pain at the site may persist for a longer period (158).

Psychosocial health risks related to body art procedures include:

1. Disappointment and embarrassment with results, especially if the decision was impulsive (9, 155).
2. Sense of rejection due to negative family or public responses (8).
3. Embarrassment and stigma from setting off metal detectors if the person has a lot of hardware (8, 76).
4. Regret because of an impulsive decision to have a body art procedure (about 50% of persons with tattoos) (158).
5. If branding is done, the smell of burning flesh is unforgettable, causing anxiety and later panic attacks and phobias (158).

Professional or responsible piercers view **intimate piercing** (*piercing of the genital area*) as a form of child abuse. They do not carry out the procedure on anyone under age 18 years.

Removal of tattoos is difficult. It may take from 4 to 12 treatments over a year, and there is no guarantee of success (9). Various methods are described by Schnare (158).

Prior to the procedure is a time to explore, counsel, and teach. Establish rapport, trust, and a therapeutic relationship. Body art always has a story. Explore reasons for the teen seeking body art, surrounding events, the desired art procedure, and the desired design. The adolescent is concerned about appearance, which is a rationale for further counseling and teaching. Explore other issues: religious prohibitions, possible reactions of future employers, and possible future effects on relationships (102).

Ask where the person will have the procedure done. Encourage finding a professional body artist with a good reputation who uses sterile technique. Emphasize that the teen is in control not only of the art form but also the selection of artist. Encourage the teen to avoid a hasty decision ("Will you be happy with the art in a month, a year, 10 years?"). Emphasize to avoid an art procedure when drunk or high on drugs.

A history of diabetes, allergies, or skin disorders demands use of sterile technique in the procedure or, preferably, no artwork. Teach signs of infection: redness, edema, discharge, discomfort or pain, and elevated body temperature.

Teach about aftercare, depending on the type of art form, to avoid complications. Refer the teen to comprehensive and published aftercare resources (158). Internet referrals or testimonials may be unreliable. Emphasize the importance of seeking medical attention if symptoms last more than 24 to 48 hours postprocedure. Tell the person there is a 12-month automatic deferral for blood donation after obtaining body art due to the possibility of transmitting bloodborne disease (102). Inform the person that piercing is more easily undone than tattoos if the artwork is no longer desired. Tattoo removal requires laser treatment, takes considerable time, and is expensive (102, 158). Discourage branding. It is extremely painful, and the infection risk is high. Disfigurement may occur.

If the adolescent comes *after the procedure with physical or emotional negative effects, do a thorough physical and mental examination.* Do not focus only on the site that is the chief complaint. Some complications of these procedures can be life threatening physically. Refer as necessary.

Assess for location of body art—tattoos, piercings, and permanent cosmetics—prior to the client undergoing magnetic resonance imaging (MRI). Metallic substances in tattoo compounds and permanent cosmetics, especially iron oxide, distort the magnetic image of structures within the body and can create an electric current that causes second-degree burns. Body piercing jewelry causes burns, and the stronger magnets in MRI equipment increases risk of dislodging the body piercing jewelry and tearing of the skin. Prior to MRI, all metal objects must be removed. Protective goggles should be worn to cover permanent cosmetics around the eyes. If MRI cannot be used, alternative tests are used (8).

You may have the opportunity to counsel or educate parents in relation to their teen and body art. The Case Situation, Relating to a Teen's Request, gives an example of the use of behavioral principles.

Sexuality, Self-Concept, and Body Image

Sexuality *encompasses not only the individual's physical characteristics and the act of sexual intercourse but also the following* (29, 73): (a) *search for identity as a whole person, including a sexual person;* (b) *role behavior of males and females;* (c) *attitudes, behaviors, and feelings toward self, each gender, and sexual behavior;* (d) *relationships, affection, and caring between people;* (e) *the need to touch and be touched;* and (f) *recognition and acceptance of self and others as sexual beings.* One of the greatest concerns to the adolescent is sexual feelings and activities. Because of hormonal and physiologic changes and environmental stimuli, the adolescent is almost constantly preoccupied with feelings of developing sexuality.

Increasing hormone levels precede rapid arousal of emotions and correlate with mood shifts. In males, hormone levels precipitate masturbation and thoughts about sex. In females, changing hormone levels are more tied to emotional changes from happiness midcycle to sadness or anger a day or two before menstruation begins (16). Hormones have their greatest impact indirectly by producing visible signs of sexual maturation, such as breast and beard development and adult size and shape. Peers and adults react emotionally to these changes. The effects of the sociocultural context are dramatic, shaping thoughts, fantasies, preoccupations, impulses, and actions (16, 73).

Sexual desire is under the domination of the cerebral cortex (73). Differences in sexual desire exist in young males and females, and desire is influenced by cultural and family expectations for sexual performance. The female experiences a more generalized pleasurable response to erotic stimulation but does not necessarily desire **coitus,** *genital sexual intercourse.* The male experiences a stronger desire for coitus because of a localized genital sensation in response to erotic stimulation, which is accompanied by production of spermatozoa and secretions from accessory glands that build up pressure and excite the ejaculatory response. The male is stimulated to seek relief by ejaculation.

Menarche is experienced by the female as an affectively charged event related to her emerging identity as an adult woman with reproductive ability. Often information in classes is not assimilated because of high anxiety during the class. She is likely to turn to her mother for instruction at the time of menarche, even if the two of them are not close emotionally.

Family and cultural traditions mark the menarche as a transition from childhood to adulthood (5). Menarche is anticipated as an important event, and in some cultures, there are definite rites of passage (5, 58). In the United States, no formal customs mark it, and no obvious change in the female's social status occurs. Nocturnal emissions are often a great concern for the boys. They are also a sign of manhood.

Both genders are concerned about development and appearance of secondary sex characteristics, overall appearance, awkwardness, and personal sex appeal, or lack of it. A common form of

Case Situation

Relating to a Teen's Request

Jane begged her mother to get her hair colored. Her hair was an unusually beautiful color for which she was often complimented. She wanted to be like all her 14- to 15-year-old friends who were frequently changing their hair color or getting some part of their body pierced. Jane especially wanted her belly pierced. Her mother said, "NO" to all of these requests. In desperation, her mother decided that she would allow Jane to get her belly button pierced if she would put in writing that she would never ask to have her hair colored in any way or have any

other part of her body pierced. Jane willingly wrote the statement, dated it, and signed it. Jane now displays a cute ornament hanging from her belly button. The mother decided that this would eliminate the constant arguing and was the least noticeable for when Jane got older and no longer wanted the piercing. However, she forgot to have Jane include tattoos in the statement and is hoping it will not come up. She will handle that situation in a collaborative way if it arises.

Contributed by Carole Piles, PhD, MSN, RN.

sexual outlet, especially for males, is **masturbation,** *manipulation of the genitals for sexual stimulation.*

Statistics indicate that genital coitus may have decreased among adolescents. However, a casual alternative in the form of oral sex is on the rise. Such experimentation is not considered sexual intercourse by some people because it is pregnancy-safe. However, the risk of sexually transmitted diseases is still present and often unrecognized (16, 140, 155). Premarital sexual activity is often used as a means to get close, even with strangers, and may later result in feelings of guilt, remorse, anxiety, and self-recrimination. The feelings associated with the superficial act may be damaging to the adolescent's self-concept and possibly to later success in a marital relationship. Adolescent males and females often report that the initial coitus was not pleasurable. Unintentional pregnancy occurs despite the availability of sexual education and birth control methods.

For adolescents who are gay or lesbian, formation of overt romantic attachments may be slower because they are reluctant to acknowledge their sexual orientation to others, or may deny their sexual urges (16). Some teens avoid mention of the subject due to their feelings about a parent who has "come out" and the family and community reverberations (34). These individuals may engage in mixed group activities to avoid social isolation, to sort out their own identity, and to avoid questions they cannot or do not want to answer. Some may seek same-gender groups and places where homosexuals meet for fun.

Present sex education information. Share with parents and adolescents that they and other people are not like disposable plastic cartons and that an intimate and important experience is cheapened and coarsened when it is removed from feelings of caring and love. Explain that teens are likely to get emotionally involved in the sexual act, and feelings will be bruised when the act leads nowhere. A wide variety of sexual experiences before marriage may cause the person to feel bored with a single partner later.

Explain that some sexual tension can be endured; in fact, it can be useful to become mature, creative, and self-disciplined. Reinforce to parents that how they live is the most critical teaching. Sex education should be directed toward the parents as much as toward their offspring, for what they teach—or do not teach—is the main factor in their child's eventual behavior.

Educate parents and teachers about the growing influence of the Internet on development of identity, self-concept, and sexuality. Encourage parents to continue to monitor computer and Internet use and maintain open communication lines with their teens. Be prepared to help the teen and the parents sort out the false from real self in identity formation.

Adaptive Mechanisms

The **ego** is the *sum total of those mental processes that maintain psychic cohesion and reality contact; it is the mediator between the inner impulses and outer world.* It is that *part of the personality that becomes integrated and strengthened in adolescence. Ego functions include to:*

1. Associate concepts or situations that belong together but are historically remote or spatially separated.
2. Develop a realization that one's way of mastering experience is a variant of the group's way and is acceptable.
3. Subsume contradictory values and attitudes.
4. Maintain a sense of unity and centrality of self.
5. Test perceptions and select memories.
6. Reason, judge, and plan.
7. Mediate among impulses, wishes, and actions and integrate feelings.
8. Choose meaningful stimuli and useful conditions.
9. Maintain reality.

When a strong ego exists and the person can do these tasks, he or she has entered adulthood psychologically. Adolescence provides the experiences necessary for such maturity, which is demonstrated cross-culturally, as depicted by **Figure 13-3**.

Ego changes occur because of (a) broadening social involvement, (b) deepening intellectual pursuits, (c) close peer activity, (d) rapid physical growth, and (e) social role changes (188). Teenage females faced with stressful life events tend to place the needs of others before their own needs and are more likely to develop an exaggerated physiologic stress response. Thus, when faced with additional or continued stress, they become overwhelmed and display poor coping strategies. This cycle continues until interrupted with counseling intervention (90, 197).

Males generally demonstrate less self-regulation and less control over emotions and behavior than females. Yet, the differences in expression of emotion may be culturally as well as biologically influenced. Males are expected by U.S. society to be more physically aggressive than females. Females are often more verbally aggressive than males and demonstrate more **relational aggression,** *being negative, ignoring, rejecting, starting rumors of dislike, teasing, or being manipulative toward another* (90, 155). However, females are becoming more open in violent expression of aggression and violence toward others, especially other females. Excessive viewing of some violent media and use of violent video games also heighten aggression in both genders (14).

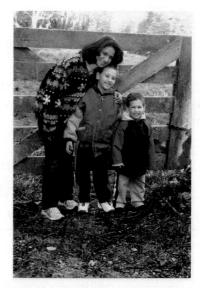

FIGURE ■ **13-3** The adolescent international student has become a family friend and is a favorite friend of the family's children.

The adolescent encounters a number of stressors and crises during this life era related to home life, peers, school and extracurricular activities, societal expectations, driving the car, leisure pursuits, and employment challenges (90). **Frustration** is the *feeling of helplessness and anxiety that results when stresses and crises occur and one is prevented from getting what one wants or needs.* Adaptive mechanisms leading to resolution of frustration and reconciling personal impulses with social expectations are beneficial because they permit the self to settle dissonant drives and to cope with strong feelings. All adaptive mechanisms permit one to develop a self, an identity, and to defend the self-image against attack. These mechanisms are harmful only when one pattern is used to the exclusion of others for handling many diverse situations or when several mechanisms are used persistently to cope with a single situation. Such behavior is defensive rather than adaptive, distorts reality, and indicates emotional disturbance.

The adaptive mechanisms used in adolescence are the same ones used (and defined) in previous developmental eras, although they now may be used in a different way. *Compensation, sublimation,* and *identification* are particularly useful because they often improve interaction with others. They are woven into the personality to make permanent character changes, and they help the person reach appropriate goals.

Teach parents that adaptive abilities of the adolescent are strongly influenced by inner resources and resilience built up through the years of parental love, esteem, and guidance. The parents' use of adaptive mechanisms and general mental health will influence the offspring (78). Even with mature and nurturing parents, the adolescent will at times find personal adaptive abilities taxed. But the chances for channeling action-oriented energy and idealism through acceptable adaptive behavior are much greater if parents and other adults set a positive example.

Mahoney describes interventions that enhance adaptive mechanisms in the African American male (95). *Group sessions that* (a) reinforce Afrocentric values, such as connectedness and spirituality, (b) build self-esteem and empathy, (c) teach problem solving and stress management, and (d) focus on avoiding drug use, school dropout, and unsafe sexual practice have been found effective (95). Adolescents generally could benefit from similar group sessions.

Moral-Spiritual Development

According to Kohlberg (93), the adolescent probably is in the conventional level most of the time. Refer to Kohlberg's Theory of Moral Development presented in Table 1-10. ∞ The adolescent may at times show regressive behavior appropriate to the second stage of the preconventional level, or maturity typical of the first stage of the postconventional level. There is no clear relationship between the teen's moral reasoning and moral behavior. The teen can talk about social justice, individual rights and freedoms, and whether a law should be obeyed. Behavior may not match the talk. Emotion, such as guilt, empathy, distress, and the internalization of prosocial norms, as well as cognition enter into moral decisions and behaviors (16, 85, 155).

The early adolescent typically is in the conformist stage. Structure and order of society take on meaning for the person, and rules are followed because they exist, as described in Kohlberg's conventional level. The young adolescent examines parental moral and religious verbal standards against practice to decide if they are worth incorporating into the personal life. The teen may appear to discard standards of behavior previously accepted, although basic parental standards likely will be maintained (16, 85).

The late adolescent is in the conscientious stage. The person develops a set of principles for self that is used to guide personal ideals, actions, and achievements. Rational thought becomes important to personal growth, as described in Kohlberg's Stage 1 postconventional level (85, 145). The teen must compare the religious versus the scientific views. Although moral-spiritual views of sensitivity, caring, and commitment may be prevalent in family teaching, the adolescent in the United States is also a part of the scientific, technologic, industrial society that emphasizes achievement, fragmentation, and technologic answers to life's problems. Often adolescents will identify with one of the two philosophies (47). These two views can be satisfactorily combined, but only with sufficient time and experience, which the adolescent has not had. Late adolescents question their earlier views about morality as they encounter people from different cultures, backgrounds, and occupations. They begin to understand that every society evolves its own definitions of right and wrong (47, 140).

Gilligan found a difference between adolescent males and females in moral reasoning. Males organize social relationships in a hierarchical order and subscribe to a morality of rights. They view morality in terms of justice and fairness (59, 140). Females value interpersonal connectedness, care, sensitivity, avoiding harm, and responsibility to others. Thus, adolescent males and females view the dating relationship differently and approach aggressive or violent situations from a different perspective (59, 115). Garmon et al. (56) also found gender differences in moral development.

INTERVENTIONS FOR HEALTH PROMOTION

Parents play a major role in the moral, cognitive, and emotional development of the teen. *Parents can help advance the teen's moral behavior in the following ways* (158):

1. Use humor in conflictual situations.
2. Use praise to reinforce desirable decisions and behaviors.
3. Listen to the teen; ask his or her opinion.
4. Ask clarifying questions; reword answers.
5. Validate to be sure the teen understands the issues.

Teens who advance least are those whose parents lecture, criticize sharply, or challenge or contradict the person's behavior without giving relevant rationale (140).

Case Situation

Dawn, Aku, and their two sons decided to sponsor a foreign exchange student through the Youth Exchange and Study (YES) Program sponsored by the U.S. Department of State. Saba is a 16-year-old Sunni Muslim from Pakistan. Dawn is a Caucasian Christian. Aku is Hindu, and his family is from India.

Saba attends high school and also practices daily to achieve her goal of finishing a 31-mile, cross-country run in the high altitude near the Rocky Mountains. She has continued practice during Ramadan, a month of prayer, fasting, and charity. Her host family and coach monitor her physical condition closely. Her coach encourages her by saying, "As long as she is improving her own record, that's what counts." Saba admits that the hardest part of fasting during the day is having no water to drink, but her faith sustains her.

Each family member practices the individual faith beliefs daily. The love and mutual respect in this family is shared throughout the community. Dawn, Aku, and Saba state this is their effort, on a small scale, toward world peace. Saba, on return to her country, believes she will be a role model for girls as she shares her experience as an exchange student. Further, this experience is a strong model for the two sons and their friends.

Submitted by Judith Zentner, MA, BS, FNP-BC.

The adolescent who matures in religious belief must comprehend abstractions. The teen is capable of deep commitment and insightful discussion. Refer to Case Situation, The Power of Faith. By age 15 or 16, the teen can make a decision. He or she will accept or reject the family religion.

If the parents represent two faiths, the teen may choose one or the other, or neither. He or she may be influenced by a friend or someone who is admired. There may be a religious experience in the form of a **conversion,** or **being saved.** *This connotes an emotional and mental decision to conform to some religious pattern.* The form may be a definite but not dramatic decision at a Confirmation or First Communion. Another form is the gradual awakening, one that is not completely accomplished in adolescence.

The adolescent who finds strength in the supernatural, who can rely on a power greater than self, can find consolation in this turbulent period of awkward physical and emotional growth. If he or she can pray for help, ask forgiveness, and believe he or she receives both, a more positive self-image develops. In this period of clique and group dominance, the house of worship is also a place to meet friends, to share recreation and fellowship, and to sense a belonging that is difficult to find in some large high schools. The faith, prayers, and efforts of parents and teachers to focus on spiritual and moral formation, not just physical and intellectual development, are important.

Some families believe that if their teen has a faith mixed with respect for God, the teen is less likely to experiment in harmful behavior. An example is presented by Brown and Wells (19). Adolescents who have been taught that they are part of a divine plan and who have been given a specific moral code may better answer the essential questions, "Who am I?" "Where am I going?" "What meaning is there in life?" Adolescents who have been raised very strictly, however, may instead develop a **reaction formation pattern of adjustment**—*rebelling and pursuing the previously forbidden activities.*

Work with parents, teens, and teachers to use an approach that promotes analytic thinking. Use the value clarification exercises described in Chapter 2. ∞ Avoid dogmatic statements about rules of conduct. Practice the therapeutic principles of communication described in Chapter 2 ∞ to foster moral, ethical, and spiritual decision making. Your behavior can be a significant model.

LATE ADOLESCENCE: TRANSITION PERIOD TO YOUNG ADULTHOOD

In some cultures parents select their offspring's schooling, occupation, and marriage partner. In the United States, adolescents are usually free to make some or all of these decisions. *In late adolescence, most teens are interested in* (a) moving out of the parental home to greater independence, (b) future and career planning, (c) stabilizing self-identity, and (d) establishing a close relationship with another.

Establishing a Separate Residence

This step is one marker of reaching young adulthood. The late adolescent often spends less time at home and prepares for separation from parents. If there is intense intrafamily conflict, if the adolescent feels unwanted, or if the adolescent is still struggling with dependence on parents or identity diffusion, a different mode of separation may occur.

In an effort to find self and think about the future or to escape abuse, incest, or other home problems, the adolescent may become either a walkaway or a runaway. The **teen walkaway** *leaves home before finishing high school or before reaching legal age. Parents generally know where the child is and are resigned to the child's new living arrangements* (20). The **teen runaway** *leaves home without overt notice and his or her whereabouts are unknown to parents, friends, or police.* Some walkaways may continue high school or get some type of job while living with relatives, friends, or a boyfriend or girlfriend. The runaway is likely to be homeless; the walkaway also is at high risk (20, 152). The **homeless adolescent** faces great challenges in a stressful environment. Besides no regular way to meet basic physical or emotional needs, there are multiple barriers to continuing the education, finding a job, and meeting health care needs. The youth engages in prostitution or juvenile offenses to meet survival needs. The female is especially likely to be victimized because of low self-esteem and exposure to predators. Out-of-home placement is an alternative to homelessness; foster home care can be difficult to obtain and may have limitations (182).

You may have an opportunity to discuss residence situations with the adolescent. If you can get to the person before he or she walks or runs away, help the teen consider the parental demands and the family situation. Discuss alternative ways of handling the problem and the importance of family support. You may contact a high school counselor or potential employer. Although either the walkaway or runaway situation should be avoided if possible, the teen should be encouraged to report incest or abuse so that the teen's parents and other siblings can receive proper therapy and an appropriate, healthy living situation can be found for the teen.

Health care is a problem for the adolescents who are homeless or runaways. Health concerns include pregnancy, sexually transmitted diseases, prostitution, alcohol and drug abuse, and child abuse and incest. *The following intervention strategies should be instituted* (73, 148):

1. Establishment of trust and rapport with the youth.
2. Ability to provide maximum medical treatment and information when the youth presents self for care.
3. Use of effective interviewing skills in order to help the youth work through issues related to family, independence efforts, safe and stable lifestyle, and ideas about future pursuits.
4. Provision of culturally competent care.
5. Establishment of a foundation for future interactions and care. Outreach programs or offering health care in nontraditional settings can be helpful.
6. Referral to other agencies as needed and as acceptable to the teen.

Career Selection

This selection has often been haphazard. Often youth are influenced by parental wishes or friends' choices. Changes in societal role expectations for males and females foster jobs or college study programs that are open to both genders. The selection is vast and thus confusing to adolescents.

For many youth, the college years are a time to consider various careers, the type of people to associate with, and how self measures against others with similar aspirations. Although college attendance and pursuit of a profession are still the ideal of many, more emphasis and opportunity exist for vocational and technical training. Many enter jobs right out of high school.

Practice Point

You are a role model to the adolescent. As you practice your profession, you may explain what you do and why you chose your profession. Direct them to members of various professions who can tell them about their jobs. Current fads should not dictate career choices that do not coincide with the person's skills.

Help adolescents clarify values and attitudes related to occupational selection. Talk with parents about their concerns. Guide teens to testing centers in which their skills and interests are measured and jobs are recommended.

Defining a Self-Identity and Close Relationship

Emotional and moral-spiritual development may take on a special significance if the adolescent period is extended into the 20s because of college education. Instead of settling into the tasks coexistent with job and family, the adolescent has time to reflect. Time and energy formerly spent in making the transition into physical adulthood can be turned toward philosophy of life and self-awareness, decisions about a desired future partner, and whether to marry and have children.

The mid-20s apparently is the least religious period in life. College youth and late adolescents often reject affiliation with their childhood church. Perhaps it is part of their break from dependence to independence. They are secure in pursuing their ambitions; they are not yet aware that their goals may not be met. They may not yet have children whom they want to educate into a religion. They may not have a perspective about the importance of their own upbringing. Yet these late adolescents are often altruistic. They wish to help others and do not hesitate to devote many hours to their goals.

Veterans, especially combat returnees or former prisoners of war, are in a difficult position. The protective family values and/or childhood religion are forcibly challenged as they experience violence, torture, hatred—the worst of human nature. If they maintain a faith, a positive attitude, and positive behavior, it is based on their maturity and supportive others.

Explore identity and moral-spiritual development with adolescents and parents. Your own behavior may be the best teacher. Explore the person's sense of self approaching a new life era and the people and support systems who will be a part of his or her life.

DEVELOPMENTAL TASKS

The *following developmental tasks are to be achieved by the end of adolescence* (37, 70):

1. Accept the changing body size, shape, and function and understand the meaning of physical maturity.
2. Learn to handle the body in a variety of physical skills and to maintain good health.
3. Achieve a satisfying and socially accepted feminine or masculine role; recognize how these roles have similarities and distinctions.
4. Find the self as a member of one or more peer groups and develop skills in relating to a variety of people, including those of the opposite gender.
5. Achieve independence from parents and other adults while maintaining an affectionate relationship with them.
6. Select an occupation in line with interests and abilities (although the choice of occupation may later change) and prepare for economic independence.
7. Prepare to settle down in a close relationship with another, by developing a responsible attitude, making appropriate deci-

sions, and forming a relationship based on love rather than infatuation.

8. Develop the intellectual and work skills and social sensitivities of a competent citizen.
9. Achieve socially responsible behavior in the cultural setting.
10. Develop a workable philosophy, a mature set of values, and standards of morality.

Until these tasks are accomplished, the person remains emotionally an adolescent, regardless of chronologic age.

How you interact with, educate, and counsel the adolescent or teach other adults to interact with him or her will contribute to the adolescent's maturity. Discuss with parents their role and concerns during this transition.

Health Promotion and Health Protection

IMMUNIZATIONS

Immunizations are a part of health protection for the adolescent, although they may be overlooked. Take a careful health history. The current recommended adolescent immunization schedule is updated annually or more frequently.

1. American Academy of Pediatrics, www.aap.org
2. American Academy of Family Physicians, wwww.aafp.prg
3. Advisory Committee on Immunization Practices, www.cdc.gov

Your actions and teaching in relation to immunizations are important for the teenager's health now and in the adult years. *If immunizations have not been received in prior age groups, they should be given as indicated.*

SAFETY PROMOTION: AN ECOLOGICAL SYSTEMS APPROACH

Being safe at any age is an issue, not just in the United States. Safety and security measures involve an **ecological systems approach**, *in that the adolescent, an individual system, develops within other systems—family/home, school/peers, and community* (16). All of these systems are interdependent and interactive as described in Chapter 1. ∞

Individual safety measures include (a) having stable and prosocial friendships and peer groups, (b) having a strong sense of self-worth and maturing identity, (c) avoiding alcohol and drug use, or enrolling in refusal-skills training classes (21), (d) and using personal protective measures previously discussed in Chapter 12, as applicable. ∞

Family/home safety measures include having parents:

1. Be interested in and involved with the adolescent's educational and social activities.
2. Monitor teen driving and recreational activities.
3. Monitor peer relationships during their visits in the home.
4. Monitor and limit access to lethal weapons.
5. Install and test smoke alarms; maintain rules that apply to the latchkey child, as described in Chapter 12. ∞
6. Follow the suggestions presented earlier in this chapter that relate to teen parties.

School safety measures include (a) offering instruction in alcohol and drug refusal skills, stress and anger management, and problem solving, and (b) enforcing safety policies related to firearms and entry of people. Maintaining a clean environment and hallway and classroom safety is also essential.

Community approaches to safety for the adolescent include (16):

1. Commitment to environmental safety related to housing, neighborhoods, parks, streets, and transit systems.
2. Low availability of lethal weapons, alcohol, and illicit drugs.
3. Availability of safe places for adolescents to socialize.
4. Policies that support enforcement of safety laws.
5. Effective emergency medical services and trauma care.

SAFETY PROMOTION AND INJURY CONTROL

The leading causes of injury-related morbidity are vehicular crashes, firearms, drownings, poisonings, burns, and falls (73). The incidence is related to developmental characteristics and risk-taking behavior.

The main threat is death due to injury, either by vehicle accidents (unintentional), violent deaths (intentional or homicide), or suicide (16, 73, 90, 140, 148, 155). Motor vehicle collisions are the leading cause of death among 15- to 19-year-olds in the United States (155). The higher rate of crashes among teen drivers is due to lack of driving experience and maturity, following too closely, driving too fast, or use of alcohol while driving. Collisions when the teen is driving with peer passengers may result when the teen wants to "show off" (63, 148). Caucasian males are more likely to die from motor vehicle accidents. African American and Latino males are more likely to die from homicide involving firearms (22, 73, 82), which are likely to occur among friends or gang members (140).

One of the biggest adolescent–parent hurdles comes with learning to drive. The adolescent needs to learn this skill; yet the arguments between parents and their children concerning how to drive, what vehicle to drive, and where to go or not to go often keep parents in a state of anxiety and children in a state of rebellion.

Head and spinal cord injuries, skeletal injuries, abrasions, and burns may all result from an accident involving a car, motorcycle, motor scooter, moped, all-terrain vehicle, snowmobile, or minibike, or from the work site. Sports-related accidents such as drowning; football, hockey, gymnastic, and soccer injuries; and firearm mishaps are also common. Contusions, dislocations, sprains, strains, overuse syndromes, and stress fractures occur frequently (73). In the adolescent, the epiphyses of the skeletal system have not yet closed, and the extremities are poorly protected by stabilizing musculature. These two physical factors, combined with poor coordination and imperfect sport skills, probably account for the numerous injuries (73).

Safety education is part of your role as an informed citizen in the community or in relation to your job. Initiate and teach safety programs with the school, church, clinic, industry, Red Cross, or other civic organizations. If you do not teach, you can insist on qualified and objective instruction. Advocate that safety courses, including driver education, knowledge of safety programs in the community, instruction in water safety, routine safety practices, and emergency care measures, be required for every adolescent. Many accidents and deaths could be avoided if adolescents were better equipped to handle their new freedom.

Inform parents and youths about safety measures and the risks and prestige value involved with the car, certain sports, and privileges. The importance of a physical examination before participation and how to prevent sports injuries should be emphasized.

Because of the sports activities in which adolescents are involved, they may sometimes experience musculoskeletal chest pain, minor strains or sprains to a joint, and minor ankle strain (49).

Musculoskeletal chest pain *arises from the bony structures of the rib cage and upper-limb girdle, along with the related skeletal muscles.* Age does not automatically rule out heart-related problems. Although musculoskeletal pain is usually aggravated by activity that involves movement or pressure on the chest cage rather than by general exertion (such as stair climbing), a thorough lung and cardiac examination is merited. Apply heat to the area (unless it is a fresh injury) and rest the area (49).

Minor strains and sprains to a joint involve a *mild trauma that results in minimal stretching of involved ligaments and contusion of the surrounding tissues.* Health promotion involves RICE: rest, ice, compression, elevation of the affected joint. Use an ice pack for 24 to 36 hours; local heat can then be used if needed (49).

A **minor ankle sprain** involves *stretching of the ligament without tearing.* Health promotion involves use of RICE, an elastic bandage, and possibly keeping weight off the ankle longer than 24 to 36 hours through the use of crutches (49).

Refer to the **Box**, *Healthy People 2010:* Example of Objectives for Adolescent Health Promotion, for health concerns and prevention strategies in the United States, formulated by the Department of Health and Human Services (179). The initiative is directed to improving quality of life for youth through health education, improved screening for disease prevention, and reduction of disease prevalence and death (179). For more information, refer to the Website www.health.gov or call 1-800-367-4725.

COMMON HEALTH PROBLEMS: PREVENTION AND PROTECTION

Health care for the adolescent includes attention to a schedule of health screening measures, immunizations, counseling, and high-risk categories. Several references describe how to conduct physical assessments with the adolescent (73, 114, 148).

Adolescence can be a healthy time. The minor illnesses of childhood, such as colds, earaches, and other childhood diseases, become less common. Inoculations, bouts of illness, and years of exposure have increased immunity. Because of the relationship between some diseases and socioeconomic status, low-income adolescents from

African American, Puerto Rican, Mexican American, and American Indian populations may have a higher than normal incidence of infectious diseases, orthopedic and visual impairments, dental caries, and mental illness. They are also more likely to live in areas where health care services are inadequate. Health problems in turn affect development of positive body image, sexual and personal identity, value system, and independence from parents (5).

About 10% to 15% of adolescents engage in multiple problem behaviors. For example, heavy substance abuse is related to early, unprotected sexual activity, lower grades, dropping out of school, and delinquency. Early sexual activity is associated with use of cigarettes and alcohol, use of marijuana and other illicit drugs, lower grades, dropping out of school, and delinquency. Many high-risk youth "do it all" (16, 73, 140, 148, 155). These behaviors negatively affect health and will be discussed in the following section about risk-taking behaviors.

In addition to the hazards of accidents and teenage pregnancy, other health problems are also apparent among adolescents.

Adolescents may develop a variety of other disorders or diseases. Inner ear damage from exposure to rock music is increasing and can be assessed by pure tone audiometry. The adolescent is also subject to postural defects, fatigue, anemia, and respiratory problems. Health problems related to body artwork are becoming more common. Other diseases include hypertension and cardiovascular disease, diabetes, various cancers, and sexually transmitted diseases. Dysplasia of the cervix, a precursor of cervical carcinoma, is a sexually transmitted disease that is occurring with increased frequency in adolescent females. Sexually active females should receive annual Pap smears. Teens should be taught breast or testicular self-examination (49, 73, 148).

Teach adolescents and parents about threats to health and preventive measures. Health-related topics include physical changes, nutrition, exercise, rest, weight control, and abstinence. Recommend that parents talk with the teen about health concerns related to genetics and lifestyle. Refer to community resources for additional counseling or education related to family or offspring health conditions. Some teens are chronically ill.

Risk-Taking Behaviors: Health Promotion Implications

The developmental changes, environmental stresses, and societal influences contribute to teens in Western societies engaging in risk-taking behaviors (16, 73, 83, 140, 155). Adolescents may experience emotional distress and depression and attempt to cope by being rebellious to parents or running away from home. Those who are particularly vulnerable and have limited coping skills attempt to self-medicate, join peer groups that may be destructive eventually, or engage in self-destructive or risk-taking behavior. Some teens experiment with smoking tobacco, excess use of alcohol and drugs, having unprotected sex, or engaging in truancy and delinquent behaviors (16, 92, 140, 155). Generally, risk-taking behavior leads to depression, not vice versa (35, 96). The depressive teen may not have sufficient energy to initiate risk-taking activity, although the person will try to comfort self through self-medication (35). If depression and hopelessness are severe enough, suicide attempts may result.

DEPRESSION AND SUICIDE RISK

Most adolescents have short bouts with suicidal preoccupations in the presence of stresses. Sometimes even a small disappointment or frustration can lead to suicidal ideas or an impulsive suicidal attempt. Often the impulsive acts are committed to force parents to pay attention to the adolescent's pleas for help and get needs met. Because the adolescent often feels great ambivalence toward parents, he or she rejects parents and yet solicits love, sometimes by attempting suicide. In reality, the parents may be giving all the love they can (31). Hurting self is a way to get even and make the other sorry for not treating the person right or to punish self for guilt over actions or thoughts (real or imagined). Death is not seen as irreversible (31). If there is a history of family suicide, the adolescent may attempt reunion with the deceased, often on the anniversary of the suicide (89).

Signs of suicide are often subtle to detect, but a composite of behaviors should be a clue that the teen is experiencing severe stress. See **Box 13-6**, Warning Signs for Adolescent Suicide and Interventions for Prevention, for a list of behaviors associated with or indicators of suicide attempts and intervention principles (16, 73, 140, 148, 155). If peers state that a friend is suicidal, investigate their concerns. No threat should be ignored.

Listen to the emotionally distressed adolescent and *ask about problems. Take a careful history to identify the underlying stresses:* family and school indicators, personality traits, and danger signs. Instruments to assess depression in youth include the Children's Depression Inventory, Diagnostic Interview for Children and Adolescents, Reynolds Adolescent Depression Scale, Center for Epidemiological Studies Depression Scale, and Risk of Suicide Questionnaire (6, 52, 73, 99).

If you believe you are unable to handle the situation, discuss it with the teen and refer him or her to a guidance counselor, nurse therapist, clergy, school psychologist, or private or school physician or psychiatrist. Frequently the adolescent will turn to an adult with whom he or she has had a personal relationship or sees as an advocate for teens, which may help the adolescent through the crisis. Accept, support, inform, and serve as an advocate, working with parents and the adolescent. *Follow-up care with the family and adolescent after suicidal gestures* is important.

If the adolescent makes a suicide attempt, after the necessary medical and physical care is given it is essential to give crisis intervention as described in Chapter 2. ∞ The goals, once life is ensured, are to help the person work through feelings related to the suicide attempt, feel hope, identify the problem, see alternative ways of handling it, and mobilize supportive others to continue caring contact with the client. The family also needs your support and help in working through their feelings of anxiety, shame, guilt, and anger. Care of the surviving family, friends, and peers of a successful suicide victim is essential.

ALCOHOL ABUSE AND ALCOHOLISM RISK

Alcohol, tobacco, and marijuana are considered the **gateway drugs** *in that they are easily accessed, are popular, and may lead to use of more addictive substances,* including cocaine and heroin. The U.S. media depicts use of these substances in prime-time network television dramas, movies, videos, and music, which makes this behavior look

BOX 13-6	**Warning Signs for Adolescent Suicide and Interventions for Prevention**

LOSS OF SOMEONE OR SOMETHING IMPORTANT

(The greater the number of losses in a short period, the higher the risk)

1. Death
2. Divorce
3. Move to new school or geographic location
4. Job
5. Self-esteem related to poor relationship or loss of status
6. Prolonged family disruption
7. Pet
8. Health

FEELINGS AND BEHAVIORS OF DEPRESSION

1. Change in daily habits
2. Changed eating or sleeping patterns
3. Lack of energy; fatigue; weakness; extreme lethargy
4. Problems of concentration; slow speech or movements
5. Drop in grades or work performance
6. Neglecting appearance more than usual
7. Lack of friends or interests
8. Truancy at school or poor work attendance
9. Increase in drug or alcohol use; excessive smoking
10. Appearing sad, angry, sullen, irritable most of time; mood swings
11. Accident proneness
12. Increase in promiscuity
13. Continuous acting out that masks other behavior
14. Negative self-concept; feeling unloved, rejected, guilty, hopeless

STATEMENTS ABOUT SUICIDE

1. Direct or indirect statements about a plan
2. Thought + Action = Suicide Attempt or Success

BEHAVIORAL ACTIONS OR CHANGES

1. Subtle or abrupt, different than norm
2. History of suicide attempt
3. Giving away prized possessions
4. Withdrawal from activities and friends
5. Writing, artwork, or talking about suicide and death
6. Accident proneness
7. Crying for no apparent reason
8. Depressed mood quickly lifts
9. Value physical complaints
10. Listening only to music about death

HIGH-RISK SYMPTOMS

1. A clear plan with time and details, using a lethal method
2. Intoxication with drugs or alcohol
3. Anniversary of the death of a loved one by suicide
4. Auditory hallucinations telling the teen to die
5. Extreme isolation and no support systems
6. Feelings of hopelessness, helplessness, and worthlessness
7. A previous suicide attempt using a lethal method and continued suicide ideation

INTERVENTIONS

1. Determine lethality
2. Encourage communication with family, teachers, or other supportive adults
3. Encourage appropriate expression of feeling, especially guilt and anger
4. Use self-esteem building activities
5. Encourage positive statements about self
6. Assist the child to cope with the situation that is causing despair or sense of helplessness

---

inviting or "cool." Negative short- or long-term health effects are rarely presented. Most teens have tried one or more of these substances, although alcohol use is most common and begins earlier in the teen years (92). It is easily accessible, acceptable, part of the home and meals, inexpensive, and frequently purchased legally by adults to be shared with minors (6, 16, 73, 92, 140, 155).

Heavy drinking is *consuming five or more drinks at one occasion on each of five or more days in the past month* (21% of adolescents between ages 12 and 20 years). **Binge drinking** is *consuming five or more drinks on the same occasion in the past month* (42% of adolescents, mostly late teens; age 21 is peak) (73). Binge drinking is common on the college campus. Alcohol use is on a continuum; the spectrum extends from abstinence, to low- to high-risk problem drinking, to alcohol abuse, and to alcohol dependence (6, 73).

Ethanol, the type of alcohol present in alcoholic beverages, is absorbed unchanged from the stomach and small intestine into the bloodstream. The *rate of absorption depends on* (a) genetics, (b) presence of food in the digestive system, (c) ethanol concentration, (d) how fast it is consumed, and (e) the person's age, size, total body water, and tolerance. Ethanol is metabolized in the liver through a complex process involving two enzyme systems (6, 65). Alcohol use in the adolescent correlates with and causes abnormal brain behavior. Alcohol impairs long-term memory and self-control by damaging the hippocampus and the prefrontal cortex (16, 32, 186). Alcohol effects on the autonomic nervous system include changes in cognitive function, such as judgment, memory, and learning ability. Mood changes are common. Alcohol may be consumed to cope with depression and stress; in turn, the person becomes more depressed and unable to cope with stress and anxiety (6, 94, 140, 186). The national campaign of "Don't drink and drive" and having a designated driver who does not drink at the party has been effective. However, alcohol use is a common factor in motor vehicle accidents, deaths, and injuries. Alcohol is also a contributing factor in death from homicide and suicide (6, 16, 155).

A number of psychosocial factors contribute to excess alcohol ingestion (6, 16, 23, 155):

1. The teen needs to feel mature or defend against depression or anxiety.
2. There is a lack of enforcement of underage drinking laws.
3. Advertising and marketing practices glamorize drinking.
4. Alcohol is seen as a way to gain gratification and avoid problems.
5. Peer pressure and social and cultural beliefs and practices encourage underage drinking.
6. Parental drinking patterns or encouragement by parents to drink at home constitute a model.

Genetic factors interact with the environment to increase vulnerability to the disease (6, 92).

Avoid lecturing to adolescents about the hazards of drinking and driving and the medical effects of drinking. Help the person to clarify values about healthful activities and see the detrimental effects of drinking—physically, emotionally, mentally, and socially. Teach adolescents how to identify hazards and to act responsibly to avoid injury to themselves and others.

Drug Abuse Resistance Education (DARE) continues in the schools. The program does not necessarily reduce alcohol use in teens (16). **Dialectical Behavior Therapy**, *which integrates cognitive, behavioral, and psychodynamic or insight-oriented principles,* is effective with individuals and groups. Refer to support groups, such as Alateen, Al-Anon, and Alcoholics Anonymous, which are effective for the teen, the siblings, and parents in a variety of ways: to overcome the addiction, gain information, and reduce social isolation. The Relapse Prevention Model is useful for adolescents who are addicted and relapse (142).

Refer parents, teachers, and adolescents for information and other services to a local branch of the National Council on Alcoholism and Drug Dependence (12 West 21st St., New York, NY, 10010; phone 212-206-6770, fax 212-645-1690). If the teen is medically ill, the teen and family should be referred to appropriate medical care services. The National Institute on Alcohol Abuse and Alcoholism presents information on its Website, www.niaaa.nih.gov.

NICOTINE USE—CIGARETTE SMOKING RISK

Nicotine is one of the most addictive substances known (16, 129). Early or teenage smoking, in contrast to initial smoking when the person is in the 20s, causes permanent genetic changes in the lungs, which increase the risk of lung cancer, even if the smoker quits. The age of onset is more important than the number of cigarettes the person smokes (155, 183). Use of tobacco and nicotine, including smokeless tobacco, is the largest preventable cause of premature death and disability in the adult (42, 129).

Risk factors for teen smoking and initiation include (16, 42, 73): (a) low self-esteem and self-efficacy, (b) limited social skills, (c) limited understanding or denial of consequences, (d) vulnerability to peer pressure and media, (e) poor academic achievement and limited school involvement, (f) desire to look more adult, and (g) having parents who smoke (16).

Early-age smoking causes a reduced height and size and decreases food intake and nutrient absorption, which has physical

consequences at puberty (16). There are a number of other consequences of active or passive smoking to the pregnant teen or adult, as described in Chapter 8. ∞

Intervention guidelines with the adolescent include:

1. Work with teens to keep nonsmokers from starting and help smokers to stop through school and media education programs.
2. Use anticipatory guidance. Initiate discussion about tobacco use at home, of friends, and of self.
3. If the teen admits smoking, explore convictions about staying healthy (values clarification).
4. Encourage the teen to pursue activities that would make the person feel good about self and improve health and physical activity.
5. Explore health risks and financial cost of smoking.
6. Discuss smoking cessation strategies. Also refer to Chapter 14 for strategies. ∞
7. Follow up with the teen to provide support.

DRUG USE AND ABUSE RISK

Drug experimentation is perceived by some as a normal part of growing up in the United States. Such experimentation is a health risk and can lead to harmful consequences from excessive use. Prevention is a major goal of parents, educators, law enforcement agencies, health care professionals, and society at large (92).

By high school graduation or late adolescence, 80% to 85% of youth will have experimented with the **gateway drugs** *(alcohol, tobacco, and marijuana)* (6, 16, 22, 92, 140, 155, 176). Some will have proceeded to other substances or illicit drugs (92).

Drug abuse is the *use of any drug in excess or for the feeling it arouses.* A **drug** is a *substance that has an effect on the body or mind.* Excessive use of certain drugs causes **drug dependence**, a *physical need or psychological desire for continuous or repeated use of the drug.* **Addiction** is *present when physical withdrawal symptoms result if the person does not repeatedly receive a drug and can involve* **tolerance,** *having to take increasingly larger doses to get the same effect.*

System factors contribute to individual protection from drug use (92):

1. **External** —Family supervision; positive school, neighborhood, and community environment and activities.
2. **Internal** —Family bonding, connectedness to school, and self-confidence, self-control, and **self-efficacy,** *confidence that engaging in meaningful tasks has successful outcomes.*
3. **Contextual and interpersonal** —Societal values, norms, and laws; attitudes and modeling by family and other adults, media presentations, and peer relationships.

Absence of these factors contributes to risk for excess drug use. *Other factors that protect against drug use include* (a) teaching an active, problem-solving coping style (16, 188); (b) promoting a sense of competence, self-esteem, and well-being (16, 64); and (c) fostering cognitive maturity (16, 64). Families can enhance these skills while not engaging in drug use. Parent-teen conversations (not necessarily about drugs) (16), their involvement in community and religious organizations, and the teen's involvement in after-school sports, drama, music, or other extracurricular or volunteer activities

MediaLink Alcoholism and Alcohol Abuse

may be the best protective measures. The DARE (Drug Abuse Resistance Education) programs have been most effective in imparting knowledge. There is inconsistent evidence related to reduced drug use (16). Other approaches have to be tried. Mennick (109) reports preventive measures related to methamphetamine abuse in youth.

Reasons for drug abuse include (16, 73, 140, 148, 155):

1. Curiosity; attempt at maturity or sophistication.
2. Peer pressure or to gain entry to group.
3. Need to overcome feelings of insecurity and aloneness and be accepted in the group.
4. Demonstration of autonomy; easy availability and ability to obtain.
5. Imitation of family patterns; cultural acceptance.
6. Rebellion or to challenge authority.
7. Need for a crutch, escape, exhilaration.
8. Unhappy home life, to relieve tension and stress.
9. Sense of alienation or identity problem.

Gradually the drug subculture replaces interest in family, school, church, hobbies, peers, or other organizational activity. The beliefs and attitudes of the drug subculture are learned from experienced drug users and are fortified by the media, music, and celebrities (16, 73, 140, 148, 155).

Addictive drugs provide a shortcut to the *brain's reward system* by flooding the nucleus accumbens, a cluster of nerve cells below the cerebral hemisphere, with dopamine, which produces a sense of pleasure and euphoria. The hippocampus lays down memories of the rapid sense of satisfaction, and the amygdala creates a conditioned response to certain stimuli. The person repeats the drug taking reward system unless there is a block to dopamine releases or damage to the nucleus accumbens (15, 65). Repeated drug use causes a reduced dopamine production, reducing pleasurable or euphoric feelings. Thus the need persists as the person seeks these feelings. Finally, drug taking gives no real sense of pleasure; motivation for or ability to continue the normal life patterns no longer functions. If the person quits taking the drug, stressors or any stimuli or situation previously associated with the substance use can cause a relapse because the dopamine reward system has had time to rejuvenate. The amygdala and hippocampus receive the message that evokes memories and feelings, and the person can relapse into addiction again (6, 12, 15, 65, 86, 172).

Ingestion depresses the cerebral cortex and releases inhibitions in the limbic system (15, 65), the center of love, pleasure, anger, pain, and other emotions. The limbic system seeks instant and constant gratification or stimulation and contributes to the adolescent's sense of boredom. Thus some adolescents go to extremes in seeking alcohol, hard drugs, hard rock, and aggressive outlets.

See **Box 13-7**, Signs and Symptoms of Drug Abuse Among Adolescents, for assessment information. All clients and patients, especially adolescents, should be questioned about marijuana use when the person comes to a health care agency for treatment (122, 153). Assessment must keep abreast of the repeating and changing trends in drug abuse, such as use of heroin (125), methamphetamine (101, 130), inhalants (104, 126), ecstasy (72, 120), PCP (123), or LSD (127). Open-ended questions, reflecting feelings

and possible behaviors, and then more directive questions can be an effective sequence. Further, they should be offered screening for HIV and other sexually transmitted diseases since these diseases are often associated with drug abuse (154).

Therapy is usually entered into as a result of family pressure—or a crisis event such as attempted suicide or arrest. The behavior and illness of the young drug abuser control the entire family, causing family illness. Love and care in a family are essential, but that alone will not cure the drug abuse problem. Professional treatment, including psychoeducation of the patient and family about risks and options for change, should be obtained in a facility that treats the whole person and family, using an interdisciplinary team approach, and that provides after-discharge care to the teen and family. Intensive treatment over time to the entire family system creates the attitude change that is essential for remaining healthy and functional. A combination of drug detoxification and emotional, cognitive, didactic, and experiential therapies is helpful to reduce symptoms and work through underlying emotional and interactional pathology.

If, after discharge, the adolescent returns to the drug-using friends, there will likely be a return to drug abuse and all the consequences. The change in attitudes, self-concept, and body image must be total enough so the person feels like a new person. He or she must be strong enough in that identity that the new self is maintained in the face of the inevitable peer, school, family, and other stressors. *The person must feel that he or she is gaining more than what is being lost to maintain the changes begun in treatment, to move forward in maturity, and to stay healthy* (3).

Support groups in the school, community, and church (19) for teens who do not want to use alcohol or drugs are essential to prevent the loneliness and ostracism some teens feel when they go against peers. Illicit drug trade can be stopped best by community action, which reduces supply to individuals.

Refer to the drug tables in **Appendix B** ∞ about Legal and Illicit Drugs, Marijuana, and Club Drugs. The tables summarize names and descriptions of commonly abused drugs, physical and emotional complications, withdrawal characteristics and nursing interventions. **Club drugs**, *are relatively inexpensive substances* currently popular *as enhancers of the party atmosphere of raves, dance clubs, and bars.* Many youthful users falsely believe that these drugs are safe. Some youth are now attending New Age Raves, parties which ban alcohol and drugs but use music, lights, and meditation or yoga to create the euphoria that is safer than drug-induced euphoria (163). Many of these drugs are manufactured in clandestine laboratories; it is difficult to determine the effects of the drug itself and the substances with which it is mixed. Drugs such as Rohypnol, GHB, and ketamine (see **Appendix B**) ∞ have also been implicated in sexual assault or "date rape" due to their sedative effects and ability to impair memory (162). Club drugs tend to be used more by adolescents and by those experiencing difficulties with the law than by young adults (72, 121, 164, 195).

Often the youth is taking a mixture of these drugs, as use of any of them is likely to increase use of other drugs. Assessment becomes more complex. At times neither the person nor friends know for sure what drugs have been used. Further, assessment is

BOX 13-7	**Signs and Symptoms of Drug Abuse Among Adolescents**

1. Decrease in quality of schoolwork without a valid reason. (Reasons given may be boredom, not caring about school, or not liking the teachers.)
2. Personality changes; lack of empathy; becoming more irritable, less attentive, less affectionate, secretive, unpredictable, uncooperative, apathetic, depressed, withdrawn, hostile, sullen, easily provoked, insensitive to punishment
3. Less responsible behavior; not doing chores or school homework; school tardiness or absenteeism; forgetful of family occasions such as birthdays
4. Change in activity; lack of participation in family activities, school or church functions, sports, prior hobbies, or organizational activities
5. Change in friends; new friends who are unkempt in appearance or sarcastic in their attitude; secretive or protective about these friends, not giving any information
6. Change in appearance or dress, in vocabulary, in music tastes to match those of new friends, imitating acid, thrasher, heavy metal, or industrial rock-and-roll stars
7. More difficult to communicate with; refuses to discuss friends, activities, drug issues; insists it is all right to experiment with drugs; defends rights of youth, insists adults hassle youth; prefers to talk about bad habits of adults
8. Rebellious, resistant to authority, antisocial behavior, persistent lying; seeks immediate gratification; feels no remorse

9. Irrational behavior, frequent explosive episodes; driving recklessly; unexpectedly stupid behavior
10. Loss of money, credit cards, checks, jewelry, household silver, coins from the home, when losses cannot be accounted for
11. Addition of drugs, clothes, money, albums, tapes, or stereo equipment suddenly found in the home
12. Presence of whiskey bottles, marijuana seeds or plants, hemostats, rolling papers, drug buttons, and marijuana lead buttons; also may be unusual belt buckles, pins, bumper stickers, or T-shirts and magazines in the car, truck, or home
13. Preoccupation with the occult, various pseudoreligious cults, satanism, or witchcraft; evidence of tattoo writing of 666, drawing of pentagrams on self or elsewhere, or misrepresentation of religious objects
14. Signs of physical change or deterioration, including pale face, dilated pupils, red eyes; chewing heavily scented gum; using heavy perfumes; using eyewash or drops to remove the red; heightened sensitivity to touch, smell, or taste; weight loss, even with increased appetite (marijuana smoking causes the "munchies"—extra snacking)
15. Signs of mental change or deterioration, including disordered thinking or illogical patterns, decreased ability to remember or to think in rapid thought processes and responses; severe lack of motivation

Adapted from References 2, 22, 32, 52, 89, 92, 93, 96, 135, 140, 172, 176, 186.

complicated by the symptoms that result from the drug use, including psychosis, which occurs with persistent use of marijuana and other illicit drugs (122, 195). Use of cocaine (or crack) is a serious health and social problem.

SEXUAL ACTIVITY

Adolescence is a time of intense sexual feelings, fantasies, exploration, experimentation, and incorporation of sexuality into identity. Sexual physical development and sexuality as a part of self-concept and body image have been discussed earlier. Sexual behavior includes necking, petting, mutual masturbation, **intercourse** or **coitus,** *genital penetration,* and sometimes **oral sex** (16, 140, 155). Multiple partners add to risk (67).

Sexual decision making and premarital coitus were controlled in the past by family, social, and religious rules and restrictions. Today sexual activity is almost completely regarded as an individual responsibility. Because of the emotional and social characteristics of adolescents, the individual may not have the readiness, decision-making or value-clarification skills, or ego strength to behave counter to the peer group in order to abstain. There is not much educational help for the adolescent. Add to that the stimulating influence of mass media, and the adolescent may feel caught. Growing up in poor neighborhoods seems to increase teenage pregnancy rates, especially for African Americans (5).

The areas related to adolescent sexual activity that influence health are those involving sexually transmitted diseases and the use of contraceptives, pregnancy, and abortion. Sexual abuse and incest, discussed earlier, are also related. A careful history is essential. Case finding and reporting according to state law is necessary for all STDs.

Sexually Transmitted Diseases

Sexually transmitted diseases (**STDs**) are *infections grouped together because they spread by transfer of infectious organisms from person to person during sexual contact, through sexual intercourse, oral sex, or anal sex.*

Often pubertal maturation precedes psychological and cognitive maturity. The absence of future planning is often evident in failure to see implications of current behavior on future outcomes. Adolescents perceive themselves at low risk ("it can't happen to me") even when infection is present, since some STDs are asymptomatic (73).

Statistics for sexual intercourse among adolescents may have decreased. However, a casual alternative, sexual activity in the form of oral sex, is on the rise. Such experimentation is not considered sexual intercourse and is considered pregnancy-safe. However, the risk of STDs is still present and often unknown (73, 152). Women and children bear an inordinate share of the problem—sterility, ectopic pregnancy, fetal and infant deaths, and birth defects, as well as cancer of the cervix (73).

Adolescents have many reasons for wanting to be sexually active, including to (7, 16, 73, 133, 148, 155):

1. Enhance self-esteem; feel "grown-up."
2. Have someone care about them; love and be loved.
3. Experiment; follow changing cultural norms.
4. Be accepted by peers.
5. Be close to and touched by another.
6. Feel pleasure or have fun.
7. Seek revenge or rebel against authority.
8. Determine normality.
9. Gain control over another.

Interventions for health promotion with the teen who has an STD must be easily accessible, show sensitivity to the teen, and provide confidential services and privacy (100). Respond in a way to avoid feelings of embarrassment and stigma. Be nonintrusive. A dialogue can be initiated with the teen about pubertal changes (menstrual period, wet dreams). Then guide the discussion to sexuality and sexual behavior. Or initiate a discussion about use of leisure time and friendships. Then move into asking about sexual behavior of friends. It then seems natural to ask about the teen's own sexual experience. It is imperative to interview the teen alone for a portion of the visit. It is equally important to have a discussion with the parent and adolescent together so that opinions can be expressed. Counsel and educate about the human papilloma virus vaccine. Encourage the teen to discuss STD risk with the partner. Role play with the teen can give a communication model to the teen. Teach the importance of abstinence or safe-sex practices. A group can be formed at school, a community agency, or a church (19) to explore feelings, values, and coping strategies related to sexual behavior; increase self-efficacy; provide education; and convey support. The Health Belief Model, described in Chapter 2, ∞ provides a foundation to explore feelings and attitudes and to predict health behavior (142). At times it may be effective to present in-depth physiologic information (157). Follow the state statutes for reporting the STD and for the teen's right to confidentiality while providing the necessary tests and treatments.

Contraceptive Practices

Contraception, or **birth control,** is the *use of various devices or chemicals to prevent or terminate pregnancy.* Although contraceptives may prevent pregnancy, they have unwanted side effects or disadvantages; only the condom prevents STDs. **The only way to avoid pregnancy, STDs, and the unwanted side effects is sexual abstinence or use of protective measures. Table 13-3** presents information about contraception (11, 73, 148).

Some youth do not use contraceptives for the following reasons (28, 73, 154, 155):

1. Misconceptions or ignorance about them
2. Inability to secure appropriate contraceptives

3. Inability to plan ahead for their actions
4. Belief that using contraceptives marks them as promiscuous
5. Rebelliousness against authority or rules

Males are less likely to recognize risk of pregnancy as a result of sexual activity, have less information about contraceptives, and are less supportive of contraceptive use than females. The attitude of the male may indeed influence the female toward sexual activity without contraceptive use, even though she realizes the hazards and wishes to avoid them (73, 155).

Effective contraceptive education and counseling involves taking a thorough history, screening to identify method of choice, and discussion about effectiveness. Your approach is key to the teenager's adherence to instructions about use of contraceptives, as well as the practice of abstinence. McNamara found that use of behavioral therapy—contingency management—increased abstinence behavior (105).

Adolescent Pregnancy

Adolescent pregnancy in the United States has been on the decline, except for Latinos. African American incidence is higher than that for Caucasians (140). Teen birth is higher in the United States than in other Western countries because of more teen sexual activity, less or inconsistent use of contraceptive measures, and fewer abortions (16, 155). There are cultural differences in age of onset of sexual intercourse and acceptability of teen, unmarried pregnancy (5, 16, 58). The gay or lesbian couple does not have the risk of unintended pregnancy, but the risk of STDs is present unless a barrier such as a condom is used (18, 155).

Unintended pregnancy carries health and physiologic risks for the pregnant teen, problems for her family, and risks for the offspring. Effects on the teen father are less well known (7, 73, 91, 155). Teenage motherhood may slow educational achievement and restrict personal development and employment opportunities. If a pregnant teen marries, she is more likely to be abused, abandoned, or divorced than is a nonpregnant teenage bride (16, 140, 155, 158, 173). Health hazards from teenage pregnancy increase as education, employment, and income opportunities fall, even among older teens (16, 140). Teen pregnancy may also be the result of sexual abuse or incest (21). Teenage pregnancy has implications for the future care and health of the baby and for future intimate relations. If teenagers do marry, the marriage is more likely to end in separation and divorce than is true for the general population (16, 140, 155).

Various factors and combinations of factors may contribute to the teen becoming pregnant. **Box 13-8,** Factors Influencing Incidence of Adolescent Pregnancy, summarizes them (16, 67, 73, 140, 148, 155).

The early adolescent is not physically, socially, emotionally, educationally, or economically ready for pregnancy or parenthood. The late adolescent is physically mature but may not be ready for pregnancy emotionally, socially, or economically.

Neonatal risks associated with teenage maternity are not uniform but are common. The risks vary by age of the adolescent mother, amount of prenatal care, and ethnic identification. See Chapter 8 for effects on the offspring. ∞

Risks are highest for 11- to 14-year-old adolescents. Early fertility implies early menarche, which is associated with short

TABLE 13-3

Contraceptive Measures: Effectiveness and Disadvantages

Name	Description	Effectiveness	Disadvantages
Oral contraceptives	Pills used to chemically suppress ovulation; new low-dose pill available, with one-tenth amount of hormones, thus fewer side effects	Highly effective, 2 pregnancies in 100	Fewer serious effects than previously seen; screen for nausea, edema, weight gain, depression, anemia, yeast infections, blood clots, myocardial infarction, liver cancer; smokers have increased triglycerides, total cholesterol, and lipoproteins and greater cardiovascular disease risk
Intrauterine device (IUD)	Metal coil inserted in uterus, preventing implantation of fertilized ovum	Very effective, 5 pregnancies in 100 Remains in place up to 5 years	Cramping and bleeding between periods, heavy periods, anemia, perforation of uterus, pelvic infection
Spermicidal chemicals	Chemical substances inserted in vagina before intercourse	Less effective, 5 to 24 pregnancies in 100; effective if used with diaphragm or barriers	Irritation of penis or vagina
Billings' ovulation method	Changes in cervical discharge show presence of ovulation	Very effective when followed and abstinence maintained during fertile time	Accurate observation by the woman is necessary
Diaphragm or cervical cap	Small occlusive device inserted over cervix before intercourse	Very effective when properly placed and checked often	Irritation of cervix; aesthetic objections Requires proper fitting
Condom	Occlusive device placed over penis before ejaculation	Effective when properly used, 9 to 10 pregnancies in 100 Protects against STD	Aesthetic objections; possibly impaired sensation in male during sexual activity
Rhythm	Abstinence of intercourse before and during ovulation; increased body temperature during fertile days	Less effective, 5 to 24 pregnancies in 100	Pregnancy unless menstrual periods regular, ovulation closely observed, and abstinence adhered to
Estrogen-progestogen contraceptive ring (nuvaking)	Ring inserted around cervix, in place 3 weeks, removed 1 week for menses to occur	Slowly releases hormones; effects similar to other hormonal contraceptives	Use with oral contraceptive increases side effects Cigarette smoking increases risk of cardiovascular side effects
Injections	150-mg injection of a progestogen, medroxyprogesterone acetate (Depo-Provera); 200-mg injection of a progestogen, Norigest	Injections 98% effective for 3 months	Intermittent vaginal bleeding Apply EMLA (lidocaine and prilocaine) 2½ hours preinjection to reduce discomfort
Implants	Levo-Norgestrel (progestin) inserted via silicone rubber, matchstick-size tubes into woman's arm	Implants last average of 1 year, continual release of synthetic hormone inhibits ovulation, thickens cervical mucus, and impedes sperm passage; removed if woman desires pregnancy	Contraindicated in women with liver disease, breast cancer, blood clots, unexplained vaginal bleeding. Side effects: headaches, dizziness, weight gain, nervousness, nausea Medication not immediately available; need another method for 2 weeks

continued

TABLE 13-3

Contraceptive Measures: Effectiveness and Disadvantages—continued

Name	Description	Effectiveness	Disadvantages
Hysterectomy	Surgical removal of uterus; usually done for pathologic condition of uterus rather than for sterilization only	Completely effective; ovum and hormonal production unchanged; menstruation ceases	Mortality rate higher than after tubal ligation; possible postoperative complications; irreversible procedure
Tubal ligation	Surgical interference with tubal continuity and transport of an ovum	Effectiveness depends on type of procedure done, 0.5 to 3 pregnancies in 100; ovum maturation, menstruation, and hormonal production unchanged	Occasional recanalization (fallopian tube ends regrowing together) causing fertility; adhesions, infection, or swelling of tubes postoperatively
Vasectomy	Surgical severing of the vas deferens (sperm duct) from each testicle	Effectiveness depends on type of procedure done; failure rate low; less expensive and time consuming and easier to obtain than female sterilization, no risk to life; no effect on hormone production of testes or sexual functioning	Bleeding, infection, and pain postoperatively in 2%–4%; occasional recanalization of severed ends of vas deferens causing fertility; uncertain reversibility

Note: A combination of contraceptive practices may be used by the couple.

BOX 13-8 Factors Influencing Incidence of Adolescent Pregnancy

DEVELOPMENTAL FACTORS

1. Low self-esteem
2. Need to be close to someone; to relieve loneliness
3. Recent experience of significant loss or change
4. Early physical sexual maturation
5. Egocentrism
6. School dropout or truancy, school underachiever
7. Personal fable (feeling that "it won't happen to me")
8. Responsiveness to peers' sexual behavior
9. Independence from family
10. Need to prove own womanhood
11. Denial of personal sexuality or sexual behavior
12. Self-punishment for earlier sexual activity or pregnancy for which teen feels shame, guilt

SOCIETAL FACTORS

1. Variety of adult sexual behavior values
2. Implied acceptance of intercourse outside of marriage
3. Importance of involvement in heterosexual relationships stressed by the media
4. Inadequate access to contraception
5. Access to public financial support for teen parents and offspring

FAMILY AND FRIENDS

1. Difficult mother–daughter relationship
2. Desire to break symbolic tie between self and mother
3. Lack of religious affiliation
4. Mother, sister, or close relative pregnant as teen
5. Sexually permissive behavior norms of the larger peer group
6. Sexually permissive behavior of close friends; immediate peer group sexually active
7. Inadequate communication in heterosexual relationships
8. Fulfillment of mother's prophecy if she expects such behavior
9. History of sexual abuse or incest
10. Few, if any, girlfriends
11. Older boyfriend
12. Substance abuse or use in family or peer group

stature, a risk factor for poor neonatal outcome. The excessive rates of short gestation, low birth weight, and neonatal mortality may result from a variety of physiologic consequences of environmental or sociocultural disadvantage, not primarily from biological developmental limits. The teen may drop out of school; she may not have achieved well in school prior to the pregnancy. Often she is from a low-income background. She is more likely to encounter complications in the pregnancy than the late adolescent or early adult (16, 73, 148).

The late adolescent male is more likely to be involved in the pregnancy and be supportive to the female than his younger counterpart. Urban teenage African American fathers are more involved with their children and the children's mothers than stereotypes suggest (16). The more mature the adolescent female and male when they become parents, the more likely they will manifest the positive parenting characteristics described in Chapter 9. ∞ The younger the adolescent, the more likely it is that negative parenting behaviors will occur. Often the adolescent parent expects behavior beyond the developmental ability of the baby, which creates intense frustration and anger that result in child abuse or neglect. Assess these behaviors. The ultrasound procedure and education using visual aids can foster attachment feelings. Agencies that have adolescent pregnancy programs should provide both teen fathers and mothers with parenting classes, support, and child development information.

Often teens who become mothers have themselves come from single-parent homes or homes in which active participation by the father is lacking. Further, the teenage father often gives no real support—emotional or financial. The maternal grandmother is the one who is expected to raise the child. If she cannot, the adolescent single parent is likely to lack the emotional maturity or knowledge to demonstrate positive parenting characteristics. If the teenage couple marries, divorce often occurs within the first or second year (16, 73, 91).

Yet, motherhood can provide a pathway to adulthood. Some teen mothers, even if single, return to school and become better students. They become a nurturing mother, mature, and overcome adversity (165).

Refer to Chapter 9 ∞ for ways to help the teenage mother be a more effective and loving mother and feel more secure and comfortable with parenting. Support and assist the teen mother to continue education, secure competent day care, and plan for the future in relation to child care and occupational opportunities. Decision making and life skills should be taught. Refer the teen to a drop-in center where she can take her baby to be free of child care for a few hours and to gain emotional support and information. Advocate for the teen parent to receive multiple support from family, school, peers, church, the media, the community, and the legal system.

Abortion

Abortion is a *method of terminating a pregnancy through expulsion or extraction of the fetus,* usually for economic, emotional, or social reasons. Teens who cannot economically take care of a child may resort to this form of birth control when they believe they cannot possibly meet the demands of parenting. Abortion carries risks to the physical and psychological health of the female (81). More

widespread use of abstinence or contraception would reduce the need for abortion, according to research by Haglund (66).

More people are choosing to keep the baby rather than have an abortion; abortion rates have dropped. You may be involved in helping the female who is pregnant, the parents, and even the father of the baby to determine their values and feelings about remaining pregnant versus having an abortion. Give full information, including the effects of abortion and alternatives. Counsel the pregnant adolescent about options following state law (73). Time and support from a mature adult are essential; an immediate decision should not be made. Be nonjudgmental and listen. If the decision is not to have an abortion, refer to an agency that gives holistic assistance to help the pregnant teen. The pregnant teen has an alternative to abortion if the biological father has withdrawn and her family is unsupportive.

If she has had an abortion, you may be the one who is sought for support. Counsel to help her resolve feelings of loss, trauma, guilt, and isolation, and sometimes physical aftereffects as well (50, 151, 166). Teens are more likely to experience cervical lacerations compared to older women because of a smaller cervix. They are at higher risk for postabortion complications: hemorrhage, endometritis or pelvic inflammatory disease (the immune system is not as mature as in adult women), Rh sensitization, and genital tract injury (73, 166). An increased risk for breast cancer exists long term since a full-term pregnancy at a young age reduces breast cancer risk (166).

Implications of this decision should be discussed with a support system. It is important that she feels accepted as a person, not judged, and is given a sense of hope and mastery over her life. A postabortion group experience may be helpful (30), and follow-up counseling is useful.

COMPUTER AND INTERNET EXCESSIVE USE

For today's teens, electronic media have always been a part of life, starting in the preschool years. Cell phones may have been standard by the first or second grade to assist parental monitoring and assurance of the child's safety. The accessible, affordable media allows increasing anonymity for the teen (17, 27, 60, 149). Excess use involves the same physiologic reward system in the brain and the psychosocial processes that occur with other addictive substances (6, 12, 15, 65, 172).

Excessive use of the computer and Internet can be a risk behavior to health, including use during leisure time and with peers. Cyberdating and use of the Internet to construct an identity and sexuality follows (17). The teen may become the object of harassment or be the one to harass or bully another (167). The Internet may be used to obtain illicit drugs or harmful substances; unknown contacts may strongly encourage risk-taking behaviors. Finally, excessive use, at first overlooked, becomes a dependent or addictive process (24, 61, 137, 138, 149, 159, 187).

Persistent and recurrent misuse of the computer/Internet (or **computer addiction**) *is indicated by the presence of at least five of the following* (6, 137, 138, 159):

1. Engages in computer activities to experience emotional gratification and relief.

2. Manifests restlessness, irritability, insomnia, increased anxiety, depression, or hostility when not engaged in computer activity.
3. Is preoccupied with computer activities, thinks continually about being online, newest hardware or software.
4. Spends money or time on computer to improve mood.
5. Neglects social, family, educational, or work obligations.
6. Denies to family, co-workers, or peers about the amount of time spent on computer.
7. Risks loss of significant relationships and achievement, career, and financial opportunities.
8. Fails at repeated attempts to control computer/Internet activities.
9. Shows physical signs, such as carpal tunnel syndrome, backache, migraine headache, poor hygiene and self-care, eating and exercise irregularity.
10. Continues computer activity despite recurrent problems.

Treatment involves the same goals as are formulated with abuse of alcohol or other substances: prevention or treatment, resolution, and return to health.

HEALTH PROMOTION INTERVENTIONS FOR RISK-TAKING BEHAVIOR

General Concepts

Some teenagers, especially those with understanding and helpful families, go through adolescence with relative ease. It is a busy, happy period. But the increases in teenage suicide and in escape activities, such as drugs and alcohol, speak for those who do not have a positive experience. Adolescents are looking for adults who can be admired, trusted, and leveled with and who genuinely care. Parents are still important as figures to identify with, but teenagers now look more outside the home—to teachers, community leaders, and entertainment celebrities. Health care providers can be one group of community leaders with the opportunity, through lifestyle and teaching health promotion, to influence the impressionable teen.

Allow the teen to handle as much personal health care and business as possible; yet, be aware of the psychosocial and physical problems with which he or she cannot cope without help. Watch for hidden fears that may be expressed in unconventional language. For example, the high school junior may state concern about the figure or physique. Underlying this statement may be a fear that he or she will not adequately develop secondary sex characteristics. The female may believe she is not physiologically normal or sexually attractive or may have an eating disorder. With adequate assessment, you may discover the male is simply physically slow in developing. Explaining that not all adolescents develop at the same rate may rid the mind of great anxiety. Today's adolescent is bombarded with information, knows more about life than did former generations, but lacks the maturity to handle it. Do not assume that because of apparent sophistication, the teen understands the basis of health promotion. Give specific information.

Education and Counseling of the Adolescent and Family

Use information from this chapter to counsel parents and the teen about preventing risk-taking behaviors. Use *value-clarification ex-ercises* to foster analytic thinking. Reinforce that an authoritative parenting style (described in Chapter 11) ∞ is more effective in prevention than are authoritarian, permissive, or inconsistent parenting styles. Teach parents techniques for building the teen's self-esteem and competence in problem solving, coping, and social skills. Explain how *these measures promote health and protect the teen from engaging in risky behavior.* Emphasize the *importance of open communication* between the teen and parents. Emphasize that *parents set limits and adhere to the stated consequences,* regardless of the adolescent's protests. *Establishing a contract* with the teen about the who, what, when, and where of behavior is effective.

Teach parents signs and symptoms that indicate substance use or abuse. If parents request drug testing, the teen should be involved in the decision to test and in the interpretation of results. Alternatives should be explored about how a teen will get home rather than ride in a car with someone who had abused alcohol or drugs.

Teach the adolescent and family effective decision-making skills so that the person learns how to develop a plan of action toward some goal. *The Decision-Making Model involves* (a) defining the problem; (b) gathering and processing information; (c) identifying possible solutions and alternatives of action; (d) making a decision about action; (e) trying out the decision; (f) evaluating whether the decision, actions, and consequences were effective or desirable; (g) rethinking other alternative solutions with new information; and (h) acting on these new decisions. Have the adolescent write out answers when setting goals, think of possible solutions, and analyze consequences to make an abstract process more useful. Some teens and parents may resist health promotion suggestions but respond to this model.

Promote warm, accepting, supportive, nonjudgmental feelings and honest feedback as the adolescent struggles with decisions. Help him or her make effective choices by *fostering a sense of self-importance* (*he or she is a valuable and valued individual*). *Help the teen look ahead to the future in terms of* (a) values, goals, and consequences of behavior; (b) a sense of what is significant in life; and (c) a resolve to live so the values and goals are fulfilled and positive consequences are achieved.

Both individual and group counseling are useful. In the group setting, the adolescent may be asked to bring a close friend or parent to share the experience. *Group sessions are effective for the following reasons:*

1. The person realizes concerns, feelings, and a sense of confusion are not unique to him or her.
2. Experiences and successful solutions to problems can be shared with others who are at different points of development.
3. Ideas and roles can be tried out in the group before being tried in real life.
4. Questions are explored; reasonable argument refines problem solving and assertive behavior.
5. Values can be clarified and decisions made with support and feedback from others.

Working with the Youth Who Uses Alcohol or Drugs

PERSONAL ATTITUDES Work through your attitudes about alcohol and drug use and abuse in order to assess the person accurately or intervene objectively. Do you believe alcohol and drugs are the answer to problems? How frequently do you use either? Have you ever tried illicit drugs? What are the moral, spiritual, emotional, and physical implications of excessive alcohol or drug use, whether the drugs are illegal or prescribed? What treatment do alcohol and drug abusers deserve? Work through these questions with a counselor, if necessary.

An accepting attitude toward the drug abuser and alcoholic as a person is essential. At the same time, help the youth become motivated and able to cope with stresses without relying on drugs or alcohol. Use effective communication and assessment. Because these problems are complex, you need to work with others. The treatment team should consist of various health care professionals and members of self-help groups who have been rehabilitated and are qualified to help rehabilitate others.

PROMOTING EDUCATION Teach in the schools and community about drugs—prescription drugs and current ones available on the street, their symptoms, and long-term effects—as well as the effects of alcohol. Know local community agencies that do emergency or follow-up care and rehabilitation with people who abuse drugs and alcohol.

All drugs and chemical substances have a potential for harm from allergy, side effects, toxicity, or overdosage. Give information verbally, through literature, and through other media. Different drugs taken simultaneously may have an unpredictable or increased effect. Taking unprescribed drugs may mask signs and symptoms of serious disease, thus postponing necessary diagnosis and treatment. Adolescents may not realize that drugs obtained illegally have an unknown purity and strength and are frequently produced under unsanitary conditions. They may not realize that when injections are given without sterile technique, infectious hepatitis, AIDS, tetanus, or vein damage may result. Help parents realize the impact that their behavior and attitudes toward drug and alcohol use have on their children. Refer the teen and parents to community resources, such as the National Council on Alcoholism and Drug Abuse.

Education should be directed to the broader community as well as to individual clients. *Help teenagers understand that problems of alcohol and drug abuse can be avoided in several ways:* (a) make decisions based on knowledge rather than on emotion, (b) have the courage to say "no," and (c) know and respect the laws. Encourage teens to participate in worthwhile, satisfying activities, have a constructive relationship with parents, and recognize that the normal, healthy person does not need regular medication except when prescribed by an authorized practitioner. *Help teens realize the unanticipated consequences of drug and alcohol abuse:* (a) loss of friends; (b) alienation from family; (c) loss of scholastic, social, or career opportunities; (d) economic difficulties; (e) criminal activities; (f) legal penalties; (g) poor health; and (h) loss of identity rather than finding the self. Refer to the Case Situation.

Working with the Youth Related to Sexuality

PERSONAL ATTITUDES Examine personal attitudes toward yourself as a sexual being, the sexuality of others, family, love, and changing mores regarding sexual intercourse before you do any sex education through formal or informal teaching, counseling, or discussion. How objective are you? Can you talk calmly about biological reproduction and use the proper anatomic terms? Can you relate biological information to the scope of family life? Can you emotionally accept that masturbation, homosexuality, intimacy between unmarried persons, unwed pregnancy, sexually transmitted diseases, and various sexual practices exist? Can you listen to others talk about these subjects? Can you listen to the adolescent who is trying to understand sexual experience in his or her own family? For example, some adolescents have to deal with the formerly hidden primary sexual orientation of a parent who announces a same-gender preference. In addition to working out a personal sexual identity, the identity of the parent must be reworked. If you cannot handle these issues, let some other professional do sex education and counseling.

PROMOTING EDUCATION Work with parents, school officials, and community leaders and agencies so that objective, accurate information about sexuality, family, pregnancy, contraceptives, and sexually transmitted diseases can be given. Most adults favor sex education in school as one way to reduce the problem of teenage pregnancy.

Teenagers need the opportunity to identify what they consider to be important problems and a chance to discuss feelings, attitudes, and ideas and to obtain factual information and guidance. The sex act should be discussed as part of a relationship between individuals requiring a deep sense of love, trust, and intimacy and not just as a means of sensory gratification. Sexual behavior is not solely a physical phenomenon but one of great psychosocial significance. The consequences of sexual activity must be explored honestly. Parent-child communication, trust, and closeness are predictors of less sexual activity (16). If parents talk *only* about avoiding pregnancy and STDs, the teen may infer that parents approve of "safe" sexual activity. The best parental strategy is to include information about social, emotional, familial, and moral consequences of sexual activity when discussing physiologic aspects of sex (16). Sex education courses given outside the home supplement the influence of parental guidance and teaching. Such sex education and related discussions can also be offered through church youth groups, the Red Cross, local YMCA or YWCA, or other public organizations. You can initiate and participate in such programs.

Encourage the teenager and family to talk together. Teach the parents how and what to teach, where to get information, and the significance of formal sex education beginning in the home.

CARE AND COUNSELING You may work directly with a pregnant teenager or one with a sexually transmitted disease as a school or clinic nurse or in your primary care practice. That person needs your acceptance, support, and confidentiality as you do careful interviewing to learn the history of sexual activity, symptoms, and contacts. Because of the problems associated with unwed pregnancy, abortion, and sexually transmitted diseases; fear of reprisals; and the quixotic personality of the adolescent, your behavior at the first meeting is crucial. You may not get another chance for thorough assessment or beginning intervention. Use *effective interviewing, communication, and crisis intervention* as described in Chapter 2. ∞

The teen with an STD wants your help and comfort. Information is needed about the disease, symptoms, contagious nature,

Case Situation

Jess, 17, was taken for treatment to an adolescent chemical abuse unit. "My parents, when they put me in [the hospital], they thought I was just drinking and using pot. When they got my tox screen back, my mom almost fainted."

The drug-screening analysis showed that marijuana, Valium, Demerol, Dilaudid, and codeine all had been ingested within a week. "All I did was live to get high—and, I guess you could say, get high to live," he said.

"I used to work at the home of a doctor who had a medicine cabinet full of everything anybody could dream of. He had a bunch of narcotics and stuff, and I thought I was in heaven. But I could go out right now and get drugs in about 15 minutes if I wanted. People, they're waiting for you to buy it. Around [age] 10, I started drinking a little bit—just tasting it, and getting that warm feeling. The first time I got high, I was 12, and I loved it. There wasn't no stopping me then. I got high all I could. I used to wake up and think, 'How can I get high today?'"

His friends put pressure on him to try other drugs. "I told myself I'd never do any pills, never drop any acid, but those promises went by the wayside." He first took Quaaludes in the ninth grade and dropped acid that year at a concert. Soon he was drinking a lot and taking speed and Valium and other depressants.

"If I drank any beer, I'd want another one. If I got drunk, I'd want to get high; if I got high, I'd want to get pills. When I started out, I thought it was just cool, and that feeling was great. Instead of dealing with normal, everyday problems, I'd run off and get high. It got so I was picking fights just so I could stomp out of the house and get high."

He became a connoisseur. "I didn't buy dope at school. There's no good dope at school."

He also became more difficult to handle at home and at school, "I started fighting a lot with my parents. My grades dropped. I got into fistfights at school. I was real rebellious. I usually was high during class."

"I think it was real obvious to my teachers, because of the way I dressed and the way I acted in class. All the guys I hung around with had real long hair, moccasin boots, heavy metal T-shirts, and leather pants."

"I was pretty much an A student, and they [grades] dropped to low Cs and Ds. I was really withdrawing into myself. I've left home a few times."

"I wasn't myself when I was stoned. For years, I didn't even know how to feel [emotions]."

"One time I was on LSD and I took a razor blade and cut my leg up. I still have the scars from that. I blanked out a lot. I'd come home beaten-up looking, and didn't know why."

Jess spent 8 weeks in treatment and now says he's been straight for over a year.

"It's a dependency," he said. "There's no way to eliminate it. You just try to control it. If I smoked a joint today or took a drink, I'd be right back."

Jess agrees with other former addicts: part of the problem is the naiveté of the parents.

"My parents, when I started getting in trouble, weren't going to admit it." Advice for parents who uncover a drug problem is simple: "Get some help. Not just for your kids, but for the parents and siblings also, because the whole family gets crazy. It's a family disease."

"I'll have to be on the lookout for the rest of my life to avoid falling back into drug use. I've learned just to be myself, and people will like me—and I never would have believed that before."

Contributed by Ruth Murray, EdD, MSN, N-NAP, FAAN.

---

consequences of untreated disease, and where to get treatment. In all of these diseases, both male and female partners (along with any other person who has had sexual contact with these partners) should be treated by medication, as appropriate, use of hygiene measures, and counseling and teaching. Teach about the importance of continued body hygiene and avoiding self-medication, the danger of reinfection from continued sexual intercourse, and the long-term damage to genital tissue from any sexually transmitted disease or repeated abortions. Remind your clients that the *symptoms* of the disease *may go away*, but the *disease may not*. Hence a complete course of treatment is essential. Reinforce that there are two reliable ways to prevent infection or reinfection: abstinence or use of a condom. One brief sexual contact is all that is necessary to acquire sexually transmitted diseases.

The female who thinks she is pregnant wants to find out and talk about personal feelings, family reactions, and what to do next. Explain what services are available and answer her questions about the consequences of remaining pregnant, keeping or placing the baby for adoption, or terminating pregnancy. Refer to comprehensive maternity services that can reduce maternal and neonatal complications.

An adolescent female may want to know about methods of abortion and services available. Reputable abortion clinics do counseling before the abortion. The questions you raise and guidance you give can help her make necessary decisions and avoid complications.

When caring for the sexually assaulted teen, there are several areas of concern in addition to the physical examination, saving of specimens, documenting and reporting, and determining if a date rape drug was used. Refer to **Appendix B**. ∞ Care, including complex physical care, must be given accordingly. Several references will be helpful (49, 73, 148). Realize that the male, as well as the female, may be a victim of sexual attack. *Other areas of concern include* (a) the emotional crisis and mental status; (b) the relationship of the perpetrator to the teen (dating partner, acquaintance, stranger); (c) prior sexual assault or a history of abuse in the home; (d) relationship with parents and other support systems; (e) cultural considerations; and (f) emotional and social consequences. Post-traumatic stress disorder may occur (3).

In many states, a minor can be treated for sexually transmitted diseases and other conditions without parental consent. Although this law prevents parents from being with their child in a serious situation, it does enable minors to receive treatment without fear of parental retribution and without having to wait until parents feel ready. Encourage the adolescent to confide in the parents, if at all possible, and to seek their support. In turn, encourage the parents to be supportive. Consent and confidentiality are key concerns in all areas of health care of the adolescent: emergency care and treatment for alcoholism and drug abuse, sexually transmitted disease, pregnancy, and other problems. Be familiar with local and state legislation and policies dealing with legal age and treatment of minors.

Health Promotion and Nursing Applications

ASSESSMENT

Information in this chapter will assist you in holistic assessment of the adolescent and the family. Information includes normative characteristics and strengths, behaviors that indicate the teen's struggles during this era, common health problems, and risk-taking behaviors that have health consequences. Astute assessment involves use of therapeutic communication techniques and a relationship approach that fosters trust and willingness to engage in discussion. Utilize references at the end of the chapter to increase holistic assessment and competence.

NURSING DIAGNOSES

Based upon your assessment, relevant nursing diagnoses are presented in the **Box**, Nursing Diagnoses Related to the Adolescent (118). Other nursing diagnoses can be formulated related to direct care of the ill adolescent (135) or health promotion measures that could be instituted.

INTERVENTION

Interventions to promote and maintain health and prevent physical or mental disorders have been discussed throughout the chapter. A summary is often presented; you will find additional necessary information in the references at the end of the chapter as well as in other resources. Refer to **Box 13-9**, Considerations for the Adolescent and Family in Health Promotion, for a summary of key intervention considerations.

Keep abreast of research findings that can guide assessment and intervention. For example, the Child and Adolescent Trial for Cardiovascular Health (CATCH) was one of the largest intervention school-based studies conducted in the United States in an effort to decrease risk for heart disease in children. The study included specific information from the youth and family, such as planned physical exercise, nutrition and meal service, and smoke-free school policies. Results 5 years later indicated that interventions can be maintained by the school. However, adherence to the interventions by students was less than desired. Family lifestyle and attitude affect ongoing adherence to healthful changes in family patterns in the home as well as the student's willingness to comply with healthful changes at school (142).

EVALUATION

Analysis of personal knowledge, beliefs, and attitudes toward the adolescent and his or her developmental changes and risk-taking behaviors is essential to **evaluate** the health care provider's

---

Nursing Diagnoses Related to the Adolescent

Anxiety	Deficient **K**nowledge
Disturbed **B**ody Image	Risk for **L**oneliness
Readiness for Enhanced **C**ommunication	Imbalanced **N**utrition: Less than Body Requirements
Ineffective **C**oping	Imbalanced **N**utrition: More than Body Requirements
Readiness for Enhanced **C**oping	Chronic Low **S**elf-Esteem
Compromised Family **C**oping	**S**elf-Mutilation
Fatigue	Risk for **S**piritual Distress
Delayed **G**rowth and Development	Risk for **S**uicide
Ineffective **H**ealth Maintenance	Risk for Other-Directed **V**iolence
Health-Seeking Behaviors	Risk for Self-Directed **V**iolence
Risk for **I**njury	

Source: Reference 118.

BOX 13-9	Considerations for the Adolescent and Family in Health Promotion

1. Family, cultural background and values, support systems, and community resources for the adolescent and family
2. Parents as identification figures, able to guide and to allow the adolescent to develop his or her own identity
3. Relationship among family members or significant adults and its impact on the adolescent
4. Behaviors that indicate abuse, neglect, or maltreatment by parents or other significant adults
5. Physical growth patterns, characteristics and competencies, nutritional status, and rest, sleep, and exercise patterns that indicate health and are within age norms for the adolescent
6. Completion of physical growth spurt and development of secondary sex characteristics that indicate normal development in the male or female; self-concept and body image development and integration related to physical growth
7. Nutritional requirements greater than for the adult
8. Immunizations, safety education, and other health promotion measures
9. Cognitive development into the stage of formal operations, related value formation, ongoing moral–spiritual development, and beginning development of philosophy of life
10. Peer relationships, use of leisure time
11. Overall appearance and behavioral patterns at home, school, and in the community that indicate positive identity formation, rather than role confusion or diffusion, or negative identity
12. Use of effective adaptive mechanisms and coping skills in response to stressors
13. Behavioral patterns in late adolescence that indicate integration of physical changes; cognitive, emotional, social, and moral-spiritual development; effective adaptive mechanisms
14. Behavioral patterns and characteristics that indicate the adolescent has achieved developmental tasks
15. Parental behavior that indicates they are achieving their developmental tasks

approach. **Evaluation of use of culturally competent care** can be determined through validation with the client, as well as by keeping abreast of knowledge development. Responses of the teen and family, as well as critiques by other professionals, also assist in the **evaluative process.** *Various instruments have been mentioned throughout the chapter* and may be **useful for evaluation of care,** depending in part on the mood and developmental status of the teen at the time, as well as the rapport established with the investigator or professional, which can affect responses to surveys or other tools. Refer to **Box 13-9,** Considerations for the Adolescent and Family in Health Promotion, for criteria that can be formulated into ongoing or end-of-care evaluation. Johnson et al. (81) is a reference to assist in developing evaluation criteria.

Summary

1. Adolescence is the final period of rapid physical growth, as well as a time of considerable cognitive and emotional change.
2. Relationships with the family remain basically important, but the peer group is dominant and exerts considerable influence on the adolescent's behavior.
3. This is the time during which the individual works to develop his or her identity or sense of uniqueness, to become independent of and separate from parents while retaining basic ties and values.
4. Because of the many available options, determining one's identity, value systems, and career or life path can be difficult, take time, and sometimes be detoured by various societal forces or acquired habits, such as substance abuse.
5. A number of health problems may arise in the physical, psychological, or social dimensions.
6. **Box 13-9,** Considerations for the Adolescent and Family in Health Promotion, summarizes recommendations to consider in assessment and health promotion. The family is included in considerations.
7. The home situation affects emotional and physical health, adaptive ability, school performance, social skills, later job and marital adjustment, and the type of citizen and parent the adolescent will become.
8. Health promotion—individual, family, and a community-wide program—continues the foundation laid earlier for adult health.

Review Questions

1. A parish nurse is counseling the parents of an adolescent. The parents express concern that the child is refusing to attend church services, which they believe is a crucial part of their family life. The nurse recognizes by refusing to participate in religious services, the child is probably:
   1. Attempting to establish an identity by rejecting parental values.
   2. Punishing the parents for their rigid limits.
   3. Exhibiting behaviors of substance use by the child.
   4. Attempting to tell the parents of a desire to join another church.

2. A client tells the nurse that since her children have left home, she and her husband are finding that they really do not know each other anymore. Which task of family development is this couple struggling with at this time?
   1. Establish a sharing of responsibilities.
   2. Reestablish a mutually satisfying marriage relationship.
   3. Rework relationships with relatives, friends, and associates.
   4. Formulate a workable philosophy of life.

3. A 12-year-old boy expresses he is upset about not having grown much in the last year. Also, his female classmates are now taller than he is. The nurse should base the response to the child on the fact that:
   1. Height is genetically determined.
   2. He has likely reached his full adult height.
   3. He will likely continue to grow for several more years.
   4. Short stature in a male in this age group should be evaluated by a specialist.

4. When discussing hypertension with a group of adolescents, the nurse should include which of the following relevant facts about this condition? Select all that apply.
   1. Hypertension is not usually a concern in adolescents.
   2. High diastolic blood pressure is associated with smoking.
   3. Stress is a factor in development of hypertension.
   4. Exercise has no impact on blood pressure.
   5. Caucasian females are most likely to be affected by hypertension.

References

1. Amar, A., & Alexy, E. (2005). "Dissed" by dating violence. *Perspectives in Psychiatric Care, 41*(4), 162–171.

2. American Psychiatric Association. (1994). *Diagnostic and statistical manual of mental disorders—IV*. Washington, DC: Author.

3. Ammerman, R., Lynch, K., Donovan, J., Martin, C., & Maisto, S. (2001). Constructive thinking in adolescents with substance use disorders. *Psychology of Addictive Behaviors, 15*, 89–96.

4. Anderson, S., Griesemer, B., Johnson, M., Martin, T., McLain, L., Rowland, T., et al. (2000). Medical concerns in the female athlete. *Pediatrics, 106*(3), 610–613.

5. Andrews, M., & Boyle, J. (2003). *Transcultural concepts in nursing care* (4th ed.). Philadelphia: Lippincott Williams & Wilkins.

6. Antai-Otong, D. (2007). *Psychiatric nursing: Biological & behavioral concepts.* Clifton Park, NY: Delmar Learning.

7. Armistead, L., Kotchick, B., & Forbrand, R. (2004). Teenage pregnancy, sexually transmitted diseases, and HIV/AIDS. In L. Rapp-Paglicci, C. Dulmus, & J. Wodarski (Eds.), *Handbook of preventive interventions for children and adolescents* (pp. 227–254). Hoboken, NJ: John Wiley & Sons.

8. Armstrong, M., & Elkins, L. (2005). Body art and MRI. *American Journal of Nursing, 105*(3), 65–66.

9. Armstrong, M., Owen, D., Roberts, A., & Koch, J. (2002). College students and tattoos: Influence of image, identity, family, and friends. *Journal of Psychosocial Nursing, 40*(10), 21–29.

10. Aroian, K. (2006). Children of foreign-born parents. *Journal of Psychosocial Nursing, 44*(10), 15–18.

11. Aschenbrenner, D. (2006). Over-the-counter access to emergency contraception. *American Journal of Nursing, 106*(11), 34–36.

12. Bailey, K. (2004). The brain's rewarding system & addiction. *Journal of Psychosocial Behavior, 42*(6), 14–18.

13. Bates, B. (2005). Delusions of parasitosis a sign of crystal methamphetamine use and possible HIV. *Clinical Psychiatry News, 33*(12), 64.

14. Begany, T. (2005). Violent video games heighten aggression, literature review confirms. *NeuroPsychiatry Reviews, 6*(9), 10–11.

15. Begany, T. (2006). Systems of balance: The neurobiology of addiction and dependence. *NeuroPsychiatry Reviews, 7*(8), 12–13.

16. Berger, K. (2005). *The developing person through the life span* (6th ed.). New York: Worth.

17. Berson, M. (2000). The computer can't see you blush. *Kappa Delta Pi Record, 32*(4), 158–162.

18. Borden, C. (2004). Lesbian and gay youths at risk. *American Journal of Nursing, 104*(10), 13.

19. Brown, E., & Wells, S. (2006). A faith-based integrated substance abuse and HIV prevention program for rural African American adolescents. *Journal of American Psychiatric Nurses Association, 11*(6), 349–356.

20. Burgess, A., & Birnbaum, H. (1982). Youth prostitution. *American Journal of Nursing, 82*(5), 832–834.

21. Butler, J., & Burton, L. (1990, January). Rethinking teenage childbearing: Is sexual abuse a missing link? *Family Relations*, 73–79.

22. Centers for Disease Control and Prevention. (2004). Youth risk behavior surveillance—United States, 2003. *Morbidity and Mortality Weekly Report, 53*(SS02), 1–96.

23. Children of alcoholics are at greater risk of substance abuse. (2006). *NeuroPsychiatry Reviews, 7*(4), 10–11.

24. Christenson, M., Orzack, M., Babington, L., & Patsdaughter, C. (2001). Computer addiction: When monitor becomes control center. *Journal of Psychosocial Nursing, 39*(3), 40–47.

25. Collins, A. (2003). More than myth. The developmental significance of romantic relationships during adolescence. *Journal of Research on Adolescence, 13*, 1–24.

26. Confronting suicide: Part II. (2003). *Harvard Mental Health, 19*(12), 1–4.

27. Cooper, A., & Griffin-Shelley, E. (2002). A quick tour of online sexuality: Part I. *Annals of the American Psychotherapy Association, 5*(6), 11–13.

28. Cromwell, P., & Daley, A. (2005). Effective contraceptive counseling with adolescents in a nurse-based setting. *Nursing Clinics of North America, 37*, 499–512.

29. Dacey, J., & Margolis, D. (2006). Psychosocial development: Adolescence and sexuality. In K. Thies & J. Travers (Eds.), *Handbook of human development for health care professionals* (pp. 191–218). Sudbury, MA: Jones and Bartlett.

30. Daly, J. (2004). Postabortion groups: Risk reduction in a school-based health clinic. *Journal of Psychosocial Nursing, 42*(10), 49–54.

31. Daly, P. (2005). Mothers living with suicidal adolescents: A phenomenological study of their experiences. *Journal of Psychosocial Nursing, 43*(3), 22–28.

32. DeBellis, M., Clark, D., Beers, S., Soloff, P., Boring, A., Hall, J., et al. (2000). Hippocampal volume in adolescent-onset alcohol use disorders. *American Journal of Psychiatry, 157,* 737–744.

33. Deering, C., & Jennings, D. (2002). Communicating with children and adolescents. *American Journal of Nursing, 102*(3), 34–41.

34. Deevy, S. (1989). When Mom or Dad comes out: Helping adolescents cope with homophobia. *Journal of Psychosocial Nursing, 27*(10), 35–36.

35. DeFranco, C. (2005). Risky adolescent behavior leads to depression, not vice versa. *NeuroPsychiatry Reviews, 6*(10), 1, 15.

36. Dudek, S. (2007). *Nutrition essentials for nursing practice* (5th ed.). Philadelphia: Lippincott Williams & Wilkins.

37. Duvall, E., & Miller, B. (1986). *Marriage and family development* (6th ed.). New York: Harper & Row.

38. Duyff, R. (2002). *American Dietetic Association complete food and nutrition guide* (2nd ed.). Hoboken, NJ: John Wiley & Sons.

39. Eberly, M. (2005). It's **NOT** about food: Getting to the heart of eating disorders. *Journal of Christian Nursing, 22*(2), 15–19.

40. Echrick, J., & Strohmeyer, S. (2006). Motor development. In K. Thies & J. Travers (Eds.), *Handbook of human development for health care professionals* (pp. 161–189). Sudbury, MA: Jones and Bartlett.

41. Elder, G., & Conger, R. (2000). *Children of the land: Adversity and success in rural America.* Chicago: University of Chicago Press.

42. Elder, J., Iniguez, E., & Larios, S. (2004). Tobacco use. In L. Rapp-Paglicci, C. Dulmus, & J. Wodarski (Eds.), *Handbook of preventive interventions for children and adolescents* (pp. 255–274). Hoboken, NJ: John Wiley & Sons.

43. Elliot, D.L., Moe, E.L., Goldberg, L., DeFrancesco, C.A., Durham, M.B., & Hix-Small, H. (2006). Definition and outcome of a curriculum to prevent disordered eating and body-shaping drug use. *Journal of School Health, 76,* 67–73.

44. Ely, G. (2004). Dating violence. In L. Rapp-Paglicci, C. Dalmus, & J. Wodarski (Eds.), *Handbook of preventive interventions for children and adolescents* (pp. 415–457). Hoboken, NJ: John Wiley & Sons.

45. Erikson, E. H. (1963). *Childhood and society* (2nd ed.). New York: W. W. Norton.

46. Erikson, E. H. (1968). *Identity: Youth and crisis.* New York: W.W. Norton.

47. Erikson, E. H. (1975). Memorandum on youth. In W. Sze (Ed.), *Human life cycle* (pp. 351–359). New York: Jason Aronson.

48. Eron, L. (1998). What becomes of aggressive school children. *Harvard Mental Health Letter, 14*(10), 8.

49. Fenstermacher, K., & Hudson, B. (2004). *Practice guidelines for family nurse practitioners* (3rd ed.). Philadelphia: Saunders.

50. Fergusson, D., Harwood, L., & Ridder, E. (2006). Abortion in young women and subsequent mental health. *Journal of Child Psychology and Psychiatry, 47*(1), 16–24.

51. Foley, S. (2006). Health problems in teen girl athletes. *American Journal of Nursing, 106*(5), 22.

52. Folse, V., Eich, K., Hall, A., & Ruppman, J. (2006). Detecting suicide risk in adolescents and adults in an emergency department: A pilot study. *Journal of Psychosocial Nursing, 44*(3), 22–29.

53. Fraser, M., & Williams, S. (2004). Aggressive behavior. In L. Rapp-Paglicci, C. Dulmus, & J. Wodarski (Eds.), *Handbook of preventive interventions for children and adolescents* (pp. 100–129). Hoboken, NJ: John Wiley & Sons.

54. Garbarino, J. (1992). *Children in danger.* New York: Jossey-Bass.

55. Garbarino, J., Guttmann, E., & Seeley, J. (1987). *The psychologically battered child: Strategies for identification, assessment, and intervention.* San Francisco: Jossey-Bass.

56. Garmon, J., Basinger, K., Gregg, V., & Gibbs, J. (1996). Gender differences in stage and expression of moral judgment. *Merrill-Palmer Quarterly, 42,* 418–437.

57. Gerdorian, K. (2005). The needs of adolescent girls who self-harm. *Journal of Psychosocial Nursing, 43*(8), 41–49.

58. Giger, J., & Davidhizar, R. (2004). *Transcultural nursing: Assessment and intervention* (4th ed.). St. Louis, MO: Mosby.

59. Gilligan, C. (1982). *In a different voice: Psychological theory and women's development.* Cambridge, MA: Harvard University Press.

60. Golden, G. (2002). *Sex and the Internet: A guidebook for clinicians.* New York: Brunner-Routledge.

61. Golden, G., & Cooper, A. (2003). A brief summary of assessment and treatment issues for compulsive online sexual activity—Part I. *Annals of the American Psychotherapy Association, 6*(1), 28–30.

62. Gormly, A. (1997). *Lifespan human development* (6th ed.). Fort Worth, TX: Harcourt Brace College Publishers.

63. Gregory, R. (2003). Finding effective strategies for working with adolescents. *Journal of Psychosocial Nursing, 41*(5), 47–51.

64. Griffin, K., Scheier, L., Borvin, G., & Diaz, T. (2001). Protective role of personal competence skill in adolescent use: Psychological well-being. *Psychology of Addictive Behaviors, 15,* 194–203.

65. Guyton, A., & Hall, J. (2006). *Textbook of medical physiology* (11th ed.). Philadelphia: Elsevier Saunders.

66. Haglund, K. (2003). Sexually abstinent African American adolescent females' descriptions of abstinence. *Journal of Nursing Scholarship, 35*(3), 231–238.

67. Harner, H. (2005). Childhood sexual abuse, teenage pregnancy, and partnering with adult men. *Journal of Psychosocial Nursing, 43*(8), 18–28.

68. Harris, M., & Cumella, E. (2006). Eating disorders across the life span. *Journal of Psychosocial Nursing, 44*(4), 22–26.

69. Harter, S., Marold, D., Whitesell, N., & Cobbs, G. (1996). A model of the effects of perceived parent and peer support on adolescent false-self behavior. *Child Development, 67,* 366–374.

70. Havighurst, R. (1992). *Developmental tasks and education* (3rd ed.). New York: David McKay.

71. Henry, D., Tolan, P., & Gorman-Smith, D. (2001). Longitudinal family and peer group effects on violence and nonviolent delinquency. *Journal of Clinical Child Psychiatry, 30,* 172–186.

72. Hess, D., & DeBoer, S. (2002). Ecstasy. *American Journal of Nursing, 102*(4), 45–47.

73. Hockenberry, M., & Wilson, D. (2007). *Wong's nursing care of infants and children* (8th ed.). St. Louis, MO: Mosby Elsevier.

74. Hoerman, L. (2006). The obese teen: The neuroendocrine connection. *American Journal of Nursing, 107*(2), 40–48.

75. Howard, D., Qui, Y., & Boekeloo, B. (2002). Personal and social contextual correlates of adolescent dating violence. *Journal of Adolescent Health, 33*(1), 9–17.

76. Howard-Ruben, J. (2002). People who pierce and the nurses who care for (and about) them. *Nursing Spectrum Metro Edition, 3*(8), 29–30.

77. Hubbard, G. (1989). Perceived life changes for children and adolescents following disclosure of father-daughter incest. *Journal of Child and Adolescent Psychiatric and Mental Health Nursing, 2*(2), 78–82.

78. Hunter, A., & Chandler, G. (1999). Adolescent resilience. *Journal of Nursing Scholarship, 31*(3), 241–247.

79. *Ice: Speed, smoke, and fire.* (1991). Phoenix, AZ: D.I.N.

80. Jancin, B. (2006). Piercing and tattoos possibly linked to suicidality. *Clinical Psychiatry News, 33*(8), 63.

81. Johnson, M., Bulecheck, G., Butcher, H., Dochterman, J., Maas, M., Moorhead, S., & Swanson, E. (2006). *NANDA, NOC, NIC linkages: Nursing diagnoses, outcomes, and interventions* (2nd ed.). St. Louis, MO: Mosby Elsevier.

82. Juszezak, L., & Cooper, K. (2005). Improving the health and well-being of adolescent boys. *Nursing Clinics of North America, 37,* 443–447.

83. Kelley, A., et al. (2004, June). Risk-taking and novelty seeking in adolescence. *Annals of the New York Academy of Sciences, 102,* 27–32.

84. Kim, T. (2005). Adolescent use of drugs, tobacco, continues decline. *Clinical Psychiatry News, 33*(2), 1, 4.

85. Kohlberg, L. (1976). Moral stages and moralization: The cognitive development approach. In *Moral development and behavior.* New York: Holt, Rinehart, & Winston.

86. Koob, G. F. et al. (2004). Neurobiological mechanisms in the transition from drug use to drug dependence. *Neuroscience and Biobehavioral Reviews, 27*(8), 739–749.

87. Krepcio, D., Foell, K., Folta, S., & Goldberg, J. (2003, August). The vegetarian teen. *Nursing Spectrum, Midwestern Edition,* 22–25.

88. Kritek, K., Birnbaum, A., & Levinson, D. (2004). A schematic model for focusing on youth in investigation of community design and physical activity. *American Journal of Health Promotion, 19*(1), 33–38.

89. Krysinska, K. (2003). Loss by suicide: A risk factor for suicidal behavior. *Journal of Psychosocial Nursing, 41*(2), 34–41.

90. Ladd, G. (2006). Adolescent anxiety: Developmental context and cognitive perspectives. In K. Thies & J. Travers (Eds.), *Handbook of human development for health care professionals* (pp. 339–354). Sudbury, MA: Jones and Bartlett.

91. LaRossa, R. (1988). Fatherhood and social change. *Family Relations, 37*, 451–457.

92. LeCroy, C., & Mann, J. (2004). Substance abuse. In L. Rapp-Paglicci, C. Dulmus, & J. Wodarski (Eds.), *Handbook of preventive interventions for children and adolescents* (pp. 198–236). Hoboken, NJ: John Wiley & Sons.

93. Liu, X. (2004). Sleep and adolescent suicidal behavior. *Sleep, 27*, 1351–1358.

94. Lynskey, M., Heath, A., Bucholz, K., Slutski, W., Madden, P., Nelson, E., et al. (2003). Escalation of drug use in early-onset cannabis users versus co-twin controls. *Journal of the American Medical Association, 289*, 427–433.

95. Mahoney, D. (2005). Interventions empower African American boys. *Clinical Psychiatry News, 33*(1), 54.

96. Mahoney, D. (2005). Teen sex, drug use may bring on depression. *Clinical Psychiatry News, 33*(11), 7.

97. Margolis, D. (2006). Gender development. In K. Thies & J. Travers (Eds.), *Handbook of human development for health care professionals.* Sudbury, MA: Jones and Bartlett.

98. Martin, H., & Ammerman, S. (2002). Adolescents with eating disorders: Primary care screening identification and early intervention. *Nursing Clinics of North America, 37*, 537–551.

99. McCarter, A., Sowers, K., & Dulmus, C. (2004). Adolescent suicide prevention. In L. Rapp-Paglicci, C. Dulmus, & J. Wodarski (Eds.), *Handbook of preventive interventions for children and adolescents* (pp. 85–99). Hoboken, NJ: John Wiley & Sons.

100. McEvoy, M., & Cowpey, S. (2002). Sexually transmitted infection: A challenge for nurses working with adolescents. *Nursing Clinics of North America, 37*, 461–478.

101. McGuinness, T.M. (2006). Emergency: Methamphetamine abuse. *American Journal of Nursing, 106*(12), 54–59.

102. McGuinness, T. (2006). Teens & body art. *Journal of Psychosocial Nursing, 44*(4), 13–16.

103. McGuinness, T. (2006). Active living for healthy youth. *Journal of Psychosocial Nursing, 44*(6), 13–16.

104. McGuinness, T.M. (2006). Nothing to sniff at: Inhalant use and youth. *Journal of Psychosocial Nursing, 44*(8), 15–18.

105. McNamara, D. (2005). Contingency management increases abstinence. *Clinical Psychiatry News, 33*(8), 60.

106. McPherson, M. (1999, April). The power of believing in your child. *Focus on the Family*, 10–11.

107. McVey, G. (2004). Eating disorders. In L. Rapp-Paglicci, C. Dulmus, & J. Wodarski (Eds.), *Handbook of preventive interventions for children and adolescents* (pp. 275–300). Hoboken, NJ: John Wiley & Sons.

108. Meininger, J., Liehr, P., Chen, W., Smith, G., & Mueller, W. (2004). Developmental, gender, and ethnic differences in moods and ambulatory blood pressure in adolescents. *Annals of Behavioral Medicine, 28*(1), 10–19.

109. Mennick, F. (2007). Preventing methamphetamine abuse in youths. *American Journal of Nursing, 107*(2), 22.

110. Messina, V., Melina, V., & Mangels, A. (2003). A new food guide for North American vegetarians. *Journal of the American Dietetic Association, 133*, 771–775.

111. Metallinos-Katsares, E., & Gorman, K. (2006). Nutrition and the behavior of children: Food for thought. In K. Thies & J. Travers (Eds.), *Handbook of human development for health care professionals* (pp. 139–159). Sudbury, MA: Jones and Bartlett.

112. Metheny, N. (2000). *Fluid and electrolyte balance: Nursing considerations* (4th ed.). Philadelphia: Lippincott.

113. Monteleone, J. (1998). *A parent's & teacher's handbook on identifying and preventing child abuse.* St. Louis, MO: G.W. Medical Publishing.

114. Muscari, M. (1999). The first gynecologic exam. *American Journal of Nursing, 99*(1), 68–69.

115. Muuss, R. (1988). Carol Gilligan's Theory of Sex Differences in the Development of Moral Reasoning During Adolescence. *Adolescence, 23*(89), 229–243.

116. Mytton, J., DiGuiseppi, C., Gough, D., Taylor, R., & Logan, S. (2007). *School-based secondary prevention programs for preventing violence (Review): The Cochrane Collaboration.* New York: Wiley.

117. Nagel, B., Medina, K., Yashii, J., Schweinsburg, A., Moadab, I., & Tapert, S. (2006). *Age-related changes in prefrontal white matter volume across adolescence, 17*(13), 1427–1431.

118. NANDA International. (2007). *NANDA-I nursing diagnoses: Definitions & classifications 2007–2008.* Philadelphia: Author.

119. National Institute on Drug Abuse. (2005, April). *Selected prescription drugs with potential for abuse.* Washington, DC, National Institutes of Health, U.S. Department of Health and Human Services.

120. National Institute on Drug Abuse. (2006, April). *MDMA (Ecstasy) abuse.* Washington, DC, National Institutes of Health, U.S. Department of Health and Human Services.

121. National Institute on Drug Abuse. (2006, April). *NIDA InfoFacts: Club drugs.* Washington, DC, National Institutes of Health, U.S. Department of Health and Human Services.

122. National Institute on Drug Abuse. (2006, April). *NIDA InfoFacts: Marijuana.* Washington, DC, National Institutes of Health, U.S. Department of Health and Human Services.

123. National Institute on Drug Abuse. (2006, April). *NIDA InfoFacts: PCP.* Washington, DC, National Institutes of Health, U.S. Department of Health and Human Services.

124. National Institute on Drug Abuse. (2006, May). *NIDA InfoFacts: Crack and cocaine.* Washington, DC, National Institutes of Health, U.S. Department of Health and Human Services.

125. National Institute on Drug Abuse. (2006, May). *NIDA InfoFacts: Heroin.* Washington, DC, National Institutes of Health, U.S. Department of Health and Human Services.

126. National Institute on Drug Abuse. (2006, May). *NIDA InfoFacts: Inhalants.* Washington, DC, National Institutes of Health, U.S. Department of Health and Human Services.

127. National Institute on Drug Abuse. (2006, May). *NIDA InfoFacts: LSD.* Washington, DC, National Institutes of Health, U.S. Department of Health and Human Services.

128. National Institute on Drug Abuse. (2006, June). *NIDA InfoFacts: Prescription pain and other medications.* Washington, DC, National Institutes of Health, U.S. Department of Health and Human Services.

129. National Institute on Drug Abuse. (2006, July). *NIDA InfoFacts: Cigarettes and other tobacco products.* Washington, DC, National Institutes of Health, U.S. Department of Health and Human Services.

130. National Institute on Drug Abuse. (2006, November). *NIDA InfoFacts: Methamphetamine.* Washington, DC, National Institutes of Health, U.S. Department of Health and Human Services.

131. National Institute on Drug Abuse. (2006, November). *NIDA Research Report: Steroid abuse and addiction.* Washington, DC, National Institutes of Health, U.S. Department of Health and Human Services.

132. National Institute on Drug Abuse. (2006, December). *NIDA-sponsored survey shows decrease in illicit drug use among nation's teens but prescription drug abuse remains high.* Washington, DC, National Institutes of Health, U.S. Department of Health and Human Services.

133. Norris, J., & Kunes-Carroll, M. (1985). Self-esteem disturbance. *Nursing Clinics of North America, 20*(4), 745–761.

134. Ohring, R., Graber, J., & Brooks-Gunn, J. (2002). Girls' recurrent and concurrent body dissatisfaction. Correlates and consequences over 8 years. *International Journal of Eating Disorders, 31*, 404–415.

135. Oldaker, S. (1985). Identity confusion: Nursing diagnoses for adolescents. *Nursing Clinics of North America, 20*(4), 763–778.

136. Ortiz, M. (2006). Staying alive: A suicide prevention overview. *Journal of Psychosocial Nursing, 44*(12), 44–49.

137. Orzack, M. (1998). Computer addiction: What is it? *Psychiatric Times, 15*(8), 2–3.

138. Orzack, M., & Ross, C. (2000). Should virtual sex be treated like any other sex addiction? *Sexual Addiction & Compulsivity, 7*, 115–125.

139. Oswald, L. (1989). Cocaine addiction: The hidden dimension. *Archives of Psychiatric Nursing, 3*(3), 134–141.

140. Papalia, D., Olds, S., & Feldman, R. (2004). *Human development* (9th ed.). Boston: McGraw-Hill.

141. Patterson, K. (2003). Counseling study paints picture of heavier college woes; more students seen with depression, suicidal thoughts. *NAMI Advocate, 1*(3), 20–22.

142. Pender, N., Murdaugh, C., & Parsons, M. (2006). *Health promotion in nursing practice* (5th ed.). Upper Saddle River, NJ: Pearson Education.

143. Pharris, M., & Nafstad, S. (2002). Nursing care of adolescents who have been sexually assaulted. *Nursing Clinics of North America, 37,* 471–497.

144. Piaget, J. (1985). *The equilibration of cognitive structures: The central problem of intellectual development* (T. Brown & K.J. Thampy, Trans.). Chicago: University of Chicago Press.

145. Piaget, J. (1972). Intellectual evolution from adolescence to adulthood. *Human Development, 15,* 1–12.

146. Piano, M. (2005). The cardiovascular effects of alcohol: The good and the bad. *American Journal of Nursing, 105*(7), 87–91.

147. Polk-Walker, G. (1990). What really happened? Incidence and factor assessment of abused children and adolescents. *Journal of Psychosocial Nursing, 28*(11), 17–22.

148. Potts, N.L., & Mandleco, B.I. (2007). *Pediatric nursing: Caring for children and their families* (2nd ed.). New York: Thomson/Delmar Learning.

149. Pritarelli, M., Browne, B., & Johnson, K. (1999). The bits and bytes of computer/Internet addiction: A factor analysis approach. *Behavior Research Methods; Instruments & Computers, 31,* 305–314.

150. Quindlen, A. (2006, March 20). The face in the crowd. *Newsweek,* 80.

151. Reardon, D., & Congle, J. (2002). Depression and unintended pregnancy in the National Longitudinal Survey of Youth: A cohort study. *British Medical Journal, 324,* 151–152.

152. Remez, L. (2000). Oral sex among adolescents. Is it sex or is it abstinence? *Family Planning Perspectives, 32,* 298–304.

153. Rey, J. (2007). Does marijuana contribute to psychotic illness. *Current Psychiatry, 6*(2), 36–47.

154. Roberts, S., & Kennedy, B. (2006). Why are young college women not using condoms? Their perceived risk, drug use, and developmental vulnerability may provide important clues to sexual risk. *Archives of Psychiatric Nursing, 20*(1), 32–40.

155. Santrock, J. (2004). *Life-span development* (9th ed.). Boston: McGraw-Hill.

156. Schapiro, N. (2002). Issues of separation and reunification in immigrant Latino youth. *Nursing Clinics of North America, 37,* 381–392.

157. Scherer, P. (1990). How AIDS attacks the brain. *American Journal of Nursing, 90*(1), 44–52.

158. Schnare, S. (2002). Tattooing, branding, and body piercing. *Women's Health Care: A Practical Journal for Nurse Practitioners, 1*(4), 23–28.

159. Shaffer, H., Hall, M., & VanderBilt, J. (2000). "Computer addiction": A critical consideration. *American Journal of Orthopsychiatry, 70*(2), 162–168.

160. Shellenberger, S. (2007, March). Cutting pain. *Focus on the Family,* 14–16.

161. Shepherd, B. (1999, August). When Moms pray. *Focus on the Family,* 3–5.

162. Smalley, S. (2003, February 3). The perfect crime: GHB. *Newsweek,* 52.

163. Smalley, S. (2003, July 7). The new age of Rave. *Newsweek,* 52–53.

164. Smith, K.M., Larive, L.L., & Romanelli, F. (2002). Club drugs: Methylenedioxymethamphetamine, flunitrazepam, ketamine hydrochloride, and gamma-hydroxybutyrate. *American Journal of Health-Systems Pharmacy, 59,* 1067–1076.

165. Smith-Battle, L. (2005). Examining assumptions about teen mothers. *American Journal of Nursing, 105*(4), 13.

166. Sobie, A., & Reardon, D. (2001). Detrimental effects of adolescent abortion, Part II. *Post-Abortion Review, 9*(1), 4–5.

167. Splete, H. (2005). Technology extends reach of the bully. *Clinical Psychiatry News, 30*(5), 51.

168. Steinberg, L. (2005). Cognitive and affective development in adolescence. *Trends in Cognitive Science, 9*(2), 68–75.

169. Strickland, C., Walsh, E., & Cooper, M. (2006). Healing fractured families: Parents' and elders' perspectives on the impact of colonization and youth suicide prevention in a Pacific Northwest American Indian tribe. *Journal of Transcultural Nursing, 17*(1), 5–12.

170. Suarez-Orozco, C., & Suarez-Orozco, M. (2001). *Children of immigration.* Cambridge, MA: Harvard University Press.

171. Szabo, J., & Goldfarb, B. (2005). Metabolic syndrome rising in adults and adolescents. *DOC News, 2*(1), 7.

172. The addicted brain. (2004). *Harvard Mental Health Letter, 21*(1), 1–4.

173. The adolescent brain: Beyond raging hormones. (2005). *Harvard Mental Health Letter, 22*(1), 1–3.

174. Thies, K. (2006). Development of children with chronic illness. In K. Thies & J. Travers (Eds.), *Handbook of human development for health care professionals* (pp. 381–410). Sudbury, MA: Jones and Bartlett.

175. Thomas, W.P., & Collier, V.P. (1999). Accelerated schooling for English language learners. *Educational Leadership, 56*(4), 46–49.

176. Tuttle, J., Melmyk, B., & Loveland-Cherry, C. (2002). Adolescent drug and alcohol use: Strategies for assessment, intervention, and prevention. *Nursing Clinics of North America, 37,* 443–460.

177. Tyre, P. (2002, March 25). Bringing up adolescents. *Newsweek,* 38–40.

178. United States Department of Agriculture, Center for Nutrition Policy and Promotion. (2005). *MyPyramid CNPP-15.* Washington, DC: Author.

179. United States Department of Health and Human Services. (2000). *Healthy People 2010. With understanding and improving health and objectives for improving health* (2nd ed.). Washington, DC: U.S. Government Printing Office.

180. Wadsworth, B. (2004). *Piaget's Theory of Cognitive and Affective Development* (5th ed.) Boston: Pearson Education.

181. Walsh, M., & Barrett, J. (2006). The roots of violence and aggression. In K. Thies & J. Travers (Eds.), *Handbook of human development for health care professionals* (pp. 355–377). Sudbury, MA: Jones and Bartlett.

182. Warren, J., Gary, F., & Moorhead, J. (1994). Self-reported experiences of physical and sexual abuse among runaway youths. *Perspectives in Psychiatric Care, 30*(1), 23–28.

183. Weincke, J., Thurston, S., Kelsey, K., Varkenyl, A., Wain, J., Mark, E., & Christiani, D. (1999). Early age at smoking initiation and tobacco carcinogen DNA damage in the lung. *Journal of the National Cancer Institute, 91,* 614–639.

184. Weisfeld, G. (1999). *Evolutionary principle of human adolescence.* New York: Basic Books.

185. Weiss, R., Taksali, S., Tamborlane, W., Burgert, T., Savoye, M., & Caprio, S. (2005). Predictors of change in glucose tolerance status in obese youth. *Diabetes Care, 28,* 902–909.

186. White, A., Ghia, A., Levin, E., & Schwartzwelder, H. (2000). Binge pattern ethanol exposure in adolescent and adult rats: Differential impact on subsequent responsiveness to ethanol. *Adolescence: Clinical & Experimental Research, 24*(8), 1251–1256.

187. Wieland, D. (2005). Computer addiction: Implications for nursing psychotherapeutic practice. *Perspectives in Psychiatric Care, 41*(4), 153–161.

188. Williams, B., Ponesse, J., Schachar, R., Logan, G., & Tannock, R. (1999). Development of inhibitory control across the life span. *Developmental Psychology, 35,* 205–213.

189. Wills, T., Ashby, D., & Yaeger, A. (2001). Time perspective and early-onset substance use: A model based on stress coping theory. *Psychology of Addictive Behaviors, 15,* 118–125.

190. Windling, P. (2005). Tattoo taboos? Swiss law will soon regulate pigments, parlors, removals. *Clinical Psychiatry News, 33*(11), 70.

191. Winsler, A., Diaz, R., Espinosa, L., & Rodriguez, J. (1999). When learning a second language does not mean losing the first: English language development in low-income, Spanish-speaking children attending bilingual preschool. *Child Development, 70*(2), 349–362.

192. Witt, R. (2006). Emerging epidemic of lympho-granuloma venereum. *Clinician Review, 16*(5), 56–64.

193. Wodarsky, L., & Wodarsky, J. (2004). Obesity. In L. Rapp-Paglicci, C. Dulmus, & J. Wodarski (Eds.), *Handbook of preventive interventions for children and adolescents* (pp. 301–320). Hoboken, NJ: John Wiley & Sons.

194. Wolfe, J. (2006). How the tobacco industry targets children. *American Journal of Nursing, 106*(11), 13.

195. Wu, L., Schlenger, W.E., & Galvin, D.M. (2006). Concurrent use of methamphetamine, MDMA, LSD, ketamine, GHB, and flunitrazepam among American youths. *Drug and Alcohol Dependence, 84,* 102–113.

196. Yaziga, R., Odem, R., & Polakoski, K. (1991). Demonstration of specific binding of cocaine to human spermatozoa. *Journal of the American Medical Association, 266*(14), 1956–1959.

197. Young, E., & Korzum, A. (1999). Women, stress, and depression: Sex differences in hypothalamic-pituitary-adrenal axis regulation. In E. Leibenluft (Ed.), *Gender differences in mood and anxiety disorders: From bench to bedside* (pp. 31–52). Washington, DC: American Psychiatric Association.

UNIT IV

The Developing Person and Family Unit:
Young Adult Through Death

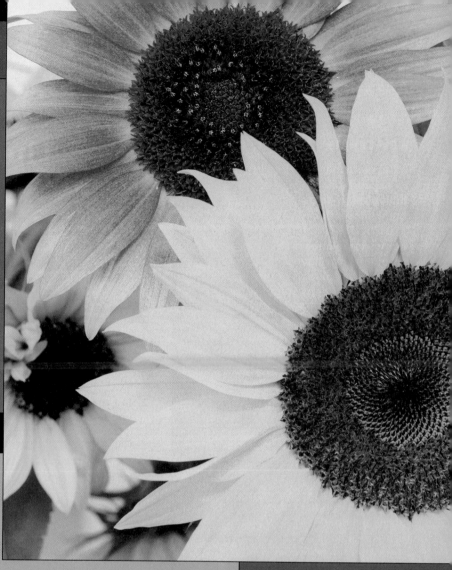

CHAPTERS

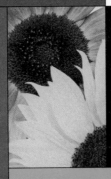

CHAPTER 14

The Young Adult: Basic Assessment and Health Promotion

OBJECTIVES

Study of this chapter will enable you to:

1. Discuss young adulthood as a developmental crisis and how and why the present young adult generation differs from earlier generations.

2. List the developmental tasks of the young adult's family, and describe your role in helping families to meet these tasks.

3. Assess the physical characteristics of a young adult.

4. Teach nutritional requirements to the young adult male and female, including the pregnant and lactating female.

5. Describe factors and health promotion measures that influence biological rhythms and illness, and the dyssynchrony that may result.

6. Relate the stages of the sleep cycle, effects of deprivation of the different sleep stages, and the need for balance in rest, sleep, exercise, and leisure.

7. Analyze the developmental crisis, emotional characteristics, self-concept, body image development, and adaptive mechanisms of a young adult, and determine health promotion implications.

8. Contrast lifestyle options, and describe their influence on the health status of the young adult and health promotion measures.

9. Analyze how cognitive characteristics, social concerns, and moral, spiritual, and philosophic development influence the total behavior and well-being of the young adult.

10. Describe the developmental tasks of the young adult, and relate your role in helping him or her achieve them.

MediaLink **www.prenhall.com/murray**

Go to the Companion Website for interactive resources that accompany this chapter.

Glossary
Review Questions
Challenge Your Knowledge
Learning Activities

Critical Thinking
Tools
Media Link Applications
Media Links

When does young adulthood begin in the United States? Physiologically, growth has ended. A person must be age 18 to vote, 30 to be a senator, and 35 to be president. A female may have her first child at 15 or at 35, or she may have none. Even with these variations, young adulthood in the United States is about 25 to 45 years or later. The *age range for young adulthood may begin* in the *late teens* for members of the middle and lower economic levels who begin a career and support themselves. For those who attend college, young adulthood tasks *may be delayed until the mid-20s, or even later.* Some continue living at home like late adolescents, whether employed or job seeking, into the *late 20s. The age range is being extended past the earlier established 35 or 40 years because* (14, 202):

1. Duration of adult eras is extended as life span is statistically lengthened.
2. Physiologically, more people maintain young adult characteristics longer, on the average, with the practice of health promotion behaviors.
3. More youth delay beginning the multidimensional tasks of young adulthood in order to pursue college-level education.
4. More families delay having children until the mid-30s, which delays achieving developmental tasks of young adulthood.
5. The age for the physiologic marker for the end of young adulthood, menopause, is in the early 50s, in contrast to earlier generations.
6. Cosmetic surgery is utilized to maintain the physical appearance of young adulthood.

Childhood and adolescence are the periods for growing up; adulthood is the time for settling down. The changes in young adulthood relate more to sociocultural forces and expectations and to value and cognitive changes than to physical development. The principles of development described in Chapter 3 apply to this era. ∞

The young adult is expected to enter new roles of responsibility at work, at home, and in society and to develop values, attitudes, and interests in keeping with these roles. The young adult may simultaneously handle work, school, marriage, home, and child rearing. Or he or she may work primarily at one of these tasks at a time, neglecting the others. Related to changing roles, the young adulthood era may be divided into **young-young adulthood**, *age early 20s or 25 years to age 30 or late 30s;* and **late-young adulthood**, *age 35 or late 30s to 45, late 40s, or even 50 years of age* (14, 202).

The definition, expectations, and stresses of young adulthood are influenced by socioeconomic status, urban or rural residence, ethnic and educational background, various life events, the historical era, and the country of residence. This generation of young adults is unique. Many young adults in the United States and other countries have experienced economic growth and related abundance of material goods and technology, the changing roles of females and males, rapid social changes, and sophisticated medical care. They have never known a world without the threat of nuclear war, pollution, overpopulation, and threatened loss of natural resources. Young adults in countries experiencing war, poverty, and underdevelopment may have never known anything but a subsistence or survival mode of life, and their life era may be cut short.

Instant media coverage of events has made the world a small and familiar place (14, 202). Some people are concerned about societal and global issues and are active in political initiatives, Amnesty International, Habitat for Humanity International, medical and health services in other countries, as well as in the local community or church. Some are uninvolved and concerned primarily about themselves. Some offspring of the Baby Boomer generation in the United States have been taught and now live the same values of self-gratification and expectations of empowerment, as described in the section about the Baby Boomers in Chapter 15 ∞ (201, 202). The timing of developmental milestones for many people is being modified.

Family Development and Relationships

The major family goal of the parents of young adults is the reorganization of the family into a continuing unity while releasing maturing young people into lives of their own. Most families actively prepare their children to leave home.

Use the following information for assessment and health promotion with parents of young adults and the young adult family members. Help parents of young adults to understand that, although they are releasing their own children, new members are being drawn into the family circle through their offspring's marriage or close relationships. That the young adult is ready to leave home indicates the parents have done their job. Use the following knowledge to educate and counsel families as they work through concerns about family relationships.

FAMILY RELATIONSHIPS: PARENTS AND OFFSPRING GENERATIONS

In the United States, the young adult is expected to be independent from the parents' home and care, although if the person has an extended education, he or she may choose to remain living with the parents to save expenses. Sometimes the young adult does not leave the parents' home as quickly as parents would like. With the increasing number of separations and divorces, the uncertain job market, and the cost of establishing a residence/home, the young adult offspring may move back home, sometimes with children and spouse. Emancipation from parents may not occur for years. Parents may resent the intrusion. More than one mother has said, "My child is 30, and I don't think he's ever going to leave home. I'm tired of being his cook, his cleaning maid, his laundress, his therapist, and his bank." If the young adult does live at home, he or she should expect (and be expected) to assume a share of the home responsibilities and to adjust lifestyle to that of the parents, to whom the home belongs. Sometimes the adult offspring can be a real help to the parents. Eventually the parents may have to ask the adult offspring to move out so that both parents and offspring can resume achieving their developmental tasks.

Some parents delay this emancipation process because of their own needs to hold onto their offspring. They may have a strong desire to be needed by or wish to continue living vicariously through their children. However, families have much less control over the lifestyle, vocational choice, and friends or eventual mate of their offspring than they did in earlier generations. For emancipation to occur, the parents must trust their offspring, and the offspring must feel the parents' concern, support, and confidence in his or her ability to work through situations.

In a family with several children, the parents may anticipate having the older children leave. The parents then have less responsibility, and the remaining children get the benefit of a less crowded home and more parental attention. At the same time, the emancipated offspring can still use home as a place to return during times of stress. The younger children may be more reluctant later on to leave home.

Often family expenses are at a peak during this period as parents pay for education and weddings or finance their offspring while they establish their own home or profession. Young adults will earn what they can, but they may not be able to be financially independent even if they are no longer living at home. Both parents may work to meet financial obligations. As young adult offspring establish families, parents should take the complementary roles of letting go and standing by with encouragement, reassurance, and appreciation.

Often the main source of conflict between the parents and young adult offspring is the difference in philosophy and lifestyle between the two generations. The parents who sacrificed for their children to have a nice home, material things, education, leisure activities, and travel may now be criticized for how they look, act, and believe. In fact, the young adult may insist that he or she will *never* live like the parents.

Help the parents resolve that their grown children will not be carbon copies of themselves. Validate for parents that they can take solace in knowing that usually the basic values they instilled within their children will remain their basic guidelines, although outward behavior may seem different. (Often behavior will not be that much different.) Help parents realize the importance of their acceptance and understanding of their offspring and of not deliberately provoking arguments over ideologies.

Reinforce the parents as they provide a secure home base, both as a model for the young adult and to reduce feelings of threat in the younger children. Although the parents are withstanding the criticism from their grown children, validate that younger children in the home will be feeling conflict, too. The parents are still identification models to them, but young children and adolescents value highly the attitudes and judgments of young adult siblings, who, in turn, can have a definite influence on younger children. Explore how the parents can help the younger children realize that there are many ways to live and that they will encourage each to find his or her own way when the time comes.

PARENTAL FAMILY DEVELOPMENTAL TASKS

Gradually the parents themselves must shift from a household with children to a couple again as the last young adult establishes a home. Family structure, roles, and responsibilities change, and use of space and other resources change. In summary, *the tasks to be accomplished by the family of the young adult include to* (61):

1. Rearrange the home physically and reallocate resources (space, material objects) to meet the needs of remaining members.

2. Meet the expenses of releasing the offspring and redistribute the budget.

3. Redistribute the responsibilities among grown and growing children and finally between the husband and wife or between the adult members living in the household, on the basis of interests, ability, and availability.

4. Maintain communication within the family to contribute to harmony and happiness while remaining available to the young adult and other offspring.

5. Enjoy companionship and sexual intimacy as a couple while incorporating changes.

6. Widen the family circle to include the close friends, partners, or spouses of the offspring and the entire family of in-laws. This task may be reworked more than once (in case of offspring divorce) or in nontraditional ways (in case of same-sex partners, adoptive families, or multicultural families).

7. Reconcile conflicting loyalties and philosophies of life.

Your listening, teaching, and counseling may assist parents of adult offspring to achieve their developmental tasks. Explore their feelings related to challenges. Encourage the family to seek support from their elder family members, as well as from friends.

Physiologic Concepts and Physical Characteristics

Use the following information to educate the young adult about normal characteristics, expected changes in this era, and measures to maintain physiologic stability and health. Use this information in your assessment and health promotion intervention.

Although body and mind changes continue through life, physical growth is completed. Changes that occur during adult life are different from those in childhood; they occur more slowly and in smaller increments. The average life expectancy in the United States today is 77 years (201). Life expectancy at birth is currently 75 in males and 80 years in females. The X chromosome is protective of longevity (101). Young adulthood is the life era when most people are in their peak for strength, energy, and endurance (181). All body systems are at the optimal level of function (26, 66, 181, 201). **Organ reserve**, *the capacity each organ has for responding to unusually stressful events or conditions that require intense or prolonged effort,* is high (26, 201).

Observe and remember racial physiologic differences (80). For example, in a Black person's skin, a red glow is typically present. Color changes due to illness, such as anemia or jaundice, are difficult to detect in very dark-skinned people, as they may also have darkly pigmented lips and nail beds. Sunlight is the best for skin assessment, or assessment should be done in a well-lighted room with no glare. *Pallor, cyanosis, or jaundice can be assessed by inspecting the conjunctiva and oral membranes. Jaundice appears as yellowish discoloration of the palms, the soles of feet, and the sclera* (80).

WEIGHT AND HEIGHT
Calculation of Body Mass Index: Health Implications

Weight, a measurement of mass, is expressed as kilograms (kg) or pounds (lb). Females have usually reached full height by 16 to 18 years. Males may reach full height by 18 years; some grow another inch before age 25 (26, 39, 181, 201). **Norms** *denote a set standard of development or the average achievement of a group. However, there is probably no average adult person. Each person is an individual. Normal values cover a wide range of healthy individuals. Height and weight depend on many factors* (26, 39, 181, 201): (a) heredity, (b) gender, (c) socioeconomic level, (d) childhood and adult food habits and preferences, (e) level of activity, and (f) emotional and physical environments. Weight loss or gain and norms for height and weight are difficult to determine. Most height and weight tables do not consider the individual and specific influencing factors; they usually record either average weight for a given height and age or ideal or desirable weight for a specific height. The **average weight** is a *mathematic norm, found by adding the weights of many people and dividing by the number in the sample* (26, 39, 181, 201). The body has a **set point**, *the weight that is maintained when no effort is made to gain or lose weight,* and the weight that is felt as most comfortable by the person (201).

Obesity is an epidemic in the United States. The average weight for all ages, sex, and races is increasing. Adult males and females are about an inch taller than they were in 1960 but are nearly 30 pounds heavier on average. Average weight for males ages 20 to 74 years rose from 166.3 pounds in 1960 to 191 pounds in 2002. Average weight for females ages 20 to 74 years increased from 140 pounds in 1960 to 164.3 pounds in 2002 (38). Females have twice as much body fat as men. In females, adipose is concentrated in the breasts and hips. In males, there is more adipose in the abdomen (90, 201). Desirable weight for height is now calculated by utilizing body mass index formulas rather than actuarial tables for height and weight (38).

Body mass index (BMI) *is a single number representing the ratio of height to weight, without regard for gender, and the risk for health problems associated with weight.* The measurement system is replacing the insurance tables for height and weight. There are several formulas to determine BMI (38, 60, 62). One formula is (62):

$$\text{Body mass index (BMI)} = [\text{Weight in kilograms} \div (\text{Height in cm} \div \text{Height in cm})] \times 10,000$$

Another formula to determine BMI follows (60, 62):

$$\text{BMI} = \frac{703 \times \text{weight in pounds}}{(\text{height in inches})^2}$$

The BMI is also calculated by dividing weight in kilograms by height in meters squared (38). For example, a person who weighs 180 pounds and is 5 feet 5 inches would have a BMI of 30. The following depicts a calculation:

Body Mass Index (BMI), kg/m²

1. **Convert body weight to kilograms.**
   (1 kilogram = 2.2 pounds)

   Body weight (pounds) ÷ 2.2 = weight (kilograms)
   Example: 132 pounds ÷ 2.2 = 60 kilograms

2. **Convert height to meters.**
   (1 meter = 39.37 inches)

   Height (inches) ÷ 39.37 = height (meters)
   Example: 65 inches ÷ 39.37 = 1.65 meters

3. **Calculate BMI.**

   Weight (kg) ÷ height (m)² = BMI
   Example: 60 kg ÷ (1.65 m × 1.65 m) = 22.03 BMI

4. **Check BMI against risk for health problems related to body weight.**

   See **Figure 14-1**, which depicts another formula for **calculating BMI in overweight and obese children/adolescents and adults** (38).

   Health risks increase as the BMI increases (60, 62). A source of comprehensive information about BMI and risk factors is the Centers for Disease Control (CDC) Website, www.cdc.gov.

   The World Health Organization (WHO) estimates that, worldwide, over 1 billion people are overweight. If current trends continue, that number will increase to 1.5 billion by 2015 (170). People with a higher percentage of body fat tend to have a higher BMI than those who have a greater percentage of muscle. *A BMI of 25 is considered* **overweight.** *A BMI of 30 is* **obese.** During 1999 to 2002, the mean weight for young adults about 20 years old was 190 pounds in males 5 feet 9 inches, and 163 pounds in females 5 feet 4 inches (170, 178, 247).

   Overweight and obesity are risk factors for cardiovascular disease, the number-one cause of death (over 17 million deaths every year). There is a global shift in diet toward increased energy (fat

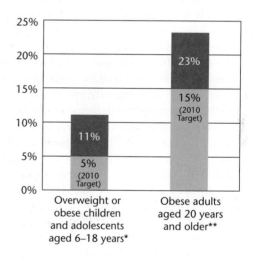

* In those aged 6 to 19 years, overweight or obesity is defined as at or above the sex- and age-specific 95th percentile of body mass index (BMI) based on CDC Growth Charts: United States.

** In adults, obesity is defined as a BMI of 30 kg/m² or more; overweight is a BMI of 25 kg/m² or more.

Body mass index (BMI) is calculated as weight in kilograms (kg) divided by the square of height in meters (m²) (BMI = weight[kg]/height[m²]). To estimate BMI using pounds (lbs) and inches (in), divide weight in pounds by the square of height in inches. Then multiply the resulting number by 704.5 (BMI = weight[lbs]/height[in²] X 704.5).

FIGURE 14-1 Body mass index formula calculation to define overweight and obesity in children/adolescents and adults.

Source: Centers for Disease Control and Prevention, National Center for Health Statistics. National Health and Nutrition Examination Survey. 1988–94. *Health People 2010.*

and sugar), increased salt, and a trend toward decreased physical activity due to the sedentary nature of modern work, better transportation, and increasing urbanization (60).

The WHO estimates more than 75% of females over 30 years are now overweight in countries as diverse as Barbados, Egypt, Malta, Mexico, South Africa, Turkey, and the United States. Estimates are similar for males, with over 75% now overweight in, for example, Argentina, Germany, Greece, Kuwait, New Zealand, Samoa, and the United Kingdom. The people in the Western Pacific islands of Nauru and Tonga have the highest global prevalence of overweight, with nine out of every ten adults being overweight (170).

Overweight and obesity-related health problems substantially raise the risk for hypertension, high cholesterol, type 2 diabetes, heart disease and stroke, pulmonary and gallbladder disease, arthritis, sleep disturbances and problems breathing, and certain types of cancers. In addition, the risk for osteoarthritis, joint problems, and back pain increases with obesity (195, 201). Weight increase with age may increase risk of premature death from heart disease, diabetes, and certain cancers. Physical diseases are coupled with lower self-esteem from social stigma and discrimination (201).

Over 50% of adults in the United States are estimated to be overweight or obese. Obesity is more prevalent in selected populations, such as among African American and Mexican American females with lower incomes, in contrast to Caucasian females, with lower incomes. Among African Americans, the proportion of females who are obese is 80% higher than the proportion of males who are obese (236).

Spontaneous losses in body weight following low-fat diets with a reduction of the carbohydrate-to-protein ratio show promising outcomes. Exercise training increases energy expenditure, promoting changes in body composition and body weight while keeping dietary intake constant. Research suggests exercise, with dietary restriction and strength training, has even greater implications in decreasing body fat percentage (224). The new guidelines do not allow a weight gain in the late 30s, early 40s, or middle age. It is recommended that the weight of the mid-20s be maintained as the baseline for life, if that weight was normal (224).

Body Fluids: A Component of Weight

Total body water content varies with age, gender, and body fat content. For the typical male, 60% of body weight is constituted of intracellular or extracellular fluids, in contrast to 50% in the typical female. **Extracellular fluid (ECF)** *is divided into two components:* **plasma** *(intravascular)* and **interstitial** *(tissue fluid or fluid that exists between cells).* Part of ECF is also the **transcellular fluids,** *secretions from epithelial cells,* such as found in the respiratory tract, salivary glands, gastrointestinal and biliary tracts, pancreas, liver, sweat glands, eye cavities, and cerebrospinal fluid. Of the total body fluids, 66% exists in the intracellular space, primarily in skeletal muscle mass, and 33% of body fluids are in the plasma space. Adipose (fat) cells contain little water compared to lean tissue. Thus, females and the elderly typically have less fluid-related body weight than males because they have proportionately more body fat. Obese females have considerably less fluid (160). After age 40 years, total body fluid decreases for both males and females. The gender differentiation remains (160). Electrolyte composition and the homeostatic mechanisms of body systems, kidneys, heart, lungs, and the pituitary, adrenal, and parathyroid glands involve complex processes. Several texts present in-depth information (90, 160).

The young adult typically maintains fluid and electrolyte balance. However, illness or extreme stress on the body may contribute to dehydration. *Signs and symptoms of dehydration—less severe to more severe—include* (160):

1. Thirst, desire to drink, decreased tear production.
2. Vital sign changes: elevated body temperature, tachycardia, decreased pulse volume, decreased blood pressure.
3. Dry mouth and loss of tongue **turgor** *(elasticity)* with mouth breathing. Gums and cheeks remain moist even when lips and tongue are dry. Tongue turgor is not affected by age; loss of turgor is a reliable sign.
4. Pinched facial expression, sunken eyes caused by decreased intraocular pressure.
5. Decreased skin turgor, which is best measured by picking up a pinch of the skin over the forehead, sternum, or inner aspects of the thighs.
   a. In children, skin turgor decreases after 3% to 5% of body weight is lost or if there is severe malnutrition.
   b. In people over 60 years of age, skin turgor is normally less taut or decreased.
6. Complaints of fatigue; behavioral changes.
7. Pale, cool skin due to vasoconstriction, a compensation for hypovolemia.
8. Neuromuscular changes, unsteady gait, uncoordinated movements.
9. Changes in filling of neck veins, if the person is not in heart failure.
10. Slow capillary refill when pressure is applied for 5 seconds and then released. Normal color should return in 1 to 2 seconds in a healthy person.
11. **Oliguria,** *reduced urine output.*
12. Loss of body weight.
13. **Edema,** *excess accumulation of interstitial fluid,* either localized or general, due to electrolyte changes or a concurrent disease state.

MUSCULOSKELETAL SYSTEM

Babies are born with 270 soft bones—about 64 more than an adult. By the age of 20 to 25 years, many of these are fused together into 206 hard, permanent bones (195). Skeletal growth for the young adult is completed by age 25, or sooner, when the epiphyseal line calcifies and fuses with the main shaft of the long bones. The vertebral column continues to grow until the individual reaches age 25 years; 3 to 5 mm may be added to an individual's height, especially in males. Males grow 10% taller than females. Male hormones promote growth of the long bones (90, 201). Smaller leg bones, the sternum, pelvic bones, and vertebrae attain adult distribution of the red marrow by approximately 25 years of age. By the early 40s, the bones will begin to lose some mass and density unless the person practices preventive diet and exercise measures (60, 62). The process begins earlier in females than males. With increasing age, the cartilage in all joints has a more limited ability to regenerate itself. Normally, posture is erect (181, 195).

Body systems are functioning at their peak efficiency, and the individual has reached optimum physiologic and motor function and stamina. Muscle growth is complete at age 30. Peak muscle strength is attained, and maximum physical potential occurs between the ages of 19 and 30. However, the young adult can extend this "biological window" of peak performance to a later age, as evidenced by professional athletes (201) and by people who work in manual labor (e.g., farmers, dock hands, construction or building trades). A 10% loss of strength occurs gradually between the ages of 30 and 60. This loss usually first occurs in the back and leg muscles. A person can maintain peak performance through the 30s and much of the 40s, however, with regular exercise and dietary moderation (26, 60, 62, 181). Social history is very relevant to bone and joint development. Anorexia and bulimia increase the risk of fractures. Tobacco and alcohol delay wound healing (195).

SKIN

The skin is the largest organ of the human body. The skin of the young adult is smooth, and skin turgor is taut. *The functions of the skin include* (181, 195): (a) prevention of fluid loss; (b) barrier to invading organisms; (c) sensations of touch, temperature, and pain; (d) regulation of body temperature and blood pressure; (e) synthesis of vitamin D; and (f) excretion of sweat, urea, and lactic acid. In late-young adulthood the skin begins to lose moisture, becoming more dry and wrinkled. Smile lines and lines at the corners of the eyes are usually noticeable.

Acne usually disappears in the young adult because sex hormones have less influence on secretion of oils from sebaceous glands of the skin. The skin of the African American may manifest some conditions that are not seen or are manifested differently in Caucasians, such as hypopigmentation, keloids, pigmentary disorders, **pseudofolliculitis** *(razor bumps),* and alopecia (8).

CARDIOVASCULAR SYSTEM

Maximum physical potential is reached in young adulthood so far as muscles and internal organs are concerned. Heart and circulatory changes occur gradually with age, depending on exercise and diet patterns. During young adulthood, the total blood volume is 70 to 85 ml/kg of body weight. **Cardiac output** is defined as *the volume of blood pumped by the heart (the total blood flow in the body) to the systemic circulation.* Cardiac output is dependent on the heart rate and the stroke volume (cardiac output = heart rate × stroke volume). **Normal cardiac function** is defined as *the volume of blood ejected per unit time and is described as the product of the heart rate and stroke volume* (148).

Maximum cardiac output is achieved and peaks between 20 and 30 years of age. The male's heart weighs an average of 10 oz and the female's an average of 8 oz. Heart rate averages 72 beats per minute. The blood pressure gradually increases, reaching 100 to 120 mmHg systolic and 60 to 80 mmHg diastolic. Heart and blood vessels are fully mature, and cholesterol levels increase (90, 249).

Blood pressure *is the conducting force of blood flow in organs and tissues* (148). Maintaining **normal blood pressure** *(120/80 mmHg)* *is considered optimal and reduces risk for later heart disease and strokes* (148). Functional classification and management of normal blood pressure is now recognized as less than 120/80 by the New York Heart Association (44, 237, 249). **Prehypertension** *is recognized as a systolic blood pressure between 120 and 139 and a diastolic blood pressure between 80 and 89* (166). A blood pressure of 140/90 mmHg or higher is an indicator of need for prescribed medication and lifestyle changes (166, 237). Unfortunately, due to unhealthy lifestyles (smoking, obesity, drug use), hypertension associated with heart failure is now seen in the young adult (237).

The Coronary Artery Risk Development in Young Adults (CARDIA) study indicated that time urgency/impatience and hostility were the most significantly associated with risk of developing hypertension at 15-year follow-up (254). No relationship was found for achievement striving/competitiveness, depression, or anxiety. Race and gender were not associated with long-term risk of hypertension (254). However, females have more elastic blood vessels than males related to estrogen (90, 201), which has implications for cardiovascular health. However, the study by Peters (186) indicated relationship between racism, chronic stress, emotions, and blood pressure. The National Heart, Lung, and Blood Institute releases guidelines for normal blood pressure and hypertension. The Website is www.nhlbi.nih.gov.

Caucasian norms do not consistently apply to people from other racial backgrounds. For example, in Caucasian diagnostic norms, an inverted T wave is a pathologic cardiac finding. However, in African Americans, especially males, it is to be expected (80).

B-type natriuretic peptide (BNP) is a substance secreted from the ventricles or lower chambers of the heart in response to changes in pressure that occur when heart failure develops and worsens. The level of BNP in the blood increases when heart failure symptoms worsen, and decreases when the heart failure condition is stable. The BNP level in a person with heart failure—even someone whose condition is stable—is higher than in a person with normal heart function and has potentially important diagnostic, therapeutic, and prognostic implications (40, 41, 168).

Arteries become less elastic as we age. Hemorrhoids and other varicose veins may become health problems, especially in the childbearing female (70).

RESPIRATORY SYSTEM

Since birth, the lungs have increased in weight 20 times. Breathing becomes slower and deeper, 12 to 20 breaths per minute (195). The maximum breathing capacity decreases between ages 30 and 60. Breathing rate and capacity will differ according to the size of the individual. Larger people have a slower rate (70).

GASTROINTESTINAL SYSTEM

The *digestive organs* function smoothly during this period of life. Stomach capacity is 2,000 to 3,000 ml. The amount of ptyalin decreases after 20 years of age, and digestive juices decrease after 30 years of age. *Dental maturity* is achieved in the early 20s with emergence of the last four molars (wisdom teeth) (90, 201). Some people must have their wisdom teeth extracted because they become impacted and cause pain.

NEUROLOGIC SYSTEM

The *brain* continues to grow into adolescence and young adulthood and reaches its maximum weight and size during adulthood.

MediaLink National Heart, Lung and Blood Institute

Practice Point

Some young adults wear corrective glasses, contact lenses, or hearing aids. Assess for them when you are giving emergency care, especially if the person is unconscious, so that they are not lost or the person does not suffer eye or ear injury. Information on how to remove contact lenses from another person's eyes can be obtained from your local optometry association, optometrist, or ophthalmologist.

Mature patterns of brain wave activity do not appear until age 20; maturation continues to age 30. Dendrites continue to branch or be pruned (lost) as in earlier years, depending upon use of various skills. Nerve conduction velocity is at maximum functional capacity (90). The sensory status changes little (201).

Visual and auditory sensory perceptions should be at their peak (e.g., 20/20 vision). Gradually during late-young adulthood the lenses of the eyes lose elasticity and begin to have difficulty changing shape and focusing on close objects. However, by age 30 the changes are seldom sufficient to affect function of the eye (181, 201). Kemper & McDowd (119) used eye-tracking technology to examine young and older adults' online performance in reading. Participants read target sentences and answered comprehension questions following each sentence. Online measures revealed no age differences in text processing. However, young adults did have an advantage over older adults in overall reading time and text comprehension. Older adults are less able than young adults to distinguish target and distracter information held in working memory (119). Hearing remains constant for the individual. Females in this age group can detect high auditory tones better than males (201).

Although the *human brain is similar in males and females, gender differences exist in the neurologic system* (90, 201):

1. The part of the *hypothalamus* responsible for sexual behavior is larger in males than females.
2. Part of the **corpus callosum,** *bands of tissue through which the two brain hemispheres communicate,* is larger in females than males.
3. Areas of the *parietal lobe* responsible for vision and spatial skills are larger in males than females.
4. Areas of the brain (*cerebrum, limbic tissue*) involved in emotional responses are more active in females than males.

Implications are apparent for differences in what is considered traditional role behavior.

ENDOCRINE SYSTEM

Adrenal secretion of cortisol decreases approximately 30% over the entire adult life span. Because plasma cortisol levels remain constant in young adulthood the person maintains good response to stress. **Basal metabolic rate (BMR),** the *body's consumption of oxygen and minimum calories required to fuel the involuntary or metabolic life processes of the body at rest after a 12-hour fast,* is at maximum functional capacity at age 30. BMR decreases gradually, which is related to decrease in the mass of muscle tissue, which is

a large oxygen-consuming tissue (60, 62). A gradual decrease in *thyroid hormone* is an adjustment to the progressively slower metabolic rate. The blood level of thyroxine (T_4) falls approximately 15% over the adult life span. The blood level of triiodothyronine (T_3), the active thyroid hormone, declines only when the person is ill and not eating. In females, *estrogen* and *progesterone* levels fluctuate. Changes are indicated by the monthly menstrual cycle (90).

SEXUALITY AND SEXUAL DEVELOPMENT
Sexual Maturity

Sexual maturity for males is usually reached in the teens, but sexual drive remains high through young adulthood. The Leydig cells, the source of male hormones, decline in number after age 25 (90). In healthy females, menstruation is well established and regular. Female organs are fully matured; the uterus reaches maximum weight by age 30. The optimum period for reproduction is between 20 and 30 years of age (90).

Sexuality may be defined as a *deep, pervasive aspect of the total person, the sum total of one's feelings and behavior as a male or female, the expression of which goes beyond genital response.* Sexuality includes **sex** or **gender identity,** the *sense of self as male, female,* **bisexual** *(feeling comfortable with both sexes),* homosexual, or **ambivalent** *(transsexual).* Gender identity also includes **sex** or **gender role,** *what the person does overtly to indicate to self and others maleness, femaleness, bisexuality, or ambivalence* (253). Throughout the life cycle, physiologic, emotional, social, and cultural variables influence sexuality. Today's society offers many choices in sexual behavior patterns. Personal sexual values are shaped by social class and culture (8, 80). The greatest change in sexuality has been its growing openness (26, 181, 201).

During adulthood *a number of sexual patterns may exist*—ranging from heterosexuality, bisexuality, and homosexuality, to masturbation and abstinence. Most people feel attracted or sexually responsive at some time to both genders. Within each of these patterns the person may achieve a full and satisfactory life or be plagued with lack of interest, impotence, or guilt. Changes in sexual interest and behavior occur through the life cycle and can be a cause of conflict unless the partners involved can talk about their feelings, needs, and desires. Many misunderstandings arise because of basic differences between the male and female in sexual response. The more each can learn about the other partner, the greater will be the chance of working out a compatible relationship for successful courtship, marriage, and intimacy. The person cannot assume that the partner knows his or her wishes or vice versa. Each must declare personal needs.

Sexuality Assessment

Follow these guidelines when you are taking a sexual history:

1. Ensure privacy and establish confidentiality of statements.
2. Progress from topics that are easy to discuss to those that are more difficult to discuss.

Sexuality assessment includes the gynecologic examination, breast screening, and Papanicolaou (Pap) smear in the female, and a genital-rectal examination in the male. A history is also part of assessment.

The general sexual assessment plan for the female follows (123):

1. Breast self-examination by the woman monthly after age 19 or 20. Clinical breast exam:
   a. Every 2 to 3 years for women ages 19 or 20 to 40.
   b. Annually for women over age 40.
2. Mammogram every year beginning at age 40.

Klingman discusses in-depth examination of the female external and internal genitalia, the Pap smear procedure and result categories, and the rectovaginal examination (123). Klingman also discusses *in-depth assessment of the male* (122), *the physical procedure, comfort and emotional considerations, and normal findings.* Health assessment is also discussed by Rhoads (195).

As you conduct a sexual assessment, begin with general statements about the assessment to reassure the person and reduce anxiety, shame, and evasiveness. Observe nonverbal behavior while you listen to the person's statements. Do not ask questions just to satisfy your curiosity.

The *following are topics to include in the sexual history:*

1. How sex education was obtained
2. Accuracy of sex education
3. Menstrual history if female, or nocturnal emission history if male
4. Past and present ideas on self as a sexual being, including ideas on body image, masturbation, coitus, childbirth, parenting
5. Sexual experiences—with males, females, or both
6. Number of partners in past year

Practice Point

Respect the person's desire not to talk about sexual matters and moral, spiritual, or aesthetic convictions. Know the terminology and have a nonjudgmental attitude when the person talks about sexuality concerns. Your matter-of-fact attitude helps the adult feel less embarrassed. Be aware of how illness and drugs can affect sexual function. Do not assume that chronic or disabling disease or mutilating surgery ends the person's sexual life.

7. Use of condoms, when started, consistency of use
8. Ability to communicate sexual needs and desires
9. Partner's (if one exists) sexual values and behavior
10. Sexual partners who have AIDS
11. History of sexually transmitted disease in self or partners

Sexuality Education

Because people feel freer now to discuss sexual matters, you may be questioned by the person recuperating from an illness, by the husband or wife after delivery, or by the healthy young adult who feels dissatisfied with personal knowledge or sexual pattern. Be prepared to give accurate information.

Educate that menstruation is a part of sexuality. Refer to **Figure 14-2** to educate about the normal menstrual cycle. Validate that discomforts associated with menstruation may be caused

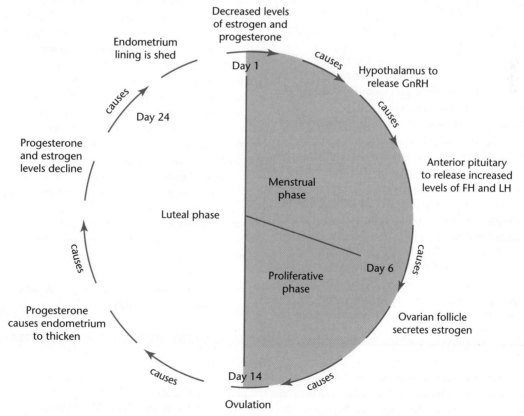

FIGURE ▪ 14-2 The menstrual cycle.
Source: Reference 217, p. 323.

INTERVENTIONS FOR HEALTH PROMOTION

The following are facts about sexuality that you can teach young adults based on research (19, 26, 51, 89, 132, 181, 201, 226):

1. Sexual mores and norms vary among ethnic and cultural groups, socioeconomic classes, and from couple to couple. Sexual activity that is mutually satisfying to the couple and not harmful to themselves and others is acceptable.
2. Sexual activity varies considerably among people in relation to sex drive, frequency of orgasm, or need for rest after intercourse.
3. Various factors and feelings are as influential on males as on females in determining sexual expression. Sexual function is not an uninhibited, mechanical, automatic act requiring only appropriate stimulus and intact physical equipment.
4. Heterosexual intercourse is a reproductive act, but people do not engage in sexual intercourse only for reproduction. Many sexual acts are nongenital in nature but involve people sharing touch, affection, and pleasure.
5. The more sexually active person maintains the sex drive longer into later years.
6. The human sexual drive has no greater impact on the total person than any other biological function. Sex is *not* the prevailing instinct in humans, and physical or mental disease does *not* result from unmet sexual needs.
7. Erotic dreams that culminate in orgasms occur in 85% of males at any age and commonly in females, increasing in older females.
8. The female is not inherently passive and the male aggressive. Maximum gratification requires that each partner is both passive and aggressive in participating mutually and cooperatively in sexual intercourse.
9. Females have as strong a sex desire as males, sometimes stronger.
10. Females have greater capacity than males with regard to duration and frequency of orgasm. The female can have several orgasms within a brief period.
11. Female orgasm is normally initiated by clitoral stimulation, but orgasm is a total body response rather than clitoral or vaginal in nature.
12. The female may need stimulation to the clitoris other than that received during intercourse to achieve orgasm. The female may not have orgasm during sexual intercourse. Overall sexual response is enhanced for the female when there is warm, loving behavior from the

partner before, during, and after intercourse, when foreplay between partners increases arousal, and when she has worked through strict parental admonitions against touching self, enjoying her body, masturbation, or sexual intercourse.
13. Simultaneous orgasm of both partners may be desired, but is an unrealistic goal and occurs only in the most ideal circumstances. It does not determine sexual satisfaction.
14. No physiologic reason exists for abstinence during menses as menstrual flow is from the uterus, no tissue damage occurs to the vagina, and the female's sex drive is not necessarily diminished.
15. No relationship exists between penile size and ability of the male to satisfy the female. Little correlation exists between penile and body size and sexual potency. The female's reaction to penile size or her feelings with penile penetration, however, do affect the male's ability for orgasm and satisfaction.
16. No single most accepted position for sexual activity exists. Any position is correct, normal, healthy, and proper if it satisfies both partners.
17. Achievement of satisfactory sexual response is the result of interaction of many physical, emotional, developmental, and cultural influences and of the total relationship between the partners.
18. Chronically ill or disabled persons learn to live with physical changes and to adapt to express their sexual interests. Underlying fantasies, anxiety, guilt, attitudes toward self, and history of relationships with people affect sexual functioning.
19. In the normal male, spermatozoa are produced in optimum numbers and motility when ejaculation occurs two or three times weekly. A decreased or increased frequency of ejaculation is associated with deceased number of sperm.
20. Decreased sexual desire for either males or females may be related to physical or emotional illness, prescribed medications, use of alcohol or other drugs, changed behavior in the partner, or fatigue from the stress and demands of employment or professional life.
21. Making love and having sex are not necessarily the same, although ideally they occur together.
22. *Avoid the risk of sexually transmitted disease (STD) through* (a) use of abstinence, (b) obtaining honest disclosure from a sexual partner, or (c) obtaining immunization when available (167).

by social, cultural, and emotional factors and hard physical labor, not just by changing hormone levels. Validate females of different sociocultural backgrounds who express different responses. Validate that periods of emotional stress, either happy or upsetting, can cause irregular menses. Emphasize that irregularities in the

menstrual cycle should be checked with the primary care provider or a gynecologist.

Give accurate information and counseling when the person or family asks questions or indicates concerns. Prepare instructional units for a specific teaching plan to share with patients with various conditions, especially chronic diseases, and to be shared with their partners to help them better understand how to meet sexual needs. Give information related to sexual activity rather than personal advice or judgment. Know community resources for consultation or referral when necessary.

Educate about the importance of avoiding sexually transmitted diseases. There are two strategies: abstinence or mechanical protection such as condoms.

Human Sexual Response Cycle

You may be asked to discuss the following information. The **sexual response cycle** *involves physiologic reactions, psychological components, and psychosocial influences or behavior.*

The *two main physiologic reactions of the cycle are* (a) **vasocongestion**, *engorged blood vessels*, and (b) **myotonia**, *increased muscular tension.*

The **four phases of the cycle** are *excitement, plateau, orgasm, and resolution* (150). The phases vary with each person and from time to time. The **excitement phase** *develops from any source of body or psychic stimuli.* If adequate stimulation occurs, the intensity of excitement increases rapidly. This phase may be interrupted, prolonged, or ended by distracting stimuli. The **plateau phase** *is a consolidation period that follows excitement, during which sexual tension intensifies.* **Orgasm** *is the climax of sexual tension increase* that lasts for a few seconds during which vasocongestion and myotonia are released through forceful muscle contractions. Contractions force **semen**, *the milky fluid that contains sperm*, out of the vas deferens, through the prostate, and out of the body via the urethra. The **resolution phase** *returns the body to the preexcitement physiology.* The woman may begin another cycle immediately if stimulated, but the man is unable to be restimulated for approximately 30 minutes (150).

Physiologic requisites for the human sexual response include (a) an intact circulatory system to provide for vasocongestive responses, and (b) an intact central and peripheral nervous system to provide for sensory appreciation and muscular innervation and to support vasocongestive changes. There are detailed accounts of changes that occur in both the genital system organs and other body systems during the four phases of the human sexual response (150, 253).

Sexual Response During and After Pregnancy

Intercourse can continue during pregnancy, although either partner may prefer other intimate behaviors: the female because of discomfort and fear that her appearance may be displeasing to the male, and the male because of concern about discomfort to the female or fetal distress, or because he finds her body less attractive as pregnancy progresses. Although infection from intercourse is a possibility during pregnancy, this problem also applies to the nonpregnant state. Genital cleanliness is always an important measure in preventing infection. Concern for the partner's well-being is also important. Signs of infection should always be reported early to a physician so that treatment can be given.

Sexual response during and after pregnancy varies slightly from the usual pattern. During orgasm, spasm of the third-trimester uterus may occur for as long as a minute. Fetal heart rate is slowed during this period, but normally there is no evidence of prolonged fetal distress. Vasocongestion is also increased during sexual activity in genital organs and the breasts. During the resolution phase, the vasocongested pelvis often is not completely relieved; as a result, the woman has a continual feeling of sexual stimulation. Residual pelvic vasocongestion and pressure in the pelvis from the second- and third-trimester uterus cause a high level of sexual tension (150).

Teach couples that coital activity is prohibited if there is any threat to fetal viability throughout the pregnancy, and during the postpartum period if there is concern about episiotomy breakdown or endometriosis. If there is potential aggravation by the physical nature of coitus with penile penetration, only that form of sexual activity need be avoided. If the problem is one of potential uterine contractility, abstinence from all orgasmic sexual activity, including masturbation of the female, should be recommended. If prostaglandins in semen contribute to the problem, the male should wear a condom during intercourse. If the problem is a combination of the above, all sexual activity with the female is contraindicated; however, sexual activity directed at the male may continue. Couples should always receive specific instruction about continuing sexual intercourse during the last month of pregnancy, depending on the condition of the woman.

Teach couples that such orogenital sexual activity as blowing air into the vagina should be avoided during pregnancy and for at least 6 weeks postpartum. Inflation of air into the vagina may cause air embolism; death may occur. Air embolism is also the reason that douching is avoided during pregnancy and postdelivery (70). By the fourth or fifth week postpartum, sexual tensions are similar to nonpregnant levels, but physiologically the female has not returned to the nonpregnant state. By the third postpartum month, physiologic status has returned to prepregnancy levels (150).

Premenstrual Phenomena

Premenstrual syndrome (PMS) *is a group of signs and symptoms occurring approximately a week before menses and associated with hormonal changes and fluid retention:* mild cerebral edema and edema of fingers, feet, thighs, legs, hips, breasts, abdomen, and around the eyes. Utilize information in **Box 14-1**, Common Signs and Symptoms of Premenstrual Syndrome, to teach physiologic symptoms and signs and emotional reactions that are reported by some females. Not all these signs and symptoms appear together. They are variable in degree, and they decrease after menses begins (70, 139, 181, 249, 253). Symptoms are more likely to appear or increase as females enter their 30s or reach age 40. PMS is not the same as **dysmenorrhea**, *painful or severely uncomfortable menstruation.*

PMS symptoms may appear because of how neurochemicals and hormones interact with estrogen and progesterone (90), and these interactions are affected by nutrition and stress (60, 62). Other factors may be emotional conflicts related to femininity or other emotional stress. Negative attitudes toward menstruation and a stressful social milieu increase PMS symptoms. Females with PMS have more psychological distress and often a mother who had premenstrual symptoms (181). Regardless of cause, symptoms are not evidence of biological or emotional inferiority. For the majority of females, the menstrual cycle is an ongoing part, but not a

BOX 14-1	Common Signs and Symptoms of Premenstrual Syndrome

PHYSIOLOGIC SYMPTOMS AND SIGNS

1. Fatigue, increased need for sleep
2. Appetite change, craving for salty or sweet foods
3. Abdominal distension, swollen hands or feet, puffy eyes
4. Headache or backache
5. Breast tenderness, swelling, increased nodularity just before menstrual period
6. Weight gain
7. Nausea
8. Constipation or diarrhea
9. Acne or hives
10. Dizziness
11. Menstrual cramps
12. Clumsiness
13. Sex drive changes
14. Thirst
15. Proneness to infection
16. Lower alcohol tolerance

PSYCHOLOGICAL REACTIONS

1. Apprehension or anxiety
2. Confusion
3. Forgetfulness
4. Frequent crying
5. Indecisiveness
6. Irritability
7. Restlessness
8. Mood swings
9. Sadness or depression
10. Suspiciousness
11. Tension
12. Withdrawal
13. Difficulty with concentration

Adapted from references 70, 139, 181, 249, 253.

focus, of their lives—one that causes little discomfort. No consistent relationship between premenstrual mood and cognitive function has been found, although some late-young-adult females describe difficulty with concentration. The magnitude of the premenstrual mood change is not typically great enough to affect intellectual functioning (181, 211).

Treatment for PMS may be symptomatic, including hormones to curtail production of estrogen and progesterone, diuretics, antidepressants and antianxiety medications, and serotonin-reuptake inhibitors. Some of the time these medications are not necessary. Dietary measures and exercise are encouraged (60).

Be empathic to the female who describes these symptoms or feelings. Educate the spouse and other family members about their significance, the possible need for medical treatment, and that their caring and reduction of stress may contribute to a decrease in symptoms. Teach measures to affect PMS symptoms.

Ovulation and Natural Family Planning

Educate the couple who seeks information about natural family planning as an option for birth control. Refer to **Figure 14-2** and **Figure 14-3**■, Relationship of menstrual cycle to use of Billings Ovulation Method (natural family planning). Knowledge of the cycle helps the couple to plan for avoiding or achieving pregnancy. Ovulation normally occurs in every menstrual cycle but not necessarily midcycle. The ovum is capable of being fertilized for 24 to 96 hours after ovulation. Sperm survive in the female reproductive tract for 3 to 4 days (90). Share the following information about ovulation, especially with couples who desire natural family planning (195, 242, 249, 253).

The mucus cycle by which to predict ovulation is as follows:

1. The cycle begins with menstruation. The period is usually followed by a few "dry days," variable in number, when no mucus is seen or felt. Intercourse may occur during menstruation if the couple desires and is safe for avoiding pregnancy during the dry days.
2. As the ovum begins to ripen, some mucus is felt at the vaginal opening and can be seen if the female wipes the vaginal area with toilet tissue. This mucus is generally yellow or white, but definitely opaque and sticky. If pregnancy is to be avoided, abstinence from unprotected intercourse should be planned.
3. When the blood estrogen level (derived from the ripening ovum) reaches a critical point, the glands of the cervix respond with a different mucus. This "fertile mucus" starts out cloudy and not sticky and then becomes very clear, like raw egg white. Pregnancy may occur with unprotected intercourse during the period that fertile mucus is developing, is at a peak, and is diminishing.
4. After ovulation, progesterone causes the abrupt cessation of the clear, slippery, fertile mucus and produces a change in mucus, which is sticky, much less preponderant, and sometimes not present at the vagina. Progesterone prepares the uterine lining for the reception of the egg if the egg has been fertilized. Usually the egg is ovulated within 24 hours of the peak of wetness, but this interval may be as long as 48 hours or longer in some females.
5. Although the sticky mucus does not allow a sperm to live very long, the sperm could possibly survive long enough to reach a freshly ovulated egg through a lingering fertile mucus channel.

Teach the following information to the couple who plans spacing of children, or none. If this method is used to avoid pregnancy, there should be abstinence from intercourse from the beginning of the slippery fertile mucus until the height of wetness ("peak day" when there may be so much wetness that mucus is not seen but moisture is noted on the underclothing) *plus a full 72 to 96 hours* to ensure that the ovum will not be impregnated (90, 242). Because the lifetime of the sperm depends on the presence of the fertile mucus, all genital contact between the partners must be avoided if pregnancy is not being planned. The first drop of semen (the one that escapes before ejaculation) has the highest concentration of sperm. The average ejaculation of about 1 teaspoon of semen contains 200 to 500 million sperm. A female may conceive

INTERVENTIONS FOR HEALTH PROMOTION

Teach women that the following **measures can offset PMS symptoms** (60, 62, 139, 181, 249):

1. Consume less caffeine in beverages, colas, and over-the-counter drugs and less sugar, alcohol, and salt.
2. Eat four to six small meals a day rather than two or three meals to minimize the risk of hypoglycemia that accompanies PMS.
3. Snack on complex carbohydrates, such as fresh fruits, vegetable sticks, and whole wheat crackers, which provide energy without excessive sugar.
4. Drink six to eight glasses of water to help prevent fluid retention by flushing excess sodium from the body.
5. Limit fat intake (especially in red meats), which increases levels of hormones that cause breast tenderness and fluid retention. Choose dairy products low in fat.
6. Eat more whole grains, nuts, and raw greens, which are high in vitamin B, magnesium, and potassium, and add vitamin B_6 and calcium to reduce symptoms.
7. Develop a variety of interests, including maintaining exercise routines, so that focus is not on self and body symptoms during this period.
8. Walk and perform other physical exercise at least five times weekly to reduce symptoms of mood swings, increased appetite, crying, breast tenderness, craving for sweets, fluid retention, and depression. Exercise raises beta-endorphin levels, which in turn increases feelings of well-being and improves the glucose tolerance curve.
9. Get extra rest and use relaxation techniques, meditation, and massage. Treat yourself to a relaxing and creative activity.
10. Discuss your feelings with family and friends so that they can be more understanding of your behavior.
11. Join a self-help group to hear other ideas on how to more effectively cope with symptoms.

even if only one drop of semen touches her external genital organ; sperm are powerful, and the fertile mucus is equally potent.

Teach that spotting or bleeding may occur between menses and may be associated with ovulation, a cervical polyp, postintercourse in the presence of cervicitis, or carcinoma (70, 249). Any abnormal pattern of bleeding should be investigated by a gynecologist.

Female Circumcision

Female circumcision, *female genital cutting,* or *female genital mutilation,* is a widespread culturally and religiously based practice in some parts of the world, such as some countries in the Middle East, Africa, Indonesia, and Malaysia. The circumcision may occur the eighth day after birth, the tenth day after birth, at 3 or 4

Menstrual Cycle

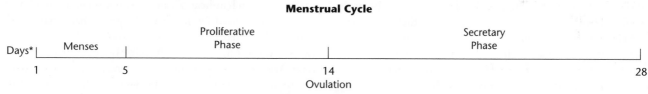

*1st day **menses** (menstruation) = 1st day menstrual cycle

Billings Ovulation Method

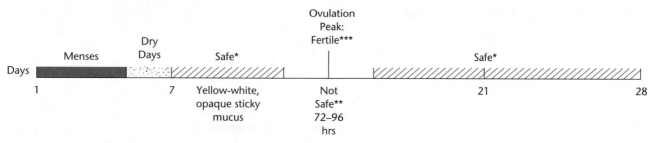

*Safe = Fertilization will not occur.
**Not Safe = Fertilization can occur.
***Fertile Mucus: Clear, slippery, like raw egg white, peak of secretions, moisture felt.

FIGURE ■ **14-3** Relationship of menstrual cycle to use of Billings Ovulation Method (natural family planning).

years, or at 8 or 10 years as part of prepuberty rites to womanhood. In most countries where female circumcision occurs, it is a way to control females sexually, economically, and religiously and to control the heritage line and inheritance. The tradition is practiced among Christians, Muslims, and Jews in some parts of Africa (209).

There are several types of circumcision, classified on the basis of severity. All types of this practice usually are followed by a variety of complications. Initially there is shock, hemorrhage, sepsis, and lacerations to surrounding tissue. Shortly thereafter retention of urine, urinary tract infections, and tetanus may occur. Dysmenorrhea, pelvic inflammatory disease, and infertility are common. After marriage, painful intercourse, perineal lacerations, infections, hemorrhage, frigidity, and severe anxiety occur. During childbirth the scar tissue must be cut during the second stage of labor, or mother and baby may die because of obstruction to delivery, sepsis, or hemorrhage (27, 209, 223).

Some nurses in other parts of the world report their efforts to stop this practice. They report that Western approaches will not work in eliminating this problem because the practice is so traditional. It is generally accepted by females because in countries where it is practiced, the uncircumcised female would not be considered for marriage. These nurses report that as the population becomes generally better educated, traditional practices, including circumcision, decline. Thus, the nurses are heavily committed to promoting general and health education so that a better educated population will pass legislation prohibiting the practice. The media have told of females who emigrated from their homeland to avoid this practice.

You may, in the emergency, maternity, and gynecologic departments, care for circumcised females who have migrated to this country. When you care for females from the non-Western part of the world, assess for circumcision and its effects. Be nonjudgmental. Focus on care that will prevent further complications. Help her gain understanding why this practice may be harmful to her daughters. As the male is the decision maker in these cultures, you will have to establish a working relationship with him if any changes are to be made for the female children. Be aware that female circumcision may be practiced in this country outside of the traditional health care system. Work through your own feelings with a supervisor or counselor. This woman needs a sensitive caretaker.

Variations in Sexual or Gender Behavior

The identity crisis that occurs during adolescence may not be completely resolved by the time the person enters young adulthood chronologically. Identity confusion may lead to confusion over sexual identity and may precipitate homosexual and heterosexual experimentation and arouse homosexual fears and curiosity. Sexual or gender orientation exists on a continuum, from exclusively heterosexual, to **bisexual** (*attracted to both genders*), to exclusively **homosexual** (*attracted to same gender*) behavior. The bisexual person may have a heterosexual family relationship and undisclosed gay or lesbian orientation.

SAME-GENDER RELATIONSHIPS **Homosexuals** are *people who are regularly aroused by and who engage in sexual activity with members of their own gender.* Being a **homosexual man** (*gay*) or a **homosexual woman** (*lesbian*) was accepted by many ancient cultures and is becoming more socially accepted in the United States and Canada.

Views on homosexual behavior vary. Members of some religious groups believe that the biblical scriptures provide the standard for human sexuality, prohibiting homosexuality, as well as premarital intercourse, adultery, and prostitution. Political and legal changes are occurring so that there is less criticism of homosexuality (26, 113, 140, 181, 201). Legal positions vary from state to state in the United States on the rights of gays and lesbians. In Canada, same-sex marriage is legal. Attitudes about homosexuality also vary from culture to culture (8, 80).

Various theories attempt to explain the developmental, emotional, or physiologic causes of homosexual behavior. A number of factors may be involved (4, 26, 120, 165, 201, 228, 258). Same-gender experiences are a part of normal growth and development in childhood and early adolescence (228). Sullivan (228) theorized that the normal homosexual period in life is the chum stage in preadolescence as explained in Chapter 12, ∞ *when the person first cares for someone as much as he or she cares for self.* Although the chum stage involves a very close emotional experience, it may include some touching between the two chums. Sullivan (228) believed that if the person did not have a chum in preadolescence or adolescence, he or she would enter young adulthood still seeking a chum of the same gender. At this point, however, the societal expectation is heterosexuality, and the person's behavior may be interpreted in a sexual rather than emotional way. If the person is rejected by, or is uncomfortable with, persons of the opposite gender, he or she may receive the greatest acceptance (friendship) from others of the same gender. That reinforces the same-gender preference (228).

Some research indicates sexual orientation in males is largely innate and influenced by heredity. The genes that drive homosexuality are inherited from mothers. In one study among identical twins, if one brother was gay, the other brother was gay 52% of the time. Among fraternal twins, the rate was 22%. The numbers were nearly the same for lesbians. How the genes that determine homosexuality interact is undetermined (120).

A physiologic (neurologic and hormonal) basis for homosexuality is being emphasized. An early critical period *in utero* may influence sexual orientation. Exposure of the fetus during the second to fifth months to hormone levels characteristic of females may cause the individual (male or female) to later be attracted to males (90, 181, 201). Research shows that clusters of neurons in the hypothalamus govern sexual behavior. An oval cluster thought to be responsible is twice as large in heterosexual as in homosexual males that were studied (90, 133, 201).

Some scientists theorize that in males a testosterone release starts around age 4 that organizes brain cells toward the opposite-gender orientation. Genes in homosexual boys prompt the same urge in a different direction. Further, environmental, psychological, or cultural triggers may affect physiologic expression (90, 181).

According to Masters and Johnson, the sexual response in homosexuals is the same as that of heterosexuals (149). Family interactions of homosexual partners and heterosexual partners without children are similar (26, 149).

The emphasis is on the relationship between the two people and their love and care for each other. Typically, friends include homosexuals and heterosexuals. If the lesbian couple decide to have a child by artificial insemination, or if the gay or lesbian couple adopt a child, considerable planning is done before the child arrives in the home (140), just as occurs in heterosexual couples. Becoming parents may create emotional problems with each partner's family of origin. Long-term effects on the child are unknown. Some researchers say there are no negative effects on the child raised by two females or two males (140, 201). Others believe every child should be raised by a female and male because each brings a different perspective to child rearing (26, 129, 130, 181, 201, 228). Developmental tasks for the couple during the childbearing and childrearing experience are similar to those of heterosexual couples (26, 61, 201, 253). Gays and lesbians may be able to relate to their biological children as they did before if they decide to leave a heterosexual marital relationship for a stable gay or lesbian relationship (26, 201).

The process of coming out, *openly disclosing one's homosexual orientation,* occurs in four stages, as follows (4, 31, 113, 181):

1. Recognition of being homosexual happens as early as age 4 or as late as adolescence, or later. This time of trying to find self can be lonely, confusing, and painful.
2. Getting to know other homosexuals and establishing romantic and sexual relationships with them diminishes feelings of isolation and improves self-image.
3. Telling family and friends may not be done at all, or at least not for a long time. This revelation can bring disapproval, rejection, isolation, stigma, and conflict. Family members may feel a sense of betrayal, mistrust, and anger.
4. Complete openness involves telling colleagues, employers, and anyone else. In this stage, there is healthy acceptance of sexuality and the self. The person risks negative reactions. Support and acceptance comes from same-gender friends and is likely to come from firm friendships formed with the opposite gender.

People who identify themselves as homosexual evidence a complexity of emotional and social adjustment and diversity of lifestyles, interests, problems, and relationships comparable to those of heterosexuals. There is also a wide spectrum of emotional experience on the homosexual-heterosexual continuum. Contrary to the stereotype, sexual intercourse is not the predominant concern; meaningful relationships with love and companionship are the key (31, 89, 92, 113, 181, 201, 217). Some people demonstrate a homosexual orientation only under extreme conditions, such as imprisonment. Some have their total life adjustment dominated by homosexuality and live in a homosexual subculture. Some remain discreet and secretive about their homosexuality. Others seek out organizations that minister to gays and lesbians who seek heterosexual activity, to marry, and to have families.

The lesbian has not been studied as much as the gay male. It is still more socially acceptable for two females to live together in one household than for two males. There may also be less societal fear of lesbians than of gays. As a result, less is known about the feelings, reactions, lifestyles, or health problems of lesbians (131, 217, 222, 258).

The occurrence among homosexuals of sexually transmitted diseases, such as pediculosis, gonorrhea, syphilis, urethritis, anorectal warts and infection, herpes genitalis (type 1, HSV-1, and type 2, HSV-2), AIDS, intestinal infections, shigellosis, and hepatitis, has been publicized. The rapidly increasing incidence of AIDS has caused some homosexuals to change their sexual practices, to limit the number of sexual partners, or to increase use of condoms. Heterosexual partners also get these diseases through sexual intercourse, and not all homosexuals get them.

Convey a nonjudgmental attitude as you care for, educate, or counsel the person who is gay or lesbian. Often this person feels discriminated against by health care providers (102). This person may be a business executive, minister, inventor, health care professional, delivery person, artist, homemaker, or parent with children. Explore feelings and reactions of children who learn that a parent is gay or lesbian. Give support; discuss coping strategies.

Parents of homosexual offspring are often not considered; they may also need help in coping with the homosexuality. Parents of gay or lesbian offspring may feel too embarrassed or guilty to talk about their feelings. Some believe that they have lost a child. Some grieve at the prospect of not having a grandchild. Some fear meeting a same-sex lover. Acceptance of the fact that their child is a homosexual may be a long time in coming, but most parents eventually reach that point. Listen to feelings and concerns. Help them focus on a wholesome relationship. Caution against punitive behavior toward the offspring, and refer them to a counselor to work through spiritual and emotional conflicts related to the situation. Refer the parents to a local chapter of Parents of Lesbian, Gay, Bisexual, and Transgender Persons (PFLAG) (113).

Consider cultural values as you care for clients and educate or counsel people about sexuality concerns. African American adolescents believe that being gay or adopting a nonheterosexual sexual identity is either wrong, a "White" phenomenon, or a failure to acknowledge the ethnic/cultural community. Asian American youths are least likely to report sexual and romantic relationships. Among Caucasian, African American, and Latino youths, heterosexual dating is projected as normative and promoted as healthy for development (59, 89).

RELATIONSHIPS OUTSIDE OF MARRIAGE Sexual activity outside of marriage may include homosexuality, group sexual experiences, premarital intercourse, cohabitation, or infidelity. Separation or divorce from the married spouse may occur. Refer to Chapter 6 ∞ for more information about the family who has experienced divorce and about stepfamilies. Sexual intimacy without a sense of commitment and love, responsibility, and care for the other person means using another to meet one's needs, taking the other as an object rather than as a person (154, 180, 181, 201). Compatibility between two people is in the head, not the pelvis. The idea of finding a compatible lifetime partner through premarital or extramarital sexual intimacy is not proven.

Cohabitation, *a consensual informal union between two persons of the opposite sex who live together without being married,* is not unusual in the United States. Sometimes the arrangement of the young adult male and female living together is asexual. They are friends and for economic, companionship, or convenience reasons wish to share an apartment. They may perceive themselves as

androgynous, *not tied to traditional gender roles*. Sometimes the person may have had no siblings or no siblings of the opposite gender, and the person wants the experience of living with someone of the opposite gender who would be like a sibling. In such a situation both work to keep the relationship asexual. Most decide whether or not to marry or separate within several years (26, 180, 181, 201, 245).

Young adults sometimes live together in an effort to avoid some of the problems they saw in their parents' marriage or to test the degree of the partner's commitment before actually becoming married. Those goals may be achieved for some, but the danger is that one partner may take the commitment very seriously and the other may use the situation only as a convenient living arrangement. The uncaring person may suddenly decide to leave, an easy process because no legal ties are involved. The other person is left with much the same hurt as a married person going through a divorce. Marriages preceded by cohabitation are not consistently happy and may end in divorce (26, 181, 201, 245). Living together before marriage does not solve problems that might arise after marriage (181). Cohabitation varies from culture to culture, depending on traditional customs and socioeconomic pressures. In the United States, there is an acceptance of the lifestyle (26, 181, 201).

The idea of finding a compatible partner through extramarital sexual intimacy is also unfounded. These arrangements are short-lived, usually less than one year (201). Yet, in this time of high divorce rates, such activity is not unusual. *Various factors contribute to infidelity or cohabitation:* (a) the need to prove masculinity or femininity; (b) difficulty in maintaining a steady and continuing relationship; (c) feelings of insecurity, rejection, or jealousy; (d) a sense of loss when heightened passions of the initial stages of love do not remain constant; (e) getting great satisfaction from doing something different, forbidden, or secretly; or (f) wishing to recapture one's youth.

You may counsel that marriage to one person and living with the frustrations, conflicts, and boredom that is part of any close and lengthy relationship requires constant work by both parties. The person may feel physically attracted to another at times and will have to resolve the feelings within self, through discussion with and understanding from the partner, or with the help of a counselor. Refer to the section on marriage presented later in the chapter.

Nutritional Needs

As the nutrition of childhood set the stage for the health of the young adult, so now the stage is being set for health in middle and old age. Growth is essentially finished by young adulthood. Activity level may stabilize or diminish. Caloric intake should be based on occupation, amount and duration of physical activity or mental effort, emotional state, age, body size, climate, individual metabolism, and presence of disease. A **calorie** or **kilocalorie (kcal)** *is a unit of measure of the amount of energy required to raise 1 kg of water 1 °C* (60, 62).

Basal metabolic rate or **basal energy expenditure (BEE)** *includes the energy spent on digesting, metabolizing, and absorbing food*. BMR accounts for up to 70% of total energy requirements in most people (60, 62). Voluntary physical activity accounts for 25%

to 30% of total calories used. Lean tissue (muscle mass) contributes to a higher BMR than adipose tissue. Females have a 5% to 10% lower metabolism than males of comparable height and weight. In the healthy, nonpregnant state, females need fewer calories than males. The greater the body surface, the higher is the BMR. The obese person, however, requires fewer calories for size because adipose tissue consumes less oxygen and calories than muscles (1 lb muscle burns 35 calories/day; 1 lb body fat burns 2 calories/day); thus less energy is expended comparatively. Calorie consumption depends not only on type of activity but also on duration of activity and weight of the person (60, 62).

NORMAL NUTRITION

Refer to the MyPyramid Website (mypyramid.gov) for nutritional guidelines to make healthy food choices based on gender, age, and activity patterns. Pregnant women should move caloric requirements one to two channels higher. There is no specific plan for everyone. Food guide graphics relevant to other cultures' foods and style of eating are available (62), for example, for African American, Asian American, and Latino populations, and people in Great Britain, Canada, and the Mediterranean area.

There are five major food groups, and some foods from each group should be consumed every day. *Overall the diet should* (60, 62): (a) have plenty of grain products, fruits, and vegetables; (b) contain a moderate amount of protein (about 10% to 12% of total calories); (c) contain limited amounts of sugar and salt; and (d) be low in fat, saturated fat, and cholesterol (20% to 25% of total calories). Trans fat must be avoided as much as possible, as it increases LDL (bad) cholesterol and triglycerides and decreases HDL (good) cholesterol. *Replace fat with fiber foods.*

Eight to ten 8-oz glasses of water daily have traditionally been recommended. New guidelines by the Institute of Medicine state that water intake should be guided by thirst. Water needs vary with activity level, the weather, physical status, age, and gender. Water comes not only from drinking water but from milk, juice, coffee, and tea. About 70% of total water comes from beverages and some food (60, 62).

Potassium requirements have been set at 4,700 mg daily; the average intake is 1,000 to 2,000 mg less. The sodium intake is typically too high (3,000 to 4,000 mg daily); recommended intake is 1,500 mg daily (66). Diet pills should be avoided, unless prescribed (60, 62).

To maintain bone density, the daily dietary intake for women should be 1,000 mg calcium, 700 mg phosphorus, 400 to 420 mg magnesium, 200 IU vitamin D, and 3 mg fluoride (60). Food sources for these nutrients are presented in **Appendix A, Major Sources and Functions of Primary Nutrients.**

Pregnancy

During pregnancy, the BMR increases by the fourth month of gestation. By term, the BMR is 15% to 20% above normal due to increased oxygen demands of the fetus and maternal tissue. At least an additional 300 *calories* daily are needed. Since metabolism nutrients are altered, the primary fuel for fetal needs is glucose. *Fat* becomes the major maternal source of available glucose to the fetus. (Insulin efficiency decreases in later pregnancy to increase glucose availability for the fetus. Thus some females develop gestational diabetes, which usually does not remain.) Seafoods with omega-3 fatty acid are recommended (62). *Protein* intake after the first trimester should be 1.1 g/kg/day, or a daily increase of about 25 g above normal (total about 70 g). Inadequate protein intake increases risk for anemia, poor uterine muscle tone, miscarriage (spontaneous abortion), reduced resistance to infection, and a newborn with shorter length, lower weight, and a lower Apgar score (60, 62). *Vitamin and mineral supplements* are necessary and should contain 30 to 60 mg of elemental *iron*, 0.2 to 0.4 mg of *folacin* (62), and 800 g *folic acid* the first trimester and 400 g thereafter. *Herbal supplements should not be taken* (60). Weight gain during pregnancy is recommended, depending on baseline weight. If underweight, or tall, the woman should gain 28 to 40 pounds. Overweight or shorter-stature women should gain 15 to 25 pounds. Teens and African Americans should gain at the upper end of weight because of the greater risk for low-birth-weight babies. If pregnant with twins, the female should gain 35 to 45 pounds (60).

Lactation

During lactation, the mother's *calorie* intake should increase by 500 to 650, her *protein* intake by 30 g (total 65 g/day), and *calcium* intake should be 1,200 mg for optimum health (60). **Box 14-2**, First-Rate Snack Pack, can be used to teach about ways to maintain energy and nutrition (60, 62).

Fluid intake is critical; 2 to 3 quarts should be consumed daily—preferably water, milk, and unsweetened fruit juice. The mother should drink a glass of water every time the baby nurses. If the mother is a vegan, vitamins B$_{12}$ and D, calcium, and iron supplements are essential. A multivitamin/mineral supplement is recommended (62).

Certain foods should be avoided during lactation because they pass through breast milk and negatively affect mother and baby (60, 62): (a) fish from water contaminated by dioxin, PCBs, or mercury (see Chapters 4 and 8); ∞ (b) alcoholic beverages; (c) caffeine beverages; and (d) foods with an allergy history. Common allergen foods are peanuts, tree nuts, almonds, eggs, fish, and cow's milk. Foods with oils from onions or garlic may cause a taste to the breast milk that is not tolerated by the infant.

Competitive Athletics

Recommended requirements for people who are competitive or elite athletes are (47, 48):

1. Females—at least 3,000 to 3,500 calories/day.
2. Males—at least 2,500 to 4,000 calories/day.
3. Caloric components: protein, about 15%; fat, about 30%; and carbohydrate, 55% to 60%.
4. Protein sources are meat, poultry, fish, legumes, eggs, nuts, seeds, and dairy foods.
5. Fat sources are meat, cheese, eggs, nuts, seeds, oils, butter, margarine, and desserts/snacks.
6. Carbohydrate sources are grains, pastas, rice, bread, cereal, fruits, vegetables, and beverages.

On rest days and short runs, caloric requirements should be closer to the lower end. Refer interested young adults to the Boston Marathon Website, www.bostonmarathon.org.

BOX 14-2 **First-Rate Snack Pack**

Air-popped popcorn seasoned with herbs
Bagels
Breadsticks
Broth-based soups
Cereals, low-sugar, low-fat
Cocoa, low-sugar, low-fat
English muffins
Fresh fruit
Frozen fruit juice bars
Gingersnaps
Graham crakers
Low-fat or nonfat frozen yogurt
Matzoh
Milk shake of low-fat milk and frozen fruit
Pita chips with salsa
Plain nonfat yogurt with fruit and cinnamon or other seasonings
Pretzels
Raw vegetables
Rice cakes
Rye crisps or rice cakes thinly spread with peanut butter or low-fat cheese
Sorbet
Tabbouleh
Unsalted nuts
Vanilla wafers
Vegetables marinated in vinegar or dipped in low-fat yogurt and seasoned with herbs
Whole wheat crackers and cereals
Zwieback crackers

Adapted from Health Information Card, Supplement to Health, Health Magazine, Boulder, Co.: 1999. By Health Magazine. Reprinted with permission from HEALTH, © 1999.

NUTRITION ASSESSMENT

Incorporate nutritional status into nursing assessment and the health history. The oral cavity should be included in a nutritional assessment and at other times of nursing care. **Figure 14-4**☐ presents a form that can be used to assess eating habits and nutritional state. *Ask questions related to the following list to guide your assessment with the person or family* (60, 62, 93):

1. Knowledge of nutrients, food groups, nutrient requirements, and their relationship to health.
2. What increases or decreases appetite.
3. Cultural background, including religious beliefs, ethnic patterns, and geographic area, and the influence on food intake and preference.
4. Relationship of lifestyle and activity to food intake.
5. Influence of income on dietary habits.
6. Knowledge of alternatives to high-cost foods.

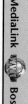

MediaLink Boston Marathon

Record all foods and drinks that you had during the day and during the night.

Day of Week (Circle)   Mon   Tues   Wed   Thurs   Fri   Sat   Sun

Breakfast
Foods/Amounts (cup, tbsp)   Drinks/Amounts (cup, glass)

_____

_____

Lunch
Foods/Amounts (cup, tbsp)   Drinks/Amounts (cup, glass)

_____

_____

Dinner
Foods/Amounts (cup, tbsp)   Drinks/Amounts (cup, glass)

_____

_____

Snacks
Time   Foods or Drinks   Amount (cup, glass, tbsp, or pieces)

_____

Do you take vitamin or mineral supplements?   Yes ___ No___
If yes, please list kind and how many per day.

_____

_____

Do you take any other nutritional supplement?   Yes ___ No___
(e.g., yeast, protein bran)
If yes, please list and describe.

_____

_____

FIGURE ■ 14-4 Form for assessing eating habits and nutritional state.

7. Usual daily pattern of intake: times of day, types, amounts; main meal of day. Evidence of eating disorders.
8. Eating environment.
9. Special diet requirements; food allergies.
10. Relationship of eating patterns of family or significant others to individual's habits and patterns.
11. Medications and methods used to aid digestion and nutrition intake; influence of medications on nutritional intake.
12. Condition of teeth and chewing ability; use, condition, and fit of dentures, if any.
13. Types of food individual has difficulty chewing or swallowing.
14. Condition of oral cavity and structures.
15. Disabilities that interfere with nutritional intake.
16. Assistance or special devices needed for feeding.

Assessment must consider nutrition and disease relationships. Recommend to young adults to *avoid* excess sugar and salt, an abundance of animal products and red meats, and a steady diet of foods in which there are additives and preservatives (especially nitrates and nitrites). Suggest an *increase* in fiber through eating bran or other foods (whole wheat bread, whole grain cereals, raw fruits or vegetables) so that young adults can cut down on disease proneness and improve their elimination pattern. Teach that eating the recommended food groups, exercising, and losing weight are ways

to increase the level of high-density lipoproteins that remove cholesterol from the arterial walls and to decrease low-density lipoproteins that contribute to disease.

OBESITY

Refer to the earlier discussion of obesity in the section on body mass index (BMI). Physiologic effects and consequent diseases were described. Obesity is an epidemic in the United States. In fact, 65% of Americans are overweight (29, 33, 60, 62, 236).

One of the biological factors, in addition to genetics, that is related to obesity is the chemical **leptin**, *produced and released by adipose cells.* Leptin decreases food intake and increases energy expenditure and weight loss when normal concentrations are present. It is involved in the sensation of **satiety**, *being full,* and the percentage of body fat. A reduced concentration may interfere, so that the person eats past the satiety point (leptin concentration). Activity level is also critical. Often the active adolescent becomes the sedentary young adult but does not lower caloric intake. Thus more calories are eaten than are needed for energy (60, 62).

A major psychological factor is how the person thinks about food. Food fills emotional, not just physical, needs (24, 60, 62). Food preferences and amounts are based on childhood and past eating patterns and related emotional needs. Body image—

meaning of body size—is also related. Lower family income contributes to obesity; carbohydrate foods or those high in empty calories are often less expensive and more immediately satisfying (29).

In an attempt to lose weight, the young adult may try a variety of approaches. The most basic approach is to lower calorie intake and increase exercise. A weekly deficit of 3,500 calories is needed to lose 1 pound (60, 62). Cognitive and behavioral individual and group therapy and a support system or group are effective.

Many people can lose weight, but they gain it back as soon as they abandon their diets. An *increase in exercise is recommended rather than a continual decrease in calories, for the following reasons* (60, 62):

1. Appetite is decreased after exercise because of lowered blood supply to the gastrointestinal tract.
2. Exercise may decrease tension and stress, resulting in less frequent eating for nonnutritive purposes.
3. Adequate energy or caloric intake is necessary for efficient use of protein for growth and tissue maintenance.
4. Basal metabolic rate decreases after a period of caloric restriction.
5. Caloric restriction combined with mild exercise can result in greater fat loss and reduced loss of lean body mass than caloric restriction alone.
6. Nutritional adequacy of diets low in energy value is questioned; many of the essential nutrients, especially minerals, are in relatively low concentrations.

According to a survey by the National Weight Control Registry, *the following behaviors help the person lose weight and keep it off for at least a year* (13):

1. Caloric intake of 1,300 to 1,500 calories daily, of which 23% to 24% came from fat. A low-fat, high-carbohydrate diet helps weight maintenance.
2. Eating breakfast, a morning meal, daily.
3. Monitoring weight once weekly, preferably daily.
4. Physical exercise weekly to expend 2,500 calories/kcal in females and 3,300 calories/kcal in males, equal to 60 to 90 minutes of moderate exercise daily.

For more information, refer to the Registry Website, www.nwcr.ws.

The trend is for more obese or overweight females to seek cosmetic surgery to remove excess body and adipose tissue or to remove folds of skin or tissue after massive weight loss (60). These types of procedures carry risk. Careful holistic assessment and an ethical, highly skilled surgeon and health care team are essential for effective outcome. Differentiation must be made: Is the surgery necessary for health or is it related to cosmetic appearance trends primarily?

Generally, a low-potency vitamin-mineral supplement is recommended for persons on calorie-restricted diets. Treatments for the obese person are discussed by several authors (60, 62, 249).

Educate dieters that any special diet must be analyzed for its nutritional value and overall effect on the body. Additionally, suggest a group approach and behavior modification techniques to achieve weight loss.

VEGETARIANISM

The vegetarian is seldom obese. **Vegetarianism,** *abstinence from animal products,* is popular with young adults, but it is not new. Certain religious groups (e.g., the Seventh-Day Adventists) have been effectively practicing a form of vegetarianism for years. In addition to religious reasons, people are vegetarians for moral reasons (opposed to killing animals for food), for economic reasons (cannot afford animal protein), and for health reasons (may believe that a significant amount of animal food is detrimental or that a large amount of plant food is beneficial). Young adults probably fall mainly into the last category.

Vegetarians can be defined as (60):

1. **Pure vegetarians** or **vegans:** *people who eat only plant foods.*
2. **Lacto vegetarians:** *people whose diet includes milk and milk products.*
3. **Lacto-ovo vegetarians:** *people whose diet includes both milk and egg products.*

Utilize nutritional management and education guidelines explained in Chapter 13. ∞ Refer to **Figure 13-1,** Vegetarian food guide rainbow, for information on recommended foods and servings (159). Refer to **Table 13-1,** Modifications in the vegetarian food guide for children, adolescents, and pregnant and lactating women (159). Other recommendations should be taught. Supplementary calcium, iron, zinc, vitamins B_2 and B_{12}, and vitamin D may be needed. Vegans who consume no milk and no eggs must have vitamin B_{12} supplements. If caloric and protein intake is minimal, serum albumin and total serum protein may be low (60, 62, 159).

Eight amino acids are essential nutrients that must be obtained daily in the diet: isoleucine, tryptophan, threonine, leucine, lysine, methionine, valine, and phenylalanine. Cystine and tyrosine are quasi-essential. In addition, infants must have arginine and histidine. The bioavailability of protein depends on proper balance of essential amino acids. Dietary deficiency of any substance may enhance vulnerability to herpes, anxiety, overeating, high blood pressure, insomnia, and other disorders. There is increasing evidence that specific amino acids play important roles in central nervous system function and therefore behavior (60, 62).

Teach about specific dietary inclusions. A wide variety of legumes, grain, nuts, seeds, vegetables, milk, and eggs can supply adequate amounts of required nutrients. Although the proteins in many foods are considered incomplete (in contrast to the complete proteins—meat, fish, poultry, and dairy products—which contain all essential amino acids), certain proteins such as those found in cereals (lysine) and those in legumes (methionine) complement each other when eaten together (60, 62, 159). For example, peanut butter or chili beans (high in lysine but low in methionine) can be served with whole-wheat bread or corn bread (low in lysine but high in methionine). Other complementary combinations are beans and wheat in baked beans and brown bread or refried beans and rice or corn tortillas, lentils and rice in soup, beans and rice in casseroles, bean curd and rice, peas and rye in split pea soup and rye bread, and peas and rice in black-eyed peas and rice. Further, amino acids in milk products and eggs complement plant proteins. Such combinations are cereals and milk in breakfast cereal with milk, pasta and cheese in macaroni and cheese, bread and cheese in a cheese sandwich, rice and milk in rice cooked in milk instead of water, bread and egg in poached egg on toast, and peanuts and milk in a peanut butter sandwich and yogurt (60, 62, 159).

Young adults may idealize about being a vegetarian. Share the information from this chapter. Caution them that being a vegetarian is not necessarily healthy. A meal of soda, cheese pizza, and ice cream is "vegetarian," but as such, it is not healthy. Whether it is healthy depends on the foods ingested—quality, quantity, and type.

CULTURAL INFLUENCES ON NUTRITION

Recommended daily nutrients are depicted differently by different cultures. For example, the traditionally healthy Mediterranean diet pyramid reflects the eating style of people living in Greece, southern Italy, parts of Portugal and Spain, Morocco, Tunisia, Syria, Turkey, and Lebanon. It is high in nonsaturated fat (40% of calories) but is associated with long life expectancy and low rates of heart disease, certain cancers, and other diet-related chronic illnesses. This may be due to high levels of exercise, different lifestyle patterns, and lean body weights (60).

African Americans are frequently **lactose intolerant,** as described in Chapter 5. ∞ The level of consumption of dairy products is low and calcium intake must be monitored. *Foods and cooking patterns and ingredients based in Africa, the Caribbean, and southern United States* are popular with some African Americans. These foods are economical and are well seasoned with salt and fat. For example, chitlins are made by scrubbing pig intestines, boiling them with vinegar for several hours until tender, and serving them with spicy hot sauce. Collard, turnip, and mustard greens contain fiber, calcium, and vitamin A. However, if overcooked, foods may lose fiber and nutrition, especially if the **pot liquor,** *the cooking liquid,* is discarded. The dietary fat and salt intake may create health problems, especially for the pregnant female (8, 29).

Because pregnancy in some cultures is classified as **hot** (*hot-cold theory*), the pregnant female believes she has **high blood,** *excess blood in the body.* Astringent and acidic foods, such as lemons, pickles, and vinegar, or the medicine Epsom salts are used to treat the condition because it is believed that these substances open pores and allow heat to escape. Meats and high-calorie foods are avoided and foods high in sodium are increased, based on hot-cold theory. Thus, the pregnant female may become more iron deficient, and the high-sodium diet may increase the risk for eclampsia. African American females who follow traditional food patterns may have too little intake of calcium, magnesium, iron, zinc, vitamins B and E, and folic acid unless adequate supplements are used (8, 80).

Latino females often follow traditional eating patterns and select foods based on **hot-cold theory,** as described in Chapter 5. ∞ They may have inadequate intake of vitamins A and C, iron, and calcium, depending on specific cultural patterns and supplementation (8).

To the *American Indian,* food has religious, cultural, tribal, social, and family meanings. Tribal/nation-specific rules may be followed to maintain health or balance. Three staples are considered basic or sacred by most of the 550 recognized tribes or nations in the United States: corn, squash, and beans. Many American Indi-

ans are lactose intolerant. Depending on the geographic area and tribe, game, fish, berries, roots, wild greens, and fruits are important food sources. Lack of accessibility or refrigeration may limit consumption of meat and fresh fruits and vegetables. If nonperishable foods are the bulk of the diet, they may be deficient in key nutrients and too high in refined sugar, cholesterol, fat, and calories. Diets on some reservations supply less than 66% of the recommended calories, calcium, iron, iodine, riboflavin, and vitamins A and C. Diets tend to be high in carbohydrates, saturated fat, sodium, and sugar (8, 53, 54).

The health risk for many American Indians is undernutrition with obesity and type 2 diabetes, associated with a loss of traditional food practices and reduced physical activity. There is increased mortality from chronic diseases (53, 54). Conti describes how nutrition models were developed for American Indians in California and the Three Affiliated Tribes in North Dakota. Each model tells the story of food system change and health consequences, using cultural imagery and emphasizing traditional food patterns (54). Such education and support for values and traditions can be effective in nutrition, weight control, and disease prevention.

More young adults are interested in "organic foods" for themselves and their children because of general use of pesticides, herbicides, hormones, and antibiotics in food production systems. For example, nonorganic apples are sprayed up to 16 times with 36 different pesticides to ensure a picture-perfect appearance. **Organic-grown meats, poultry, eggs, and dairy products** *come from animals that received no antibiotics or growth hormones.* **Organic-grown produce and grains** *are produced without use of conventional pesticides, synthetic fertilizers, bioengineering, or radiation.* Farms and companies that process or handle organic foods must be certified that they meet U.S. Department of Agriculture standards. *Two Websites are helpful:*

1. National Organic Standards Board
2. U.S. Department of Agriculture National Organic Program, both found at www.ams.usda.gov.

Cultural food traditions affect females during pregnancy, for example, causing anemia or affecting fetal development. Some females believe cravings must be satisfied, for example, through **pica,** *eating nonfood substances.* Chapter 8 presents additional information. ∞ Other folklore is also followed. One example is to avoid eating craved-for strawberries, because it is believed they will cause a red birthmark. If the female believes the *third trimester of pregnancy is hot* (**hot-cold theory**), foods and medications with iron may be avoided. Cultural food patterns also affect the *postpartal diet. Latino* and *Asian females* may prefer to avoid cold foods (certain fruits, vegetables, and juices) for 1 to 2 months after delivery because they are believed to slow the flow of blood and prevent emptying of the uterus (8).

Discuss that iron (hot) may be taken with fruit juice (cold balance). Teach about the importance of certain nutrients and foods to the baby's and mother's health. Explore foods that are acceptable to her, analyze their nutritional content, and emphasize the importance of their intake. Share up-to-date information. Refer to Chapter 5 for more information. ∞

MediaLink Organic Foods

INTERVENTIONS FOR HEALTH PROMOTION

The following suggestions contribute to nutritional health:

1. Keep a specific record of intake for one week to determine eating patterns (use Figure 14-4).
2. Increase consumption of fiber from fruits, vegetables, and whole grains. Eat a variety of foods and drink plenty of water.
3. Decrease consumption of foods or beverages high in refined sugars or caffeine. Drink more water and fruit juices.
4. Do not add salt to foods during cooking or at the table. Avoid snack foods with visible salt or foods prepared in brine. Instead use herbs, spices, and lemon for seasoning.
5. Decrease consumption of foods high in total fat and animal fat. Replace, at least to some extent, saturated fats (beef, pork, butter, fatty meats) with polyunsaturated fats (fish, poultry, veal, lean meats, margarine, vegetable sources). Keep fat total intake to no more than 20% of daily calories. Limit saturated fats to less than 10% of total fat calories. Avoid trans fats.
6. Substitute low-fat and nonfat milk for whole milk, and substitute low-fat dairy products, for example, cheeses, for high-fat products. Limit cholesterol intake to less than 300 mg daily.

7. Reduce use of luncheon or variety meats (e.g., sausage, salami).
8. Avoid deep fat frying. Use baking, boiling, broiling, roasting, and stewing, which help remove fat.
9. Avoid excessive intake of any nutrient or food. Overconsumption or deficiency of any substance can contribute to disease.
10. Avoid more than a minimum intake of alcohol and caffeine.
11. Educate about use of supplemental vitamins and minerals. Nutrients team up in complex ways. Each food has a variety of these compounds that are synergetic in the natural states, which synthetic vitamin/mineral tablets cannot give (66).
12. Answer questions about the use of **probiotics,** *beneficial microorganisms formed in foods* such as yogurt or probiotic beverages. Supplements are available in the United States. They help to treat or prevent certain diseases because they prevent harmful organisms from getting a foothold (e.g., in the gastrointestinal tract) (98).

NUTRITION EDUCATION

You may be able to advise young adults about nutrition in a variety of settings. Adjust your information to the vegetarians or those who have allergies or specific ethnic or cultural preferences.

Teach about the adverse effects of caffeine. (See Appendix B, Table 1.) ∞ Effects of caffeine can be detrimental to health. Warn also that herbal teas may contain strong drugs that can cause severe problems. Those containing catnip, juniper, hydrangea, jimsonweed, lobelia, nutmeg, and wormwood can be toxic to the central nervous system and can cause severe reactions, including hallucinations (60). People with allergies should stay away from teas containing chamomile, goldenrod, marigold, and yarrow (60). Warn that some herbal teas have twice as much caffeine as a regular cup of coffee (60).

Biological Rhythms

DEFINITIONS

Time structure unfolds as a beginning, middle, and end. **Chronobiology** *is the study of the rhythms of life.* **Entrainment models of timing** *embody the view that the rate and rhythm of everyday events, such as the sleep-wake cycle, engage people on a moment-to-moment basis through attentional synchrony* (152). Rhythms occur throughout the life cycle of each individual.

From the time of birth different body structures and functions develop rhythmicity at different rates. By the time the individual reaches young adulthood, biological rhythms are established by body chemistry and by the **suprachiasmatic nucleus,** *a tiny cluster of cells buried in the anterior hypothalamus* (90). **Biological rhythms** *are self-sustaining, repetitive, rhythmic patterns found in plants, animals, and humans.* The rhythms are found throughout our external and internal environment and can be exogenous or endogenous (10, 76, 152).

Exogenous rhythms *depend on the rhythm of external environmental events,* such as seasonal variations, lunar revolution, and the night-and-day cycle, that function as time givers. These events help to synchronize internal rhythms with external environmental stimuli and establish an internal time pattern or biological clock (76, 152).

Endogenous rhythms, such as sleep-wake and sleep-dream cycles, *arise within the organism.* Endogenous and exogenous rhythms are usually synchronized. Many internal rhythms do not readily alter their repetitive patterns, however, even when the external stimuli are removed. For instance, when a person shifts to sleeping by day and waking at night, as frequently happens with nurses, a transient or temporary desynchronization occurs. Body temperature and adrenal hormone levels are usually low during the sleep cycle. With the shift in sleep and waking, the person is awake and making demands on the body during the usual sleep period. Thus, physical and mental function is not optimal. Three weeks may be needed before internal rhythms adapt to the shift. A similar period of desynchronization occurs when a person makes a flight crossing time zones (25, 76, 128, 152).

Within any 24-hour period, physiologic and psychological functions reach maximum and minimum limits. When a physiologic function approaches a high or low limit, the body's feedback mechanisms attempt to counterregulate the action. *This* **circadian or endogenous rhythm** *reoccurs in a cyclic pattern within a 20- to 28-hour period, even when external factors are held constant.* Body temperature, blood pressure, pulse, respirations, urine production, reproduction, and hormone, blood sugar, hemoglobin, and amino acid levels demonstrate this rhythmic pattern. Similar variations or rhythms in the levels of alertness, fatigue, tenseness, and irritability can also be demonstrated. *When rhythms reach their maximal level or peak,* they are **in phase.** *When various rhythms peak at different times,* they are **out of phase** (10, 25, 76, 215).

Mental efficiency and performance apparently are related to the rhythms of body temperature and catecholamine excretion in the adult. The body temperature rises and drops by approximately 2 °F over each 24-hr period. The body temperature begins to decline near 10 p.m., is lowest on awaking, gradually rises during the morning, levels off in the afternoon, and then drops again in the evening. **Figure 14-5** depicts the diurnal cycle of temperature variations. The level of adrenocortical hormone secretion appears correlated with body temperature rhythms and the individual's state of alertness and wakefulness. The level of adrenocortical hormones rises early in the morning, peaks around the time we typically awaken, and then drops to a low point by late evening (215). Usually the best mental and physical performances coincide with peak temperature, and the least desirable performances coincide with intervals of lowest body temperature. In addition, studies have shown that the lowest excretory rates of epinephrine in day-active people correlate with the time of maximum fatigue and poorest performance. Physical strength crests at different times of the day (76, 215).

Infradian rhythms refer to *biological variations that have a longer, slower cycle than circadian rhythms.* **Ultradian rhythms** are *biological variations with a frequency less than the circadian 24-hour rhythm.* **Masking** *refers to processes that alter the biological rhythms, such as drinking coffee on a regular basis to stay awake* (10).

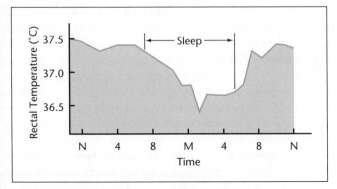

FIGURE 14-5 Diurnal cycle of temperature variations.

Source: From Berger K. J., & Williams, M. B. (1992). *Fundamentals of Nursing: Collaborating for Optimal Health* (p. 446). Stamford, CT: Appleton & Lange.

WORK SCHEDULES

Work schedules should be developed with biological rhythms in mind. You can determine your own circadian patterns to help you gain insight into physical feelings and behaviors and can use this information to plan your days to advantage. You might choose to cope with the most difficult patient assignment or daily task during the time of peak mental and physical performance, for example.

There are increased health risks related to shift work (109, 110, 215). Almost every body system may be affected (76, 215). Nurses, many industrial and law enforcement personnel, and other workers are frequently required to change shifts every week or month. Night and rotating shift workers are at excessive risk for accidents and injuries on the job because of disrupted circadian rhythms. Sleep cycles are interrupted, and persistent fatigue exists. Alertness and other physiologic processes suffer. Eating habits and digestion are disrupted. Constipation, gastric and peptic ulcers, and gastritis develop. Social activities and interactions essential to physical and mental health are interrupted. Family life and relationships are interfered with; shift workers have difficulty fulfilling family and parental roles. Rotating shift assignments are thus relevant to workers' health and quality of work performance (109, 110, 234). Altering the sleep-wake sequence requires time for the person to make adjustments and regain synchrony.

If shift rotation cannot be eliminated, individuals should be required to rotate no more frequently than once a month. Consistently working at night allows a person to acquire a new sleep-wake rhythm. Therefore, night work should be made more attractive to persons who can adapt to the shift and are willing to remain on it permanently. Those who cannot adapt should be exempt from rotation (76, 215).

Educate about the possible consequences of routine rotating shift work in nursing and other occupations. Night workers taking medications should be aware that the effects of medications may vary somewhat from those they usually experience when working days. Drug metabolism varies throughout the day but even more when a person is experiencing jet lag or the early phase of shift rotation. Educate individuals with a chronic illness, such as diabetes, epilepsy, or hypertension and cardiac problems, about the effects of biological rhythms when they plan their medication regimen. Obtain more information about biological rhythms from the National Institute of Mental Health Website, www.nimh.nih.gov.

NURSING ASSESSMENT AND INTERVENTION FOR CIRCADIAN RHYTHM HEALTH

Nursing care should be planned with biological rhythms in mind. With 1-day surgery or the 1- or 2-day hospitalizations, this is difficult or unlikely. However, for the patient who is in the hospital for a longer period of time, for rehabilitation in a long-term care setting, or for repeated admissions due to chronic illness or treatment (e.g., with cancer, uncontrolled diabetes), using knowledge about body rhythms is effective. *Transient desynchronization may occur whenever a person is exposed to the hospital or nursing home stimuli.*

Because cyclic functioning is synchronized with environmental stimuli, physiologic disequilibrium occurs whenever patients are confronted with environmental or schedule changes. New noise levels; lighting patterns; schedules for eating, sleeping, and personal hygiene; and unfamiliar persons intruding on the person's privacy may all contribute to this desynchronization. Disturbed mental and physical well-being and increased subjective fatigue reflect the conflict between the internal time pattern and external events. Several days usually are required before the person adapts to the environment and thereby regains synchronization—normal biological rhythms.

The *nursing history* should be directed at getting information about the patient's pre-illness or prehospitalization patterns for sleep, rest, food and fluid intake, elimination, and personal hygiene. The following questions are a useful guide: Do you consider yourself a "day" person or a "night" person? Do you feel cheerful when you first wake up? What time of day do you feel most alert? What hours do you prefer to work? Why do you prefer these hours? How do you feel when something causes you to change your routine? Answers to these questions will provide you information about the patient's daily patterns. Once this information has been obtained, nursing actions can be initiated that support these established patterns and possibly prevent total disruption of body rhythms during hospitalization.

A *daily log* of sleep and waking hours, preferred mealtimes, hunger periods, voiding and defecation patterns, diurnal moods, and other circadian rhythms *recorded for 28 days before admission to a long-term care facility* can help determine the person's cyclic patterns. Diagnostic tests and certain forms of therapy can then be prescribed by using the person's own baseline rhythm measurements. After a few days in the care center, certain objective data are available that will assist you in further assessment of the person's circadian patterns. You might be able to identify peaks and lows in the vital signs. An intake and output record that shows both the time and the amount voided will aid in determining the patient's daily urinary-excretory pattern.

Vital signs routines should be based on circadian rhythm patterns rather than on tradition or convenience of the agency staff. Both internal and skin temperatures show a systematic rise and fall over a 24-hour period, a cycle difficult to alter in normal adults. *Body temperature* usually peaks between 4 and 6 p.m. and reaches its lowest point around 4 a.m. in people who are active by day and sleep by night. When the internal temperature is normally peaking, other body functions such as pulse rate, blood pressure, and cardiac output (volume of blood pumped by the heart) are also changing. *Pulse rate* is high when the temperature is highest and drops during the night. The human heart rate will vary as much as 20 or 30 beats per minute in 24 hours. *Blood pressure* shows a marked fall during the first hour of sleep, followed by a gradual rise throughout the daily cycle, with a peak between 5 and 7 p.m. *Cardiac output* reaches minimum levels between 2 and 4 a.m., the period of lowest temperature findings (25, 76, 215).

Control some external factors, such as meals, baths, and various tests, to make them more nearly similar to the patient's normal routine. This lessens the stress to which the patient is subjected. Obtaining and using a nursing history constitutes one method of lessening this stress. Monitor medication effects and suggest altered timing for administration. Modify the care plan for the patient's sleep-wake cycle.

REST AND SLEEP

Sleep is a *complex biological rhythm, intricately related to rest and other biological rhythms* (25, 76, 215). Emotional and physical status, occupation, and amount of physical activity determine the need for rest and sleep. For example, workers who alternate between day and night shifts frequently feel more exhausted and may need more sleep than people who keep regular hours. Surgery, illness, pregnancy, and the postpartum state all require that the individual receive more sleep. Mothers of infants, toddlers, and preschoolers may need daytime naps. *Young adults should have 7 to 8 hours of sleep* to maintain physiologic and mental functions, maintain ability to connect memories, enhance performance on difficult tasks, and enhance relationship skills (1, 251). Specific sleep needs are individualized.

Some young people find themselves caught in a whirlwind of activities. Jobs, social activities, family responsibilities, and educational pursuits occupy every minute. The young adult can adjust to this pace and maintain it for a length of time without damaging physical or mental health. The person may think he or she is immune to the laws of nature and can go long periods without sleep. If the person is not functioning well on a certain amount of sleep, the schedule should be adjusted to allow for more hours of rest, utilizing knowledge of personal biological rhythms for rest and activity. Setting aside certain periods for quiet activities, such as reading and various hobbies, is restful but not as beneficial as sleep.

NORMAL SLEEP PATTERN

Sleep is a complex pattern and essential for health (5, 10, 90, 198). Educate young adults to better understand their individual pattern.

The circadian rhythm opposes the sleep drive for about 16 hours daily, which promotes wakefulness. The **reticular activating system (RAS)** is the *functional component of the brain stem that exerts influence on consciousness and the wake-sleep cycle.* The RAS activates the state of consciousness and functions to decrease alertness and to produce sleep. **Electroencephalograms (EEGs),** *recordings of brain wave activity,* vary with the awake and asleep states and at different intrasleep cycles. **Figure 14-6☐ depicts** *changes in electroencephalogram and brain activity during sleep and intrasleep cycles.* When a person is wide awake and alert, the EEG recordings show rapid, irregular waves. High-frequency beta and alpha waves predominate. As the person begins to rest, the wave pattern changes to an **alpha rhythm,** *a regular pattern of low voltage, with frequencies of 8 to 12 cycles per second.* During sleep, a **delta rhythm,** *a slow pattern of high voltage and 1 to 2 cycles per second,* occurs. At certain stages of sleep, **sleep spindles,** *sudden short bursts of sharply pointed alpha waves of 14 to 16 cycles per second,* and **K complexes,** *jagged tightly peaked waves,* occur.

Sleep is divided into stages: (a) **NREM** (*non–rapid eye movement) sleep is divided into four stages—light to deep;* (b) **REM** (*rapid eye movement) sleep follows the deepest NREM sleep as the person ascends to stage II sleep and occurs before repeated descent through stages II, III, and IV* (5, 10, 128, 198, 259).

In **NREM stage I sleep,** the *person makes a transition from wakefulness to sleep in approximately 5 minutes.* The alpha rhythm is present, but the waves are more uneven and smaller than in later

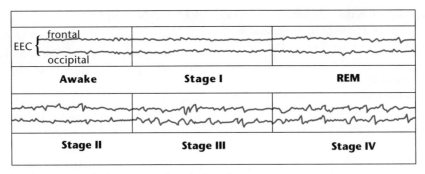

FIGURE ■ 14-6 Changes in electroencephalogram tracing during sleep.

stages. The person is drowsy and relaxed, has fleeting thoughts, is somewhat aware of the environment, can be easily awakened, and may think he or she has been awake. The pulse rate is decreased.

NREM stage II sleep is the *beginning of deeper sleep and fills 40% to 50% of total sleep time.* The person is more relaxed than in the prior stage but can be easily awakened. Sleep spindles and K complexes appear in the brain waves at intervals.

NREM stage III sleep is a *period of progressively deeper sleep and begins 30 to 45 minutes after sleep onset.* EEG waves become more regular. Delta (slow) waves appear, and sleep spindles are present. Muscles are more relaxed. Vital signs and metabolic activity are lowered to basal rates. The person is difficult to awaken.

NREM stage IV sleep is *very deep sleep, occurs approximately 40 minutes after stage I, comprises 10% to 15% of sleep, and rests and restores the body physically.* This stage is of as great importance as REM sleep in healthy young adults. Delta waves are the dominant EEG pattern. The person is very relaxed and seldom moves, is difficult to arouse, and responds slowly if awakened. Physiologic measures are below normal. Sleepwalking and enuresis may occur during this stage. After strenuous physical exercise, this stage is greatly needed. Deep sleep is less deep the last half of the night.

REM sleep is called *active or paradoxic sleep and is the stage of rapid eye movements and dreaming that occurs before descending to the deeper sleep of stages II, III, and IV.* This stage is of great importance. In REM sleep the EEG readings are active and similar to those of stage I sleep, but various physiologic differences from other sleep stages are present. *Physiologic differences, in addition to rapid, side-to-side eye movements, occur:*

1. Muscles relax, and tendon reflexes are absent. Occasional twitching occurs; the body is in immobility-like paralysis.
2. Respiratory rate increases 7% to 20%, alternating between rapid and slow with brief apneic periods.
3. Pulse rate is irregular and increases 5%; cardiac output decreases.
4. Blood pressure fluctuates up to 30 mmHg.
5. Body temperature lowers.
6. High oxygen consumption by the brain and a change in cerebral blood flow occur.
7. Metabolism increases.
8. Blood may become thicker resulting from autonomic instability and temperature changes.
9. Production of 17-hydroxycorticosteroids, posterior pituitary hormones, and catecholamines increases.

10. Gastric secretions increase.
11. Penile erections occur in males of all ages.

REM sleep occurs in 70- to 90-minute cycles that increase as the night progresses. Duration of REM sleep is longer and more intense just after minimum body temperature, around 5 a.m. It rests and restores mentally and is important for learning and psychological functioning. It allows for review of the day's events, categorizing and integrating of information into the brain's storage systems, and problem solving. During psychological stress this stage is vital. Dreams that occur during REM sleep allow for wish fulfillment and release of potentially harmful thoughts, feelings, and impulses so that they do not affect the waking personality.

In a 7- or 8-hour period, the person will have 60- to 90-minute cycles of sleep descending from stage I to IV and back to REM sleep. After 10 to 15 minutes of REM sleep, the person again descends to stage IV. The person may ascend to REM sleep three to five times a night, but each time he or she spends a longer period in it. In the first third of the night, more time is spent in stage IV sleep; in the last third of the night more time is spent in REM sleep. Dreams in the early REM stages are shorter, are less interesting, and contain aspects of the preceding day's activities. As the night progresses, the dreams become longer, more vivid and exciting, and less concerned with daily life. Stages III and IV together constitute approximately 20% of sleep time until old age, when deep sleep almost disappears.

The neurotransmitter most involved in sleep regulation is gamma-aminobutyric acid (GABA), produced by neurons in the hypothalamus. These cells inhibit cholinergic neurons' arousal function, especially histamine and norepinephrine (10, 259). Serotonin, dopamine, and l-tryptophan also play a role in sleep (10). Sleep circuits are affected by other neurobiological circuits: metabolism, motor function, executive function and attention, cardiovascular function, and emotional status (10, 81).

VARIATIONS IN SLEEP PATTERNS

The percentage of time a person spends in sleep differs with age, circadian rhythmicity, medical and psychiatric illness, use of medications, job, environmental conditions, and body temperature at the time of falling asleep (25, 76, 215, 259). If the person's body temperature is at its high point in the biological rhythm, he or she will sleep two times longer than if the temperature is at a low point in the biological rhythm. REM sleep remains constant throughout adult life, constituting 20% to 25% of sleep, in contrast to 40% to

50% of sleep for babies. But the percentage of time spent in stage IV sleep decreases 15% to 30% with age so that the aged person sleeps less time and awakens more frequently. Patterns of sleep for elderly females change approximately 10 years later than for males. The aged person's adjustment to sleep seems dependent on arteriosclerotic changes so that the alert aged person sleeps about the same as the young adult. The aged person with cerebral arteriosclerotic changes sleeps 20% less than the young adult (10, 249, 259).

REM sleep is related to the onset of certain diseases. Convulsions are more likely to occur in the epileptic individual just before awakening, which is during REM sleep. Because the pulse is irregular during REM sleep, myocardial infarctions and arrhythmias are more likely to occur. Gastric secretion is increased during the REM state. The person with a peptic ulcer has more pain at these times (259).

Sedatives, antidepressants, and amphetamines significantly decrease REM sleep. If the person continually takes a sedative, there is a gradual return to the usual amount of REM sleep. But when the drug is withdrawn, REM sleep is markedly withdrawn, causing insomnia and nightmares, irritability, fatigue, and sensitivity to pain, all of which persist up to 5 weeks. Thus sedatives should be given sparingly, including to the young adult, although different sedatives cause different effects, and effects differ from person to person. Assess if the person is regularly taking sedatives. If so, continue them during hospitalization, if possible, to avoid withdrawal symptoms while receiving health care. Taper dosage down gradually (10, 25, 249, 259).

If REM deprivation and the rebound of more REM sleep later occur because of administration of sedatives, the patient with any health problem, but especially cardiovascular disease, should have sedative administration stopped before hospital discharge. At home the person will not have the close observation needed during the prolonged periods of REM sleep when myocardial infarction is more likely to occur.

Educate clients that alcoholic beverages should not be used to promote sleep. Alcohol speeds the onset of sleep but interferes with REM sleep, which may contribute to hangover feelings.

SLEEP DEPRIVATION

Sleep deprivation, *chronic lack of the required amount of sleep or less than 6 hours of sleep for three or more nights,* should be avoided by the young adult. The person may feel rested if he or she awakens after 4 or 5 hours of sleep, but there has been insufficient time for REM sleep. If the person is awakened frequently, the sleep cycle must be started all over again. **Box 14-3**, Physical and Psychological Changes with Sleep Deprivation, presents information for client education (16, 20, 94, 251, 259).

Various conditions interfere with sleep and contribute to sleep loss or sleep deprivation:

1. Medical illness, including pain, fibromyalgia, chronic fatigue syndrome, Parkinson's disease, rheumatoid arthritis (249), fever, obesity (20), impaired glucose tolerance (20, 249), restless legs syndrome (55), and sleep apnea (103).
2. Circadian rhythm disturbances (25, 103, 128, 218, 225).
3. Depression, anxiety states, and emotional distress (10, 16, 57, 147).

| **BOX 14-3** | **Physical and Psychological Changes with Sleep Deprivation** |

PHYSICAL CHANGES

1. Lack of alertness
2. Feeling pressure on head
3. Nystagmus; ptosis of eyelids
4. Lack of coordination; tremors
5. Slowed reflexes
6. Fatigue
7. Bradypnea
8. Cardiac arrhythmias
9. Poorer performance
10. Increased errors; injury prone
11. Physical discomfort; hypochondriasis

PSYCHOLOGICAL CHANGES

1. Anxiety; insecurity; irritability
2. Introspective; unable to respond to support from others; irritable
3. Apathy; withdrawal; decreased motivation
4. Depression
5. Increased aggressiveness
6. Suspiciousness
7. Decreased mental agility
8. Decreased creativity
9. Decreased spontaneity
10. Illusions
11. Decreased concentration
12. Poor judgment, risk taking
13. Memory failure
14. Confusion; disorientation
15. Hallucinations
16. Bizarre behavior; psychosis

Adapted from references 16, 20, 94, 251, 259.

---

4. Various medications, including antidepressants, decongestants, antihypertensives (REM sleep), and caffeine (10, 249, 259).
5. Alcoholic beverages (NREM sleep) (259).
6. Environmental conditions, such as noise or work schedules or conditions (1, 50, 109, 110, 127).
7. Demands upon parents from young children.

Hyperthyroidism, urinary problems, chronic gastrointestinary problems, cardiovascular problems, respiratory problems, pregnancy, and menstrual hormone cycle symptoms also interfere with sleep.

Sleep apnea *is a breathing-related sleep disorder caused by upper airway obstruction interfering with airflow to the lungs.* The hypoxemia briefly awakens the person, often hundreds of times a night, as the respiratory center is stimulated to resume breathing (9, 90). Refer to Chapter 15 for more information. ∞ Sleep apnea, if it exists, should be diagnosed early, including in the pregnant woman. Sleep apnea in pregnancy is a risk to the mother and fetus.

Educate the young adult that when the person decides to recover lost sleep by sleeping longer hours, he or she will spend more time in REM sleep. Twelve to 14 hours of sleep help to overcome brief periods of sleep deprivation. Studies indicate a minimum of 5 hours of sleep daily is needed. For most people 7 to 8 hours are needed to avoid sleep deprivation (10). After 48 hours of sleep loss, the body produces a stress chemical related structurally to LSD-25, which may account for behavioral changes. After 4 days of sleep deprivation, the body does not produce adenosine triphosphate (ATP), the catalyst for energy release, which may be a factor in fatigue (25). With longer sleep deprivation, confusion, hallucinations, and psychosis occur (10).

Being frequently awakened during the night, such as happens to parents with young children, produces the same effects as sleeping fewer hours, even if the total length of time asleep is the usual amount. Blocks of uninterrupted sleep are a definite physical and psychological need. Help parents work out a system that responds to the baby's needs but also allows each parent to get as much uninterrupted sleep as possible.

Use the preceding information on sleep stages and effects of sleep interruption and deprivation to teach young adults. The patient, who needs all stages of sleep for physical and psychological restoration, should not be awakened during the night if at all possible. Observe the person before awakening by studying eye move-

ments under the lids. If he or she is in REM sleep, wait a few minutes for it to end before awakening the person, as this is a short and important stage. Sleep has priority over most procedures. Shift workers need to advocate for themselves or through a group or collective bargaining to ensure that they remain safe and effective workers by not being subjected to changing work schedules too frequently. Educate about the need for regular breaks at work. Educate that fatigue is a critical factor for nurses: undesirable outcomes in addition to physiologic dysfunction include decreased mental acuity, medication errors, and personnel and personal problems (127).

SLEEP DISTURBANCES

Millions of people in the United States do not get normal sleep daily. They either sleep too much or not enough, suffer night terrors, or stop breathing for a minute or two periodically during sleep. The cost of sleep disorders is enormous; some people pay a great deal for pills and potions to maintain normal sleep. Health and safety risks are also considerable.

Insomnia, a *disorder of initiating and maintaining sleep*, is sometimes a problem for young adults. **Primary insomnia** is a *sleep problem that exists in the absence of any major medical or psy-*

INTERVENTIONS FOR HEALTH PROMOTION

Teach the following **sleep hygiene measures** *to help the person with sleep disorders:*

1. Get enough exercise, at least 20 to 40 minutes, 3 to 5 days a week.
2. Maintain a regular schedule of pre-bedtime relaxation, sleep, and wakefulness to keep biorhythms in synchrony. Avoid daytime napping.
3. Reduce caffeine intake (coffee, tea, chocolate candy or milk, soft drinks). Caffeine can remain in the blood for 20 hours.
4. Avoid strenuous activity for 3 to 4 hours before retiring. Use soothing, enjoyable stimuli, such as a back rub for muscular and emotional relaxation, quiet music, a warm bath, deep breathing and progressive relaxation to loosen tight muscles, or a nonstimulating book or hobby. With monotony or boredom, the cerebral cortex does not respond to the reticular formation.
5. Try a glass of warm milk, which contains l-tryptophan, a chemical that increases brain serotonin and induces sleep.
6. Limit alcohol intake. It reduces quality of sleep by causing a light sleep and more wakening and reduces REM sleep.
7. Limit cigarette smoking. Nicotine causes the person to take longer to fall asleep, wake more often, and have less REM and deep NREM sleep.
8. Avoid large meals and high-fat or hard-to-digest meals near bedtime. Gastric secretions regurgitate into the esophagus, causing heartburn. This may be relieved by raising the head of the bed on blocks.

9. Avoid medications that cause sleeplessness as a side effect.
10. Improve the sleeping environment. Make the bedroom dark (or use a dim light), quiet, and as comfortable as possible so it is associated only with pleasurable feelings. Use earplugs and eyeshades if necessary.
11. Purposefully relax after going to bed. Stretch out, get comfortable, let the body become heavy and warm. Avoid television or work tasks.
12. Use pleasant imagery, meditative thoughts, or prayer. Let the mind "float."
13. If you lie awake worrying, about an hour ahead, write in a worry journal, making a list of worries and the next day's tasks. The journal is a place to put things while you sleep.
14. Sleep on your back on a firm mattress. If possible, obtain a mattress that conforms to body contours. When sleeping on your side, tuck a small pillow between your waist and the mattress to provide proper support. Sleeping on the abdomen is not recommended because the head is turned sharply to one side, affecting neck joints and the lower back. In addition, pressure on one side of the face can irritate the jaw. Sleeping with one arm under the pillow stresses the jaw and may interfere with circulation or pinch a nerve in the wrist.
15. If not asleep in 20 minutes, get out of bed and go to another room. Stay calm. Do something boring or relaxing until you are sleepy.

chiatric condition. Other types of insomnia are **sleep onset** (*difficulty falling asleep*), **sleep maintenance** (*awakening in the middle of the night*), and **terminal insomnia** (*early-morning awakening*). Factors that may lead to insomnia include those discussed with sleep deprivation.

Sleep disturbances can also be categorized as follows (64, 127):

1. Primary sleep disorders, which include insomnia, sleep problems due to nightmares (such as sleepwalking), breathing-related disorders, and sleep-wake cycle (circadian rhythm) disorders previously discussed.
2. Secondary sleep disorders, which are related to mental illness or excess use of alcohol or drugs (prescribed or illicit) and other substances.

The cause may be unknown, or sleep disturbances may be caused by habits of daily living. Neuroanatomical studies link sleep disorders to dysregulation in the hypothalamic-pituitary-adrenal (HPA) axis, which affects cortisol release and growth hormone activity. There may also be a genetic link (10, 64). Referral to a sleep research center, with electronic monitoring of the sleep cycle and close surveillance, ensures the problem can be identified and treated.

Assess the quantity and quality of sleep in determining the existence of insomnia. Individual sleep requirements vary, and an individual's satisfaction with the length and quality of sleep is the basis for assessing the presence of insomnia.

Melatonin, *a metabolite of serotonin, is produced by the pineal gland during darkness. It is regulated by the degree of light and darkness.* There is no conclusive evidence that melatonin supplements are effective for sleep disorders. The larger dose in pills is 3 mg, in contrast to the 0.1 to 0.3 mg secreted by the body, and may actually have harmful long-term effects. Sleeping pills, even prescription, may cause unusual dreams, rebound insomnia, or extreme drowsiness the next day. Tranquilizers and sedatives are a last resort to treat insomnia, as they may produce sleep problems (10, 249).

The following resources present more information about sleep and sleep disorders.

Cleveland Clinic Health Information Center *Brain Basics: Understanding Sleep*   www.clevelandclinic.org

American Sleep Disorders Association   www.adsa.org

American Sleep Apnea Association   www.sleepapnea.org

NAPS: New Abstracts and Papers on Sleep   www.websciences.org

Respiratory Problems and Sleep (Dr. John Stradling—United Kingdom)   www.u-net.com

Restless Legs Syndrome Foundation   www.rls.org

Physical Fitness and Exercise

RECOMMENDED ACTIVITY AND BENEFITS

Physical fitness is a *combination of strength, endurance, flexibility, balance, speed, agility, and power and reflects ability to work for a sustained period with vigor and pleasure, without undue fatigue, and with energy left* for enjoying hobbies and recreational activities and for meeting emergencies. Fitness relates to how the person looks

and feels, both physically and mentally. Basic to fitness are regular physical exercise, proper nutrition, adequate rest and relaxation, conscientious health practices, and good medical and dental care. Young adults have a high interest in physical fitness programs but sometimes have difficulty maintaining a regular fitness schedule.

Benefits of exercise in adulthood add to those cited for youth and lay the foundation for increased longevity and better health through the life span. The following **Box**, Client Education, presents information on the benefits of exercise in adulthood, even for people with some level of disability (60, 62, 173, 181, 185).

Stretching is an important element of any exercise program. **Figure 14-7** depicts an example.

Recommendations for exercise follow. After the person has had a thorough physical examination and has been cleared by a physician, daily sessions of 30 to 60 minutes on 4 to 5 days each week of moderate-intensity exercise are recommended for maintaining health, muscle tone, and strength. For conditioning the cardiovascular system, increasing lung capacity, enlarging capillaries in the muscles and heart, or raising metabolic rate, 30 minutes of aerobic or sustained exercise, and conditioning 3 to 5 times a week is necessary (60, 62, 181, 185, 201). The *formula to achieve the desired energy output is* (60, 62):

$$220 - \text{(age of person)} \times 65\% \text{ to } 85\%$$
$$\text{(multiplied by 0.65 to 0.85, depending on}$$
$$\text{desired amount of energy expenditure)}$$

Very fast walking or other activity that increases the heart rate 70% to 85% of maximum heart rate (MHR) or increases the heart rate to approximately 150 or more beats per minute is considered the best exercise of all. To lose weight, 90 minutes of exercise daily is recommended, at least walking. Exercise intensity is monitored by assessing MHR during exercise. Utilize **Box 14-4**, Estimated Target Heart Rates for Exercise, for health promotion education (60, 62). People who cannot engage in aerobic exercise can usually walk 20 to 30 minutes or participate in other exercise daily (60,

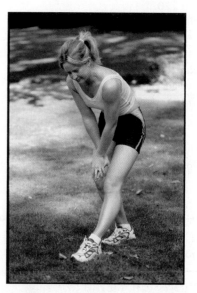

FIGURE ■ 14-7 Stretching is an important element of any exercise program. (John Davis © Dorling Kindersley)

Client Education

Benefits of Exercise in Adulthood

1. Reduce risk of cardiovascular disease and hypertension.
   a. Reduce systolic and diastolic blood pressure.
   b. Reduce low-density lipoproteins (LDLs), triglycerides, and total cholesterol; increase high-density lipoproteins (HDLs).
   c. Increase stroke volume, reduce resting heart rate.
   d. Increase blood supply to heart muscle, blood vessels, and capillaries.
   e. Increase peripheral blood circulation and return.
2. Increase respiratory system function, lung elasticity, and blood oxygen content.
3. Improve musculoskeletal system function.
   a. Increase lean muscle mass, reduce adipose tissue mass.
   b. Maintain or lose weight.
   c. Maintain bone mass, prevent osteopenia or osteoporosis.
   d. Improve muscle strength and endurance.
   e. Improve balance and coordination.
   f. Increase joint flexibility.
   g. Reduce chronic muscle, joint, neck, and back pain and muscle tension.
4. Improve endocrine system and metabolic function.
   a. Improve glucose tolerance and insulin function.
   b. Increase metabolism rate.
   c. Enhance oxidation of fatty acids.
5. Improve immune system function.
   a. Reduce incidence of selected types of cancers.
   b. Increase speed of general body healing (about 25%).
6. Improve sexual function.
   a. Reduce impotence in males.
   b. Reduce premenstrual syndrome, reduce hot flashes in menopausal women.
   c. Enhance sexual satisfaction.
7. Improve psychological status.
   a. Improve cognitive function, short-term memory, and learning; increase alertness.
   b. Improve emotional state and mood; reduce stress, anxiety, depressive feelings.
   c. Improve body image and self-concept.
   d. Improve personality characteristics such as persistence, self-confidence, and composure.

Source: Adapted from references 60, 62, 113, 181, 185.

BOX 14-4 Estimated Target Heart Rates for Exercise

1. Estimate *maximum heart rate (MHR)* by subtracting your age from 220.
   Example: $220 - 60 = 160$
2. Estimate *heart rate reserve (HRR)* by subtracting resting heart rate (RHR) from MHR.
   Example: $160 - 70 = 90$
3. Multiply HRR by 0.5 and add resting heart rate. This is the *target heart rate that is 50% of your maximum capacity.**
   $$90 \times 0.5 = 45$$
   $$70 + 45 = 115$$
4. Multiply HRR by 0.8 and add resting heart rate. This is the *target heart rate that is 80% of maximum capacity.*†
   $$90 \times 0.8 = 72$$
   $$90 + 72 = 162$$

---

*50% of maximum capacity is considered optimum for most people.
†60% to 80% of MHR corresponds to 60% to 80% of recommended aerobic capacity.

Source: Adapted from Bortz, W. (1998). Exercise: The Master Medicine. Diabetes Wellness Letter, 4 (4), 1–5.

62, 181, 201). Utilize **Box 14-5**, Levels of Exercise, to educate about various activities based on intensity of the activity and time of participation, which indicate an index energy expenditure (60, 62, 181, 185, 201). A health self-appraisal program can help the person determine the present state of health and fitness and implications for the years ahead.

Strength training can reduce, even reverse, some natural age-related declines in muscle mass and strength. Such exercise for 20 minutes two or three times a week is effective (181, 185).

Jogging is effective for joints that are already in good condition. Jogging as a regular form of exercise can aggravate old injuries of the back, hips, knees, and ankles because it puts as much as five times normal body weight on lower joints and extremities. Jogging can cause abnormal wear on joints and muscles. The person who jogs must also engage in exercise for the upper extremities and other muscles. *Aerobic exercise* such as brisk walking, jumping rope, and bicycling may actually be better exercise than jogging. *Weight lifting* can strengthen muscle. These activities stress bone to promote bone building, thickness, and strength and increase circulation throughout the body (60, 62, 185).

Swimming is probably the best overall activity because it increases strength and endurance and stimulates heart and blood vessels, lungs, and many muscle groups without putting excess stress on the person because of less gravity pull in the water. Further, swimming keeps joints supple, aids weight loss or weight control,

BOX 14-5	Levels of Exercise

LIGHT-INTENSITY ACTIVITIES

Increases oxygen consumption to about 3 times the level for body at rest. Provides some health benefits.

Walking, strolling
Home care, vacuuming
Pet care
Gardening indoors
Stationary cycling, low-to-moderate pedaling, low resistance
Swinging
Bowling
Fishing (sitting)
Boating, sailing
Horseback riding

MODERATE-INTENSITY ACTIVITIES

Increases oxygen consumption 3 to 6 times the level of body at rest. If done for 30 minutes, 5 days weekly, has life-prolonging value.

Walking briskly, 3–4 mph
Conditioning calisthenics, yoga
Home care, general cleaning
Gardening outdoors (weed, use of power mower)
Grounds improvement
Playing Frisbee or catch
Ping pong, table tennis, racket sports
Bicycling, up to 10 mph
Fishing, fly casting
Hunting

Canoeing, leisurely, at 2–4 mph
Social dancing
House painting
Carpentry
Golfing, carrying clubs
Swimming

HEAVY-INTENSITY ACTIVITIES

Increases oxygen consumption to more than 6 times that burned while body at rest. Duration and frequency determines reduction in death rate.

Moving heavy furniture
Walking briskly uphill 4–5 mph for 45 minutes, 5 days weekly
Jogging
Mowing lawn, push mower
Fast cycling, 10 mph for 1 hour, 4 times weekly
Classes in body movements, calisthenics
Aerobic dance
Jumping rope
Cardiovascular exercise, stair climbing or ski machine, 2–3 hours weekly
Fishing, wading in rushing stream
Canoeing, more than 4 mph
Team sports
Racquetball or singles tennis for 1 hour, 3 days a week
Skating, skiing
Swimming 3 hours vigorously per week
Golf practice at driving range

Adapted from references 60, 62, 181, 185, 201.

and reduces hypertension. Perhaps more important, it is an enjoyable activity, either alone or with others (60, 62, 185).

During pregnancy, exercise routines can be continued unless they are contraindicated medically. The guidelines are as follows (60, 62, 181, 185):

1. Avoid competitive exercise; do not push excessively.
2. Avoid workouts in hot, humid weather.
3. Strenuous exercise should not last longer than 15 minutes.
4. Pulse rate should not exceed 140 beats per minute.
5. Body temperature should not rise above 100.4 °F (38 °C) during exercise.
6. After the fourth month of pregnancy, no exercises should be performed while lying on the back.

Review benefits of exercise with the person. The Health Promotion and Health Belief Models (see Chapter 2), the Behavioral Model (see Chapter 1), ∞ and the Transtheoretical Model (189, 190) can be used to help the young adult make lifestyle changes to integrate more activity and exercise. Refer to **Box 14-4**, Estimated Target Heart Rates for Exercise, to help the person determine aer-

obic capacity during exercise. Explore barriers to an exercise plan and ways to minimize or eliminate them (e.g., some child care responsibilities could be assumed by the partner to allow the other to schedule an exercise program). If exercise occurs outdoors, emphasize the importance of using an appropriate sunscreen agent. Refer to **Box 14-6**, Suggestions for an Exercise Program, and **Box 14-7**, Principles of Body Mechanics (60, 62, 185). An informative Website is the U.S. Department of Health and Human Services, www.aspi.hhs.gov.

Physical activity and exercise programs can be established at the work site, local YMCA or YWCA organizations, community recreation centers, or commercial gymnasiums and health clubs. The exercise program should be easily accessible, enjoyable, and appropriate to the person's lifestyle and physical condition.

GENDER DIFFERENCES

Females and males sometimes share the same physical exercise activities; sometimes interests and energy levels are different. Partners may engage in exercise activities separately. Some females may have as much, or more, endurance as males, especially with

MediaLink US Department of Health and Human Services

BOX 14-6 Suggestions for an Exercise Program

1. Get a pre-exercise physical examination that includes the feet.
2. Make exercise a part of your lifestyle: errands, stairs instead of elevator, parking distance.
3. Start in small increments, keep it fun, and avoid injury.
4. Avoid exercising for 2 hours after a large meal and eating for 1 hour after exercising.
5. Avoid exercise in extremes of weather.
6. Include at least 10 minutes of warm-up and cool-down exercises in an exercise program.
7. Use proper equipment, footwear, and clothing when exercising.
8. Post goals, pictures of the ideal self, and notes of encouragement in a readily seen place for self-encouragement.
9. Use visualization daily to picture successful attainment of exercise benefit (e.g., looking toned or graceful, ideal weight).
10. Keep records of weekly measures of weight, blood pressure, and pulse.
11. Focus on the rewards of exercise; keep a record of feelings and compare differences in relaxation energy, concentration, and sleep patterns.
12. Work with a peer or join a structured exercise class, running club, or fitness center. Spend more time with people dedicated to wellness.
13. Stop exercising or at least slow down and consult with a practitioner if any unusual, unexplainable symptoms occur.
14. Reward self for working toward exercise goals and for attaining them. For example, after a month in an exercise program, buy a new pair of running shoes or treat yourself to a special wish.

Adapted from references 60, 62, 73, 181, 185.

BOX 14-7 Principles of Body Mechanics

1. The wider the base of support and the lower the center of gravity, the greater is the stability of the object.
2. The equilibrium of an object is maintained as long as the line of gravity passes through its base of support.
3. When the line of gravity shifts outside the base of support, the amount of energy required to maintain equilibrium is increased.
4. Equilibrium is maintained with least effort when the base of support is broadened in the direction in which movement occurs.
5. Stooping with hips and knees flexed and the trunk in good alignment distributes the work load among the largest and strongest muscle groups and helps to prevent back strain.
6. The stronger the muscle group, the greater is the work it can perform safely.
7. Using a larger number of muscle groups for an activity distributes the work load.
8. Keeping center of gravity as close as possible to the center of gravity of the work load to be moved prevents unnecessary reaching and strain on back muscles.
9. Pulling an object directly toward (or pushing directly away from) the center of gravity prevents strain on back and abdominal muscles.
10. Facing the direction of movement prevents undesirable twisting of spine.
11. Pushing, pulling, or sliding an object on a surface requires less force than lifting an object, as lifting involves moving the weight of the object against the pull of gravity.
12. Moving an object by rolling, turning, or pivoting requires less effort than lifting the object, as momentum and leverage are used to advantage.
13. Using a lever when lifting an object reduces the amount of weight lifted.
14. The less the friction between the object moved and surface on which it is moved, the smaller is the force required to move it.
15. Moving an object on a level surface requires less effort than moving the same object on an inclined surface because the pull of gravity is less on a level surface.
16. Working with materials that rest on a surface at a good working level requires less effort than lifting them above the working surface.
17. Contraction of stabilizing muscle preparatory to activity helps to protect ligaments and joints from strain and injury.
18. Dividing balanced activity between arms and legs protects the back from strain.
19. Variety of position and activity helps maintain good muscle tone and prevent fatigue.
20. Alternating periods of rest and activity helps prevent fatigue.

training, but there are some physiologic differences that account for differences in performance in physical exercise activities or athletic events (185).

Males have greater upper-body strength, primarily because of their longer arms, broader shoulders, and higher muscle-fiber counts. Muscle can be conditioned by exercise, but muscle-fiber count cannot be increased. Whether or not males exercise, their muscle fibers gain bulk from the hormone testosterone. In males, the heart and lungs, which average 10% larger than those of females, provide more powerful and efficient circulation. The delivery of oxygen to male muscles, a factor crucial to speed, is further enhanced by the higher concentration of hemoglobin in the blood. Finally, the longer limbs provide them with greater leverage and extension (90, 185).

The aspects of female physiology that result in their athletic advantages are not as self-evident as in males. The female's body contains an average of 9% more adipose tissue than the male's body. This tissue is deposited not only on the thighs, buttocks, and breasts, but in a subcutaneous layer that covers the entire body. It is this adipose tissue that makes the female more buoyant and better insulated against cold, both of which can be advantages in long-distance swimming or running. Body adipose tissue may also be one of the reasons few female runners report the pain and weakness that most male runners encounter. The body is conditioned to call on stored fats once its supply of glycogen, which fuels the muscles, has been exhausted. As females have greater reserves of body fat, they are able to compete in an athletic event longer. Females perspire in smaller amounts and less quickly than males. Perspiring is the body's way of avoiding overheating. Yet females may tolerate heat better than males. Not only can body temperature rise in a female several degrees higher before she begins to sweat, but she sweats more efficiently because of the even distribution of the sweat glands. In females, **vascularization**, *capacity for bringing blood to the surface for cooling*, is also more efficient. Females also have certain structural advantages for all types of running and swimming events. In swimming, narrower shoulders offer less resistance through water. Even at identical heights (and ideal weights), female bodies are lighter than male bodies, leaving them with less weight to carry while running (90, 185).

FOOT CARE

Foot care is important in an exercise program as well as in daily living. The feet, during walking, will meet the surface at 1 to 2 times the body weight and up to 3 times its weight when running.

Educate about proper shoe fit, which includes heel height, stability, cushioning, wedge support, and forefoot cushion. Proper-fitting and absorbent socks are important. Thorough washing and careful drying of feet after exercise and as part of normal hygiene is essential.

Psychosocial Concepts

COGNITIVE DEVELOPMENT

The young adult continues to learn and engages in the Formal Operations Stage described by Piaget (244). Other cognitive processes include use of emotional intelligence, the **Problem-Finding Stage** or **Post-Formal Thought** (11), and dialectical and triarchic thought processes (220, 221). Your health promotion interventions are rendered more or less successful, depending upon the cognitive abilities and processes of the person.

Theories About Cognitive Development

Cognitive theories are described here; refer also to Chapter 1. ∞ Erikson (65) theorized that the basis for adult cognitive performance is laid during the school years when the child accomplishes the task of industry, learns how to learn and win recognition by producing and achieving, and learns to enjoy learning. The child learns an attitude that lasts into adulthood: how much effort a task takes and how long and hard he or she should work for what is desired or expected. The sense of industry is useful in adult life, both in coping with new experiences and in functioning as a worker, family member, citizen, and lifelong learner.

Schaie proposed a **Life-Span Model of Cognitive Development**: *different abilities are required in different life stages* (202). The child and youth is in the **acquisitive stage**, *acquiring knowledge and skills for their own sake and to prepare for adulthood.* The young adult spans the **achieving stage**, *pursuing knowledge to achieve a goal,* and the **responsible stage**, *solving practical problems associated with responsibilities to others.* The responsible stage is a major focus and deepens in middle age. The later years or old age is the stage of reintegration (202).

Learning continues throughout the adult years. Dendrites in the brain continue to branch as they are used. Longitudinal studies indicate that the brain continues to change in structure and complexity until age 40 or 50. The brain shows increasing myelination through middle age, which permits more integrated modes of social response and stable or increasing intellectual functions (26, 90, 181, 201).

Becoming mature in young adulthood involves intellectual growth, becoming more adaptive and knowledgeable about self, forming values, and developing increasing depth in analytic and synthetic thinking, logical reasoning, and imagination. The multiple and different intelligences described in Chapter 12 are applied or more fully developed, ∞ depending on individual talents and interests (220, 221). Developing social and interpersonal skills and personal friendships may have a powerfully maturing effect on intellectual skills (66, 67).

Table 14-1, Major Ego (Cerebrum) Functions or Tasks of the Adult is based on the Analytic Theory discussed in Chapter 1 ∞ (10, 26, 66, 115, 228). **Table 14-2**, Assessment of Reality Testing Function of Ego (Cerebrum): Distinction Between Inner and Outer Stimuli, is based on psychosocial research. Both tables will assist you in assessing reality thinking processes and levels of impairment (10, 26, 115).

Influences on Learning

Influences differ somewhat from childhood to adulthood. *Influences include* (11, 181, 233, 244): (a) level of knowledge in society generally, (b) personal values and perceptions and previously learned associations, (c) level of education, (d) available life opportunities, (e) interests, (f) participation by the person in the learning activity, (g) the learning environment, and (h) life experiences. As a result of these influences, the person maintains a preferred

TABLE 14-1

Major Ego (Cerebrum) Functions or Tasks of the Adult

1. **Reality testing**
   a. Distinguishes inner and outer stimuli
   b. Perceives accurately: time, place, and events that relate to self or are familiar
   c. Is psychologically minded and aware of inner states
   d. Has accurate sense of body boundaries
2. **Judgment**
   a. Anticipates probable dangers, legal limits, and social censure or disapproval of intended behavior
   b. Is aware of appropriateness and consequences of behavior
   c. Behaves in a way that reflects judgment
3. **Sense of reality of the world and self**
   a. Distinguishes external events that are real and those that are embedded in familiar context, such as déjà vu, trance-like states
   b. Experiences the body and its functions and one's behavior as familiar, unobtrusive, and belonging to the self
   c. Develops a sense of individuality, uniqueness, self, self-esteem
   d. Develops a sense that the self is separate from the external environment
4. **Regulation and control of drives, affects, and impulses**
   a. Directs impulse expression to indirect forms of behavioral expression
   b. Balances delay and control behavior
   c. Demonstrates frustration tolerance
   d. Maintains self-esteem independent of daily occurrences and others' opinions
   e. Does minimal acting out
5. **Interpersonal relationships**
   a. Relates to and invests in others, taking account of one's own needs
   b. Relates to others in an adaptive way and based on present mature goals rather than past immature goals
   c. Perceives others as separate rather than as an extension of self
   d. Sustains relationships over long period and tolerates absence of the person
   e. Lists own assumptions against objective data or others' opinions
6. **Thought processes**
   a. Sustains processes for attention, concentration, anticipation, concept formation, memory, and language

   b. Controls unrealistic, illogical, loose, or primitive thinking
   c. Thinks clearly
   d. Has no association or communication problems
7. **Adequate regression in the service of the ego**
   a. Relaxes perceptual and conceptual acuity and other ego controls with concomitant increase in awareness of previously preconscious and unconscious contents
   b. Increases adaptive potentials as a result of creative endeavors
8. **Defensive functioning**
   a. Uses adaptive mechanism for ideation and behavior effectively
   b. Controls anxiety, depression, or other behavioral affects of weak defensive operations
9. **Stimulus barrier**
   a. Maintains a threshold for, sensitivity to, or awareness of stimuli that impinge on senses
   b. Uses active coping mechanisms in response to levels of sensory stimulation to prevent or minimize disorganization, avoidance, withdrawal
10. **Autonomous functions**
    a. Maintains function or prevents impairment of sight, hearing, intention, language, memory, learning, or motor function
    b. Maintains function or prevents impairment of habit patterns, learned skills, work routines, and hobbies
11. **Synthetic-integrative functioning**
    a. Reconciles or integrates potentially contradictory attitudes, values, affects, behavior, and self-representations
    b. Relates together and integrates psychic and behavioral events, whether or not contradictory
    c. Identifies chronologic order of events
    d. Integrates good and bad aspects of self
12. **Mastery-competence**
    a. Is motivated with sufficient energy to meet daily demands
    b. Plans goal-directed behavior
    c. Performs in relation to existing capacity to interact with and master the environment
    d. Expects success in performance of tasks
    e. Maintains autonomy
    f. Evaluates self and resources, as well as expectations of others
    g. Is open to and capable of change
    h. Has diversity of interests

Adapted from references 10, 26, 66, 115, 228.

TABLE 14-2

Assessment of Reality Testing Function of Ego (Cerebrum): Distinction Between Inner and Outer Stimuli

1. **Maximal impairment**
   a. Hallucinations and delusions pervade
   b. Minimal ability to distinguish dreams from waking life
   c. Inability to distinguish idea, image, and hallucination
   d. Perception disturbed, e.g., moving objects appear immobile and vice versa
2. **Severe impairment**
   a. Hallucinations and delusions severe but limited to one or more content areas
   b. Difficulty distinguishing events as dream or reality
3. **Medium impairment**
   a. Illusions more common than hallucinations
   b. Aware of experiencing illusions and others do not
   c. Projects inner states onto external reality more than having hallucinations or delusions
4. **Minimal impairment**
   a. Possible confusion about inner and outer states when awakening, going to sleep, or under severe stress
5. **No impairment**
   a. Distinguishes inner and outer stimuli accurately
   b. Denies external reality occasionally as part of adaptive behavior
   c. Is aware whether events occurred in dreams or waking life
   d. Identifies source of thoughts and perceptions as being an idea or image and from internal or external source
   e. Distinguishes between inner and outer prescriptions even under extreme stress
   f. Checks perceptions against reality automatically

Adapted from references 10, 26, 108.

way of learning or cognitive style—a characteristic way of perceiving, organizing, and evaluating information, as described in Chapter 12 ∞ (26, 115, 181, 238, 244). These influences will affect your ability to do health education with the person.

Formal Operations Stage

According to Piaget (244), the young adult remains in the **Formal Operations Stage**. *The adult is creative in thought, begins at the abstract level, and compares the idea mentally or verbally with previous memories, knowledge, or experience.* In *formal operational thinking, the person* (a) combines or integrates a number of steps of a task mentally instead of thinking about or doing each step as a separate unit; (b) considers the multiplicity and relativism of issues and alternatives to a situation; (c) synthesizes and integrates ideas or information into the memory, beliefs, or solutions so that the end result is a unique product; and (d) differentiates among many perspectives, and is objective, realistic, and less egocentric. The person can imagine and reason about events that are not occurring in re-

ality but that are possible or in which he or she does not even believe. Hypotheses are generated, conjectures are deduced from hypotheses, and observations are conducted to disconfirm the expectations. The thought system can be applied to diverse data. The person can evaluate the validity of reasoning. A concrete proposition can be replaced by an arbitrary symbol such as p or q. Probability, proportionality, and combining of thought systems occur (244). These cognitive characteristics are especially useful to the person who is pursuing advanced education or is engaged in a complex or demanding career.

Emotional intelligence (EI) is *the ability to understand and regulate personal feelings and respond empathically and effectively to the feelings of others.* Emotional intelligence is a part of, not the opposite of, cognitive knowledge and is involved in acquiring and using tacit knowledge (42, 83, 84).

Arlin (11) proposed that some people continue to develop cognitively beyond the Formal Operations Stage proposed by Piaget into a *fifth stage* of cognitive development that progresses through adulthood. The Formal Operations Stage describes strategies used in problem solving (244). The **fifth stage, Problem-Finding Stage,** or **Post-Formal Thought** (11, 214), *goes beyond the problem-solving stage and is characterized by creative thought in the form of discovered problems; relativistic thinking; the raising of general questions from ill-defined problems; use of intuition, insight, and hunches; and the development of significant scientific thought* (11, 181, 214). The person is better able to handle uncertainty, inconsistency, contradictions, imperfection, and compromise.

Dialectical thought *builds on post-formal thought and involves the ability to consider a thesis and its antithesis, and arrive at a synthesis.* Such thinking considers pros and cons, advantages and disadvantages, and possibilities and limitations simultaneously (21, 26, 197).

There are *four criteria for post-formal thought* (11, 181, 214):

1. **Shifting gears.** *Going from abstract reasoning to practical, real-world considerations.*
2. **Multiple causality, multiple solutions.** *Awareness that most problems have more than one cause and more than one solution and that some solutions are more likely to work than others.*
3. **Pragmatism.** *Choosing the best of several possible solutions and recognizing criteria for the choice.*
4. **Paradox recognition and awareness.** *Understanding that a problem or solution has inherent conflict.*

Sternberg, in his Triarchic Theory of Intelligence, stated that IQ tests do not measure creative insight and practical intelligence. He proposed *three elements in his theory of adult intelligence* (220, 221):

1. **Componental or analytic.** *How efficiently people process information, solve problems, monitor solutions, or evaluate results.*
2. **Experiential, insightful.** *How people approach novel and familiar tasks, compare new information to old, and think originally while automatically performing familiar operations.*
3. **Contextual, practical.** *How people deal with the environment, size up a situation, adapt to or change a situation, or find a new, more suitable setting.*

The person may use different thinking for scientific operations, business transactions, artistic activities, and intimate interpersonal interactions. At times, the adult will of necessity engage in thinking typical of Concrete Operations (244). The adult may regress to the Preoperational Stage (some never get beyond this stage), as shown by superstitious, egocentric, or illogical thinking (244). The adult may not have the ability to perform formal operations.

The young adult continues to learn both formally and informally to enhance cognitive and job skills and self-knowledge. Environmental stimulation is important in continued learning. Increasingly young adults are changing their minds about their life work and change directions after several years of study or work in the original field. An important aspect of late-young-adult intelligence is **tacit knowledge,** the *information, "know-how," or "savvy" not formally taught or openly expressed but acquired by the individual through use of experience and "common sense"* (181, 221).

Gender Differences

Males and females with equivalent IQ scores use the brain differently according to magnetic resonance imaging (MRI) studies (118):

1. Females have more white matter and less gray matter cells related to IQ than do males.
2. In males, the strongest correlation between gray matter and IQ is in the frontal and parietal lobes.
3. In females, the strongest correlation between gray matter and IQ is in the frontal lobes and Broca's area.
4. In males, a significant relationship exists between mathematical reasoning and temporal lobe activity. No such correlation exists in females.

The left hemisphere is dominant in most people for language, logical reasoning, and mathematical calculation. The right hemisphere processes spatial and visual abstractions, recognition of faces, body image, music, art forms, and intuitive, preconscious, and fantasy thinking. At birth, asymmetry in the left hemisphere is more marked in the male. Female infants have a somewhat larger area of visual cortex in the right hemisphere than male infants, which implies an anatomic advantage for nonverbal ideation. The female's brain matures earlier; the two hemispheres are more integrated in the female as indicated by less impairment of intellectual function in females who have suffered either right or left hemisphere damage. Males are more vulnerable to brain damage (90). On tests, females use verbal strategies to solve spatial problems because of the greater interplay between the two hemispheres. In adulthood, females are better able to coordinate activities of both hemispheres; thus, they can think intuitively and globally (78, 181). Males are better at activities in which the two hemispheres do not compete, such as problem solving and determining spatial relationships (181).

Cognitive abilities have often been related to personality traits and interpersonal orientation. Sex-role socialization has been related to cognitive style. The level of information processing a person attains may exert a profound influence on personality and on ability to integrate and differentiate in problem solving (26, 181, 201).

Claims about gender differences in other cognitive abilities, such as creativity, analytic ability, and reasoning, apparently are the result of differences in verbal, quantitative, or visual-spatial abilities, or the opportunity to develop such abilities—in either gender

(26, 181). The confident young adult takes pride in being mentally astute, creative, progressive, and alert to events. He or she normally has the mental capacity to make social and occupational contributions, is self-directive and curious, and likes to match wits with others in productive dialogue.

Both males and females have similar basic needs, their own unique cognitive abilities and talents, and often unspoken ideas and feelings longing for self-expression. From young childhood on, both females and males should be considered cognitively capable and have the opportunity, including in the adult years, to meet the maximum potential.

Teaching the Adult

Information on cognitive development should be considered whenever you are teaching adults. **Table 14-3**, Principles of Adult Learning, presents information to assist you with client teaching (124). You, the teacher, are the authoritative facilitator. Emphasize a sharing of ideas and experiences, role play, and practical application of information. In some cases you will help the person to unlearn old habits, attitudes, or information in order to acquire new habits and attitudes.

If you teach young adults who have not achieved literacy, you must compensate for their inability to read and write. Slow, pre-

TABLE 14-3

Principles of the Learning Process

1. Learning is an active, self-directed process. Adults learn at their own pace and their own style.
2. Learning is central to ongoing development and behavioral changes—person centered and problem centered.
3. Learning is influenced by readiness to learn, abilities, potential to learn, and emotional state.
4. Learning is facilitated when the content or behaviors to be learned are perceived as relevant and related to needs.
5. Learning proceeds from simple to complex and known to unknown.
6. Learning is facilitated when the learner has opportunities to take risks, test ideas, make mistakes, question, and be creative. Threat to self is minimal.
7. Learning is facilitated when the person has knowledge of progress and feedback that serves as a measure for further learning.
8. Learning transfer occurs when the person can recognize similarities and differences between past experiences and the present situation.
9. Learning is effective when it can be immediately applied and reinforced.
10. Learning occurs best when the teaching methodology is relevant to the content to be learned.
11. Learning occurs best in an environment that is nonthreatening, comfortable, and free of distractions.
12. Learning occurs best and is continued when the learner feels satisfied and successful.

cise speech and gestures and the use of pictures and audiovisual aids are crucial. Demonstration and return demonstration ensure learning. Do not underestimate the importance of your behavior and personality as a motivating force, especially if some members of the person's family do not consider learning important. Some adults have attention deficit/hyperactivity disorder (ADHD). They demonstrate difficulty with concentration, attention, initiating and completing tasks, and ego or executive functions (3, 5, 6, 10). Females with the diagnosis, in contrast to males, have lower self-esteem and more psychological distress. Modify teaching strategies accordingly.

Helpful resources include:

1. Children and Adults with Attention Deficit/Hyperactivity Disorder (CHADD); phone: 800-233-4050, www.chadd.org.
2. National Center for Gender Issues and ADHD; phone: 202-966-1561, www.negiadd.org.

WORK AND LEISURE ACTIVITIES

Although the following discussion focuses on work outside of the home, implying paid employment, we do not demean or overlook the young adult female or male who chooses to stay at home and rear a family. *Homemaking and child rearing are essential and important work;* each is fatiguing and stressful in its own way. In fact, *working at home has its own hazardous to health.* Noise and air pollutants or chemical toxins come from appliances, building materials, cleaning products, and combinations of materials or supplies used in a home. (See Chapter 4.) ∞

Work Options and Attitudes

Work has a powerful role in life as it (a) defines self, self-esteem, and roles; (b) gives a sense of purpose; (c) provides opportunities for mastery and creativity; (d) structures life rhythms, financial standing, and residence; (e) contributes to friendships; and (f) affects exercise and leisure activities. It may contribute to physical or emotional health problems and poor family relationships, even divorce. The workload may interfere with participation in the broader community, church, or family/friendship activities.

Factors that reduce job satisfaction include (201): (a) lack of job clarity, (b) control by or conflicts with supervisors or colleagues, (c) inadequate managerial support, (d) heavy schedules and time pressures, (e) changing shift schedules, (f) unsafe environment or potential for violence, (g) inadequate salary for job demands, and (h) sexual harassment. Nurses often face some or many of these factors in their work site and suffer physical and emotional health problems, injury, and disability as a result (7, 109, 147, 155, 173, 175, 234, 235). Some nurses and other health care workers experience violence from patients in their workplace (7, 121, 173). The American Nurses Association works actively on advocacy and legislation for protection of the nurse as well as the patient; go to www.ajn.com.

There are many work options and attitudes. For example, the young adult "workaholic" executive may put in 70 to 80 hours weekly at the job, feel guilty when not working, and channel much anger and aggression through work. In contrast, a factory worker, while feeding a certain part into the assembly line, may be planning what to do after work. The blue-collar worker may have more

job stress than the executive. The young adult may, after several years, lose interest in the job and decide to go into another field that appears challenging. Personality structure or type may indicate optimal career choice. There are six *basic career-related personality types* (104, 201):

1. **Realistic:** Like outdoors, manual activities; prefer to work alone.
2. **Investigative:** More interest in ideas than people, aloof; prefer intellectual or research rather than social occupations.
3. **Artistic:** Creative, enjoy working with ideas and materials, value nonconformity, ambiguity; may work in a job of second choice and pursue artistic interests in leisure or hobby.
4. **Social:** Like working with people, have a helping orientation; careers in education, social work, counseling.
5. **Enterprising:** Oriented toward people more so than things; persuasive; careers in sales, management, politics.
6. **Conventional:** Like well-structured situations, work well as accountant with details and numbers, clerical or secretarial tasks, computers.

Most people combine characteristics of several types, which promotes flexibility and the ability to survive in a changing job market. They may be able to incorporate interests and talents into leisure activities, if not a career. These personality types are incorporated into the Strong Campbell Interest Inventory used in career guidance (201).

In many countries in Europe, Central America, and South America, and in Hawaii and the Pacific Islands, leisure is considered a healthy part of the lifestyle. "Hurry" is not (106). In addition to the usual types of jobs, a new classification exists—the knowledge worker or the creative class (75), as described in Chapter 5. ∞ Because of expanding technology, rapid change, the burgeoning size of industries and mega-industries, and the knowledge explosion, the **knowledge worker** is *hired to do job planning and to create, innovate, and make decisions within the organization.* The ultimate goal of the knowledge worker is cost containment for the company, improved efficiency of the worker, a more marketable product, and a more willing buyer. You may fall into this group. You may be involved in or help the health care agency develop long-range plans and goals, or be a consultant. You might observe nurses or other health care providers at work to determine a more effective way to deliver care. You would cope with unanticipated changes, predict changes, and collaborate with others in this role.

The worker—all the way from the executive level to the delivery person—may be engaged in **substance abuse,** *ingesting excessive alcohol or drugs or engaged in pushing illicit drugs* on the job. The implications of substance abuse are grave, including job errors, accidents to self or others, poor job performance, a product that does not meet standard results, and increased insurance and workers' compensation costs. Thus, products and services cost more to consumers. The lives of family, friends, and co-workers are affected.

The majority of young adult females are in the workforce. Sometimes the job is a necessity (e.g., she is single, divorced, and has children; her husband has only seasonal work or a low-paying job). Many females are working to maintain occupational skills,

MediaLink Attention Deficit Hyperactivity Disorder

MediaLink American Nurses Association

self-esteem, and independence. If she is trying to work in addition to carrying on the traditional roles of wife, mother, and housekeeper, she will likely feel conflict and fatigue (1). Finding day care facilities for young children can be a problem. Yet there are advantages. The family, whether single parent or two parents/two careers, can learn to work together on various home roles. The working wife-mother can convey an attitude of self-confidence and satisfaction. The children will probably be more adaptive as they mature if they learn various household responsibilities and see their mother and father in a variety of roles. Further, the children will learn that it is essential to become well prepared for adult work roles. Employers, to attract and keep competent workers, are offering flexible work schedules, job sharing, on-site child care, and both paternity leave and extended maternity leave.

Job satisfaction is important to health. Work remains a central part of the adult self-concept in most Americans. A close relationship exists between occupational and family satisfaction. If the person is dissatisfied in one, either work or family life, he or she will try to compensate in the other (66, 181, 201, 219). The person can take steps toward job satisfaction.

Because the nurse views the person holistically, you may be asked for assistance by the manager or the employer. They may find it difficult to understand the young adult worker who acts differently than the middle-aged or older worker. The behavior of the young adult worker who has newly achieved an executive position may be poorly understood by employees who are middle-aged and near retirement. Help them understand that workers from different generations or from diverse cultural groups may have their own value systems and respond to different motivational stimuli.

You may assist with safety and health problems, listen to and counsel about job problems, and assist in resolving conflicts related to the work setting, or the homemaker, career, and mother roles. Through counseling and education, foster feelings of self-respect in relation to employment. Low self-esteem and feelings of stress in the worker lower productivity, morale, and profits. Consult with the work system to promote workers' feelings of self-esteem and belief in the importance of their work.

In cases of substance abuse on the job, work with the personnel director, safety director, employee assistance program, administrative personnel, and the affected individual (and family if possible) to help the person get the necessary medical treatment. Refer to the discussion about alcoholism and drug abuse later in this chapter. Refer to tables in Appendix B.

You may also become an advocate for the female who is undergoing sexual harassment on the job. Increasingly female employees are gaining the courage to talk publicly about and to seek legal aid for sexual harassment. Harassment can range from a passing caress to threats of or actual rape. Yet people who are harassed on the job may not complain, whether it is about the hug that the supervisor gives everyone daily—wanted or not—or about actual body contact, because of fear of lack of confidentiality, fear of greater or more subtle harassment or retaliation, and fear of poor evaluations, loss of pay raises, or job loss.

You may have a role in the workplace to develop policies and procedures to handle complaints of sexual harassment on the job. Ideally the work atmosphere should be such that, first, harassment would not occur, and second, everyone would be concerned about the problem and know how to handle it. You can foster such an atmosphere.

Leisure

Some young American adults focus on leisure (101, 181). As job hours per week are being cut (especially in automated jobs), the time for leisure increases. Additionally, the work ethic is decreasing in importance. Socialization of current young adults has fostered a leisure ethic, which can promote health and longevity (201).

Leisure is *freedom from obligations and formal duties of paid work and opportunity to pursue, at one's own pace, mental nourishment, enlivenment, pleasure, and relief from fatigue of work.* Leisure may be as active as backpacking up a mountain or as quiet as fishing alone at a huge lake. Some people never know leisure, and others manage an attitude of leisure even as they work. *Various factors influence the use of leisure time:* (a) gender; (b) amount of family, home, work, or community responsibilities; (c) mental status; (d) income and socioeconomic class; and (e) past interests.

Leisure gadgetry has invaded the marketplace. Electronic games have replaced household appliances as America's favorite gadgets. Technology affects leisure through changes in both products and values. The electronic games that reward aggressive and competi-

---

INTERVENTIONS FOR HEALTH PROMOTION

Share the following **suggestions for building job satisfaction**:

1. Cultivate a positive attitude.
2. Identify priorities. Discuss with the spouse, or the children if they are old enough, what tasks must be done, what can be delegated (either on the job or to a service company in the home), and who can take on which responsibilities to even the load. Communicate needs.
3. Allocate tasks. Design a system for assigning tasks, based on skill, age, availability, and fairness. Rotate tasks, if possible, or assign tasks that are especially requested.

4. Use a support network. Family, friends, neighbors, and child care providers can be asked for assistance on a regular basis or for help in emergencies.
5. Rechannel emotional investments. Having multiple roles gives an opportunity to excel in one realm if you have problems in another.
6. Assess progress. Be willing to change and take risks. Discuss effectiveness of the plan and problem areas.

tive behavior teach values and behavior that will be carried over to other leisure activities and the workforce. The result may be contradictory to the meaning of leisure and even to meaning in life.

The real answer to the work–leisure dilemma is that the worker and the player are one. The unhappy worker will not automatically become happy in leisure. Challenging work makes leisure a time of refreshment. Successful leisure prepares the worker for more challenge. The young adult has to learn how to work and how to pursue pleasant events (201).

Maintaining friendships is a healthy use of leisure time. It takes time, self-disclosure, and sharing of interests to form friendships. Friendships involve mutual respect, agape love, enjoyment of each other, acceptance, trust, assistance, emotional support, confidentiality, spontaneity, and a buffer from stress (26, 78, 92, 201, 252). Some conflict may surface and is natural as intimacy deepens. Getting closer to friends, rather than making more friends, is the way to reduce loneliness. In a world in which people juggle career and family, time may limit the size of the friendship circle. Several close friendships should be made. Successful friendship combines the freedom to depend on one another with the freedom to be independent. If free time is too limited, fewer friendships may be formed.

Gender differences exist in forming and maintaining adult friendships, as summarized in **Table 14-4** (26, 78, 92, 181, 201, 252). All males and females do not specifically fit these descriptors, however. In cross-gender friendships, the female may become upset by the way the male talks to her (which is like he talks to males), and vice versa. The female may not like his good-natured bantering. The male gets frustrated because she won't take his practical advice; she just talks about her problem. Sexual boundaries may also be a problem in cross-gender friendships. It is healthy to have a variety of types of friendships (26).

Counsel about the importance of leisure as a part of balanced living. Emphasize that the young adult needs to develop a variety of interests as preparation for the years ahead to maintain physical and mental health. Recommend that the person should avoid developing all the friendships at the workplace. In today's competitive world and with frequent job changes, people at work may not be able to form lasting friendships. It is wiser to start out being more formal and distant until the trusting relationship evolves.

EMOTIONAL DEVELOPMENT

Emotional development in young adulthood is an ongoing, dynamic process, an extension of childhood and adolescent developmental influences and processes. Development is still influenced by the environment, but the environment is different. The fundamental developmental issues continue but in an altered form. Thus trust, autonomy, initiative, industry, and identity all are reworked and elaborated, based on current experiences (36, 65–67).

The young adult is expected to demonstrate (a) increased clarity and consistency of personality, (b) stabilization of self and identity, (c) established preferences of interests and activities, (d) increased coping ability, (e) less defensiveness, (f) decrease in youthful illusions, fantasy, and impulsiveness, (g) more responsiveness to and responsibility for self and others, (h) more giving than taking, and (i) more appreciation of surroundings. It is a time to develop expanded resources for happiness. Young adults do not consistently develop or demonstrate these characteristics. In contrast, there is an increasing emphasis on narcissism in the U.S. society. Young adults believe they are special and must be given special consideration on the job, in various community services, and even in church. They are teaching their offspring the same attitude, which children and adolescents regularly convey. The young adult should expect, but often has difficulty facing, restrictions and demands not previously experienced, some sacrifice of freedom and spontaneity, and less opportunity for variety, novelty, and impulsive adventure. There is more challenge to develop **empathy** *(depth of feeling and understanding of another's feelings),* to learn in detail

TABLE 14-4

Gender Differences in Adult Friendship

Female	Male
1. Form close emotional relationships; are more intimate and emotional.	1. Form competitive relationships; disagree with each other more often.
2. Engage in friendly conversation as a major activity.	2. Engage in physical exercise or activity—work, play, or roughhouse, especially outdoors.
3. Share intimate ideas, self-disclose, talk openly, share confidences and secrets from the past.	3. Keep conversation more distant, superficial, less intimate, present oriented.
4. Express feelings.	4. Talk about ideas, information, activities, sports.
5. Reveal weaknesses or limits.	5. Avoid talking about own weaknesses or limits.
6. Discuss problems, including health, at length; seek assistance with solutions.	6. Seek solutions; avoid discussion of problems or health.
7. Anticipate listening ear, empathy, expressions of understanding. Give practical assistance.	7. Anticipate answers, practical solutions. Avoid listening or expressions of empathy.
8. Interact with people, career, and technology/computer.	8. Interact first with career and technology/computer, then people.

Adapted from references 26, 32, 36, 78, 181, 201, 252.

how systems work, and to reevaluate self and the world. The narcissistic individual cannot focus or handle these challenges but will remain self-focused and place great demands on others. If behavior is not too heavily bound by defenses against anxiety, the person's behavior becomes more varied as experience accumulates (65–67).

Theories of Emotional Development

Various theorists are referred to in Chapter 1 ∞ to foster understanding of adult personality development. Selected concepts of the theorists Jung, Vaillant, Gould, Sheehy, Levinson, Sullivan, and Erikson are summarized in the following pages.

Jung (115) *defined personality development along different lines during the first and second halves of the life cycle. Outward expansion is the first period, until approximately age 40 to 45.* Maturational forces direct the growth of the ego and the unfolding of capacities for dealing with the external world. Young people learn to get along with others, establish careers and families, and try to be successful. Thus, it is usually necessary to combine the traditional feminine and masculine traits into a unique, nonthreatening whole. The young person dedicates self to the task of mastering the outer world confidently and assertively, without being too preoccupied with self-doubts, fantasies, and inner nature. Extroverts, rather than introverts, may have an easier time in adjusting during this period.

From his longitudinal study of adult males, **Vaillant** (238–240) *defined development that continues through adulthood in a number of ways, emotionally, mentally, socially in relationships, and in a career. Simultaneously, the developing and successful adult also demonstrates what Freud called the psychopathology of everyday life.* All have special adaptational problems and mechanisms. Vaillant believed that emotional health and development are evolutionary, not static. Isolated traumatic events rarely mold individual lives. Development comes from continued interaction between choice of adaptive mechanisms and sustained relationships with others. Poor adaptation, which lowers the threshold for perceiving or handling stress, leads to anxiety, depression, and physical illness. Vaillant's study identified *mature defenses*—altruism, humor, suppression or minimization of discomforts, anticipation, and sublimation—that promote adaptation (238). *Successful adapters* (a) have had good relationships with parents, (b) are energetic and alert, (c) feel good about themselves, (d) love their work, (e) have very close relationships with the spouse and friends, and (f) sublimate aggression into enthusiastic pursuits of projects, work, or competitive sports. His findings about males seem applicable to adult females as well (238–240).

Gould (85, 86) *defined life stages and key issues or tasks in late adolescence and young adulthood. The direction of change through adulthood is becoming more tolerant of self and more appreciative of the surrounding world.* Although Gould did not list specific assumptions about adult development, he described adulthood as a time of thoughtful confrontation with the self—letting go of an idealized image, the desire to be perfect, and acknowledging the realistic image of self and personal feelings. Conflicts between past and present beliefs are resolved. Through constant examination and reformulation of beliefs embedded in feelings, the person can substitute a conception of adulthood for childhood legacy and fan-

tasies. Whereas children mark the passing years by their changing bodies, adults change their minds, deepen their insights about self, and mature emotionally. **Table 14-5**, Gould's Developmental Stages of Adulthood, is a summary.

Sheehy (210, 211) *defines development as occurring throughout adulthood, influenced by external events or crises, the historical period, membership in the culture, social roles, and the internal realism of the person*—values, goals, and aspirations. Sheehy ties development in late adolescence and young adulthood to Erikson's developmental stage.

Levinson (134–138) *describes adult developmental stages as age-linked and universal, including biological, psychodynamic, cultural, social, and other timetables that operate in only partial synchronization.* **Life structure** *refers to a pattern of the person's life at a specific time and is used to focus on the boundary between the individual and society.* **External life structure** *refers to roles, memberships, interests, conditions or style of living, and long-term goals.* **Internal life structure** *includes the personal meanings of external patterns, inner identities, care values, fantasies, and psychodynamic qualities that shape the person.* Like Vaillant, this research focused on males and findings are also applicable to females. **Table 14-6**, Levinson's Theory of Early Adulthood, is a summary.

Sullivan (228) *defines young adulthood as the time when the sexuality of human development is powerful, and there is a need to find adequate and satisfying expression. This era is the time of intimate love and expanding experiences and collaboration with people.* If for some reason the person is thwarted in expression of sexual feelings, perhaps because of illness or injury that causes a felt or imagined change in

TABLE 14-5

Gould's Developmental Stages of Adulthood

Stage	Age Range (yr)	Developmental Task
1	16–18	Preadulthood; desire to escape from parental control. May perceive self as adult in some cultures.
2	18–22	Leave family. Establish peer friendships.
3	22–28	Develop greater independence. Commit self to career and family.
4	28–34	Transition; question life goals. Reevaluate marriage and career commitments.
5	34–43	Sense of time running out. Realign life goals.
6	43–53	Settle down. Accept personal life situation.
7	53–60	Accept past. Greater tolerance for others; general mellowing.

Adapted from references 85, 86.

TABLE 14-6

Levinson's Theory of Early Adulthood

Era	Age Range	Life Structure
Preadulthood	0–22	Preparing for adulthood. Transition to early adulthood. Begin novice phase; person is
	17–22	guided out of adolescence.
Early adulthood	17–45	Combine social and occupational roles that are adapted to personality and skills.
	22–28	Enter young adulthood. Novice phase tasks: a. Form dream for life b. Establish or enter relationship c. Select occupation d. Establish love relationship
	28–33	Age 30 transition: reappraise life plan and modify it.
	33–40	Culminating life plans and structure for early adulthood: seek to realize goals.
	40–45	Transition to or preparation for midlife.

Adapted from reference 135, 136.

body image, sexual concerns may become paramount. Sublimation is an effective adaptive mechanism. (See Chapter 1.) ∞

Developmental Crisis: Intimacy Versus Isolation

According to **Erikson** (65–67), **the psychosexual crisis is in intimacy versus self-isolation. Intimacy** is *reaching out and using the self to form a commitment to and an intense, lasting relationship with another person or even a cause, an institution, or creative effort* (65–67). *In an intimate experience there is mutual trust, sharing of feelings, and responsibility to and cooperation with each other. The physical satisfaction and psychological security of another are more important than one's own. Involvement with people, work, hobbies, and community issues is an expansion of personal intimacy.* He or she has poise and ease in the lifestyle because identity is firm. There is a steady conviction of who he or she is, a self-acceptance, and a unity of personality that will improve through life (65–67, 108). **Intimacy,** according to Sullivan (228), *is a situation involving two people that permits acceptance of all aspects of the other, self-disclosure, and a collaboration in which the person adjusts behavior to the other's behavior and needs in pursuit of mutual satisfaction.* A person's mental health is dependent on the ability to enter into a relationship and experience self-disclosure. In so doing, the support and maintenance of the relationship alleviates feelings of loneliness.

In the intimate relationship, as in friendships, females are more concerned than males with the relationship and are interested in the process rather than the product of something. Females also recognize their vulnerability and can self-disclose and acknowledge the need to change more readily than males. Interpersonal dependency, an element of the normal adult personality, encompasses attachment and dependency. Anxious or insecure attachment develops when a natural desire for a close relationship with another is accompanied by apprehension that the relationship will end. If anxiety is transferred to the other person, the response may be a withdrawal from the relationship, contributing to feelings of loneliness. If a healthy balance between dependence and independence exists, social relationships and intimacy are maintained more eas-

ily, and the risk of experiencing loneliness and isolation decreases (66, 67, 108, 201).

Although intimacy includes sexual intercourse and orgasm, it means far more than physical or genital contact. With the intimate person, the young adult is able to regulate cycles of work, recreation, and procreation (if chosen), and to work toward satisfactory stages of development for offspring and the ongoing development of self and the partner. Intimacy is a paradox. Although the person shares his or her identity with another for mutual satisfaction or support (via self-abandon in orgasm or in other shared emotional experiences), he or she does not fear loss of personal identity. Each does not absorb the other's personality (65, 67, 108).

Many in late adolescence or early-young adulthood do fear a loss of personal identity in an intimate relationship. In an increasingly complex society the search for self-definition is a difficult one. Identity is not always solidly possessed by the time one is 20, 25, or 30 years old. Achieving a true sense of intimacy seems illusive to many of this generation. Movies, novels, plays, and pornographic media glorify sex for self-gratification. Many are puzzled, hurt, or dismayed when they find such sexual encounters are disappointing.

Isolation, or **self-absorption,** is the *inability to be intimate, spontaneous, or close with another, thus becoming withdrawn, lonely, and conceited, and behaving in a stereotyped manner.* The isolated person is unable to sustain close friendships. The person may not marry; there is avoidance of a bond with another. If he or she does marry, the partner is likely to find personal emotional needs unmet while giving considerably of the self to the isolated, self-absorbed person (65, 66). **Box 14-8**, Consequences of Isolation, summarizes behavior and feelings of the person (65, 66) to utilize in assessment and intervention strategies.

Love and Marriage

LOVE The feeling that is the basis for intimacy is love (65, 66, 228), and love and intimacy change over time (51, 181, 228). The young adult often has difficulty determining what is love. A

BOX 14-8	Consequences of Isolation

1. Is pessimistic, distrustful, ruthless
2. Is lonely; may rationalize why being alone is enjoyed
3. Avoids close relationships, especially with person of the opposite sex
4. Lives a facade
5. Has experienced a number of unsuccessful relationships
6. Insists on having own way in a relationship
7. Lacks empathy for others; cannot see another's perspective
8. Is naively childlike
9. Is easily disillusioned, embittered, cynical
10. Overextends self without any real interest or feeling
11. Is unable to reciprocate feelings or behavior in a relationship; makes demands but cannot give in a relationship
12. Participates readily in encounter groups or forced fellowship to temporarily relieve loneliness, alienation
13. Avoids real issues in life
14. May be overtly friendly but drops a relationship when it becomes intimate; unable to sustain a relationship; may become engaged but never marry
15. May spend considerable time on the computer or Internet but is actually alienated from people

Adapted from references 65–67.

classic description of love, as stated by the apostle Paul in I Corinthians 13:4–7, has been the basis for many statements on love by poets, novelists, humanists, philosophers, psychiatrists, theologians, and common people.

> *Love is patient and kind; love is not jealous or boastful; it is not arrogant or rude. Love does not insist on its own way; it is not irritable or resentful; it does not rejoice at wrong, but rejoices in the right. Love bears all things, believes all things, hopes all things, endures all things.*

One of the most important things the person can learn within the family as a child and adolescent is to love. By the time the person reaches the mid-20s, he or she should be experienced in the emotion of love. If there was deprivation or distortion of love in the home when he or she was young, the adult will find it difficult to achieve mature love in an intimate relationship. By this time, the person should realize that *one does not fall in love; one learns to love; one grows into love.*

There are several aspects of intimate love: passion, intimacy, and commitment. **Passion,** *falling in love, an ecstatic excitement fueled by risk and unfamiliarity,* is strong at the beginning of a relationship. Friendship, affectionate love, attachment, caring, and intimacy follow. **Consummate love** *involves passion, intimacy, commitment, and a cognitive appraisal of the relationship.* **Commitment** *grows through a series of day-to-day decisions to spend time together, care for each other, share possessions, and overcome problems* (26, 92, 96, 201). This developmental pattern is common for cou-

ples in the Western world but may not be observed in cultures where marriages are arranged (8, 80).

Discuss with young adults the concept of intimacy in a holistic sense. Explore their ideas about marriage, establishing a home, the relationship between spouses, the role of motherhood and fatherhood, and the relationship between parents and children. When you help people sort through feelings about life and love, you are promoting health and stability in them and their offspring.

MARRIAGE Attachment is a concept that applies across the life span and is manifested in several layers of relationship in adulthood (216). The traditionally accepted way for two people in love to be intimate is in marriage, a social contract or institution implying binding rules and responsibilities that cannot be ignored without some penalty. Marriage in some form is endorsed by all cultures because it formalizes and symbolizes the importance of family and social stability. Marriage is more than getting a piece of paper. The spouse in the United States is expected to be a lover, friend, confidant, counselor, career person, and parent—simultaneously (201). According to **Social Exchange Theory,** *each person contributes something useful to the other without excessive cost to self* (26, 226). *There is equity in the relationship—shared contributions—not absolute equality* (26, 226). Refer to the Case Situation for an example.

There are norms in every society to prevent people from entering lightly into the wedded state (e.g., age limits, financial and property settlements, ceremony, witnesses, and public registration and announcement). *Marriage gives rights in five areas* (201, 226, 256): (a) sexuality; (b) psychosocial attachment, support, and commitment; (c) birth and rearing of children; (d) domestic and economic services; and (e) property and realistic expectations. For some, either before marriage or after divorce and before remarriage, **cohabitation** is like a *"trial marriage."* More than half of all U.S. couples who marry have lived together (181). In the United States, cohabitation does not protect marital rights and can contribute to relationship and legal problems (26, 181, 201, 245). Cohabitating unions are less stable than marriages. Abuse is common among cohabitating couples (26). Couples who have a child together are less likely to break up (181). Refer to the discussion on cohabitation under the sexuality section earlier in this chapter.

The pattern and sequence of a person's life history influence whether, whom, when, and why he or she marries. The problems of marital adjustment and family living have their roots and basis in the choice of the partner (181). The personality of each partner will affect personality development and maturity of the other. The person chooses someone for an intimate relationship whose lifestyle and personality pattern strengthen and encourage personal development. One couple invited others to a celebration of their 25th wedding anniversary with the following words (260):

> *We continue to adjust to each other, an adjustment that started 25 years ago, and will never stop because we each continue to grow and change. We will always be different. Don't mistake it for a solid marriage. There is no such thing. Marriage is more like an airplane than a rock. You have to commit the thing to flight, and then it creaks and groans, and keeping it airborne depends entirely on attitude. Working at it, though, we can fly forever. Only the two of us know how hard it has been or how worthwhile. Celebrate with us . . .*

Case Situation

Young Adult Development: Marriage and Commitment

James Chaney, 26 years old, received his bachelor's degree in nursing this year after combining full-time employment as an attendant at a local hospital and part-time school attendance for 5 years. He has recently accepted a position at the hospital as a nurse in the surgical intensive care unit. James and his wife, Mary, have been married for 2 years. Mary, 25 years old, is finishing her bachelor's degree in accounting while she continues employment with an insurance firm. James and Mary plan to wait a few years before starting a family as both realize the importance of graduate education in their fields. They would also like to move from their apartment to a home with more space and a yard.

To save money to achieve their future plans, both James and Mary work extra hours when asked. This has frequently inter-fered with their studies. They also find they have little time for leisure activities and less time together. Communication is sometimes in the form of memos posted on the refrigerator. Increasingly, the stresses of balancing school, work, and home demands have resulted in arguments, often over minor issues.

When a long-anticipated vacation must be canceled because of unexpected expenses, James and Mary are disappointed and angry; however, they decide to plan a week of inexpensive activities in the local area that will allow them to spend time together uninterrupted. They decide to tell no one that they have remained at home. The resulting vacation is truly restful and meaningful as they share favorite activities and explore their dreams and goals for the future.

Contributed by Judith Zentner, MA, BS, FNP-BC.

In the United States, an increasing number of mixed marriages are occurring, as depicted by Figure 14-8 ▨. A number of *factors influence the success of the marriage that crosses religious, ethnic, socioeconomic, or racial boundaries* (26, 114, 181, 201):

1. Motive for marriage
2. Desire, commitment, and effort to bridge the gulf between the couple and their families
3. Ability and maturity of the two people to live with and resolve their differences and problems
4. Reaction of the parental families, who may secretly or openly support **homogamy** (*marriage between a couple with similar or identical backgrounds*)
5. More liberal social attitudes that override parental objections

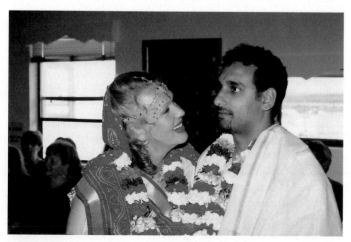

FIGURE ▨ **14-8** The Christian bride and Hindu groom exchange vows.

You may have opportunity to counsel and educate the young adult family about their relationship. You may ask certain questions to ascertain readiness for a healthy marriage: Can you take responsibility for your own behavior or do you rely primarily on your parents/others? Have both of you thought about what lies ahead: disagreements and agreements, sickness and health, sadness and happiness, financial difficulties? Have you considered whether or not to have children and what it entails? Do you understand female and male sexuality—the differences and similarities? What can you each give to marriage?

MORAL-SPIRITUAL DEVELOPMENT

The young adult may be either in the Conventional level or beginning the Postconventional level of moral development (see **Table 1-10**). ∞ In the Postconventional level he or she follows higher ethical principles and a unified philosophy of life. There are two stages in this level (125). In both stages the person has passed beyond living a certain way just because the majority of people do. In Stage I of this level, the person adheres to the legal viewpoint of society. The person believes, however, that laws can be changed as people's needs change, and he or she is able to transcend the thinking of a specific social order and develop universal principles about justice, equality, and human rights. In Stage II, the person still operates as in Stage I but is able to incorporate injustice, pain, and death as an integral part of existence (125) and engage in efforts to correct injustice and diminish pain. There is deepening empathy for others and their value systems (66, 81). The young adult is unlikely to be consistently in Stage II of the Postconventional level.

Kohlberg (125) espouses that the reason for the behavior indicates the level of moral development and that for a person to be at any level, the reasons for behavior should be consistent to the stage

INTERVENTIONS FOR HEALTH PROMOTION

Teach the following guidelines for a healthy relationship:

1. Spend time together. Establish themselves as a collaborative pair in their own eyes and in the eyes of mutual friends and both families.
2. Give priority to the spouse and home. If friends of either husband or wife are offensive to the partner, be prepared to minimize this friendship. Build new friendships together.
3. Be faithful to the spouse. If one person engages in an extramarital affair, it is possible to repair the brokenness, but a feeling of mistrust may remain and is difficult to overcome.
4. Remember that a good marriage promotes health and longevity and reduces stress.
5. Work through intimate systems of communication: exchange of confidences, feelings, empathy, and ability to predict each other's responses.
6. Plan ahead for a stable relationship and arriving at a consensus about how their life should be lived. Be committed to each other.
7. Be mindful of sensitive areas, those that are sources of irritation in each other's life. Each needs to work at coping with the other's idiosyncrasies or habits and try to meet the other's preferences to keep love in the relationship. Agree to disagree.
8. Give each other positive reinforcement. Express praise, appreciation, and affection to release love rather than focus on problems.
9. Manage money and material possessions together. Money and things are important, but focus on the person. Share power.
10. Maintain a spirit of courtship, spontaneity, and freshness to keep love in a marriage.
11. Deal with crises in a positive way. Always be respectful.

50% of the time. Therefore it would appear difficult for the average young adult, concerned about family, achieving in a career, paying the bills, and so on, to be in the Postconventional level. Although the person may follow principles some of the time, conflicting situations and demands arise. To be consistently in the Postconventional level takes considerable ego strength, a firm emotional and spiritual identity, and a willingness to stand up to societal forces. It may take years of maturing before the adult can be that courageous and consistent in Western society. For example, how does the young adult handle the dishonesty seen on the job? How does the mother or father handle the child viewing violence on television or video games at a friend's home? How does the couple react when a friend brags that he is having extramarital sexual experiences?

Today's young adults have grown up with the influence of science and technology. Some are **postreligious,** *disinterested in other worlds, and concerned only in the secular existence or technology/electronic media of the present.* Some reject the institutional church. Some have retained a desire and ability to apply spiritual and moral principles in this world. Parents with young children may join a faith family (church or synagogue), seeking a way to instill values and a religious faith in their children.

The spiritual awakening often experienced during adolescence, which might have receded with seeking of success, may now take on a more genuine and mature aspect. The young adult searches for a new connectedness with others, nature, the universe, or a higher being. The mystery of life, of faith, of belief in God is explored actively by some young adults. The young adult may seek to enhance personal spirituality through various methods of stress management presented in Chapter 2, ∞ group activities (church or nonchurch sponsorship), or worship experiences. Currently, there appears to be more focus on the spiritual dimension in young adulthood; young adults seek friends and leisure activi-

ties within a faith community. If the young adult has children, he or she must rear them with some underlying philosophy. Their moral-spiritual questions must be answered. The young adult's religious teaching, perhaps previously rejected, may now be accepted as "not so bad after all." Or the young adult may build a new version of spirituality: individual, comprehensive, dynamic, flexible, searching, combining basic standards of morality and conduct with new attitudes and ideas.

One of the dilemmas for the interfaith or intercultural couple is what values and religion, if any, to follow in the home and to teach the children; how to celebrate holidays; and what rituals and traditions to follow (e.g., Hanukkah or Christmas). Even when the couple makes a choice, there may be conflicts with relatives. Grandparents often have difficulty accepting that their child married someone of another faith or culture. Such marriages can work, and the children can have a firm moral and spiritual development. It is important for both spouses and their families to discuss feelings openly from the beginning. The couple should learn as much as possible about each other's religion or culture and talk to their families and friends about their experiences. It is critical that each family group remain open and accepting of the other. In turn, the children can learn deeper dimensions of spirituality, moral values, and their cultural background.

Although spiritual development and moral development are often thought of simultaneously, there is no significant link between specific religious affiliation or education and moral development. Moral development is linked positively with empathy, the capacity to understand another's viewpoint, and the ability to act reciprocally with another while maintaining personal values and principles.

You may discuss spiritual or moral issues with the young adult. Your own behavior is important. Being with people who are at a higher moral level stimulates the person to ask questions, consider his or her actions, and move to a higher moral level. You are a role model. Research shows that more patients, including young adults, welcome the opportunity to talk about spirituality concerns or religious beliefs during illness of self or a family member (192).

ADAPTIVE MECHANISMS

The young adult seeks stability while he or she is adapting to new or changing events. When the young adult is physically and emotionally healthy, overall functioning is smooth (66, 142, 177, 243). Adaptation to the environment, satisfaction of needs, and social interaction proceed relatively effortlessly and with minimum discomfort. The mature young adult's behavior demonstrates control of impulses and drives and is in harmony with superego ideals and demands. He or she can tolerate frustration of needs and is capable of making choices that seem best for total equilibrium. The person is emotionally mature for this life stage. Yet the adult can experience considerable stress and situational crises. **Stress overload**, *a feeling of pressure or tension, difficulty in functioning as usual, problems with decision making, feelings of anger and impatience, and physical symptoms, may occur* (243).

Emotional maturity is not exclusively related to physical health. Under stress, the healthiest people might momentarily have irrational impulses; in contrast, the extremely ill have periods of lucidity. Emotional health and maturity have an infinite gradation of behavior on a continuum rather than a rigid division between healthy and ill (228). Concepts of maturity are generated by culture. What is normal in one society may be abnormal in another.

In coping with stress in the environment, the young adult uses many of the previously discussed adaptive mechanisms. Use of these mechanisms, such as *denial* and *regression,* becomes abnormal or maladaptive only when the person uses the same mechanism of behavior too frequently, in too many situations, or for too long a duration. Refer to **Table 1-6** to review adaptive mechanisms for assessment and intervention strategies. ∞

Active listening and support to the adult in his or her decision making are effective. Refer also to principles of intervention for stress and crises discussed in Chapter 2. ∞

SELF-CONCEPT AND BODY IMAGE DEVELOPMENT

Definitions

The person's **self-concept,** *perception or definition of self physically, emotionally, and socially, is now defined and expanded to fit the young adult perspective. Perception is based on* (35, 73, 181, 205):

1. Reactions of others that have been internalized.
2. Self-expectations and self-evaluation.
3. Perceived abilities—physically, mentally, emotionally, and socially.
4. Knowledge, attitudes, values, and spiritual insights.
5. Habits, occupation, and lifestyle.
6. Physical appearance and body function.
7. Health status: physical and mental.

These factors affect self-concept and affect how that person will handle situations and relate to others. How the person behaves de-

pends on positive or negative feelings about self, whether the person believes others view him or her positively or negatively, and beliefs about others' expectations for behavior in a situation. The reactions of family members, including spouse, and the employment situation are strong influences on the young adult's self-concept. Additionally, the person discloses different aspects of self to various people and in various situations, depending on needs, what is considered socially acceptable, reactions of others, and past experience with self-disclosure (35, 73, 181, 205).

Body image, *a part of self-concept, is a mental picture of the body's appearance integrated into the parietotemporal area of the cortex. Body image includes the surface, internal, and postural picture of the body and values, attitudes, emotions, and personality reactions of the person in relation to the body as an object in space, separate from others.* This image is flexible, subject to constant revision, and may not be reflective of actual body structure. Body image shifts back and forth at different times of the day and at different times in the life cycle (73, 181, 205).

Under normal conditions, the body is the focus of an individual's identity, and its limits more or less clearly define a boundary that separates the person from the environment. One's body has spatial and time sense and yields experiences that cannot be shared directly with others. A person's body is the primary channel of contact with the world, and it is a nucleus around which values are synthesized. Any disturbance to the body influences total self-concept.

Contributing Influences

Many factors contribute to the body image (35, 73, 181, 205):

1. Parental and social reaction to the person's body.
2. The person's interpretation of others' reactions to him or her.
3. The anatomic appearance and physiologic function of the body, including sex, age, kinesthetic and other sensorimotor stimuli, and illness or deformity.
4. Attitudes and emotions toward and familiarity with the body.
5. Internal drives, dependency needs, motivational state, and ideals to which the person aspires.
6. Identification with the bodies of others who were considered ideal (a little bit of each person significant to the person is incorporated into the self-concept and personality).
7. Perception of space and objects immediately surrounding the body, such as a chair or car; the sense of body boundaries.
8. Objects attached to the body such as clothing, a wig, false eyelashes, a prosthesis, jewelry, makeup, or perfume.
9. Activities the body performs in various roles, occupations, or recreation.

The kinesthetic receptors in the muscles, tendons, and joints and the labyrinth receptors in the inner ear inform the person about his or her position in space. By means of perceptual alterations in position, the postural image of the body constantly changes. Every new posture and movement is incorporated by the cortex into a **schema** (*image*) in relation to or association with previously made schemata. Thus the image of the body changes with changing movements—walking, sitting, gestures, changes in appearance, and changes in the pace of walking (35, 205).

Self-produced movement aids visual accuracy. When a person's body parts are moved passively instead of actively (e.g., sitting in a wheelchair instead of walking), perceptual accuracy about space and the self as an object in space is hindered (246). Athletes, ballet dancers, and other agile people are more accurate than most in estimating the dimensions of the body parts that are involved in movement. Activity appears to enhance sensory information in a way that passive movements do not. If a person undergoes body changes, he or she must actively explore and move the involved part to reintegrate it (35, 162, 205, 246).

Self-Knowledge: Professional and Client Applications

To intervene effectively you must know yourself. How do you visualize your body or feel about yourself as you go through various motions? What emotions are expressed by your movements? How do you think others visualize you? Movement of the body parts, gestures, and appearance communicate a message to the observer, the client, or family member that may or may not be intended. The message you convey about yourself to another may aid or hinder the establishment of a therapeutic relationship. Be realistically aware of the posture and movement of your body and what you may be conveying to another. Self-knowledge is not necessarily the same as knowledge gained about the self from others. Key concepts for assessment and intervention are emphasized in italics in the following section. These concepts provide a theoretical, yet practical, foundation.

Each person sees self differently from how others see him or her, although the most mature person is able to view self as others do. New attributes or ideas are integrated into the old ones, but all ideas received are not necessarily integrated. Before any perception about the self can be integrated into one's self-concept, the perceptions must be considered good or necessary to the self (228). *If the person believes that he or she is competent* (a **positive self-image,** "*good me*"), *a statement about incompetence will not be integrated into the self-image unless he or she is repeatedly told. If, however, the person has a* **negative self-image** *("bad me"), it will also take many statements of his or her worth before they can be accepted and integrated into the self-concept* (228).

A person has definite ideas and feelings about his or her own body, what is satisfying and what is frustrating. The person discovers that he or she has certain abilities and disabilities, likes and dislikes, and ways of affecting others. What the person thinks of self has remarkable power in influencing behavior and the interpretation of others' behavior, the choice of associates, and goals pursued.

Feelings about certain self-attributes vary according to the importance placed on them and how central or close they are to the essence of self. Events such as illness or injury involving the face and torso are usually more threatening than those involving the limbs, as the face and the torso are integrated first into the young child's self-perception. The extremities are seen as part of the self later and may therefore be less highly valued in comparison (35, 58).

Feelings about one's characteristics also depend on whether a characteristic or body part is viewed as a functional tool for living or as a central personal attribute. For example, teeth can be viewed as a tool for eating or as central to the face, smile, youth, and personality. Dentures can be accepted and integrated as part of the body image more easily if they are viewed as a tool rather than if they are thought of as a sign of decline and old age. The person's work may

also be viewed as a tool, function, or way to earn a living and help others or as central to the self. Age and gender are also characteristics that differ in degree of centrality or importance to the person (35, 58).

Involved in self-concept and body image are the body parts supposedly considered strategically important in the character of the ethnic group or race (e.g., the German backbone, the Jewish nose, or the dark skin of the Black person). The body part with special significance, which would also include the afflicted limb in a disabled person, is believed heavier, larger, or more conspicuous and is perceived to be the focus of others' attention, although it may not be.

Location and history of family residence, religion, socioeconomic background, and even attempts at moving to a higher social class level are integrated into the adult self-concept but not the body image. The *occupation* or *profession* may be integrated into body image, as well as self-concept, depending upon the work performed. The person who uses the body or a specific body part, such as the hands, limbs, or back muscles, consistently as part of the job will link occupation into body image.

Body image in the adult is a social creation. Normality, judged by appearance, and ways of using the body are prescribed by the culture (8, 73, 80). Approval and acceptance are given for normal appearance and proper behavior. Self-concept continually influences and enlarges the person's world, mastery of and interaction with it, and ability to respond to the many experiences it offers. This integration, largely unconscious, is constantly evolving and can be identified in the person's values, attitudes, and feelings about self. The experiences with the body are interpreted in terms of feelings, earlier views of the self, and group or cultural norms (35, 58, 73, 162). *In the adult there is a close interdependence between body image and personality, self-concept, and identity.* Females have a more clearly defined and stable body concept than males. The differences seem related to different anatomic structures and body functions but also to the contrasts between males and females in their upbringing, style of life, and role in culture (35, 58, 73).

Use information about self-concept and body image as you promote health and intervene with the well, ill, or injured client. Your feedback to others is important. If you are to help another elevate self-esteem or feel positively about his or her body, you must give repeated positive reinforcement and help the person overcome unrealistic guilt, shame, and "bad me" feelings. Saying something positive or recognizing abilities once or twice will not be enough. The self-concept, whether wholesome or not, is difficult to change, as the person perceives others' comments and behavior in relation to an already established image to avoid conflict and anxiety within self.

You will encounter many young adults with body image distortions or changes as a result of accidental or war injuries, disease, weight gain or loss, pregnancy, or identity problems. You can make a significant contribution to the health of this person for the remainder of life by giving assistance through physical care, listening, counseling, teaching, rehabilitation, and working with significant others.

Be aware that health care professionals and certain treatment practices may contribute to a negative self-concept. Often the health care system treats the client (well or ill) as an unthinking, incompetent object. Although there may be some attitudinal changes occurring, many people still hold traditional stereotyped beliefs about gender-related behavior. Advocate for policies, procedures, and practices that promote a healthy environment and a healthy approach to the client in any care environment. Educate staff about need for change.

Your behavior, use of problem solving, and verbal facility can change negative or sexist attitudes. Your efforts are important for your own positive self-concept and for unbiased care of each person, thus promoting a positive, healthy self-concept and body image.

DEVELOPMENTAL TASKS FOR THE YOUNG ADULT

In this postmodern age, developmental tasks may be difficult to achieve in the rapidly changing society. There is a sense of fragmentation. Yet, the core of the developmental tasks relate to the stability of the individual and close relationships. **Figure 14-9**☐, Developmental tasks of the young adult center around the family unit, conveys a sense of health and that love is the foundation. See also the Case Situation. The developmental tasks will be accomplished in a variety of ways, depending on the individual and culture (8, 61, 80, 101).

The young adult is expected to achieve the following tasks during this era (61):

1. Accept self and stabilize self-concept and body image.
2. Acknowledge and resolve conflicts between the emerging self and conformity to the social order.
3. Establish independence from parental home and financial aid; resolve difficulty of home ownership.
4. Become established in a vocation or profession that provides personal satisfaction, economic independence, and a feeling of making a worthwhile contribution to society; update skills as necessary.
5. Learn to appraise and express love responsibly through more than sexual contacts.
6. Establish an intimate bond with another, either through marriage or with a close friend.

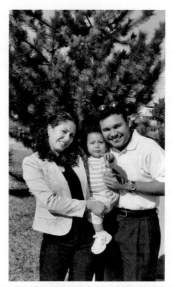

FIGURE ☐ **14-9** Developmental tasks of the young adult center around the family unit.

7. Establish and maintain a home and manage a time schedule and life stresses.
8. Find a congenial social and friendship group.
9. Decide whether to have a family and carry out tasks of parenting.
10. Resolve changed relationships with the couple's parental families.
11. Formulate a meaningful philosophy of life and reassess priorities and values.
12. Become involved as a citizen in the community.
13. Achieve a more realistic outlook about other cultures, mores, and political systems.

Use therapeutic communication and relationship principles, counseling, and education about healthy lifestyle choices to assist the person in exploring options to achieve these tasks. Such exploration may occur with the healthy adult during a routine

Case Situation

Father-Son Relationship

John, a 35-year-old, spends as much time as possible with his 13-year-old son, Mike. Some of the time is spent doing tasks together, including yard work. Mike enjoys the outdoors and the exercise. John has taught Mike various tasks, including cutting the grass, using appropriate safety measures. Mike gets paid a small amount and earns extra money cutting the neighbor's yard. Mike knows the joy of earning and saving money, using some to help others (buying toys to be given to poor children locally and overseas), and spending some on himself. Thus, he is

following his parents' teachings. John and Mike also spend some time on the church sports teams. Mike's parents believe ordinary activities develop self-confidence, develop a work ethic, and teach how to use leisure. They do not "brag" about or give meaningless praise to Mike, but both parents reinforce him verbally. Mike realizes all his behavior is not always positive, but he knows that as a person, he is accepted, worthy of recognition, and loved.

Contributed by Carole Piles, PhD, MSN, RN.

screening, during a crisis situation, or in a situation when health care services are being provided. The partner, if available, should be included in the discussion. If there are children, meeting individual tasks and parenting tasks can contribute to either a sense of stress or accomplishment. Assist the person or family in clarifying values and decision making.

Lifestyle Options

In the United States, the young adult has many options. He or she may decide to base the style of living around age, work or leisure, profession, or marriage and family.

SINGLEHOOD

Singlehood, *remaining unmarried and following a specific lifestyle,* is not new. Maiden aunts, bachelors, and those whose religion calls for singlehood are traditional. Others never marry but are in some form of committed relationship. Remaining unmarried is increasingly an option.

The single person can accomplish the task of intimacy through emotional investment of self in others. Many are extroverts, have several very close friends with whom they share activities, have a meaningful career, and have a harmonious relationship with parents. If they marry, they want to feel that they have chosen the right partner and have spent time living just for themselves so that they do not resent the responsibilities of marriage (26, 181, 201).

Many prefer to remain single as they pursue prolonged education and strive to become established in their occupational field. Others find that being free of relationships, to sample a variety of lifestyles, and to travel as they please before settling down to raise a family is an important part of establishing identity. They avoid living out their lives in the same manner and location as their parents and may live in an apartment complex or loft for singles only, following a lifestyle that conveys freedom. For whatever reasons, the number of single people in this country is on the rise, especially in the 20- to 34-year-old age group (181, 201).

The single person may be in emotional isolation, unable to establish a close relationship and alienated from self and others, or depressed about the life situation. However, most singles do not fit this description.

The single person may need help in resolving feelings about being a single person and validation about the choice. If the person is single because of isolation and self-absorption, mental health counseling may be needed, not for singlehood, but because of feelings about self and others. For additional information on singlehood, refer to Chapter 6. ∞

FAMILY PLANNING: THE EXPECTANCY AND PARENTHOOD STAGES

Parenthood and family planning are options for either the couple or a single person. Couples may use natural family planning, discussed earlier in the chapter. There are challenges, but the couple tends to form a closer bond and communication (242). Contraceptives for the female and vasectomy procedures for the male are other options. These methods make it possible for couples to say: "We don't want children now," "We don't want children ever," or "We want to try to have two children spaced 3 years apart."

Reasons for Childbearing

The couple may have a child for a variety of reasons (14, 26, 61, 101, 181, 199, 201):

1. Psychological and spiritual fulfillment of having a child
2. Extension of self
3. Sense of pride or joy
4. Offset loneliness
5. Have someone to love self
6. Attempt to hold a marriage together
7. Feeling of power, generated by ability to create life
8. Representation of wealth
9. Have an heir for family name and wealth or family business
10. Religious convictions

Whether the couple chooses to have only one child or more children is related to more than fertility and religious background. Lifestyle, finances, career, available support systems, and emotional maturity are factors.

Information presented in Table 13-3, ∞ which summarizes contraceptives, will help you teach about family planning. Chapter 6 provides information useful for understanding the family with whom you are working.

Developmental Tasks for the Couple During the Expectant Stage

You are in a position to assist the couple in understanding the changes that childbearing will create and the following developmental tasks for this stage of family life.

Review Chapter 6 for a summary of the expectant and parenthood stages, including developmental tasks presented in Table 6-2. ∞ *Additional developmental tasks include* (61, 199):

1. Rearrange the home to provide space, facilities, and supplies for the expected baby.
2. Rework the budget and determine how to obtain and spend income to accommodate changing needs and maintain the family unit financially.
3. Evaluate the changing roles, division of labor, how responsibilities of child care will be divided, who has the final authority, and whether the mother should continue working outside the home if she has a career or profession.
4. Adapt patterns of sexual behavior to the pregnant status.
5. Rework the communication system between the couple, explore feelings about the pregnancy and ideas about child rearing, and work to resolve the differences.
6. Acquire knowledge about pregnancy, childbirth, and parenthood.
7. Rework the communication system and relationships with family, friends, and community activities, based on the reality of the pregnancy and their reactions.
8. Use family and community resources as needed.
9. Examine and expand the philosophy of life to include responsibilities of childbearing and child rearing.

Developmental tasks that must be mastered during pregnancy and the intrapartum period to ensure readiness for the maternal role are (199):

1. **Pregnancy validation:** *Accepting the reality of the pregnancy, working through feelings of ambivalence.*
2. **Fetal embodiment:** *Incorporating the fetus and enlarging body into the body image.*
3. **Fetal distinction:** *Seeing the fetus as a separate entity, fantasizing what the baby will be like.*
4. **Role transition:** *After birth, an increasing readiness to take on the task of parenthood.*

Transition to parenthood, feelings, symptoms, body image changes, and needs for social support during pregnancy all affect family functioning and child care after birth (26, 69, 181, 201).

Father's Response

Some research indicates that attachment of the father to the baby begins during pregnancy, rather than after birth, and that a strong marital relationship and vicariously experienced physical symptoms resembling pregnancy (and sometimes the couvade syndrome [49]) strengthen attachment (69, 71, 112, 129, 130, 145, 151, 227). Refer to Chapter 6 for an explanation of the couvade syndrome. ∞

Studies indicate a characteristic pattern of development of subjective emotional involvement in pregnancy among first-time expectant fathers. Three phases occur: announcement phase, moratorium, and focusing period (151). These phases may be seen in subsequent pregnancies as well.

The **announcement phase** is *when pregnancy is suspected and confirmed.* If the male desired the pregnancy, he shows desire and excitement. For many males, fatherhood represents adulthood, sexual adequacy, and normalcy. If he did not want the pregnancy, he shows pain and shock (151).

During the **moratorium period,** the *male suppresses thoughts about the pregnancy.* This period can last from a few days to months and usually ends when the pregnancy is obvious. This period is characterized by emotional distance, a feeling the pregnancy is not real, concentration on himself and other life concerns, and sometimes leaving home. The emotional distance allows him to work through ambivalence and jealousy of the female's ability to bear a child, but his distance causes her to feel unloved, rejected, angry, and uncared for. Marital tension exists. Pregnancy often emphasizes the disparity in the couple's life pace and focus. Gradually the male faces the financial and lifestyle implications of the pregnancy. If he feels financially insecure or unstable with his partner, or wishes to extend the childless period, he resents pregnancy and spends a longer time in the moratorium stage. Most males eventually become enthusiastic about the pregnancy and baby when they feel the baby move or hear the heartbeat. If he does not become enthusiastic and supportive, the couple may be at risk for marital and parenting problems (151).

The **focusing period** occurs *when the male perceives the pregnancy as real and important in his life.* He redefines himself as a father; he begins to feel more in tune with and is more helpful to his partner. He begins to read or talk about parenting and child development, notices other children, and is willing to participate in childbirth classes and purchase baby supplies. He constructs a mental image of the baby, sometimes different from her mental image of the baby. The circle of friends may change to those who have children. He may feel fear about the coming labor and birth

and feel responsible for a successful birth (151). The male who participates in pregnancy and birth experiences greater closeness with the infant and spouse and heightened self-esteem and esteem for the spouse. His readiness for pregnancy may significantly influence emergence of the father's involvement (129, 130). The father's concept of his role varies with the culture. For example, in Japan (112), the historical view has been of wage earner for the family, friend to the children, and authority figure. The perception of the role is expanding to be more involved in nurturing the children, more supportive and helpful to the wife/mother, and a decision maker for the family (112).

Mother's Response

An even stronger attachment occurs in the female as she physically experiences the fetus and physical symptoms related to pregnancy. Feelings for the child are stronger if she has a loving, supportive partner. Some males have difficulty accepting the responsibility implied by a pregnant partner and do not want to be involved in care of her during pregnancy or postpartum, or the child (71, 107, 129, 130). Refer to Chapter 9 about the attachment relationship between mother and child. ∞

Encourage the pregnant female and her partner to attend childbirth education classes during pregnancy. During the labor and delivery process, give support and acceptance. Be flexible. Help the couple to use what they learned and practiced in prenatal classes. Let them assume responsibility for decisions when possible. Teaching during the postpartum period is crucial to family-centered care. Cultural considerations are also important. More information about natural childbirth preparation and delivery can be obtained from the Lamaze International Website, www.lamaze.org.

Be aware that in contrast to the societal romanticized view of pregnancy and care of the pregnant female, *she may be a victim of physical, emotional, and mental abuse* (17, 68, 158, 193). Refer to the later section Intimate Partner Violence for information on ways to promote the female's safety and to empower her to achieve well-being (153, 163). Refer to a maternity nursing book for specific information on prenatal care, the labor and delivery process, and postpartum care—for both the normal and high-risk pregnancy and delivery.

OTHER APPROACHES TO PARENTHOOD

Some couples delay childbearing until they are in their 30s or early 40s. The female may wish to pursue her education, a career, or a profession. The couple may choose to travel, start a business, become financially established, or have a variety of experiences before they settle down with one or two children. With genetic counseling, the surgical ability to undo vasectomy and tubal ligation, improved prenatal and neonatal care, and reduced risk of maternal or neonatal complications, pregnancy is usually safe for the mother in her 30s and even early 40s. Many of the risks of late parenthood are related to preexisting disease. Of equal concern are the emotional and social implications, especially after birth when the couple's life revolves around the baby rather than work or earlier interests. Maternal role behaviors and the sense of challenge, role strain, and self-image in the mother role are similar during the first year for childbearing women of all ages (23).

MediaLink   Lamaze International

The single person may desire to be a parent. The single female may, through pregnancy or adoption, choose to have a child. Some are well-educated, professional women in their late 30s or 40s who believe they have no chance of becoming married, for various societal reasons, but who wish to have the experience of motherhood. Some single males who will not be biological fathers are also choosing to experience fatherhood through adoption.

You are in a key position to help the single person think through the wish to have a child, including the following: (a) child care responsibilities and the need for the child to have both male and female caregivers, (b) whether the person has or plans a relationship with someone of the opposite gender to be in the nurturing parent role, (c) presence of a support system and response of the family of origin, and (d) considerations for the child during the school-age and adolescent years. Through values clarification, help the person consider religious, cultural, societal, economic, and lifestyle factors.

Family planning is sometimes made difficult by **infertility,** *inability to conceive after one year of regular, unprotected intercourse or the inability to carry a pregnancy to a term, live birth.* Both partners should be given diagnostic tests together, as 50% of infertility factors are in females and 50% are in males. Infertility can create great psychological problems for each individual, between the couple, and between families of each partner (212, 213, 242). The problem becomes compounded by the increasing difficulty in adopting a healthy baby in most communities, as most single mothers retain their babies. *There are several methods of assisted reproduction from which couples may choose* (212, 213, 253): (a) in vitro fertilization, (b) artificial insemination, and (c) surrogate parent. *Information about these methods is available from the following Websites:*

1. American Society of Reproductive Medicine, www.asrm.org.
2. National Infertility Association or RESOLVE, www.resolve.org
3. Communicable Disease Centers, for a report on fertility clinics, www.cdc.gov.

Counsel and educate about methods of assisted reproduction. Explore values and feelings about having a child. Explore ethical considerations, including the possibility of having multiple births or a child with a congenital deformity. Explore legal ramifications if a surrogate parent is utilized. Through values clarification, have the partners explore spiritual, cultural, religious, societal, economic, and lifestyle factors. Use a decision tree: What are the pros and cons of each method, related factors, and the balance of benefits and risks? Couple counseling may be indicated.

Health Promotion and Health Protection

IMMUNIZATIONS

The young adult should continue immunizations. The CDC recommends that colleges and universities require student documentation of immunity (including tuberculin testing) to preventable diseases as a prerequisite to registration. Adults should be vaccinated each fall against influenza. A tetanus-diphtheria (Td) booster is needed every 10 years. Pregnant women and the chronically ill should be vaccinated for influenza. Recommended immunizations and revaccination, including for adults with uncertain immunization histories and for the chronically ill, are listed in the CDC Website. Those at risk for tuberculosis and in need of the annual two-step skin testing should also refer to the CDC Website.

Educate about the importance of maintaining recommended immunizations and a personal record of type and date. Refer clients to the Websites for updated and changing information and answers to questions about safety concerns.

SAFETY AND HEALTH PROMOTION
Safety and Accident Prevention

Safety suggestions presented earlier in Chapters 9 through 13 are relevant for the young adult family and their children. ∞ The stress related to daily living and occupations can contribute to accidental injury. Motor vehicle accidents, industrial accidents, and drownings rank high as major causes of accidental death in young adults. Other injuries typical in young adulthood are fractures, dislocations, lacerations, abrasions, and contusions (70). These injuries require restriction of activity, which also presents the young adult with social and economic problems.

Some accidental injuries and deaths result from leisure activities. Swimming, diving, boating, and scuba diving can contribute to death, especially if the young adult has been ingesting alcohol or drugs. Head injuries are responsible for most of the deaths related to bicycle and motorcycle accidents. Hang gliding, parachuting, flying small aircraft, mountain climbing in poor weather conditions, and other mountain sports are responsible for a large number of injuries and fatalities, especially if the person is an amateur.

Caution young adults, especially males, who are the greater risk takers, about safety precautions: (a) drive defensively, (b) avoid alcoholic beverages or drugs while driving or engaged in water, mountain, or other sports, and (c) observe the safety precautions for the specific activity. Educate about home safety. Discuss stresses associated with work and how negative attitudes can contribute to accidents. Explore factors that increase anger and aggressive feelings, which can contribute to risk taking, accidents, and injuries or death. Work with occupational settings to promote periodic health screenings. Initiate safety programs in various settings.

Educate people about hearing protection, described as an environmental health problem in Chapter 4. ∞ Eye protection, such as wearing sunglasses or use of goggles in certain occupations or home activities, is also necessary. McNeeley (155) describes risks to health care workers from airborne microbes and chemicals that come in contact with the eyes and stick to the mucous membranes and produce conjunctivitis. Employees in any occupation should be taught ways to protect the eyes, whether performing technologic, manufacturing, manual, or other labor.

Health Promotion Screening

In young adulthood, regular screening tests should be done (self-examinations and clinical testing) as a way to obtain baseline data. After that, consistent records help detect changes in early stages, if any. The screening promotes health by giving direction for lifestyle

TABLE 14-7

Routine Screening for Health and Early Cancer Detection

1. Female: Breast, Uterine, Cervical
   a. Breast self-examination monthly **(see Table 14-8)**.
   b. Clinical breast examination at least every 2 to 3 years during the 20s and 30s and annually after age 40 years.
   c. Mammogram annually beginning at age 40 years.
   d. Papanicolaou smear test annually, or every 2 years with liquid-based Pap test, especially if history of genital warts, multiple sexual partners, or abnormal results. After age 30, if three normal tests in a row, testing may be done every 3 years.
   e. Cervical cancer testing every 3 years after beginning sexual intercourse or after 21 years of age.
2. Male: Scrotum, Penis, Prostate
   a. Testicular self-examination monthly.
   b. Clinical examination if one testicle seems much larger or harder than the other, or if a lump is present.
   c. Prostate examination through digital rectal by professional exam and blood test for prostate-specific antigen (PSA), beginning at 50 years of age.
3. Males and Females: Skin
   a. Self-examination monthly after bath or shower to become familiar with general appearance of skin and pattern of spots, blemishes, color.

b. Observe all sides of arms and legs, tops and palms of hands, between fingers and toes, finger- and toenails, bottom of feet, genital area.
c. Have someone else check top of head if bald or thin hair, back of neck, torso, buttocks, and thighs.
d. Use mirror to complete observation if exam must be done completely by self.
4. Males and Females: Colon and Rectum
   a. Observe daily color of feces or other changes.
   b. Note any changes in bowel elimination pattern.
   c. Fecal occult blood test (FOBT) annually.
5. Males and Females: Mouth
   a. Observe appearance of tooth-gum margins daily while brushing and flossing.
   b. Check at least monthly tongue, palate, and inner cheeks for color changes or any lumps or swelling.
   c. Check daily any sore in mouth that is healing slowly.
   d. Use brush biopsy kit after instruction by dentist.
   e. Use product such as VigiLite Plus to screen inside mouth; blue dye shows on tissues that need professional examination.

Adapted from References 169, 185, 241, 249.

patterns, thereby preventing major health problems. Screening tests are presented in **Table 14-7**, Routine Screening for Health and Early Cancer Detection.

Other screening measurements include (169, 249):

1. Blood pressure measurement baseline and periodically, unless hypertension or cardiac disease exists. Measurement should have begun in childhood and should continue throughout life.
2. Calculation periodically of BMI and estimated target heart rate for exercise.
3. Blood glucose every 1 to 3 years to diagnose prediabetes or type 2 diabetes, more often if necessary.
4. Lipid panel at least every 4 years to determine total cholesterol, triglycerides, and ratio of LDL (bad) to HDL (good or protective) cholesterol.
5. Dental examination and cleansing twice annually to check effectiveness of twice-daily brushing and flossing and to detect and prevent **caries** (*tooth decay*) and periodontal disease.
6. Bone density index (BDI) every 1 to 3 years, beginning in late-young adulthood, 45 to 50 years, to determine early onset of osteopenia, and later osteoporosis.
7. Magnetic resonance imaging (MRI), in addition to mammography, for females over age 25 at high risk of developing breast cancer (known lifetime genetic risk of 20% to 25% or more) (188). A known genetic risk is determined by a positive test for mutations in the BRCA1 or BRCA2 genes or a first-

degree relative (parent, sibling, child) who tested positive for these mutations (188), refer to www.cancer.gov. for more information.
8. Chest x-ray and electrocardiogram (EKG) once as a baseline in adulthood, and then as needed.

Testing may be necessary for allergies; 54.3% of the U.S. population have a positive skin response to one or more allergens. Allergens include pollen, dust mites, mold, food, latex, medications, stinging insects, substances found in processed food or manufactured products, and environmental pollutants. If the young adult or the offspring presents with respiratory, dermatologic, or gastrointestinal symptoms, screening should be directed toward potential allergens. The process may continue over a period of time (249).

More information about recommendations and rationale for screening for common physical diseases can be obtained through the U.S. Preventive Services Task Force, Agency for Healthcare Research and Quality in Rockville, Maryland, www.ahrg.gov.

Refer to the **Box** *Healthy People 2010:* Example of Objectives for Young Adult Health Promotion for health concerns and prevention strategies in the United States. Objectives and strategies include concerns with primary health care and screening; health education, including for college students; physical and mental illness prevention and intervention; partner assault; and work safety (236). For more information refer to the Website, www.health.gov, or call 1-800-367-4725.

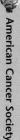

1. Decrease suicide rate.

2. Decrease proportion of homeless adults with severe mental illness.

3. Increase number of persons in primary health care who receive mental health screening and assessment.

4. Increase proportion of adults with mental health disorders who receive treatment.

5. Increase proportion of persons with co-occurring substance abuse and mental disorders who are treated for both diseases.

6. Increase the number of states, territories, and including Washington, D.C., that develop an operational mental health plan to address cultural competency.

7. Increase the number of states, territories, and including Washington, D.C., with an operational mental health plan that addresses mental health crisis intervention.

8. Increase the proportion of persons appropriately counseled about health behaviors.

9. Increase the proportion of adults with disabilities reporting satisfaction with life.

10. Increase the proportion of college and university students who receive information from their institution on each of the six priority health-risk behavior areas (tobacco use, alcohol and illicit drug use, sexual behaviors that cause unintended pregnancies, and sexually transmitted diseases, dietary patterns that cause disease, and inadequate physical activity).

11. Reduce the number of cases of HIV infection among adolescents and adults.

12. Reduce the rate of physical assault by current or former intimate partners.

13. Promote the health and safety of people at work through prevention and early intervention.

14. Reduce periodontal disease.

15. Increase the proportion of adults who engage regularly, preferably daily, in moderate physical activity for at least 30 minutes per day.

16. Increase the proportion of people (75% of adults 18 years and older) who use at least one sun protective measure.

17. Reduce the proportion of adults who exceed guidelines for low-risk drinking.

18. Reduce tobacco use by adults.

Adapted from reference 236.

COMMON HEALTH PROBLEMS: PREVENTION AND HEALTH PROMOTION
Other Health Problems

Young adults in the United States are typically healthy (177). Many have no disease. Young adults can draw on physical reserves and bounce back easily from physical stress. Thus, they may push their bodies too far. The negative effects may not appear for a decade or longer (201). Gender and ethnicity are related to health beliefs and behaviors. Females are longer-lived than males and, in general, healthier with fewer physical or mental diseases (201). Females have more resistance to infections than males because of estrogen's effect on the immune system (90, 201). Males engage in riskier behavior than females during the college years (201). Asian Americans report more cigarette smoking but less consumption of dietary sugar, salt, and fat. Latinos report the highest fat intake (8, 201).

The leading causes of death are motor vehicle accidents, homicides, and suicides. Deaths from cancer and AIDS are more common after 35 years of age. Heart disease and complications of hypertension and diabetes are increasing as causes of death due to overweight, lack of exercise, and tobacco smoking. The foundation for health in later years is laid in young adulthood (177). Males in this life era are slain (75% of the killings involve guns) at higher rates in the United States than in countries with more stringent gun control (181).

Globally, many people die from preventable illnesses, and for millions of people survival is a daily struggle. *Worldwide killers are* (117): (a) AIDS, (b) ischemic heart disease, (c) acute lower respiratory infections, mainly pneumonia, (d) cerebrovascular disease, (e) diarrhea and dysentery, (f) chronic obstructive pulmonary disease, (g) tuberculosis, (h) malaria, (i) measles, and (j) infections. In the United States, health problems and risks, preventive behavior, and response to illness are influenced by gender, lifestyle, environment, and other factors Sections on infectious communicable diseases, including AIDS, HVP and tuberculosis can be found in the Companion Website.

Malignancies

Cancer is a major cause of death in the United States and in some other countries of the world. Regular screening, education about risks and signs and symptoms, use of preventive measures, and lifestyle changes are strategies to reduce incidence in young adulthood and throughout the adult years. Yet some people avoid screening on any level and educational materials especially if genetic studies are involved (182, 192). **Table 14-7** summarizes routine screening for early detection of cancer. **Table 14-8** sum-

MediaLink   Common Health Problems

TABLE 14-8

Breast Self-Examination (BSE)

There are many good reasons for doing breast self-examination (BSE) each month. One reason is that breast cancer is most easily treated and cured when it is found early. Another is that if you do BSE every month, it will increase your skill and confidence when doing the exam. When you get to know how your breasts normally feel, you will quickly be able to feel any change. Another reason, is that it is easy to do.

The best time to do BSE is right after your period, when breasts are not tender or swollen. If you do not have regular periods or sometimes skip a month, do BSE on the same day every month.

1. Lie down and put a pillow under your right shoulder. Place your right arm behind your head.
2. Use the finger pads of your three middle fingers on your left hand to feel for lumps or thickening. Your finger pads are the top third of each finger.
3. Press firmly enough to know how your breast feels. If you're not sure how hard to press, ask your health care provider. Or try to copy the way your health care provider uses the finger pads during a breast exam. Learn what your breast feels like most of the time. A firm ridge in the lower curve of each breast is normal.
4. Move around the breast in a set way. You can choose either the circle (A), the up and down line (B), or the wedge (C). Do it the same way every time. It will help you make sure that you've gone over the entire breast area, and remember how your breast feels each month.
5. Now examine your left breast using right-hand finger pads.
6. Repeat the examination of both breasts while standing, with one arm behind the head. You may want to do BSE while in the shower. If you find any changes, see your doctor right away.

Remember: BSE could save your breast—and save your life. Most breast lumps are found by women themselves, but, in fact, most lumps in the breast are not cancer. Be safe, be sure.

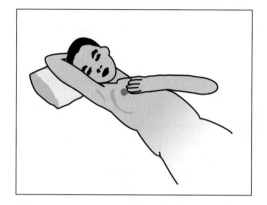

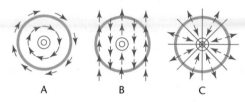

A   B   C

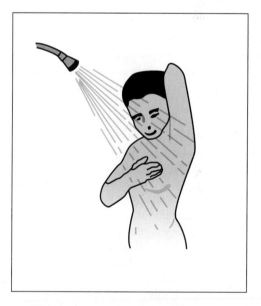

Source: From *How to Do Breast Self-Examination.* No. 2088, Atlanta: American Cancer Society, 1998.

marizes and depicts breast self-examination. Breast cancer risk can also be detected by genetic testing.

All young adult females should be taught to do breast self-examinations since most breast cancers are first detected by the individual. Teach the information described and depicted in **Table 14-8**, Breast Self-Examination. Demonstration on a model can be useful to show the client the correct technique. Utilize **Table 14-7** to emphasize the need for screening and health promotion measures.

Teach the male to examine his scrotum and penis by palpating for unusual nodules. Klingman describes in detail the examination

of the penis, scrotum, rectum, and prostate, and detection of inguinal and femoral hernias (122). Utilize **Table 14-9**, which describes self-examination of the scrotum and penis.

Skin cancer is one of the most common cancers among young adults. The incidence of melanoma continues to increase, as do melanoma mortality rates. Substantial sun exposure usually occurs before age 20 years and plays an important role in the development of skin cancer. Therefore, sun-safe behaviors play a vital role in preventing skin cancer (82, 241).

Teach about the risks for skin cancer and melanoma utilizing **Table 14-10.** Teach mothers to protect their children from

TABLE 14-9

Procedure for Examination of the Scrotum and Penis

1. Perform the examination immediately after a shower or a warm bath. Both the scrotum and examiner's hands should be warm.
2. Hold the scrotum in the palms of the hands and palpate with thumb and fingers of both hands. Examine in a mirror for swelling.
3. Examine each testicle individually, using both hands. Gently roll testicle between thumbs and fingers. (One testicle should be larger.)
4. Locate the epididymis (found on top of and extending down behind the testicle); it should be soft and slightly tender.
5. Examine the spermatic cord next; it ascends from the epididymis and has a firm, smooth, tubular texture.
6. Become familiar with the consistency of normal testicular structures so that changes can be detected.

Adapted from references 70 and 248.

TABLE 14-10

Risk Factors for Melanoma and Other Skin Cancers

Severe sunburn in childhood (3 or more before age 14).

Fair skin that freckles easily.

Family history; parent or sibling, especially if family member had history of atypical moles. (Dermatologist examination recommended every 3 months.)

Atypical moles that are benign between puberty and age 40 may be cancer precursors.

Chronic overexposure to intense sunlight.

Age: more common in young adults.

Appearance of lesion:
  Asymmetrical;
  Border irregular: ragged, notched, blurred;
  Color uneven: black, brown, or tan; areas of white, gray, red, or blue;
  Diameter: changes in size.

Size of lesion: good prognosis if lesion invades skin no more than 0.75 mm deep (95% of patients survive 5 years; 90% survive 15 years); poorer prognosis if lesion is 1 mm deep or deeper (50% survive 5 years).

Adapted from references 70 and 248.

damaging effects of sun. *Safe-sun habits for children and adults include* (a) staying in the shade, especially 10 a.m. to 4 p.m., (b) covering with a hat to shade face, neck, and ears, (c) wearing shirts and slacks that are lightly woven, and (d) using sunscreen. People should avoid tanning booths and sun lamps; sunglasses should be worn.

The article by Van Beuge is a useful resource that gives information about the disease, photos of lesions, the Clark and Breslow classification or staging for severity of the lesion, and treatment and nursing care (241).

Educate that, in general, *cancer risk is reduced by daily* (a) eating 4 to 5 servings of vegetables and fruits, and whole-grain bread products rather than white or refined grain bread products; (b) limiting red or fatty meats, pastries, and sweetened juices or soft drinks; (c) avoiding fried or charbroiled meats; and (d) limiting daily alcohol intake to no more than one drink (60, 62, 249). Risks for lung, oral, esophageal, and pancreatic cancers are reduced by avoiding tobacco in any form (28, 39, 60, 164, 199, 231, 249).

Educate that **dipping**, *chewing tobacco or holding tobacco in the mouth to get nicotine effects, can cause oral cancer.* Dipping is addictive; the nicotine content in the product is high. Gum disease, with receding and bleeding, tooth decay, and grayish white patches on the inner cheek, appears. The cancer develops quickly at the area where dipping most frequently occurs. Educate that *this product is not a safe alternative to smoking.* Addiction increases use; use speeds onset of cancer. Nearly 90% of oral cancers begin from dipping, and the prognosis is poor.

Emphasize that daily habits may contribute to risk for cancer (77). Risks for lung and hematopoietic cancers apparently are increased in adulthood after childhood exposure to parental smoking. Incidence of breast cancer or fibrocystic disease is higher in females who consume increased amounts of caffeine. Consuming two or more cups of caffeinated coffee a day may be associated with in-

INTERVENTIONS FOR HEALTH PROMOTION

Teach signs that should be considered suspicious of **skin cancer or melanoma** *and reported to a physician* (70, 241, 249):

1. Changes in a dark-colored mole or spot
2. Pink or flesh-colored nodule that slowly grows larger
3. Open or crusted sore that does not heal
4. Red, rough patch, orange-peel skin, or bump that persists
5. Mole that grows, changes, hurts, bleeds, or itches

6. Mole that is larger in size than a pencil eraser and has irregular borders or variegated colors with shadings of red-white or blue-black
7. Elevation or bulge in a mole that was flat
8. Mole on the bottom of the feet or in an area of repeated trauma
9. Changes in body contours

MediaLink Transtheoretical Model

creased risk of colon or bladder cancer (60). Explore with members of various cultural groups their risk for specific types of cancer (8, 80). Explain that environmental and cultural factors, lifestyle stress, and exposure to pollutants contribute significantly to increased incidence of cancer. Chapter 4 describes some of these environmental pollutants. ∞ Further, hormones (e.g., cortisol) secreted by the brain and adrenal glands in response to emotional stress may inhibit the immune system and enhance growth of cancerous tumors. Explore how stressful times often reduce the person's pursuit of healthy habits as well (e.g., exercise, nutrition), which may contribute to cancerous growth. Educate the need for stress management. Immune substances affect activity of the hypothalamic-pituitary-adrenal axis, the neuroendocrine system that regulates stress responses. Demonstrate relaxation methods and discuss lifestyle habits to show that physical, emotional, social, and spiritual circumstances are highly interdependent.

LIFESTYLE EFFECTS ON HEALTH AND ILLNESS

Life is rooted in and organized around a person's changing culture and society, whether the changes are dramatic or subtle. Coping with extreme change taxes the person physically and psychologically, affects achievement of developmental tasks, and may be responsible for physical disease. Research shows relationships between physical adaptation and illness and sociocultural experiences (96, 97, 141, 156, 186, 192, 249). Stresses of poverty may be a cause of disease (8, 34, 80, 186).

The adult is most likely to fall ill, whether from a sinus infection, cold, or something more serious, when feeling lowered self-esteem, discouragement, despair, humiliation, depression, powerlessness to change or cope with a situation, imagined helplessness, or loss of gratifying roles. Apparently such feelings modify the capacity of the organism to cope with concurrent pathogenic factors. Biologically, the central nervous system undergoes an inflammatory process with chronic stress, increasing risk for degeneration (156). It fails in its task of processing the emergency defense system so that the person has a higher statistical tendency toward illness or death. Conversely, contentment, happiness, faith, confidence, and success are associated with health (32, 97).

One lifestyle that involves geographic mobility, lack of consistent public education, transient and inadequate housing, hard work, poor nutrition, and inadequate immunizations or other health promotion measures is that of the *migrant farm worker. The migrant worker has unique and numerous health care needs because* (a) the opportunity for prevention of certain illnesses is nonexistent, (b) prenatal and maternal care is lacking, (c) chronic health problems are numerous, (d) economic resources are scant, and (e) contacts with the health care system are sporadic and temporary. *Homeless individuals and families* also have similar health care needs and problems. Be attuned to cultural differences, including language difficulties, definitions of health and illness, food preferences, lines of authority, health practices, job-related diseases, and general lifestyle of your clients. Chapter 5 presents information about the migrant person and family. ∞

The young adult is likely to be interested in and benefit from relaxation methods, such as first formulated by Benson (24) and

biofeedback training, *learning to control body functions once considered involuntary.* Teach that biofeedback technique (explained in Chapter 2) ∞ is much like learning other skills of muscular coordination and physical activity. It involves controlled production of alpha waves, the brain waves typical of relaxation and reverie (10, 24, 90).

EMOTIONAL HEALTH PROBLEMS AND PHYSICAL EFFECTS
Stress Reactions

Stress reactions *are physiologic and psychological changes, including the Alarm, Resistance, and Exhaustion stages* (refer to Chapter 2), ∞ *resulting in illness, unusual or disturbed adaptive behavior patterns,* or *depression* (5, 6, 10, 141). Mate selection, marriage, child rearing, college, job demands, social expectations, and independent decision making are all stressors that carry threats of insecurity and possibly some degree of failure. Stress reactions may take the form of physical illness (5, 6, 141). The culture defines what is considered stressful or traumatic and also ways to cope. Yet some of the same stressors or crises are defined in every culture (8, 9, 34, 80). Young adults may experience a variety of illnesses in response to stress.

The ability to cope with stressors can be challenging. Depression may be experienced by anyone. Assessment and health promotion are essential. Even the young adult in any setting—home or community—who appears healthy may be contemplating suicide. Or the person may try to comfort self through other self-destructive behaviors, such as alcoholism, drug use or abuse (prescribed or illegal), eating disorders, or smoking.

INTIMATE PARTNER VIOLENCE

Family violence is a social, emotional, and physical health problem of all cultural groups and socioeconomic levels. Wife beating has always been a problem. Historically a woman was the man's property and beating was (and still is) accepted behavior in some cultures (8, 50, 56, 89, 216). Traditionally the female was too ashamed or too helpless to admit the problem or seek help. Further, no help existed.

Intimate partner violence or **domestic violence** *is a pattern of assaultive and coercive behaviors that the person uses against current or former intimate partners, those living together, married, or divorced. Abuse is intentional behavior to establish power and control over another through fear and intimidation.* Abusive relationships are not violent all the time. Abusers weave intimacy and abuse to control their partners, which creates additional hurt and confusion for the abused person (163). Such abuse or violence is unlike other abuse, in that it distorts what is expected to be a partnership based on mutual respect. Neither partner has a legitimate role in discipline or control of the other (163). Most domestic violence is perpetrated against the female (85%), although female abuse against the male partner exists (15%) (163). Same-gender abusive relationships also exist (185).

Some stresses predispose to family violence and male abuse of the female and children. These stresses are listed in **Box 14-9** (26, 56, 144, 163).

Attempts continue to make the police and legal system more protective of the female who has been treated violently, and more

MediaLink Reactions to Stress

MediaLink Family Violence

BOX 14-9	**Stresses that Predispose to Family Violence**

1. Financial pressures, low pay, high cost of living
2. Family separation
3. Geographic mobility, loss of friends, social supports, and familiarity
4. Isolation and communication barriers
5. Cultural differences; living in a strange environment or with unfamiliar customs, creating higher mutual dependence
6. Lack of family support
7. Living abroad such as in military families
8. Inability to separate administrative or work roles from home life (Behavior that is functional at work may not be at home.)
9. Lack of privacy at work or at home
10. Job pressures or competitiveness, lack of support from supervisor

Adapted from references 26, 56, 144, 163.

restrictive to the violent male. Emergency shelters for mothers and their children have been established in urban areas. The shelter may be a resource so they are not at home when the male, who is released shortly after arrest following a police intervention, returns home—even more violent than before. Crisis telephone lines have been established and publicized by the media. *A variety of services are necessary:* (a) drop-in centers for the day to get respite and assistance, (b) special programs that provide apartments for the abused mother and her children, (c) programs that assist the female with employment or continued education and child care, and (d) referrals to health care, counseling, and other social services. Many programs or services for the abused mother and children focus on the broader issue of family violence and conduct community education and advocacy programs. Assistance to females seeking divorce is inadequate in most cities because of the cost and bureaucratic red tape.

Assessment of the Abused Female

Assessment of a family and female suffering adult abuse often reveals the following typical characteristics (10, 17, 56, 68, 91, 144, 158, 163, 184, 193, 194, 255):

1. The family and the abused female are isolated socially or physically from neighbors, relatives, and friends.
2. The female feels increasing helplessness, guilt, isolation, and low self-esteem. She feels trapped and has been forced to be dependent on the male.
3. The person may range in age from teens to old age and may suffer violent injury for months or years.
4. The female's educational and occupational status is often higher than that of the male. The female in a professional, executive, or highly respected position may be too embarrassed to admit abuse to self or anyone and may rationalize why she deserves abuse.

5. Most beatings begin early in marriage and increase in frequency and intensity over the decades. If the couple cohabitated before marriage, there may have been warning signs, such as threats and verbal abuse or controlling behavior. Usually shortly after marriage, various forms of abuse are direct—economic control, emotional, verbal, social isolation, and physical.
6. Most violence occurs in the evening, on weekends, and in the kitchen.
7. Generally there are no witnesses, although children in the home directly or indirectly witness the event.
8. The female is frequently unable to leave the home because of child care responsibilities or concern for possible child abuse, lack of money or transportation, no place to go, and lack of support people or support agencies in the community. Further, she has learned helplessness behaviors and feels unable to try to escape.
9. The injuries from abuse may not be visible, but if abuse is present, the female usually talks about the problem freely when asked directly if abuse is occurring.
10. With increasing incidence of abuse and the physical and emotional consequences of abuse, the female may become more passive, less flexible, less able to think logically, more apathetic, depressed, and possibly suicidal. She may also be quite creative and flexible to de-escalate anger or violent situations against self or the children. She may realize it is safer to stay than leave.
11. Abusive behavior may include destroying property, breaking favorite possessions, and harming pets as well as the children.
12. Abuse often involves stalking behavior, being followed, harassed, and terrified by the partner or ex-partner. The abuser monitors the partner's whereabouts, phone conversations, and mail to prove nothing can be concealed (255).
13. Abusive partners are often addicted to alcohol, drugs, or other substances. More violence occurs when the abuser is drunk or high on illicit drugs. The abuser rationalizes that he was not responsible because of "the booze" or "the drugs."
14. Sexual abuse and marital rape are typical, including insistence on sex right after a beating, when she is ill or injured, or immediately after childbirth (61).
15. Spiritual and religious abuse occurs as the partner uses scripture or religious teachings to create guilt in the abused person, justify abusive behavior, enforce obedience, and emphasize that she must forgive him but is not forgiven of her behavior (83, 161, 179).
16. Economic abuse is common. All earnings have to be given to the abusive partner. Often bank accounts and financial or legal documents have only the abusive person's name on them, often unknown to the abused partner.
17. Eventually the frustration, stress, and anger may be externalized into physical behavior that is more than protective of the self or the children; she may in turn become violent to the point of killing the abusive partner.

Incest, *sexual intercourse between biologically related persons,* is another form of abuse that may affect either the adult male or the female, but more commonly the female. Incest is considered one form of sexual abuse, although adult family members may convey that incestuous behavior is normal (88). Chapter 13 discusses incest with the child/adolescent. ∞ *Symptoms and problems in adulthood resulting from childhood or adolescent sexual abuse and incest include* (17, 68, 88): (a) chronic depression, hopelessness related to shame and guilt; (b) drug and alcohol abuse; (c) various physical complaints, including panic attacks, headaches, hysterical seizures, and symptoms in all major organ systems; (d) problems with trusting or intimate relationships with the opposite sex; (e) character disorders, such as borderline or narcissistic states; (f) multiple personality disorders; and (g) sexual dysfunction and gynecologic problems. This problem is expected to affect more young adults in the future, based on the current statistics of childhood and youth sexual abuse.

Women remain in a threatening situation for many complex and interrelated reasons, as described in **Box 14-10**, Reasons Why Women Are Unable to Leave a Violent Situation. An astute assessment will uncover at least some of these characteristics and factors if present. **Box 14-11**, Identification of Partner Violence in the Health Care Setting, describes some "red flags" for assessment that can help you identify a battered adult in an emergency room or intensive care, occupational, or other medical setting (10, 68, 144, 158, 163, 193, 255).

Why does the person leave the violent situation? Often the mother leaves when she feels suicidal but does not want to kill herself because of concern about the children's welfare; fear for the life of the unborn child, if pregnant; or concern for the lives of her children. Fear of being killed is a motivator. Acknowledging that the situation will never improve is important. The shock of a particular beating or the horror of being beaten while pregnant may be the turning point. The female realizes she has no power to make her partner change. At some point she may have received enough subtle or overt encouragement to leave or a new vision of what marriage and family life should be, coupled with a renewed sense of self-worth and the feeling she "doesn't have to take it anymore." She realizes the point at which the male no longer asks for forgiveness, shows no remorse (as he might have after the first beating), and denies he behaved violently. There comes a decision point, and then a plan may be made (144, 153, 163, 174). Some females, however, leave abruptly to avoid being murdered (153, 163, 174). However, the abused female who leaves the partner is at high risk for homicide from the partner. **Do not casually recommend she leave the home site or the relationship. A plan must be foolproof.**

Despite the desperate situations and the difficulty in finding aid, the abused female is not typically helpless. She is a survivor.

| BOX 14-10 | **Reasons Why Women Are Unable to Leave a Violent Situation** |

1. Lacking economic independence and being without money
2. Being forbidden to leave the house or visit or call others
3. Fear of being alone, being unable to support self and children, or the man's finding and harming her after she left him (Personal safety is a continual issue.)
4. Lacking emotional or social support (Often parents encouraged her to return to the abusive partner.)
5. Believing that she is unworthy of anything better
6. Having nowhere to go or being turned away from a public shelter
7. Believing traditional norms related to women's role, marriage, religion, and violence; believing the woman is less than human
8. Believing there are positive aspects of the relationship that are worth preserving; emotional dependency in the relationship
9. Desiring a father for her children; wanting to protect the children from greater harm
10. Feeling disbelief, sense of horror, and shock about the man's violent behavior to her and denial or rationalizations that it would happen again
11. Believing the man's promise that he will not hit again; thinking she can change him
12. Finding the police unresponsive to calls for help (Many women have kept extensive records of the number of times legal action was taken with unsatisfactory results.)
13. Taking responsibility for the violence, feeling guilty and that this behavior is her fault (Often the man would say, "Look what you made me do.")
14. Feeling helpless; being unable to counter the power, authority, and threats of the man (Often the women were forced out or locked out of the home in the middle of the night in winter without clothing or money.)
15. Increasing force or violence, which was condoned by police or society, from failing to comply with the husband's wishes or demands
16. Relying on the sexual relation to punish him, to prevent battering, and to prove self-worth (Sexual enjoyment lessened as battering increased.)
17. Wanting to protect the man's reputation in the community or in the job
18. Having several small children and the related child care responsibility, often coupled with need to protect the children against the man's violence
19. Fearing what would happen after leaving the home and man (welfare, homelessness, unemployment, single parenting) (Often there is a predictability about his behavior versus the unpredictability of the future.)
20. Introjecting the societal attitude that the victim is to blame
21. Believing that all marriages are like this (violent), especially if the woman grew up in a violent home

Adapted from references 10, 68, 144, 158, 163, 193, 258.

BOX 14-11 — Identification of Partner Violence in the Health Care Setting

MULTIPLE INJURIES

Multiple abrasions and contusions to different anatomic sites should alert health care providers. There are relatively few ways of sustaining such injuries.

BODY MAP

Many incidents of abuse involve injury to the face, neck, chest, breasts, or abdomen, whereas most accidents involve the extremities.

RAPE

Most female rape victims are raped by a male intimate partner, and many times rape is yet another incident of ongoing physical abuse.

SEVERITY OF INJURY

Severity varies among abused victims. Presentation of medically insignificant trauma to the emergency service may alert medical personnel that ongoing assault and impending danger constitute the real emergency for which she is seeking aid.

PREGNANCY

Abused women are more likely to be beaten when pregnant. There is a higher rate of miscarriage among battered women.

Adapted from references 68, 144, 158, 163, 193, 255.

TRAUMA HISTORY

Frequent visits to the emergency department or physician
A history of trauma can be the key indicator! Both asking about previous injuries and looking at her medical records are important. Records may indicate repeated visits and injuries to the same site.

SUICIDE ATTEMPTS

Studies indicate that battering is a frequent precipitant of female suicide attempts; conversely, women who attempt suicide are likely to have a history of domestic violence.

INCONSISTENT DESCRIPTION OF INJURIES

Injuries do not fit with the woman's description of the genesis of injury.

VAGUE AND NONSPECIFIC COMPLAINTS

Complaints include, for example, anxiety, depression, and sleeplessness and many indicate intrafamilial crisis.

HEAVY USE OF ALCOHOL AND DRUGS

Victims are more likely than nonvictims to use alcohol and drugs, and partners are much more likely to use alcohol and drugs excessively.

Generally, she continually schemes how to stop the battering, either by examining personal behavior or planning ways to escape and how to get and keep some money. She takes steps to please the partner and to satisfy the demands while protecting and caring for the children. She may be the primary wage earner in the home. She may describe how she actively defends self. If she did not, it was not because she felt helpless but because other negative consequences or a worse beating would ensue.

Assessment of the Abusive Male

Typical adult and parental behavior of the male who is abusive indicates that he (17, 111, 144, 163, 193):

1. Has battered a previous partner.
2. Is employed, and frequently under stress at work.
3. Has children who have viewed the domestic violence and his battering behavior.
4. Was under the influence of alcohol or drugs at the last battering incident.
5. Uses physical punishment on the children.
6. Has been violent with others not in the family, outside the home.

7. Has a family history of suicide (attempted and completed).
8. Has been violent only when under the influence of alcohol and drugs, or only when not under the influence of alcohol or drugs.
9. Lacks close friends or someone with whom to talk.

Psychological violence by the male against the female includes (26, 111, 163, 193):

1. Explicit threats.
2. Extreme controlling type of behavior: taking her everywhere; saying when she must come home; knowing her whereabouts, companions, and life activities; and timing the duration of any activity away from home.
3. Pathologic jealousy: continually questioning her about her behavior, making accusations without cause, highly suspicious.
4. Mental degradation: calling her names or telling her she is incompetent, stupid, and no good.
5. Isolating behavior because of his jealousy, suspicion, and dependence, whereby he controls the female's behaviors so that she in turn becomes extremely isolated and dependent on him.

The male who abuses the female partner has a typical childhood history (17). He is likely to have:

1. Received physical punishment as a child.
2. Witnessed his mother abused or treated violently by his father.
3. Attacked one of the parents during childhood or adolescence.
4. Suffered physical abuse as a child.
5. Suffered sexual abuse as a child.

In his perception, his childhood experiences taught him how to live and legitimizes his behavior.

The male batterer comes from all walks of life and cultures. *Typical personality characteristics of the male abuser or perpetrator* include (17, 26, 111, 144, 163, 181):

1. Denying or minimizing the violent behavior and its effects. (He may actually lose memory of the event because of his rage.)
2. Blaming the behavior of the female or others as the cause of the violent scenes.
3. Demonstrating uncontrollable anger and rage in physical and verbal behavior (intermittent explosive disorder) (5, 6, 111).
4. Depending on the partner as sole source of love, support, intimacy, and problem solving, resulting from the controlling and isolating behavior that entwined him and the partner and children.
5. Feeling alienation from others and society. (He considers himself a loner and therefore his "own boss"—means he can do whatever he wants in his home.)
6. Expressing jealousy and suspiciousness of his partner, children, and finally everyone else.
7. Expressing low self-esteem, lack of confidence in his ability to keep his partner, lack of skill or ability to ask for what is wanted in a nonthreatening way.

Intervention Guidelines

Intervention involves the entire family and may include supportive relatives or friends. A multidisciplinary team approach is essential.

Group therapy and individual therapy are effective for the female (10, 144). Group therapy may be more effective than individual therapy for the male, as it helps him recognize angry and frustrated feelings in himself, realize it is not acceptable to vent feelings through violent behavior, and learn alternative coping and behavior patterns from other males (10, 144). Work also with the children, if possible. Research shows that children (ages 2 to 12) of abused mothers have deep feelings of fear about safety and abandonment, anger, confusion, social isolation, and aggression. Utilize play and art therapy. Children's play reveals conflicts about overpowering adults and identification with the same-sex parent. Children are learning, and need to unlearn and resolve, abnormal behavior and roles that could be carried into their adult relationships and lifestyle.

Explore social support and the meaning the person attaches to stressful events. These influence whether the person becomes ill or remains healthy—physically and emotionally—in a situation. The abused female who extricates herself from her violent situation has strengthened her ability to survive, to resolve crisis, and to move forward. Validate her decisions. Explore alternatives and options. Reinforce thoughtful, safe, effective decisions. Reinforce her spiritual insights.

Work with others to establish emergency centers, crisis phone lines, housing accommodations, and other services for the abused female and her children and to exert pressure to reform the current legal and judicial system so it will be more equitable to females. Educate the public. Engage in advocacy.

You may be in a position to work with the female on a continuing basis. Continuing assessment for a history of trauma and its sequelae is necessary. Physical, emotional, social, and economic

---

INTERVENTIONS FOR HEALTH PROMOTION

Intervention guidelines include to:

1. Make a thorough and holistic assessment, using the prior content.
2. Provide necessary emotional crisis and emergency physical care.
3. Encourage the abused female to share her secret with you, another nurse, a social worker, a confidante, or a religious leader.
4. Help her secure help from social service agencies, legal aid societies, counselors, health centers, and the welfare office.
5. Encourage formulating a plan for separation from her husband or partner if her life is in danger.

6. Work with the individual to encourage her to talk through feelings of shame, guilt, embarrassment, anger, and fear, either in individual or group sessions.
7. Be sensitive in the reporting process (196).
8. Help her gain courage to make decisions, including decisions on how to protect herself and her children, how to leave the partner, and where to go.
9. Assure continuing intervention to resolve the physical and emotional trauma, including post-traumatic stress disorder. Time and therapy are needed for resolution (254).

INTERVENTIONS FOR HEALTH PROMOTION

Foster empowerment, *the core of advocacy, in the following ways:*

1. Reinforce the female to perceive herself as competent, able to make decisions and take charge of her life.
2. Believe what she says. Acknowledge her feelings. Affirm her experience.
3. Emphasize that other females have successfully moved beyond the abusive experience.
4. Validate with her the injustices she has suffered.

5. Respect her confidentiality and autonomy—the right to make her own decisions. Reaffirm she is an expert on her life.
6. Review what she has done to survive, to keep herself and her children as safe as possible.
7. Help her plan for future safety—what she can do and where she can go to escape.
8. Educate her about community services—a housing hotline, a crisis counseling hotline, a shelter for victims.
9. Promote her access to community services.

---

effects of family or interpersonal violence, or spouse/partner abuse, are more likely to result in a complex reaction of post-traumatic stress disorder (PTSD) if crisis and continuing intervention is not implemented. The female may have gained freedom from the battering partner, but effects on health necessitate your ongoing counseling and education and various support services in the community to prevent or treat disorders of extreme stress (DESNOS) or PTSD (91).

Advocate for effective legal and community services for the female who is abused and her children. These services must be sensitive to the needs of people from various cultural groups. Check with the legal services in your area for information.

Refer the female to local relevant Websites. She may need to use the computer at her work site, a local library, or the health care setting to access information.

The following national Websites may be helpful:

1. Battered Women's Justice Project, www.bwjp.org
2. Family Violence Prevention Fund, www.endabuse.org
3. National Coalition Against Domestic Violence, www.neadv.org
4. National Domestic Violence Hotline, www.ndvh.org
5. National Electronic Network on Violence Against Women, www.vawnet.org
6. National Network to End Domestic Violence, www.nnedv.org
7. National Resource Center on Domestic Violence, www.nredv.org
8. National Stalking Resource Center, www.neve.org
9. U.S. Centers for Disease Control and Prevention Family and Intimate Violence Prevention Team, www.cdc.gov

The problems of partner abuse—like those of child abuse discussed in Chapters 9 through 13, ∞ violent television programming discussed in Chapters 12 and 13, ∞ and elder abuse discussed in Chapter 16—are part of overall societal violence. ∞ Each professional, as a citizen and health care provider, must work in whatever way possible to decrease violence, its cause, and its effects.

SOCIAL HEALTH PROBLEMS
Divorce

Divorce is the *termination of marriage, preceded by emotional distress in the marriage, separation, and legal procedures. Divorce is a crisis for those involved and can affect society, in general, as well as the physical and emotional health of the persons involved* (114, 154, 180). Divorce is frequently a factor in poverty and homelessness. Yet, there are times when separation and divorce in a relationship may improve the mental and physical health of one or both persons. An example is the abusive or battering situation.

Some young people enter marriage to escape the problems of young adulthood. Marriage provides them with a ready-made role, and it supposedly solves the problem of isolation. If marriage takes place before the individual has developed a strong sense of identity and independence, true intimacy cannot be achieved.

Marriage often breaks down because of the partners' inability to satisfy deep mutual needs in a close demanding relationship. One of the partners may be overly dependent and seek in the other a mother or father figure. Dependent behavior may at first meet the needs of the more independent partner. But as the dependent person matures, the relationship is changed. If the stronger partner neither understands nor allows this change, divorce may follow.

Emotional deprivation in childhood is also a poor foundation for marriage. Children of divorce are more likely to get divorced and to see divorce as a way to resolve marital conflict. Separation from the father in early life has adverse effects for children (26, 129, 130, 181, 201). There may be insufficient experience of feeling acknowledged, wanted, appreciated, or loved. Low self-esteem may interfere with being responsive to acceptance, approval, or any form of appreciation and love. The person from a home in which the parents' marital relationship was one of detachment or conflict or in which abuse or divorce occurred is poorly prepared for marriage. There is no healthy or loving marital model to follow. However, the person may intentionally work to model the marriage after another's happy and healthy marriage. Considerable effort and time is needed.

The divorce rate reflects the ease with which a divorce can be obtained. The lack of commitment to people and relationships when the going gets tough, seen also in other areas of life, and the dichotomy between the romanticized ideal of marriage and the reality of married life contribute to separation and divorce. Further, our youth are not educated for family life in any formal sense. What they learn in the home may be poor preparation for marriage and good preparation for the divorce court.

When marriage fails and bonds are broken, aloneness, anger, mistrust, hostility, guilt, shame, a sense of betrayal, fear, disappointment, loss of identity, anxiety, and depression, alone or in combination, may appear both in the divorcee and the one initiating the divorce. Eventually there may be a feeling of relief. There must be an interval of adjustment to the physical and emotional loss, to the crisis of divorce.

The offspring also experience a life crisis. Thus, expression and control of aggressive and sexual impulses, dependency-independency issues, de-idealization of the parents, peer problems, and premature responsibilities of adulthood may intensify (26, 201). The adolescent is likely to blame both parents or feel closer to only one.

Often a second marriage is a rebound affair. A partner may be selected as soon as possible to help ease the feelings from the divorce and relieve the loneliness. Ideally, the second marriage should be entered into with time (at least one year) and thought so that needs of both partners are met. *Second and subsequent remarriages can be successful, but they carry a higher risk of instability* (26, 201).

Remarriages are more likely to end in divorce because of:

1. The person's lack of ability to form a mutually satisfactory new relationship.
2. The past experiences, vulnerability, guilt, and insecurity that cannot be easily removed.
3. The hassles of her kids, his kids, and their kids.
4. Child and wife support from the male's former marriage.
5. Interference from the ex-spouse.

Give emotional support to the parents and children if the divorce cannot be prevented. Mothers and children may need help to meet physical and economic needs. The losses must be resolved, a new identity must be formed, and the children involved should have the option of continued close relationships with both parents.

Help divorced females or males to identify and pursue personal goals. Primary needs of divorced females are economic independence, education, managing parenting, maintaining friendships, and obtaining adequate housing, school, and environment for self and children. Goals for the male may be the same, although typically there is less economic difficulty. Mental health goals are also a priority. Support groups for the divorced person can assist in meeting needs and securing goals. Such groups can also assist with custody rights and with obtaining child support.

Establish groups for children of divorcing and divorced parents to help them work through the feelings of loss, anger, guilt, and ambivalence about relationships with parents and often, eventually, stepparents and stepsiblings. The key is for the parents to continue showing love to their children and to maintain open communication between them about the offspring.

> ### Practice Point
>
> You may experience considerable emotional turmoil when you think about the abortion issue. If you feel incapable of providing counsel, refer the person to someone who can give counseling and who knows community resources.

Educate the family. The child should be given honest information at whatever level he or she can understand. The child must know that he or she did not cause the divorce. Contact with both parents is preferable for the child; safety must be considered.

Abortion

Young adult females, married and unmarried and of all socioeconomic classes, may have an **abortion** to *terminate an unwanted pregnancy.* Increasingly, unmarried females are choosing to have and keep their babies. Induced abortion may be done because of fetal abnormality (126).

Educate that abortion should not be considered lightly. Abortion induces physical complications such as hemorrhage and later cervical incompetency, risk of preterm delivery with a later pregnancy (232), and increased risk of breast cancer because full-term pregnancy reduces risk of later breast cancer (232). Emotional anguish, guilt, unhappiness, or self-directed anger may follow the decision to have an abortion. Long-term follow-up of women who had an induced abortion reveal psychological consequences, such as increased incidence of grief and depression (126, 232, 248) and increased risk for substance abuse (52). Through education, counseling, and values clarification, assist the young adult to consider consequences of sexual activity. Explore ethical and moral issues, the female's reactions, the consequences, preabortion and postabortion counseling received by the female, and avenues of assistance.

Health Promotion and Nursing Applications

ASSESSMENT: A HOLISTIC APPROACH

Information pertinent to assessment of the healthy adult or the adult who has the goal of health promotion and maintenance is presented throughout the chapter. Assessment is ongoing. Additional information gained as you intervene assists in formulating additional nursing diagnoses, revising therapy goals and intervention strategies, and establishing additional evaluation criteria.

New assessment data may arise from:

1. Astute observation related to daily practices (183, 207).
2. Being sensitive to and noting cultural differences (8, 9, 34, 63, 80, 187, 206).
3. Using information from research tools described in a number of listed references (208).
4. Utilizing models for specific situations or health concerns (9, 45, 56).

5. Engaging, empathic, careful, and confidential interviewing (15).
6. Using alternatives to face-to-face interviewing, such as written or computerized self-report methods (158).
7. Using established tools such as the Alcohol Use Disorders Identification Test (AUDIT) developed by Kopeka, as described in Antai-Otong (10).

Realize that your assessment questions may remind the client of a prior traumatic event or unresolved illness, or of a negative experience with a health care provider. Reluctance to answer, withdrawal from the provider, or expressions of anger are cues of negative reminders. Conveying empathy, establishing rapport, and building a trust relationship with the client sounds easy and redundant. These are always uniquely individual with each client, and even with prior clients in new situations (for example, pregnancy, domestic violence).

Young adult clients are concerned about genetic effects on health. In your assessment it is impossible to calculate the exact probability of anyone developing disease. The *following principles for risk are a guide* (249):

1. *Genetic makeup or family history* is a strong determinant of risk for some diseases. The Human Genome Project may help better predict risk profile in the future.
2. *Magnitude or a slight elevation* (10% to 30%) in risk for a given disease has a minor effect on the person. A marked increase in risk (80% to 100%) would serve as an alarm.
3. *Repetition* or independently researched risk factors, such as cigarette smoking, excess alcohol intake, obesity, sedentary lifestyle, and diet high in saturated fats, are risks for everyone.

NURSING DIAGNOSES

Refer to the **Box**, Nursing Diagnoses Related to the Young Adult, which reflects assessments (171). The nursing diagnoses guide nursing goals and interventions. You may also formulate other diagnoses as you work with well or ill clients.

INTERVENTIONS TO PROMOTE HEALTH

Health promotion interventions to assist the young adult and the family to meet physical, cognitive, emotional, social, and spiritual needs and developmental tasks are described throughout the chapter. Utilize **Box 14-12**, Considerations for the Young Adult in Health Promotion, as you plan interventions. *Foster culturally congruent care, which includes four constructs* (34, 206):

1. **Cultural diversity, commonalities, and differences** *involves acknowledging that contributions of people from many populations and backgrounds enrich the United States and our lives even as health care services are being challenged.* More than one million people, immigrants from around the world, come to the United States annually. You cannot be ethnocentric as you care for clients, as explained in Chapter 5. ∞
2. **Cultural awareness** *is consciously rethinking facts, beliefs, and attitudes, learning more about the client's life patterns, and avoiding assumptions or stereotypes about clients based on group membership.*
3. **Cultural sensitivity** *is openness to learning about others, seeking cross-cultural encounters, and treating others as they would want to be treated.*
4. **Cultural competence** *involves effective, consistent actions based on understanding of diversity, cultural norms and lifeways of self and others, and sensitivity in action or behavior.* No one is fully competent with everyone or every group.

Cognitive-behavioral therapy is effective to learn new coping skills, manage stressful lifestyles, be more creative and productive, and control distressing thoughts (10, 34). Healthful patterns affect all dimensions of the person and foster family health as well. The Abstract for Evidence-Based Practice describes testing an intervention to reduce negative thinking and depressive symptoms to overcome chronic stressors.

Educate the client about self-help or consumer-operated services (229). In some organizations, consumers use their experiential knowledge gained from working through their own recovery

---

Nursing Diagnoses Related to the Young Adult

Latex **A**llergy Response	Imbalanced **N**utrition: More Than Body Requirements
Anxiety	Impaired **P**arenting
Disturbed **B**ody Image	**P**ost-trauma Syndrome
Parental Role **C**onflict	Ineffective **R**ole Performance
Ineffective **C**oping	Chronic Low **S**elf-esteem
Adult **F**ailure to Thrive	**S**exual Dysfunction
Dysfunctional **F**amily Processes: Alcoholism	**S**leep Deprivation
Ineffective **H**ealth Maintenance	**S**ocial Isolation
Deficient **K**nowledge	**S**piritual Distress
Sedentary **L**ifestyle	Risk for **S**uicide

Source: Reference 171.

BOX 14-12 **Considerations for the Young Adult in Health Promotion**

1. Cultural and family background, values, support systems, community resources
2. Relationships with family of origin, extended family, family of friends or spouse
3. Behaviors that indicate abuse by spouse or significant other
4. Physical characteristics, nutritional status, and rest/sleep and exercise patterns that indicate health and are age-appropriate
5. Integrated self-concept, body image, and sexuality
6. Immunizations, safety education, and other health promotion measures used
7. Demonstration of continued learning and use of formal operations and concrete operations competencies in cognitive ability

8. Overall appearance and behavioral patterns that indicate intimacy rather than isolation
9. Behavioral patterns that demonstrate a value system, continuing formation of philosophy of life, and moral-spiritual development
10. Established employment, vocation, or profession, including homemaking and child care
11. Behavioral patterns that reflect commitment to parenting, if there are children
12. Relationships with work colleagues, coping skills for work stress
13. Demonstration of integration of work and leisure and avoidance of physical or emotional illness
14. Behavioral patterns and characteristics indicating the young adult has achieved developmental tasks

---

Abstract for Evidence-Based Practice

Interventions with Mothers to Reduce Depression and Chronic Stressors

Peden, A., Ragens, M., Hall, L., & Grant, E. (2005). Testing an intervention to reduce negative thinking, depressive symptoms, and chronic stressors in low-income single mothers. *Journal of Nursing Scholarship, 37*(3), 268–274.

KEYWORDS

depression, single mothers, negative thinking, chronic stressors.

Purpose ➤ To test effectiveness of using cognitive-behavioral group sessions as intervention with low-income mothers at risk for depression, and who experienced negative thinking and chronic stressors.

Conceptual Framework ➤ Poverty, chronic stressors, and negative thoughts increase risk for depression in low-income, single mothers. Cognitive-behavioral therapy prevents onset of and relapse of depression.

Sample/Setting ➤ The sample of 205 single mothers with at least one child age 2 to 16 years old and who were 185% or below poverty level were recruited from Women, Infants, and Children (WIC) sites and public health clinics. The mothers were not receiving psychiatric treatment or medication and were not suicidal or pregnant.

Methods ➤ The Beck Depression Inventory (BDI) and Center for Epidemiologic Studies Depression Scale (CES-D) were administered. Of the 205 women, 136 were identified as at risk for depression and agreed to participate. Participants were randomly assigned to either a control or an intervention/experimental group. Women in the intervention group partic-

ipated in 6 hours of cognitive-behavioral group sessions over 4 to 6 weeks. The modifiable risk factor targeted was negative thinking. The intervention included frequent use of positive affirmations. In the intervention group, 91 of the 136 completed all three interviews: baseline, 1 month, and post-intervention 6 months.

Findings ➤ No significant difference was found in demographic data or for BDI or CES-D scores for the control ($n = 74$) and experimental ($n = 62$) groups. Analysis of the 1-month and 6-month post-intervention scores revealed less prevalence of depressive symptoms in the experimental than in the control group. The level of negative thinking and chronic stressors scores continued to decline between 1 and 6 months after intervention for the control and experimental groups but were lower for the intervention compared to the control group.

Implications ➤ The Hawthorne effect could have influenced results; using an attention control group in future research would eliminate this potential effect. Findings indicate that the mental health benefits of a nursing intervention, altering negative thinking and using positive affirmations, is a way to improve mood in at-risk people. Such interventions may not remove the chronic stressors but can assist single mothers to better cope with them.

to help others recover (e.g., Alcoholics Anonymous, Narcotics Anonymous, Overeaters Anonymous). In some organizations, consumers and professionals plan, implement, and evaluate services (e.g., National Alliance of Mental Illness). *Self-help groups foster* (229): (a) consumer operation and collaboration, (b) empowerment, (c) peer support, (d) education about self-help activities, (e) social and recreational activities, (f) advocacy, and (g) community outreach and public relations. You may be involved as a collaborator in a self-help group.

You may use interventions that do not involve direct face-to-face intervention or individual or group education or counseling sessions. The young adult seeks information and care in programs that are compatible with expectations and lifestyle. Thus, you may utilize telephone intervention—crisis or long term. One study showed that safety-promoting behaviors by abused women increased with an 18-month telephone intervention for victims of intimate partner violence (153). Increasingly, interventions for any health problem, physical or psychological, will be electronic-related. For example, treatment for the person who is alcoholic may be Web based (72). Use of *Internet* intervention may not be feasible for some people, for example, the homeless, the migrant worker or others in rural areas, those who are marginal in society, or those who have difficulty utilizing a computer. Initiate interven-

tion services that are aimed specifically for young adults. Seek their input in the planning of such services. Teach clients how to evaluate Internet-based treatment and to identify the best treatment options (72). Some clients need the motivating factor of face-to-face, personalized counseling and education.

EVALUATION

Obtain feedback from young adult clients to **evaluate** the services you provide. Utilize statements from **Box 14-12**, Considerations for the Young Adult in Health Promotion, to formulate evaluation criteria. Scrutinize your own beliefs and attitudes in relation to the needs, behaviors, and reactions. You may develop evaluation criteria based on information presented in this chapter or derived from cited instruments or references at the end of the chapter. Evaluation may be based on research studies, or on questions raised by other professionals or the clients (87). Feedback from referral agencies, community resources, or the agency's ethics committee may give further evaluative data to either maintain or revise intervention strategies. The example given by O'Connor on the effects of mandatory reporting of domestic abuse presents a practice dilemma that you and other professionals will face and need to analyze or evaluate (176). Your belief system and the belief systems of your colleagues will also guide evaluation (87).

Summary

1. Young adulthood is a time of stabilization personally and in society. Physical growth is completed.
2. Young adulthood is a time of peak function and health.
3. The person has established independence from parents but maintains a friendly relationship with them.
4. The person is settling into a committed intimate relationship and friendships and into a career or profession.
5. The couple may choose to become parents or remain childless.
6. The person may choose to remain single.
7. Development continues in the cognitive, emotional, social, and moral-spiritual dimensions.
8. Philosophy of life and knowledge of what he or she can make out of life is being formulated.

9. Efforts at teaching and counseling can enhance the young adult's awareness of health promotion and establish a program to make that position more stable.
10. Behaviors, whether at home, on the job, at leisure, or with family, friends, or strangers, are adaptive in response to stressors.
11. Stress effects may result in unhealthy habits or physical or emotional illness.
12. **Box 14-12**, Considerations for the Young Adult in Health Promotion, summarizes what you should consider in assessment and health promotion of the young adult. The family is included in considerations.

Review Questions

1. When explaining assessment findings to a young adult female, the nurse should include which of the following points when talking about gender differences in weight?
   1. Females typically have about half as much body fat as males.
   2. Females typically have about twice as much body fat as males.
   3. Females typically store fat in the abdomen.
   4. Males typically store fat in the hips.

2. The nurse in the college health office is counseling a female student. The student tells the nurse that her boyfriend is angry because she refuses to have intercourse during her menstrual period. Which of the following research findings can the nurse provide to the student?
   1. Intercourse during menses can cause tissue damage and is contraindicated.
   2. Intercourse during menses is not contraindicated, but sex drive is diminished.

3. Intercourse during menses is not contraindicated, but the student should do what she is comfortable with.

4. Intercourse during menses may cause increased cramping and discomfort.

3. A 21-year-old healthy, moderately active male, weighing 170 pounds at 5 feet 10 inches, asks the nurse about the appropriate daily calorie intake to maintain his current weight. Taking into account BMI, physical activity, and digestion and absorption needs, which is the best response for the nurse to offer this student?
   1. 1,870 calories/day
   2. 2,618 calories/day

3. 2,880 calories/day
4. 3,500 calories/day

4. A young adult who recently started rotating between the day and night shift at his job came to the clinic nurse with symptoms that are consistent with depression. The nurse concluded that the recent onset of depression is likely related to:
   1. The client being overwhelmed by new adult responsibilities.
   2. Genetic factors that increase risk of depression.
   3. Disruption in body rhythms of diurnal cycles.
   4. Substance abuse that the client is not admitting.

References

1. Aaronson, L., Pallikkathoyll, L., & Crighton, F. (2003). A qualitative investigation of fatigue among healthy working adults. *Western Journal of Nursing Research, 25*(4), 419–433.

2. Addiction and the problem of relapse. (2007). *Harvard Mental Health Letter,* (1), 4–5.

3. A lifetime of distractions. (2004). *Harvard Health Letter, 29*(123), 1–3.

4. Allen, M., & Burrell, N. (2002). Sexual orientation of the parent. The impact on the child. In M. Allen, R. Preiss, B. Gayle, & N. Burrell (Eds.), *Interpersonal communication research: Advances through meta-analysis* (pp. 125–143). Mahwah, NJ: Erlbaum.

5. American Psychiatric Association. (1994). *Diagnostic and statistical manual of mental disorders* (4th ed.). Washington, DC: Author.

6. American Psychiatric Association. (2000). *Diagnostic and statistical manual IV-TR.* Washington, DC: Author.

7. Anderson, C., & Parish, M. (2003). Report of workplace violence by Hispanic nurses. *Journal of Transcultural Nursing, 14*(5), 237–243.

8. Andrews, M., & Boyle, J. (2003). *Transcultural concepts in nursing care* (4th ed.). Philadelphia: Lippincott.

9. Antai-Otong, D. (2002). Culture and traumatic events. *Journal of American Psychiatric Nurses Association, 8,* 203–208.

10. Antai-Otong, D. (2003). *Psychiatric nursing: Biological & behavioral concepts.* Clifton Park, NY: Thomson/Delmar Learning.

11. Arlin, P. (1975). Cognitive development in adulthood: A fifth stage? *Developmental Psychology, 11*(5), 602–606.

12. Bailey, K. (2004). The brain's rewarding system & addiction. *Journal of Psychosocial Nursing, 42*(6), 14–18.

13. Baker, R. (2006). Weight loss and diet plans. *American Journal of Nursing, 106*(6), 52–59.

14. Baltes, P. (2000). Life span development theory. In A. Kazdzin (Ed.), *Encyclopedia of psychology.* Washington, DC: American Psychological Association.

15. Balzac, F. (2005). Effective alcohol abuse screening means asking the right questions. *NeuroPsychiatry Reviews, 6*(4), 1, 22.

16. Balzac, F. (2006). Sleep deprivation impairs memory, skews risk taking. *NeuroPsychiatry Reviews, 7*(12), 14.

17. Bancroft, L., & Silverman, T. (2002). *Batterer as parent: Addressing the impact of domestic violence on family dynamics.* Thousand Oaks, CA: Sage.

18. Bandura, A. (2002). Social Cognitive Theory. In A. Kazdin (Ed.), *Encyclopedia of psychology.* Washington, DC: American Psychological Association.

19. Barnard, A. (2005). Effects of sexuality on lesbian experiences. *Journal of Psychosocial Nursing, 43*(10), 36–43.

20. Bass, J., & Turek, F. (2005). Sleepless in America: A pathway to obesity and the metabolic syndrome? *Archives of Internal Medicine, 165,* 15–16.

21. Basseches, H. (1984). *Dialectical thinking and adult development.* Norwood, NJ: Ablex.

22. Beard, B. (2007). The faces of AIDS. *Journal of Christian Nursing, 24*(1), 22–25.

23. Beck, C. (2006). Postpartum depression: It isn't just the blues. *American Journal of Nursing, 106*(5), 40–50.

24. Benson, H. (1988). *Beyond the relaxation response.* New York: William Morrow.

25. Bentley, E. (2000). *Awareness: Biorhythms, sleep, and dreaming.* New York: Routledge.

26. Berger, K. (2005). *The developing person through the life span* (6th ed.). New York: Worth.

27. Berggren, V., Bergstrom, S., & Edberg, A. (2006). Being different and vulnerable: Experiences of immigrant women who have been circumcised and sought maternity care in Sweden. *Journal of Transcultural Nursing, 17*(1), 50–57.

28. Bialous, S., & Sarna, L. (2004). Sparing a few minutes for tobacco cessation. *American Journal of Nursing, 104*(12), 54–60.

29. Blixen, C., Singh, A., & Thacker, H. (2006). Values and beliefs about obesity and weight reduction among African-American and Caucasian women. *Journal of Transcultural Nursing, 17*(3), 290–297.

30. Boschert, S. (2005). Gay men: Therapy curbs risky sexual acts, HIV. *Clinical Psychiatry News, 33*(12), 48.

31. Bozett, F. (1987). *Gay and lesbian parents.* New York: Praeger.

32. Cacioppo, J. (2000). Emotion and health. In R. Davidson, K. Sherer, & H. Goldsmith (Eds.), *Handbook of affective sciences.* New York: Oxford University Press.

33. Calonge, N. (2004). U.S. Preventive Services Task Force screening for obesity in adults: Recommendations and rationale. *American Journal of Nursing, 104,* 94–100.

34. Campingha-Bacote, J. (2007). Becoming culturally competent in ethnic psychopharmacology. *Journal of Psychosocial Nursing, 45*(9), 27–33.

35. Cash, T., & Pruzinsky, T. (Eds.). (1990). *Body images: Development, deviance, and change.* New York: Guilford Press.

36. Caspe, A. (1998). Personality development across the life course. In W. Damon (Ed.), *Handbook of child psychology* (Vol. I). New York: Wiley.

37. Cataldo, J. (2001). Helping our clients with smoking cessation. *Journal of American Psychiatric Nurses Association, 7,* 26–30.

38. Centers for Disease Control. (2004). Mean body weight, height, and body mass index, United States 1960–2002. Advance data no. 347 (PHS2002-1250).

39. Centers for Disease Control and Prevention. (2005). QuickStats from the National Center for Health Statistics: Mean weight and height among adults aged 20–74 years, by sex and survey period—United States, 1960–1962. *MMWR: Morbidity and Mortality Weekly Report, 54*(31), 771.

40. Chen, H. H., & Burnett, J. C. (2000). Natriuretic peptides in the pathophysiology of congestive heart failure. *Current Cardiology Reports, 2*(3), 198–205.

41. Cheng, V., Kazanagra, R., Garcia, A., et al. (2001). A rapid bedside test for B-type peptide predicts treatment outcomes in patients admitted for decompensated heart failure: A pilot study. *Journal of the American College of Cardiology, 37*(2), 386–391.

42. Cherniss, S. (2002). Emotional intelligence and the good community. *American Journal of Community Psychology, 30,* 1–11.

43. Cherpes, T. L., Meyn, L. A., & Hillier, S. L. (2005). Cunnilingus and vaginal intercourse are risk factors for herpes simplex virus type 1 acquisition in women. Sexually transmitted diseases. *Journal of the American Sexual Transmitted Diseases Association, 32*(2), 84–89.

44. Chobanian, A., Bakris, G., & Black, H. (2003). The seventh report of the Joint National Committee on prevention, detection, evaluation, and treatment of high blood pressure: The JNC 7 report. *Journal of the American Medical Association, 289*(19), 2560–2572.

45. Choi, M., & Harwood, J. (2004). A hypothesized model of Korean women's responses to abuse. *Journal of Transcultural Nursing, 15*(3), 207–216.

46. Cibulka, N. (2005). Mother-to-child transmission of HIV in the United States. *American Journal of Nursing, 105*(7), 56–63.

47. Clark, N. (2002). *Nancy Clark's food guide for marathoners.* Boston: Sports Nutrition Publishers.

48. Clark, N. (2003). *Nancy Clark's sports nutrition guidebook* (3rd ed.). New York: Human Kinetics.

49. Clinton, J. (1986). Expectant fathers at risk for couvade. *Nursing Research, 35*(2), 290–294.

50. Cmiel, C., Karr, D., Gasser, D., Olyphant, L., & Neveau, A. (2004). Noise control: A nursing team's approach to sleep promotion. *American Journal of Nursing, 104*(2), 40–47.

51. Coentz, S. (2006). *Marriage, a history: From obedience to intimacy—How love conquered marriage.* New York: Viking.

52. Coleman, P. (2005). Induced abortion and increased risk of substance abuse: A review of the evidence. *Current Women's Health Reviews, 1,* 21–34.

53. Compher, C. (2006). The nutrition transition in American Indians. *Journal of Transcultural Nursing, 17*(3), 217–233.

54. Conti, K. (2006). Diabetes prevention in Indian country: Developing nutrition models to tell the story of food-system change. *Journal of Transcultural Nursing, 17*(3), 234–245.

55. Cook, L. (2004). Educating women about the hidden dangers of alcohol. *Journal of Psychosocial Nursing, 42*(6), 24–31.

56. Copel, L. (2006). Partner abuse in physically disabled women: A proposed model for understanding intimate partner violence. *Perspectives in Psychiatric Care, 42*(2), 111–129.

57. Criellar, N., Ratcliffe, S., & Chien, D. (2006). Effects of depression on sleep quality, fatigue, and sleepiness in persons with restless legs syndrome. *Journal of American Psychiatric Nurses Association, 12*(5), 262–271.

58. Cronan, L., & Gloucester College of Higher Education. (1993). Management of the patient with altered body image. *British Journal of Nursing, 2*(5), 257–261.

59. Dube, E. M., & Savin-Williams, R. C. (1999). Sexuality identity development among ethnic sexual-minority male youths. *Developmental Psychology, 35*(6), 1389–1398.

60. Dudek, S. (2007). *Nutrition essentials for nursing* (5th ed.). Philadelphia: Lippincott Williams & Wilkins.

61. Duvall, E., & Miller, B. (1984). *Marriage and family development* (6th ed.). New York: Harper & Row.

62. Duyff, R. (2002). *American Dietetic Association complete food and nutrition guide* (2nd ed.). Hoboken, NJ: John Wiley & Sons.

63. Ehrmin, J. (2005). Dimensions of cultural care for substance-dependent African-American women. *Journal of Transcultural Nursing, 16*(2), 117–125.

64. Epstein, D., & Bootzen, R. (2002). Insomnia. *Nursing Clinics of North America, 37,* 611–631.

65. Erikson, E. (1963). *Children and society* (2nd ed.). New York: W.W. Norton.

66. Erikson, E. (Ed.). (1978). *Adulthood.* New York: W.W. Norton.

67. Erikson, E., & Erikson, J. (1997). *The life cycle completed* (pp. 66–72). New York: W.W. Norton.

68. Esposito, N. (2006). Women with a history of sexual assault. *American Journal of Nursing, 106*(3), 69–73.

69. Fawcett, J., et al. (1986). Spouses' body image changes during and after pregnancy: A replication and extension. *Nursing Research, 35*(4), 220–223.

70. Fenstermacher, K., & Hudson, B. (2004). *Practice guidelines for family practitioners* (3rd ed.). Philadelphia: Saunders.

71. Ferketich, S., & Mercer, R. (1995). Predictors of role competence for experienced and inexperienced fathers. *Nursing Research, 44,* 89–95.

72. Finfgeld-Connett, D. (2006). Web-based treatment for problem drinking. *Journal of Psychosocial Nursing, 44*(9), 20–27.

73. Fontaine, K. (1991). The conspiracy of culture: Women's issues in body size. *Nursing Clinics of North America, 26*(3), 669–676.

74. Flikhema, M. (2007). Sexual practices and HIV: How can nurses respond? *Journal of Christian Nursing, 24*(1), 26–29.

75. Florida, R. (2002). *The rise of the creative class.* New York: Basic Books.

76. Foster, R., & Kreitzman, L. (2005). *Rhythms of life: The biological clocks that control the daily lives of every living thing.* New Haven, CT: Yale University Press.

77. Gaffney, K. (2006). Postpartum smoking relapse and becoming a mother. *Journal of Nursing Scholarship, 38*(1), 26–30.

78. Garner, P., & Estep, K. (2002). Empathy and emotional expressivity. In J. Worell (Ed.), *Encyclopedia of women and gender.* San Diego, CA: Academic Press.

79. Geralamo, A. (2004). State of the science: Women and the nonpharmacological treatment of substance abuse. *Journal of American Psychiatric Nurses Association, 10*(4), 181–189.

80. Giger, J., & Davidhizar, R. (2004). *Transcultural nursing: Assessment and intervention* (4th ed.). St. Louis, MO: Mosby.

81. Gilligan, C. (2002). *The birth of pleasure.* New York: Alfred A. Knopf.

82. Glanz, K., Saraiya, M., & Wechsler, H. (2006). Guidelines for school programs to prevent skin cancer. *MMWR: Morbidity and Mortality Weekly Report, 51*(RR04), 1–16.

83. Goleman, D. (1995). *Emotional intelligence: Why it can matter more than IQ.* New York: Bantam.

84. Goleman, D. (1998). *Working with emotional intelligence.* New York: Bantam.

85. Gould, R. (1975). Adults' life stages: Growth toward self-tolerance. *Psychology Today, 8*(7), 74–78.

86. Gould, R. (1978). *Transformations: Growth and change in adult life.* New York: Simon & Schuster.

87. Graham, K. (2006). Evaluating addiction treatment in light of scripture. *Journal of Christian Nursing, 23*(2), 18–24.

88. Greenfield, M. (1990). Disclosing incest: The relationships that make it possible. *Journal of Psychosocial Nursing, 28*(7), 20–23.

89. Guarnero, P. (2007). Family and community influences on the social and sexual lives of Latino gay men. *Journal of Transcultural Nursing, 18*(1), 12–18.

90. Guyton, A., & Hall, J. (2006). *Textbook of medical physiology* (11th ed.). Philadelphia: Elsevier Saunders.

91. Hagedorn, K., Lasuick, G., & Coupland, J. (2006). Post-traumatic stress disorder Part III: Health effects of interpersonal violence among women. *Perspectives in Psychiatric Care, 42*(3), 163–173.

92. Harris, C. R. (2002). Sexual and romantic jealousy in heterosexual and homosexual adults. *Psychological Science, 13,* 7–12.

93. Harris, M., & Curmella, E. (2006). Eating disorders across the life span. *Journal of Psychosocial Nursing, 44*(4), 20–26.

94. Harrison, Y., Horne, I., & Rothwell, A. (2000). Prefrontal neuropsychological effects of sleep deprivation in young adults—a model for healthy aging. *Sleep, 23,* 1067–1073.

95. Hastings, J. (2007). Addiction: A nurse's story. *American Journal of Nursing, 107*(8), 75–79.

96. Harvey, J., & Weber, A. (2001). *Odyssey of a heart* (2nd ed.). Newark, NJ: Erlbaum.

97. Haylock, P., Mitchell, S., Cox, T., Temple, S., & Curtiss, C. (2007). The cancer survivor's prescription for living. *American Journal of Nursing, 107*(4), 58–70.

98. Health benefits of taking probiotics. (2005). *Harvard Women's Health, 12*(9), 6–7.

99. Heiner, R. (2002). *Social problems: An introduction to critical constructionism.* New York: Oxford University Press.

100. Hertz, R. (2006). *Single by chance, mothers by choice.* New York: Oxford University Press.

101. Hill, D. (2006). Sense of belonging as connectedness, American Indian worldview and mental health. *Archives of Psychiatric Nursing, 20*(5), 210–216.

102. Hitchcock, J., & Wilson, M. (1992). Personal risking: Lesbian self-disclosure of sexual orientation to professional health care providers. *Nursing Research, 41,* 178–183.

103. Hobson, J., & Silvestri, L. (1999). Parasomnias. *Harvard Mental Health Letter, 15*(5), 3–5.

104. Holland, J. (1987). Current status of Holland's Theory of Careers: Another perspective. *Career Development Quarterly, 36,* 24–30.

105. Holmes, R., & O'Byrne, P. (2006). Bareback sex and the law. The difficult issue of HIV status disclosure. *Journal of Psychosocial Nursing, 44*(7), 26–33.

106. Honore, C. (2004). *In praise of slowness.* New York: Harper Collins.

107. Horn, B. (1990). Cultural concepts and postpartal care. *Journal of Transcultural Nursing, 2*(1), 48–51.

108. Houre, C. (2002). *Erikson on development in adulthood. New insights from the unpublished papers.* New York: W.W. Norton.

109. Hughes, R. (2004). The perils of shift work. *American Journal of Nursing, 104*(9), 60–63.

110. Hughes, R., & Rogers, A. (2004). Are you tired? *American Journal of Nursing, 104*(3), 36–37.

111. Intermittent explosive disorder. (2006). *Harvard Mental Health Letter, 23*(3), 5–6.

112. Iwata, H. (2003). A concept analysis of the role of fatherhood: A Japanese perspective. *Journal of Transcultural Nursing, 14*(4), 297–302.

113. Izrael, J. (2003, July–August). Support groups help parents when children "come out." *United Church News,* Sec B5.

114. Jewell, A. (2003, August–September). Two roads. *Focus on the Family,* 12–13.

115. Jung, C. (1971). Psychological types. In G. Adler, et al. (Eds.), *Collected works of Carl G. Jung, Vol. 6.* Princeton, NJ: Princeton University Press.

116. Karnath, B. (2003). Smoking cessation: How to make pharmacotherapy work. *Consultant, 43*(6), 665–674.

117. Katz, J., & Hirsch, A. (2003). When global health is local health. *American Journal of Nursing, 103*(12), 75–79.

118. Kelley, J. (2005). Men and women achieve intelligence differently. *NeuroPsychiatry, 6*(2), 1, 22.

119. Kemper, S., & McDowd, J. (2006). Eye movements of young and older adults while reading with distraction. *Psychology & Aging, 21*(1), 32–39.

120. Kendler, K., Thorton, I., Gilman, S., & Kessler, R. (2000). Sexual orientation in a U.S. national sample of twin and nontwin sibling pairs. *American Journal of Psychiatry, 157,* 1843–1847.

121. Kindy, D., Peterson, S., & Parkhurst, D. (2005). Perilous work: Nurses' experience in psychiatric units with high risks of assault. *Archives of Psychiatric Nursing, 19*(4), 169–175.

122. Klingman, L. (1999). Assessing the male genitalia. *American Journal of Nursing, 99*(7), 47–50.

123. Klingman, L. (1999). Assessing the female reproductive system. *American Journal of Nursing, 99*(8), 37–43.

124. Knowles, M. S. (1984). *Androgogy in action.* San Francisco: Jossey-Bass.

125. Kohlberg, L. (1971). *Recent research in moral development.* New York: Holt, Rinehart, & Winston.

126. Korenramp, M., Cluislieens, M., vandan Bout, J., Mulder, E., Hunfeld, J., Bilardo, C., et al. (2005). Long-term psychological consequences of pregnancy termination for fetal abnormality: A cross-sectional study. *Prenatal Diagnosis, 25,* 253–260.

127. Kunert, K., King, M., & Kolkhorst, F. (2007). Fatigue and sleep quality in nurses. *Journal of Psychosocial Nursing, 45*(8), 31–37.

128. Labyak, S. (2002). Sleep and circadian schedule disorders. *Nursing Clinics of North America, 37,* 599–610.

129. Lamb, M. (1987). The emergent father. In M. E. Lamb (Ed.), *The father's role: Cross-cultural perspectives* (pp. 1–26). Hillsdale, NJ: Lawrence Erlbaum.

130. LaRossa, R. (1988). Fatherhood and social change. *Family Relations, 3,* 451–457.

131. Leifer, C., & Young, E. (1997). Homeless lesbians: Psychology of the hidden, the disenfranchised, and the forgotten. *Journal of Psychosocial Nursing, 35*(10), 28–33.

132. Levant, R. (2002). Men and masculinity. In J. Worell (Ed.), *Encyclopedia of women and gender.* San Diego, CA: Academic Press.

133. Levay, S. (1991). A difference in the hypothalamus structure between heterosexual and homosexual men. *Science, 253,* 1034–1037.

134. Levinson, D., et al. (1976). Periods in the adult development of men: Ages 18–45. *Counseling Psychologist, 6*(1), 21–25.

135. Levinson, D. (1978). *The seasons of a man's life.* New York: Ballantine Books.

136. Levinson, D. (1986). A conception of adult development. *American Psychologist, 41,* 3–13.

137. Levinson, D. (1990). A theory of life structure development in adulthood. In K. N. Alexander & E. J. Langer (Eds.), *Higher stages of human development* (pp. 35–54). New York: Oxford University Press.

138. Levinson, D. (1996). *Seasons of a woman's life.* New York: Alfred Knopf.

139. Lewis, L. (1995). One year in the life of a woman with premenstrual syndrome: A case study. *Nursing Research, 44,* 111–115.

140. LoBaugh, E., Clements, P., Averill, J., & Olguin, D. (2006). Gay-male couples who adopt: Challenging historical and contemporary trends toward becoming a family. *Perspectives in Psychiatric Care, 42*(3), 184–194.

141. Lunney, M. (2006). Stress overload: A new diagnosis. *International Journal of Nursing Terminologies and Classifications, 17*(4), 168–175.

142. Lyon, B. (2002). Cognitive self-help skills: A model for managing stressful lifestyles. *Nursing Clinics of North America, 37,* 285–294.

143. Mabunda, G. (2004). HIV knowledge and practices among rural South Africans. *Journal of Nursing Scholarship, 36*(4), 300–304.

144. Mahoney, D. (2005). Getting to the root of domestic violence. *Clinical Psychiatric News, 33*(12), 49.

145. Maloni, J., & Ponder, M. (1997). Fathers' experience of their partner's antepartum bed rest. *IMAGE: Journal of Nursing Scholarship, 29*(2), 183–188.

146. Martinez-Schallmoser, L., Telleen, S., & MacMullen, N. (2003). The effect of social support and acculturation on postpartum depression in Mexican-American women. *Journal of Transcultural Nursing, 14*(4), 329–338.

147. Mason, D., & Kary, K. (2005). The state of science: Focus on work environments. *American Journal of Nursing, 105*(3), 33–34.

148. Masse, L., & Antonacci, M. (2005). Low cardiac output syndrome: Identification and management. *Critical Care Nursing Clinics of North America, 17,* 375–383.

149. Masters, W., & Johnson, V. (1979). *Homosexuality in perspective.* Boston: Little, Brown.

150. Masters, W., & Johnson, V. (1981). *The human sexual response.* New York: Bantam.

151. May, K. (1982). Three phases of father involvement in pregnancy. *Nursing Research, 31*(8), 337–342.

152. McAuley, J. D., Jones, M. R., Holub, S., Johnston, H. M., & Miller, N. S. (2006). The time of our lives: Life span development of timing and event tracking. *Journal of Experimental Psychology: General, 135*(3), 348–367.

153. McFarlane, J., Malecha, A., Watson, K., & Hall, I. (2004). Increasing the safety-promoting behavior of abused women. *American Journal of Nursing, 104*(3), 40–50.

154. McGuinness, T. (2006). Marriage, divorce, and children. *Journal of Psychosocial Nursing, 44*(2), 17–20.

155. McNeeley, E. (2005). The consequences of job stress for nurses' health: Time for a check-up. *Nursing Outlook, 53,* 291–299.

156. Meagher, M. (2007). Chronic stress may worsen neurodegenerative disease course. *NeuroPsychiatry Reviews, 8*(9), 8.

157. Men and depression. (2006). *Harvard Mental Health Letter, 23*(5), 1–3.

158. Merriman, J. (2006). Screening for intimate partner violence—What's the best approach? *NeuroPsychiatry, 7*(10), 1, 18.

159. Messina, V., Melina, V., & Mangels, A. (2003). A new food guide for North American vegetarians. *Journal of the American Dietetic Association, 103*(6), 771–775.

160. Metheny, N. (2000). *Fluid & electrolyte balance: Nursing considerations* (4th ed.). Philadelphia: Lippincott.

161. Miles, A. (1999). When faith is used to justify abuse. *American Journal of Nursing, 99*(5), 32–35.

162. Miller, K. (1991). Body image therapy. *Nursing Clinics of North America, 26*(3), 727–736.

163. Missouri Coalition Against Domestic & Sexual Violence. (2006). *A framework for understanding the nature and dynamics of domestic violence.* Jefferson City, MO: Author.

164. Mitchell, A., & Parish, T. (2005). Using combination therapy for smoking cessation. *Clinical Review, 15*(5), 40–45.

165. Moberly, E. (1992). Can homosexuals really change? *Journal of Christian Nursing, 8*(4), 14–17.

166. Moore, J. (2005). Hypertension, catching the silent killer. *Nurse Practitioner, 30*(10), 16–35.

167. Moore, S., & Seybold, V. (2007). HPV vaccine. *Clinical Reviews, 17*(1), 36–40.

168. Morrison, L. K., Harrison, A., Krishnaswamy, P., et al. (2002). Utility of a rapid B-natriuretic peptide assay in differentiating congestive heart failure from lung disease in patients presenting with dyspnea. *Journal of the American College of Cardiology, 39*(2), 202–209.

169. MRI's emerging role in breast cancer screening. (2007). *Harvard Women's Health Watch, 15*(2), 1–3.

170. Munro, A., & Epping-Jordan, J. (2004). The World Health Organization warns of the rising threat of heart disease and stroke as overweight and obesity rapidly increase: WHO urges healthy diet, physical activity, no tobacco use. *WHO: Department of Chronic Diseases and Health Promotion.* Retrieved June 1, 2006.

171. NANDA International. (2005). *NANDA nursing diagnosis: Definitions and classification 2005–2006.* Philadelphia: Lippincott.

172. National survey sharpens picture of major depression among U.S. adults. (2005). *NeuroPsychiatry, 6*(10), 1, 10.

173. Nelson, R. (2005). Nurses with disabilities. *American Journal of Nursing, 105*(6), 25–26.

174. NiCarthy, G. (2004). *Getting free: You can end abuse and take back your life.* Seattle, WA: Seal Publisher.

175. O'Brien-Pallas, L., Shamean, J., Thornsen, D., Alksma, C., Koehoorn, M., Kerr, M., & Bruce, S. (2004). Work-related disability in Canadian nurses. *Journal of Nursing Scholarship, 36*(4), 352–357.

176. O'Connor, A. (2004). Dying to tell? Do mandatory reporting laws benefit victims of domestic violence? *American Journal of Nursing, 104*(10), 75–79.

177. Oelbaum, C. (1974). Hallmarks of adult wellness. *American Journal of Nursing, 74*(9), 1623–1625.

178. Ogden, C. L., Fry, C. D., Carroll, M. D., & Flegal, K. M. (2004). Mean body weight, height, and body mass index: United States 1960–2002. *Advanced data from vital and health statistics. No. 347.* Hyattsville, MD: U.S. Department of Health and Human Services, CDC, National Center for Health Statistics. Retrieved June 1, 2006. www.cdc.gov/nehs/data/ad/ad3471.pdf

179. Ortiz, C. (2005). Disclosing concerns of Latinas living with HIV/AIDS. *Journal of Transcultural Nursing, 16*(3), 216–217.

180. Ortman, P. (2005). Post-infidelity stress disorder. *Journal of Psychosocial Nursing, 45*(10), 47.

181. Papalia, D., Olds, S., & Feldman, R. (2004). *Human development* (9th ed.). Boston: McGraw-Hill.

182. Pasacreta, J., Jacobs, L., & Cataldo, J. (2002). Genetic testing for breast and ovarian cancer risk: The psych-social issues. *American Journal of Nursing, 102*(12), 40–47.

183. Paskawicz, J. (2005). Latex allergy revisited: Clinicians stay alert. *Clinical Reviews, 15*(11), 66–75.

184. Patzel, B. (2006). What blocked heterosexual women and lesbians in leaving their abusive relationships. *Journal of American Psychiatric Nurses Association, 12*(4), 208–215.

185. Pender, N., Murdaugh, C., & Parsons, M. (2006). *Health promotion in nursing practice* (5th ed.). Upper Saddle River, NJ: Pearson Education.

186. Peters, R. (2006). The relationship of racism, chronic stress, emotions, and blood pressure. *Journal of Nursing Scholarship, 38*(3), 234–240.

187. Posmontier, B. (2004). Postpartum practices and depression prevalence: Technocentric and ethnokinship cultural perspectives. *Journal of Transcultural Nursing, 15*(1), 34–43.

188. Price, B. (1995). Assessing altered body image. *Journal of Psychiatric and Mental Health Nursing, 2,* 169–175.

189. Prochaska, J., & DiClemente, C. (1984). *The Transtheoretical Approach: Crossing traditional boundaries of change.* Homewood, NJ: Dow Jones-Irwin.

190. Prochaska, J., Norcross, J., & DiClemente, C. (1994). *Changing for good: A revolutionary six-step program for overcoming bad habits and moving your life positively forward.* New York: Avon.

191. Quit smoking for good. (2006). *Focus on Healthy Aging, 9*(7), 4–5.

192. Rancour, P. (2002). Catapulting through life stages: When younger adults are diagnosed with life-threatening illnesses. *Journal of Psychosocial Nursing, 40*(2), 33–37.

193. Recognizing domestic partner abuse. (2006). *Harvard Women's Health Watch, 14*(1), 6–7.

194. Renck, B. (2006). Psychological stress reactions of women in Sweden who have been assaulted: Acute response and four month follow-up. *Nursing Outlook, 54,* 312–319.

195. Rhoads, J. (2006). *Advanced health assessment and diagnostic reasoning.* Philadelphia: Lippincott Williams & Wilkins.

196. Richard, E., & Shepard, A. (1981). Giving up smoking: A lesson in loss therapy. *American Journal of Nursing, 81*(4), 755–757.

197. Riegel, K. (1975). Toward a dialectical theory of development. *Human Development, 18,* 50–64.

198. Roth, T. (2004). Characteristics and determinates of normal sleep. *Journal of Clinical Psychiatry, 65,* 8–11.

199. Rubin, R. (1975). Maternal tasks in pregnancy. *Maternal-Child Nursing Journal, 4*(3), 143–153.

200. Sandelowski, M., Lambe, C., & Barroso, J. (2004). Stigma in HIV-positive women. *Journal of Nursing Scholarship, 36*(2), 122–128.

201. Santrock, J. (2004). *Life-span development* (9th ed.). Boston: McGraw-Hill.

202. Schaie, K., & Willis, S. (2001). *Adult development and aging* (5th ed.). Upper Saddle River, NJ: Prentice Hall.

203. Scherer, P. (1990). How AIDS attacks the brain. *American Journal of Nursing, 90*(1), 41–52.

204. Scherer, P. (1990). How AIDS attacks the peripheral nervous system. *American Journal of Nursing, 90*(5), 66–70.

205. Schilder, P. (1951). *The image and appearance of the human body.* New York: International University Press.

206. Schism, D., Doorendos, A., Benkert, R., & Miller, J. (2007). Culturally competent care: Putting the puzzle together. *Journal of Transcultural Nursing, 18*(2), 103–110.

207. Scholler-Jaquish, A., Weiss-Raffasi, C., Ashcraft, A., & Diaz, S. (2003). The latex allergy psychiatric patient. *Journal of Psychosocial Nursing, 41*(2), 28–36.

208. Seshadri, S., Beiser, A., Kelly-Hayes, M., Kase, C., Au, R., Kannel, W., & Wolf, P.A. (2006). The lifetime risk of stroke: Estimates from the Framingham study. *Stroke, 37*(2), 345–350.

209. Shaw, E. (1983). Female circumcision. *American Journal of Nursing, 83*(6), 684–687.

210. Sheehy, G. (1976). *Passages: Predictable crises of adult life.* New York: Bantam Books.

211. Sheehy, G. (1992). *The silent passage: Menopause.* New York: Random House.

212. Sherrod, R. (2004). Understanding the emotional aspects of infertility. *Journal of Psychosocial Nursing, 42*(3), 42–47.

213. Sherrod, R. (2006). Male infertility: The element of disguise. *Journal of Psychosocial Nursing, 44*(10), 31–37.

214. Sinnott, J. (1996). The developmental approach: Postformal thought as adaptive intelligence. In F. Blanchard-Fields & T. M. Hess (Eds.), *Perspectives on cognitive change in adulthood and aging* (pp. 358–386). New York: McGraw-Hill.

215. Smolensky, M., & Lamberg, L. (2000). *The body clock: Guide to better health.* New York: Henry Holt and Company.

216. Sperling, M., & Berman, W. (1994). *Attachment in adults: Clinical and developmental perspectives.* New York: Behavioral Science Book Science.

217. Spinks, V., Andrews, J., & Boyle, J. (2000). Providing health care for lesbian clients. *Journal of Transcultural Nursing, 11*(2), 137–143.

218. Splete, H. (2005). Biological rhythms are key to assessing sleep. *Clinical Psychiatry News, 32*(2), 60.

219. Steiner, L. (2006). *Mommy wars: Stay-at-home and career moms face off on their choices, their lives, their families.* New York: Random House.

220. Sternberg, R. (1988). *The triarchic mind: A new theory of human intelligence.* New York: Viking Press.

221. Sternberg, R. (2003). *Wisdom, intelligence, and creativity synthesized.* New York: Cambridge University Press.

222. Stevens, P., & Hall, J. (1988). Stigma, health beliefs & experiences with health care in lesbian women. IMAGE: *Journal of Nursing Scholarship, 20,* 69–73.

223. Stewart, R. (1997). Female circumcision: Implications for North American nurses. *Journal of Psychosocial Nursing, 35*(4), 35–38.

224. Stiegler, P., & Cunliffe, A. (2006). The role of diet and exercise for the maintenance of fat-free mass and resting metabolic rate during weight loss. *Sports Medicine, 36*(3), 239–262.

225. Stong, C. (2006). Blue light special. Treating circadian rhythm sleep disorders. *NeuroPsychiatry, 7*(9), 1, 16, 18–19.

226. Streil, J. (2002). Marriage: Still "his" and "hers"? In J. Worell (Ed.), *Encyclopedia of women and gender.* San Diego, CA: Academic Press.

227. Strickland, O. (1987). The occurrence of symptoms in expectant fathers. *Nursing Research, 36*(3), 184–189.

228. Sullivan, H. S. (1953). *The Interpersonal Theory of Psychiatry.* New York: W.W. Norton.

229. Swarbrick, M. (2006). Self-help services. *Journal of Psychosocial Nursing, 44*(12), 27–35.

230. Swift, B. (2005). Symptoms, circuits, and stress. *Clinical Psychiatry News, 33*(10), 2–4.

231. The truth about smoking cessation. (2007). *Johns Hopkins Medical Letter: Health After Fifty, 19*(8), 8.

232. Thorpe, J., Hartmann, K., & Shadigian, E. (2002). Long-term physical and psychological health consequences of induced abortion: Review of the evidence. *Obstetric and Gynecological Survey, 58*(1), 67–79.

233. Tobias, C. (1995, October). How do we understand? *Focus on the Family, 13.*

234. Trinkoff, A., Geiger-Brown, J., Brady, P., Lipscomb, J., & Muntaner, C. (2006). How much and how long are nurses now working? *American Journal of Nursing, 106*(4), 60–72.

235. Trossman, S. (2005). Who you work with matters. *American Nurse, 37*(4), 1, 11–12.

236. United States Department of Health and Human Services. (2000). *Healthy People 2010: With understanding and improving health and objectives for improving health* (2nd ed.). 2 Vols. Washington, DC: U.S. Government Printing Office.

237. United States Preventive Services Task Force. (2004). Screening for high blood pressure: Recommendations and rationale. *American Journal of Nursing, 104*(11), 82–87.

238. Vaillant, G. (1977). *Adaptation to life.* Boston: Little, Brown.

239. Vaillant, G. (1977). How the best and the brightest came of age. *Psychology Today, 11*(9), 34ff.

240. Vaillant, G. (1997). The normal boy in later life: How adaptation fosters growth. *Harvard Magazine, 55*(6), 234–239.

241. Van Beuge, S. (2007). Making a stand against malignant melanoma. *American Nurse Today, 2*(8), 18–21.

242. Vande Vusse, L., Hanson, L., Fehring, R., Newman, A., & Fox, J. (2003). Couples' views of the effects of natural family planning on marital dynamics. *Journal of Nursing Scholarship, 35*(2), 171–176.

243. Wachs, T., & Kohnstamm, G. (Eds.). (2001). *Temperament in context.* Mahwah, NJ: Erlbaum.

244. Wadsworth, B. (2004). *Piaget's Theory of Cognitive and Affective Development: Foundations of constructivism* (5th ed.). Boston: Pearson.

245. Warren, N. (2003, June–July). The cohabitation epidemic. *Focus on the Family,* 10–11.

246. Weisskopf, M. (2007). *Blood brothers: Among the soldiers of Ward 57.* New York: Henry Holt.

247. WHO (World Health Organization). (2006). Health situation analysis in Americas 1999–2000. *The World Health Report 2006.* Retrieved June 1, 2006. www.who.inf/whr/2006/annex/06_annex1_en.pdf

248. Williams, G. (2001). Short-term grief after an elective abortion. *Journal of Obstetric, Gynecologic, and Neonatal Nursing, 36*(2), 174–183.

249. Williams, L., & Hopper, P. (2007). *Understanding medical-surgical nursing* (3rd ed.). Philadelphia: F.A. Davis.

250. Willis, K. (2007). Kick the cigarette habit. *American Nurse Today, 2*(4), 58–60.

251. Wilner, A. (2007). Sleep improves relational memory. *NeuroPsychiatry Reviews, 8*(9), 6.

252. Winstead, B., & Griffin, J. (2002). Friendship styles. In J. Worell (Ed.), *Encyclopedia of women and gender.* San Diego, CA: Academic Press.

253. Wismont, J., & Reame, N. (1989). The lesbian childbearing experience: Assessing developmental tasks. *IMAGE: Journal of Nursing Scholarship, 21*(3), 137–142.

254. Woods, S., & Wineman, N. (2004). Trauma, posttraumatic stress disorder symptom clusters, and physical health symptoms in post-abused women. *Archives of Psychiatric Nursing, 18*(1), 26–34.

255. Wright, J., Burgess, A. G., Burgess, A. W., McCrary, G., & Douglas, J. (1995). Investigating stalking crimes. *Journal of Psychosocial Nursing, 33*(9), 38–46.

256. Wynd, C. (2005). Guided health imagery for smoking cessation and long-term abstinence. *Journal of Nursing Scholarship, 37*(3), 245–250.

257. Yan, L., Liu, K., Matthews, K., Davighus, M., Ferguson, T., & Kiepe, C. (2003). Psychosocial factors and risk of hypertension: The coronary artery risk development in young adults study. *Journal of the American Medical Association, 290*(16), 2138–2147.

258. Young, M. (1993). Leaving the lesbian lifestyle. *Journal of Christian Nursing, 8*(4), 11–13.

259. Zunkel, G. (2005). Insomnia: Overview of assessment and treatment strategies. *Clinician Reviews, 15*(7), 38–42.

Interview

260. Heuerman, P., & J. Interview—Twenty-fifth Wedding Anniversary Invitation.

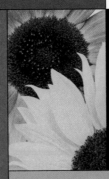

CHAPTER 15

The Middle-Aged Person: Basic Assessment and Health Promotion

OBJECTIVES

Study of this chapter will enable you to:

1. Discuss family relationships, generational differences, and sexual development of the middle-aged adult, conflicts that must be resolved, and your role in helping the family work through concerns and conflicts.

2. Examine the developmental tasks for the middle-aged family, and give examples of how these can be accomplished to promote healthy relationships.

3. Relate the emotional, social, economic, and lifestyle changes usually encountered by the widow or widower.

4. Describe the hormonal changes of middle age and the resultant changes in appearance and body image, physiologically and emotionally.

5. Analyze the nutritional, rest, leisure, work, and exercise needs of the middle-aged adult, factors that interface with meeting those needs, and your role in helping the person meet these needs.

6. Contrast the middle-aged adult's cognitive skills and emotional and moral development to that of young adulthood.

7. Analyze the developmental crisis of this era, related adaptive mechanisms, and significance to social welfare and health.

8. Describe the developmental tasks for this person and your role in helping him or her accomplish these tasks.

9. Explore with a middle-aged adult ways to avoid injury and health problems and to promote health.

10. Assess the body image and physical, mental, and emotional characteristics of a middle-aged person.

MediaLink   www.prenhall.com/murray

Go to the Companion Website for interactive resources that accompany this chapter.

Glossary
Review Questions
Challenge Your Knowledge
Learning Activities

Critical Thinking
Tools
Media Link Applications
Media Links

Historical Changes Related to this Era

Middle age does not exist in every country. It is attributed to improved nutrition, control of communicable disease, discovery and control of familial disease, and other medical advances. In the United States, life has been stretched in the middle. What used to be old age is now middle age. Most non-Westernized and preindustrial cultures recognize only mature adulthood, followed by old age. In some countries, the average life span is shorter than the age span that constitutes early middle age in the United States.

Work structure, roles, and technologic development have become more complex. Family life and childrearing patterns have changed toward smaller families and a longer postparental period. Thus, the periods of childhood and youth have lengthened. Middle age has lengthened as a life era. Midlife development implies growth of the personality to encompass some characteristics that had stereotypically been assigned to the opposite gender. Individuals may also work out more flexible adaptations. The family becomes increasingly oriented to its responsibility to the greater society.

DEFINITIONS

Defining middle age is a nebulous task. Chronologically, **middle age** *covers the years of approximately 45 to 65 and even 70 or 75, but each person will also consider the physiologic age condition of the body and psychological age*—how old he or she acts and feels (17, 135, 148). Point of view alters definition: a child or a young adult of 20 may think age 45 is old. The 45-year-old may consider himself or herself young. Many people today consider themselves young until age 50 and middle-aged until 70 years or later. About half of the U.S. population defines itself as middle-aged until 75 years (17, 95, 135, 148). Middle age in the United States is increasingly a state of mind (115). However, definitions of and expectations for middle age vary with the cultural group, especially if the person is a recent immigrant (7). There are also gender differences (73). Females in the United States tend to think of themselves as middle-aged sooner than do males (16, 73). Age assignment varies according to social class. The person living in poverty perceives the prime or midpoint of life to vary from the late 20s to 40.

Culture, ethnicity, lifestyle, genetics, and illness also affect age assignment and reactions to the changing appearance that denotes life in the middle. Images portrayed in the media and literature also affect personal and societal reactions and age assignment; they change over time (135, 144). As more people lead healthier lifestyles and medical discoveries slow aging effects and increase life expectancy, the boundaries of middle age are being pushed upward, especially because of the increasing productivity and achievement being demonstrated.

Some couples in this age bracket may actually be middle-aged chronologically but be pursuing the developmental tasks of young adulthood that are described in Chapters 6 and 9∞. If the couple first has children or the person remarries and has stepchildren in the 40s, the couple will have teenagers in their late 50s or early 60s. They may have less time for middle-aged tasks and may want to retire when their children need college money and are still living at home.

An increasing number of Americans are considered middle-aged. They earn most of the money, pay a major portion of the bills and most of the taxes, and make many of the decisions. Thus, the power in government, politics, education, religion, science, business, industry, and communication is wielded not by the young or the old, but by the middle-aged.

Middle age is a time of relatively good physical and mental health, new personal freedom, and maximum command of self and influence over the social environment. At work the person has increasing potential and ability to make decisions, hold high-status positions, and earn a maximum income. The person has expanding family networks and social roles, and married life for postparental couples can be as harmonious and satisfying as the early married years.

A middle-ager has the ability to see personal strengths and limits and to accept, with a sense of humor, those normal changes that are part of development. For the female, middle age and the postmenopause is a time of health and zest, a "second adulthood" (156). That also applies to middle-aged males (157).

THE BABY BOOMER GENERATION

The **Baby Boomer cohort** *is the largest generation in U.S. history*—76 to 80 million middle-agers. This group has been referred to as *Boomers, Zoomers, active adults, lifelong experimenters, aging hipsters,* and the *Me Generation* (3, 70, 79, 80, 112). The group as a whole do not want to be called Boomers, at least not by marketing ads (75). This generation consider themselves young (younger than they are), deny aging effects, and practice a distinct value system and experimental lifestyle. They grew up in unparalleled affluence, opportunity for education, and social mobility—all of which fostered individual path-seeking and attitudes of "doing things my way," and "I want it all and I want it now" (2, 46, 82).

This population cohort has generally been characterized as self-centered or narcissistic (6), highly self-confident, expecting immediate gratification of every need and wish. They are sensuous, highly verbal and expressive, and defiant against tradition and parental values. They "want it all": meaningful work, lots of time for pleasure and play, and happy, close-knit families. They expect products to be made especially for them, their convenience, and unique tastes. In turn, they have taught these values and attitudes to their children, known as the "Mini-Me Generation" (3, 46, 79, 80, 82, 112).

This cohort of people does not wish to identify themselves with anyone who is old. They plan to work past the traditional retirement age of 65 to 70 years of age. They may be forcibly retired early from their workplace. If so, they begin a second career, start their own business, work out of the home, or return to college to prepare for a career change. They may enter professions or jobs that offer less pay but are perceived as meaningful to themselves and society (3, 82, 98, 112, 114, 148).

Despite their years of self-gratification, this generation expresses an underlying desire to be useful. Members of the upper economic levels are philanthropic, donating money and time to worthwhile causes and community service organizations. The wealthy enter politics, seeking ways to make worthwhile societal contributions—a mix of idealism and self-centeredness. They are confounded by their comfort and real-world challenges, such as racial conflict, worldwide poverty and disease, and war. Some members of this group may be involved in corruption at all levels of management and society in the United States (3, 46, 148); others demonstrate integrity and generativity. The leaders in this cohort have been the role models for the young, whether positive or negative (46, 98).

This generational cohort has been highly visible as described and presented in the media. Yet there are millions of middle-agers who do *not* fit the Baby Boomer characterization and do *not* live those values or lifestyle. *There is as much uniqueness in this as in any generation.* This age cohort represents all socioeconomic levels, social and ethnic groups, and geographic and religious backgrounds. *Some deliberately follow a lifestyle to refute the "Baby Boomer" image.* They have life values, circumstances, experiences, and norms that do not allow self-absorption and immediate gratification. Many are ordinary citizens of middle or lower economic levels, working at jobs necessary to our society, even if in prior years they considered them boring. They do not seek societal recognition. Some suffer from poor health. Some have died early. Their idea of perfect and continuing health was not realized.

Health care providers must understand the media portrayal of this generation and also the unique individuals. Life expectancy, statistically, for the current 60-year-old is 82.3 years. Yet 30% of this generation are obese, which statistically shortens life. This cohort "reinvents" itself every 5 years. They want to be on the cutting edge of everything, and they want to be fashionably young. Thus, eyeglasses and walkers may be necessary, but they will have to appeal to the person's idea of youth and beauty (3). Illness and accidental injury occur to individuals; the body image changes and life crises will have to be treated psychologically as well as physically (3, 70, 112).

Work with the denial about illness and developmental changes, such as decline in vision, hearing, or strength, and gradually decreasing organ reserves. This cohort is well educated; present research-based information. Teach about *effective use* of the Internet to find *accurate* health-related information. Reinforce health promotion practices, and educate about necessary lifestyle changes. Explore inevitable aging changes, and reinforce positive aspects of continuing maturity. Validate concerns about the caregiver role to elder parents and share information from that section of this chapter. Recognize personal achievements and strengths, reinforce realistic ideas about future planning, and make recommendations when ideas are unrealistic about self-care, future plans, or individual pursuits.

Family Development and Relationships

GENERATIONAL DIFFERENCES AND RELATIONSHIPS WITH CHILDREN

The **generation gap**, the *distance between adolescent and adult generations in values, behaviors, and knowledge, marked by a mutual lack of understanding,* is not necessarily wide but may have always existed to some degree (16, 96, 129). The experience of the parent generation, and therefore their values and expectations, differs from that of their offspring. **Table 15-1**, Assessment of Generational Differences, summarizes generational differences in values and motivations of several generations (36, 90, 158, 190, 197). In some ways, the generational lines are blurring. Some presently middle-aged adults, perhaps out of fear of their own mortality, are looking and acting more like their children. These adults would rather think of themselves as carefree, innocent, and young. The changing attitudes, values, behavior, and dress of middle-aged persons (the Baby Boomers) reflect our cultural emphasis on youth and beauty, versus tradition and wisdom, and our more informal society (3, 80, 148). Yet, each generation is concerned about the other, although for different reasons. In fact, the younger and older generations can successfully combine efforts to work for legislation, policy changes, or social justice.

There is a difference in values and lifestyle between the early and late middle-agers, as presented in **Table 15-1**. Refer to **Table 5-4**, Values of Dominant or Mainstream Culture in the United States, which contrasts traditional and current values of mainstream culture. See also **Table 5-5**, Comparison of Selected African American Values and Dominant Cultural Values in the United States. ∞ In contrast to the Baby Boomers, the late middle-aged adult was born sometime in the early 1940s. Values and behavior have been influenced by growing up with inadequate material resources after the Great Depression and during World War II and by the rapid social and technologic changes that occurred during the late 1940s and the 50s and 60s. *The generation gap may be as much between early and late middle-agers as between middle-agers and their offspring.*

The nuclear family is no longer as prominent in the United States, and we discount learning from elders. The offspring cannot be fully prepared for the future by the parent generation. They must develop new patterns of behavior based on the changing world, their own experience, and that of peers. The present affluence, emphasis on age differences and independence, and insistence on a unique lifestyle that is characteristic of today's younger people add to the value conflicts for late middle-agers and may be better understood by younger middle-aged persons. The addition of innate parental feelings of affection, admiration, and compassion for youth to the negative feelings produces an ambivalence (135, 148).

Social mobility, *in which the offspring moves away from the social position, educational level, economic class, occupation, or geographic area of parents,* causes offspring overtly to forsake parental teaching and seek new models of behavior. The mass media and societal trends help to set standards and expectations about behavior that may be counter to parental teaching or wishes. Rapid social changes and awareness that much about the future is unknown threaten established faiths and stimulate attraction to new ideologies and exceptional behavior. This is particularly difficult for immigrant and refugee families, both in relation to the social changes around them and their own children's social mobility.

Discuss with middle-aged persons what they as adults have to offer their children. They are the only generation to ever know, experience, and incorporate such rapid technologic and scientific changes into daily life and the job. They can give their offspring

TABLE 15-1

Assessment of Generational Differences

Generational Birth Years	Generational Name	Generational Values	Generational Motivations
Pre-1946	Traditionalists Silent Generation	Duty, tradition. Loyalty. Rise above enormous challenges by sublimating individual needs to greater good of society or family. Family. High achievement. Leadership. Fiscally conservative. Patriotic.	Satisfaction of job well done. Transition to change rather than abrupt changes. Recognition by others of the individual's talent, ability, and potential. Flexibility in job demands and schedules.
1946–1964	Boomers Baby Boomers Zoomers Active adults Me Generation	Individuality, self-absorption. Question authority, argumentative. Immediate gratification. Narcissistic. Youthful appearance and behavior. Competitive. Meaning in work and leisure. Conveniences in life/living. Contribute to causes; donate money and time based on ideals and self-centeredness. Protest societal issues. Can achieve anything; optimistic.	Whatever defies tradition in society or the workplace. Products made specifically for expressed desires and unique tastes. Challenge status quo. Fast changes. Balance in busy life; "more time off." Desire to be close to their children; offspring's positive response.
1965–1981	Generation X Mini-Me Generation	Independence. Entrepreneurial. Cynical or skeptical about others or situations. Achievement. Diversity. Pragmatism. "Being savvy."	Media of all types. Planning for education and careers. Education, especially via media. Innovative work culture. Recognition for ability, contribution. Accomplishments that pave way for future promotions, change.
1982–2001	Generation Y "Echo-boomers" Millennial Generation Millennials	Technology (dislike reading). Global awareness. Meaningful life; "make a difference." Progressive thinkers; eager to embrace change. Sense of entitlement; expect others to take care of things for them. Truth-telling. Authenticity. Integrity; trust. Autonomy. Family oriented, team oriented. Pluralistic—no distinctions of race, ethnicity, gender. Success; perceive self as always doing well. Accepting (not cynical). Religion. Community participation. Practical problem solving; realistic. Inclusion in decisions.	Digital products. Easily bored. Overlook differences (positive or negative); everyone treated the same. Realistic goals. Stable marriage, children. Close relationships with parents, families, older people. Avoid "glitzy" marketing. Trustworthy teachers and other adults. Not politically active. Lack of work experience; need orientation to rules and job; want flexible, individualized time schedule; need mentor. Have fun with work. Debriefing; time to talk about feelings, concerns, experiences. Feedback and suggestions.

imaginative, innovative, and dedicated adult care. Reaffirm that it is up to the parents to teach *how to learn and the value of commitment*. Explain to parents that the continuity of values from generation to generation typically exists within a family. This is true in American society as well as in other societies.

Educate middle-aged parents to reduce conflict with their offspring through several intentional strategies:

1. Emphasize listening and open communication. Suggestions have been presented in previous chapters.
2. Encourage support of each other, and foster ability to rely on each other. Help youth realize parents do rely on them and vice versa.
3. Foster connectedness between the generations through shared activities, yet allowing independence as the youth matures.
4. Avoid excessive control or fostering undue dependency, such as doing school homework, college applications, or chauffeuring. Explore with parents how they encourage or limit autonomy, gradual independence, a sense of responsibility, and identity formation in offspring.
5. Explore differences between monitoring, being a "guiding hand," and asserting control over and making decisions for the offspring. The goal is to guide, to be a consultant, not to control or live the offspring's life for them.
6. Educate offspring how they can assume more adult responsibility rather than being too dependent on parents.

Encourage the middle-aged parent to exchange information and ideas honestly and with a sense of humor. As parent and offspring learn together to cope with the future, the parent assists youth to reach responsible, independent adulthood without a false maturity or alienation. The adult cannot abdicate the role of parent. If the parent works to maintain open communication, the generation gap can be minimal. Your work with families can promote greater harmony and health.

Divorce in Offspring

An increasing concern for middle-aged parents is lifestyle options of their offspring. Cohabitation may lead to marriage; divorce following these marriages is common. Divorce after marriage is common in the United States, usually within the first 10 years. Divorce is discussed in Chapters 6 and 14. ∞ The parents may feel shock (or relief if they did not like the child's spouse). The stages of crisis and related grief described in Chapter 2 that accompany divorce and loss of a family member are keenly felt. ∞ They may believe that their effort and help in getting the child "out of the nest" through marriage or helping the couple set up a home were to no avail. This feeling may be especially strong if the divorced family member decides to live at the parents' home again. The parents may blame their child or the in-laws and may criticize the couple for not working on the marital problems as the middle-aged parents have done (16, 80, 135, 148).

If younger children are still at home, their needs and desires may be temporarily neglected because the emphasis is on the divorce crisis. The younger children may have to give back a room to the returning divorced brother or sister. The parents, in an attempt to make the divorced family member feel comfortable, may negate their own new patterns of freedom. If the divorced son or daughter is in a financial crisis, the parents' money may also go to help him or her instead of being used as originally planned. If the divorcing couple has children, additional strain will be felt.

Return of Young Adult Offspring to the Parental Home

Young adults may return home to live with parents for reasons other than separation or divorce. Some new college graduates cannot find a job of their choice or are finding that their first jobs are not paying enough for them to cover high rents along with other costs of living. Thus, they live with their parents until they can accumulate some money or can move to higher-income jobs. Some young adult children return home more than once until they finally become independent.

This may cause stress, as most middle-aged parents look forward to having children leave the home—the so-called empty nest (16, 127, 135, 148). The middle-aged adult wants space, time, and financial resources to pursue personal, organizational, and civic goals rather than to continue child care responsibilities. Freedom to frolic, to invigorate the marriage with renewed closeness, and to share activities is achieved in ways that reflect the individual personalities and the culture (16). Prolonged dependence of young adult offspring may also create conflict with grandparents and other children who are still at home.

The Grandparent Role

The grandparent role has a different dimension in middle age than in later adulthood, although people become grandparents during the middle-aged era, or even in late-young adulthood. The middle-aged person is not necessarily happy about being a grandparent, because that may indicate old age.

If the offspring has established his or her own home and has a family, grandparenthood is a happy status and role. The relationship to the grandchild is informal and playful. The child is a source of fun, leisure activity, and self-indulgence. Emphasis is on mutual satisfaction. Authority lines are irrelevant, and the child is seen as someone for whom to buy gifts.

Younger grandmothers, especially, face major stressors (30): (a) adjustment to the caregiver role, possibly with young children while caring for the parental generation and their own children; (b) financial stress; (c) lack of living space to accommodate the children and their toys and belongings; (d) role restriction; and (e) special problems with discipline and child rearing. If the adult offspring is divorced and brings young grandchildren into the middle-aged adult's home or if the offspring is unmarried and has children, the sense of responsibility and loss of independence are heightened. The middle-aged female, especially, may resent the demands and constraints placed on her by having young children, including grandchildren, in the home full-time. The carefree relationship is less likely if the grandchild lives in the home with the middle-aged person. Further, having extra children and grandchildren in the home interferes with the spousal relationship. It is difficult to meet the usual developmental tasks. The return of children to the home and the resultant demands may also serve to prevent the female from pursuing new career goals.

In the case of divorce, the middle-aged grandparents wonder about their future relationship with their grandchildren. Relations may be strained between the in-laws as each family wonders how to interact with the other. Recent cordiality and affection may turn to anger and criticism. There are instances of grandparents seeking legal custody of the grandchildren because of their concern about the apparent lack of parenting and about the other set of grandparents. A growing number of grandparents are raising their grandchildren because their offspring are dead, divorced, or incapacitated from drugs or another devastating problem. Middle-aged parents may be threatened emotionally or have social or financial problems because of their children's separation or divorce.

Use principles of crisis intervention and principles of communication (review Chapter 2). ∞ Caution middle-aged parents to proceed carefully with financial assistance. Few young adults pay back family loans. The middle-aged grandparents may also need encouragement in securing visitation rights when divorce or death has severed the relationship. Help the middle-aged couple regain a sense of confidence in setting limits so that they can pursue their own life goals and a method of working through decisions and problems with the young adult offspring.

RELATIONSHIP WITH SPOUSE
Positive Marital Adjustment

Predictors of a successful, long-term marriage include (a) similar identity perceptions and styles (26), (b) congruence of perceptions between spouses of the marriage and each other, and (c) sexual satisfaction (16, 148). Equally important as rearing the children and establishing wholesome affectional ties with them, and later with the grandchildren, is the middle-aged adult's relationship with the spouse. There tends to be a gradual rise in marital happiness during middle adulthood (16, 135, 148, 176). Romantic love is less strong; affectionate or companionate love is stronger. Physical attraction, romance, and passion are more important in new and young adult relationships (148). Security, loyalty, and mutual emotional interests are more important in mature relationships (148). Couples stay together because they have built up **marital capital**, *emotional, social, and financial benefits of marriage that are difficult to give up* (135, 143, 148).

A happy marriage has security and stability, although there are also struggles. The couple knows each other well; they no longer have to pretend with each other. Children can be a source of pleasure rather than concern. Each partner knows that the way of life and well-being depends on the other. Each has become accustomed to the behavior of the other. There is increased shared activity, including household chores. The sexual relationship can be better than ever before. Middle-aged adults are likely to have roots firmly planted in the community of choice. Warm friendships are likely with members of their own generation and with parents, the family of the spouse, and families of married children. Marriage can be secure economically; the middle-aged working wife contributes. The median income annually is often above the national average. Nationally, many working women are middle-aged (16, 36, 135, 143, 148, 176).

Although there has been much discussion in the literature about the crisis of menopause and the "empty nest," menopause and middle age usually bring both men and women an enriched sense of self and enhanced capacity to cope with life. It may be a transition in that behavioral changes are necessary but not a crisis in the negative sense of incapacitation. It may be like a second honeymoon. However, the empty nest may be felt more by single parents.

The years before retirement are anticipated as promising. Responsibility for the children is over; adultlike peer relationships are sought with the children. Parents realize that if they have done their job as parents, the children should be ready to leave the nest. Their independence is what parenting is about. The emotionally close relationship between husband and wife is culturally defined and thus varies from group to group. For example, in the Latino culture (7), wives develop more intense relationships with their children or other relatives than with their husbands. Latino males form close bonds with siblings or friends—ties that meet needs for companionship, support, and caring that might otherwise be expected from the wife (7). In the U.S. mainstream culture, females are more likely than males to have self-disclosing friendships. In the Middle East, males express friendship to each other with words and embraces (which would be attributed to homosexuality in the United States) and may be less affectionately expressive with the spouse (7).

Sexuality in the Relationship

Females may equate ability to bear children with capacity to enjoy sexual relationships, although they have nothing to do with each other. She needs the male's support to reinforce her femininity. The middle-aged male is also undergoing a crisis. He believes that he is losing his vigor and virility, which are products primarily of psychological reactions rather than physiologic inabilities. In the 50s, there may be a reduction of male potency triggered by fears of impotence and feelings of inability to satisfy his partner, who may be sexually more active after menopause. He may equate success on the job with success as a husband and believe that he is losing both. He may covet his son's potency and youth.

The middle-ager is an active sexual being. Physical changes in appearance and energy and the multiple stresses of daily living may result in an increased desire for physical intimacy and the need for reassurance of continuing sexual attractiveness and competency. Intercourse is not valued for procreation but for body contact, to express love and trust, and to reaffirm an integral part of the self-concept. The person may fear loss of potency and rejection by the partner, but talking with the spouse about feelings and preferences related to sexual activity can promote increased closeness.

Males and females differ in their sexual desire and behavior. Males reach their peak in their late teens and young adulthood. Females peak in desire in the late 30s or 40s and maintain that level of desire and activity past the menopause into late middle age, and beyond. The enjoyment of sexual relations in younger years, rather than the frequency, is a key factor for maintenance of desire and activity in females, whereas frequency of relations and enjoyment are important factors for males (16, 36, 67, 107, 135, 148).

Disenchantment in any or all areas of life, with lack of enthusiasm for self and each other and for their physical relationship, may threaten the sexual relationship and marriage in the middle years. Husband and wife are no longer distracted by daily activities of raising a family, and children are no longer present to act as buffers. There is increasing awareness of aging parents, aging friends, and signs of their own aging. Each may become preoccupied with the self and anxious about losing youthfulness, vitality, sex appeal, and the partner's love. Each needs the other but may hesitate to reach out and demonstrate affection or intimacy. The end result may be for one or the other to reach outside the marriage to prove youthfulness, masculinity, or femininity.

Negative Marital Relationship

Negative, critical feelings can gradually erode what was apparently a happy relationship. At some point the husband and wife may feel they are each living with a stranger, although the potential still exists for a harmonious marriage. With everything seeming to go well for them, the middle-aged couple may now feel that the zest has gone out of their love life. Their relationship is changing because they are changing.

Marital crisis may result from (39, 135, 148):

1. Having little or no laughter with, love for, or interest in each other.
2. Experiencing increasing distance or coolness in the relationship.
3. Feeling disappointment with self, that life is empty.
4. Feeling depleted emotionally because of lack of communication with the spouse.
5. Seeking rebirth or changing directions.
6. Seeking escape from reality and superego pressures.

Often the couple overlook that they still do really love each other. They simply have to become reacquainted. It may be difficult to "tune in" to each other because both are encountering problems peculiar to their own gender. Divorce, separation, or cohabitation have generally been less common in middle adulthood, although they are becoming more common with the Baby Boomer generation. Divorce in this era has more impact than for marriages of shorter duration. Income is usually reduced for both the male and female. Family ties are weakened when long-term social support systems become more essential. Prior friendly relationships with in-laws are typically halted. Parent-child relationships may become more distant or conflicted. If young children are still at home, child care and custody can be issues. Relationships with the grandchildren, if any, can be curtailed, depending upon feelings of the adult offspring toward either parent (16, 85).

Some middle-agers are in a second or third marriage if they were divorced in young adulthood. If the couple divorce, the person initiating the divorce typically wants to escape an untenable situation. The partner being divorced feels betrayed (148). If the offspring are adults, they may be more able to cope with the parents' divorce, especially if they realize this had been a conflictual or abusive relationship and if the parents' resources are divided fairly between the two. If there are younger children in the home, the mother, now a single parent, may experience financial difficulty that affects the care of and opportunities for the children, even if she continues her job/career or initiates employment (40, 148).

The middle-ager is often more adaptable in the face of separation and divorce than is the young adult. The male is more likely than the female to remarry (16). The midlife female may have more friends and better social relationships, a greater sense of personal mastery, and less depression and hostility than the young

adult female who is divorced. After 5 years, she is likely to feel a greater sense of autonomy. The midlife divorced male is more self-accepting and less depressed and hostile than the young adult divorced male but demonstrates less personal development (135).

Remarriage after divorce can bring initial happiness—another honeymoon. Males become healthier and more sociable. Females become more financially secure. If a new baby is born to this unit, relationships with children from his or her prior marriages are likely to be strained. A child with the new spouse strengthens the second marriage and usually loosens remaining emotional bonds to the first marriage, and to offspring from that marriage. The second marriage is statistically likely to end in divorce. Children suffer each time a parent's marriage ends (16, 85).

Extramarital Relationship

Relationships with work colleagues and the feelings of marital crisis may set the stage for an extramarital affair. This tendency is increased when the younger woman finds the company of an older male more interesting than that of males in her own age group. Although divorce occurs during these years, the extramarital affair does not necessarily lead to the divorce courts. Divorce is major surgery, and the male may be reluctant to cut that much out of his life. Besides, he may find, having aroused the ardor of the younger female, that he is no match for her physical demands. With increased consciousness of his age, he may return to his wife, particularly if she has in the meantime assessed her own situation, remained committed, and changed behavior (3, 135, 148). Midlife crisis is discussed further in another section. The crisis may be physical as well as emotional, especially if the affair resulted in sexually transmitted disease.

Reducing Marital Stress

Counsel or educate the middle-aged adult who is having difficulty in relating to his or her spouse. Work with the couple or refer them to couple counseling. Share information from this chapter and from the section on midlife crisis to assist the couple. Validate that their effort to resolve issues is worthwhile. The mature years can be regarded as the payoff on an investment of many years together, many problems shared, and countless expressions of love exchanged. Encourage a willingness to change outlook, habits, and lovemaking, if necessary, to enhance their marriage. Explore ways to promote such changes.

Gay and Lesbian Relationships

Many homosexuals do not come out until well into young adulthood. Middle-aged gays and lesbians may be associating openly for the first time. Many are working out conflicts with their parents or families. Some continue to hide their homosexual relationships. The homosexual may live alone even though in a committed relationship (135).

Gay males who do not come out until middle age often go through a long search for identity, with feelings of guilt and secrecy. They may have been in a heterosexual relationship and fathered children. The males who earlier accepted their sexual orientation often cross racial, socioeconomic, and age barriers within the gay community. Some move to cities with large gay populations in order to more easily find a relationship (135).

INTERVENTIONS FOR HEALTH PROMOTION

The following *guidelines for couples may help them reduce stress and maintain health in the marriage:*

1. Talk daily to each other about feelings so that small problems are solved continually, rather than allowing emotional tensions to accumulate, creating a breaking-point scene.
2. Explore with each other feelings and ideas about possible, even if unlikely, life events that may occur—"what if" conversations. Such anticipatory problem solving helps the couple expand the repertoire of ideas and behavior so that if unexpected events occur, each will have more adaptive resources.
3. Vary schedules and chores, family goals or expectations, and roles and rules, or make other periodic changes, just to stay comfortable with change and to be prepared to adapt if a crisis requiring flexibility occurs.
4. Use each other as a resource. Talk to each other about individual problems, validate solutions, or ask each other

about options for dealing with problems. Each must be willing to disclose about self to the other and be willing to support and help the other.
5. Maintain contact with others, including the extended family, who can help during a crisis. Sometimes the family does not exist or cannot be supportive. Seek friends or other resources, such as a church or a support group.
6. In times of high stress or crisis, each should express the feelings of anger, grief, or helplessness to the other and to others who are caring. Expressing feelings about the circumstance, not about the spouse, allows conflict to surface and be handled.
7. Keep active with each other and with others, which prevents feelings of either stagnation during routine times or helplessness during stressful times.

Principles that apply to sustaining a heterosexual relationship apply to sustaining gay and lesbian partnerships. When family and friends are supportive, the partner relationship quality tends to be higher than if there is lack of validation and support by family. If both partners are relationship oriented, they tend to be happy and can balance demands of work or career and the partnership. Friends are important and may be more supportive than family (135).

Be supportive to the gay or lesbian couple. Explore how they can strengthen their own relationship as well as relationships with family members or friends. Refer them to faith communities that are inclusive, such as the United Church of Christ and similar denominations, that in turn will foster friendships. Validate their advocacy efforts. Present an accepting, welcoming attitude in the health care setting.

INTIMATE PARTNER VIOLENCE OR ABUSE

Physical, verbal, emotional, or economic abuse, if present during the young adult years of marriage or committed relationship, may persist. Information presented in Chapter 14 about the abusive relationship is relevant. ∞ The abused female may feel trapped for economic or social reasons, or by a desire to keep a home together for the children. When the last child leaves home, she may initially believe the spousal relationship will improve. If the abusive partner remains or becomes more abusive, the other may consider options for leaving, especially if a support system—family, friends, agency for abused women—is available. The employed female may also feel more empowered and make plans to safely leave the relationship. **Divorce may be pursued. The female is at great risk during this process.**

Use listening and counseling principles discussed earlier. Interventions presented in Chapter 14 are relevant. ∞ Refer the abused person to community resources, as appropriate.

DEATH OF SPOUSE OR LONG-TERM PARTNER

Widowhood or widowerhood, the *status change that results from death of the husband or wife,* or of a long-term gay or lesbian partner, is a major crisis in any life era, but it is more likely to occur first in middle age. There are about four times as many widows as widowers. Females generally take better care of their health, so they live longer: 2 years in Kenya, 6 years in the United States, and 12 years in Russia (16). In the United States, the husband is usually about 3 years older than the wife, so wives average about 10 years of widowhood (16).

The death may be sudden due to an accident, follow a relatively short but acute illness, or occur after a longer period of illness and one or more hospitalizations. Sudden death and acute grief can be very difficult. Prolonged illness and hospitalizations allow for anticipatory grieving, described in Chapter 17. ∞ During hospital or home care of the ill partner, the person who is about to become a widow or widower usually appreciates being able to participate in care of the spouse. However, emphasize that the ill partner will not suffer lack of care or support if a few hours are taken for personal rest (153).

In the health care setting, listen to feelings of anger, sadness, and guilt. You may be better able to listen, support, and encourage than family or friends. Gently test reactions to determine if he or she is ready for the shock of death by offering to call a member of the clergy or by asking if family members need to be prepared for decline in the spouse's condition. If the person appears brave and strong, accept the veneer of courage if that is holding the person together. Realize the person may feel much ambivalence—not wanting the partner to suffer pain and yet wanting him or her to be alert and to talk, or praying that death will relieve suffering and yet hoping for survival. After death the person may linger on the nursing unit—a place of support—rather than leaving for home, a very empty place. Remain available and supportive.

The person's reaction to death of a spouse depends on personality and emotional makeup, the relationship between the couple (how long they have been married, how long the mate has been ill), and religious, cultural, and ethnic background. It is also determined by other factors that existed in the relationship; for example, there may be less sorrow, or even relief, if the dead spouse was abusive, or severely or chronically disabled, either physically or mentally.

The *death of a spouse may mean many things* (4, 16, 97, 135, 148–150, 154, 186, 189):

1. Loss of a sexual partner and lover, friend, companion, caretaker.
2. Loss of an audience for unguarded spontaneous conversation and expressing sense of humor.
3. Loss of a "handy man," helper, housekeeper, accountant, plumber, or gardener, depending on the roles performed by the mate.
4. Financial problems, especially for the widow.
5. Secondary losses involving reduced income, which frequently means change in residence, environment, lifestyle, leisure, and social involvements.
6. Return to the workforce, especially for the widow if previously not employed outside the home.
7. Giving up any number of things, such as activities, traditions, or gifts, previously taken for granted.
8. Continuing loneliness and fear of the future.

Widowhood is a threat to self-concept and sense of wholeness; now the person is seen as "only one." The role of spouse is gone, even if the marriage was not a happy one. The woman's identity may be so tied to that of her husband that she feels completely lost, alone, and indecisive and a nonperson after his death. If the person has no one else close with whom to talk or from whom to receive help, he or she may become suicidal. The widow or widower misses having someone with whom to share both happy occasions and sad news and problems. He or she can dial a crisis line to talk about a problem; it may be more difficult to tell about a source of happiness. The emotional burden is increased if there are still children in the home to raise. The remaining parent has a hard time helping them work through their grief because of personal mourning. Friendship patterns and relations with in-laws also often change.

The *widow* is a threat to females with husbands; they perceive her as competition, and she is a reminder of what they might experience. With friends the widow is the odd person in number, so social engagements become stressful and are a constant reminder of the lost partner. The widow also becomes aware that she is regarded as a sexual object to males who may offer her their sexual services at a time when she has decreased sexual desires but a great need for companionship and closeness. Yet in contrast to assumptions, most widows are quite competent in managing their lives (16, 135, 148).

Although the *widower* is more accepted socially, he too will have painful gaps in his life. If the wife concentrated on keeping an orderly house, cooking regular and nutritious meals, and keeping his wardrobe in order, he may suddenly realize that what he had taken for granted is gone. Even more significant is the loss if his wife was a "sounding board" or confidante in business matters and if she was actively involved in raising children still in the home.

The bereavement of widowhood affects physical health; somatic complaints related to anxiety are not unusual. The person may experience symptoms similar to those of the deceased spouse (16, 148). The symptoms of acute grief and the mourning process, which are a part of the crisis of loss, are discussed in Chapter 2, and Tables 2-7 and 2-8. ∞

Widowers are more vulnerable to depression than widows, possibly because males are less likely to have formed close friendships with a number of people. Because of the ratio of widowers to widows, males are more likely to remarry or to have female companionship. Mortality rates, based on risk factors, are approximately the same for widowed and married females, but significantly higher for widowed than married males. Mortality rates among widowed males who remarry are lower than among those who do not remarry. Physical health of the survivor is often jeopardized because of immune, neurologic, and endocrine system response to the caregiving responsibilities and grief. Grief and loneliness are risks for poor nutrition, sleep disorders, overuse of prescription or over-the-counter drugs, and alcohol consumption. Death, including from suicide, is more likely to occur during the first year of widowhood, especially in late middle age (16, 135, 148–150).

Tasks for the widow or widower following death of a spouse or long-term partner are to (148):

1. Recognize the reality of the loss.
2. Express feelings about the loss.
3. Find significant methods to manage emotional pain.
4. Incorporate prior relationships that included the deceased.
5. Sustain or reestablish supportive relationships with others.
6. Maintain or develop a positive self-image.
7. Maintain or reestablish physical and mental health.

In one study, widows reported supportive and nonsupportive experiences. *Widows reported that supportive behavior from others include* (150):

1. Listening to the widow's feelings and stories.
2. Avoiding judgmental statements about the widow's behavior.
3. Avoiding shallow or unwanted advice or control of the conversation.
4. Doing practical tasks, such as delivering meals, or helping with shopping, lawn, or household tasks or child care.
5. Continuing to ask what additional help is needed in order to give specific assistance, such as help with financial concerns.
6. Expressing feelings of loss through empathic statements, holding or hugging the person, sharing tears, and demonstrating caring and emotional closeness.

Nurses and other professionals who gave explanations about what was happening during the terminal illness and who also gave thorough, high-quality care were described appreciatively.

Nonsupportive behaviors from others include (150):

1. Avoiding mention of the spouse, as if death never happened.
2. Distancing, not continuing a social life with the survivor, even though there had been a close friendship or work relationship (a way to avoid facing personal mortality).
3. Acting fearful around the person, as if she would "steal" the woman's husband, or as if the disease that caused the husband's death may be contagious and others may become ill also.
4. Receiving hurtful, irritating, or insensitive comments, or the tone of voice or timing of comments being inappropriate.
5. Being told choices, related to the husband's prior care or the funeral or memorial service plans, were poorly made or inadequate.
6. Being neglected by own or spouse's family, or others relating to the children but not the widow or mother.

Your contact with the widow (or widower) can help to resolve the crisis. *Assist the person in the following ways to promote crisis resolution:*

1. Express your empathy; validate the person's feelings.
2. Encourage the bereaved to talk about feelings, and help the person to find a supportive relationship.
3. Build up the widow's confidence and self-esteem, especially if she had lived a protected life.
4. Help her (or him) identify people other than the children who can assist in a practical way with various tasks to avoid feelings of burden in any helper.
5. Encourage getting a medical checkup and following healthful practices in response to physical complaints. Educate about the somatic aspects of grief and mourning.
6. Encourage her (or him) to try new experiences, expand interests, join community groups, do volunteer work, and seek new friends. Now is a good time for the person to pursue activities formerly not done because the mate did not enjoy them.
7. Encourage the person to utilize various resources, such as books for the person resolving grief or specific for the widow or widower. Browsing through the local library or bookstore can be a reason to get out of the home, briefly interact with others, use leisure time, or meet a friend. The book or video can also be a source of useful messages.
8. Refer the person to community agencies that offer services and friendships. Refer to Chapter 17 for information about resources. ∞
9. Explore spiritual, religious, or cultural resources—the belief system, being a member of a faith community, and traditions or rituals that help resolve grief, mourning, and bereavement. Refer to Chapters 7 and 17 for information. ∞
10. Emphasize the importance of taking time to grieve and to seek help from supportive others.

You may want to offer group crisis intervention or a support group through a local community agency, church, or school. Many of the problems that confront the widow or widower also confront the divorced person. Your intervention principles will be similar, although the words will be different.

RELATIONSHIP WITH AGING PARENTS AND RELATIVES

Because people are living longer, parents in later maturity and their adult offspring may expect more than 50 years of overlap. There is an increase in the number and duration of intergenerational linkages. The middle-aged person is the **"sandwich generation,"** *in the middle in many ways, including in the middle of two demanding generations.* Although child care responsibilities may be decreasing, considerable care of or involvement with offspring may remain at the same time there is increasing care of, involvement with, and responsibility for aging parents, aunts, uncles, siblings, or grandparents. The adult daughter and elderly mother may have remained in a close relationship through the years. If so, that daughter is likely to become more involved in that parent's life as the years pass. The friendship and interdependency of the younger years develop into a relationship with an increasingly dependent mother. The middle-aged female may be in additional close relationships with elderly relatives more than the middle-aged male or son. Culture and ethnicity influence the relationship with parents, siblings, other relatives, and ultimately the caregiver role (7, 16, 191).

Caregiving refers to *the prolonged assistance given to meet the physical and emotional needs of a person with functional limitations or incapacity with or without payment toward 24-hour care.* The caregiver may be family or nonfamily (outside) help. The care receiver may be living alone in his or her own home, with a spouse, or with the caregiver. The **primary caregiver** *usually is a relative and has the most responsibility.* The **secondary caregiver** is *less involved (even if a relative) and offers support or gives assistance to the primary caregiver.* Sometimes assistance is indirect, such as shopping, transportation, and other home tasks. The **informal caregiver** and **family caregiver** *are family members, friends, and neighbors who provide care, either primary or secondary caregivers, full-time or part-time* (178).

The literature about middle-aged caregiving focuses on the caregiving to parents. However, sometimes the middle-aged adult is the caregiver for the grandparents or other elderly relatives, a disabled or chronically ill spouse, and the child (e.g., when the adult offspring has a chronic illness or an injury causing permanent loss of some function). More frequently, the middle-ager is carrying out several caregiving roles simultaneously. Hainsworth et al. (64) discuss the chronic sorrow that wives experience when they care for a chronically mentally ill husband. Chronic sorrow may be felt by the other caregivers also (37).

Responsibility for Elderly Relatives

Cultural trends affect the dilemma of caring for older dependent relatives (7, 16, 52, 135, 191):

1. Long-term societal emphasis on personal independence and social mobility of middle-aged and young adults creates physical separateness of generational households and new kinship patterns of intimacy at a distance.
2. Dynamics of the marriage bond and socialization of young children, with the emphasis on affection, compatibility, and personal growth of each person in the nuclear family, are considered the most important aspects of family life.

3. Longer life spans of older people and the problem of caring for the older generations when they become dependent add to concerns of elders and middle-agers.

Filial responsibility is an *attitude of personal responsibility toward the parents that emphasizes duty, protection, care, and financial support,* which are indicators of the family's traditional protective function (109). Middle-class Caucasian culture in the United States believes that good relationships between the aged and their adult children depend on the autonomy of the parents, which interferes with satisfactory role reversal between generations. Yet, older persons do assist their children and younger family members in many ways and as long as possible. However, they are likely to expect children to assume responsibilities when they can no longer maintain their independence (104).

Families provide nurturance and companionship through:

1. Visits and telephone calls.
2. Providing information.
3. Assistance in decision making.
4. Assistance with shopping, laundry, household chores, and transportation.
5. Immediate response to crisis.
6. Being a buffer against bureaucracies.
7. Help in searching out services.
8. Facilitation for continuity of individual–bureaucracy relations.

In many ethnic or racial cultures, structure and style for the younger generations have evolved through an extended family system to provide support, assistance, protection, and mobility. Often inadequate family economic reserves and inadequate health insurance necessitate the middle-aged adult having to be the caregiver (7, 16, 52, 135).

Middle-aged children of various racial and ethnic groups are more likely than Caucasians to provide a home for elderly parents or other relatives. There are some differences within groups. For example, elderly Japanese are more likely to live with a spouse or alone than occurs with other Asian groups. Elderly Southeast Asians are more likely to live with family members (7).

Many families have four or five generations. The young middle-aged person may have parents, grandparents, and great-grandparents. Further, elderly siblings, aunts, uncles, or cousins may also be living and need and expect help from the middle-aged adult. The person who is in his or her 40s, 50s, or early 60s may be seen as possessing energy, free time, and money. Older relatives become more demanding just when the middle-aged adult believes he or she deserves time for self, a vacation, and an opportunity to pursue additional education or a social cause. The additional stress occurs when the older relatives want their needs met right now. They can create considerable guilt and frustration in middle-aged adults.

Certainly the older and middle-aged generations can give a great deal to each other. Older generations can share insights and wisdom about life. Sometimes they can give assistance financially or with various tasks. The older generation can be a source of joy, pride, and inspiration. If they live long enough, however, the middle-aged adult will have someone who is increasingly dependent and in need of help. Many people in the Baby Boomer generation have not yet accepted this possibility (5, 46). Sometimes the middle-aged adult realizes the dependence and need for help before the elderly person is ready to admit the need, and that can become a source of frustration and stress.

Caregiver Role

Care of a parent is a normative but challenging, even stressful, experience. However, most people willingly help the parent and derive satisfaction from doing so. Various *factors that influence the caregiving role* include (4, 5, 7, 70, 139, 140, 171):

1. Cultural and ethnic background.
2. Seriousness of the elder's health status.
3. The caregiver–care recipient relationship and living arrangement.
4. Duration of the caregiving experience.
5. Other roles and responsibilities of the caregiver.
6. Overall coping effectiveness of the caregiver.
7. Caregiver sex and age.
8. Number of generations needing care.
9. Help and support from others—family, employer, or social agencies.
10. Information needed to carry out tasks related to physical care of the parent.

Meeting parents' or other elders' dependency needs may have many adverse effects (16, 47, 109, 135, 140, 151, 162, 171, 178, 191):

1. Financial hardship, including effects on current wages and pension or retirement benefits from the workplace.
2. Physical symptoms such as sleeplessness and decline in physical health, especially in the primary caregiver.
3. Emotional changes and symptoms in the caregiver and other family members, including frustration, inadequacy, anxiety, helplessness, depression, guilt, resentment, lowered morale, and emotional distance.
4. Emotional exhaustion related to restrictions on time and freedom and increasing responsibility.
5. A sense of isolation from social activities.
6. Conflict because of competing demands, with diversion from care of other family members.
7. Difficulty in setting priorities.
8. Reduced family privacy.
9. Inability to project future plans.
10. Sense of losing control over life events.
11. Interference with job responsibilities through late arrival, absenteeism, or early departure needed to take care of emergencies or even routine tasks.
12. Interference with lifestyle and social and recreational activities.

Thus the whole family and its relationships are affected.

The dilemma of care for elderly parents, siblings, or other relatives inevitably has an emotional impact. The caregiver role is a major one, especially for the female. The middle-ager who is the older daughter is most likely to do the caregiving, which is seen as a female role. Care of the dependent parent is only one phase of the caregiving role or career. The female often is caring for many people and several generations simultaneously, either in her own home or in their homes. Interestingly, females who work outside the home provide as much caregiving as those who do not. Unemployed daughters provide more tangible help, but employed daughters contribute in other ways (135, 178, 200). Some may reduce their working hours; others quit their jobs, especially if the aged parent lives with them. For some, adult day care services may be available to use while the daughter is at work, as described in Chapter 16. ∞ Parent care makes the wife feel tied down and competes for time with the husband. Relations between husband and wife are affected because of financial or other help one person may give to an elderly parent, especially when done without consulting the other spouse. The needs of elderly parents may cause discord among their sons and daughters by recalling childhood rivalries and jealousies. The middle-aged person often resents those siblings who will not help care for the elderly parents or other relatives. Further, if the middle-aged adult believes he or she was not well cared for by the parents as a child, continued resentment, anger, or hate may inhibit a nurturing attitude or even minimum assistance.

The meaning of caring for the dependent parent is different from caring for the dependent child. The child's future holds promise for reducing dependency needs; the older parent will have increasing dependency needs. Parent care also fosters reflection about the final separation from the parent and of one's potential dependence on one's own children. The way filial care is negotiated depends on the past and has implications for the future when the adult child is old.

Sometimes the adult child continues to care for the parent beyond physical and psychological means to do so, rather than to use formal support systems. *Various dynamics are at work:* (a) symbiotic ties, (b) gratification from being the burden bearer, (c) a fruitless search for parental approval that has never been received, and (d) expiation of guilt for having been a favorite child.

Some cultural, ethnic, or religious groups promote the caregiver role because of a value or belief system, or a sense of responsibility (52). African American caregivers rely on religious beliefs to help them cope with the stress of caregiving. The belief in and intense daily relationship with God provides support during the time of a relative's illness or death. Close extended family and spiritual ties within the African American family and community and belief in the power of prayer support the caregivers. Females are the main caregivers in the African American family (7, 139, 200).

The middle-aged adult may perceive caregiving as an acceptable permanent, full-time role that is altruistic and enhances self-esteem. Because this role gives meaning, a job or other roles may be discontinued, or this role may be a substitute for a failed marriage or for being widowed. Thus, successful resolution of this crisis may be acceptance of what cannot be done, as well as of what can and should be done. Refer to **Box 15-1**, Danger Signals Indicating Caregiver Needs Assistance, for information pertinent to client education. For elders, successful adaptation to dependence includes accepting what adult children cannot do (16, 109, 135, 139, 153, 162, 178, 200).

A kind of psychological distancing between parents and their caregiving children may occur. The adult children may feel little affection for the parent, feeling rather a kind of grief, and may hesitate to cancel the caregiving burden out of a sense of respect and

---

BOX 15-1 | **Danger Signals Indicating Caregiver Needs Assistance**

1. Your relative's condition is worsening despite your best efforts.
2. No matter what you do, it is not enough.
3. You believe you are the only person in the world enduring this.
4. You no longer have any time or place to be alone for even a brief respite.
5. Things you used to do occasionally to help are now part of your daily routine.
6. Family relationships are breaking down because of the caregiving pressures.
7. Your caregiving duties are interfering with your work and social life to an unacceptable degree.
8. You are going on in a "no-win situation" just to avoid admitting difficulty.
9. You realize you are alone and doing all the work because you have shut out everyone who offered to help.
10. You refuse to think of yourself because "that would be selfish" (even though you are unselfish 99% of the time).
11. Your coping methods have become destructive; you are overeating or undereating, abusing drugs or alcohol, or being harsh or abrasive with your relative.
12. There are no more happy times; loving and caring have given way to exhaustion and resentment and you no longer feel good about yourself or take pride in what you are doing.

---

loyalty to the parent. The adult child, often a married daughter, may not feel enough gratification from the caregiving to offset the sense of burden, yet the cultural expectation of closeness and love for family members leads her to pursue the role. The person may question whether she can care for the parent if she does not feel love and may be concerned about the cost of caregiving to personal emotional stability (152, 162, 171).

Some of the impatience, aggravation, and desire to see less of the older person comes from the middle-aged adult's dawning realization that the older person is a picture of what the middle-aged person may become. The person who is in the prime of life may fear greatly the physical disabilities, illness, personality eccentricities, intellectual impairments, or social changes that old age may bring.

One of the most difficult decisions when parents become aged and dependent concerns the housing arrangement. The older daughter is usually the one to take the dependent parent into her home. Or the unmarried adult child may move into the parent's home. When one or both of the parents cannot manage living alone, the middle-aged person may not have the room to take the parent into his or her home. Even if there is adequate space, if all members of the household are working, finding someone to stay during the day may be difficult, although such an arrangement or the use of adult day care may be less cost prohibitive than placing the parent who is in poor health in a care facility. Most communities do not have adequate, or any, day care facilities for elderly adults. Placing the parent in an institution may be the only answer, but it is typically considered the last resort. Refer to Chapter 16 for more information on what to consider in housing alternatives. ∞

Counsel the middle-aged adult to work through the conflicts, feelings of frustration, guilt, and anger about the increased responsibility and past conflicts or old hurts from parents or siblings. Commend the family as the main provider of health and social services. Validate that caregiving is strenuous. Discuss with the middle-aged adult ways to gain a sense of satisfaction from the help given. Promote greater understanding of the person being helped. Negative feelings that exist between the middle-aged adult and elderly person can be overcome with effort: love, realistic expectations, a sense of forgiveness, and the realization that sometimes it is all right to say "no" to the demands of the elders.

Educate about physiologic, emotional, cognitive, and social needs, changes, and characteristics of the elder care recipient, utilizing information from Chapter 16. ∞ Teach the caregiver stress management, utilizing information from Chapter 2. ∞ Share information about time management techniques described in Chapter 14 that may reduce the sense of burden. ∞ Encourage participation in a support group. Encourage the caregiver to maintain other roles outside of caregiving and family roles. A change of scene and pace may increase the sense of caregiver well-being and health. Refer to a counselor or spiritual leader as necessary. Counseling can promote a resolution of feelings that in turn fosters a more harmonious relationship between the middle-aged adult and parents.

One way to help the adult child to continue the caregiving role, set aside guilt, and gain more positive feedback is to offer a **relabeled perspective**, that *being a good child means not feeling great affection but showing concern for the well-being of the parent and giving care to the limits of one's ability.* Helping the adult child internalize this perspective helps him or her begin to cope with the stresses without being overwhelmed. Thus, the parent can be cared for in the adult child's home and has the advantage of a home environment. Although some adult children are helped through this relabeling process, some ethnic or racial groups do not respond to this technique. For example, African Americans have maintained a kind of behavioral closeness between generations that produces a different pattern of attitudes and less social and emotional distance between middle-generation adults and their parents. Reinforce and validate their perspectives.

Outside resources can be used to support the adult child in the caregiving role. Often a little help will enable the person to make changes and use inner resources in a distressing situation. Have the caregiver keep a daily list of the care recipient's helping behaviors and of negative behaviors (not feelings). This can assist the caregiver to see the role and behavior in a realistic or positive light and to gain reinforcement from the caregiving, because almost always the helping behaviors outnumber the negative behaviors. Such a log can provide a base for talking with the middle-ager about the interaction with the parent and ways to resolve feelings and improve the interaction.

Advocate for caregivers. You may be the occupational nurse or physical therapist for the factory or business office site. You could organize lunchtime support groups for employee caregivers, offer individual counseling through employee assistance programs, or refer the employee to community resources that teach about or assist with elder care. Resources that are available to assist with elder care are described in Chapter 16, including the geriatric case manager. ∞ You may be the case manager to assist with long-distance caregiving, housing options, and financial issues. Refer the middle-ager to the American Association of Retired Persons (AARP) Website about caregiving, www.aarp.org.

DEATH OF PARENTS IN ADULTHOOD

A critical time for the adult is when both parents have died, regardless of whether the relationship between parents and offspring was harmonious or conflictual. The first death of a parent signals finiteness and mortality of the self, the other parent, and other loved ones. Memories of childhood experiences are recalled. The person may wish deeply, even though simultaneously realizing it is impossible, to be able to relive some of those childhood days with the parent, to undo naughty behavior, be a good child just once more, sit on the parent's lap and be cuddled one more time, return to relatively carefree days, and relive holidays. Further, more recent memories are recalled—the joys that were shared and the disharmonious times that are normal in any relationship but that are likely to engender guilt. There may be deep yearning to hold the parent one more time. Mourning may be done not only for the parent but for previously lost loved ones. Some mourning is in anticipation of future losses of the other parent, other beloved relatives and friends, and self. When the other parent dies, the adult is an orphan. Now he or she is no longer anyone's "little boy" or "little girl." The person may feel forlorn and alone, especially if there are few other relatives or friends. Sometimes there are no other living relatives and no sons so that the adult offspring represents the last of the family line or family name. The person may question who and what will be remembered and by whom. This is a time of spiritual and philosophic searching whether the adult child is alone, has siblings, or has other relatives.

If there was conflict between the adult offspring and parents to the point of one-sided or mutual hate and unforgiveness, grief feelings may be denied or repressed or may be especially guilt laden. Consequently, the mourning process is delayed and not resolved as effectively. There is a yearning that life experiences with the parents could have been better or different, a wish that harsh feelings could have been smoothed, and a sadness over what was never present more than a sadness over what has been lost. The adult survivor may fear that he or she in turn may have similarly parented children, if any, and anxiety may arise about how the third generation will feel when their parent dies. Will the scene and feelings be replayed? Can that be prevented? Certainly this can be a time for the adult to take stock, undo past wrongs with his or her children (and others), resolve old conflicts, and become motivated to move ahead into more harmonious relations with family members and others.

You may be a key person in helping the adult survivor or adult orphan relive, express, and sort out feelings; accept that any close relationship will not always go smoothly; and finally achieve a balance between happy, sad, and angry memories and feelings in regard to the parent who has died. Through such counseling, the person can mature to accept and like self and other significant persons better and to change behavior patterns so that future relationships are less thorny.

FAMILY DEVELOPMENTAL TASKS

The *following developmental tasks are to be accomplished by the middle-aged family in order to achieve health, happiness, harmony, and maturity* (34):

1. Maintain a pleasant and comfortable home.
2. Ensure security for later years, financially and emotionally.
3. Share household and other responsibilities, based on changing roles, interests, and abilities.
4. Maintain emotional and sexual intimacy as a couple or regain emotional stability if death or divorce occurs.
5. Maintain contact with grown children and their families.
6. Decrease attention on child care tasks and adapt to departure of the children.
7. Meet the needs of elderly parents or other relatives in such a way as to make life satisfactory for both the elderly and middle-aged generations.
8. Participate in community life beyond the family, recommitting energy once taken by child care.
9. Use competencies built in earlier stages to expand or deepen interests and social or community involvement.

As you care for the middle-aged client, work through the meaning of midlife changes and ways to cope with them to prevent or minimize negative effects. Incorporate a discussion of effects of illness upon achievement of developmental tasks when caring for the ill client.

Physiologic Concepts and Physical Characteristics

The growth cycle continues with physical changes in the middle years, and different body parts age at different rates. One day the person may suddenly become aware of being "old" or middle-aged. Not all people decline alike. How quickly they decline depends on the stresses and strains they have undergone and the health promotion measures that were maintained. If the person has always been active, he or she will continue with little slowdown. People from lower socioeconomic groups often show signs of aging earlier than people from more affluent socioeconomic groups because of their years of hard physical labor, poorer nutritional status, limited access to health care, and lack of money for beauty aids to cover the signs of aging.

Now the person looks in the mirror and sees changes that others may have noticed some time ago. Gray, thinning hair, wrinkles, coarsening features, decreased muscular tone, weight gain, varicosities, and capillary breakage may be the first signs of impending age.

HORMONAL CHANGES: FEMALE CLIMACTERIC

This is the era of life known as the *menopause* for the female or the *climacteric* for either gender. The terms are often used interchangeably. The **menopause** is *the permanent cessation of menstruation preceded by a gradually decreasing menstrual flow.* The term **perimenopausal years** denotes *a time of gradual diminution of ovarian function and a gradual change in endocrine status from before the menopause through one year after the menopause.* The **climacteric** is *the period in life when important physiologic changes occur, with the cessation of the female's reproductive ability and the period of lessening sexual activity in the male.* Basic to the changing physiology of the middle years is declining hormonal production (63, 135, 148, 198).

Contrary to the myths about the menopause described in **Table 15-2,** depression or other psychiatric symptomatology is neither inevitable nor clearly related to the perimenopausal or climacteric years (16, 17, 23, 36, 40, 86, 135, 148, 197). Most females feel relieved or neutral about menopause; only a small percentage view it negatively. Attitudes toward menopause improve as females move from before to after menopause. Perception of health becomes more positive as menopause proceeds. The worst part about the menopause or climacteric may be not knowing exactly what to expect about this *normal period of life.*

In the United States menopause is viewed in the mainstream culture as a biomedical or psychiatric event, but sociocultural and feminist views are also found in the literature. **Table 15-3** lists assumptions about menopause from the biomedical and sociocultural perspectives (16, 17, 36, 102, 126, 148, 196).

In the biomedical view, menopause is a cluster of symptoms or a syndrome. The ovarian failure, with a hormone deficiency, is the cause of various physical and psychological symptoms, such as hot flashes, vaginal atrophy, and depression. The syndrome can be treated by hormone replacement although recent studies suggest this should only be done on a short-term basis (10, 36, 87).

In the psychiatric view, the changes of menopause cause anxiety and depression, which can be treated with psychotropic medication (6). Females who think of menopause primarily in these terms may feel negatively about themselves during the climacteric period, because the emphasis is on the body's deficiency or loss. Thus traditional homemakers in the United States may experience greater difficulty with menopause because the reproductive role has passed (36, 197).

In societies in which females rise in status after menopause or generally enjoy high status regardless of reproductive stage, a menopausal syndrome is nonexistent (7, 52). Perception of the menopause experience is largely based on perceptions of the physical, social, and psychological changes she undergoes (40, 88, 102, 148).

The sociocultural view has emerged over several decades in reaction to the biomedical and psychiatric view, in response to the feminist movement, and especially in response to greater understanding of females from various cultures in the United States or of females in other societies. In the sociocultural view, menopause has little or no effect on the individual. Instead, role changes or

TABLE 15-2

Myths About the Menopause

Myth	Fact
1. Menopause is a deficiency disease and catastrophe.	1. Menopause is a normal developmental process.
2. Most women have serious disability during the menopause.	2. Most women pass through it with a minimum of distress. Some have no noticeable symptoms or reactions and simply stop menstruation.
3. Menopause is the end of life.	3. The average life expectancy for today's 50-year-old woman is 81 years; one third of her life is post-menopausal. Postmenopause is a time of new zest.
4. Menopausal women are more likely to be depressed than other people (older men are handsome, distinguished, and desirable; older women are worn out and useless).	4. Menopausal depression in middle age is likely to be caused by social stressors: a. The double standard of aging b. Caregiver demands c. Loss of loved ones d. Loss of roles e. Other health problems (the decreased level of estrogen affects neurotransmitters that regulate mood, appetite, sleep, and pain perception)
5. Numerous symptoms accompany the menopause.	5. Predictable manifestations of menopause are: a. Change in menstrual pattern b. Transient warm sensations or vasomotor instability (hot flashes) to some degree (47%–85% of women) c. Vaginal dryness in some women
6. Hot flashes are "in the woman's head."	6. Vasomotor instability results from hemodynamic compensatory mechanisms. Until the body adjusts to less estrogen, hypothalamic instability causes dips in the body's core temperature. The flash is the body's adaptive response to equalize peripheral and core temperatures through dermal heat loss.
7. The woman may have a heart attack during a hot flash.	7. The tachycardia that occurs during a flash is the body's adaptive response to skin temperature changes.
8. The woman loses sexual desire during and after the menopause.	8. Vaginal changes may cause some discomfort, which would reduce libido. Psychosocial concerns about the empty nest, partner's loss of sexual capacity, or expectation of loss of libido are more likely the cause than reduced estrogen.
9. The indicators of the menopause are the various symptoms women experience.	9. Women may have regular menstrual cycles with decreased estrogen levels; hot flashes may occur before the menopause begins.
10. Only women have to worry about osteoporosis.	10. By age 70, osteoporosis risk is equal in men and women.

cultural attitudes toward aging are identified as the cause of any discomforts (36, 102, 197).

In the feminist view, menopause has been a taboo subject, veiled in secrecy and myths, in which rights of females are suppressed in the name of biology. This view has become marginal, but in the late 1970s and early 1980s, feminists were the force behind initiation of research about the perimenopausal years and the menopause event (102).

The sociocultural view explains the difference between an estimated 2 million females in the United States with severe menopausal symptoms, and the absence of incapacitation during the menopause in females in other cultures. In other cultures, there is a role beyond the menopause (7, 16, 41, 52). In the United States, most females and males, and a growing number of researchers, also see that there are life roles beyond the menopause (7, 52, 102, 156).

Menopause

The average age for onset of menopause is 51 or 52 years (10, 45, 195, 198). The range may be from 45 to 55 years, although it may occur as early as age 35 in approximately 1% of females (10, 36,

TABLE 15-3

Biomedical vs. Sociocultural Assumptions About Menopause

Biomedical

1. Science, which is objective and precise, provides the true knowledge about a condition.
2. Women are products of their reproductive systems and hormones.
3. Women's behavior is caused by their biology and hormones.
4. Menopause can be studied as biomedical variables, treatments, and outcomes.
5. Menopause is a disease that causes psychological distress, and outcome of the handicap of menstruation.
6. Women are considered medically old and socially useless when menopause occurs.
7. Norms of the male are the baseline for considering norms for the woman.
8. Menopause can be treated as a disease of decreased hormones.
9. Treatment will restore the woman to the premenopausal, and desirable, state.

Sociocultural

1. Science is an important model for research, but view of women is less negative than in the biomedical model.
2. The world, and therefore womankind, is dynamic and cannot be fully understood from experimental studies.
3. Social and cultural variables are basic to understanding people, their behavior, and reactions to their bodies.
4. Attitudes, relationships, roles, and interactions are important variables in understanding people.
5. Positions of women and societal conditions contribute to women's reactions to the menopause.
6. The meaning of an event is critical to the person's reaction to the event.
7. There is no consistent relationship between the biochemical or physiologic processes and the person's perception of an event or behavior.
8. *Menopause is a natural developmental phase, not a disease process,* based on changes in the endocrine system.
9. *Menopause is a part of natural life transitions,* and views include cultural ideas about life and nature.

135, 148). The process of aging causes changed secretion of follicle-stimulating hormone (FSH), which brings about progressive and irreversible changes in the ovaries, leading to the menopause and loss of childbearing ability. The primordial follicles, which contain the ovum and grow into vesicular follicles with each menstrual cycle, become depleted, and their ability to mature declines. Finally, ovulation ceases because all ova have either degenerated or been released. Thus, the cyclic production of proges-

terone and estrogen fails to occur and levels rapidly fall below the amount necessary to induce endometrial bleeding. (The adrenal glands continue to produce some estrogen.) The menstrual cycle becomes irregular; periods of heavy bleeding may alternate with amenorrhea for 1 or 2 years, eventually ceasing altogether (45, 63). Consistent or regular excessive bleeding may be a sign of pathology, not of the approaching menopause.

The pituitary continues to produce FSH and luteinizing hormone (LH), but the aging ovary is incapable of responding to its stimulation. With the pituitary no longer under the normal cyclic or feedback influence of ovarian hormones, it becomes more active, producing excessive gonadotropins, especially FSH. Increased FSH acts as a vasodilator. A disturbed endocrine balance influences some of the symptoms of menopause. Progesterone affects moods; it binds to the neurotransmitter gamma-aminobutyric acid (GABA). Reduced progesterone contributes to mood changes and depression. Although the ovaries are producing less estrogen and progesterone, the adrenals may continue to produce some hormones, thus helping to maintain younger feminine characteristics for some time (63).

During the perimenopausal period (approximately 5 years), some discomforts may occur in a small percentage of females, the most common being vasomotor and urogenital changes. Vasomotor changes cause hot flashes associated with chilly sensations, dizziness, headaches, perspiration, palpitations, water retention, nausea, muscle cramps, fatigability, insomnia, and paresthesia of fingers and toes. Hot flashes have been reliably associated with cigarette smoking, but their relationship to other factors, such as surgically induced menopause, physical activity, and alcohol consumption, has been inconsistent. Urogenital changes include dryness and discomfort in the vagina (81). Many symptoms, including irritability, depression, emotional lability, and palpitations, are frequently attributed to menopause but are not as commonly associated (98). Some females may experience a first episode of depression during the menopausal transition due to fluctuating estradiol levels (23, 49). Most females experience no symptoms, only a decrease, then cessation, of menses. The great majority of females experience no effect in their sexual relationships from the menopause. Most find menopause a time of integration, balance, liberation, confidence, and action (135, 148, 156).

Difficulties experienced during menopause may be associated with concurrent life change or recent loss, or marital, psychological, or social stress. The cause of the symptoms apparently is more complex than simple estrogen deficit. Psychological factors such as anger, anxiety, and excitement are considered as important in precipitating hot flashes in susceptible females as conditions giving rise to excess heat production or retention, such as a warm environment, muscular work, and hot food. However, the symptoms may arise without any clear psychological or heat-stimulating mechanism (10, 36, 156, 195, 198).

HORMONAL CHANGES: MALE CLIMACTERIC

This comes in the 50s or early 60s, although the symptoms may not be as pronounced as in the female climacteric. Sheehy describes the **"MANopause,"** *a 5- to 12-year period during which males go through hormonal fluctuations and physical and psychological changes*

(157). Other authors also describe the male menopause (36, 43, 67, 74, 135, 148) and andropause (15).

A male's "change of life" may be passed almost imperceptibly, but he usually notices it when he makes comparisons with past feelings and performance. A few males may even complain of hot flashes, sweating, chills, dizziness, headaches, and heart palpitations. Unlike females, however, males do not lose their reproductive ability, although the likelihood diminishes as age advances. The output of sex hormones of the gonads does not stop; it is merely reduced about 1% a year (9, 43, 63, 67). Testosterone level usually is lower in the middle-aged man who has high stress, lowered self-esteem, and depression. Testosterone therapy should be used cautiously because administration may increase libido, muscle mass, and strength, but also increase the risk for prostatic hypertrophy and cancer, and diabetes (9, 99, 172, 195, 196). Medications to treat erectile dysfunction are not the entire answer either (122, 135, 146, 172, 180, 187). The physical and emotional changes may be indicative of other health problems, such as diabetes and heart disease (183). Thorough health assessment is advised.

In addition, the male may be dissatisfied at work, which adds to the sense of midlife crisis. Other losses in this period, including death of loved ones, will add to the sense of crisis and aging. The Baby Boomer generation has, overall, a denial of inevitable aging changes (2, 65, 82, 112).

Interventions offered for erectile dysfunction progress from those that are least to most invasive. Healthy lifestyle changes, such as quitting smoking, losing weight, and increasing exercise, are the first-line recommendations for this condition. The next step is to identify drugs that may have this side effect (e.g., blood pressure medications) and find alternatives. Various psychotherapies and behavior modification techniques may be appropriate for some men whose impotence is tied to stress, body image, self-esteem, or relationship issues. Lastly, medications such as Viagra (sildenafil citrate), Levitra (vardenafil HCl) or Cialis (tadalafil), locally injected drugs, vacuum, or surgically implanted devices may be recommended (122, 180).

PHYSICAL CHANGES

Table 15-4 summarizes physical changes that occur in middle age, physiologic reasons for the changes, and characteristics that are commonly seen. Implications for health promotion and client teaching are summarized (16, 17, 36, 45, 63, 116, 135, 148, 198).

Utilize knowledge from **Table 15-4** to educate the middle-ager about normal physiology and the changes that occur over several decades. Help the person focus on strengths rather than be overwhelmed by the societal youth orientation in the United States.

HORMONE REPLACEMENT THERAPY

The benefits of hormone replacement therapy (HRT), as well as the side effects or drawbacks, have been widely discussed and continue to be studied. Until 2002, HRT had been standard therapy in the United States for managing menopausal symptoms. It relieved unpleasant symptoms, such as hot flashes and vaginal dryness, and also appeared to protect against postmenopausal conditions such as osteoporosis and heart disease. However, in 2002, the Women's Health Initiative (WHI), a large, multisite clinical trial,

posed that HRT caused more health risks than offered benefits (24). Consequently, health care providers began to seriously reconsider HRT as routine treatment. The number of HRT prescriptions sharply declined from 26.5 million in 2001 to 16.9 million in 2003 (110, 159).

The most alarming results occurred with the combination estrogen-progestin therapy. This combination was found to increase heart disease, breast cancer, stroke, blood clots, and dementia. Mammography abnormalities also increased, resulting in an increased number of false-positive results due to the increased breast tissue density caused by estrogen. Combination therapy did not seem to improve quality of life measures, such as sleep, emotional health, general health, physical functioning, or sexual satisfaction (24, 110, 159).

For females taking estrogen-alone therapy, the WHI found no increased incidence of breast cancer or heart disease as with combination therapy, but did find a slightly increased risk of stroke. Estrogen-alone therapy increased false-positive results on mammograms due to increased breast tissue density. Typical adverse reactions for any type of estrogen therapy were uterine bleeding and breast tenderness. However, the WHI found that some former HRT claims remained valid, irrespective of type of therapy. For example, females on HRT showed a decreased risk of osteoporosis-related hip fractures and colorectal cancer (24, 110, 159).

The WHI did show some critical limitations (24). The average age of participants was 63 at the beginning of the study. This may indicate that results were biased toward older postmenopausal women more likely to be in poorer health, especially those having preexisting cardiovascular disease. This bias raises questions about generalizing the findings to younger females, particularly those who start estrogen early in menopause. The study suggests there is less risk of heart disease if estrogen is taken early in the postmenopausal period (142). Participants age 50 to 59 who took estrogen experienced fewer heart attacks and deaths from coronary heart disease than those on placebo. Results from the Nurses Health Study also support that HRT does not increase cardiovascular risk unless it has already been established (24, 142). To answer such questions about HRT in early postmenopause, the Kronos Early Estrogen Prevention Study (KEEPS) and the Early Versus Late Intervention Trial with Estradiol (ELITE) have been started, but results will not be available for several years (57, 61, 110, 123, 159).

Despite the warning posed by these studies, HRT remains the treatment of choice for symptoms such as hot flashes, night sweats, and vaginal discomfort (including dryness, itching, burning, and discomfort with intercourse) (159). HRT should be considered for osteoporosis prevention only after other medications have been tried (109, 110). Therapeutic trials are conclusive only for estrogen because this therapy is the one most frequently studied. Other medications may prove effective given further research (57, 61, 88, 110, 123, 159).

For females already taking HRT, it is important to consider benefits versus risks and whether the reasons for originally taking the therapy are still valid. For example, hot flashes decrease within 3 to 5 months within 30% to 50% of females and resolve in 85% to 90% within 4 to 5 years. Females should thus be evaluated every 6 months to a year to see if they still require medication. Lowering

TABLE 15-4

Physical Changes and Characteristics of Middle Age and Health Promotion Implications

Body System or Physical Parameter	Change/Characteristic	Implications for Health Promotion
Endocrine and Reproductive Systems		
Women	Decline in production of neurotransmitters that stimulate hypothalamus to signal pituitary to release sex hormones	Reproductive cycle is ended; this may represent sexual liberation or loss of femininity.
	Less estrogen synthesized	Counsel about meaning of femininity.
	No estrogen produced by ovaries; menses stops	Support group may be helpful.
	Aging oocytes (eggs) destroy necessary genetic material for reproduction	Instruct in Kegel exercises.
	Uterine changes make implantation of blastocyte unlikely	Hormone replacement therapy may be prescribed.
	Gradual atrophy of tissues:	Artificial (water-soluble) lubrication can be used during intercourse to reduce discomfort.
	Uterus and cervix become smaller	Regular sexual intercourse maintains lubrication and elasticity of tissue.
	Vulvar epithelium thins	
	Labia majora and minora flatten	
	Vaginal mucosal lining thinner, drier, pale (20%–40% women; some never experience this)	
	Natural lubrication during intercourse decreases	
	Neuroendocrine symptoms, such as hot flashes and night sweats followed by chilling, fatigue, nausea, dizziness, headache, palpitations, and paresthesias may occur.	Avoid precipitating factors such as hot drinks, caffeine, alcohol, stress, and warm environment.
Men	Testosterone production gradually decreases, which eventually causes:	Counsel to stop smoking.
	Degeneration of cells in tubules	Sperm production continues to death, so man is capable of producing children.
	Production of fewer sperm	Premature ejaculation is less likely, which may contribute to more enjoyable intercourse.
	More time needed to achieve erection	Practice Kegel exercises for firmer erections.
	Less forceful ejaculation	
	Testes less firm and smaller	
Basal Metabolism Rate (BMR)		
Minimum energy used in resting state	BMR declines 2% per decade	If eating pattern is maintained, 3 to 4 pounds are gained per decade.
	Gradually reduces as ratio of lean body mass to adipose tissue decreases (metabolic needs of fat are less than for lean tissue)	Fewer calories (2%) need to be consumed, even if the person exercises regularly, to avoid weight gain.
Weight	Gain should not occur; weight gain occurs if as many calories consumed as earlier: wider hips, thicker thighs, larger waist, more abdominal mass	Overweight contributes to a number of health problems: crash diets should be avoided.
Integumentary System		
Sebaceous oil glands	Produce less sebum secretions, skin drier and cracks more easily	Protect and lubricate skin with lotion or moisturizer.
	More pronounced in women after menopause than in men of same age	Avoid excess soap and drying substances on skin. Avoid excessive strong sun and wind exposure.
Sweat glands	Decrease in size, number, and function	Ability to maintain even body temperature is affected; dress in layers to maintain comfort.

continued

TABLE 15-4

Physical Changes and Characteristics of Middle Age and Health Promotion Implications—continued

Body System or Physical Parameter	Change/Characteristic	Implications for Health Promotion
Skin	Skin wrinkles, tissue sags, and pouches under eyes form because: Epidermis flattens and thins with age, collagen in dermis becomes more fibrous, less gellike Elastin loses elasticity, causing loss of skin turgor Loss of muscle tone causes sagging jowls	Wrinkles are less apparent with use of moisturizer or lotion. Wrinkled appearance of skin is made worse by excess exposure to sun or sunburn; use sunscreen. Skin is more prone to injury; healing is slower. Use humidifier in home.
Women	Estrogen decrease gradually causes skin and mucous membranes to lose thickness and fluids; skin and mucous membranes thinner, drier, and begin atrophy Estrogen decrease gradually causes breasts to sag and flatten	Avoid burns and bruises. Use lotions. Maintain support with correctly fitted brassiere. Maintain erect posture.
Hair	Progressive loss of melanin from hair bulb causes gray hair in most adults by age 50; hair thins and growth slows; hair rest and growth cycles change	Slow hair loss by gentle brushing, avoiding excess heat from hair dryer, and avoiding chemical treatment.
Women	Estrogen decrease may gradually cause increased growth of facial hair Hair loss not as pronounced as in male	Accept change. Manage cosmetically.
Men	Testosterone decrease causes gradual loss of hair Hereditary male-pattern baldness occurs with receding hairline and monk's spot area on back of head	Accept change. Manage with styling, hairpiece, or hair transplant.
Muscular System	Slight decrease in number of muscle fibers; about 10% loss in muscle size from ages 30 to 60 Gradual loss of lean body mass Muscle tissue gradually replaced by adipose unless exercise is maintained Most loss of muscle occurs in back and legs Grip strength decreases with age Gradual increase in subcutaneous fat	Physical exercise and fitness, proper nutrition, and healthy lifestyle can improve or sustain muscle strength during middle age. Variations in peak muscular activity depend on type of exercise.
Skeletal System	Gradual flattening of intervertebral disks and loss of height of individual vertebrae cause compression of spinal column	Maintain erect posture. Maintain adequate calcium intake (1,000–1,200 mg daily). Exercise maintains bone mass and joint flexibility, improves balance and agility, and reduces fatigue. Loss of height occurs in later life.
Men and women	At age 70, osteoporosis risk equal in men and women unless vitamin D has been taken to increase bone density	Vitamin D decreases risk of fractures.

TABLE 15-4

Physical Changes and Characteristics of Middle Age and Health Promotion Implications—continued

Body System or Physical Parameter	Change/Characteristic	Implications for Health Promotion
Women	Estrogen reduction increases decalcification of bones, bone resorption, decreased bone density, and gradual osteoporosis Cultural differences: Caucasians and Asians more likely than Latinos and African Americans to suffer bone porosity because their bones are less dense and they lose mass more quickly	Maintain exercise and calcium intake. Maintain erect posture. Maintain calcium and good nutrition intake. Teach safety factors; forearms, hips, and spinal vertebrae are most vulnerable to fractures. Supplemental vitamin D and regular small amounts of exposure to sunlight improve calcium absorption. Avoid smoking, high alcohol intake, and high caffeine intake, all of which interfere with nutrition. Caffeine causes calcium loss. Women may eventually be 3 in. shorter if they have vertebral osteoporosis. Dowager's hump will form in cervical and upper thoracic area if osteoporosis occurs. Women who have taken oral contraceptives for 6 or more years have higher bone density in lumbar spine and femoral neck.
Neurologic System		
	Speed of nerve conduction, nerve impulse traveling from brain to muscle fiber, decreases 5% by age 50, and only 10% through life cycle Brain structural changes minimal; gradual loss of neurons does not affect cognition	Sensation to heat and cold and speed of reflexes may be impaired. Teach safety factors. Functional abilities are maintained, and learning from life experiences enhances functional abilities.
Vision	Average 60-year-old requires twice the illumination of 20-year-old to do close work Eyes begin to gradually change at about 40 or 50, causing **presbyopia** (farsightedness) Lens less elastic, loses accommodation Cornea increases in curvature and thickness, loses luster Iris responds less well to light changes; pupils smaller Retina begins to lose rods and cones Optic nerve fibers begin to decrease	Wear brimmed hat and sunglasses that block UV rays to protect vision. Person eventually needs bifocals or trifocals to see small print or focus on near objects. Eyes do not adapt as quickly to darkness, bright lights, or glare (implications for safety and night driving). More light is needed to see well.
Hearing	Auditory nerve and bones of inner ear gradually change Gradual decrease in ability to detect certain tones and certain consonants Loss of hearing from high-pitched sounds	Reduce exposure to loud work machinery or equipment; wear ear protectors. Reduce exposure to loud stereo, radio, or electronic music. Cross-cultural studies show our high-tech culture contributes to increasing and earlier impairment. Hearing aids, correctly chosen, or surgery may correct hearing impairment.

continued

TABLE 15-4

Physical Changes and Characteristics of Middle Age and Health Promotion Implications—continued

Body System or Physical Parameter	Change/Characteristic	Implications for Health Promotion
Voice		
Women	Estrogen decrease gradually causes lower pitch of voice	
Men	Testosterone decrease gradually causes higher pitch of voice	
Cardiovascular System		
	Efficiency of heart may drop 80% between 30 and 50	Regular aerobic exercise maintains heart function and normal blood pressure.
	Decreased elasticity in muscles in heart and blood vessels	Inactivity affects system negatively.
	Decreased cardiac output	Quit smoking.
	Cardiovascular disease risk for women equal to that of men by age 70 because reduced estrogen causes lipid changes, increase in low-density lipoproteins (LDLs), decrease in high-density lipoproteins (HDLs), and gradual increase in total serum cholesterol.	Maintain healthy diet. Take regular low doses of aspirin. Maintain low-cholesterol diet.
Respiratory System		
	Gradual loss of lung elasticity	Regular exercise enhances respiratory efficiency.
	Thorax shortens	Inactivity affects system negatively.
	Chest cage stiffer	
	Breathing capacity reduced to 75%	
	Chest wall muscles gradually lose strength, reducing respiratory efficiency	
Urinary System		
Women	Glomerular filtration rate gradually decreases	Maintain adequate fluid intake; drink 8 glasses of water daily.
	Loss of bladder muscle tone and atrophy of supporting ligaments and tissue in late middle age causes urgent urination, possibly cystocele, rectocele, and uterine prolapse.	Instruct in Kegel exercises as follows: Draw in perivaginal muscles (pubococcygeus muscle) and anal sphincter as if to control urination, without contracting abdominal, buttock, or inner thigh muscles. Maintain contraction for 10 seconds. Follow with 10 seconds of relaxation. Perform exercises 30–80 times daily.
Men	Hypertrophy of prostate begins in late middle age; enlarging prostate around urethra causes frequent urination, dribbling, and nocturia	Urinary stasis may predispose to infections. Drink adequate amount of water. Surgery may be necessary.

the dose of estrogen and decreasing the duration of use may decrease risks. For isolated vaginal symptoms, administering estrogen in a vaginal cream, tablet, or ring may decrease risks since the estrogen remains localized and does not circulate throughout the body (61, 110, 123).

HRT should not be used (123) (a) if there is a history of breast cancer or blood clots, or (b) as a preventative measure of memory loss, heart attacks, or strokes. Other medications or lifestyle modifications can prevent these conditions. For women with breast cancer, consider the use of medications such as clonidine, venflaxafine, and megestrol, which are associated with significantly decreased hot flashes. Vitamin E, black cohosh, isoflavones (soy), magnets, and the antidepressant fluoxetine appear to have no statistical effect. Results for nonvasomotor symptoms are mixed (123).

Menopausal symptoms may also be managed by (33, 35, 61, 110, 123):

1. Increasing physical activity and exercise.
2. Eating a low-fat, high-fiber diet, and keeping blood sugar, cholesterol, and triglyceride levels within healthy limits.
3. Smoking cessation and limiting alcohol intake.
4. Maintaining normal weight and blood pressure.

Prevention of osteoporosis in both males and females includes ensuring adequate intake of calcium and vitamin D, exercise (39, 41), and nonhormonal medications called bisphosphonates, such as alendronate (Fosamax) and risedronate (Actonel) (61, 110, 123).

Educate the female on HRT about all aspects of the treatment. Monitor regularly to determine dosage adjustment. If exogenous estrogen is given, schedule serial mammograms and annual gynecologic examinations. Assess for bleeding. (Estrogen alone or unopposed estrogen is usually prescribed only for females who have had hysterectomies.) How long HRT must be continued to maintain benefits is unknown. Explain that when HRT is withdrawn, symptoms of menopause reappear. Later reduced bone density may occur if other treatment is not given.

Schedule females who are receiving estrogen replacement therapy because ovaries were surgically removed or to relieve menopausal symptoms every 6 to 12 months for a Papanicolaou (Pap) test, breast examination, and blood pressure reading. Blood and liver function tests should be done. Teach all menopausal females that any abnormal bleeding (if receiving estrogen-progestin therapy) or spotting 12 months after cessation of menses indicates an increased risk of carcinoma and should be reported immediately to a physician.

Reinforce in the midlife female that hormonal changes are normal and to ignore commonly presented myths. Emphasize that she ask questions and be aware of the possibility of false-positive mammogram results in order to query the validity of findings.

Various therapies can be effective to reduce or cope with symptoms, such as regular exercise and massage. Demonstrate relaxation and meditation methods. Teach about use of biofeedback as described in Chapter 14. ∞ Other complementary and alternative methods are presented with Websites in Chapter 2, Table 2-9. ∞

You may organize or lead a support group for females in midlife related to discussion about physical changes and individual reactions or concerns. Refer them to Websites such as the North American Menopause Society (www.menopause.org) and the Agency for Healthcare Research and Policy (www.ahrp.gov) for educational materials. Information about the Kronos Early Estrogen Prevention Study is available at 866-878-1221 www.keepstudy.org.

EMOTIONAL CHANGES RELATED TO PHYSICAL CHANGES

Varying levels of estrogen and progesterone across the menstrual cycle appear to affect mood, vulnerability to addictive drugs, and sensitivity to pain. Motivated behavior, through alterations in the brain's reward system (amygdala, orbitofrontal cortex, striatum, and midbrain), may also be affected by menstruation (36, 63, 195). Depression, irritability, and a change in sexual desire may oc-

cur in response to physical changes and their meaning, but they do not automatically occur. Some females fear loss of sexual identity. Earlier personality patterns and attitudes are more responsible for the symptoms than the cessation of glandular activity. Previous low self-esteem and life satisfaction are likely to contribute to difficulties with menopause. Reactions to menopause are consistent with reactions to other life changes, including other reproductive turning points such as puberty. Females with high motherliness scores and heavy investment in childbearing react more severely to the menopause (136, 156, 195).

Reactions to menopause vary across social classes and according to the availability of alternative roles. Females in the middle and upper economic levels appear to find the cessation of childbearing more liberating than females of lower economic levels. Perhaps more alternatives are open to the more affluent. Younger females anticipating menopause express the most concern. Postmenopausal females, in contrast to those who are premenopausal, take a more positive view, agreeing that the menopause creates no major discontinuity in life. Except for the underlying biological changes, women have a relative degree of control over their symptoms and need not inevitably have difficulties. In general, menopausal status is not associated consistently with measurable anxiety in any group (151, 155, 156).

Females in middle age from working- and middle-class backgrounds who are in good physical health, are married, and have at least one child consistently indicate that menopause is a normal life event rather than a threat to feminine identity (16, 87, 126, 195). They regard it as unlikely to cause much anxiety or stress. Some believe health improves after menopause; 65% believe there is no effect on sex life. Any change in sexual activity during the climacteric period is seen as a function of the couple's attitudes. Sexual relations are reported by 50% as more enjoyable because menstruation and fear of pregnancy are removed. Few report having symptoms sufficient to seek medical treatment, although 75% report minor discomforts. A majority believe change in health or emotional status during the menopause reflects individual differences in coping with stress or idiosyncratic factors. In general, 80% attribute little or no change in their lives to menopause. Most believe they have control over the symptoms and need not have symptomatic difficulties (16, 87, 126, 135, 148, 195). Those responses contrast with the current medicalization of menopause in the United States.

Females in various cultures experience menopause differently. A study of Japanese, American, and Canadian females revealed that Japanese females experience menopause differently than Western females. Fewer than 10% reported hot flashes and they reported little or no physical or psychological discomfort. This was substantiated by physician survey. There is no Japanese term for "hot flash" although their language makes many subtle distinctions about body states. In Japan, menopause is regarded as a normal life event, not a medical condition requiring treatment, in contrast to beliefs in the United States and Canada. Hot flashes are rare among Mayan and Indonesian females, North African females in Israel, and Navajo Indian females (102, 135).

Cultural attitudes affect interpretations of menopausal physical sensations and menopause as a life event. Childbearing and nutritional practices may influence the experience of menopause.

MediaLink Menopause and Midlife Changes

Mayan females, who are almost constantly pregnant or breastfeeding, look forward to menopause as the end of a burden. Far Eastern diets (tofu, soybeans) have more phytoestrogens, an estrogen-like compound, which may lower premenopausal hormone levels. When natural estrogen levels fall, the phytoestrogens may act like estrogen in inhibiting menopausal symptoms. Further, Japanese females, the longest-lived females in the world, have a lower incidence of osteoporosis than Caucasian females in the United States, despite their lower average bone mass. They are also about 25% as likely as females in the United States to die of coronary heart disease and breast cancer. Besides phytoestrogens in the diet, Japanese females eat well-balanced diets, exercise throughout life, and seldom smoke or drink (7, 33, 35, 52, 102, 115, 135).

There are minimal cross-cultural studies of the male climacteric. Male ratings of their physical health, in contrast to female ratings, have a greater influence on their perception of physical decline. Females tend to focus more on psychological considerations (146). The African American male apparently experiences a midlife crisis much like that of the Caucasian male. Bachelors and widowers who may be lonely and lack the warmth of family ties frequently suffer at least temporary loss of libido in the middle years (4). Some males may experience again a long dormant homosexual interest (74).

NUTRITIONAL NEEDS

Basal metabolic rate (BMR) *gradually* decreases every decade after age 20. For each decade after age 25, there should be a reduction in caloric intake proportionate to activity level and to decreasing BMR (33). The reduced basal energy requirements caused by losses in functioning protoplasm and frequently reduced physical activity combine to create less demand for calories. Refer to the MyPyramid Website mypyramid.gov for client education about calorie calculation and nutritional recommendations.

Protein intake daily should be 0.8 g/kg of body weight and contribute 10% to 20% of total calories. At least two servings of fish should be eaten weekly (33).

Intake of *carbohydrate* and *foods with trans fat, high fat, saturated fat, and cholesterol content should be reduced.* A low-saturated fat (use of plant oils and canola oil), low-cholesterol diet may decrease low-density lipoprotein (LDL or bad cholesterol) by 15% to 20%. Man-made trans fat should be avoided because it decreases high-density lipoprotein (HDL or good cholesterol) and increases LDL. *Monounsaturated fats* should constitute about 20% of calorie intake (33, 35). It is recommended to broil or bake rather than fry foods and cook with monounsaturated fats (164). Foods with "empty" calories, such as rich desserts, candies, fatty foods, gravies, sauces, and alcoholic and nondiet cola beverages, should be reduced or avoided. Substitute sparkling waters or reduced-calorie wines or beers; half of any previous intake of alcoholic beverage is desirable. Intake of salty food should be limited; herbs, spices, and lemon juice can be used for flavoring. Overweight is not just a genetic factor (33, 35) and should be avoided, because it is a factor in diabetes, cardiovascular and hypertensive disease, and problems with mobility, such as arthritis (33, 35, 196).

Adequate *calcium* intake, preferably from food rather than supplements, is essential for both males and females (1,200 mg/day; 1,500 mg/day for the postmenopausal female who is not treated with estrogen). Note that one glass of milk contains 300 mg of calcium, although there are many other sources of calcium (33, 35). *Vitamin D* (800 to 1,000 IU) is necessary for calcium absorption (33). *Other minerals* that are necessary daily for bone health are phosphorus (700 mg), magnesium (320 mg for females and 420 mg for males), and fluoride (3 mg for females and 4 mg for males). Iron, iodine, and other minerals remain at the recommended daily intake for young adults (33).

After 60 years of age, the percentage of total body fluid may decrease from about 55% or 60% to 52% in males and from about 50% to 40% in females. Total body fluid loss is greater in obese persons (116). Plenty of *fluids*, especially water and juices, along with an adequate diet, will control weight and maintain vigor. Fluids help prevent "heartburn," constipation, and other minor discomforts caused by physiologic changes. Snacks of *fiber* (total 25 to 30 g/day) and protein maintain energy (33). Equally important, the person should chew food well, eat smaller portions throughout the day to maintain a consistent blood glucose level metabolism, eat in a pleasant and unhurried atmosphere, and avoid eating when overtired.

Drinking too much coffee or tea can be a real problem in middle age. Intake should be limited to 1 or 2 cups daily, between meals, including decaffeinated forms. The tannins in coffee and tea at mealtime can reduce the body's ability to absorb nutrients such as calcium. There may also be an association between coffee and high blood cholesterol levels. Coffee and tea, other than green tea, should be avoided if there is a family history of heart disease or if the person is overweight, eats a high-fat diet, and does not exercise (33, 35).

There is no evidence that use of commercial vitamin-mineral preparations is necessary unless they are prescribed by a physician because of clinical signs of deficiency and insufficient diet. Calcium supplements should be avoided if there is existing kidney disease, because high calcium intake increases the risk of kidney stones (33).

Health teaching must begin with understanding cultural concepts and values before a significant trend toward wise eating habits can begin. Teach that the daily diet should contain all of the food groups found in a variety of foods, with emphasis on protein, minerals, vitamins, low-cholesterol and low-calorie foods, and fiber. Joining self-help groups, such as Weight Watchers or Take Off Pounds Sensibly (TOPS), is effective for many people. It is possible to change habits of overeating and to lose weight in middle age.

Teach the middle-aged person about the risks of osteopenia and osteoporosis, and the importance of integrating healthy nutrition, exercise, and erect posture for prevention of these and other health risks. Emphasize to avoid using extreme diets to decrease weight quickly and to avoid repeatedly losing weight that is then regained. Each gain–lose cycle reduces the total muscle mass with weight loss and increases body fat, as regained weight is in the form of adipose tissue. Adipose tissue burns fewer calories than muscle, so each round of dieting makes it more difficult to lose weight and maintain weight loss. Extreme low-calorie diets should also be avoided because with them, the basal metabolic rate becomes lower so that, even with restricted calories, little weight is lost. Thus, to lose weight it is essential to exercise—at least moderately—and eat a healthy high-fiber, low-fat diet. Share information from **Box 15-2**, Healthy Eating Plan for the Middle-Aged Adult (33, 35, 164), and from this section as you educate the client.

MediaLink MyPyramid

BOX 15-2 | **Healthy Eating Plan for the Middle-Aged Adult**

GO NUTRIENT DENSE AND HIGH FIBER

1. Buy cereals that give you a larger portion for the calories.
2. Serve meals loaded with complex carbohydrates such as pasta, rice (brown for more fiber), barley, and potatoes.
3. Be creative with your potato toppings—plain yogurt mixed with herbs, picante sauce, or melted low-fat cheese.
4. Use meals such as lean beef and skinless turkey and chicken, not as the biggest part of the meal, but more as condiments. Serve them in 2- to 3-oz portions.
5. Use romaine lettuce in salads instead of the pale, anemic-looking variety. Romaine lettuce has approximately eight times more vitamin A and double the iron of iceberg lettuce.
6. Serve an iron-rich plant food such as a legume or dried fruit with a vitamin C-rich food such as citrus fruit. Vitamin C helps your body use the iron more efficiently.
7. Chop fruits and vegetables as little as possible, cook them just a short time, and minimize standing time. A number of vitamins are destroyed by air, light, and heat.
8. Choose dark green and bright orange vegetables and fruits. They tend to have more nutrients than the paler plant foods. One half cup of cooked, chopped broccoli, for instance, has more than double the vitamin A and eight times more vitamin C than the same amount of lighter green beans.
9. Choose plain, low-fat yogurt and add your own fruit.
10. Steam foods rather than cook them in large amounts of water, which can leach away important nutrients.
11. Select whole grain products more often than refined ones.
12. Try to avoid empty calories (those giving you few nutrients) such as those found in alcohol or in desserts such as cake and pie.
13. Work more fiber into your meals with peas and beans: mix them with rice or pasta, use them in meatless chili, or sprinkle them on salads.

EASE MORE FISH INTO MEALS

1. Try fish in your favorite meat and chicken recipes.
2. Do not overcook fish. Cook fish for approximately 10 minutes per inch of thickness, be it on the grill, under the broiler, or in an oven preheated to 450°F.
3. Be creative: serve fish and shellfish in soups, salads, stews, pasta, and stir-fry dishes.

CUT THE FAT

1. Reduce fat in the diet by eating ordinary foods and cutting back on just four things: fat used in prepared foods and in cooking, oils, red meats, and whole milk dairy products. These measures will reduce fat intake to approximately 20% of caloric intake.
2. Avoid fried foods. Simulate the crunch of fried foods by oven frying. For instance, dip fish or chicken in egg whites and then in bread or cracker crumbs and bake on a nonstick cookie sheet at 300°–350°F until done; or slice potatoes into spears and bake in the oven at 350°F for 30 minutes.
3. Invest in cookware that uses little or no oil when sautéing or pan frying. Lightly coat regular pans and casseroles with nonstick vegetable spray.
4. Experiment with low-fat, low-calorie flavor enhancers such as Dijon mustard, horseradish, chopped green or red peppers, onions, and seasonings such as tarragon, dry mustard, dill, and curry powder.
5. Chill sauces, gravies, and stews ahead of time so the hardened fat can be skimmed from the surface.
6. Make sauces without fat by slowly mixing cold liquid directly into the flour or cornstarch. Stir until smooth and bring to a boil, stirring frequently.
7. Use evaporated skimmed milk instead of cream in coffee and recipes.
8. In place of sour cream, use nonfat sour cream, low-fat or nonfat yogurt, or lowfat cottage cheese that has been mixed in a blender with a little milk and lemon juice.

BOOST MILK INTAKE (WITHOUT DRINKING A DROP)

If your system is not lactose intolerant, but you prefer not to drink milk as a beverage:

1. Sneak nonfat dry milk powder into anything you can: soups, sauces, casseroles, meat loaf, and stews. Add a few teaspoons of it to coffee; this blend will taste like café au lait.
2. Treat yourself to low-calorie puddings made with skim or low-fat milk.
3. Make milk-based soups with skim milk.
4. Use a blender to make a low-fat milk shake with a few ice cubes, skim or low-fat milk, fresh fruit, and low-calorie sweetener.
5. Experiment with fun flavorings in low-fat milk: vanilla, rum extract, or even cocoa with a little artificial sweetener.
6. Have cold breakfast cereals with milk and fresh fruit.

REST AND EXERCISE

Exercise

Exercise and erect posture may not increase longevity but they will enhance quality of life by keeping people healthy and independent. **Figure 15-1** ■ depicts one popular form of exercise. A combination of the following activities appears optimum: consistent brisk walking, stretching, weight bearing, bicycling, gardening, strenuous housecleaning, dancing, rowing, swimming, aerobics, and resistance activities. *Moderate constant exercise of 30 minutes daily, or at least 5 days a week, is recommended.* Alternatively there should be vigorous or aerobic exercise for a minimum of 20 minutes three times a week. Any activity that accelerates cardiac and respiratory rates is considered beneficial (18, 98).

Various physiologic changes occur with exercise (18, 19, 21, 98, 117, 124, 137, 174):

1. Blood supply and oxygen are increased to the brain and other body systems.
2. Genes in nerve cells signal production of proteins called neurotrophic or growth factors. Thus, branching, more connections, and new cell formation occur; neurons become more robust.
3. Cell growth in the hippocampus is stimulated, which prevents depression, lifts mood, and improves cognitive function.
4. Osteoblast production is increased.
5. Improved neurologic and circulatory function speeds reaction time.
6. Lean muscle mass is maintained or restored by strength training exercises; loss of lean muscle mass is not an inevitable consequence of aging (33, 35).
7. Lean muscle mass contributes to a higher metabolic rate than adipose tissue. People with more muscle mass (usually males)

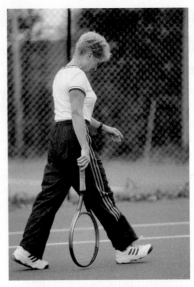

FIGURE ■ **15-1** Middle-aged adults should be encouraged to participate in healthy behaviors such as exercising.
(Guy Drayton © Dorling Kindersley)

have a higher metabolic rate than do people with proportionately more adipose tissue (usually females) (33, 35).
8. Endorphin production increases, which enhances mood.
9. Increased circulation removes infiltration of wastes from the brain and fosters excretion of wastes from the body.

Educate administrators in the occupational setting and the public that the middle-aged adult is generally healthy and invests considerable energy in occupational or professional, home, and organizational activity, and in leisure time pursuits to the extent possible. Although chronic disease is more prevalent than in the

---

INTERVENTIONS FOR HEALTH PROMOTION

Educate the public and clients that exercise has positive effects for the middle-ager because it (16, 18, 19, 21, 33, 35, 63, 98, 117, 148, 193):

1. Maintains or improves strength (by as much as 170% with weight-lifting routines).
2. Maintains or improves muscle mass, which also stabilizes joints.
3. Maintains or improves coordination, agility, flexibility, balance, and endurance.
4. Stimulates bone formation and increases bone density and size.
5. Maintains collagen tissue elasticity and prevents shortening of connective tissue. Stretching exercises, hatha yoga, and floor exercises put joints and muscles through range of motion.
6. Improves cardiovascular function and circulation, increases pulse rate between 85 and 120 beats per minute,

and lowers blood pressure, which reduces heart disease risk by 30% to 50%.
7. Promotes deeper respirations and lung elasticity.
8. Improves abdominal muscle tone and posture, aiding gastrointestinal function.
9. Maintains weight or promotes weight loss by increasing metabolism, reducing appetite and the percentage of body fat by "burning off" calories.
10. Improves sleep, which enhances immune function.
11. Improves alertness, mental function, memory, and overall intellect.
12. Fosters positive self-concept, self-esteem, and life satisfaction.
13. Improves resilience in response to stress.
14. Reduces depressive mood, anger, and emotional tension.

young, there is ordinarily good resistance to communicable diseases, superior emotional stamina, and a willingness to work despite minor illnesses. The person brings economy of effort, singleness of purpose, and perseverance to various roles. Judicious exercise may modify and retard the aging process. Teach people with sedentary jobs that doing back exercises can prevent loss of muscle tone and discomfort. Utilize **Figure 15-2**■, Back exercises for daily sitters, for your teaching.

Suggest that the person may benefit from enrolling in an exercise program that is directed by a health professional. Emphasize that physical activity can prevent risk for at least six diseases: cardiac disease, hypertension, obesity, diabetes, osteoporosis, and depression (4, 196).

Foot problems may occur in middle age. **Foot balance**, *the ability to alter one's position so that body weight is carried through the foot with minimum effort*, is essential to prevent strain, foot aches, and pain during exercise as well as when walking or standing. Foot imbalance may result from contracted toes, improper position, size or shape of one or more bones of the foot, weak or rotating ankles, muscle strain, weak ligaments, poor body posture, overweight, arthritis, injuries, and improperly fitted or shaped shoes. Treatment by a podiatrist consists of careful assessment of the posture and provision of balance inlays for insertion into the shoes (132).

Other common foot problems in middle age are bunions and corns. A **bunion** is *a sore, swollen bump at the base of the big toe, caused by heredity or poorly fitting shoes.* A **corn** is *a hard callus that forms on the toes, caused by the function of toe bones rubbing against each other or against the shoe* (196).

Teach that these or other foot problems should be treated by a podiatrist. Scraping or cutting a callus is a risk for infection.

Given that back pain is unpredictable, a daily dose of preventive exercises will help keep your back strong. Here are several exercises you can do at home.

The first rule of exercising is to warm up. Shake out the arms and legs. Stretch the arms, reaching up with one, then the other. March in place for several minutes to circulate the blood and loosen leg muscles.

(1) The pelvic tilt can be done in any position. Lie on your back, knees bent, feet flat. Press your waist and lower back to the floor, tightening the abdominals, tucking the buttocks under the pelvis, and relaxing the upper body. Release. Tuck again. Release. Repeat.

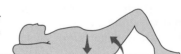

(2) Tightening the abdominal muscles will strengthen the back. Begin by lying on your back on a carpeted floor. Bend the knees and keep the feet flat on the floor. Arms are on the floor with palms down. Slowly bring one knee to your chest and face. Slowly return the leg, knee still bent, to the starting position. Repeat this exercise with each leg 5–10 times.

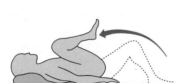

(3) Kneel on the floor on all fours. Extend the left leg out from the buttocks so that there is a straight horizontal line from the heel to the head. Now bend the knee so the bottom of the foot is facing the ceiling. Raise the leg carefully and evenly several times. Straighten the leg again and start over. Repeat with the opposite leg.

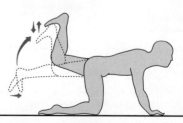

While the exercises illustrated here are considered comparatively safe, if you suffer from back or joint problems, extreme overweight, or chronic heart, circulation, or respiratory problems, check with your doctor or chiropractor before starting any exercise program. If any exercise selected becomes painful, stop immediately.

FIGURE ■ **15-2** Back exercises for daily sitters.

Source: From Back Protection for Daily Sitters, Staying Well Newsletter, *May–June (1991), 2. Publication produced by the Foundation for Chiropractic Education and Research, Des Moines, Iowa.*

Teach the person to observe for the following *common signs of need for diagnostic evaluation and possible treatment* (196):

1. Circulation to the feet; changed color, temperature, and sensation in feet and toes.
2. Swelling of the feet and ankles.
3. Cramps in the feet and the calf while walking or at night.
4. Inability to keep the feet warm even when wearing socks or when covered.
5. Loss of the fat tissue on the padded surfaces of the feet.
6. Chronic ulcers on the feet that fail to respond to treatment.
7. Absence of or bounding pulse in the arteries of the feet.
8. Burning in the soles of the feet.

Teach foot care or foot hygiene measures:

1. Keep feet covered with socks, slippers, or shoes, even indoors.
2. Clean the feet with soap and water at least once daily. Dry feet and between toes thoroughly.
3. Use a moisturizer if feet are dry or cracked.
4. Exercise the feet, extend the toes, and then flex rapidly for 1 or 2 minutes. Rotate the feet in circles at the ankles. Try picking up a pencil or marble with the toes.
5. Walk barefoot on uneven surfaces, such as thick carpet, grass, or a sandy beach. Observe for hazards on outdoor surfaces that could cause cuts.
6. Walk daily and properly. Keep toes pointed ahead and slightly outward; lift rather than push the foot, letting it come down flat on the ground, placing little weight on the heel.
7. Massage the feet to rest them after a tiring day.
8. Lie down with feet higher than head for approximately one-half hour daily.
9. Avoid wearing poorly fitted shoes or shoes with high heels and pointed toes.
10. Seek help with trimming toenails if poor vision, arthritis, or mobility-limiting conditions exist.

More information on walking fitness is available from the AARP Website (www.aarp.org) and the Step Up to Better Health Program (www.walking.org).

Sleep

Most middle-aged adults sleep without difficulty; 7 to 8 hours of sleep constitute a recommended and normal pattern. Rest and sleep must be balanced with physical activity to maintain optimum function. Refer to Chapter 14 for more information on normal sleep patterns. ∞ Between 20 and 60 years of age, waking hours and duration for quiet sleep and rapid eye movement (REM) sleep remain comparable. However, the middle-ager may awake several times during the night, in contrast to the young adult, and duration of deep or stage IV sleep is shorter (1, 45, 148). Insomnia may be a sign of a more serious underlying medical condition, for example, cardiac or thyroid disease or depression. Some medications interfere with sleep, such as some antidepressants, antihypertensives, thyroid medication, and corticosteroids (196).

Present information from the **Box** Client Education: Sleep Hygiene Recommendations to promote better sleep. Explore factors that may contribute to sleep difficulties. Refer to the physician as necessary.

Parasomnias *are conditions in which sleep is disrupted by inappropriate activation, either in the brain centers that control body movements or in the autonomic nervous system that governs physiologic and emotional functions.* Some are characteristic of non-REM (NREM) sleep and occur in the first third of the night. Others are typical of REM sleep and occur in the last two thirds of the night (1, 6, 71). Hobson and Silvestri describe various disorders and treatment (71). However, one kind of sleep disturbance—sleep apnea—in middle age is being studied to a greater extent (1, 6, 71).

Sleep apnea, *more than five episodes of cessation of airflow for at least 10 seconds, up to 2 minutes, each hour of sleep,* is a problem that is being increasingly recognized (35% to 40% of middle-agers or elders). This syndrome is found primarily in males over 50 and

Client Education

Sleep Hygiene Recommendations

1. Avoid daytime inactivity or social isolation.
2. Establish presleep routines, for example, a warm bath, reading, or relaxing activities.
3. Maintain a regular time for sleep and awakening. Use the bed only for sleeping.
4. Go to bed when feeling sleepy, or do something boring to become drowsy.
5. Get regular exercise, but avoid the hours just before bedtime.
6. Avoid caffeine (coffee, tea, cola, chocolate) within 6 hours of bedtime.

7. Avoid alcohol within several hours of bedtime.
8. Avoid daytime naps.
9. Avoid sleep medications, if possible, since they interfere with deep sleep and have a detrimental effect if taken for too long.
10. Some herbal remedies, such as valerian root (sedating effect) and leava (anti-anxiety effect), may promote sleep (these have not been evaluated by the FDA). Melatonin may promote sleep; pills have far higher amounts than occur naturally (unevaluated by FDA). Being outdoors in sunlight is more effective for melatonin release.

Client Education

Sleep Apnea

PATHOPHYSIOLOGY

1. Airway collapses or is restricted during sleep
2. Continued effort to breathe, respiratory difficulty
3. Hypoxia caused by intervals of not breathing
4. Sleep disturbed

MANIFESTATIONS

1. Excessive daytime sleepiness
2. Frequent nocturnal awakening
3. Chronic heavy, loud snoring
4. Severe morning headaches, sleepiness
5. Unrefreshing daytime sleep
6. Irritability and personality changes
7. Poor concentration, impaired memory
8. Hypertension
9. Cardiac arrhythmias
10. Depression
11. Impotence, sexual dysfunction
12. Right-sided heart failure

DIFFERENTIAL DIAGNOSIS: NARCOLEPSY

1. Manifestations of unexpected falling asleep, sudden loss of muscle tone, REM sleep disturbed, temporary paralysis of muscles when falling asleep or awakening, hallucinations

CLIENT CARE

1. Maintain sleep diary, including hours in bed, hours slept, and sleep quality
2. Avoid daytime napping
3. Schedule rest time before bedtime
4. Establish regular bed and wakeup times
5. Avoid caffeine, nicotine, alcohol, and stimulants such as decongestants
6. Avoid pharmacotherapy
7. If no improvement, schedule sleep laboratory referral for evaluation

TREATMENT

1. Weight loss of 10% of body weight
2. Dental appliance worn during sleep
3. Ventilation therapy such as continuous positive-airway pressure (CPAP)
4. Surgery, if severe case

---

postmenopausal females, especially in people who are obese and have short, thick necks. Often it is first detected because the person snores loudly or dozes during the daytime. Morning headaches are common due to carbon dioxide retention. A large European study reported that people diagnosed with depression were more likely to have a sleep-related breathing disorder. It is unknown which comes first (138). It can be life-threatening. *There are three types* (1, 12, 45, 71):

1. **Obstructive.** *Respiratory effort continues despite pharyngeal obstruction to airflow.* The hypoxemia stimulates the respiratory center to initiate breathing.
2. **Central.** *There is no respiratory effort with airflow;* the respiratory center fails to initiate breathing.
3. **Mixed.** *Episodes of no respiratory effort initially are followed by respiratory effort and then airflow.*

The person may have the symptoms or manifestations listed in the **Box**, Client Education: Sleep Apnea (1, 71, 138).

Educate the person and family member who sleeps with the person, or nearby, to keep a sleep diary, on which treatment and teaching can be based. Incorporate information from the Client Education: Sleep Apnea Box about pathophysiology, manifestations, self-care measures, and treatment options in your teaching plan. The client will need special instruction on using the continuous positive-airway pressure (CPAP) device in order to use it comfortably while sleeping.

Health Promotion and Health Protection

IMMUNIZATIONS

Middle-aged adults should have been immunized for tetanus/diphtheria, measles, mumps, and rubella. Tetanus diphtheria (Td) toxoid should be administered every 10 years as a booster. Influenza, hepatitis B, and pneumonia vaccines are recommended for health workers and those with chronic disease or heart or lung disease. Hepatitis B vaccine should be administered if the person or partner has had other sexual partners in the past 6 months, has a sexually transmitted disease, or has injected illegal drugs. Recommended immunizations and revaccination, including for middle-agers with uncertain immunization histories and for the chronically ill, are presented in the Centers for Disease Control (CDC) Website, www.cdc.gov. Those at risk for tuberculosis and in need of the annual two-step skin testing should also refer to the CDC Website.

Educate about the need to maintain recommended immunizations and a personal record of type and date. Refer clients to the Websites for updated and changing information and answers to questions about concerns.

GENDER HEALTH ISSUES

Female health issues *refer to prevention, diagnosis, and management of female health concerns that are* (33, 196):

1. Unique to females: menstruation, pregnancy, and reproductive diseases.
2. More prevalent in females than males: eating disorders, breast cancer, autoimmune diseases, some gastrointestinal diseases, osteoporosis, and depression.
3. Manifested differently in females than males, such as cardiac disease and AIDS. Cardiac disease and cancer are the first and second leading causes of death in females in the United States.

Other leading causes of death are obesity and consequent diseases, such as diabetes and strokes. Osteoporosis and consequent fractures also contribute to cause of death, beginning in late middle age (196).

Male health issues *relate to the male's shorter life span, partly because males are greater risk takers.* Rates of accidental death and disability from accidents are greater among males than females, whether from voluntary (e.g., driving) or involuntary (e.g., serving in combat) causes. Males, generally, smoke tobacco and drink alcoholic beverages more than females, and seek medical care or preventive services less than females. Males tend to define themselves by their work; they may feel more stress and express it more in physical illness than do females (33, 148).

Lifestyle may be a major basis for gender differences in health and longevity. For example, Mormon males live as long as females, generally (33).

INJURY AND ACCIDENTS

The gradually changing physical characteristics and preoccupation with responsibilities may contribute to the middle-aged person having accidents. Accidents, either motor vehicle or job related, may occur, causing injury or death.

Fractures and dislocations are leading causes of injuries for both genders. More males are affected than females, probably because of occupational differences. Occupation-related accidents and falls in the home are causes of injury and death.

Accidents that disable for one week or more increase for the worker after age 45. Because of interest in accident protection legislation, industries and other occupational settings are increasingly health and safety conscious. Efforts must continue in this direction (88, 94, 165).

Teach about safety as it relates to remodeling a home, maintaining a yard, or establishing a work center: (a) install handrails for stairways, and a handgrip in the shower or the bathtub; (b) place electric outlets in convenient locations; (c) use indirect, nonglare, and thorough lighting; (d) keep tools, equipment, and home or yard

machines in proper working condition; (e) install smoke detectors in various locations in the home (batteries should be checked monthly and changed twice annually); (f) keep guns separated from ammunition and both locked to be inaccessible to children; (g) remove or secure anything that would predispose to a fall, such as rugs, electrical cords, or small objects; (h) clean up spills on the floor promptly and avoid slippery waxes; and (i) keep medications in a safe place and ensure the label is readable. Reinforce the personal/family planning for gradual failing of physical abilities by making the home as safe, convenient, and comfortable as possible as they rethink homemaking functions for the coming decades. In addition to home safety, you can be instrumental in initiating or strengthening a safety program in an occupational or educational setting.

ILLNESS PREVENTION

Middle age is not automatically a period when the body fails or a time of physical or psychological hazard or disease. No single disease or mental condition necessarily is related to the passage of time, although the middle-aged person requires better maintenance than was necessary in earlier years. Assess the middle-ager carefully for signs of illness. Recommend the screening tests described in Chapter 14. ∞ In addition, after age 50, a bone density index (BDI) should be done every 2 years to determine calcium density in bone and presence of osteopenia and osteoporosis in females and at-risk males (33, 35, 196). Beginning at age 50, *one of the following screening tests should be done to screen for colon and rectal cancer or colon polyps:*

1. Fecal occult blood test (FOBT) or fecal immunochemical test (FIT) annually.
2. Flexible sigmoidoscopy or contrast barium enema every 5 years, even if annual FOBT is normal.
3. Colonoscopy every 5 years.
4. Virtual colonoscopy every 3 years if unable to get a colonoscopy due to a medical condition.

Refer to the American Cancer Society Website, www.cancer.org, for more information.

Major health problems of this era are cardiovascular disease, cancer, pulmonary disease, diabetes, obesity, alcoholism, anxiety, depression, and glaucoma (52, 196). The **Box** *Healthy People 2010: Example of Objectives for Midlife Health Promotion* presents health concerns and strategies for this life era, formulated by the U.S. Department of Health and Human Services (179). Objectives include to reduce risks to injuries, chronic illness, disabilities, and deaths due to avoidable situations and to improve health for more people (179). For more information, refer to the Website www.healthypeople.gov or call 1-800-367-4725.

Assist the person to maintain energy and improve health by teaching the information presented in this section and throughout the chapter. The person can learn to change eating, drinking, or smoking habits and to use only medically prescribed drugs. *Measures to promote health include* (a) obtaining regular physical examinations, (b) participating in leisure activity, (c) using relaxation techniques, (d) working through the emotional and family concerns related to middle age, (e) affirming the worth of self as a

Healthy People 2010

Example of Objectives for Midlife Health Promotion

1. Increase the proportion of persons appropriately counseled about health behaviors.

2. Prevent disease, disability, and death from infectious diseases, including vaccine-preventable diseases.

3. Reduce injuries, disabilities, and deaths due to unintentional injuries and violence.

4. Promote the health and safety of people at work through prevention and early intervention.

5. Reduce periodontal disease.

6. Improve health, fitness, and quality of life through daily physical activity.

7. Increase smoking cessation attempts by adult smokers.

8. Improve the visual and hearing health of the nation through prevention, early detection, treatment, and rehabilitation.

9. Reduce deaths and injuries caused by alcohol- and drug-related motor vehicle crashes.

10. Reduce illness, disability, and death related to tobacco use and exposure to secondhand smoke.

Adapted from reference 179.

---

middle-aged person, (f) preparing for the later years, and (g) confronting developmental tasks. The person also needs to prepare for possible accidents or illness through self-assessment, medical checkups, family discussion, and insurance planning.

Educate clients to stay up-to-date on recommended screening by using a new tool, Stay Healthy at Any Age: Your Checklist for Health, developed by the Agency for Healthcare Research and Quality. The Website www.ahrq.gov has a different link for the male and female checklists.

Teach that the mounting statistical, experimental, and autopsy findings point to cigarette smoking as a causative factor in breast and lung cancer, cardiovascular disease, chronic obstructive pulmonary disease, and peptic ulcer. For the person who feels trapped, depressed, frustrated, or isolated, easily accessible escapes are alcohol, drugs, and excess food intake. Assist the person in finding other ways to cope with stressors.

Review content of the medicine cabinet, which may look like a pharmaceutical display. Explain why old injuries become bothersome and new injuries do not heal as quickly. Consider whether illness or accident proneness can also be a means of resolving serious difficulties or of escaping responsibilities. If understanding and help from others is negligible or nonexistent and the possibility of recouping losses or rearranging one's life seems unlikely, the brief care and attention given during illness or after injury may not offer sufficient gratification. Determine presence of suicidal thoughts and any attempted or actual suicide attempts, which are a call for help or an escape from problems. The prop of ill health should not be removed without study and caution, for removing one syndrome may result in discharge of emotional tension through another physical or emotional syndrome. Thus nursing intervention and medical treatment must be directed toward both physical and emotional factors.

Because nursing care is holistic, you can meet emotional and spiritual needs of the person while giving physical care and doing health teaching related to common health problems discussed in the following pages. Special screening and education sessions should be established for the male who may not readily follow health promotion measures or seek health care. Discuss medication rationale and actions. Teach about medication management. The person should keep, easily retrievable, a list of prescribed and over-the-counter medications and daily administration times. Review how to effectively read labels and package inserts and how to detect adverse drug effects. Discuss measures to prevent side effects or toxicity. Emphasize the importance of discarding outdated medications. Reinforce notifying the primary health care provider if there are any symptoms, unanticipated changes, or questions. Emphasize that all medications should be inaccessible to children and adolescents. Warn that teens often use parental medications, particularly benzodiazepines and pain relievers, for their own drug abuse.

Refer the client to consumer-friendly drug information Websites:

1. Consumer Drug Information and Medical Product Safety Information, both at www.fda.gov
2. MedlinePlus, www.nlm.nih.gov
3. SafeMedication.com, www.safemedication.com

COMMON HEALTH PROBLEMS: PREVENTION AND HEALTH PROMOTION

A variety of health problems may occur, although many middle-aged adults remain healthy. Common health problems in middle age are: atherosclerosis, hypertension, coronary artery disease, stroke, various kinds of cancer, asthma, impaired vision and hearing, AIDS, obesity (gaining 20 pounds in adulthood increases illness risk by 60%), arthritis, and osteoporosis (44, 165, 196). These health problems can contribute to disability; the disabled worker often has to cope with challenging work conditions that interfere with health and employment.

Cardiac Disease

Gender differences exist for disease incidence (148) and presentation, for example, in females with a heart attack (51, 84, 124, 130, 131, 159, 160, 194, 199). Psychological status and emotional stress also contribute to cardiovascular disease (9, 20, 25, 62, 108, 134, 177).

Educate both females and males to take aspirin daily to reduce risk of a heart attack. The American Heart Association recommends low-dosage aspirin therapy of 83 mg daily or 100 mg every other day for females over 65 years. The maximum dosage for high-risk females of any age is 325 mg daily to reduce risk of stroke, provided there is no risk of bleeding (130). *There has been much media publicity about the need to take an aspirin immediately when a person is having a heart attack.*

Educate middle-agers about psychosocial as well as physical risk factors for cardiovascular disease. Validate with the person that dietary changes, exercise, control of weight and waist size, leisure activities, relaxation techniques, smoking cessation, and drinking less alcohol are achievable and reduce risk. The Baby Boomer's value system responds to a challenge and reinventing self. Assist the client in developing a plan for positive lifestyle change. Utilize concepts from the Transtheoretical Model of Change discussed in Chapter 14 ∞ to better understand the client and to foster effective change. Refer the person to a counselor to resolve emotional or family concerns. For the female, joining the Red Hat Society may be a useful leisure and psychosocial activity.

Cognitive behavioral therapy, augmented with pharmacotherapy, is effective for prevention, during illness, and in rehabilitation. The middle-ager, especially one who follows the Baby Boomer lifestyle, may respond well to telemonitoring, telecounseling, and computer counseling.

Educate about smoking cessation methods. The premenopausal female may not respond as effectively and may get inconsistent results from nicotine replacement, such as patches. Apparently menstrual cycle hormones affect tobacco withdrawal symptoms (51).

Educate about effects of the metabolic syndrome, characterized by large waist sizes, hypertension, glucose intolerance, low HDL cholesterol, and high triglycerides. Exercise should be focused to restructure waist size, which can be as important as other exercise and diet. The female with metabolic syndrome, hyperglycemia, or diabetes is at greater risk than the male for early cardiac disease and early death (51, 196).

Refer the midlife person and family to the American Heart Association Website for more information, www.americanheart.org.

Refer to the Framingham Heart Study Website for information on risk factors and to calculate a person's 10-year risk of having a heart attack, www.nhlbi.nih.gov.

Refer the midlife person and family to the following Websites for more information:

Centers for Disease Control and Prevention, Division for Heart Disease and Stroke Prevention (DHDSP), www.cdc.gov

World Health Organization, Cardiovascular Diseases www.who.int

Cancer

In males the primary sites for cancer are the prostate, lung, colon, rectum, and bladder. In females, the common sites are lung, breast, colon, and rectum (105, 145, 196).

See the **Box**, Client Education: Risk Factors for Breast Cancer for more detail (29, 33, 35, 44, 105, 196). Chapter 14 gives information on breast self-examination. (See Table 14-8.) ∞

The Nurses' Health Study, which obtained information from 115,000 females in the United States over a 20-year period, analyzed a wide-ranging assortment of risk factors. Their findings indicate that 1 in 8 females will eventually develop breast cancer and 1 in 2 will develop cardiovascular disease. Long-term HRT increases the likelihood of breast cancer in females by 40%. Annual mammography screening has been found to reduce cancer deaths by one third in females 50 to 60 years of age; mammography should not be eliminated on the basis of cost (24). The Abstract for Evidence-Based Practice **Box** presents research findings about other factors besides cost that influence whether the female seeks mammography screening.

Colorectal cancer, the second greatest cause of death in the United States, affects males and females about equally and increases steadily after age 50. A variety of screening tests can detect the precancerous polyps. Surgical removal in the early stages is curative. Regular screening for colorectal cancer should begin at age 50. The prognosis for colorectal cancer is good if diagnosed and treated in the precancerous or early stages (88, 94, 149).

Educate about risk factors and the importance of regular screening for cancer, which was summarized earlier. *Educate the public and clients about ways to lower the risk of colon cancer, including to* (a) reduce consumption of red and processed meat; (b) engage in regular exercise; (c) stay slender, avoid overweight or obesity (a BMI of 25 or above); and (d) ingest 1,000 mg of calcium daily (33, 35).

Explore emotional concerns about being a cancer survivor, which is a lifelong battle (29, 68, 72, 77, 78, 106, 133). Explore

Client Education

Risk Factors for Breast Cancer

- Family history: first-degree relatives (mother, sister).
- BRCA-1 or BRCA-2 gene mutation present.
- Early menarche (before age 12).
- Late menopause (after age 55).
- Late first live birth (after age 30).
- No children.

- Oral contraceptive use before age 20 and after age 35.
- Estrogen replacement therapy.
- Postmenopausal obesity.
- Dietary fat, increasing pituitary prolactin and estrogen production.
- Lack of exercise.

Abstract for Evidence-Based Practice

Decision Making About Mammography Screening

Fowler, B. (2006). Social processes used by African American women in making decisions about mammography screening. *Journal of Nursing Scholarship, 38*(3), 247–254.

KEYWORDS

African American, decision making, mammography screening, social processes, women.

Purpose ➤ To describe social processes that influence African American women to make a decision about use of mammography screening.

Conceptual Framework ➤ Concepts of social referents or supports and decision making and findings from research about breast cancer and mammography screening were utilized. Grounded theory proposed by Glaser and Strauss (1967), Glaser (1978), and Strauss and Corbin (1998) was utilized for data collection and analysis.

Sample/Setting ➤ African American women, 50 years or older, were recruited from two African American churches ($n = 16$). A theoretical sample of African American women age 50 years or older was recruited from influential African American professional or social organizations ($n = 14$). The combined sample of 30 participants ranged in age from 52 to 71 years ($M = 63.4$ years) and had no history of breast cancer. The theoretical sample had mammography screening within the past 2 years and no household income limitations, in contrast to the church sample, which had no mammography screening in the past 2 years. Almost half of the church sample had a total household income at 100% of poverty level. No differences in decision-making styles were found between the two groups.

Method ➤ Data were collected through two audiotaped interviews, utilizing an interview guide and written field notes. The first interview of 1 to 1.5 hours was followed within 2 months by an interview of 2.5 to 3 hours to discuss and verify findings. Constant comparative analysis was used, beginning with the first interview, transcribed verbatim. Confidentiality was maintained throughout.

Findings ➤ Social processes used to make decisions about mammography screening were labeled "taking charge," "enduring," and "protesting."

The "taking charge" group ($n = 5$; age range 52 to 62 years) had an education ranging from associate to master's degrees. These women were employed at least part-time (average annual income $27,000). They were assertive and proactive about breast health decisions (100% screening) and had prior positive experiences with health care providers. They knew negative effects of breast cancer and benefits of adherence to breast health recommendations, and they identified with influential women in the media.

The "enduring" group ($n = 10$; age range 54 to 70 years) had at least a high school education and a median annual income of $41,000 from full-time employment. They were reactive to opinions of the congregation and health care providers, balanced fears and fatalistic beliefs, and relied on the church ministry authority (100% screening).

The "protesting" group ($n = 15$; age range 58 to 71 years) had completed high school and had an average annual income of $17,000 from retirement, disability, and Social Security benefits. They had reactive and confrontational attitudes about breast health. Media information was perceived as threatening and biased against African American women, thereby not trustworthy (33% screening). They were fatalistic and fearful and held strict beliefs about God's power, which lessened perceived need for screening.

All groups were involved as caregivers, which influenced decision making. The "taking charge" group believed in preventive action as a result. The "enduring" group believed caretaking was a responsibility and a way of serving God. The "protesting" group fulfilled the caregiver's role but felt it was a burden and that it interfered with preventative action.

Implications ➤ Health care providers can approach and work with the African American church ministry to reach the congregation for health education. Providers must be respectful and positive in approach related to screenings and health care. Health care education must be sensitive to religious beliefs of clients. Advocacy for media messages appropriate to this population, as well as other population groups, is essential related to breast health and mammography screening.

MediaLink Nursing Center

the client's support system. Educate and counsel family or significant others and other support systems, such as the church, school, professional groups, and organizations for middle-agers (Red Hat Society, local chapters of AARP, school or university alumni associations). Topics include prevention, risk factors, treatment options, and survivor fitness. Professional groups, as well as survivors and their families, may seek information about long-term sequelae of cancer and cancer therapies (77, 78, 106, 133). Comprehensive information is available at www.nursingcenter.com.

Refer the person and family to the following resources:

1. American Cancer Society (phone: 800-227-2345), www. cancer.org
2. American Lung Association (phone: 800-586-4842), www. lungusa.org
3. Cancer Information Service, National Cancer Institute (phone: 800-422-6237) cis.nci.nhi.gov
4. National Tobacco Quitline (phone: 800-784-8669), www. smokefree.gov
5. Tobacco Information and Prevention Source (TIPS), Office on Smoking and Health, CDC (phone: 770-488-5705), www.cdc.gov

Mind-Body Connections

Research over the decades shows the connection between mind and body (9, 19, 20, 25, 42, 108, 118, 119). Some personality traits carry more risk than others for heart attack and stroke (17, 118). Type A traits, such as aggressiveness, competitiveness, and anger, top the list (9, 25). Type D traits, such as depression, despair, or negative attitudes, also carry risk (19, 42, 49, 177).

One study of anger levels in 1,623 heart attack patients found the risk for heart attack was 2.3 times greater during the 2 hours following an anger episode (118). Another study of 2,074 middle-aged males in Finland found that strokes were twice as common in those with high anger scores (118). A study of 541 premenopausal females found that high anger increased the likelihood of plaque formation in the carotid arteries of middle-aged women (118). Other studies also link anger, hostility, resentment, depression, and heart disease (108, 173, 195).

Research shows that negative thoughts and feelings, such as depression, have been linked with cancer (72, 78, 105, 133). One study found that males in their 40s who were depressed were more likely to develop cancer in the next 20 years, even after correction for background and other variables (4, 187).

Teach individuals about the mind-body connection, constructive coping skills, relaxation techniques, exercise, and anger and stress management. Low-dose aspirin therapy, sound diet, and exercise can protect the heart. Diet and not smoking can reduce cancer risk. Explain that strengthening self-esteem, taking control over cognitive distortion, and developing positive thinking strategies are equally powerful in improving the immune system and thereby improving health and preventing disease. Validate that establishing close friendships and leisure activities promote positive physiologic as well as emotional effects. Chapters 2 and 14 ∞ also present information about the effect of emotional status on physical health.

Psychosocial Concepts

INFLUENCES ON COGNITIVE ABILITY

The brain is the physical foundation or substrate of the mind, the sense of self, and personality. It is capable of growing, adapting, and becoming more complex and integrated throughout life. As the brain matures and evolves, the consequent knowledge, emotions, and expressive abilities promote more brain development, new connections (branching), and ongoing further growth and psychological development (22, 36, 63). Each person has enormous potential for growth, change, and maturation, for positive feelings and love, and for happiness.

Throughout life, the brain encodes thoughts and memories by forming new connections among neurons. Neurons become more intertwined although they lose some processing speed. The brain of a mentally active 50-year-old looks like a dense forest of interlocking branches, which reflects both deeper knowledge and better judgment. This acquired knowledge is a real asset in most occupations and all professions. Positron emission tomography (PET) scans and magnetic resonance imaging (MRI) reveal that the right and left hemispheres become less bifurcated or less separated in their function. See Chapter 1 ∞ for major functions of each hemisphere. Both hemispheres are increasingly used for logical reasoning and intuitive tasks. Apparently, healthy brains compensate for aging changes by expanding neural networks across the corpus callosum which divides the two hemispheres (63). For example, the 20-year-old may say, "My brain says to do this; my heart says to do that." The 50-year-old says, "I trust my gut on this decision and I'm comfortable with it." Intuition or emotion and logical reasoning have been integrated as the foundation for behavior (22, 36).

The middle-aged adult scores higher on tests that require general information or vocabulary abilities. At age 60, intelligence quotient (IQ) test results are equal to or better than those of young adults. Only arithmetic reasoning shows a plateau through the adult years if skills are not used. Speed requirements of the test may mitigate against the IQ test scores; adults show a peak in speed of performance in the 20s and a gradual decrease in overall speed of performance through the years. Adults usually value accuracy and thoroughness more than speed (135, 148). In fact, IQ tests may be irrelevant. What should be tested is how people identify problems and use reason and intuition to solve them. In various studies, physically fit and active people are found to have a higher IQ score than those who engage in little physical activity (18, 22, 88, 135).

More middle-aged people are returning to college for baccalaureate, graduate, doctoral, and postdoctoral degrees. They have shown themselves capable scholastically and in applying intellectual ability in the workplace. Some have pursued additional education to begin their own business or a new career, to pursue a hobby, or for fun (3, 36, 48, 119). Universities and community colleges have adapted courses and curricula accordingly to meet the educational needs and characteristics of the Baby Boomers (82). Past studies of the American Association of University Women indicated that females were at an educational disadvantage after the early elementary years. Females in midlife currently perform academically as well as, or better than, males.

COGNITIVE DEVELOPMENT

Cognitive processes in adulthood include reaction time, perception, memory, learning and problem solving, and creativity. These are performed through characteristics of both Concrete and Formal Operations, depending on the situation (16, 135, 148, 161, 188).

Reaction time, *speed of performance or response,* is individual and generally stays the same or diminishes during late middle age. The speed of response is important primarily in test situations, because much of the problem solving necessary in adulthood requires deliberation and accuracy rather than speed. Reaction time is related to complexity of the task, the habitual pattern of response to stimuli, and familiarity with the task. Time for new learning increases with age, but adults in their 40s and 50s have the same ability to learn as they did in their 20s and 30s (36, 135).

Memory, or *recall,* is maintained through young and middle adulthood; no major age differences are evident. Some quantitative changes may occur. For example, a person in early adulthood who could recite a 10-digit span of numbers as a series of discrete units may be able to recite only 8 grouped or categorized digits in late middle age. The ability to categorize or group information, to sharpen observational skills and give more attention to the phenomenon, to relate meaning to that to be remembered, and to use **interactive imagery**, *imagining events in a story form with self in the interaction,* are all ways to strengthen memory and aid learning. The middle-aged adult memorizes less readily material that is not well organized and seems to retain less from oral presentation of information than younger persons (16, 135, 148).

There are different types of memory. **Sensory memory,** *information stored in a sense organ, is transitory, a few seconds.* **Short-term memory** *may be based on recall for days or weeks.* **Long-term memory** *may last a lifetime.* Memory is not reliable in the adult years or at any age. Most people forget or ignore episodes that do not fit the self-image or that are considered unimportant. People who think they remember an event from childhood or a number of years previously may be making up plausible scenarios, fantasies, or confabulations based on earlier reports or stories. The middle-aged adult who continues to use memory will retain a keen memory (17, 89, 135, 148).

Learning, *acquisition of knowledge formally or informally through life experiences,* occurs in adults of all ages. The highly intelligent person becomes even more learned. The capacity for intellectual growth is unimpaired and is enhanced by interest, motivation, flexibility, a sense of humor, confidence, and maturity attained through experience. Learning means more; it is not just learning for learning's sake. Knowledge is applied; motivation to learn is high for personal reasons. Reluctance to learn occurs if the new material does not appear relevant or does not serve the person as well as current information (16, 135, 148, 188).

Problem-solving abilities, *working through the complexities of a situation or a task, through integration of cognitive skills and experience, with consideration of the context,* remain throughout adulthood. There are no significant differences between 20-, 40-, and 60-year-olds in learning a task. Generally, better educated people perform better than less educated people in any age group. When there is no time limitation, there are no differences in complex task solutions although young and middle-aged adults use different strategies. Young adults, knowing they can function quickly, may be more likely to use less efficient reasoning strategies, including trial and error. In late middle age, because people know they are becoming slower, they tend to think a problem through first so they can solve it in fewer tries. Thus, they appear to be slower in grasping and solving a problem. But the wider life experiences prompt recognition of more variables in a situation and thus enhance problem solving (89, 135, 148, 188).

The middle-aged adult is able to do all the cognitive strategies of **Piaget's Stage of Formal Operations** (188) as explained in Chapters 13 and 14. ∞ Sometimes the practicality of a situation will call forth use of the Concrete Operations Stage, because not all problems in life can be solved by abstract reasoning. The middle-aged adult does both operations realistically in problem solving. He or she also engages in the **Problem-Finding Stage,** *the fifth stage of cognitive development,* proposed by Arlin (8). The person seeks not only answers but the underlying problems in a situation, as described in Chapter 14. ∞ Societal, occupational, and general life experiences are crucial to cognitive operations of the middle-aged person. Thus, perceptions about the same situation, problem, or task can vary considerably in a group of middle-aged adults.

Cognitive characteristics that are developed in the young adult are used throughout middle age as well. Various patterns mark the development and use of multiple intelligences (167–169), such as to symbolize experience and behave in a way that shows organization, integration, stability, and unity in the cognitive process. Representing experience symbolically as hunches, words, thoughts, or other symbols is part of being middle-aged. The person can reflect on past and current experience and can imagine, anticipate, plan, and hope. The person develops an inner private world that gives him or her resources for happiness and potential for anxiety. The person can recall past defeats and triumphs and monitor ongoing thoughts for consistency and logic. When the person solves a problem, he or she can explain how it was solved. Because the middle-ager is more imaginatively productive, he or she is capable of producing more images, thoughts, and combinations of ideas; is able to use reflection to gain perspectives about life; and is aware of personal beliefs, values, motives, and powers. The mature middle-ager is increasingly interested in other persons and warm, enduring relationships and is adaptable, independent, self-driven, conscientious, enthusiastic, and purposeful. The person reflects about personal relationships, the ups and downs or contradictions in relationships, and their sources of strain and satisfaction. The person empathizes more deeply, and concomitantly understands why other persons feel and act as they do (8, 39, 89, 135, 148). These characteristics of cognition are part of contextual, social, and emotional intelligence or postformal intelligence (8, 55, 56, 101). Chapter 14 presents additional information. ∞

Riegel proposed that adult thought is characterized by **dialectical thinking:** *seeking intellectual stimulation and even crisis, welcoming contradictions and opposing viewpoints, creating a new order, and discovering what is missing.* Adults struggle cognitively with morality, ethics, philosophy, religion, and politics; yet, they do not necessarily need to resolve the contradictions they face. Dialectical thought increases with age (16, 36).

Knowles proposed that another characteristic of adult thought is **meta-analysis,** *to integrate or synthesize information from numerous sources* (89). *The person does not look for one answer but looks at any experience, situation, or data from multiple perspectives* (8, 17, 50). Thus, knowledge is ever-changing.

Cognitive development in middle age implies maintenance and change. **Maintenance,** *through satisfying needs and upholding one's internal order,* is necessary for cognitive function to occur. **Change,** *involving adaptation and creative expansion,* is part of the cognitive development of the adult. Maintenance and change occur with different emphases in various life stages. The child develops adaptation mechanisms as he or she learns. The adolescent and adult move into creative expansion. After middle age, the person assesses the past and self and wants to restore inner order. In old age, the person either continues to follow previous adaptive and creative drives or regresses to need-satisfying tendencies.

The intellectually curious, whether or not a self-acclaimed Baby Boomer, have an increased need and ability to spin new syntheses and theories, to make meaningful that which seems meaningless, to coordinate hypothesis formation and testing, to be systematic at problem solving, to seek environmental diversity, and to become more subtle, differentiated, integrated, and complex. The mature person has a progressive integration; that is, he or she is continually open to ideas, flexible, curious, and actively engaged. If cognitive efficiency becomes disrupted, a mature person is able to recover from such disorganization more quickly than an immature person, even though the two do not differ in intelligence. The mature person becomes discriminating in decisions based on the facts at hand and can postpone, suppress, or ignore. The person can analyze and judge information, without being influenced by either personal desires or persuasive opinions of others. Thought becomes objective and judgment independent (17, 36, 39, 89, 136, 148).

Neugarten (125–129) found that the person changes both cognitively and emotionally over time as the result of accumulated experience. The person abstracts from experiences and creates more encompassing and more refined categories for interpreting events. The middle-aged person differs cognitively from the young adult in that he or she was born in a different historical era and thereby has different formative experiences. The middle-aged adult thus has a greater apperceptive mass or store of past experience by which to evaluate events or make decisions. Through the adult years, perspectives and insights broaden and deepen, and attitudes and behaviors change (125–129).

Gould (58–60) focused more on personality than cognitive development. However, he described adulthood as a time of thoughtful confrontation with the self—letting go of the idealized image and the desire to be perfect, and acknowledging the realistic image of self and personal feelings. The adult continues to gain new beliefs about self and the world. Conflicts between past and present beliefs are resolved (58–60).

Assist the middle-aged adult (and others) in understanding the cognitive changes and strengths of cognitive ability. Reinforce a positive self-image related to cognitive abilities. Utilize this information as you assess and educate about health promotion practices to maintain effective cognitive function. Relate information about physical status to cognitive health. Have the middle-ager identify personal cognitive style and multiple intelligences, which are described in Chapter 12, ∞ and characteristics that are cognitive strengths as a way to affirm positive self-concept. Emphasize that the best years are still ahead in cognitive function.

CREATIVITY

Because of better integration of the two hemispheres of the brain, the person becomes more flexible, more creative, and less negative in emotional response (22). *Creative thinking and creativity involves* (13): (a) developing alternative solutions, (b) engaging in divergent thinking or bringing together two or more ideas that were previously isolated, and (c) combining different forms of knowledge and cognitive strategies which are mediated by the two brain hemispheres. Providing a cognitively and socially stimulating, enriched home environment and formal education fosters brain development and encourages divergent thinking.

Dennis (31) found an age pattern for creative output. Research indicates a peak activity in early and middle adulthood. Unique, original, and inventive productions are more often created in the 20s, 30s, and 40s than later in life. The more a creative act depends on accumulated experience, the more likely it is to occur in middle age or later life. People are less productive in total creative output in their 20s than in their 30s and 40s. Poets, novelists, and scholars gain in productivity in middle and old age. Quality increases as a greater proportion of contextual, intuitive, and social intelligence is used (31, 135). Some creative works cannot be produced without the benefit of years of experience and living, absorbing the wisdom of the culture, and the resultant development of new insights. Increasingly, we see scientists, researchers, professors, artists representing all fields, authors, craftspersons, and others maintaining creative cognition and activity into the 80s and beyond. Creativity is seen not only in famous people or young people. The average middle-aged adult may have many responsibilities and stresses. However, typically he or she approaches a situation, task, or learning experience in a creative way.

Encourage the middle-aged adult to pursue creative ideas and activities and to approach roles, responsibilities, and tasks in a creative way. Help the middle-aged adult overcome self-consciousness about the unique cognitive response to a situation. Reinforce efforts to begin new ventures in life. Emphasize continued learning, in various courses, either for college credit or noncredit courses. Continued learning can deal with specific problems or specific content. It can also be fun. An academic program may be necessary for changing a profession or occupation. Review that creativity and continued learning can promote personal satisfaction; relieve boredom, loneliness, or an unhappy situation; and broaden the mind for the sake of learning. Validate that rapid technologic changes in business or the professions cause obsolescence of knowledge and skills, which also forces middle-aged persons to continue to learn.

Reaffirm to the Baby Boomer cohort that continued learning and creativity helps them find a place in the changing workplace and society and helps to reinvent the self, a value of the cohort (3, 111, 166).

When you are teaching, use methods that capitalize on the learning strengths of mature adults, including:

1. Active discussion and role play.
2. Less emphasis on memorization.
3. Presentation of large amounts of new information.
4. Suggestions to develop cognitive strategies that will help him or her synthesize, analyze, integrate, interpret, and apply knowledge.
5. Validation with the middle-aged adult and others that he or she can learn, because myths to the contrary are prevalent.
6. Provision of a conducive environment, one that considers sensory changes.
7. Consideration of the sensory changes discussed previously.

WORK AND LEISURE ACTIVITIES RELATED TO COGNITIVE FUNCTION

Work

Middle-agers are good workers. In comparison to young adults, they are more inclined to:

1. Resolve job conflicts and try to work out what is wrong (120, 148).
2. Participate in challenges and changes in the workplace (120, 148).
3. Have a lower avoidable absenteeism rate (148).
4. Become expert at what they are doing and be willing to mentor or teach others (16, 120, 184, 185).
5. Use life experience and maturity on the job (14, 16, 120, 184, 185).
6. Be less emotionally labile (16).
7. Value work, but also value being a good parent, a loving spouse, and involved with the children (14, 16, 148).

Work is viewed differently by different middle-agers, as well as by different generations, as summarized in **Table 15-1.** Consider that the older middle-aged person grew up under the influence of the Great Depression and with the Protestant ethic. Both stressed the economic and moral importance of work. Thus, work became respected and sought. Being without a job or idle was a harbinger of problems and meant being lazy and worthless. How has this middle-aged adult adjusted to mechanization, waning of the work ethic, and the demise of a full day's work for a full day's pay? For the young middle-ager, what was a promising career or lifetime employment may have ended in being laid off permanently by the company, forced early retirement, or forced job hunting. Finding different work could be difficult.

Educate and counsel the client who is unemployed and job hunting. Utilize **Box 15-3**, Suggestions for Someone Who Is Unemployed, to educate and stimulate discussion. Or you may want to educate the client about career options described in the **Box** Client Education: Career Track Options in Late Middle Age.

The person may be fortunate enough to be in a business or profession in which he or she works successfully for self or is allowed freedom within a specialized area of work. That person will experience the dignity of being productive and will enjoy increasing self-esteem, autonomy, and sense of achievement. However, many middle-aged adults are employed in a system in which the value is on production, not the person. Often, in contrast to union-set rules, whereby no more than a specified amount can be done within a specified time, ever-greater output is demanded on the job.

The Information Revolution is pulling people apart similar to the way the Industrial Revolution brought people together. There is a greater variety of job choices, but there is less loyalty to one workplace or one boss. Middle-aged Americans are creating a new style of employment and more flexible careers. Midlife for some is a time of career change. More people than ever plan to work past retirement age. Workers age 55 through 64, the Baby Boomer generation, are the fastest-growing segment of the workforce (11, 36, 48, 114).

There are several categories of workers that are different from the past. They have been described as follows (48, 114):

BOX 15-3	**Suggestions for Someone Who Is Unemployed**

1. Offer hope and encouragement, but guard against sounding "superior." This may be a dark valley, emotionally, economically, philosophically, and spiritually.
2. Remind the person that unemployment is a reflection of current economic conditions and social trends, not of personal worth.
3. Seek opportunities to affirm the person's talents and positive attributes.
4. Help him or her consider all the options, including launching a business from home, changing careers, and working part-time.
5. Allow the person to express feelings, but do not encourage self-pity. Your time with the person should leave him or her feeling uplifted and hopeful. Pray with the person if he or she desires.
6. Offer to hold him or her accountable to a specific job-hunting schedule. It is often hard to stay motivated and organized without a friendly nudge.
7. Talk about subjects other than unemployment.
8. Encourage the person/family to relax and have fun. If you are a friend, invite them to your home or give them a gift certificate for dinner and a movie.
9. If the person is a friend or relative, provide practical, but discreet, help, including food, clothing, and finances.

1. **Free agents.** *They seek and find professional and financial independence in a variety of entrepreneurial occupations. Many work alone, out of a home office, and are involved in community services as well as business ventures.* They know how to market talents to the highest and most interesting bidder.
2. **Nomads.** *They have no real loyalty to the job or the boss as they move from one geographic area and job to another. They spot the next trend, find a job at a company, and are ready to move with it.* In their job hopping and hunting, they develop useful contacts and a variety of skills. They take advantage of job opportunities as they arise.
3. **Globalists.** *They travel from time zone to time zone around the world as they work in a borderless economy with their laptop computers. They constantly network, scout out opportunities, and improvise as necessary.*
4. **Niche finders.** *They spot new markets emerging from recent social and economic trends and build, market, and manage a company to capitalize in it.* They are the leaders in the new industry.
5. **Retreads.** *They relish learning and stay abreast of technologic change. Because of their maturity and experience, they will never be without a job.* Self-improvement, helping peers adapt, and reminding younger workers that computer skills are only one facet of the job guarantee that they will never become obsolete.

Client Education

Career Track Options in Late Middle Age

COAST INTO RETIREMENT

Do the job but no more; collect the paycheck; enjoy the final years.

GO FOR LAST PROMOTION

Campaign to obtain final reward for all that was contributed to receive public acknowledgment of the importance of work done.

TRY FOR GREAT ACHIEVEMENT

Work to outdo the present record and others' records so that others will see you saved the best for last.

SURVIVE DIFFICULT PERIOD

Recognize the company's difficult period; learn to survive and even prosper in the challenging time.

RETIRE EARLY

Take the attractive package being offered by the company so that the years of later maturity can be enjoyed.

START YOUR OWN BUSINESS

If tired of working for others, go into business for self (e.g., consulting in work arena, turning hobby into business).

6. **Corporate leaders.** *New-age bosses redesign jobs to incorporate new skills and ventures. They give workers freedom to maneuver as needed to keep valuable employees. They expand responsibilities for self and others as they dream up new projects.*

But whatever the category, for employed Americans, a lot of time goes to working for a living. The time spent at the full-time job has increased over the past two decades. There is a decline in leisure for some people. Many feel that they are overworked and have insufficient time for family. For some, the ideal playground is the workplace. All sorts of workers carry cell phones or pagers; business-related calls come in constantly. It can be difficult in some jobs to keep up with voice mail and e-mail, let alone necessary reading. The Baby Boomers declared their contempt for "the man in the gray flannel suit": the company-oriented worker. However, they have done more than any other generation to erase the line between work and private life in many professions, managerial jobs, or careers. Work has forced the middle-ager to develop and expand skills beyond what was considered possible to accomplish (16, 148).

Many middle-aged females work outside of the home. Thus, they are especially in the middle (the "sandwich generation") in terms of the demands of various roles on their time and energy: wife, mother, homemaker, grandmother, worker, and organization member. Females who are caregivers may have quit their jobs or have work conflicts. *The middle-aged female is often in the middle in terms of two competing values:* (a) traditional care of elders as a family responsibility and (b) autonomy, to be free to work outside the home as desired. Each family member feels the repercussions as the balance of roles and responsibilities changes.

Most middle-aged females are working today for a variety of reasons (16, 135, 148):

1. Inflation and the rising cost of living
2. Changes in attitudes about gender-appropriate roles
3. The rising divorce rate that forces females to become economically independent

Practice Point

As a professional person, you will have to resolve conflicts related to your work role. Hence, you are in a position to assist the middle-aged person in talking about and resolving feelings and values related to work and other activity. As a professional, you may integrate a sense of leisure and enjoyment with work, as described in Chapter 14. ∞ Share that attitude with the middle-aged client.

4. Fewer children in the home
5. Use of labor-saving devices for the home
6. Increasing educational levels that stimulate career interests or the desire to remain in the profession
7. Expectancy of a higher standard of living
8. Assistance with costs of sending children to college

Discuss the degree of work stability, extent to which work is satisfying, and emotional factors that have operated in the person's concept of work and in the self-concept. Explore the middle-aged person's view of personal mental and physical health. Because the demands on middle-aged adults are often overwhelming—work, home, family, church, and social and civic organizations—teach steps for effective time management. Utilize the **Box** Client Education: Guidelines for Time Management for counseling and education of the middle-ager.

Retirement

Some people in this era retire early by plan. The life decade of the 50s is a point of transition in development of consciousness about retirement. *Baby Boomers perceive themselves working well beyond the usual retirement age, related to* (3, 70): (a) views of self and society, (b) desire to contribute and avoid boredom, and (c) being financially prepared for later life.

Client Education

Guidelines for Time Management

1. Establish priorities; maintain a log if necessary. *Write goals.*
2. *Do it now.* Do not procrastinate with small tasks; schedule large projects.
3. Recognize *unpleasant tasks; work on them first.*
4. *Clear the decks and desks.* Eliminate clutter; organize the workplace for efficiency.
5. *Stick to the job.* Avoid distractions.
6. *Do one thing at a time.* Finish one major task before beginning another; however, *there are times you can do two things at once,* for example, planning while waiting in line.
7. *Plan ahead.* Assemble what is needed for a task before initiating it; set aside relaxation time.
8. *Consider limitations—your own,* equipment not available for a project, and other responsibilities that will interfere.
9. *Learn to say "no" and suggest someone else* who would be able to handle the situation. Delegate low-priority jobs to others.
10. *Anticipate delays* that are inevitable in every task; plan for interruptions and unforeseen events.
11. *Plan on alternative way* to do the job; have backup activity if a selected task cannot be done as scheduled.
12. *Use odd times.* Shop when stores are not crowded; carry a notebook to jot ideas while you wait.

Middle-aged persons least likely to anticipate retirement include those who (10, 36, 135, 148):

1. Work in a company that is prospering.
2. Have unfinished agendas at work.
3. Have high job satisfaction.
4. Perceive retirement as unfeasible because they have not done advance financial (or emotional) planning.
5. Retain their health.

Retirement will have to come eventually. Utilize **Box 15-4**, Suggestions for Planning for Early Retirement, for client education.

Explore with the person various options to prepare for retirement—at age 55, 62, 65, 70, or 75. Assist the person to examine risks or the worst possible scenario if an option is chosen. Examine what it will take in effort and ability to make the option happen, strategies to fall back on if the option is not successful, and the support system (financial, emotional, and social) to ensure success. Discuss personal willingness both to take the risks and to enjoy the benefits. A part of planning for retirement is to study the financial plans that go with each option to ensure, to the extent possible, financial security in old age.

Leadership Role

The middle-aged adult's cognitive stage is in favor of him or her being a formal or informal leader, if other factors are favorable. Usually middle-aged leaders have developed necessary qualities from childhood on, but occasionally a person does not believe that he or she has this ability until there is a measure of success in life work.

The leader demonstrates the following characteristics (36, 192):

1. Utilizes socioeconomic resources; accurately assesses resources.
2. Attains higher level of education or success than majority of group to be led.
3. Sets a good behavioral example.
4. Expresses realistic self-concept, self-confidence, and optimism.

BOX 15-4 Suggestions for Planning for Early Retirement

1. Start planning early. Most successful early retirees have long-range plans in place before they reach 40.
2. Stay with a good employer. Unless you are sure you can strike it rich on your own, work for secure companies with generous pension plans. Avoid excessive job hopping so you can accrue substantial pension benefits.
3. Make use of employer-sponsored investment programs. Place a percentage of your paycheck into tax-deferred plans. Participate to the maximum. You will have age restrictions to begin withdrawing without penalty.
4. Save and invest wisely in other plans—bonds, stocks, property, other annuities, IRAs. You cannot count on Social Security or a company pension. You may have to live off savings. You will need between 60% and 80% of pre-retirement income.
5. Plan for medical bills. Unless you have an early retirement package that extends your health coverage, you will need to factor in high insurance premiums until Medicare begins to cover costs.
6. Scale back your lifestyle. There are many ways to do this. You might buy a smaller house, forgo extravagant vacations, or send your children to public colleges instead of Ivy League schools.
7. Explore career directions you can pursue later in life. You may want to work a few months a year or hours a week. Some individuals have turned a hobby into a way to make money.
8. Mentally prepare yourself. Assess your values, goals, and aspirations and relate them to how you would like to live given more time and sufficient income.

5. Expresses realistic goals and a vision; has ability to encourage others toward those goals.
6. Exudes high frustration tolerance; has high energy level.
7. Praises and reinforces others' behavior and ideas.
8. Expresses negative thoughts tactfully; establishes trust.
9. Accepts success or failure gracefully.
10. Delegates authority; inspires risk taking and making hard decisions.
11. Understands group needs; creates atmosphere of positive energy.
12. Is flexible in meeting group needs.

The middle-aged person may demonstrate this leadership ability on the job or in community or church organizations. Females who are most successful in leadership careers are those who have little conflict in the multiple roles of career woman, mother, wife, and organizational/church member. Their husband's support and encouragement are major assets, but they are also assertive on their own behalf about their roles outside the home.

Single females are frequently in professional or career and community leadership roles, if they desire. Or they may be supportive to designated leaders or an informal leader in the work or social group.

Leisure time can be devoted to volunteer activities. Regular volunteer activity contributes to physical, emotional, and social health. Volunteer activities may have to be focused for the busy middle-ager, but such activity is useful to the community as well as the individual (170). There are multiple needs and opportunities in any community from which the middle-ager can choose. Such activity is preparation for the use of time in the retirement years.

Encourage or reaffirm the middle-aged person in the leadership role. Assist the person to work through feelings or conflicts related to the work setting or the job itself.

Leisure

Leisure *refers to the pleasant times when the person can pursue his or her choice of activities, hobbies, and interests* (165). The midlife couple may pursue some leisure activities together, and each may engage in personal interests separately.

Leisure time has useful functions (22, 36, 63):

1. Foster branching of dendrites and neurons, through neuronal use, as shown by MRI.
2. Enhance mental clarity, especially through challenging cognitive activities, games, and other leisure activities at least 4 times a week.
3. Promote a sense of mastery, self-control, positive outlook, and sense of accomplishment, which strengthens the immune system.
4. Lower blood pressure; improve physical functions by reducing stress responses.
5. Reduce anxiety and depression through effect on neurotransmitters.
6. Improve quality of life perceptions.

The middle-aged person, taught little about how to enjoy free time, may be faced with increasing amounts of leisure time because of advances in technology, earlier retirement, and increased

longevity. The average midlife adult who has moved up the pay scale and whose children may be grown will have more money and more time to take trips or try new hobbies.

Factors that hinder the late middle-ager in use of these new opportunities include the following (135, 148):

1. The value of work rather than leisure was learned in younger years.
2. The cultural emphasis is on intellectual pursuits. Play is considered childish and a poor use of time and talents.
3. The person was taught at home, in school, or on the job to at least appear busy.
4. The person may fear that leisure will create regression, reducing the desire to return to work.
5. A lack of previous opportunity prevented learning creative pursuits or hobbies.
6. There may be hesitation to try something new because of fear of failure.

In an **age-integrated society,** such as in the United States, *all kinds of roles—learning, working, and playing—are open to adults of all ages.* In midlife, these roles are increasingly integrated (135). In a study of 12,338 males, ages 35 to 57 years, over a 5-year period, data were collected about use of vacation time. Analysis of medical and death records over 9 years for males who lived at least one year past the last vacation, compared to males who never took vacations, revealed that males who took annual vacations were 31% less likely to die within the 9-year period and 32% less likely to die of coronary heart disease (108, 148).

Help the person avoid feelings of alienation that result from inability to use leisure time. Review functions of leisure. Explore social networks. Use the suggestions in **Box 15-5,** Teaching Use of Leisure in the Daily Schedule, for education of middle-aged clients. Emphasize that leisure activities can be good preparation for retirement.

EMOTIONAL DEVELOPMENT

Emotions are rooted in the neural structures known as the limbic system. Strong negative emotions originate in the **amygdala,** *a pair of almond-shaped limbic structures near the center of the brain* (63). The amygdala function seems to change with age. The late middle-ager demonstrates less evidence of fear, anger, and hatred than does the young adult. As the person matures, the behavior is less impulsive in response to emotion and the focus is less on negative feelings. Thus, the person becomes a better leader and mentor and less a loner (22).

The middle years, the climacteric, are a period of self-assessment and greater introspection—a transitional period. In middle age (and beyond) the person perceives life as time left to live rather than time since birth (39, 125, 127–129). Time is seen as finite; death is a possibility. Middle-aged adults clock themselves by their positions in different life contexts—changes in body, family, career—rather than by chronologic age (166). *Time is seen in two ways* (76, 125, 137): (a) time to finish what the person wants to do, and (b) how much meaning and pleasure can be obtained in the time that is left. The person makes the often agonizing reappraisal of how achievements measure up against goals and of the entire sys-

BOX 15-5	Teaching Use of Leisure in the Daily Schedule

1. Emphasize that play and recreation are essential to a healthy life.
2. Stress the indispensability of leisure as a part of many activities, whether work or creative endeavors. Leisure is both a state of mind and use of time away from work.
3. Have the person analyze leisure activities, whether they bring pleasure, work off frustration, make up deficits in life, or create a sense of pressure or competition.
4. Help the person recognize the interplay of physical and intellectual endeavors and their contribution to mental health.
5. Differentiate compulsive, competitive, and aggressive work and play from healthy, natural work and play. Intrinsic in play are spontaneity, flexibility, creativity, zest, and joy.
6. Recognize the person's creative efforts to encourage further involvement in leisure activities.
7. Educate the person about the importance of preparing for retirement.
8. Inform the person of places, courses, or workshops at which he or she can learn new creative skills and use of talents.
9. Encourage the person to enjoy change, to participate in organizations, and to initiate stimulating contacts with others.
10. Encourage the person to stop the activity when it no longer meets personal needs.

Information taken from references 37, 93.

tem of values. He or she can no longer dream of infinite possibilities. The person is forced to acknowledge personal capabilities. Goals may or may not have been reached. Aspirations may have to be modified. The person will have to go on with ever-brighter, ever-younger people crowding into the competitive economic, political, and social arena (113). In the United States, success is highly valued and is measured by prestige, wealth, or power. To be without these by late middle age causes stress, and the likelihood of achieving them diminishes with age. However, the middle-aged adult is perceived as a valuable worker and volunteer because of the experience and knowledge he or she can contribute (36).

Educate the person and family about normal changes and benefits of interpersonal relationships. Emphasize exercise and leisure strategies previously discussed that can enhance intellectual power and emotional development, and thereby the branching of neurons. Reinforce the importance of social relationships.

Developmental Crisis: Generativity Versus Stagnation or Self-Absorption

The psychosexual crisis of middle age, according to Erikson (38, 39, 163), is generativity versus self-absorption and stagnation. **Generativity** *is a concern about providing for others that is equal to*

the concern of providing for the self. *It is a sense of parenthood and creativity; of being involved in establishing and guiding the next generation, the arts, or a profession; and of feeling needed and being important to the welfare of humankind* (39). The person can assume the responsibility of parenthood. As a husband or wife, each can see the strengths and weaknesses of the other and combine their energies toward common goals. A biological parent does not necessarily get to the psychosocial stage of generativity, and the unmarried person or the person without children can be very generative.

The **generative middle-ager** *takes on the major work of providing for others, directly or indirectly. There is a sense of enterprise, productivity, mastery, charity, altruism, and perseverance. The greatest bulk of social problems and needs falls on this person who can handle the responsibilities because of personal strengths, vigor, and experience. There is a strong feeling of care and concern for that which has been produced by love, necessity, or accident* (38, 39). He or she can collaborate with others to do the necessary work. Ideas about personal needs and goals converge with an understanding of the social community, and the ideas guide actions taken on behalf of future generations.

The **generative person** *feels a sense of comfort or ease in lifestyle. There is realistic gratification from a job well done and from what has been given to others. He or she accepts self and the body,* realizing that although acceptance of self is originally based on acceptance from others, unless there is self-acceptance, he or she cannot really expect acceptance from others.

The generative middle-aged adult may be a mentor to a young adult. A **mentor** *is an adult with experience, wisdom, patience, and understanding who befriends, guides, and counsels a less experienced and younger adult in the work world or in a social or an educational situation.*

The mentor has the following roles (28, 113, 120, 184, 185):

Advisor	Tutor	Protector
Guide	Advocate	Friend
Sponsor	Role model	Evaluator

Mentoring *involves developing a long-term relationship with many roles.* The mentor is usually approximately 10 years older; is confident, warm, flexible, and trustworthy; enjoys sharing knowledge and skills; and promotes psychosocial development and success of the younger person. The mentor is found in business, management, nursing, or other careers or professions. The mentor sponsors the younger person as an associate, creates a social heir, teaches him or her as much as possible for promotion into a position, or recommends the one being mentored for advancement. The current middle-aged mentor is also aware that some younger people are resistive to the idea of being mentored. *The young adult may* (113): (a) highly value autonomy, (b) believe he or she knows more than the mentor or perceive self as capable of learning what is required and achieving without help, or (c) perceive that the mentor is too traditional and inflexible for the current demands. Several authors present more information on mentoring (28, 113, 120, 158, 184, 185).

With midlife generativity, there is an expansion of interests and investment in responsibilities. The image of one's finite existence is in view; the person consciously reappraises and uses self. With introspection, the self seems less important, and the words *service, love of others,* and *compassion* gain new meaning. These concepts motivate action in church work, social causes, community fund drives, cultural or artistic efforts, a profession, or political work. The person is often a leader. The person's goal is to leave the world a better place in which to live. Thus, the person must come to terms with violations of the moral codes of society (e.g., tax loopholes used by some adults) and, with superego and ego in balance, develop a constructive philosophy and an honest method of operation.

Some middle-aged adults believe the most important work of the person begins after parenthood ceases. *Contributions are cognitive and emotional in nature:* (a) preserving culture, (b) maintaining the annals of history, (c) keeping alive human judgment, (d) maintaining human skills, (e) preserving and skillfully contriving the instruments of civilization, and (f) teaching all this to oncoming generations. Although young and middle-aged adults are involved in such functions, these qualities of the human mind are best manifested in the late middle years or thereafter.

The mature and generative middle-aged person has tested ways of doing things. He or she draws on experience, and may have deep sincerity, mature judgment, and a sense of empathy. A sense of values or a philosophy underlying life gives a sense of stability, reflection, and caution. The person recognizes that one of the most generative things he or she can give to society is the way life is led. Consider the following statement by a 50-year-old male:

> *Those were full years—raising the kids with all its joy and frustration. I'm glad they're on their own now. This is a new stage of life. I can go fishing; Mary can go out to lunch. We have more time together for fun, and now we have more time for working at the election polls and in volunteer activities.*

A sense of **stagnation** or **self-absorption** enshrouds the person if the developmental task of generativity is not achieved (38, 39). He or she regresses to adolescent or younger behavior, characterized by physical and psychological decline or invalidism. This person hates the aging body and feels neither secure nor adept at handling self physically or interpersonally. He or she has little to offer even if so inclined. He or she operates on a slim margin and soon burns out. See **Box 15-6**, Assessment of Consequences of Self-Absorption. Consider the following statement by a 50-year-old female:

> *I spent all those years raising the kids and doing housework while Bob moved up the professional ladder. We talked less and less about each other, only about the kids or his job. Now the kids are gone. I should be happy, but I'm lost. I can't carry on a decent conversation with Bob. I don't have any training for a job. And I look terrible! I sit around and eat too much. I wear high collars to hide my wrinkled neck, and no cosmetics really hide the dark circles under my eyes.*

Immature adults have impaired and less socially organized intellectual skills and value systems. The immature person seeks self-absorption and avoids concern about the problems of others (38, 39, 125, 163). Yet the characteristics of the self-absorbed person are health-endeavoring attempts and reparative efforts to cope or

---

BOX 15-6 | **Assessment of Consequences of Self-Absorption**

1. Denial of signs of normal aging
2. Unhappiness with advancing age, desire to stay young, fear of growing old
3. Regression to inappropriate youthfulness in dress or behavior, rebelliousness, foolish behavior
4. Preoccupation with self, self-indulgence
5. Physical, emotional, social, and interpersonal insecurity
6. Attempts to prove youthfulness with infidelity to spouse
7. Resignation, passivity, noninvolvement with societal or life issues
8. Isolation or withdrawal from others
9. Despair about signs of aging (considers self old, life is over)
10. Either overcompliance or excessive rigidity in behavior
11. Intolerance, cynicism, ruthless attitude
12. Lack of stamina, chronic health problems that are not coped with
13. Chronic defeatism, depression

---

adapt. These characteristics may or may not work well, depending on the intensity of personality characteristics and the social and physical environment.

Maturity

Because **maturity**, *being holistically developed as a person,* is not a quality of life reached at any one age or for all time, the characteristics described as generativity are general guidelines. *Maturity is doing what is appropriate for age, situation, and culture.* As the person grows older, the ideal level of maturity and autonomy may recede further into the future and never be fully achieved (38, 39, 69). *Maturity is the achievement of efficiently organized psychic growth predicated on integration of experiences of solving environmentally stimulated conflicts.* The external environment is a potent force on the person; conflicts are primarily socially incurred. The psychosocial organization in maturity shows a cultural direction. As one ages, the psychic interests broaden and are less selfish. Part of maturity is **staying power**, *the power to see it through, which is different from starting power.* Seeing it through is to use faith and persistence, to continue even against great odds to stand firm in the face of opposition at a crucial time.

Characteristics of staying power include to:

1. Demonstrate integrity of consciousness and personhood.
2. Remain loyal to values, faith, philosophy, and beliefs.
3. Hold to a cause greater than self, being intolerant of negative or evil forces.
4. Give up something worthwhile rather than worrying about present risks.

The **mature adult** *is reflective, restructures or processes information in the light of experience, and uses knowledge and expertise in a directed way to achieve desired ends.* No one reaches the highest ideal of self-actualization described by Maslow and summarized in

Assessment Criteria of Emotional Maturity

1. Ability to deal constructively with reality
2. Capacity to adapt to change
3. Relative freedom from symptoms that are produced by tensions and anxieties
4. Capacity to find more satisfaction in giving than receiving
5. Capacity to relate to other people in a consistent manner with mutual satisfaction and helpfulness
6. Capacity to sublimate, to direct one's instinctive hostile energy into creative and constructive outlets
7. Capacity to love
8. Ability to use intuition, a natural mental ability associated with experience, to comprehend life events and formulate answers.

Chapter 1. ∞ Yet each can reach his or her own ideal and peak of well-being, functioning relatively free of anxieties, cognitive distortions, and rigid habits and with a sense of the uniqueness of the self and others (128).

In adulthood there is no one set of appropriate personality characteristics. You will work with many personality types as you promote health. Explore generativity and maturity with middle-aged clients and others in the community. Relate to a definition of health. Utilize information in this section. Refer also to **Box 15-7**, Assessment of Criteria of Emotional Maturity.

Personality Development

Emotional or personality development has also been described by the stage theorists: Jung (76, 83), Sheehy (155–157), Gould (58–60), Levinson (99–101), and Vaillant (181, 182). Other authors have also described aspects of personality development (22, 32, 39, 69, 95, 111, 126, 136, 166).

Jung *divided personality development to correspond to the first and second halves of the life cycle.* In the **first half**, *until the age of 35 or 40, the person is in a period of expansion.* Maturational forces direct the growth of the **ego** (*the conscious or awareness of self and the external world*). Capacities unfold for dealing with the external world. The person learns to get along with others and tries to win as many of society's rewards as possible. A career and family are established. To achieve, it is usually necessary for males to overdevelop their masculinity and for females to overemphasize their feminine traits and skills. The young person dedicates self to mastery of the outer world. Being preoccupied with self-doubt, fantasy, and the inner nature is not advantageous to the young adult, for the task is to meet the demands of society confidently and assertively (76, 83). In the **second half**, *beginning in the late 40s, the personality begins to undergo a transformation. The person begins to become introspective, to turn inward, to examine the meaning of life.* Earlier goals and ambitions have lost their meaning. The person may feel stagnant, incomplete, or depressed, as if something crucial is missing, even if the person has been quite successful, because success has often been achieved at the cost of personality develop-

ment. Separating self from ordinary conformity to the goals and values of mass society and achieving a measure of psychic balance are accomplished through **individuation**—*finding one's individual way* (76, 83).

Jung recognized that *although middle-aged persons begin to turn inward, they still have much energy and resources for the generativity described by Erikson and for making personal changes.* The person may begin new or long-forgotten projects and interests or even change careers. Males and females begin giving expression to their opposite sexual drives. Males become less aggressively ambitious and more concerned with interpersonal relationships. They begin to realize that achievement counts for less and friendship for more. Females tend to become more aggressive and independent. Such changes can create midlife marital problems. Although ongoing development may create tension and difficulties, Jung believed that the greatest failures come when adults cling to the goals and values of the first half of life, holding on to the glories and beauty of youth (76, 83).

Neugarten (126–128) found personality characteristics in middle age similar to those described by Jung (76).

Sheehy (155–157), **Gould** (58–60), **Levinson** (99–101), and **Vaillant** (181, 182) also describe *midlife stages of development.* See **Table 15-5**, Levinson's Theory of Mid-Adulthood. These stage theorists confirm many of the characteristics already described and emphasize that this is a time of new stability and authenticity.

As you work with the middle-aged person, use the concept of generativity versus self-absorption in assessment of the client's developmental level. Promote generative or altruistic behavior through your listening, support, encouragement of activities, teaching, counseling, and referral to organizations and causes that can use the person's contribution of talents, time, and financial resources. The generative person or mentor needs to hear that what he or she is doing is indeed a worthwhile contribution. Your reinforcement of another's strengths facilitates further emotional development and maturity. The self-absorbed person should be referred to a long-term counselor.

BODY IMAGE DEVELOPMENT

The gradually occurring physical changes described earlier confront the person and are mirrored in others. The climacteric causes realignment of attitudes about the self that cut into the personality and its definition. Other life stresses cause the person to view self and the body differently. The person not only realizes he or she looks older but subjectively may feel older as well. Work can bring a sense of stress if he or she feels less stamina and vigor to cope with the task at hand. Illness or death of loved ones creates a concern about personal health, sometimes to excess, and thoughts about one's own death are more frequent. The person begins to realize that the previous self-image of the youthful, strong, and healthy body with boundless energy does not fit. Depression, irritability, and anxiety about femininity and masculinity may result. In the United States, more than in European or Asian cultures, youth and vigor are highly valued, a carryover from frontier days. The person's previous personality largely influences the intensity of these feelings and the symptoms associated with body image changes. Difficulties are also caused by fear of the effects of the climacteric, folklore about sexuality, attitudes

TABLE 15-5

Levinson's Theory of Mid-Adulthood

Age Range	Life Structure
40–65	Reevaluate match between self-concept and achievements; are senior members in community; assume responsibility for next generation.
45–50	Enter middle adulthood bridge between past and future.
50–55	Age 50 transition; take stock of self in relation to family and occupation.
55–60	Culminate life plans and structure for middle age; new level of stability; may be peak of career.
60–65	Lake adult transition; prepare for aging.
65 and beyond	Late adulthood.

Source: Adapted from references 99–101.

toward womanhood, social and advertising pressures in our culture, and emphasis on obsolescence.

Most people gradually adjust to their slowly changing body and accept the changes as part of maturity. The mature person realizes it is impossible to return to youth. To imitate youth denies the mature person's own past and experience. The excitement of the middle years lies in using adeptly the acquired experience, insights, values, and realism. The middle-aged person feels good about self. Healthy signs are that he or she prefers this age and has no desire to relive the youthful years.

Promote integration of a positive body image through your communication skills and teaching. Reaffirm to the client the strengths of being middle-aged, using information presented in this chapter. Emphasize the specific strengths of the person in your education and counseling. Validate the person's positive self-image. Support the person's attempts to identify and work at improving attributes, as appropriate.

Emphasize that cosmetic surgery based on body-image issues should be done after careful assessment and by a highly qualified surgeon who incorporates the psychological dimension through collaboration with a multidisciplinary team. Some invasive procedures or poor surgical techniques could leave the person looking less attractive. Even worse, function or life could be jeopardized. There are no significant complications most of the time. Reinforce that the person determine, perhaps with loved ones, whether any cosmetic surgery is necessary and whether the procedure would accomplish health promotion goals. Benefits versus risks, aftereffects of surgery, long-term effects for health and appearance, and additional procedures that may be necessary should be discussed by the client with the primary care provider, surgeon, other health team members, and individuals who have had the same surgery (27).

ADAPTIVE MECHANISMS

The adult may use any of the adaptive mechanisms described in previous chapters. Adaptive mechanisms and the superego are strong but not rigid. **Adult socialization** is *the processes through which an adult learns to perform the roles and behaviors expected of self and by others and to remain adaptive in a variety of situations.* The middle-aged adult is expected and normally considers self to be adaptive. The emphasis is on active, reciprocal participation of the person. Little preparation is directed to anticipating, accepting, or coping with failure. The ability to shift emotional investments from one activity to another, to remain open-minded, and to use past experience as a guide rather than as the rule is closely related to adaptive ability (39).

The adult, having been rewarded for certain behaviors over the years, has established a wide variety of role-related behaviors, problem-solving techniques, adaptations to stress, and methods for making role transitions. These behaviors may not be adaptive to current demands or crises or to increasing role diffusion. There is a continuous need for socialization in adulthood, for a future orientation, for anticipating events, and for learning to respond to new demands (39). Ongoing learning of adult roles occurs through observation, imitation, or identification with another; trial-and-error behavior; the media and books; or formal education.

Coping or adaptive mechanisms used in response to the emotional stress depend on the person's (a) capacity to adapt and satisfy personal needs, (b) sense of identity, (c) nature of interaction with others, (d) sense of usefulness, and (e) interest in the outside world. The middle-aged adult must be able to channel emotional drives without losing initiative and vigor. *During middle age the person is especially vulnerable to a number of disrupting events:* (a) physiologic changes and illness in self and loved ones, (b) family stresses, (c) changes in job or role demands or responsibilities, (d) conflict between family generations, and (e) societal changes.

Counsel the middle-aged adult to prevent or overcome maladaptive mechanisms. Extend empathy and reinforce the person's sense of emotional maturity and health. Validate that the person is able to cope with life stressors and work through perceived failures. Use principles and techniques of stress management and implement crisis intervention described in Chapter 2. ∞ If you feel unable to listen to or work with the problems of someone who may be twice your age, refer the person to a counselor.

MIDLIFE CRISIS

Middle age can be seen as a developmental transition or a developmental crisis. **Midlife crisis** *refers to a major and revolutionary turning point in one's life, involving changes in commitments to career or spouse and children and accompanied by significant and ongoing*

INTERVENTIONS FOR HEALTH PROMOTION

Validate the healthy middle-ager by teaching that the healthy and adaptive person:

1. Copes with ordinary personal upheavals and life's frustrations and disappointments with only temporary disequilibrium.
2. Participates enthusiastically in adult work and play.
3. Experiences adequate satisfaction in a stable relationship.
4. Expresses a reasonable amount of aggression, anger, joy, and affection without unnecessary guilt or lack of adequate control.
5. Retains a sense of balance by recognizing that each life era has its unique joys and charms, and is valued as precious.
6. Appreciates what is past, anticipates the future, and maintains a sense of permanence or stability.
7. Adapts successfully to the stresses of middle age by achieving the developmental crisis.
8. Serves as a role model of maturity.

emotional turmoil for both the individual and others. The term **midlife transition** *has a different meaning; it includes aspects of crisis, process, change, and alternating periods of stability and transition* (22, 135, 148, 155).

For some, midlife is one of the better periods of life, it is a transition from youth to later maturity. Life expectancy is longer, psychologically and physically. Midlife is healthier than ever in history. Parental responsibilities are decreasing. The couple has more time to be together without the obligations of child rearing. The couple realizes that the myth of decreasing sexual powers is not true. Females in midlife may begin or continue their education, profession, or career. Males see midlife as a time of continuing achievement. Experience, assurance, substance, skill, success, and good judgment more than compensate for the disappearance of youthful looks and physical abilities.

Midlife is seen as a crisis if the person has not resolved the identity crisis of adolescence and achieved mature intimacy in young adulthood; fears the passage of time, physical changes, aging, and mortality; or cannot handle the meaning of life's routines and changes. Midlife crisis is *not* universal but is more common in the male.

The person may declare that he or she is bored. The nagging feeling that all is not right within the self and with the world can become a way to avoid facing the challenges that are presented by a deepening self-awareness and a sense of personal immaturities or failures. Although many areas of life can be a source of boredom, the two most blamed as tedious and unsatisfying are marriage and work. Leaving either one may be a practical solution to a nagging expediency that was only partially satisfying. Often, however, the joblessness or job change or the affair or divorce is a headlong flight from aging. The new freedom may be found equally stressful and full of rejection, competition, loneliness, meaninglessness, and personal dissatisfaction with the new routines. Often the structure and tedium of work or marriage look comfortable, pleasant, and meaningful only after either situation has been left behind. The identity crisis, when it is over, is seen to have been a denial of reality, not a new level of maturity.

Family experiences are undoubtedly integral to the direction of the midlife crisis. The midlife transition for males, often the husbands of menopausal females, brings new stresses. Adolescent children may be sexually and aggressively provocative, challenging, or disappointing. Children leaving home for school or marriage change the family balance. Having no children can be a keen disappointment; there are no heirs. Some females refocus on their own development. The female may exert more independence or develop occupational skills. Self-image may change after childbearing is completed. These behavioral and role changes may be very threatening to the male. In essence, the midlife crisis involves internal upheaval.

You can be instrumental in assisting the person in working through this crisis to avoid escape into psychosomatic illness, alcoholism, and psychiatric illness. It is healthier in the long range for the person to acknowledge the disruptive feelings and the diffusion of identity, to work through them rather than deny them, and to seek a healthy and constructive outlet for these feelings. You may refer the person to a counselor who can work with the individual and family.

MORAL-SPIRITUAL DEVELOPMENT

The middle-aged person continues to integrate new concepts from widened sources into a religious philosophy if he or she has gained the spiritual maturity described in Chapter 14. ∞ He or she becomes less dogmatic in beliefs. Faith and trust in God or another source of spiritual strength are increased. Religion offers comfort and happiness. For example, the person is able to deal effectively with the spiritual meaning or religious aspects of upcoming surgery and its possible effects, illness, death of parents, or unexpected tragedy.

The middle-aged person may have become alienated from organized religion in early adulthood or may have drifted away from religious practices and spiritual study because of familial, occupational, and social role responsibilities. As the person becomes more introspective, studies self and life from new perspectives, ponders the meaning of life, and faces crises, he or she is likely to return to study of religious literature, practices of former years, and organized religious groups for strength, comfort, forgiveness, and joy. Spiritual beliefs and religion take on added importance. The middle-aged adult who becomes revived spiritually is likely to remain devout and active in demonstration of faith throughout life. If the person does not deepen spiritual insights, a sense of meaninglessness and despair is likely in old age.

INTERVENTIONS FOR HEALTH PROMOTION

Utilize cognitive-behavioral statements as you counsel or educate the person or family in mid-life crisis:

1. Do not be scared by the midlife crisis. Physical and psychological changes are normal throughout life; see them as opportunities for maturing. Promote positive feelings in self and spouse.
2. Face feelings and goals realistically. If confused or depressed, see a counselor who can help sort through feelings and goals.
3. See age as a positive asset. Acknowledge strengths. Take steps to adjust to liabilities or to correct them.
4. Reconcile self to the fact that some or many hopes and dreams may never be realized and may not be attainable. Remain open to the opportunities that are available; they may exceed dreams.
5. Consider another job or another career, if the job is not satisfying, after appraising self realistically. Or be willing to relinquish some responsibility at work. Take time to make career changes; avoid being impulsive.
6. Plan for retirement financially, and for leisure and other activities.
7. Seek outlets through recreational activities or other diversions if job pressures are great. Become involved in community service, and renew spiritual study and religious affiliations.
8. Renew old friendships and initiate new ones. Invest in others and, in the process, enhance personal self-esteem and emotional well-being.
9. Try to be flexible and open-minded rather than dogmatic or inflexible in solving problems.

10. If concerned about sexual potency, realize that the problem is typically transient. Talk about sexual feelings and concerns with the spouse. The love and concern you have for each other can frequently overcome any impotency. It is important for the female to perceive sexuality apart from childbearing and menstruation and for the male to perceive sexuality apart from having children and love affairs. If so inclined, together read "how-to" sex manuals to maintain spontaneity. Seek a marriage counselor to work out problems of sexual dysfunction or seek medical treatment, if necessary.
11. Share your feelings, concerns, frustrations, and problems with the spouse or confidante. Undisclosed feelings can increase alienation and the difficulty of repairing the relationship. Be attuned to nonverbal messages of the spouse and self.
12. Examine attitudes as a parent; strike a balance between care and protection of offspring. Realize their normal need for independence.
13. Realize that frequently the middle-aged female is becoming more assertive just when the middle-aged male is becoming more passive. Talking about these changes can help the spouses better understand each other's needs and aspirations.
14. Get a physical examination to ensure that physical symptoms are not indicators of illness.
15. Seek counseling for psychological symptoms. The counselor may be a nurse, religious leader, mental health therapist, social worker, marriage counselor, psychologist, or psychiatrist.

The Baby Boomer cohort is the first U.S. generation to be born into mass societal affluence, schooled in self-importance, and generally unaware of self-sacrifice. Generally material comforts have been taken for granted. Certainly not all individuals are affluent, and many have entered professions of caring for people. Values and behavior range the full continuum from narcissism to making generative contributions to people and society. Some feel a spiritual longing which was not fulfilled by political activism, sexual freedom, and expensive tastes. Some have tried illicit drugs to gain a transcendental experience, which did not achieve maturity but did result in addictions, lost cognitive abilities, and even death. New ideas were introduced by this generation—new forms of meditation, scientology, and other spiritual movements, including forms of mass worship. Megachurches have emerged, with a variety of worship options. Most Christian denominations offer informal and traditional worship services. Christian and Jewish faith communities offer a variety of activities to accommodate the Baby Boomers' demand for autonomy, freedom of choice, and personal involvement. Late middle-age Boomers have barely begun to consider seriously the end of their own life and what prior generations called "meeting my Maker." At some point they will have to sort out who or what is their "Maker" (2, 3, 76).

Moral and spiritual development is advanced whenever the person has an experience of sustained responsibility for the welfare of others. Middle age, if it is lived generatively, provides such an experience. Although the cognitive awareness of higher principles of living develops in adolescence, consistent commitment to their ethical applications develops in adulthood after the person has had time and opportunity to meet personal needs and to establish self in the family and community. Further, the level of cognitive development sets the upper limits for moral potential. If the adult remains in the Stage of Concrete Operations, he or she is unlikely to move beyond the Conventional Level of moral development (law-and-order reasoning), because the Postconventional Level requires a deep and broad understanding of events and a critical reasoning ability (90).

Kohlberg's work (90) on moral development was done on males. Females, according to Gilligan's theory (53, 54), generally come out at Stage 3 of Kohlberg's Conventional Level. Gilligan

TABLE 15-6

Moral Development in Women

Level	Characteristics
I. Orientation of individual survival	Concentrates on what is practical and best for self
Transition 1: from selfishness to responsibility	Realizes connection to others; thinks of responsible choice in terms of another as well as self
II. Goodness as self-sacrifice	Sacrifices personal wishes and needs to fulfill others' wants and to have others think well of her; feels responsible for others' actions; holds other responsible for her choices, dependent position; indirect efforts to control others often turn into manipulation through use of guilt
Transition 2: from goodness to truth	Makes decisions on personal intentions and consequences of actions rather than on how she thinks others will react; takes into account needs of self and others; wants to be good to others but also honest by being responsible to self
III. Morality of nonviolence	Establishes moral equality between self and others; assumes responsibility for choice in moral dilemmas; follows injunction to hurt no one, including self, in all situations

Source: Reference 52.

emphasizes an interpersonal definition of morality rather than a societal definition of morality or an orientation to law and order. Perhaps the stage of moral development often seen in females, with concern for the well-being of others and a willingness to sacrifice self for others' well-being, is an aspect of Stage 5 of the Postconventional Level, according to Kohlberg's theory, which is summarized in Table 1-10. ∞

Gilligan (53, 54), whose research centered on moral development in females, found they define morality in terms of selfishness versus responsibility. Subjects with high morality scores emphasized the importance of being responsible in behavior and of exercising care with and avoiding hurt to others. Males think more in terms of general justice and fairness; females think in terms of the needs of specific individuals. Gilligan's view of moral development is outlined in **Table 15-6**, Moral Development in Women, according to three levels and the transition points (60).

Loevinger (103) sees middle age as the Autonomous Stage of Ego Development, when the person evolves principles for self apart from the social world. The person deals with the differences between personal needs, principles by which to live, and duties demanded by society.

You may counsel the midlife person or family related to spiritual, moral, or religious concerns. Utilize theoretical knowledge if appropriate. Encourage the person to express ideas and feelings. Realize findings about moral development may depend on the cohort studied.

DEVELOPMENTAL TASKS

Each period of life differs from the others, offering new experiences and opportunities and new tasks to surmount. The developmental tasks of middle age have a biological basis in the gradual aging of the physical body, a cultural basis in social pressures and expectations, and an emotional origin in the individual lifestyle and self-concept that the mature adult has developed.

The following developmental tasks are to be accomplished by the person during and at the end of midlife (34, 39, 127, 128):

1. Maintain or establish healthful life patterns.
2. Discover and develop new satisfactions as a mate or as a close friend. Give support, enjoy joint activities, and develop a sense of unity and intimacy.
3. Help growing and grown children (biological or those of family or friends) to become happy and responsible adults. Relinquish the central position in their affections. Take pride in their accomplishments, stand by to assist as needed, and accept their friends and mates.
4. Create a pleasant, comfortable home, appropriate to values, interests, time, energy, and resources. Give, receive, and exchange hospitality. Take pride in accomplishments of self and spouse, and family members and friends.
5. Find pleasure in generativity and recognition at work, if employed. Gain knowledge, proficiency, and wisdom; be able to lead or follow. Balance work with other roles, and prepare for eventual retirement.
6. Reverse roles with aging parents and parents-in-law, assist them as needed without domineering, and act as a buffer between demands of aging parents and needs of young adults. Prepare emotionally for the eventual death of parents unless they are already deceased.
7. Maintain a standard of living related to values, needs, and financial resources.
8. Achieve mature social and civic responsibility. Be informed as a citizen. Give time, energy, and resources to causes beyond self and home. Work cooperatively with others in the common responsibilities of citizenship. Encourage others in their citizenship. Stand for the welfare of the group as a whole in issues when vested interests may be at stake.
9. Develop or maintain an active organizational membership, deriving from it pleasure and a sense of belonging. Refuse

BOX 15-8	Key Interpersonal Relationships for Never-Married or Divorced Women
Blood ties:	Nieces, nephews, siblings, children, aging parents. Often the woman gives assistance, which involves sacrifice.
Constricted ties:	Affiliation with a nonkin family, establishment of a quasi-parental tie with own child or a younger person who is like a son or daughter; or a long-term relationship with a same-generation companion. These relationships are voluntary and positive, but there is no assurance of care from these individuals.
Quasi-parental relations:	Acting like a parent to younger nonrelatives. There is no biogenetic tie but the relationship is modeled on parent–child tie.
Companionate:	A marriagelike interdependency in which there is much involvement over time and a sense of obligation to care for each other.
Friendship:	A close relationship that endures and provides security. Depending on the duration and closeness, the friend may provide help in time of need.

conflicting or too burdensome invitations with poise. Work through intraorganizational tensions, power systems, and personality problems by becoming a mature statesperson in a diplomatic role, leading when necessary.

10. Accept and adjust to the physical changes of middle age. Attend to personal grooming and relish maturity.

11. Make an art of friendship; cherish old friends and choose new ones. Enjoy an active social life with friends, including friends of both genders and of various ages. Accept at least a few friends into close sharing of feelings to help avoid self-absorption.

12. Use leisure time creatively and with satisfaction, without yielding too much to social pressures and styles. Learn to do some things well enough to become known for them among family, friends, and associates. Enjoy use of talents. Share some leisure time activities with a mate or others. Balance leisure activities: active and passive, collective and solitary, service-motivated and self-indulgent.

13. Acknowledge and confront the psychological sense that the time left for cognitive, creative, emotional, social, and spiritual fulfillment is shorter and that fulfillment may never come.

14. Continue to formulate a philosophy of life and religious or philosophic affiliation. Discover new depths and meanings in God or a Creator that include but also go beyond the fellowship of a particular religious denomination. Gain satisfaction from altruistic activities or the concerns of a particular denomination. Invest self in significant causes and movements and recognize the finiteness of life.

15. Prepare for retirement with financial arrangements and development of hobbies and leisure activities, and rework philosophy and values.

The *single, divorced, or widowed middle-aged person will have basically the same developmental tasks* but must find a sense of intimate sharing with friends or relatives. Utilize **Box 15-8**, Key Interpersonal Relationships for Never-Married or Divorced Women, as you assess and intervene with middle-aged females (147).

Peck (136) sees the issues, conflicts, or tasks the person must work through in middle age as encompassing four aspects:

1. Valuing wisdom gained from living and experience versus valuing physical powers and youth. The person needs to accept his or her age, that youth cannot be regained, and that although physical strength and power may diminish, wisdom may accomplish more than physical strength.

2. Socializing versus sexualizing in human relationships. The middle-aged adult, although still active sexually, now sees and relates to people as humans rather than just on the basis of male or female. The person relates to others without the sexual self-consciousness of adolescence or young adulthood and sees the intrinsic dignity and worth of all people as social and spiritual beings.

3. Emotional flexibility versus emotional impoverishment. The middle-aged adult, although often accused of being rigid and unable to change, remains accepting of and empathic to others, open to people of different backgrounds, and open to changing personal behavior. The person becomes emotionally impoverished only if he or she withdraws from others, avoids learning from experience, refuses to change, or demonstrates the self-absorption described by Erikson (38, 39).

4. Mental flexibility versus mental rigidity. The middle-aged adult, although accused of being closed to new ideas and excessively cautious, remains open to learning and flexible in problem-solving strategies. The person becomes mentally rigid if he or she avoids new experiences or learning opportunities or denies social, educational, or technologic changes.

Through your care, counsel, and teaching, assist the client to be aware of these tasks. Validate concerns. Explore the person's feelings. Suggest options for meeting the tasks.

Transition to Later Maturity

The middle-aged adult has developed a sense of the life cycle (118). Through introspection, he or she has gained a heightened sensitivity to the personal position within a complex social environment. Life is no longer seen as an infinite stretch of time into the future. The person anticipates and accepts the inevitable sequence of events that occur as the human matures, ages, and dies. Gender differences diminish in reality and perception. Personal mortality, achievements, failures, and personal strengths and limits must be faced if the person is to be prepared emotionally and developmentally for later maturity and the personal aging process. The person realizes that the direction in life has been set by decisions related to occupation, marriage, family life, and having or not having children. Although occupation and lifestyle can be changed, at least to some extent, the results of other earlier decisions cannot be changed. The consequences must be faced and resolved. The middle-aged person realizes he or she may not achieve all dreams, but remaining open to opportunities along the way may enable the person to achieve accomplishments never fantasized that are equally meaningful.

For example, if the young adult female focused on career and did not marry and have children, at age 50 she may still marry, but having children—or adoption—is less likely. Having no children means not being a grandparent in old age. The need to be a parent or grandparent or to nurture must be met in another way. The single or childless middle-aged female may realize that she has been nurturing a larger number of people than some middle-agers who focused attention solely on their children.

The person in late midlife realizes that life's developmental markers and crises call forth changes in self-concept and sense of identity, necessitate incorporation of new social roles and behaviors, and precipitate new adaptations. But they do not destroy the sense of continuity within the person from youth to old age. This adaptability and a sense of continuity are essential for the achievement of ego integrity in the last years of life.

Health Promotion and Nursing Applications

ASSESSMENT: A HOLISTIC APPROACH

Information has been presented throughout the chapter as a basis for holistic assessment of the person and family in midlife. Assessment information is synthesized into nursing diagnoses.

NURSING DIAGNOSES

Refer to the **Box** Nursing Diagnoses Related to Middle Age (121). You will formulate other diagnoses as you care for the ill person or work with clients who present multiple health concerns.

INTERVENTIONS TO PROMOTE HEALTH

Your role in intervention with the midlife person and family has been described throughout the chapter. Interventions may involve the health promotion or direct care measures to assist the person and family in meeting physical, emotional, cognitive, spiritual, and social needs.

Focus your intervention on the fact that the momentum of life and multiple societal roles for the middle-ager may leave little time to focus on personal health unless there is an illness crisis. *Family self-care is especially important in this era.* Emphasize that middle-agers role-model and teach young adult offspring and their children about health promotion skills and resources and familial health history.

Examine socioeconomic, gender, or occupational effects on the lifestyle and health practices of the couple and the children. For example, living conditions, stressors, social support, diet, and smoking may be influenced by employment or economic status and may differ between the females and males in the family. Teach the family about the influences on health that exist outside of the home. Explore ways that the middle-ager can advocate for a healthful work environment. **Box 15-9**, Considerations for the Middle-Aged Client in Health Promotion, summarizes what you should consider in assessment, intervention, and evaluation of care with the middle-aged client and family.

EVALUATION

Feedback from clients, families, and colleagues, as well as your own observations, are ways to **evaluate** care. The functional status improvements in laboratory tests; use of tools to measure physical status improvement (e.g., sleep apnea); tools to measure mental status such as depression or anxiety; and feedback of improved relationships with the spouse, children, or other family members provide evaluation data. Combine direct and indirect or observational methods to evaluate care with members of the interdisciplinary team.

Nursing Diagnoses Related to Middle Age

Anxiety	Anticipatory **G**rieving
Disturbed **B**ody Image	Readiness for Enhanced **K**nowledge
Caregiver Role Strain	Risk for **L**oneliness
Decisional **C**onflict	Imbalanced **N**utrition: More Than Body Requirements
Parental Role **C**onflict	**P**ost-Trauma Syndrome
Defensive **C**oping	Risk for Impaired **R**eligiosity
Readiness for Enhanced Community **C**oping	**S**leep Deprivation
Compromised Family **C**oping	**S**ocial Isolation
Interrupted **F**amily Processes	**S**piritual Distress
Fatigue	Risk for **S**piritual Distress

Source: Reference 121.

INTERVENTIONS FOR HEALTH PROMOTION

Educate the middle-ager about components for self-care (134):

1. Take time to express feelings about life situations.
2. Express a supportive or positive attitude toward others.
3. Foster positive self-esteem and positive self-concept in relationships—family, friends, and work colleagues.

4. Access health education and learn self-care skills.
5. Consider relevant and safe alternative and complementary therapies.
6. Integrate health promotion activities into daily routines at home and work.

BOX 15-9   Considerations for the Middle-Aged Client in Health Promotion

1. Family and cultural history
2. Personal history
3. Preexisting illness
4. Risk factors for disease in family (e.g., cardiovascular disease, cancer, osteoporosis, developmental disability, mental illness)
5. Psychosocial evaluation (age-related stresses, distress with partner, midlife crisis issues)
6. Caregiver responsibilities
7. Knowledge of normal changes in middle age and coping strategies—adaptive capacity
8. Nutrition history—weekly diet intake
9. Complete physical examination
10. For women:
    a. Menstrual history (age onset, pattern, current pattern)
    b. History of estrogen administration
    c. Reproductive history (number of pregnancies, at what age, miscarriages or abortions)
    d. Perimenstrual history (beginning of menopausal symptoms, response, whether menopause has occurred)
    e. Interest in or current administration of hormone replacement therapy, and side effects
11. Other members of household (review 1–9)

Summary

1. The middle years are filled with challenges, pleasures, and demands.
2. The middle-ager is in the "sandwich generation," caring for children and grandchildren, and aging parents and other relatives.
3. This is the prime of life, although some physical changes occur that require adaptation.
4. The middle-ager continues to learn and, in turn, is a mentor and leader in the community.
5. This is a time of generativity, of wanting to leave the world a better place.
6. The middle-ager relies on experience, resolves value conflicts, and initiates action that is relevant to the situation.
7. For some, middle age is a time of struggle, crisis, loss, or illness.
8. Utilize content in **Box 15-9**, Considerations for the Middle-Aged Client in Health Promotion, as you assess, intervene, and evaluate interventions with the midlife person or family.
9. Health promotion behaviors are important for present and future well-being.

Review Questions

1. Participants in a local women's group ask the nurse about the benefits and risks of hormone replacement therapy (HRT) to treat menopausal symptoms. Which of the following should the nurse include in the response to the women's questions on this issue? (Select all that apply.)

1. Increase in heart disease is associated with combination HRT.
2. Use of estrogen-only replacement results in no increased risk of breast cancer.
3. Women with a history of breast cancer should use combination HRT only.

4. Women taking HRT may have false-positive mammogram results.
5. HRT is no longer used as a treatment for menopausal symptoms.

2. The nurse is reviewing a daily food journal of a 50-year-old male who is concerned with weight gain in recent years. The nurse evaluates calorie intake with the knowledge that:
   1. BMI decreases with age.
   2. Carbohydrate needs increase during middle age.
   3. BMI increases throughout the life span.
   4. Physical activity is no longer a consideration in the middle years.

3. A middle-aged female client is concerned about her risk for heart disease due to the recent death of a sibling to myocardial infarction. The client shows no significant risk factors and indicates she would like to make lifestyle changes to re- duce her risk. Which of the following strategies should the nurse suggest to this client?
   1. Take 325 mg of aspirin three times per day.
   2. Maintain a waist-to-hip ratio of 1:2.
   3. Increase intake of whole grains and fruits.
   4. Reduce intake of nuts and fatty fish.

4. A middle-aged client mentions to the nurse that he would like to return to college but is concerned that it is too late in life to complete a college degree. The nurse can advise this client that:
   1. IQ test scores decline in middle age, so college perfor- mance may be affected.
   2. Recall begins to decline in the 20s, so memorization might be difficult.
   3. Ability to learn is reduced by the time one reaches 40.
   4. Success in college has little to do with age.

References

1. A wake-up call on sleep and health. (2007). *Tufts University Health & Nutri- tion Letter, 24*(12), 1–3.
2. Adler, J., & Scelfo, J. (2006, September 18). The Boomer files: Religion— Finding & seeking. *Newsweek,* 52–56.
3. Adler, J., Wingert, P., Springer, K., Reni, J., Samuels, A., Raymond, J., & Adams, W. (2005, November 14). The Boomer files: Hitting 60. *Newsweek,* 51–57.
4. Aldwin, C., & Levenson, M. (2001). Stress, coping, and health in midlife: A developmental perspective. In M. E. Lachman (Ed.), *Handbook of midlife de- velopment* (pp. 188–214). New York: John Wiley.
5. American Association of Retired Persons. (2001). *In the middle: A report on multicultural Boomers coping with family and aging issues.* Washington, DC: Author.
6. American Psychiatric Association. (1994). *Diagnostic and statistical manual of mental disorders* (4th ed.). Washington, DC: Author.
7. Andrews, M., & Boyle, J. (2003). *Transcultural concepts in nursing care* (4th ed.). Philadelphia: Lippincott Williams & Wilkins.
8. Arlin, P. K. (1984). Adolescent and adult thought: A structural interpreta- tion. In M. L. Commons, E. A. Richards, & C. Armon (Eds.), *Beyond for- mal operations* (pp. 258–271). New York: Praeger.
9. Artinian, N. (2003). The psychological aspects of heart failure. *American Journal of Nursing, 103*(12), 32–41.
10. Avis, N. E. (1999). Women's health at midlife. In S. L. Willis & J. D. Reid (Eds.), *Life in the middle: Psychological and social development in middle age* (pp. 105–137). San Diego, CA: Academic Press.
11. Avolio, B., & Sosik, J. (1999). A life span framework for assessing the impact of work on white-color workers. In S. L. Willis & J. D. Reid (Eds.), *Life in the middle: Psychological and social development in middle age.* San Diego, CA: Academic Press.
12. Ballwin, C., & Quan, S. (2002). Sleep disordered breathing. *Nursing Clinics of North America, 37,* 633–654.
13. Balzac, F. (2006). Exploring the brain's role in creativity. *NeuroPsychiatry Re- views, 7*(5), 7, 19–20.
14. Barnett, R., & Hyde, J. (2001). Women, men, work, and family. *American Psychologist, 56,* 781–796.
15. Bates, B. (2005). Testosterone replacement a double-edged sword. *Clinical Psychiatry News, 33*(8), 79.
16. Berger, K. (2005). *The developing person through the life span* (6th ed.). New York: Worth.
17. Brim, O. (1999). *The MacArthur Foundation Study of midlife development.* Vero Beach, FL: MacArthur Foundation.
18. Brisk walking can rebuild your brain. (2007). *Tufts University Health & Nu- trition Letter, 25*(1), 1–2.
19. Brown, W., Ford, J., Burton, N., Marshall, A., & Dobson, A. (2005). Prospective study of physical activity and depressive symptoms in middle- aged women. *American Journal of Preventive Medicine, 29*(4), 265–272.
20. Can a troubled mind spell trouble for the heart? Part I. (2003). *Harvard Men- tal Health Letter, 19*(10), 1–3.
21. Carmichael, M. (2007, March 26). Stronger, faster, smarter. *Newsweek,* 38–46.
22. Cohen, G. (2006). *The mature mind: The positive power of the aging brain.* New York: Basic Books.
23. Cohen, L. S. (2006). Risk for new onset of depression during the menopausal transition: The Harvard Study of Moods and Cycle. *Archives of General Psy- chiatry, 63,* 385–390.
24. Colditz, G., & Hankinson, S. (2005). The Nurses' Health Study: Lifestyle and health among women. *Nature Review, 5,* 388–396.
25. Collins-McNeal, J. (2006). Psychosocial characteristics and cardiovascular risk in African Americans with diabetes. *Archives of Psychiatric Nursing, 20*(5), 226–233.
26. Cook, J., & Jones, R. (2002). Congruency of identity style in married cou- ples. *Journal of Family Issues, 23*(8), 912–926.
27. Cosmetic surgery: Safety first. (2004). *Johns Hopkins Medical Letter: Health After Fifty, 17*(5), 1–3.
28. Cuomo, M. (2002). *The person who changed my life.* New York: Barnes & Noble Books.
29. Curtiss, C., Haylock, P., & Hawkins, R. (2006). Improving the care of can- cer survivors. *American Journal of Nursing, 106*(3), 48–52.
30. Davidhizar, R., Bechtel, G., & Woodring, B. (2000). The changing role of grandparenting. *Journal of Gerontological Nursing, 20*(1), 24–29.
31. Dennis, W. (1966). Creative production between the ages of 20 and 80. *Journal of Gerontology, 21*(1), 8.
32. Digman, J. (1990). Personality structure: Emergence of the five-factor model. *Annual Review of Psychology, 41,* 417–440.
33. Dudek, S. (2007). *Nutrition essentials for nursing practice* (5th ed.). Philadel- phia: Lippincott Williams & Wilkins.
34. Duvall, E., & Miller, B. (1984). *Marriage and family development* (6th ed.). New York: Harper & Row.
35. Duyff, R. (2002). *American Dietetic Association complete food and nutrition guide* (2nd ed.). Hoboken, NJ: John Wiley & Sons.
36. Dychtwald, K. (2005). *The power years: A user's guide to the rest of your life.* New York: John Wiley & Sons.

37. Eakes, G., Burke, M., & Hainsworth, M. (1998). Middle-range theory of chronic sorrow. *IMAGE: Journal of Nursing Scholarship, 30*(2), 179–184.

38. Erikson, E. (1963). *Childhood and society* (2nd ed.). New York: W.W. Norton.

39. Erikson, E. (1978). *Adulthood.* New York: W.W. Norton.

40. Etaugh, C., & Bridges, J. (2001). Midlife transitions. In J. Worell (Ed.), *Encyclopedia of women and gender.* San Diego, CA: Academic Press.

41. Eun-Ok, I. (2003). Symptoms experienced during menopausal transition: Korean women in South Korea and the United States. *Journal of Transcultural Nursing, 14*(4), 321–328.

42. Exploring the depression-bone connection. (2007). *Harvard Women's Health Watch, 14*(10), 1–3.

43. Federmann, D., & Walford, G. (2007, January 15). Is male menopause real? *Newsweek,* 58–60.

44. Fenstermacher, K., & Hudson, B. (2004). *Practice guidelines for family nurse practitioner* (3rd ed.). Philadelphia: Saunders.

45. Finch, C.E. (2001). Toward a biology of middle age. In M.E. Lachman (Ed.), *Handbook of midlife development* (pp. 77–108). New York: John Wiley & Sons.

46. Fineman, H. (2006, January 23). The Boomer files. Politics—The last hurrah. *Newsweek,* 52–57.

47. Flech, C. (2006). Double bind. *AARP Bulletin, 49*(5), 18–19.

48. Florida, R. (2002). *The rise of the creative class.* New York: Basic Books.

49. Freeman, E.W. (2006). Associations of hormones and menopausal status with depressed mood in women with no history of depression. *Archives of General Psychiatry, 63,* 375–382.

50. Gardner, H. (1993). *Multiple intelligences: Theory in practice.* New York: Basic Books.

51. Gender matters: Heart disease risk in women. (2004). *Harvard Women's Health Watch, 11*(9), 1–3.

52. Giger, J., & Davidhizar, R. (2004). *Transcultural nursing: Assessment & intervention* (4th ed.). St. Louis, MO: Mosby.

53. Gilligan, C. (1997). In a different voice: Women's conceptions of self and of mortality. *Harvard Educational Review, 47*(4), 481–517.

54. Gilligan, C., Lyons, N., & Hammer, T. (Eds.). (1990). *Making connections.* Cambridge, MA: Harvard University Press.

55. Goleman, D. (1998). *Working with emotional intelligence.* New York: Bantam.

56. Goleman, D. (2001). An E-1 based theory of performance. In C. Cherniss & D. Goleman (Eds.), *The emotionally intelligent workplace: How to select for, measure, and improve emotional intelligence in individuals, groups, and organizations* (pp. 27–44). San Francisco: Jossey-Bass.

57. Goodstein, F., Manson, J., & Stampfer, M. (2006). Hormone therapy and coronary heart disease: The role of time since menopause and age at hormone initiation. *Journal of Women's Health,* 15, 35–44.

58. Gould, R. (1975). Adult life stages: Growth toward self-tolerance. *Psychology Today, 8*(7), 74–78.

59. Gould, R. (1978). *Transformations: Growth and change in adult life.* New York: Simon & Schuster.

60. Gould, R. (1979). Transformation in mid-life. *New York University Education Quarterly, 10*(2), 2–9.

61. Grady, D. (2006). Management of menopausal symptoms. *New England Journal of Medicine, 355,* 2338–2347.

62. Grant, B. (2005). National survey sharpens picture of major depression among U.S. adults. *NeuroPsychiatry Reviews, 6*(10), 1, 10.

63. Guyton, A., & Hall, J. (2006). *Textbook of medical physiology* (11th ed.). Philadelphia: Elsevier.

64. Hainsworth, M., Busch, P., Eakes, G., & Burkes, M. (1995). Chronic sorrow in women with chronically mentally ill disabled husbands. *Journal of the American Psychiatric Nurses Association, 1*(4), 120–124.

65. Handron, D. (1993). Denial and serious chronic illness: A personal perspective. *Perspectives in Psychiatric Care, 29*(1), 29–33.

66. Harris, M., & Cumella, E. (2006). Eating disorders across the life span. *Journal of Psychosocial Nursing, 44*(4), 20–25.

67. Hassan, M., & Kellick, S. (2003). Effect of male age on fertility: Evidence for the decline of male fertility with increasing age. *Fertility and Sterility, 79*(Suppl. 3), 1520–1527.

68. Haylock, P., Mitchell, S., Cox, T., Temmple, S., & Curtiss, C. (2007). The cancer survivor's prescription for living. *American Journal of Nursing, 107*(4), 58–70.

69. Heckhausen, J. (2001). Adaptation and resilience in midlife. In M. Lachman (Ed.), *Handbook of midlife development* (pp. 345–394). New York: John Wiley & Sons.

70. Herrick, T. (2005). As Baby Boomers age, who will care for them? *Clinical News, 9*(9), 1, 18–19.

71. Hobson, J., & Silvestri, L. (1999). Parasomnias. *Harvard Mental Health Letter, 15*(8), 3–5.

72. Houlden, A., Curtiss, C., & Haylock, P. (2006). Executive Summary: The state of the science on nursing approaches to managing late and long-term sequelae of cancer and cancer treatment. *American Journal of Nursing, 106*(3), 54–59.

73. Huyck, M. (1999). Gender roles and gender identity in midlife. In S. Willis & J. Reid (Eds.), *Life in the middle: Psychosocial and social development in middle age* (pp. 209–232). San Diego, CA: Academic Press.

74. Irwin, T. (1982). *Male menopause: Crisis in the middle years.* New York: Public Affairs Pamphlets.

75. Jewell, A. (2006, January). Plastic beauty. *Focus on the Family,* 14–16.

76. Jung, C. (1995). *Modern man in search of a soul.* New York: Harcourt, Brace, & World.

77. Kaelin, C. (2005). *Living through breast cancer.* Boston: McGraw-Hill.

78. Kaelin, C. (2006). *The breast cancer survivor's fitness plan.* Boston: McGraw-Hill.

79. Kalins, D., Helms, C., & Chebatoris, J. (2006, March 20). The Boomer files: Art—Design of the times. *Newsweek,* 54–58.

80. Kantrowitz, B., & Tyre, B. (2006, May 22). The Boomer files: Parenting—The fine art of letting go. *Newsweek,* 49–63.

81. Katz, A. (2007). When sex hurts: Menopause-related dyspareunia. *American Journal of Nursing, 107*(7), 34–39.

82. Keating, P. (2004, September–October). Wake-up call. *AARP Magazine,* 55–58, 60, 105.

83. Kelleher, K. (1992). The afternoon of life: Jung's view of the tasks of the second half of life. *Perspectives in Psychiatric Care, 28*(2), 25–28.

84. Kennedy, M. (2006). Focusing on female hearts. *American Journal of Nursing, 106*(5), 20–21.

85. King, V. (2003). The legacy of a grandparent's divorce: Consequences for ties between grandparents and grandchildren. *Journal of Marriage and Family, 65,* 170–183.

86. Kirasic, K. C. (2003). Introduction—Publicly and privately held myths of midlife. In K. C. Kirasic (Ed.), *Midlife in context.* Boston: McGraw-Hill.

87. Kirasic, K. C. (2003). Fertility and menopause. In K. C. Kirasic (Ed.), *Midlife in context* (pp. 1–4). Boston: McGraw-Hill.

88. Kirasic, K. C. (2003). General health in midlife. In K. C. Kirasic (Ed.), *Midlife in context* (pp. 60–78). Boston: McGraw-Hill.

89. Knowles, M. (1990). *The adult learner: A neglected species* (4th ed.). Houston, TX: Gulf.

90. Kohlberg, L. (1977). *Recent research in moral development.* New York: Holt, Rinehart & Winston.

91. Kohlberg, L., & Ryncraz, R. A. (1990). Beyond justice reasoning: Moral development and consideration of seventh stage. In C. N. Alexander & E. I. Langor (Eds.), *Higher stages of human development* (pp. 191–207). New York: Oxford University Press.

92. Kritz-Silverstein, D., & Barrett-Connor, E. (1993). Bone mineral density in postmenopausal women as determined by prior oral contraceptive use. *American Journal of Public Health, 83,* 100–102.

93. Kritz-Silverstein, D., & Barrett-Connor, E. (1993). Early menopause, number of reproductive years, and bone mineral density in postmenopausal women. *American Journal of Public Health, 83,* 983–988.

94. Lachman, M. (2001). Introduction. In M. Lachman (Ed.), *Handbook of midlife development* (pp. xvii–xxvi). New York: John Wiley and Sons.

95. Lachman, M., & Bertrand, R. (2001). Personality and the self in midlife. In M. Lachman (Ed.), *Handbook of midlife development* (pp. 279–309). New York: John Wiley & Sons.

96. Lancaster, L., & Stillman, D. (2002). *When generations collide: Who they are. Why they clash: How to solve the generational puzzles at work.* New York: Harper Business.

97. Leming, M., & Dickinson, G. (2002). *Understanding death, dying, and bereavement* (5th ed.). Belmont, CA: Wadsworth.

98. Lewis, C. (2006). *Age-defying fitness.* Atlanta, GA: Peach Tree Publisher.

99. Levinson, D. (1986). *The seasons of a man's life.* New York: Alfred A. Knopf.

100. Levinson, D. (1986). A conception of adult development. *American Psychologist, 41,* 3–13.

101. Levinson, D. (1990). A theory of life structure development in adulthood. In K. N. Alexander & E. J. Langer (Eds.), *Higher stages of human development* (pp. 35–54). New York: Oxford University Press.

102. Lock, M. (1997). Menopause in cultural context. *Experimental Gerontology, 29,* 307–317.

103. Loevinger, J. (1976). *Ego development.* San Francisco: Jossey-Bass.

104. Lower, J. (2007). Brace yourself—here comes Generation Y. *American Nurse Today, 2*(8), 26–29.

105. Lung cancer in women. (2005). *Harvard Women's Health Watch, 13*(4), 1–3.

106. Mason, D. (2006). Surviving cancer survival. *American Journal of Nursing, 106*(3), 11.

107. Masters, W., & Johnson, V. (1981). *Human sexual response.* Boston: Little, Brown.

108. Maszak, M. (2005, December 1). Hearts and minds. *U.S. News and World Report,* 68, 70.

109. Mathews, S. H. (1995). Gender and the division of filial responsibility between lone sisters and their brothers. *Journal of Gerontology, 50B*(5), S312–S320.

110. Mayo Clinic. (2006, May). *Hormone replacement therapy: Benefits and alternatives.* www.mayoclinic.com/health/hormone-therapy/w000046

111. McCrae, R., & Costa, P. (2003). *Personality in adulthood: A five factor perspective* (2nd ed.). New York: Guilford Publications.

112. McDonald, M. (2001, April 2). Forever young. *U.S. News and World Report,* 36–38.

113. McDonald, M. (2003, November 3). The mentor gap. *U.S. News & World Report,* 36–38.

114. McGinn, D. (2006, June 19). The Boomer files: Careers—Second time around. *Newsweek,* 47–54.

115. Menon, U. (2001). Middle adulthood in cultural perspective: The imagined and the experienced in three cultures. In M. E. Lachman (Ed.), *Handbook of midlife development* (pp. 40–74). New York: John Wiley & Sons.

116. Metheny, N. (2000). *Fluid & electrolyte balance: Nursing considerations* (4th ed.). Philadelphia: Lippincott.

117. Miller, M. (2007, March 26). Exercise is a state of mind. *Newsweek,* 44–55.

118. Mind and mood after a heart attack. (2006). *Harvard Mental Health Letter, 22*(8), 1–3.

119. Muirhead, R. (2004). *Just work.* Cambridge, MA: Harvard University Press.

120. Murray, R. (2002). Mentoring: Perceptions of the process and its significance. *Journal of Psychosocial Nursing and Mental Health Services, 40*(4), 44–51.

121. NANDA International. (2005). *NANDA nursing diagnoses: Definitions and classification 2005–2006.* Philadelphia: Author.

122. National Kidney and Urologic Disease Information Clearinghouse. (2007). *Erectile dysfunction.* Retrieved October 11, 2007, from http://kidney.niddk.nih.gov/kidiseases/pubs/impotence/index.htm

123. Nelson, H.D., Haney, E., Humphrey, L., Miller, J., Nedrow, A., Nicolaidis, C., et al. (2005). *Management of menopause related symptoms.* Evidence Report/Technology Assessment No. 120. AHRQ Publication No. 05-E016-2. Agency for Healthcare Research and Quality. Rockville, MD.

124. Nelson, M. (1998). *Strong women stay slim.* New York: Bantam Books.

125. Neugarten, B. (1967). The awareness of middle age. In R. Owen (Ed.), *Middle age.* London: British Broadcasting Corporation.

126. Neugarten, B. (1968). Women's attitudes toward menopause. In. B. Neugarten (Ed.), *Middle age and aging.* Chicago: University of Chicago Press.

127. Neugarten, B. (1970). Dynamics of the transition of mid-age to old age. *Journal of Geriatric Psychiatry, 4,* 71–87.

128. Neugarten, B. (1976). Adaptation and the life cycle. *Counseling Psychologist, 6*(1), 16–20.

129. Neugarten, B., & Moore, J. (1968). The changing age-status system. In B. Neugarten (Ed.), *Middle age and aging.* Chicago: University of Chicago Press.

130. New guidelines for preventing heart disease in women. (2007). *Johns Hopkins Medical Letter: Health After Fifty, 19*(5), 1–3.

131. New view of heart disease in women. (2007). *Harvard Women's Health Watch, 14*(6), 1–3.

132. Oh, my aching feet. (2005). *Focus on Healthy Aging: Mount Sinai School of Medicine, 8*(8), 7.

133. On becoming a breast cancer survivor. (2006). *Harvard Women's Health Watch, 14*(2), 1–3.

134. Ornish, D. (1999). *Love and survival.* New York: Harper Collins.

135. Papalia, D., Olds, S., & Feldman, R. (2004). *Human development* (9th ed.). Boston: McGraw-Hill.

136. Peck, R. C. (1968). Psychological developments in the second half of life. In B. Neugarten (Ed.), *Middle age and aging.* Chicago: University of Chicago Press.

137. Pender, N., Murdaugh, C., & Parsons, M. (2006). *Health promotion in nursing practice* (5th ed.). Upper Saddle River, NJ: Pearson Prentice Hall.

138. Peppard, P. E., et al. (2006). Longitudinal association of sleep-related breathing disorder and depression. *Archives of Internal Medicine, 166*(16), 1709–1715.

139. Picot, S. J. (1995). Rewards, costs, and coping of African American caregivers. *Nursing Research, 44*(3), 147–152.

140. Pohl, J. M., Boyd, C., Liang, J., & Given, C. W. (1995). Analysis of the impact of mother-daughter relationships on the commitment to caregiving. *Nursing Research, 44*(2), 68–75.

141. Pollock, S., Christian, B., & Sands, D. (1990). Responses to chronic illness: Analysis of psychological and physiological adaptation. *Nursing Research, 39*(5), 302–304.

142. Powled, T. M. (2007, October). Easing hormone anxiety: For women just past menopause, hormone pills seem safe. *Scientific American,* 32–34.

143. Previta, D., & Amato, P. (2003). Why stay married: Rewards, barriers, and marital stability. *Journal of Marriage and Family, 69,* 561–573.

144. Rancour, P. (2002). Catapulting through life stages. *Journal of Psychosocial Nursing, 40*(2), 33–37.

145. Ravdin, P., Cronin, K., Howlader, N., Berg, C., Chlebowski, R., Feuer, E., et al. (2007). The decrease in breast cancer incidence in 2003 in the United States. *New England Journal of Medicine, 356*(16), 1670–1674.

146. Rossi, A. S. (2004). The menopausal transition and aging processes. In O. G. Brim, C. D. Ryff, & R. C. Kessler (Eds.), *How healthy are we: A national study of well-being in midlife* (pp. 153–204). Chicago: University of Chicago Press.

147. Rubenstein, R. et al. (1999). Key relationships of never married, childless older women: A cultural analysis. *Journal of Gerontology: Social Sciences, 46*(5), S270–S277.

148. Santrock, J. (2004). *Life-span development* (9th ed.). Boston: McGraw-Hill.

149. Scannell-Desch, E. (2003). Women's adjustment to widowhood: Theory, research, and interventions. *Journal of Psychosocial Nursing, 41*(5), 28–36.

150. Scannell-Desch, E. (2005). Mid-life widow's narratives of support and non-support. *Journal of Psychosocial Nursing, 41*(4), 40–47.

151. Schaefer, K. (1995). Women living in paradox: Loss and discovery in chronic illness. *Holistic Nursing Practice, 9*(3), 63–74.

152. Schultz, R., & Beach, S. (1999). Caregiving as a risk factor for mortality: The Caregiver Health Effects Study. *Journal of the American Medical Association, 282*(23), 2215–2219.

153. Schulz, R., et al. (2001). Involvement in caregiving and adjustment to death of a spouse. *Journal of the American Medical Association, 285*(24), 3123–3129.

154. Shapiro, E. (1994). *Grief as a family process.* New York: Behavioral Sciences.

155. Sheehy, G. (1991). *Pathfinders.* New York: Wm. Morrow.

156. Sheehy, G. (1998). *Menopause: The silent passage* (Rev. ed.). New York: Pocket Books.

157. Sheehy, G. (1998). *Passages for men.* New York: Random House.

158. Sherman, R. Leading a multigenerational workforce: Issues, challenges, and strategies. Retrieved May 15, 2007 from www.Nursingworld.Org/Olin/Topic30/Tpe30_2thm.

159. Sherrod, M. M., Albarez, Y., Brookshire, A., & Cheek, D. J. (2007). Heart disease: A woman's worst enemy. *American Nurse Today, 2*(2), 25–29.

160. Siegler, I. C., Kaplan, B. H., Von Dras, D. D., & Mark, D. B. (1999). Cardiovascular health: A challenge for midlife. In S.L. Willis & J. D. Reid (Eds.), *Life in the middle: Psychological and social development in middle age* (pp. 148–155). San Diego, CA: Academic Press.

161. Sinnott, J. (1998). *The development of logic in adulthood: Postformal thought and its application.* New York: Plenum.

162. Skaff, M. M., & Pearlin, L. I. (1992). Caregiving: Role engulfment and the loss of self. *Gerontologist, 32*(5), 656–664.

163. Slater, C. (2003). Generativity versus stagnation: An elaboration of Erikson's adult stage of human development. *Journal of Adult Development, 10*(1), 53–65.

164. Smith, D. (2006). Lowering your cholesterol naturally. *Mount Sinai School of Medicine: Focus on Healthy Aging, 9*(2), 1, 6.

165. Spiro, A. (2001). Health in midlife: Toward a lifespan view. In M. Lachman (Ed.), *Handbook of midlife development* (pp. 156–187). New York: John Wiley & Sons.

166. Staudinger, U., & Black, S. (2001). A view of mid-life development from life-span theory. In M. E. Lachman (Ed.), *Handbook of middle development* (pp. 1–39). New York: John Wiley & Sons.

167. Sternberg, R. (1988). *The triarchic mind: A new theory of human intelligence.* New York: Viking Press.

168. Sternberg, R. (1994). *Thinking and problem solving.* San Diego, CA: Academic Press.

169. Sternberg, R., Grigorenko, E., & Oh, S. (2001). The development of intelligence in mid-life. In M. Lachman (Ed.), *Handbook of midlife development* (pp. 217–267). New York: John Wiley & Sons.

170. Streit, M. (2007, April). Do good, feel good—studies show volunteering can improve your health. *Erickson Tribune, 1,* 9.

171. Talbott, M. M. (1990). The negative side of the relationship between older widows and their adult children: The mothers' perspective. *Gerontologist, 30*(5), 595–603.

172. Testosterone supplements. (2005). *Mount Sinai School of Medicine. Focus on Healthy Aging, 8*(5), 3.

173. The broken heart: An overlooked risk factor for heart disease? (1997). *Women's Health Advocate Newsletter, 4*(10), 7.

174. Tucker, M. (2005). Recommended exercise also curbs depression. *Clinical Psychiatry News, 33*(5), 8–9.

175. Turner-Henson, A., & Holoday, B. (1995). Daily life experiences for the chronically ill: A life span perspective. *Family-Community Health, 17*(4), 1–11.

176. Twenge, J., Campbell, W., & Foster, C. (2003). Parenthood and marital satisfaction. A meta-analytic review. *Journal of Marriage and Family, 65,* 574–583.

177. Type D personality and cardiovascular risk. (2005). *Harvard Health Letter, 30*(10), 3.

178. United States Department of Health and Human Services. (1998). *Informal caregiving: Compassion in action.* Washington, DC: Author.

179. United States Department of Health and Human Services. (2000). *Healthy People 2010: With understanding and improving health and objectives for improving health* (2nd ed.). Vol. 2. Washington, DC: U.S. Government Printing Office.

180. United States National Library of Medicine and the National Institutes of Health. (2007). MedLine Plus interactive tutorial on erectile dysfunction. Retrieved October 11, 2007, from www.nlm.nih.gov/medlineplus/tutorials/erectiledysfunction/yourchoices/htm/index.htm.

181. Vaillant, G. (1977). The normal boy in later life: How adaptation fosters growth. *Harvard Magazines, 55*(6), 234–239.

182. Vaillant, G. (2002). *Aging well.* Boston: Little, Brown.

183. Vamos, M. (1993). Body image in chronic illness: A reconceptualization. *International Journal of Psychiatry in Medicine, 23*(2), 163–178.

184. Vance, C. (1989–1990). Is there a mentor in your career future? *Imprint, 36*(5), 41–42.

185. Vance, C., & Olson, R. (1998). *The mentoring connection in nursing.* New York: Springhill.

186. Vanden Hoonaard, V., & Kestin, D. (2003). Expectations and experiences of widowhood. In J. Gubrium & J. Holstein (Eds.), *Ways of aging* (pp. 182–199). Malden, MA: Blackwell.

187. Veldhuis, J., Johnson, M., Keenan, D., & Iranmanesh, A. (2003). The ensemble male hypothalamo-pituitary-gonadal axis. In P. Timeras (Ed.), *Physiological basis of aging and geriatrics* (pp. 213–231). Boca Raton, FL: CRC Press.

188. Wadsworth, B. (2004). *Piaget's theory of cognitive and affective development* (5th ed.). Boston: Pearson Education.

189. Warda, M. (1992). The family and chronic sorrow: Role theory approach. *Journal of Pediatric Nursing, 7,* 205–206.

190. Warner, J., & Sandberg, A. (2005). *The generational style assessment.* Amherst, MA: HRD Press.

191. Weisstub, D., Thomasma, D., Ganthier, S., & Tomossy, G. (Eds.). (2001). *Aging: Caring for our elders.* Dordrecht, Netherlands: Kluwer.

192. Welch, J., & Welch, S. (2005). *Winning.* New York: Harper Collins.

193. Wenrich, C. (2007). Tired of being tired? Try Pilates! *American Nurse Today, 2*(1), 58–59.

194. What becomes of the "broken-hearted." (2007). *Johns Hopkins Medical Letter, 18*(2), 5.

195. Whitbourne, S.K. (2001). The physical aging process in midlife: Interactions with psychological and sociocultural factors. In M. E. Lachman (Ed.), *Handbook of midlife development* (pp. 109–155). New York: John Wiley & Sons.

196. Williams, L., & Hopper, D. (2007). *Understanding medical surgical nursing* (3rd ed.). Philadelphia: F.A. Davis.

197. Wingert, P., & Kantrowitz, B. (2007, January 15). The new prime time. *Newsweek,* 38–54.

198. Wise, P. (2003). The female reproductive system. In P. Timiras (Ed.), *Physiological basis of aging and geriatrics* (3rd ed., pp. 189–212). Boca Raton, FL: CRC Press.

199. Women and heart disease: A unique pair. (2005). *Johns Hopkins Medical Letter: Health After 50, 16*(12), 4–5.

200. Young, R. F., & Kahana, E. (1995). The context of caregiving and well-being outcomes among African and Caucasian Americans. *Gerontologist, 35*(2), 225–232.

CHAPTER 16

Later Maturity: Basic Assessment and Health Promotion

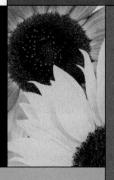

OBJECTIVES

Study of this chapter will enable you to:

1. Define terms and theories of aging related to understanding of the person.

2. Explore your role in promoting positive attitudes about growing old.

3. Contrast relationships in the late years with those of other developmental eras, including with spouse, other family members, friends, pets, and other networks.

4. Contrast the status of being single or a widow/widower in later life to that status in earlier adulthood.

5. Describe indicators of elder abuse and contrast with child and spouse abuse.

6. Describe physiologic adaptive mechanisms of aging, including in the centenarian, and influences on sexuality, health problems, and assessment and intervention to promote and maintain health, comfort, and safety.

7. Analyze the cognitive, emotional, body-image, and spiritual development and characteristics of the aged person, their interrelationship, and your role in promoting health and a positive self-concept.

8. Contrast adaptive mechanisms used by the person in this period with those used in other life eras.

9. Relate the developmental crisis of ego integrity versus self-despair, to previous life eras, and your role in helping the person meet this crisis.

10. Discuss developmental tasks, and your contribution to their accomplishment.

11. Determine changing home, family, social, and work or leisure situations of the senior and your responsibility in helping the person face these crises.

12. Describe major community programs to assist the elderly financially, socially, and in health care, and describe your professional and personal responsibility.

13. Summarize needs of the elderly, standards of therapeutic approach and health care to meet those needs, and trends in care of the person in later life.

MediaLink www.prenhall.com/murray

Go to the Companion Website for interactive resources that accompany this chapter.

Glossary
Review Questions
Challenge Your Knowledge
Learning Activities

Critical Thinking
Tools
Media Link Applications
Media Links

When does later adulthood begin? Historically, the designation of an eligible age for receipt of Social Security benefits established age 65 as the beginning age for this period in the life cycle. In reality, the age span for this period is continually changing. Images once associated with the elderly and later maturity are no longer current. The chronologic age of 65 no longer determines or predicts behaviors, life events, health status, work status, family status, interests, preoccupations, or needs. Individuals undergo aging at different rates, and their view of the aging process is influenced by many factors—genetics, culture, generation, and occupation. Not everyone 65 to 70 years old and older considers self old, but in the United States a person of that age is expected to assume roles appropriate to later maturity. Some individuals, especially members of ethnic minorities and lower socioeconomic levels, view the onset of old age as taking place earlier than age 65 (9). Younger generations, including Baby Boomers, may misperceive how this cohort views itself.

The Aging Population

Population aging is increasing worldwide, unlike any time in history. *Your professional role will be affected by these demographics.* Longevity statistics are related to decline in fertility rates and increasing life span, resulting from immunizations, advancements in technology, and effectiveness of other health care trends. There is an increase in the number of people over 60 years and a decline in people under 15 years. By 2050, the estimated number of elders (2 billion) will exceed the number of young people for the first time in history (184). This trend will affect every area of life in all countries. Economic impact will be felt in the kinds of available jobs and in the labor market; in savings, investment, and consumption; and in pensions and taxation. Social impact will be felt in health care needs and resources, family compositions, living arrangements and housing, and migration. Political impact will be felt in governmental policy, voting patterns, and representation (184).

The pace of aging trends is faster in developing than in nondeveloping countries, leaving little time for nations to adjust. In more developed countries or regions, 20% of the population was 60 years or older in 2000; by 2050, 33% will be over 60 years. In less developed regions, 8% of the population is over age 60; by 2050, nearly 20% will be over 60 years. These numbers vary by country. Yemen has the youngest population (median age 15 years). Japan has the oldest (median age 41 years) (184). In some African countries, life expectancy will be reduced by 30 years because of the AIDS epidemic (184). *In 2003, six countries accounted for 54% of the total number of people over 80 years:* (a) China, 12 million; (b) United States, 9 million; (c) India, 6 million; (d) Japan, 5 million; (e) Germany, 3 million; and (f) Russian Federation, 3 million (184).

It is predicted that *in 2050 the six countries with 10 million or more people over 80 years will be* (a) China, 99 million; (b) India, 48 million; (c) United States, 30 million; (d) Japan, 17 million; (e) Brazil, 10 million; and (f) Indonesia, 10 million (184).

The oldest-old is the fastest growing cohort worldwide. This group is increasing at 3.8% annually to comprise over 10% of the population. By 2050, an estimated 20% of older people will be over 80 years (184).

The majority of people worldwide are females, who have overall a higher life expectancy than males. In 2000, there were 63 million more females than males over 60 years. For those over 85, there were 2 to 5 times more females than males (184).

During the 20th century, the older adult population in the United States increased from 3 to over 34 million (86). By 2003, there were 35.9 million people over 65 years—12% of the total population. Of this cohort, 18.3 million were 65 to 74 years, 12.9 million were 75 to 84 years, and 4.7 million were 85 years and older (70). Most (75%) were living in metropolitan areas (70). In addition to greater longevity, there is an overall decline in disability prevalence in the United States. By 2030, an estimated 72 million (almost 20%) of the U.S. population will be over 65 years (70). The number of **centenarians**, *those 100 years or older*, has increased in the United States from 37,000 in 1990 to over 50,000 in 2000 (70).

In 2000, non-Hispanic Caucasians accounted for 8.3% of the older U.S. population. African Americans, Asian Americans, and Hispanics accounted for 8%, 3%, and 6% of the over-65 population, respectively. The older Hispanic population is projected to grow from 2 million in 2000 to 8 million in 2030, larger than the African American or Asian descent populations (70).

Females continue to outnumber males in each age group over 65 years. For example, in 2000, Caucasian life expectancy at birth was 80 years for females and 74.8 years for males (70). African American females had a life expectancy of 74.2 years; males had a life expectancy of 68.2 years (70). American Indians have the shortest life expectancy; an example is 56.5 years for males in South Dakota (138). Gender and racial differences are declining (70).

Poverty rates among the older populations differ by racial or ethnic origin. In 2003, older non-Hispanic Caucasians were less likely than older African Americans and Hispanics to be living in poverty (8% compared with 24% and 20%, respectively). Females had a higher poverty rate than males (70).

The social and economic implications of the large Baby Boomer generation entering the 65 to 70 age group in the United States, beginning about 2010 or 2011, is a concern to policy makers (2, 70). The size and longevity of this cohort will affect Social Security, Medicare, disability insurance, and retirement benefits. Various social issues are as critical, related to health care needs, caregiving (70, 81), housing (81), and social services (70, 72). This future generation is overall better educated and more health conscious than the current elder population. Perhaps this group will enter the older years in better health, with higher incomes and more wealth, and thus a higher standard of living for retirement (70). In fact, some of the Baby Boomer population have declared they plan to continue to reinvent their lives, remain active, and delay retirement. Thus, there may be more elders, but needs and characteristics may differ considerably from those of the current generation of people in later maturity.

Four-generation families, once unusual, are the norm, as depicted by **Figure 16-1** ■. Five-generation families are increasing in number. The continued aging trend in the population requires changes in all aspects of our social structure—employment, housing, education, leisure activities, transportation, industrial development, and health care.

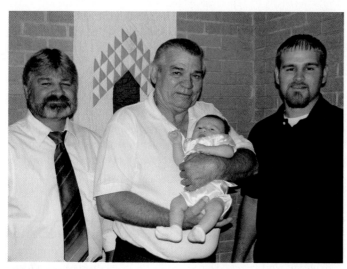

FIGURE ☐ **16-1** Four-generation families, once unusual, will become the norm as the population ages.

Definitions

Because the terms describing this age group are not consistently defined by the general public or health care professionals, it is important to clarify some of the terms used in this chapter (45, 100, 111). Utilize the following terms in your assessment.

Aging, which *begins at conception and ends at death, is a process of growing older, regardless of chronologic age.*

Biological age is the *person's present position with respect to the potential life span, which may be younger or older than chronologic age, and encompasses measures of functional capacities of vital organ systems.*

Social age, which *results from the person's life course through various social institutions,* refers to *roles and habits of the person with respect to other members of society.* Social age may be age-appropriate or older or younger than that of most people in the social group. Social age includes such aspects as the person's type of dress, language usage, and social deference to people in leadership positions.

Psychological age refers to *behavioral capacity of the person to adapt to changing environmental demands and includes capacities of memory, learning, intelligence, skills, feelings, and motivation for exercising behavioral control or self-regulation.*

Cognitive age includes the *age the person feels and looks to self, plus the fit of behavior and interests to his or her chronologic age.* The person says, "I do most things as if I were ___ years old."

Primary aging *refers to the universal changes that occur with getting older or senescence* (15, 138).

Secondary aging *refers to the consequences of particular diseases,* but these health changes may not be caused by age alone (15).

Senescence is the *mental and physical decline associated with the aging process.* The term describes a group of effects that lead to a decrease in efficient function.

Later maturity is the *last major segment of the life span. This stage begins at the age of 65, 70, or 75.* The World Health Organization categorizes this cohort in various ways: for example, young-old (60 or 65 years and over) and very old or oldest-old (80 years and older) (184). Some authors divide this group into **young-old,**

ages 65 to 74, or 65 or 70 to 80; **mid-old,** 75 to 84; and **old-old,** 80 or 85 and older (also referred to as octogenarian, and centenarian if 100 or older). The term **frail-old** or **oldest-old** is sometimes used instead of **old-old** or **very old,** depending on the functional states of the person (15, 138, 156, 184).

Functional age *refers to how well a person functions in a physical and social environment in comparison with others of the same chronologic age.* The 90-year-old may be functionally younger than the 65-year-old, related to health status (138).

Senility is a *wastebasket term still used to denote physical and mental deterioration often associated with old age. It is derogatory and should* **not** *be used.* The correct term would be related to a specific disease, such as senile dementia, Alzheimer's type (8). Often loss of function or what looks like Alzheimer's disease may be the result of drug reactions or polypharmacy, malnutrition or dehydration, delirium that is disease induced, hypothyroidism, microstrokes and hypertension, sepsis that is systemic, disorders resulting from lack of communication and sensory deprivation for physical reasons or because of institutionalization, or response to the expectations of caregivers (8, 45).

Gerontology is the *scientific study of the individual in later maturity and the aging process from physiologic, pathologic, psychological, sociologic, and economic points of view.* **Age-dependent characteristics or conditions,** *those that typically occur with advancing years,* are included in gerontological study.

Geriatrics is a *medical specialty concerned with the physiologic and pathologic changes of the individual in later maturity and includes study and treatment of the health problems of this age group.* **Age-related changes, illnesses, or diseases** *that increase in prevalence with age are the subject of study and treatment in geriatrics.*

Later maturity *is divided into three sequential segments.* The first segment may be regarded as a **sociopolitical or cultural-organizational perspective.** *Offspring are in a creative period, and the mature adult is in the ruling, protective stance as he or she assumes parental leadership over the family. The older person becomes concerned with the creation, ordering, and maintenance of a larger society.* The second segment, **reaffirmation of social, moral, and ethical standards,** is characterized by *establishment of harmonious relationships among the oncoming generations as they are involved in rendering decisions, planning, erecting social guideposts, and selecting leaders. The judgmental functions of the mind are most highly developed at this time,* created out of actual and vicarious experience with conflict situations and from cultural learning and values. The last segment of psychic maturity involves **retrospective examination,** *correlation of the present with the past to determine the true nature of accomplishments, errors, and rediscoveries. Cultural vision is at its broadest possible development. The person compares and contrasts personal values with cultural values and, through reasoning and intuition, evaluates meaning and purpose and has an increased interest in the history of human development.* Values of the adolescent are movement, agility, quantitative productivity, exhibitionistic sexual attractiveness, and artfulness. In contrast, values of the older adult are deliberation, caution, equality, modesty, and loyalty. The older adult views self with real humility as a participant in and contributor to the improvement of society (49–51).

Developmental tasks and cultural age timetables for life eras and family transitions exist for all stages of life, but they are not the same for everyone or all cultures (47). These tasks and timetables influence the life course but are likely to be flexible in the minds of individuals, especially older individuals. However, there are age "norms" in key areas of life, which have been addressed in previous chapters and are addressed in this chapter as well.

Societal Perspectives on Aging

Ageism refers to *any attitude, action, or institutional structure that discriminates against individuals on the basis of their age or that infers that elderly people are inferior to those who are younger.* Ageist attitudes toward older adults are not new in the United States. Even during colonial days, the elderly were categorized as unnecessary and burdensome. Of growing concern is the ageism of the aged; the attitudes of some older people are discriminatory toward others who are in their own age group. Generally, older females are judged more harshly than older males. Some express ageism by acting as if they do not see the elder in their midst, as if the elder is transparent (168). Children appear most positive in their perception of elderly persons (168).

Culture, ethnicity, and socioeconomic level influence the role of the older adult in family relationships and determine health practices. Differences exist among cultural populations in how they esteem and care for the elderly, how the elderly stay involved in family matters, and the types of health care services used (9, 61). Differences also exist among urban and rural families of the elderly (9). For example, African Americans view aging and death as natural processes; the older family members are held in esteem. In Asian cultures, older adults have an important role; all younger people are expected to respect them. Families in most ethnic cultures care for the elders. Westernized populations may have difficulty accepting this role. Many older adults continue to follow health practices that are linked to their cultural heritage.

In the U.S. mainstream culture, old age frequently is characterized as a time of dependence and disease. Negative presentation of older adults, especially females, in movies, books, and magazines, in jokes, and on television contributes to negative beliefs and attitudes. Society's attitude to changes associated with aging, such as gray hair, hearing loss, wrinkles, loss of muscle tone, slower movements, and approaching death, also contributes to negative attitudes.

Numerous unproven myths and age-related stereotypes pervade American culture. These myths and stereotypes obscure the truth and may prevent us from achieving our own potential as we grow older. Society stereotypes the older adult as being asexual, unemployable, unintelligent, and socially incompetent. Statements such as "You can't teach old dogs new tricks" and terms such as "dirty old men" typify the feelings of many. Instead of seeking the truth, most individuals accept myths that have been perpetuated

through the years. Some of these myths and the contrasting realities are listed in the **Box** Client Education: Myths and Misconceptions and Their Realities for the Elderly Person (15, 45, 127–129, 138, 156, 170, 196).

You have a role as educator and advocate to overcome these myths. Many of the myths and stereotypes associated with aging are culturally determined. The older adult in America lives in a culture oriented to youth, productivity, and rapid pace. Because of this orientation, older Americans may feel that they are not respected, valued, or needed. *Your approach and public education are important.*

Theories of Aging

There is no single model of longevity. Over 50,000 centenarians reached that milestone because of a unique mix of environmental, behavioral, and genetic factors. Risks for heart disease, cancer, and stroke can be reduced by eating a healthful diet, exercising, and avoiding carcinogens, such as cigarettes, sunburn, and radon, especially for people under 75 years of age (24, 45, 68, 70, 138). *Utilize knowledge of the following theories—biological, psychosocial, developmental, and sociologic—in your assessment and interventions.*

BIOLOGICAL THEORIES

Biological theories can be categorized as nongenetic cellular, physiologic, and genetic. **Table 16-1**, Theories of Physical Aging, presents definitions or explanations and applications or limitations to the theories (11, 12, 15, 45, 60, 67, 95, 138, 156).

Genetic processes that lengthen life include the following (11, 24, 45, 67, 133):

1. A gene that causes people to produce extraordinary amounts of beneficial high-density lipoprotein (HDL), which guards against atherosclerosis.
2. A gene, apo A01 Milano, that quickly clears cholesterol from the bloodstream.
3. Apolipoprotein E (apo E2, apo E3, apo E4), which has been linked to cardiovascular and Alzheimer's disease. Two copies of apo E4 increase risk for atherosclerosis and late onset of Alzheimer's disease. Two copies of apo E2 lengthen life.
4. Werner's gene produces helicase, a special enzyme that is involved in repairing DNA. Lack of the enzyme causes premature aging and death before 50.

The oldest-old are probably endowed with genes that protect them against cardiovascular diseases and with traits that keep their cells in good working order longer than expected. Having long-lived parents makes a difference, since longevity runs in families. In fact, siblings of centenarians, although not reaching 100 years, still live longer than the average person in their age cohort (11, 133, 159). Throughout the life span, females tend to have higher morbidity, or develop more diseases, whereas males tend to show higher mortality, or die from the diseases they develop (70). Gender differences emerge among supersurvivors. Females outnumber males at age 95, but males fare better in terms of mental function and physical health. Males with dementia are likely to die before 90; females with the same amount of impairment live longer (70, 111, 138).

Practice Point

Your attitude, teaching, and advocacy can diminish ageism, stereotypes, and myths. Your teaching, counseling, and practice must consider societal issues and cultural differences among the elderly and related health practices.

Client Education

Myths and Misconceptions and Their Realities for the Elderly Person

MYTH 1: AGE 65 IS A GOOD MARKER FOR OLD AGE

Fact: Factors other than chronologic age cause the person to be old. Many people are more youthful than their parents were at age 65. With increased longevity, perhaps 70 or 75 is becoming the chronologic marker (45)

MYTH 2: MOST OLD PEOPLE ARE IN BED OR IN INSTITUTIONS AND ARE ILL PHYSICALLY AND MENTALLY

Fact: Approximately 5% are institutionalized; 95% are living in the community. Although 67% of older persons outside institutions have one or more chronic conditions, 14% do not. Chronic conditions range from mild and correctable to more severe. Approximately 81% of the aged living in the community have no mobility limitations, 8% have trouble getting around, 6% need the help of another person, and 5% are homebound. The average number of restricted activity days is only twice that for young adults. Some report no physical illness, and some with physical disease processes do not consider themselves ill (45, 68).

MYTH 3: ALL OLD PEOPLE ARE ALIKE

Fact: Each older adult is unique and *quite diverse*. This segment of the life span covers more years than any other segment—sometimes more than 35 years. The older people are, the more varied are their physical capabilities, personal style, economic status, and lifestyle preferences. From birth, physical and mental elaboration continues through life to make people more and more unlike one another (45).

MYTH 4: THE NEXT GENERATION OF OLDER ADULTS WILL BE THE SAME AS THIS GENERATION

Fact: The next generation will be better educated, healthier, more mobile, more youthful in appearance, more accustomed to lifestyle change and technology, and more outspoken. The world is changing so quickly that each successive generation is vastly *different* from the ones that came before (42, 45).

MYTH 5: OLD AGE BRINGS MENTAL DETERIORATION

Fact: Approximately 5% of older adults show serious mental impairment, and only 10% demonstrate even mild to moderate memory loss. Many professionals work past 65 to 70 years (10, 45).

MYTH 6: OLD PEOPLE CANNOT LEARN AND ARE LESS INTELLIGENT.

Fact: Older adults *can* and *do* learn; however, they may need a longer period in which to respond to questions and stim-

uli. When learning problems occur, they are usually associated with a disease process. Intelligent people remain so (15, 45, 58, 158).

MYTH 7: MOST OLDER ADULTS ARE INCOMPETENT

Fact: Older people may have a slower reaction time and take longer to do psychomotor tasks. However, they have more consistent output, less job turnover, greater job satisfaction, fewer accidents, and less absenteeism (45, 196).

MYTH 8: MOST OLDER ADULTS ARE UNHAPPY AND DISSATISFIED WITH LIFE

Fact: How happy or sad the person feels reflects basic temperament throughout life, the adaptation to past and current life events, and social support. Positive social ties and realistic expectations buffer psychological distress. Older people tend to be as satisfied with their lives as middle-aged people, even when they have lower incomes and poorer health (45, 157).

MYTH 9: THE ELDERLY ARE SELF-PITYING, APATHETIC, IRRITABLE, AND HARD TO LIVE WITH

Fact: Mood is related to the present situation and past personality. The older person is as likely as a younger one to have an interesting and pleasant personality (45, 157).

MYTH 10: THE ELDERLY ARE INACTIVE AND UNPRODUCTIVE

Fact: Many young children have working grandparents. Thirty-six percent of men over 65 years are employed in some type of job. Older women often do their housework into their 80s or 90s. Older workers have a job attendance record that is 20% better than that of young workers, and they also sustain fewer job-related injuries (45, 156).

MYTH 11: THE ELDERLY DO NOT DESIRE AND DO NOT PARTICIPATE IN SEXUAL ACTIVITY

Fact: Recent research refutes this assertion. Sexual activity may decline because of lack of a partner or misinformation about sexuality in late life. The person who has been sexually active all along is able to continue sexual activity, and sexual activity involves more than intercourse between the partners (45, 110).

MYTH 12: THE ELDERLY ARE ISOLATED, ABANDONED, AND LONELY, AND THEY ARE UNLIKELY TO PARTICIPATE IN ACTIVITIES

Fact: Many elderly prefer to live in a separate household Many elderly live with someone and do not feel lonely. People over 65 years who never married have adjusted to living

continued

alone. Elderly people who do not have children often have siblings or friends with whom they live. Other elderly live in institutions or residences for the aged where they make friends. The percentage of purposefully abandoned elderly is small; often the person who is a loner in old age has always been alone (45, 82, 83).

MYTH 13: RETIREMENT IS DISLIKED BY ALL OLD PEOPLE AND CAUSES ILLNESS AND LESS LIFE SATISFACTION

Fact: Many older people look forward to retirement and are retiring before 65 so that they can continue other pursuits. More than three fourths of them have satisfying lives. Many contribute to society (45, 157, 168).

MYTH 14: SPECIAL HEALTH SERVICES FOR THE AGED ARE USELESS BECAUSE THE AGED CANNOT BENEFIT ANYWAY

Fact: At age 65 the average person can look forward to at least 10 to 15 more years of life. The elderly have fewer acute illnesses and accidental injuries, and these conditions are correctable, although older people take longer to recover than younger people do. Common chronic conditions are cardiovascular disease, cancer, arthritis, diabetes, sensory impairments, and depression, which can be treated so that the person can achieve maximum potential and comfort (45, 93).

TABLE 16-1

Theories of Physical Aging

Theory	Definition/Explanation	Applications/Limitations
Nongenetic Cellular Theories		
Wear and Tear Theory	Body systems wear out because of accumulation of stress of life and effects of metabolism. Most general and obvious explanation of aging, compares body to a machine.	Little scientific evidence. Theory does not consider self-repair mechanisms of body or differences of life span within the human species.
Cross-linkage or Faulty DNA Repair Theory	Bonds or cross-linkages develop between molecules or peptides: these bonds change the molecules' properties physically and chemically. Thus collagen in intracellular or extracellular material is chemically altered and function is affected. When collagen is cross-linked with other molecules, changes range from wrinkling, to atherosclerosis, to inelasticity of tissue. When cross-linkages occur with DNA molecules that carry genetic program, DNA is damaged and repairs slowly; mutation or death of cell occurs.	A viable theory.
Accumulation of Waste or of Senescent Cells Theory	Substances, such as metabolic waste materials and lipofuscins, which interfere with cellular metabolism and cause cell death, accumulate in cells. Examples of accumulation of metabolic waste are cataracts of the eye, cholesterol in the arteries, and bone brittleness. Cells that cannot divide anymore accumulate in older people.	These substances may be a result rather than cause of senescence.

TABLE 16-1

Theories of Physical Aging—continued

Theory	Definition/Explanation	Applications/Limitations
Accumulation of Errors Theory	*As cells die, they must synthesize new proteins to make new cells; sometimes an error occurs. When enough errors occur, organ failure results.*	Little scientific evidence.
Free Radical (or Oxidative Damage) Theory	*Oxygen-free radicals (charged or unstable molecules) or chemicals that contain oxygen in a highly activated state and react with other molecules during normal metabolism cause damage to cells and aging.* Exposure to radiation and certain enzymes may interfere with life activities.	Oxidation, as explained by theory, implicated in atherosclerosis, cancer, neurologic disease, and reduced immune function.
Deprivation Theory	*Aging is caused by deprivation of essential nutrients and oxygen to cells.*	Little scientific evidence. It is likely that deprivation is the result of aging.
Physiologic Theories		
Biological Clock or Aging by Program Theory	*Each organism contains genes or evolutionary processes that govern or control speed at which metabolic processes are performed. These genes or processes act as a genetic clock dictating occurrence of aging and dying.* Cells are genetically programmed to reproduce only a certain amount of time; human limit may be 100 to 120 years.	Humans may be able to outlive inner governing processes because of medical technology and improvements in lifestyle. Cells in nervous system and muscles do not reproduce themselves; all other cells do, at least to some extent.
	Hypothalamus may be the timer that keeps track of age of cells and determines how long they will keep reproducing.	Cells are more likely to reproduce imperfectly as they get older.
	Reproduced older cells do not appear to pass on information accurately through the DNA, which weakens functioning ability of older cells.	
Neuroendocrine Theory	*Hormonal changes produce free radicals, cross-linkages, and autoimmunity.*	Free radicals may be a special form of cross-linkage.
Immune (or Mounting Mutations) Theory	*Ability of immune system to deal with foreign organisms or processes diminishes with age.* Greatest decline is observed in thymus-derived immunity (T-cell production reduced). Production of antibodies declines after adolescence. **Autoimmune responses** may occur, *whereby normal cells are engulfed and digested*, making person more vulnerable to disease.	A viable theory. Autoimmunity may result from production of new antigens caused by (1) mutations that cause formation of altered RNA or DNA; or (2) the new antigens may have been hidden in the body earlier in life and are not recognized by body in late life. Implications for cancer.
Genetic Gene Theory	Aging is programmed; *the program exists in certain harmful genes. Genes that direct many cellular activities in early life may become altered in later years, which alters function* and may be responsible for functional decline and structural changes associated with aging.	Genetic basis exists for longevity, although environmental factors such as vaccines, nutrition, pollutants, safety factors, and medical care and technology can alter life span.

PSYCHOSOCIAL THEORIES

Just as one biological theory does not adequately address biological aging, one single psychosocial theory of aging is not adequate to explain psychological or social aging. The **Continuity Theory** proposes that an *individual's patterns of behavior are the result of a lifetime of experiences, and aging is the continuation of these lifelong adjustments or personality patterns. Personality traits remain stable, and early personality function is a guide for the retirement years. Continuity in behavioral patterns, values, and lifestyle exists over time, regardless of the actual level of activity present* (15, 45). Continuity Theory, as first proposed by Brim and Kagan, assumes neither a necessary reduction in activity levels (Disengagement Theory) nor the necessity of maintaining high activity levels (Activity Theory). They associated successful aging with the ability of the person to maintain patterns of behavior that existed before old age. Each of us has a powerful drive to maintain the sense of identity or continuity that allays fears of changing too fast or being changed against one's will by external forces. There is a simultaneous drive to develop and mature further, which fosters continuing change in at least small ways. It is theorized that adult development is not in the genes but in the intricacies of life experiences. Two psychological mechanisms, selective perception and situational reinforcement, are used to maintain a sense of continuity. **Selective perception** means that *experiences are reacted to on the basis of their relative congruence with currently held values, beliefs, and attitudes.* Noncongruent ideas are screened out of awareness, ignored, or not attended to. **Situational reinforcement** means that the *behaviors used are those that are rewarded. Previously established behavior patterns tend to have a long history of reinforcement* (15).

Five personality traits affect longevity: sociability, self-esteem and confidence, conscientiousness and social dependability, cheerfulness and optimism, and energy levels (156). A study of 1,500 people who, from 11 years of age onward, were followed every 5 to 10 years revealed that 60% lived into their late 80s. The risk of dying before age 70 was higher for people who had been optimistic, cheerful, and good-humored children. The likelihood of dying before 70 was lowest for those who had been cautious and conscientious as children. Conscientious people may practice less risky health habits (156).

DEVELOPMENTAL THEORIES

Several developmental theories have addressed psychosocial aging. **Erikson's Epigenetic Theory** (48–51) suggests that *successful personality development in later life depends on the ability to resolve the psychosocial crisis known as ego integrity versus despair.* Erikson's theory is psychodynamic, psychosocial, and a life cycle approach that emphasizes that the developmental tasks of each stage must be met before the person can work through the next tasks. The theory is discussed in detail later in this chapter.

Peck's Theory (142) hypothesizes that *there are three psychological developmental tasks of old age: ego differentiation versus work-role preoccupation, body transcendence versus body preoccupation, and ego transcendence versus ego preoccupation.* Refer to Chapter 15, ∞ and the section on adaptive mechanisms later in this chapter. Reed (149) also identified these tasks. These issues are an extension and

further development of Erikson's theory about this stage, with emphasis on change and growth in later life. According to all developmental theories, the older adult's behavior and response depend on how earlier developmental crises and tasks were handled.

Levinson theorizes that *late adulthood is characterized by a transition period that occurs between 60 and 65 years of age. The person does not become suddenly old, but physical and mental changes increase awareness of aging and mortality* (98).

SOCIOLOGIC THEORIES

Disengagement Theory, Activity Theory, and Symbolic Interaction Theory are sociologic theories. **Disengagement Theory,** proposed by Cumming and Henry (30), *suggests that all old people and society mutually withdraw, that the withdrawal is biologically and psychologically intrinsic and inevitable, and that it is necessary for aging and beneficial to society.* This voluntary withdrawal or separation from society is related to a decreased life space in the older adult, relinquishment of roles, less energy, decreased integration into society, fewer social interests, and focus on personal needs. Disengagement Theory suggests that individuals undergo a self-disengagement process during the middle and later years of life. *Studies do not support the Disengagement Theory.* The theory is referred to less and less. The older person may be alone but enjoys the solitude, is mentally alert, and is responsive socially (105, 106, 164).

Several concepts may relate to the disengagement process in late life. Sill's research (164) reveals that awareness of **finitude,** *estimate of time remaining before death,* and physical incapacity were more important than age in predicting level of activity. The person who perceives self as near death begins to constrict life space; psychological preparation for death may lead to disengagement. This type of disengagement would be similar to the depression experienced as part of the stages in the process of dying formulated by Kubler-Ross and described in Chapter 17. ∞ Further, the elder may consciously or unconsciously be aware of **terminal drop or decline,** *the period preceding the person's death from a few weeks up to 5 years,* which may account for some intellectual decline, changed verbal abilities, withdrawal from the world, and mood changes, as well as onset of physical illness (192).

Activity Theory, formulated by Maddox (105, 106) and Palmore (138) to refute Disengagement Theory, is a more popular and realistic theory. *Basic concepts of Activity Theory are that most elderly people maintain a level of activity and engagement commensurate with their earlier patterns of activity and past lifestyles and that the maintenance of physical, mental, and social activity is usually necessary for successful aging* (105, 106, 138).

Activity Theory implies that the older adult has essentially the same psychological and social needs as do middle-aged people. According to this theory, the older adult must compensate for loss of roles that are experienced. Productive activity is part of successful aging. Older people continue to be productive; some increase productivity. The older adult does not disengage but needs to maintain a moderately active lifestyle. People in their later maturity who are active with family and friends, in the volunteer role at church, in leisure such as golf, in various community organizations or projects, or in advocacy for social justice and political causes give evidence to Activity Theory. Activity fosters a sense of self-efficacy, mastery, and control (5). The most important aspect is that activity is regular and enjoyable.

Females in their 70s, 80s, and 90s are actively pursing a second adulthood. They have remained active, creative, and involved in various organizations. They are full of zest and have a passion and purpose in life. They may be returning to college or acting as consultants. They may concentrate on a few priorities intensely or volunteer in a number of projects. They demonstrate wisdom, discussed by Erikson (48–51), and ego and spiritual transcendence rather than self-preoccupation, as discussed by Peck (142).

Mead, in **Symbolic Interaction Theory,** *proposed that the person develops socially according to the continuous bombardment of self-reflections perceived from others. Biological changes, psychological changes, societal circumstances, and past and present experiences all are considered as relevant for explaining the aging process* (15, 138, 156). If ageism is strong in a culture, such as it has been in the United States, the elder perceives this attitude. It can become a self-fulfilling prophecy. People may expect to become inept and forgetful. Social and cultural expectations may strongly color self-view and consequent behavior. *Symbolic Interaction Theory explains the interrelationships of several dimensions of the aging process.*

1. Sociocultural dimensions set limits on available alternatives for the person.
2. Contextual dimensions within the individual's life course (e.g., biological change, past experiences) are an influence.
3. Personal evaluation of life experience, health status, and the future foci of energy and roles affect behavior.

Brown developed the **Urban Ecologic Model of Aging,** which is based on *person-environment interaction and the fact that human behavior and subjective well-being are reflected in the social interaction that occurs between the individual and the environment* (19). Lawton and Nahemon first proposed the Ecologic Model of Aging. Their original model characterized the *person as possessing various degrees of competence in four dimensions:* (a) biological health, including chronic medical diseases, (b) sensorimotor function and ability to perform activities of daily living, (c) cognitive ability, and (d) ego strength or emotional function. Individual adaptive behavior and subjective well-being are balanced when demands of the environment do not exceed level of ability to manage the demands. The *older person is more vulnerable than the younger counterpart, especially if the person* (19): (a) is impoverished, (b) experiences environmental stress or social problems, or (c) has multiple problems or needs. The greater the individual vulnerability, the greater the environmental impact on the person.

Brown (19) *expanded the model to include* (a) consideration of the suprapersonal environment and characteristics of the neighborhood, (b) personal characteristics of residents in the locale, (c) perceptions of the surrounding environment, (d) effects of media reports on the person's perception, (e) factual data about the surrounding environment, and (f) residential satisfaction and subjective well-being. The elder's personal experience or perception may differ from the factual reports of the neighborhood or environment, especially in urban, inner-city, or poverty-stricken areas. This model is relevant for determining health promotion strategies for the elder.

Family Development and Relationships

The changing demographic profile of developed countries has been associated with an increased number of four- and five-generation families. In such families it is common to have two generations at or near old age, with the oldest person frequently over 75 years. The "generation in the middle" may extend into retirement years in many families. Thus the "young-old," facing the potential of diminished personal resources, may be the group increasingly called on to give additional support to aged kin—the old-old and very or frail-old, as well as younger generations.

Aging in different cultures, family relationships between generations in different cultures and countries, and worldwide social changes are affecting the elderly as family members (70, 184). These changes raise issues for health care providers and affect your assessment and intervention for health promotion. *As you assess and intervene, utilize knowledge about relationships with* (a) spouse or partner, (b) offspring and other family members, (c) grandchildren and great-grandchildren, and (d) other social systems. *Educate and counsel the elder or family* in relation to the caregiver role, widowhood/widowerhood, divorce, singlehood, or same-gender relationships.

RELATIONSHIP WITH SPOUSE OR PARTNER

In 2003, older males were more likely to be married (70%) than older females (41%), and more males than females were married in each age group, even those 85 years or older. Widowhood is more common among females than males (70). Refer to Chapter 15 for information on widowhood. ∞

Married people have lower mortality than unmarried people of all ages. The survival advantage of marriage is larger for males (70). Marriage may have a protective factor; married people may be less likely to indulge in high-risk and health-damaging behaviors and more likely to receive support and care when needed (3, 70). Marriage may extend the social network of relatives and friends, who provide support at older ages (70).

In later life, responsibilities of parenthood and employment diminish with few formal responsibilities to take their place. There is usually a corresponding decline in social contacts and activities. The factors that affect the social life of the elderly are found in personal social skills and in resources available in the private life. Marital status remains a major organizing force for personal life. With children gone and without daily contact with co-workers provided by employment, the elderly lose the basis for social integration. Declining health, limited income, and fewer daily responsibilities may create greater needs for social support. Thus, having a spouse provides the possibility for increased companionship. Having a spouse also increases longevity, especially for older males (70).

Interestingly, spouses may not increase in their support of each other into late life, perhaps because of increased **interiority** (*introspection*) with aging (129). Time may erode bases of respect, affection, and compatibility. Sometimes marriages have not been filled with mutual emotional or social support in earlier years, so there is no foundation for increasing mutual emotional support. Females are often the sole support for males. Older females tend to feel the husband is not supportive emotionally or in health care; however, females tend to rely on a more extensive network of family and friends for support (45, 129).

If the female has not worked full-time outside of the home, to have her husband in the house, continually with her, wanting to share in or take over her homemaking activities, can be distressing even though it has been anticipated. The loss of privacy and solitude, doing tasks her own way and at her own pace, loss of independence, and loss of contact with friends may all be issues. If both have worked outside of the home and now are home full-time together, they have to learn to accommodate in a new way to each other's life patterns and routines, to share tasks and redefine roles, and to reaffirm and pursue individual and mutual interests. The increased accommodation to meeting each other's needs, however, is offset by increased opportunities for nurturing and being nurtured and for sharing mutual interests.

Your listening and teaching may assist the elderly person in making the necessary adjustments to the spouse. Explore with the couple the interests, activities, and hobbies they can share and those that can best be pursued individually. Validate that time alone is needed and can be enjoyable.

RELATIONSHIPS WITH OFFSPRING AND OTHER FAMILY MEMBERS

Historical trends toward smaller families, longer life spans, increasing employment of females, and increasingly high mobility of both young and old have important implications for children being a primary resource in old age.

Older females outnumber older males by nearly 3 to 2 (70). By age 85, the ratio of females to males is 2.5 to 1, which is consistent with international trends (70, 138). About 80% of centenarians are female (70). These statistics affect family relationships. At least one in four families in the United States are providing care for an older loved one (1, 70). Older African American, Asian, and Hispanic families are more likely than elderly non-Hispanic Caucasians to live with relatives. Older African American males are more likely to live alone. Older Asian males are three times more likely to live with relatives (70).

Assess the older adult's number of children, how recently the older parent has seen the children, the amount of assistance the older parent receives, and the older parent's interaction with the children. Parents with one child report fewer visits and less help received, especially if the only child is an employed daughter. Mothers with two or more children are more likely than those with only one child to see the children as a source of potential help. Interestingly, adult children with siblings are more likely to report a higher-quality relationship with the mother than are adults who are only children (138). Older parents expect children, especially daughters, to assume an appreciable level of responsibility in meeting important health, economic, and emotional needs. Assistance from children-in-law, grandchildren, siblings and siblings-in-law, and nieces and nephews increases as the number of offspring decreases. Geographic proximity is a stable predictor of older parent–child interaction, more than offspring gender or health status of the parent. Daughters who are blue-collar workers provide more assistance to older parents and have more association with

parents than the corresponding sons. Parents receive more help from offspring as the offspring's income increases (45, 138).

Older parents receive and perceive their children's help in several ways. Parents may tend to expect less help from children when they live at a distance or when they work outside the home. Further, they appreciate most the help that keeps them self-reliant or autonomous, maintains social integration, maximizes choice and expressive interactions, and forestalls reliance on more extensive services. Parents with a greater degree of ill health express less satisfaction with children's help, possibly because it symbolizes dependency and loss of social integration (45, 138). Reinforce the offspring's caregiving efforts with parents.

Some elderly people have a limited number of family members; some couples have no children. The childless couple will probably have adapted to childlessness psychologically; however, they are especially vulnerable at crisis points, such as episodes of poor health and death of spouse or housing companion. If those persons or couples cannot drive or have no transportation, they will have a greater need for help, although they may hesitate to ask for help.

The **geriatric care manager (GCM),** *a registered nurse or social worker knowledgeable about and experienced in the care of older people, is a professional caregiver to assist elders to live independently in the home as long as possible through services designed to meet their unique needs related to increasing disability, functional loss in managing activities of daily living (ADLs), or dependency consequent to chronic illness.* This is a relatively new type of caregiving service to assist offspring who are unable to care for elderly parents because they live a long distance from the parents but do care and want to be assured of their parents' diverse needs being met (1, 45). The offspring who lives at a distance may not realistically be able to return to the parental homesite or geographic area because of spousal or professional/career commitments. The GCM may be a family member or be perceived like a family member by the elder.

Educate that the role of the GCM is diverse, including to (1, 45):

1. Create a safe living environment.
2. Monitor the needs of the elder and contact and access necessary services, such as health care, legal, home maintenance, or transportation.
3. Advocate for the elder related to insurance or banking issues or health services. The GCM may assist with completing insurance forms; enrolling for Medicare, Medicaid, or Medicare Prescription D services; or paying bills, if the family so requests.
4. Make referrals to community agencies or resources that can (a) provide home services, such as home health attendant or housecleaning, or (b) eventually provide assisted living or long-term care options, when disability does not permit the elder to remain safely in the home or because the health care needs are extensive.
5. Recommend local caregiver groups or adult day care centers for the elder who is a spousal caregiver.
6. Provide consultation to the elder and to the offspring as needed, especially when physical impairment or memory disorders increase.
7. Provide support and assistance that the offspring would give to the parents if he or she were nearby and available.

BOX 16-1	Questions to Ask When Selecting Geriatric Care Management

1. What is your experience in geriatric care management?
2. Do you belong to any geriatric care managers' association?
3. Do you have a professional license (social worker, nurse, counselor)?
4. Can you provide references from clients as well as local organizations (such as hospitals or senior centers)?
5. Do you arrange for free, low-cost, or medically insured services when available and appropriate?
6. Do you personally provide any of the needed services?
7. Do you screen service providers for experience, reputation, licensing, insurance (including workers' compensation), and criminal records?
8. Are you affiliated with any service provider? If so, are you free to recommend competing providers?
9. Do you get referrals from any service provider? If so, do you receive a share of the fee?
10. Do you carry professional liability insurance? Are you bonded?
11. How often do you monitor each service personally?
12. Who covers for you when you're off duty?
13. How often can I expect routine reports? Written or phoned?
14. What are your fees and what do they include (e.g., initial assessment, expenses)?
15. Will you provide a written contract specifying fees and services?

Caution that this industry is relatively new and therefore poorly regulated. Such services can be obtained through the Visiting Nurse Association in the parental residential area, the primary care physician, or health care agency social worker. *Information and recommended GCM companies or qualified professional GCMs can also be obtained from the following sources:*

1. Administration of Aging Eldercare Locator. Phone: 800-677-1116.
2. National Association of Professional Geriatric Care Managers, which offers a national search for qualified professionals by zip code. Phone: 520-821-8008 or the Website, www.caremanager.org.

Educate elders and their offspring about GCM services, if appropriate, using the above information and referrals, and the questions listed in **Box 16-1.** Warn them to ask about the specialized knowledge base and types of elder care experience before hiring a GCM or any worker. The person should be interviewed by the offspring in parental presence, and by the parents if they are functionally able. The interaction between the GCM, or any recommended attendant, and the parents should be carefully observed and analyzed. Get feedback from the parents about their reactions to the person being interviewed.

Emphasize that the GCM should do the following:

1. Advise the family about long-term planning and how to conserve assets.
2. Be on 24-hour call and available at least by phone in an emergency.
3. Be able to communicate well and anticipate care needs.
4. Know about effective local resources such as geriatric, medical, and psychiatric specialists; senior centers, adult day care centers, and home care or hospice care agencies; and entitlements such as Medicare, Medicaid, veterans benefits, and pension plans.

Explore cost factors for such a service with the family, and whether specific or short-term services would sufficiently assist the elder and offspring. The GCM can cost from $80 to $300 hourly. Explore whether a parish nurse, described in Chapter 7, ∞ is available to carry out some of the listed functions. There may be other local senior service companies. Your teaching and referrals may enable the elderly person with few relatives or resources to manage more effectively and continue living independently. You can participate with the GCM to become politically active to improve social services and health care for the elder population.

GRANDPARENTHOOD AND GREAT-GRANDPARENTHOOD

Grandparenthood has multiple meanings for the person, depending in part on age at the initial time of grandparenthood, as is discussed in Chapter 15. ∞ The number and accomplishments of the grandchildren are probably a source of status (45, 118, 138). According to the 2000 census, there are 4.5 million children living in grandparent-headed households. More such arrangements occur in the African American population, but grandparents as primary caregivers are found in all socioeconomic and ethnic groups and in all geographic areas. Relative youth of grandparents contributes to the complex patterns of help and relationships between the generations. Older African American and Latino females are distinctive for extending their own households to children and grandchildren and assuming child care and housekeeping responsibilities into old age. However, that also helps the elder transmit values, especially grandparents who have migrated to this country and do not trust mainstream culture (9, 15, 45, 183). Traditionally, the central figure, especially in the poor African American family, has been the mother or grandmother, who has been responsible for maintenance of family stability and a source of socialization (183).

The increasing divorce rate also adds to the complexity of grandparent relationships. The child may have eight sets of grandparents.

MediaLink 🌐 National Association of Professional Geriatric Case Manager

The grandparents may be the main caretakers for the children, or there may be a part-time commitment, sharing child care with their adult children. Likewise, grandchildren have a special tie to grandparents. Research indicates that even when there is divorce in the family, adult children from divorced families continue their relationships with grandparents (27, 183).

Sometimes the grandparents are caretakers of special-needs grandchildren. The grandchild with a disability may be more taxing physically, emotionally, and economically, and there is a sense of loss and grief for what might have been. The grandparents can be a positive influence on the child, may give the parents respite, and may avoid the burdens or problems that can accompany caring for "normal" children—for example, peer pressure demands or risky behavior. Participation in play, school projects, and family gatherings are ways of building a relationship.

Grandparents increasingly are the main caretaker of the grandchild in the custodial role, although legal custody is unlikely if the child has a permanent home. Sometimes the grandparents serve as babysitter or a day care service. When the mother also lives in the home, the grandmother being the main caregiver may have a negative impact on parenting by both the mother and grandmother (45, 84, 88, 89, 130, 138). Grandparents are often happy with their role and enter into a playful, informal, companionable, and confiding relationship, as depicted in **Figure 16-2**. The grandchild is seen as a source of leisure activity, someone for whom to purchase items that are also enjoyable to the grandparent. The grandparent typically does not want to take on an authoritarian or disciplinarian role but will, and has the experience to do so, if necessary.

The number of *great-grandparents* and *great-great-grandparents* is increasing as more people live longer. The roles are emotionally fulfilling. These family members provide a sense of personal and family renewal and transcendence, add diversion to conversations if not activities, and mark longevity (37, 150).

Great-grandparents may be as active in the grandparenting role as they were as grandparents; but advanced age, geographic distance, and cohabitation, divorce, and remarriage of young adult family members tend to limit their participation (150). Great-

grandparents want to influence the younger generation with their wisdom, remain connected, share values and family stories, and give meaning to their transcendence (150).

Assess for availability and appropriateness of grandchildren, as well as adult children, to be informal caregivers of older adults when the elder needs care (183). They are the "skipped generation" in planning for care and in education and counseling interventions. Past and present relationships, as well as the elder's self-care abilities and the grown grandchild's caregiving motivations and skills, should be determined prior to the grandchild assuming the caregiver role (183). You can educate the younger generations about the importance of these elders and their roles.

SOCIAL RELATIONSHIPS

Social networks of family, friends, neighbors, former co-workers, volunteers in community support services, and service providers such as the mail carrier, police, or utility workers provide instrumental and expressive support. *They contribute to well-being of the elder* by (a) promoting socialization and companionship, (b) elevating morale and life satisfaction, (c) buffering the effects of stressful events, (d) providing a confidante, and (e) facilitating coping skills and mastery. For example, social supports buffer the effects of stressful life events and represent more than the quantity or proximity of social ties. Social ties fulfill practical needs as well. Also, the *components of informal support networks*—spouses, children, close relatives, distant kin (cousins, aunts, uncles, nieces, nephews), co-workers, close friends, neighbors, members of volunteer community support services, and acquaintances—have a variety of functions and vary in importance. Some people in the U.S. community act as lay gatekeepers. Mail carriers, veterinarians, utility workers, the sheriff's department, and farm, implement, and grain dealers provide informal social support and help look out for rural elders. Instrumental help is given in the form of advice, information, financial aid, and assistance with tasks. Socioemotional aid is given in the form of affection, sympathy, understanding, acceptance, esteem, and referral to services (16, 45, 138, 156, 179). Planning for contact between the generations (e.g., with preschoolers or adolescents) also contributes to meaningful social interactions for both generations.

Formal health-related support services include government and private agencies that provide a service. Examples include home maintenance services, chore services, home-delivered groceries or meals, pharmacies that deliver drugs or medical supplies, assistance of home health aides, home visits by professional therapists or nurses, and case management services. Formal support services that are available to elderly adults but that do not always come to the home include medical and social services, day care, respite care, and the church.

Frequency of use of social networks is not related to physical health. As income decreases, visiting with neighbors may decline. Visits to close friends or relatives are likely to increase, as does the tendency to talk to family members about feelings and to talk to friends about events. The elderly rate helpfulness of children and other family members as important. Lower income increases the senior's reliance on friends and relatives and the value placed on their help. Higher income may provide resources that facilitate social visiting and a broader network of relationships. A higher fre-

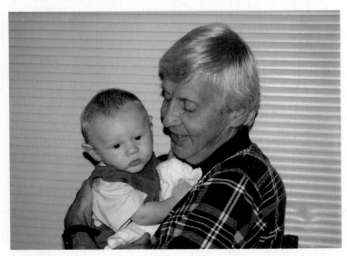

FIGURE ■ **16-2** Grandparents often look forward to their role.

quency of social contacts and greater intensity of kin and friend relationships have been found for females in comparison to males. Apparently intimacy or close friendship ties and having a confidant are less important to the male (15, 138).

Supportive ties become smaller and more unstable for the old-old. The closer the bond, the greater are the physical, emotional, and financial strains. *Burdens and costs may result* in (138): (a) being less willing or able to help, (b) manifesting physical or psychological distancing, (c) increasing the social isolation of the dependent elder, or (d) becoming enmeshed in the caregiver role to the exclusion of other relationships or roles. Informal networks ideally are integrated with formal support services.

An unregulated or informal social welfare system naturally exists in the average community or senior residence, which provides more services, security, and hope than is provided by formal agencies. This system of informal assistance is the major source of help for the elderly. *Among and for seniors, there are three neighborhood exchange types* (39, 45, 138):

1. **High helpers,** who *exhibit a more formal, quasi-professional style of helping without reciprocation.*
2. **Mutual helpers,** *who show an interdependent style of give and take.*
3. **Neighborhood isolates,** *whose social ties and help sources are primarily outside the neighborhood.*

High helpers with neighbors are those who also do volunteer work or are active in self-help groups. Often these people have been in the helping professions in their work years. They also have a spiritual or religious orientation with serving others. Mutual helpers have more neighborhood contact and are generally quite outgoing. Isolates have little contact with others and view themselves as quiet people. They may be in poor health and in need of help themselves (138).

Many of the events of later life are **exit events,** *involving continuous threat, stress, and loss, such as widowhood/widowerhood, chronic or poor health, retirement, change in residence, and lower income.* Thus, coping often becomes problem specific. It also involves **elder socialization,** *learning how to perform new roles, adjusting to changing roles, and relinquishing old roles. Socialization contributes to well-being by lending continuity and structure to the transitions encountered by people.*

Your accepting attitude and counsel assist the elderly in asking for and accepting help from others. Refer elders to community resources as needed.

CAREGIVER ROLE

The role of the middle-aged offspring in caring for the elderly parent is described in Chapter 15. ∞ Even as elders are being cared for, they are also a source of support—emotionally, socially, and financially (by providing living arrangements or direct monetary assistance)—for the adult child. Research describes the mutual caring that occurs in other cultures (3, 9, 32, 61, 160, 197) but it occurs in the United States also. In the United States, statistics about caregiving are maintained. In some cultures and countries, it is a way of life.

Family or informal caregivers (an estimated 44.4 million) constitute the greatest source of care for older adults in the United

States and will be increasingly important (7, 70). The older spouse who is the caregiver may be especially vulnerable to burden and stress because of personal health problems. *The caregiving experience depends on many variables, including* (a) the prior relationship; (b) physical, emotional, and cognitive status of the care recipient and caregiver; (c) cultural, ethnic, and religious background of the individual; (d) economic status; (e) health care and other support systems; (f) access to respite care services if desired; (g) other life changes that occur to upset balance in the caregiving system; and (h) duration of the experience. Kolanowski and Piven (93) discuss research and intervention issues in this area.

Female caregivers of spouses with dementia experience more stress and immune system responses than male caregivers, according to self-report (180). That may be related to spouse demands.

The caregiver in an elderly couple is most frequently the wife, as females live longer than males and are usually younger than spouses. If the wife is impaired, the husband is often the caregiver. The spouse is the primary source of help for married elderly with impaired capacity. Adult daughters, in contrast to sons, are the major helpers when a spouse is not present or unable to be the caregiver (45, 70). The children usually try to be caregivers (165). Siblings may share in care of the parents. Sometimes offspring change work hours or the job, or give up the job entirely (45). Some contact a geriatric care manager (1, 45). Some may arrange **Lifeline** or **MedicAlert,** *24-hour emergency response services offered by the Red Cross or hospitals.* In some cultures, the grandchild or great-grandchild may be the major caregiver, especially if they were raised by the now-frail grandparents or great-grandparents (21, 183). The probability of relying on friends is highest among impaired elderly who are unmarried and have few family members within an hour's travel. The more frail the person, the more likely a family member will be the primary caregiver rather than formal systems or nonrelated people (16, 45, 101, 179). The majority of noninstitutionalized elderly are self-sufficient (15, 70, 138, 156).

Assess the elderly person who cares for a disabled or ill spouse, who is at risk for physical and emotional stresses of caregiving superimposed on stresses of the aging process. He or she is likely to experience a barrage of feelings and role overload, including being head of the household. The spouse who is the caregiver may also be chronically ill or disabled (160). Thus, the family caregiver for the noninstitutionalized elder is in need of help from supportive services. *Refer to or establish these services for the spouse, such as* (a) a wives' support group sponsored by a senior center, (b) home health care, (c) adult day care, (d) foster home placement, (e) extended respite care, (f) homemaker services, (g) transportation and repair services, (h) visitor or "relief" services, and (i) individual counseling (35, 45).

Sometimes the elder is caregiver for an adult child with developmental disability, mental retardation, or mental illness. The gratification, frustration, and stress are related to the adult child's diagnosis and health status, size of the parent's support system, the family's social climate, and the adult child's participation in out-of-home programs.

Explore feelings of the middle-aged or elderly caregiver and the family, needs and feelings of the elderly person, issues and conflicts for the family, and ways to help families manage the caregiving experience. A number of strategies previously described—including communication and therapeutic relationships, stress management, crisis intervention, time management, and adult education methods—are useful as you intervene with the elder and the caregiver. Educate the caregiver about ways to give physical care that can involve the care recipient to the extent possible and save energy for the caregiver. Refer to **Table 16-14**, Community Resources for Older People, for *other programs that can be effective for reducing stress for caregivers of elderly family members who are emotionally or physically disabled*. **Homeshare,** *whereby a group of adults share a house or apartment and the tasks of daily living, is also an option* in some geographic regions. Selection of housemates must be done with care. Monitoring by a GCM and assistance from other providers are likely to be needed even while elders help and care for each other.

WIDOWHOOD/WIDOWERHOOD

Because death of a spouse may occur before late life, feelings, problems, and issues pertinent to the widow or widower have been discussed in Chapter 15. ∞ Bereavement does not permanently affect health status for most seniors, although the grief reaction may induce physiologic symptoms initially. Stress appears to increase as the death approaches, and then health status may deteriorate (45, 161). Regardless of the predeath mourning done by the survivor, the elderly widow or widower has a great increase in psychological distress (15, 38, 45, 156). Widowhood is more depressing for males than females. For both genders, death of a spouse affects economic resources, social support systems, and mortality (45, 50, 70, 75).

Widowhood/widowerhood disrupts couple-based relationships and obligations to a spouse and introduces emotional and material burdens on those relationships that outlive the marriage. Death of a spouse, especially after a period of caregiving, may also introduce both a measure of freedom to make new contacts and a stimulus to do so. Without the support that the spouse usually provides, the widowed may turn to friends and relatives as a source of replacement. The widowed may have greater intimacy with their friends than the married, for married people interact more with their spouses (15, 45, 156).

Elderly females have some advantage over elderly males in their ability to develop or maintain social relationships. Patterns of social relationships established among the married apparently provide the parameters within which social relationships continue among the widowed. Both married and widowed females, in contrast to males, are more likely to talk to close friends and relatives and to talk to their children about worries and crises. Loss of spouse allows for expansion or addition of new roles; frequency of contact increases. There may be greater involvement with informal social relationships than marriage (15, 31, 45, 58, 74, 101.

The widow who lives alone in her own home may be in need of a great deal of help. Neighbors often provide this help, especially if children reside out of town. The childless widow or widower, however, may not receive any more help from neighbors than a widow or widower with children, despite greater needs. Perhaps adult children are able to elicit neighbor assistance; such requests for extra help are not forthcoming if there are no children. The widower may have difficulty because he grew up in an era when the male role was more restrictive and lifeways more independent than for the female (58, 66, 156).

Your teaching, emotional support, referral to services, and encouragement to continue as active a life as possible are important as the widow or widower adjusts to losses and new roles. Refer to community educational and social groups that are of interest and accessible.

DIVORCE AND THE ELDERLY

Be prepared to give emotional support or crisis intervention to the older person who is encountering divorce or who is reworking the conflicts, dilemmas, and losses of having experienced divorce.

Those who are separated from their spouses and those who are legally divorced total slightly less than 10% of the elder population (70). The numbers of people who were ever divorced, who were divorced before age 65, and who are over age 65 when divorce occurs are increasing as elders live longer. Many divorced people remarry. In the future an increased number of seniors will fall in the ever-divorced and currently divorced categories because those entering old age will be more accepting of divorce as a solution to an unpleasant marriage. Further, in the future more elderly women will have economic independence because of their years in the workforce, and this may encourage higher divorce rates (15, 70, 156).

Being divorced in old age, or in any age, may negatively affect a person's economic position and may increase demands for social welfare support. Typically divorce is associated with a deterioration in the standard of living for females, although it has little effect for males (15, 45, 156). Further, family and kinship relationships are affected by divorce. The children or other relatives who would provide physical help and psychosocial support may not be available to one of the parents in his or her old age. The experience of being divorced can help the senior cope with later bereavement. The person knows survival is possible after a marital relationship ends.

Remarriage also establishes a new set of nuclear family relationships. To ensure economic safety, some widowed or divorced elders who want to establish a committed relationship may cohabitate and remain unmarried (6.7 million partners in 2000). The number is continuing to increase (70). Some elders establish a **prenuptial** or **antenuptial agreement**. *This contract is made before marriage to settle, in advance, respective property and financial rights of each party and the children of each person in the event of divorce or death.* In formulating a contract, the male and female should each retain their own lawyers, fully disclose all assets, and finalize the pact well before the wedding. For some people, the prenuptial contract, with all the legal work involved, becomes a reality check. The couple may decide not to marry, realizing that the relationship will not really meet each person's needs. Some elders choose to forgo a contract and formal marriage but do reside together for companionship (45, 70).

SINGLEHOOD

A small percentage (approximately 4%) of elderly people remain single and never marry (70). They have no spouse or children. They may or may not have living family members. They may or may not live alone. Never-married elders do not constitute a single "social type"; their situations are more complex. Like other elders, they are affected by social opportunities and restraints and the cultural values and changes that impinge on their life situations. Some older singles are homosexual. Some live in locations in which females outnumber males, causing an imbalance in mate selection. Others may have chosen the single lifestyle because of a career. Some have had family responsibilities that precluded marriage or were otherwise unable to break out of their families of origin. Others have been lifelong isolates and have had poor health or a stigmatized social identity. Possibly the factors for singlehood have been multiple (107, 147).

Well-being in old age can be at least partly explained by a supportive relationship with the parent in early life. Elders who had a supportive relationship are more likely to be adaptive and cope with adversity effectively in old age (147, 153, 197). There are prior relationships for never-married older females that help reduce social isolation and loneliness and increase life satisfaction and social support. Chapter 6 and Chapter 14 present information on the single "family" or adult. ∞

Having lived independently all during adult life, the person developed effective adaptive mechanisms and a supportive social network. The single person who has planned carefully for retirement may be as satisfied with self and life and as secure in all aspects as the married person. The single person may be no more lonely than the married person (107, 147, 153, 197). A decline in functional capacity greatly increases the likelihood that the unmarried older person will move in with others or become institutionalized.

Lifestyle is geared to preserving personal independence and the development of self. Privacy, self-expression through work, freedom of movement, and expanding experiences, philosophic insights, and imaginative conceptions of life are goals. Single females are happier and better adjusted than single males. Marital roles may be less beneficial and more stressful for females than for males. Lower well-being of the never married is attributable either to changes accompanying aging, which lessen the viability of single lifestyles, or to less support of single living among other older people (107, 147, 153, 197).

Friends are also important. Friendship is a process that occurs throughout life. Older adults rarely terminate friendships, though they may fade away because of lifestyle changes, geographic moves, or illness. Friends of former years who still maintain contact act as a memory for each other, a witness to another person's history. Friends can also act as family and promote health. Positive social interaction lowers the stress hormone levels, helps preserve cognitive functions, and prevents depression. Sharing ideas, talking, and listening is the main value of friendships (107, 147, 197). Refer to Chapter 14 for more information on friendship. ∞

Be alert to special emotional and social needs of the single elderly, to their reticence at times to ask for help, and to the need for information about community resources. You may become a significant confidante. Realize that living alone has different implications for people from cultures other than mainstream U.S. culture. See Abstract for Evidence-Based Practice.

GAY AND LESBIAN RELATIONSHIPS

The current cohort of people in later maturity grew up when homosexuality was rare or not acknowledged. Some elderly homosexuals may have recognized their gender preference before the Gay Liberation Movement in the late 1960s, when there was stigma attached to disclosure and the lifestyle. Others may have acknowledged their gender preference more openly after the Gay Libera-

tion Movement. The latter group view their homosexuality as a characteristic of themselves. Regardless, the homosexual elder has needs for social contact, love, and intimacy. Relationships in late life tend to be strong, supportive, and diverse. Many homosexuals have children from previous marriages or have adopted children. Friendship networks or support groups may substitute for the traditional family. The main problems for this group grow out of societal attitudes, policies, and discrimination; strained relationships with the family of origin; lack of medical or social services and social support; and bereavement and inheritance issues when a partner becomes ill or dies (45, 138, 151, 152).

ELDERS AND PETS

Pets are great companions and usually like a family member for older people. Pets are therapeutic in the home and in the center or institution for the elderly. They offer companionship and unconditional love; they soothe and lift the spirits. A specially trained dog can offer assistance and security (e.g., as a brace for the neurologically impaired). Dogs can pull wheelchairs and even help load them into cars. Pets have a beneficial effect on physical health: They lower stress response and lower blood pressure. The touch from the pet and stroking the pet offer physiologic release and lower anxiety. Pets can promote verbal communication skills; birds can even talk back (45). Although animals and birds do carry disease, healthy pets can be obtained from well-run shelters and shops or the Humane Society.

Refer the elder to Canine Companions for Independence, a national organization that supplies highly trained service dogs for helping people who use wheelchairs, who are visually impaired or deaf, or who need a social companion because of disability. Pets are chosen for temperament, not breed. There is no charge for the dog. Contact the agency at PO Box 446, Santa Rosa, CA 95402-0446 (707-528-0830).

Educate the person or family about keeping the pet immunized and cleaned and the care that prevents unnecessary decline in the pet's health. Care of pets, especially dogs, can take a lot of energy but it is essential.

Ensure that the elder has the home equipment and environment suitable for the pet, whether a dog, cat, or bird. Encourage the elder to enlist aid of family or friends and to obtain necessary instructions, supplies, and services for the pet. Explore accessible pet services. Mobile veterinarians, grooming vans, and other services are available in some areas.

You can be instrumental in promoting pet therapy. Anticipate that the death of a pet can precipitate a deep grief, and mourning will result because of the loss. Crisis counseling is useful to help the person work through the pet's death or feelings related to having to put the pet to sleep. Monitor the elder's care of the pet. Be aware that the senior who wants euthanasia for an apparently healthy pet may be contemplating suicide, or suicide may follow the death of a pet. Death of a pet can be the last straw in a series of stresses and losses. Provide social and emotional linkages to the extent possible for the person.

ELDER ABUSE AND NEGLECT

It is estimated that 500,000 to 1 million older Americans are abused annually. It is a problem that still remains hidden from the

Abstract for Evidence-Based Practice

Health of Older People Living Alone or with Relatives

You, K.S., & Lee, H. (2006). The physical, mental, and emotional health of older people who are living alone or with relatives. *Archives of Psychiatric Nursing, 20*, 193–201.

KEYWORDS

Korea; aged, psychosocial factors; adaptation, psychological; geriatric functional assessment; health status; mental health.

Purpose ➤ To compare the physical, mental, and emotional health of rural Korean older adults who live alone to those who live with relatives. The number of rural older people living alone has been increasing due to migration of younger adults to urban areas for employment.

Conceptual Framework ➤ World Organization of National Colleges, Academies, and Academic Associations of General Practitioners/Family Physicians (WONCA) Classification of Senior Health.

Sample/Setting ➤ All participants were enrolled in senior community centers in 10 randomly selected rural Korean provinces. Inclusion criteria were age 65 or older, independence and capability to perform daily tasks with minimal assistance, intact cognitive skills, and ability to communicate with the public health nurse at the senior center. Of the eligible participants who met the criteria, 110 lived alone and 102 lived with relatives. Over half (54.6%) of those living alone were 75 years or older, and 40.2% of those living with relatives fell within this age range.

Methods ➤ The Korean version of the Physical Health Assessment Scale, Mental Health Assessment Scale, and Emotional Health Assessment Scale were administered to each participant as part of a face-to-face structured interview after informed consent was obtained.

Findings ➤ Physical capabilities such as eyesight, hearing acuity, bathing, and telephone use of older adults living with relatives were significantly better than those living alone.

There was no difference in skills such as eating, dressing, using the bathroom, or taking medications. Mental capabilities such as arithmetic, writing one's name, prioritizing tasks, memory, recognition of environmental changes, and feelings of safety were better in those who lived with relatives. There were no significant differences in time orientation, ability to answer questions, giving or taking instructions, or the expression of desires. For emotional health, those elders living with relatives had significantly higher scores on almost every item, such as feeling successful, happy, interested, and satisfied with life.

Implications: ➤ Older adults who live alone may be prone to lower physical capabilities because of poorer housing conditions than those living with relatives. For example, traditional Korean houses had no bathrooms or running water, which would make bathing and laundry more difficult than for those living in more modern housing with relatives. Higher mental skills among those living with relatives suggest that family may provide the cognitive and social stimulation to maintain such skills. The better emotional health of those living with relatives also suggests the protective effect of social interactions and support upon emotional well-being.

The generalized poor emotional health of elders living alone suggests that health care service programs make emotional health a priority. The differing capabilities of those living alone versus with family suggest that different services should be tailored for people within these groups. Periodic health assessments are important for determining those capabilities that remain intact versus those that are altered, and offering appropriate interventions.

public and even professionals. The victim usually is a Caucasian female over 70 with moderate to severe physical or mental impairments. However, elder abuse occurs in all cultural groups. Usually the abuser is a relative (spouse more often than offspring) residing with her. Refer to **Box 16-2**, Types and Manifestations of Elder Abuse, for further description (10, 15, 17, 45, 119, 124, 193). Causes of elder abuse are listed in **Box 16-3**, Causes of Elder Maltreatment, Abuse, or Neglect (17, 45, 66, 119, 124, 172). Ways to prevent or reduce abuse are listed in the **Box** Client Education: Tips for the Older Person for Preventing or Reducing Abuse. These are suggestions for anticipating dependency or a change in living situation that could become an abusive relationship.

Assess for the following signs and symptoms that would indicate abuse or neglect in the elder (10, 15, 17, 20, 45, 52, 124, 193):

1. Bruises, fractures, malnourished status, burns, and other physical injuries typical of abuse, either current or in the medical history
2. Undue confusion not attributable to physiologic consequences of aging
3. Conflicting explanation about the senior's condition
4. Unusual fear exhibited by the senior in a presumed safe environment, in the home, or in the presence of the caregiver
5. Report of the daily routine that has considerable gaps in the sequence; a change in lifestyle
6. Apparent impaired functioning or abnormal behavior in the caregiver
7. Indifference, hostility, or suspicions displayed by the caregiver to the elder and in response to questions by health care providers

BOX 16-2	Types and Manifestations of Elder Abuse

PHYSICAL ABUSE

1. Neglect of physical care (food, eyeglasses, hearing aid, or information withheld)
2. Slap, bruise, push
3. Beating
4. Burns, broken bones
5. Brandishing a knife, cutting, stabbing
6. Restraint (chain to toilet or tie to bed), resulting in skin breakdown or decubitus ulcers, as well as fractures
7. Sexual molestation, rape

PSYCHOLOGICAL ABUSE

1. Verbal abuse (curse, scream, insult, demean, treat like a child)
2. Verbal threats, name calling
3. Decision making, voting denied
4. Exclusion from family activities, isolation
5. Placement in nursing home without consent or knowledge

FINANCIAL ABUSE

1. Confiscation of Social Security or other income checks
2. Person forced to sign over property or assets
3. Other financial exploitation
4. Theft of property and personal items for sale
5. Takeover of trust, guardianship
6. Exploitation of resources for profit

SOCIAL ABUSE

1. Forced isolation from family, friends
2. Constant switching of doctors
3. Refusal of home health care or other community resources (day care, home health aide, Meals-on-Wheels)
4. Inability to accept help or acknowledge difficulty with care
5. Geographic isolation, for example, rural, inner-city ghetto
6. Caregiver or client minimize injuries or situation

BOX 16-3	Causes of Elder Maltreatment, Abuse, or Neglect

1. Elder becomes more dependent or disabled.
2. Elder is cognitively impaired or has Alzheimer's disease.
3. Family is under economic stress.
4. Caregiver is exhausted or loses control; unable to cope.
5. Adult offspring is unemployed, lives in parent's home, and expects to be cared for.
6. Adult offspring is mentally ill or alcohol- or drug-addicted.
7. Family interaction pattern of screaming, hitting, and violence has existed through lifetime of marriage or child rearing.
8. Retirement and lack of role clarity for both spouses result in much frustration in retired man.
9. Man who was abusive to co-workers now abuses most available person, the wife.
10. Woman is financially dependent on spouse.
11. Elder is abandoned or seldom visited by children.
12. Victim is unwilling or unable to report the problem.

8. History of violent behavior and substance abuse or addiction in the spouse or caregiver
9. Isolated living arrangement or dependence on others, either physically or mentally, for maintenance of daily routine and health care
10. Consistent passive, withdrawn, hopeless, helpless, or unresponsive behavior toward professional caregiver in the home or health care agency
11. Excuses or rationalizations for condition of home, physical status, or unavailability of requested items or equipment for implementing home care

During assessment of potential abuse or neglect, do not let stereotypes about the elder or caregiver, an emphasis on family privacy, or denial prevent you from identifying the problem. Avoid a censuring tone of voice or judgmental expression or stance. Show a willingness to listen to the caregiver's perspective. Solicit the caregiver's early memories of relationships with the senior to learn of long-term conflicts. *Most abused seniors are reluctant and ashamed to report abuse or neglect because of* (a) fear of retaliation, (b) exposure of offspring to community censure or legal punishment, and (c) fear of potential removal from their home.

Nursing history should include the following areas: (a) present problems, (b) family history, (c) health and psychiatric history, (d) personal and social history, (e) physical examination—all systems, (f) mental status, (g) medications, and (h) communication and relational patterns (10, 20, 45, 100, 111, 119, 193). Burgess et al. (20), Muehlbauer and Crane (124), and the February 2007 issue

Client Education

Tips for the Older Person for Preventing or Reducing Abuse

1. Remain sociable and stay active in the community; enlarge your circle of friends; join local chapters of American Association of Retired Persons or Older Women's League.
2. Plan for possible disability by completing an advance medical directive and arranging for power-of-attorney.
3. Familiarize yourself with community resources that help older people remain as independent as possible.
4. Do not share a household with anyone who has a history of violent behavior or substance abuse.
5. Do not move in with a child or relative if your relationship is troubled.

6. Avoid taking into your home new or unknown people in a live-in arrangement.
7. Ask for help when you need it from a lawyer, physician, or trusted family member.
8. Call Adult Protective Services or Elder Protective Services (found in State Government section of white pages) if you or someone you know suffers abuse.
9. Call the ombudsman in State Office of Aging to investigate complaints against long-term care facilities in which you reside.

of *Archives of Psychiatric Nursing* (volume 21) present additional in-depth information on elder abuse, assessment, intervention, and evaluation components and tools.

Three questions help detect partner violence (52):

1. Have you been hit, kicked, punched, or otherwise hurt by someone within the past year? If so, when?
2. Do you feel safe in your current relationship?
3. Is there a partner from a previous relationship who is making you feel unsafe now?

Ask questions when alone with the elder and not to be overheard by the abusive caregiver in the home. Signals and other nonverbal behavior may have to be used to obtain data and avoid suspicions, which takes time, a trustworthy approach, and astute observation of the total environment. The elder must feel safe to disclose, especially if disabled or bedridden. If possible, use a multidisciplinary team approach for discussion of the problem, planning, and implementation of a safe intervention. Discuss, as appropriate, observations with the caregiver and options to reduce caregiver stress and obtaining of needed medical services for the client. Immediacy of action, especially in the home setting, depends on client status, caregiver behavior, medical care, and community resources. Analysis includes client and personal safety, accessing of emergency health and police protection services, and legal and ethical considerations.

In planning care and during intervention, be familiar with the reporting laws of your state and whether the law covers only known abuse or suspected abuse. In most states professionals who fail to report abuse may be fined, and they are accorded protection from civil and criminal liability if they report abuse.

Utilize the following checklist for topics to include when implementing psychoeducation:

1. Cycle of violence and the consequences
2. Preparations for a safe escape plan
3. Access to shelters, transportation resources, legal protection, and legal resources

Practice Point

Be aware that advocacy for the abused elder may be difficult. You may receive threats of harm from caregivers who resent the disruption of a previously convenient financial or sexual exploitation of an elderly relative. A common situation is when the elder refuses help and desires to remain in an environment that, by your standard, is unacceptable or unsafe. This can be very frustrating. Testifying in court to the nature of specific abusive situations can be anxiety provoking. You must be well prepared in the case of legal action. Thorough documentation is essential.

4. Support and safety networks that are confidential
5. Strategies to cope with stressors and threats that are a part of the abuse
6. Physical and mental health care measures, facilitation of nutrition and sleep
7. Resources or beliefs that foster hope

Such education must be given carefully, in analogies or briefly written materials or on 3 × 5 (or smaller) cards, if the abusive person is in the home or in the presence of the elder during your caregiving and education.

Because the abused or neglected senior is an adult with full legal rights, intervention is not possible without the consent of the senior if the person is legally competent. If the client is in a life-threatening situation, is competent, and chooses to remain at home, you must honor that decision after counseling the elder of the danger. If the person is legally incompetent and appears in immediate danger, report and begin appropriate procedures to ensure safety.

Physiologic Concepts: Physical Characteristics

When we are born, regardless of our genetic background or external influences, we all have one thing in common—the element of aging. From the day of birth, we begin the aging process in our unique way. There is much diversity in the aging process.

The rapidity and manifestations of aging in each individual depend on heredity, past illnesses, lifestyle, patterns of eating and exercise, presence of chronic illnesses, and level of lifetime stress. Some generalized physiologic changes do occur, however; they include a decrease in rate of cell mitosis, a deterioration of specialized nondividing cells, an increased rigidity and loss of elasticity in connective tissue, and a loss of reserve functional capacity (45, 65).

Certain other characteristics have been observed about aging (4, 15, 45, 65, 111, 138, 156):

1. Time of onset, type, and degree of aging differ between males and females and are more distinctive between the genders in middle life than in the later years.
2. Senescent alterations in one organ or in the whole organism can be either premature or delayed in relation to the body's total chronology.
3. The progression of aging in cellular tissues is asymmetric: The characteristics of old age may be displayed prominently in one system (brain, bone, cardiovascular apparatus, lungs) and be less obvious elsewhere (liver, pancreas, gastrointestinal tract, muscles).
4. **Organ reserve**, *the extra capacity of the organs that is drawn on in times of stress or illness, lessens with age.* (In young adulthood, the body can put forth 4 to 10 times its usual effort when stressed.)
5. A direct relationship exists between the sum of common aging traits and the length of survival.

GENERAL APPEARANCE

The general appearance of the older adult is determined in part by the changes that occur in the skin, face, hair, and posture. Old females have significantly more body fat, greater truncal skinfolds, and greater circumferences than old males and young adult females, and they have less fat-free body mass than young adult females (45, 138).

Skin

The overall appearance of the skin changes dramatically. See **Table 16-2**, Alterations in and Health Promotion for Integumentary System Related to Aging (45, 67, 181). Because of decreased skin elasticity, skin turgor is a poor indicator of hydration. Sweat glands atrophy and the capillary bed diminishes; thus, the skin is less effective in cooling body temperature (45).

Head

Even the appearance of the face changes as the nose and ears tend to become longer and broader and the chin line alters. Wrinkles on the face are pronounced because of the repeated stress produced by the activity of facial muscles. The predominant mood expressed by the facial muscles of the individual becomes permanently etched on the face in the form of wrinkles (smile or frown lines) above the eyebrows, around lips, over cheeks, and around the outer edges of the eye orbit. Shortening of the platysma muscle produces neck wrinkles (45).

Gray hair is the universal phenomenon associated with aging, but it is not a reliable indicator of age, as some individuals begin graying as early as their teen years. The hair gradually grays; the exact shade of gray depends on the original hair color. Eventually all the pigmented hair is replaced by nonpigmented hair, gradually the overall hair color turns pure white. Both males and females are affected. The loss of hair occurs on the scalp, in the pubic and axillary areas, and on the extremities. In most older adults there is also increased growth of facial hair due to the change in the androgen-estrogen ratio (45).

Posture

The posture of the older adult is one of general flexion. The head is tilted forward; hips and knees are slightly flexed. Muscles in the torso are held rigidly. The older adult stands with the feet apart to provide a wide base of support. He or she takes shorter steps, which may produce a shuffling gait. A shift in the center of gravity occurs as well, which affects movement and balance (45).

NEUROLOGIC SYSTEM
Nervous System

Chronic stress, inactivity, and obesity adversely affect the neurologic and endocrine systems, especially as the person ages (171). When cortisol is chronically elevated, atrophy of hippocampal cells occurs, which negatively affects a variety of body functions (67).

With aging there are major changes in the nervous system that occur normally and alter the individual's sensory response (45, 67, 97, 100, 111):

1. Shrinkage and loss of nerve cells
2. Decrease in neurotransmitter production
3. Slower nerve impulse transmission and reflex response
4. Decrease in nerve conduction velocity
5. Decline in electric activity
6. Increase in sensory threshold
7. Decline in integration of sensory and motor function

All of these neurologic changes create problems for the older adult. For example, by age 70, upper body stiffness, slower voluntary movement, slower decision making, visual changes, and slowed startle response are seen to some extent. Because of these particular neurologic changes, older adults do not respond as quickly to changes in their external environment. This slower response affects many facets of their lives (e.g., there is greater risk to overall safety, and drivers over 65 years of age are involved in a higher percentage of automobile accidents per mile driven than are drivers 25 to 54 years of age). The older adult's increase in sensory threshold affects pain and tactile perception and response to stimuli, resulting in increased susceptibility to burns or other injuries (45).

TABLE 16-2

Alterations in and Health Promotion for Integumentary System Related to Aging

Tissue/Organ	Alteration and Rationale	Implications for Health Promotion
Epidermis	Skin manufactures less collagen, elastin, and other proteins. Cellular division decreases; thus, skin cells are replaced more slowly. (Skin cells live an average of 46 days in 70-year-old, compared with 100 days in 30-year-old.)	Wounds heal more slowly. Maintain nutrition and hygiene.
	Elastin fibers are more brittle.	Use emollients and lotion to maintain moisture on skin.
	Loss of collagen fibers causes decreased turgor and loss of elasticity, wrinkles, and creases.	Avoid hot water baths, excessive soap.
	Permeability increases and cells are thinner.	Rinse skin well; pat dry.
	Ability to retain fluids decreases, causes skin to become drier, less flexible.	Some medications make skin more fragile and susceptible to bruising: aspirin, prednisone, steroid topical creams.
	Fair-skinned persons lose pink tones, become more pale.	Cosmetics may be used.
	Lentigo senilis, *irregular areas of dark pigmentation on dorsum of hands, arms, and face,* and uneven pigmentation occur.	Protect from direct sun. Use sunscreen, protective factor of 15 or higher, with UVA and UVB protection.
	Capillaries and small arteries on exposed skin surface become dilated.	Assist person in accepting appearance changes. Teach safety factors.
	Decreased response to pain sensation and temperature changes may cause accidents or burns.	Use care with heating pads or hot water bottles and ice packs.
Subcutaneous tissue (hypodermic)	Loss of fat cells, especially in face and limbs, causes sagging and wrinkles.	Assist adjustment to appearance changes.
	Lack of tissue over bony prominences contributes to decubitus ulcers.	Protect bony prominences from pressure, abrasions, injury, and decubitus ulcers.
	Lower cutaneous blood flow and loss of fat contribute to decreased insulation and susceptibility to chilling.	Provide adequate clothing and heat control for comfort.
Dermis	Decreased fat, water, and matrix content causes translucent appearance of skin.	Emollients, lotions, and cosmetics may be used.
	Larger and coarser collagen fibers decrease flexibility of collagen, reduce elasticity, and cause sags and wrinkles.	Assist person in accepting appearance changes.
	Decreased number of fibroblasts and fibers cause thinning tissue.	Avoid bumps, scrapes, and lacerations of skin. Wear protective clothing.
Hair	Reduced melanin production causes graying. Thinning, stiffness, and loss of luster are due to change in germ center that produces hair follicles. Baldness is genetic.	Use hair coloring or cosmetic techniques if desired.
	In women increased facial hair on upper lip and chin result from diminished estrogen.	Assist person in integrating appearance changes into body image.
Sebaceous oil glands	Decreased lubrication with oil causes skin to be drier, rougher, and scaly.	Use emollients/lotions. Avoid hot water, use minimal soap, rinse well. Pat dry. Use room humidifiers.
Sweat glands	Reduced number interferes with ability to sweat freely and regulate body temperature.	Prevent heat stroke. Drink adequate water. Dress in garments that allow heat transmission from body. Use fan or air conditioner as needed in hot weather.
Nails	Growth is slower. Increased calcium deposition causes ridges and thickening.	Encourage visit to podiatrist for care of toenails and cosmetologist for care of fingernails.

Brain

By age 90, the brain's weight has decreased 10% from its maximum, and reduction in size is not uniform throughout the brain. The main change is shrinkage in neuron size due to loss of connective tissue: axons, dendrites, and synapses. This occurs first in the frontal cerebral cortex, which is important to memory and cognitive functioning. The cerebral cortex shrinks more rapidly in males than females and in less educated people (67). There is a decrease in the number of functioning neurons in the gray matter, rather than in the brain stem. The white matter is not significantly different than in young people. Older brains can grow new nerve cells. Cell division occurs in the hippocampus, a portion of the brain involved in learning and memory (67, 162). The void left by these anatomic changes is filled by expanding ventricular volumes in the form of cerebrospinal fluid (67).

The amount of space between the skull and brain tissue doubles from ages 20 to 70. Reduced cerebral blood flow and oxygenation of the brain and reduced glucose metabolism may alter thought processes and perceptual function. Altered brain waves and sleep patterns, including reduced REM (dream) sleep, contribute to nighttime wakefulness. Review measures to reduce insomnia, discussed in Chapter 14. ∞ Increased activity of monoamine oxidase enzymes may contribute to depression (28, 67). Cognitive therapy, medication, and measures discussed later in this chapter prevent or reduce depression. The anatomic and physiologic changes in the brain of the older adult are not always directly related to performance abilities. Declining human performance in advanced age may be due to deficits in systems peripheral to the central nervous system or to other behavioral factors.

Vestibular and Kinesthetic Response

The response to vestibular and kinesthetic stimuli decreases with age. The vestibular division of the vestibulocochlear nerve is associated with balance and equilibrium. With aging there is a decrease in the number of nerve fibers, thus affecting balance and equilibrium. Reduction in the number of sensory cells in the utricle, saccule, and semicircular ducts further affects balance. These reductions may begin as early as 50 years of age but are especially noticeable after 70. Vestibular sense receptors are located in muscles and tendons; these receptors relay information about joint motion and body position in space to the central nervous system. Loss of neurons in the cerebellum that receive the sensory information also contributes to diminished balance (67). See **Table 16-3**, Health Promotion Implications for Neurologic Changes.

Vision

Visual changes occur. Loss of vision is gradual; fewer than 1% have extremely severe visual impairment. The number of fibers composing the optic fiber decreases over time. Lacrimal glands produce fewer tears, causing the cornea to become dry and irritated. The lens thickens and yellows, objects take on a yellowish hue, and the cells within the lens lose water and shrink. The diameter of the pupil decreases and the pupil is less able to accommodate to light changes. The lack of pupillary response, increased lens opacity, and irregular corneal surface, which causes light to scatter, together result in intolerance to glare and difficulty in adjusting from brightly

TABLE 16-3

Health Promotion Implications for Neurologic Changes

Change	Health Promotion Implication
Vestibular and kinesthetic	Teach safety factors, such as ways to maintain balance and safe walking. Canes, walking sticks, or walkers can be helpful. Make home fall-proof. Wear flat, rubber-soled, properly fitting shoes.
Tactile	Use firm but gentle pressure on hand, arm, or shoulder to indicate your presence or soothe with touch. Teach safety factors:
	1. Walk more slowly to allow feet to fully touch surface and to be cognizant of foot placement, e.g., on stairs, uneven surfaces, or outdoors.
	2. Monitor use of hot water bottles, heating pads, or ice bags to avoid burns or frostbite.
	3. Teach ways to avoid bumps or abrasions.
	A person who is confined to a bed or chair *must* have position changed frequently to prevent decubitus ulcers.
Taste and smell	Teach need for more seasoning, preferably spices and herbs rather than sugar or salt, to better enjoy food and discriminate tastes. Encourage adequate nutrition. Teach safety factors related to reduced smell, e.g., how to monitor for burning food or gas leaks.

to dimly lit areas, or vice versa. Visual contrast sensitivity for size and light decreases. These changes interfere with the ability to transmit and refract light (67). Because of loss of elasticity in the lens and slower response in accommodation, **presbyopia,** *inability to change lens shape for near vision*, is present in most adults, beginning after age 45 or 50. Even with corrective lenses, the individual may need longer to focus on near objects (45, 100).

Color vision is also altered after age 60, because of retinal changes (rods and cones), loss of rods and sensitivity of photoreceptors, and slower transmission of visual impulses to the nervous system. Cholesterol and other deposits in Bruch's membrane keep the vitamin A derivative from replenishing pigment in rods in the retina. The reception of short wavelengths (blue) is affected first, followed by middle-wavelength hues (green, greenish yellow), and, last, by the long wavelengths (red). Thus, for the older adult, colors such as green, blue, and violet are more difficult to see than are red, orange, and yellow. Pastels fade so that they are indistinguishable from each other. Monotones, whites, and dark colors are also difficult to see. Brighter colors compensate for decline in color discrimination and yellowing and opacity of the lens (67).

Night vision normally worsens with age because of smaller pupils, slower pupillary reflex, clouded lenses, reduced number of rods, and cholesterol deposits on Bruch's membrane (83). Presence of cataracts or other eye pathology adds to the problem (45).

Cataract development and glaucoma frequently occur in this age group. With **cataracts** the *lens becomes opaque, accompanied by diminished vision and increased sensitivity to glare.* **Glaucoma** is *caused by damage to the optic nerve from increased intraocular pressure.* These conditions and the other visual changes such as **arcus senilis,** the *accumulation of lipids on the cornea* (98), can be assessed during periodic eye examinations (67, 78). The elder with lens-opacifying disease has increased risk for macular degeneration, regardless of age, gender, or systolic blood pressure (45).

Age-related macular degeneration (AMD), a common, often slow-to-be-detected, eye disease in elders, *occurs when the macula, the most light-sensitive portion of the retina, begins to deteriorate.* An intact macula is necessary for good central vision and to see fine details (67). About 25% of elders over 65 and 33% over 80 experience some AMD (45).

Teach that prevention may involve an adequate diet of antioxidant vitamins or carotenoids (pigments found in yellow, orange, red, and dark green fruits and vegetables). In addition, smoking should be avoided and eyes protected from bright sunlight by wearing polarized sunglasses and a wide-brimmed hat. See **Table 16-4,** Neurologic Changes in the Eye—Implications for Health Promotion (45, 67, 78, 100, 111, 112, 134). Refer to **Box 16-4,** Guidelines for Assisting the Person Who Is Blind (134).

Hearing

With age, the pinna (external ear) becomes longer, wider, and less flexible; this change does not appear to affect hearing. **Conduction**

TABLE 16-4

Neurologic Changes in the Eye—Implications for Health Promotion

Change	Health Promotion Measure
Dry cornea	Use artificial tears if needed.
	Wear glasses to protect eyes from dust, flying debris.
Lens changes	Wear corrective glasses or contact lenses.
Presbyopia	Use hard lens to magnify print for reading.
Spatial-depth vision changes	Obtain books and periodicals in large print or tape-recorded materials.
	Teach safety considerations; take time to focus for vision.
	Teach safety factors related to doorways, space, and objects.
	It is important for institutions to place color guards on stair steps; to clearly mark doorways; to avoid having carpet, furniture, walls, and drapes all of same or similar color; walls, floor, doors, door frames, and furniture should be clearly delineated.
Pupillary and lens changes	Wear tinted glass or brimmed hat to reduce glare or bright light.
Decreased tolerance to glare	Turn on light in dark room before entering.
or light changes	Stand in doorway or at stairwell briefly to adjust to light changes from either bright light or dark.
	Teach need for more *indirect* but adequate illumination to perceive stimuli, do visual work. Avoid white or glossy surfaces.
	It is important for institutions to cover windows and avoid shiny wax on floors. Avoid glare on floors in bedroom, dining areas, lounges, or hallways.
	Teach safety considerations, especially with driving in bright sunlight or at night.
	Use night-light to allow low-lighted visibility.
Retinal changes	Teach implications for personal grooming and dress, enjoyment of colors in nature, interior decoration, and design of living environment. Brighter colors are enjoyed.
Color-vision altered	Teach family implications for selecting greeting cards and gifts.
	Adapt to yellow vision; teach implications for selecting clothing, cosmetics, or interior decor.
	It is important for institutions to use colors in interior decor that can readily be seen and enjoyed and not misinterpreted by elderly. Use sharp contrasting colors on doors, strips of contrasting color on bottom of walls, and colored or white strip at edge of each step to assist in distinguishing colors, space, and specific areas.
	Teach safety considerations to avoid misinterpretation of color or not seeing objects that are pale or light colors.

BOX 16-4	Guidelines for Assisting the Person Who Is Blind

1. Talk to the blind person in a normal tone of voice. The fact that he or she cannot see is no indication that hearing is impaired.
2. Be natural when talking with a blind person.
3. Accept the normal things that a blind person might do, such as consulting the watch for the correct time, dialing a telephone, or writing his or her name in longhand, without calling attention to them.
4. When you offer assistance to a blind person, do so directly. Ask, "May I be of help?" Speak in a normal, friendly tone.
5. In guiding a blind person, permit him or her to take your arm. Never grab the blind person's arm, for he or she cannot anticipate your movements.
6. In walking with a blind person, proceed at a normal pace. You may hesitate slightly before stepping up or down.
7. Be explicit in giving verbal directions to a blind person.
8. There is no need to avoid the use of the word *see* when talking with a blind person.
9. When assisting a blind person to a chair, simply place his or her hand on the back or arm of the chair. This is enough to give location.
10. When leaving the blind person abruptly after conversing with him or her in a crowd or where there is a noise that may obstruct hearing, quietly advise that you are leaving so that he or she will not be embarrassed by talking when no one is listening.
11. Never leave a blind person in an open area. Instead, lead him or her to the side of a room, to a chair, or some landmark from which he or she can obtain direction.
12. A half-open door is one of the most dangerous obstacles that blind people encounter.
13. When serving food to a blind person who is eating without a sighted companion, offer to read the menu, including the price of each item. As you place each item on the table, call attention to food placement by using the numbers of an imaginary clock. ("The green beans are at 2 o'-clock.") If he or she wants you to cut up the food, he or she will tell you.
14. Be sure to tell a blind person who the other guests are so that he or she may know of their presence.

hearing loss *occurs as cerumen production diminishes and the wax becomes drier. Blockage of the ear canal can occur and interfere with sound transmission.* Any auditory changes that occurred in middle age or earlier continue through later life. Males are twice as likely as females to have hearing loss. The tympanic membrane becomes thinner and less resilient and may show some sclerotic changes. In some older adults calcification of the ossicles occurs. In **sensorimotor hearing loss,** *there are changes in the organ of Corti, loss of nerve cells in the eighth cranial nerve, and an increased rate of time for passage of impulses in the auditory nerve.* Because of changes to the inner ear and cochlea, a hearing aid (many are small) or corrective surgery may partially improve hearing; however, a hearing aid magnifies all sounds. If there is sensorineural deafness, damage to the auditory nerve or the hearing center of the brain from bacterial or viral infections, head injuries, or prolonged exposure to loud noise, a hearing aid will not improve hearing (45, 189).

About 75% of people in the United States who are 75 to 79 years of age have hearing loss. Of all individuals over 65, 13% suffer severe **presbycusis,** *progressive loss of hearing and sound discrimination.* The consonant sounds, especially *s, sh, ch, th, d, g, z,* and *f,* and high-frequency sounds produce problems for the individual with presbycusis. The ability to locate the direction from which sound is coming diminishes, and older people have difficulty hearing individuals who speak rapidly or in high tones (45, 189). For helpful suggestions, utilize **Box 16-5,** Guidelines for Communicating with the Person Who Has a Hearing Impairment (45, 100, 111).

In a health care setting, the client's chart should be labeled so that all providers know the person wears contact lenses or glasses, or has a hearing loss. Always check that vision or hearing aids are

either being worn or are in a designated place and labeled container. Explore whether vision or hearing aids should be left in place during a diagnostic procedure. If they are to be removed for any procedure or surgery, teach staff how to communicate with the person, and ensure that a significant other is given the device for safekeeping. During care, provide verbal information or written materials as needed for education; determine whether the person is literate. Do not talk to the person from any position in the room except face-to-face for visually or hearing-challenged clients. If you wear a mask during care, explain what will happen before putting on the mask. Reduce distracting sounds, such as radio or television, while you are communicating with the person.

Educate the family, if necessary, about effective communication methods at home and in the community. Explore street or transportation safety factors. Suggest that the person may benefit from assistive listening devices, such as headphones or closed captioning on television. The *Internet* can be a useful tool for information. Refer the person to useful Websites.

Tactile Acuity

There is a decreased number of nerve cells innervating the skin and thus a decreased response or sensitivity to touch. Even the soles of the feet have fewer sensory receptors and less responsivity (67). Two-point threshold is one of the oldest measures to assess spatial acuity of the skin. Age-related deterioration of tactile acuity, like visual and hearing changes, begins in late middle age. Acuity of touch, however, varies with different body regions. The fingertip has more acuity than the forearm for texture and temperature in old age. Acuity is also related to space between stimuli. For example, the

BOX 16-5   Guidelines for Communicating with the Person Who Has a Hearing Impairment

1. Consider the possibility of a hearing impairment if the person appears inattentive to you. Some hearing-challenged people refuse or are unable to wear a hearing device. Some do not experience improved hearing with a device.

2. Face the person when speaking, with full light rather than shadows or candlelight on your face. If using the computer to type client information, face the person to speak, then stop to type, unless it is unnecessary for you to see content or the document that you are typing. Hearing-impaired persons usually depend on lip-reading even if they use sign language.

3. Do *not* cover your mouth with your hand as you speak. (That is applicable for anyone; it conveys you are being secretive or that what you say is unimportant.)

4. Speak in a normal voice tone. Articulate words. Move your lips and be distinct, but do not exaggerate movements. Avoid shouting. Hearing-impaired persons have learned to read lips, observe nonverbal facial expression, and glean content from the total environmental context.

Avoid speaking too quickly, but do not speak so slowly that the person cannot accurately lip-read.

5. Face the hearing-challenged person when in a group discussion. Direct conversation to him or her, using the above steps. Reduce noise to the extent possible. Converse with others in a way that the person can see your face.

6. Sit or stand next to "the good ear" when you converse if the person states hearing is better in one than the other ear. Ask when initiating conversation which ear has better sensory function.

7. Avoid abrupt onset or termination of communication. Face the person, and use appropriate nonverbal signs to let him or her know of conversation changes. Touch the hand or arm if necessary to get the person's attention.

8. Use key words or phrases to introduce a topic for assessment, education, or counseling, for example, "I have some questions about family history" or "Let's work on the best plan for you." If the person did not understand, do not repeat using the same words but substitute synonyms.

---

fingertip may be sensitive to a single nodule but not as sensitive to the dots of Braille, to the glucose testing monitor used by the person who has diabetes, or to other tactile aids used by the sensory handicapped (45, 62). Refer to **Table 16-3** for health promotion implications related to tactile changes.

Taste and Smell

With aging, there is a general decrease in taste perception because of a decline in the actual number of taste buds (about half as many as in young adulthood, but females have more than males). Diminished taste perception is linked to changes in the processing of taste sensations in the central nervous system. Taste perception may also be affected by the diminished salivation that occurs in older persons (67). Usually older adults experience an increased preference for more sugar, salt, spices, and highly seasoned foods (15, 111).

The sense of smell begins to decline in most people by middle age and continues a gradual decline into old age because the number and sensitivity of receptors decrease, especially after age 80. It is believed that the sense of smell decreases because the olfactory nerves have fewer cells. This diminished sense of smell combined with the decline in taste sensation may account for the loss of appetite experienced by many older adults (45, 100). The inability to smell also presents hazards for the individual, as he or she cannot quickly detect leaking gas, spoiled food, smoke, or burning food.

Refer to **Table 16-3** for health promotion implications related to changes in taste and smell.

CARDIOVASCULAR SYSTEM

The cardiovascular system undergoes considerable changes with aging. See **Table 16-5**, Cardiovascular Changes with Aging and

Health Promotion Implications, for changes, rationale, and strategies for health promotion and disease prevention (45, 67, 78, 100, 111). In the absence of heart disease, the heart is usually able to maintain the daily cardiac and circulatory functions of the older adult. However, the cardiovascular system may not be able to meet the needs of the body when a disease process is present or when there are excess demands caused by stress or excessive exercise. Obesity, physical inactivity, and abdominal fat distribution also reduce physiologic function.

RESPIRATORY SYSTEM

Changes produced by aging affect both internal and external respiration. The older adult has difficulty taking oxygen from the atmosphere and delivering it to internal organs and tissues. See **Table 16-6**, Respiratory System Changes and Health Promotion Implications, for information about physiologic changes (45, 67, 100, 111). Be prepared to do the Heimlich maneuver if the person chokes because of a weaker gag reflex or musculature. **Figure 16-3**□ depicts the Heimlich maneuver.

MUSCULOSKELETAL SYSTEM

How well the person is able to move the lower body is one of the best predictors of vitality in the aged person. Strength training has the greatest impact on prevention of musculoskeletal decline (15).

The major age-related change in the skeletal system is the loss of calcium from bone. Bone loss is accelerated with the loss of gonadal function at menopause. Therefore, bone loss is greater in females than in males and in older than younger females. Some studies have shown that by age 70, a woman's skeletal frame may have lost 30% or more of its calcium. With this change in bone

TABLE 16-5

Cardiovascular Changes with Aging and Health Promotion Implications

Organ/Tissue	Change and Rationale	Implication for Health Promotion
Heart Internal	At age 70, cardiac output at rest is 70% of that at age 30.	Medication may be needed to maintain adequate function. Exercise routine should be maintained.
	Number and size of cardiac muscle cells decrease, causing loss of cardiac muscle strength, reduction in stroke volume, and less efficient pumping and cardiac output.	Assess for myocardial damage, muscle damage, and congestive heart failure.
	Thickening of collagen in heart valves reduces efficiency of closure because of rigidity. Calcification of valves increases.	Assess for aortic and mitral murmurs, valve stenosis or insufficiency, and endocarditis.
	Thickness of left ventricle wall increases; left ventricle is unable to pump volume of blood in cardiac cycle.	Cognitive, visceral, and muscular functions may not be adequately maintained with less cardiac output and inadequate blood supply.
	Blood flow is maintained to brain and coronary arteries to greater extent than other body parts.	
	Pacemaker cells in sinoatrial node and atrioventricular nodes are replaced by fibrous and connective tissue, causing delay in nerve transmission and more time to complete the cardiac cycle.	Assess for ectopic activity, arrhythmias, and conduction defects.
External	Increased amount and stiffening of collagen surrounding heart, causing inelasticity. Increased fat deposits on surface of heart, reducing oxygen supply to body.	Maintain fluid balance and adequate aeration; avoid standing too long or constipation to reduce strain on heart. Straining to defecate strains right side of heart as blood suddenly pours through vena cava after pressure is decreased.
Blood vessels	Reduced elastin content and increased collagenous connective tissue in arterial walls reduce elasticity of walls of peripheral vessels, aorta, and other arteries.	Assess for increased systolic and diastolic blood pressure, abdominal pulsation, bruits, and aneurysms. Orthostatic hypotension may occur; blood pressure falls sharply on standing. Instruct person to rise to sitting position from lying position and stand slowly to allow for adjustment.
	Atherosclerosis, *increased accumulation and calcification in arterial walls*, makes smaller lumen diameter; vessel walls harder, thicker, and resistant to blood flow; and less rebound to vessel after being stretched. Blood flow is reduced to vital organs; cerebrovascular accidents (strokes) and multifarct dementia may occur.	Low-cholesterol diet should begin in early life, as these changes may occur in early life. Lifestyle: exercise, weight loss, no smoking, low-salt diet (under 3 g/day) can reduce blood pressure by 10 mmHg. Moderately elevated blood pressure may have protective effect on brain. Assess for hypertension and other circulatory problems.
	Walls of veins are thicker due to increased connective tissue and calcium deposits, decreasing elasticity.	Wear support hose to reduce varicose veins, beginning in early life. Sit with feet and lower legs elevated to enhance blood return to heart.
	Valves in large veins may become incompetent; varicose veins are common.	Avoid prolonged standing.

TABLE 16-6

Respiratory System Changes and Health Promotion Implications

Organ	Change and Rationale	Implication for Health Promotion
Nose	Reduced number and activity of cilia cause reduced bronchoelimination.	Less effective clearing of respiratory tract predisposes to infections. Avoid smoke-filled environment. Wear mask if air pollution exists. Avoid allergens. Maintain health status and avoid crowds in winter to prevent respiratory infections and pneumonia.
Throat	Cough reflex decreased. Sensitivity to stimuli decreased.	Teach safety factors, especially when eating (cut food into small portions, chew well, eat slowly).
Trachea	Flexibility is decreased; size of structure is increased.	
Rib cage and respiratory muscles	Calcification of chest wall causes rib cage to be less mobile.	Maintain exercise, deep breathing, and erect posture to enhance respiratory muscle function.
	Decreased strength of intercostal and other respiratory muscles and diaphragm impairs breathing.	
	Osteoporosis of ribs and vertebrae weakens chest wall and respiratory function.	Avoid pressure to ribs to prevent rib fracture (e.g., leaning chest on edge of bathtub).
	Calcification of vertebral cartilage and kyphosis stiffen chest wall and impair respiratory movements.	
Lungs	Capacity to inhale, hold, and exhale breath decreases with age. Vital capacity at 85 is 50%–65% of capacity at 30.	Encourage deep breathing, full exhalation, and erect posture throughout life. Maintain exercise to enhance lung function.
	Elastin and collagen changes cause loss of elasticity of lung tissue; lungs remain hyperinflated even on exhalation, and proportion of dead space increases.	Activity should be adjusted to respiratory efficiency and ventilation-perfusion ratio.
	Decreased elasticity and increased size of alveoli. Increased diffusion and surface area across alveolar-capillary membrane.	Increased difficulty in regulation of pH during illness, surgery, trauma. Monitor closely.

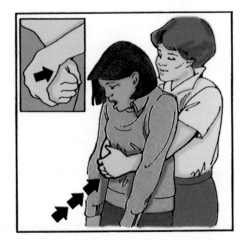

FIGURE ■ **16-3** Heimlich maneuver.
(*From Berger, K. J., and M. B. Williams.* Fundamentals of Nursing: Collaborating for Optimal Health. *Norwalk, CT: Appleton & Lange, 1992, p. 317.*)

composition comes a gradual decrease in height, on the average of 1.2 cm for each 20 years of life in both genders and all races. Decreased synthesis of bone and increased decalcification, or osteoporosis in vertebrae, cause intervertebral disk collapse (67). Loss of collagen and atrophy in intervertebral disks cause compression of the spinal column and **kyphosis,** *exaggerated curvature of the thoracic spine; the posture becomes curved in the shoulder area or the person appears stooped and shorter.* In addition to the decrease in height, bone strength is progressively lost because of loss of bone mineral content. Osteoporosis (which is discussed later) is seen as the extreme version of this universal process of adult bone loss (67, 113) and may account for the loss of 3 to 4 inches of height, depending on life span.

Decreased sensorimotor functions affect postural stability. Increased body sway is associated with reduced visual acuity, tactile sensitivity, vibration sense, joint position sense, ankle dorsiflexion strength, and quadriceps muscle strength, and increased reaction time. Peripheral sensation ability is also a factor in sway and maintenance of postural stability (45, 78).

Maintaining upright posture and balance is a complex task. As postural control mechanisms deteriorate with disease and age, the person is more susceptible to falls. Standing on one leg and tandem walking become more difficult. The center of pressure tends not to approach the edges of the base of support as closely as in younger years (78). One way to determine stability is to measure **functional reach,** *the maximum distance one can reach beyond arm's length while maintaining a fixed base of support in standing position.* Height and age affect reach, but the general ability to reach and the length of reach are related to ability to maintain stability when walking (45, 78).

The older adult experiences a gradual loss of muscular strength and endurance. Muscle cells atrophy, and lean muscle mass is lost. Studies have shown a 30% loss in muscle fiber between ages 30 and 80. In addition, as the elastic fibers in the muscle tissues decrease, the muscles become less flexible, and stiffness is noted more frequently (45, 67, 78, 138).

Changes in body weight also occur in the older adult due to loss of muscle tissue, which is dense and heavy, compared to other body tissue (45). These changes follow definite patterns. Men usually exhibit an increase in weight until their middle 50s and then gradually lose weight. Women continue to gain weight until their 60s before beginning a gradual reduction in weight. The most significant weight loss occurs near 70 years of age and is probably due to decreased number of body cells, changes in cell composition, and decreased amounts of body tissue (41, 45). See **Table 16-7,** Aging Changes and Health Promotion Implications, for information related to assessment and intervention (45, 78, 100, 111, 113).

URINARY SYSTEM

As with the other body systems, major changes in structure and function of the urinary system are associated with aging. The kidneys, bladder, and ureters are all affected by the aging process (45).

Kidney

The aging kidney suffers a decrease in renal function as one ages. There is a loss of nephrons, the size of the kidney diminishes, and there is a loss of glomeruli—as much as 30% to 50% by age 70. Vascular changes affect the blood flow. Narrowing of blood vessels and vasoconstriction often due to arteriosclerosis and hypertension produce a decreased total renal blood flow (67). This is more significant than renal tissue loss and causes reduced (40% by age 90) glomerular filtration rate and tubular function (67). See **Table 16-7** for assessment and health promotion interventions.

Bladder

The bladder of an elderly person has a diminished capacity—less than 50% that of the young adult—because of atrophy, decreased size and elasticity, and reduced tone (67). Coupled with a delayed desire to void, the elderly often have problems with frequent urination and a severe urgency to void. Aged women are especially prone to incontinence as the pelvic muscles become more flaccid (45). It is estimated that the United States spends approximately $10 billion a year on this problem. The pelvic diaphragm is the muscle mass that helps maintain bladder tone and proper closure of the bladder outlet. Weakening of the pelvic diaphragm leads to stress incontinence (67). More than 20% of admissions to geriatric facilities are due to the inability to deal with incontinence (45).

The same factors involved in the problem, reduced urinary capacity resulting in frequency and retention of residual urine, often lead to chronic cystitis, skin irritation, frequent need for antibiotics, and withdrawal from society. Urinary tract infections (UTIs) are three times more prevalent in patients who are bowel incontinent. *Escherichia coli* is the main organism found in the urine cultures of patients with bowel incontinence (45, 100, 111). Nurses need to assess for this when assisting the patient who may suffer from repeated UTIs.

Prostate hypertrophy in the older male is very common and can begin as early as age 40. Irregular changes in the smooth muscle fibers and the prostate tissue occur with age. The problem consists of frequency, especially at night, difficulty starting the stream, dribbling, and retention with overflow (45). Cancer of the prostate is the most prevalent malignancy in men. Therefore, regular physical examinations should be encouraged to screen out the possibility of a malignancy. Some males are concerned about their sexual potency if surgery is to be performed (45, 100, 111). Care should be taken to explain that although external ejaculation will be absent, erection and orgasm are likely to be unaffected.

Refer to **Table 16-7** for relevant information. Educate the client, and provide family education, about problems related to bladder and bowel incontinence. There may not be frank bowel incontinence, but there may be sufficient staining to provide contamination, and therefore more frequent hygiene may be advisable. *Measures to combat urinary incontinence include* (a) regulation of fluid intake, (b) pelvic muscle exercises (Kegel exercises), (c) a regular pattern of voiding, and (d) the use of drugs that block the hyperactivity of voiding. *Teach the female to control pelvic muscles and do the Kegel exercise as follows:*

1. Tighten the muscles at least five times each day to help strengthen the pelvic floor muscles.
2. Don't tighten other muscles, such as your hips or legs, during the pelvic floor exercises.
3. Sit, lie down, or stand during practice.
4. Practice this important exercise without anyone knowing.

Establish routines for toileting. Reinforce the client with a positive attitude; foster self-esteem and independence.

GASTROINTESTINAL SYSTEM

Changes occur throughout the gastrointestinal system. Digestion, metabolism, nutrition, and fluid and electrolyte balance are affected.

Mouth

The oral mucosa atrophies. Connective tissue becomes less elastic. Vascular tissue becomes calcified and fibrotic. Nerve cells diminish in number. Tooth decay, loss of teeth, degeneration of the jaw bone, progressive gum recession, and increased resorption of the dental arch interfere with the older adult's ability to chew food (45, 100). Saliva flow decreases and becomes more alkaline as the salivary glands secrete less ptyalin and amylase. Thirst sensation decreases, and the mouth becomes drier. All of these changes alter the digestive process at the onset (67). See **Table 16-7** for more information.

TABLE 16-7

Aging Changes and Health Promotion Implications

System/Organ	Implications for Health Promotion
Musculoskeletal	Maintain calcium intake, normal nutrition, and exercise to slow degradation of bone or osteoporosis, to overcome stiffness, and to maintain strength, endurance, and joint mobility.
	Teach safety measures related to less coordination and strength, postural and structural changes, and slower reaction time to avoid falls and fractures.
	Teach ways to arrange the home environment and needed supplies to avoid excessive reaching or climbing.
	Use devices to extend arm reach to obtain objects or supplies.
Renal	
Kidney	Avoid polypharmacy or *excessive medication intake due to slower elimination of solute load.*
	Assess for drug side effects and toxicity because kidneys are major route of excretion.
	Assess for renal insufficiency if person is dehydrated, hypotensive, feverish, or using diuretics.
Bladder	Maintain adequate fluid intake and frequent toileting.
	Avoid diuretic use in afternoon or before long travel.
	Pads may be worn in underpants or lined pants can be worn as precaution.
	Assess for urinary tract infections.
	Explore self-esteem issues related to incontinence.
	Engage in bladder retraining.
Gastrointestinal	
Mouth	Encourage drinking 8 glasses of water daily to avoid dry mouth and dehydration.
	Maintain dental hygiene and care to prevent periodontal disease and loss of teeth.
	Teach new brushing techniques, daily flossing, and use of toothpaste with fluoride additive.
	Teach safety factors related to prevention of choking and use of Heimlich maneuver if needed.
Stomach	Encourage adequate nutritional intake, adjusting food texture and taste, as necessary, and with vitamin-mineral supplements if necessary.
	Promote nutrition through programs like senior nutrition sites or Meals on Wheels, as needed.
Liver/gallbladder	Encourage adequate protein intake to overcome hepatic synthesis.
	Avoid high-fat foods.
	Avoid polypharmacy because of reduced metabolism and excretion.
Bowel	Encourage bulk, vegetables, fruits, and cereals; especially water; exercise; and regular toileting patterns to prevent constipation.
	Avoid daily laxatives if at all possible, but if self-administered for years, it will need to be continued. Mild stool softener is preferred.
Immune	Maintain nutrition, hygiene, and health status to overcome delayed immune response and trend to infections.
	Observe for masked signs of inflammation or infection; e.g., temperature or white blood cell count may not be as elevated as in middle age.
	Teach safety measures and stress management strategies to overcome delayed or inadequate body response to stress.
	Treat symptomatically for comfort if autoimmune processes occur.

Gastrointestinal Tract

Because of decreased stimuli from the autonomic nervous system, peristalsis is slowed the entire length of the gastrointestinal tract. Emptying of the esophagus and stomach is delayed. The gastric mucosa shrinks, causing decreased secretion of pepsinogen and hydrochloric acid, which delays digestion. Digestion is decreased further by the reduction in secretion of hydrochloric acid and pancreatic enzymes. Bile tends to be thicker, and the gallbladder empties more slowly. Hepatic synthesis is reduced (67). These changes result in a decreased absorption of nutrients, vitamins, minerals, electrolytes, and drugs by the gastrointestinal tract (44). Hypernatremia is related to fluid intake or increased fluid loss (44). In addition, some older adults do not have enough intrinsic factor and develop pernicious anemia. Vitamin B_{12} injections may be needed (45).

Elimination of waste products is of equal importance to gastrointestinal function in the aged. The changes in the cell, and therefore in tissue structure, and the loss of muscle tone may decrease intestinal motility. Elimination depends on fluid intake, muscle tone, regularity of habits, culture, state of health, and adequate nutrition—all of which interrelate. Alterations in many of these areas occur with aging. Poor nutrition and lack of exercise add to the problem.

In the majority of persons over age 65, there is some degree of immobility, either physical, social, or environmental. Physical changes in the tissues combine with this immobility to produce constipation or fecal impaction in circumstances that might not so affect a younger person.

Refer to **Table 16-7** for information relevant to assessment and intervention.

Fluid and Electrolyte Balance

The older adult can usually maintain homeostasis, but more time is required to return to normal after deficiency or excess occurs because of environmental stress and disease. Altered fluid and electrolyte balance frequently accompanies acute illness. The elder does not have the fluid reserves to adapt to rapid changes (117).

About a 60% decrease in total body water and a decrease in the rates of intracellular water occur as part of aging. Thirst sensation diminishes with aging, although adequate fluid may be consumed through the foods eaten (117). Yogurt, watermelon, pineapple, strawberries, apples, cooked asparagus and spinach, and lettuce are examples (41, 44, 117). With dehydration, hypernatremia occurs. A strict low-sodium diet can rapidly cause hyponatremia. Or an intravenous administration of potassium can rapidly cause hyperkalemia. Hyperthermia or fever and diarrhea can also cause fluid and electrolyte imbalance (117).

Many of the normal aging changes indirectly, if not directly, affect fluid balance. A thorough physical assessment correlated with laboratory findings is essential. Physical and cognitive impairment may result from fluid and electrolyte imbalance. Prevention of imbalance is essential.

Educate health care staff and family about the health problems with poor fluid intake or increased water loss related to illness or use of diuretics. The person's complaints, even if vague, must be carefully monitored and the treatment team should be notified.

Monitor the patient during preparation for diagnostic tests and afterward; some tests predispose to dehydration. Emphasize the need for increased fluid intake before and after gastrointestinal tests (117). Educate the care team, family, and patient about special considerations related to fluid and electrolyte balance during the perioperative period or in relation to common chronic diseases such as diabetes (117).

Teach the elder ways to avoid constipation (fluids, fiber, exercise) and to avoid abuse of laxatives, which can predispose to hypokalemia. Emphasize that during an hour of light to moderate exercise, drinking 2 to 3 cups of fluid is recommended for rehydration (41, 116, 117). Teach about the normal straw color of urine, which indicates adequate hydration. Darker urine may be a sign that more fluid should be consumed.

Recommend that the client follow physician instructions if he or she has heart, kidney, or liver disease. Overhydration may be more likely and should be avoided.

Refer staff to the article about oral hydration in older adults (111) and use the information to teach the client and family about risk factors, assessment measures, and nursing interventions for dehydration. For thorough information see the Website www.nursingcenter.com.

ENDOCRINE SYSTEM

During aging, the ability of endocrine glands to synthesize hormones appears to remain within normal limits. The imbalance between anabolic and catabolic hormones is a common marker of aging (67, 182). There are lower total body potassium and total body water levels in older than younger females (117). The number or sensitivity of hormonal receptors, however, may decrease. This means that, even though blood levels remain adequate, there is a lack of response to some hormones especially those hormones produced by the adrenal and thyroid glands. Failure to respond to these hormones decreases the individual's ability to respond to stress (67, 117, 182).

Pancreatic beta cell activity appears altered with age, although the extent varies among people. Decreased insulin response causes hyperglycemia. Aging is associated with elevated glucose levels after ingestion of glucose under the standard conditions of oral glucose tolerance testing. After ingestion of more physiologically mixed meals, a mild degree of postprandial hyperglycemia and hyperinsulinemia can still be demonstrated in the elderly compared with young adults. Postprandial elevations in glucose and insulin levels, however, are much lower after mixed meals compared with that observed during the standard glucose tolerance test. Increased circulating glucose and insulin levels are accompanied by a detectable elevation in hemoglobin A_{1c} concentration. These modest abnormalities, sustained over many years, may contribute to the development of atherosclerosis or other manifestations of aging (67, 117).

The chemical composition of fluids surrounding body cells must be closely regulated. When analysis of blood shows alterations in blood volume, acidity, osmotic pressure, or protein and sugar content, older adults require a longer time to recover internal chemical equilibrium (67, 117). Insulin, secreted by cells in the pancreas, normally accelerates the removal of sugar from the blood. In older adults given intravenous insulin with extra glucose, the glucose is removed from the bloodstream at a slower rate than in younger people because of poorer hormone production. Stress intensifies glucose intolerance. Elderly persons undergoing the stress of surgery, illness, injury, or emotional stress may manifest diabetic symptoms; the elevated blood and urinary glucose levels usually return to normal when the stressor subsides (45, 117).

There is decreased metabolic clearance rate and plasma concentration of aldosterone. An increased response by antidiuretic hormone to hyperosmolarity contributes to hyponatremia (67, 117).

Growth hormone, estrogen, and testosterone blood levels decrease in later maturity (67). Because of the decrease in estrogen levels after menopause, the breasts of the female have more connective tissue and fat and less glandular tissue. The breast tissues lose elasticity and begin to sag. The lack of estrogen causes the uterus and fallopian tubes to decrease in size. The fallopian tubes also become less motile (67). The decline of testosterone secretion is not abrupt like that of estrogen. Therefore the changes are less obvious; however, the gradual decline of hormone does increase the incidence of benign prostatic hypertrophy in the older man and affects physical reserves, as testosterone has a nitrogen-conserving effect (45).

Thyroid hormone production decreases, related to an underactive thyroid gland. This occurs more frequently as the person ages; 20% of women over 65 have the condition and need oral thyroid replacement therapy. Symptoms include cognitive impairment, emotional changes, depression, lack of energy or fatigue, cold intolerance, weight gain, constipation, slow pulse, muscular joint pain, thin and brittle fingernails and hair, and reduced sexual drive. A synthetic form of thyroid treats symptoms (100, 111). The person regains physical vitality, emotional responsiveness, and cognitive function, concentration, and memory.

IMMUNE SYSTEM

Many components of the immune system become less efficient with age, which accounts in part for the increased cancer rate. Infections and other illnesses are more serious for the elder because the immune system may be too weak to launch an effective specific counterattack. Older people with high numbers of T and B cells, natural killer (NK) cells, remain healthy. Centenarians have well-functioning immune systems. Throughout life, females have stronger and more efficient immune systems than males, and their thymus gland is larger, which may account in part for their longevity. In late life, the thymus gland starts to involute and degenerate. The total number of circulating lymphocytes decreases by approximately 15%, and antibody–antigen reactions decline. In addition, lymphoid tissue decreases, and a general decline occurs in both cell-mediated and humoral immunity (67). Production and function of T and B cells is reduced; reduced T cells may be a factor in increased malignancy rates. Autoimmune responses may increase, causing diseases such as rheumatoid arthritis and other collagen diseases (45, 67). Refer to **Table 16-7**, Aging Changes and Health Promotion Implications.

HEMATOPOIETIC SYSTEM

There are minor changes in the blood components of the older adult. Hemoglobin level, red blood cell count, and circulatory blood volume are not significantly changed. Most of the changes that occur are related to specific pathologic conditions instead of normal aging (45).

REPRODUCTIVE SYSTEM AND CHANGES THAT INFLUENCE SEXUAL FUNCTION

Although males and females experience some common changes as a result of aging, they are considered separately because of certain particular physiologic changes relating to sexual response and vigor.

Male Changes

The production of testosterone continues throughout the male's lifetime, and this hormone is available longer and at a higher level than its counterpart, estrogen, in the female. As the concentration of the male hormone diminishes, the testes become smaller and softer. The testicular tubes thicken and begin to degenerate, and sperm production decreases or is inhibited. In addition, the prostate gland enlarges, contractions weaken, force of ejaculation decreases, and volume and viscosity of seminal fluid are reduced (67). However,

males have fathered children in their 70s, 80s, and 90s; viable sperm have been found in 90-year-olds.

Masters, Johnson, and Kolodny (110) found that as a sexual partner, the older male experiences reduction in the frequency of intercourse, the intensity of sensation, the speed of attaining erection, and the force of ejaculation. The excitement phase builds more slowly, and erection takes longer to attain. With diminished vasoconstriction of the scrotum, there is less elevation of the testes. The plateau phase preceding orgasm lasts longer, with less muscle tension. There is reduced or absent secretory activity by Cowper's gland before ejaculation. The orgasmic phase is of shorter duration, and the expulsion of the seminal fluid is usually completed with one or two contractions as compared with four or more in the young male. In the resolution stage, loss of erection may take seconds as compared with the young man's minutes or hours. Refractory time, time needed for another erection, is extended from several to 24 hours (110).

Female Changes

In the older adult female, there is a decline in the blood level of estrogen and testosterone (which was lower through the prior years) because of reduced ovarian function after menopause. This reduction in hormone causes the vaginal wall to shrink and thin and the vaginal and cervical secretions to diminish and become more acid (67). These changes may produce pruritus as well as **dyspareunia** (*pain on intercourse*), which can restrict sexual activity. In addition, the size of the clitoris is slightly smaller, and lubrication from the Bartholin glands decreases. With the loss of subcutaneous body fat, the vulva and external genitalia shrink (67, 110).

The female has some testosterone as part of the sexual hormones (67). Decreased testosterone levels contribute to bone loss, fatigue, and vaginal drying, effects that are similar to those of reduced estrogen. Testosterone level decline also contributes to thinning of body hair, especially in the armpits and pubic regions, and a lower libido (67, 110).

In the excitement phase of coitus, vaginal lubrication is reduced and takes longer to appear. There is less flattening and separation of the labia majora and decreased vasocongestion of the labia minora. Atrophy or thinning of vaginal walls causes the vagina to be less elastic (less depth and breadth). Muscle tension is reduced. During the plateau phase, there is less vasocongestion and less secretion from the Bartholin glands. All of these changes make penetration more difficult and less comfortable. During the orgasmic phase, there are fewer contractions of the uterus and vagina. During the resolution phase, the vasocongestion of the clitoris and orgasmic platform quickly subsides. Burning and frequency of urination may follow intercourse as the atrophic bladder and urethra are not adequately protected. Thus, the sex act may become less satisfying and even painful. A number of diseases and some medications can cause impotence (110).

Female sexual performance in later maturity reveals no reduction in sexual desire or excitability with advancing age. Regular sexual stimulation and activity seem to overcome the effects of lower estrogen and testosterone. Masturbation relieves sexual tension in postmenopausal females into their sixth and seventh decades and for males over age 65 (23, 110).

Due to the association of continued hormone replacement therapy (HRT) with breast cancer, heart disease, and stroke, it is no longer recommended as a first-line treatment for problems of older women. Other less systemic forms of hormone therapy, such as patches, rings, and vaginal creams, are alternatives to taking oral preparations. Nonhormonal medications include the bisphosphonates, especially helpful with steroid-induced osteoporosis; raloxifene, which mimics the effect of estrogen on increasing bone density, without the hormone's side effects; calcitonin, a hormone produced by the thyroid gland; teriparatide, a parathyroid-like hormone; and tamoxifen, which has an estrogen-like effect on bone tissue (112).

Sexuality

Stress, hormonal activity, general health, and aging can each be assessed according to measurable standards. Psychological influences can be exerted to produce physiologic change in young and old alike. Because of the relationships between the mind and body and the interdependence of all body systems, societal attitudes regarding the characteristics and needs of older citizens are crucial to their quality of life.

Normal aging of the reproductive system decreases efficiency and lengthens time for response for both males and females, but unlike other organ systems that perform more specific functions, the reproductive system extends far beyond procreation. It is deeply tied to the need for interpersonal communication, and it involves that warmth and comfort found only in body contact. When one is old, the yearning for intimacy, security, and belonging becomes intensified as other privations are felt keenly: loss of friends, job status, active participation in parenting or career, and decision making.

The older person is a sexual person. *Research about sexuality in people between the ages of 60 and 91 years indicates that* (45, 110):

1. Ninety-seven percent of those engaged in sexual activity enjoy the activity.
2. Seventy-five percent think intercourse feels as good now, or better, than it did when they were young.
3. Seventy-two percent are satisfied by their sexual experiences.
4. Ninety percent think sexual activity is good for their health.
5. Females are more satisfied with activities such as sitting close to someone and talking and saying and hearing endearments if sexual intercourse is not a choice.
6. Males are more satisfied with reading or watching erotic materials and caressing another person's body if sexual intercourse is not a choice.

Educate that the person's sense of self-worth and the partner's physical health status are positively related to the continuance of sexual activity. Family caregivers and health care agency staff should arrange the environment to consider the elder's sexual needs. Privacy is essential.

HEALTHY CENTENARIANS AND SUPERCENTENARIANS

Age-related changes may not be inevitable, or may be possible to delay, according to studies of **centenarians,** *people who are 100 years or older* (32, 92) in the United States in 2000; 105 were over 110 years) (70). In the past, reports of people living well over 100 years of age in remote rural, mountainous areas were difficult to document by Western standards. However, study of *lifestyles in three isolated areas—Republic of Georgia, Pakistan, and Peru—revealed four commonalities* (15):

1. Diet consisted mostly of fresh fruits and vegetables, little meat and fat, and avoidance of overeating.
2. Work, in the home or outdoors, continued throughout life and into advanced age.
3. Integration remained in the community; there was frequent interaction with family and friends.
4. Exercise and relaxation were part of daily routine.

Geneticists are obtaining family histories and blood samples for DNA and gene study from centenarians in the United States, France, and Japan, and from American descendants of Ashkenazim (Eastern European) Jewish people (40). Genetic foundations for extreme age are being studied. Nir Barzilia has found three longevity genes in centenarians, special genes that apparently protect from diseases that kill most people earlier. Centenarians and their offspring also reveal high levels of HDL or good cholesterol (40). A study of centenarians and their siblings' ($n = 308$ pairs, 137 families) in the New England Centenarian Study identified a marker within the microsomal transfer protein gene as a modifier of human life span (61, 144, 159).

Studies of centenarians in the United States, Sweden, Germany, Italy, Japan, and Denmark reveal at least 30% are dementia-free, 90% do not show cognitive impairment until their mid- to late 90s, 80% are functionally independent at age 92, and 12% are living independently at 100 (144). **Compression of morbidity,** *delayed onset and accumulation of disease-oriented disability into the last few years of life,* is common (40, 111, 112, 144). Life-threatening disease, such as cardiac disease or cancer, occurs 20 to 30 years later than in most of the population, perhaps because of a special gene (150). Functional reserve may be greater and allow longer life despite disease presence, since some do have a long history of age-related disease with earlier mortality risk (40, 144). Most centenarians apparently escape disease, cancer, and stroke (144, 159). Yet about 30% of the centenarians are overweight and are or have been smokers (50). Functional reserve may also foster independent living (144, 159).

In the United States and other developed countries, more people are living past 100 years. There are twice as many centenarians as two decades ago, and the numbers are expected to double in every decade. Some are in excellent health (15). *Research with these individuals who are 100 years or older reveals the following characteristics* (15, 40, 71, 111, 112, 133, 159):

1. Similar or higher thyroid hormone levels as younger people
2. Similar cortisol and growth hormone levels as young adults
3. Adaptability in the face of everyday events and change
4. Avoidance of worry about the future, not giving in to negative predictions
5. Behavioral response that reflects the attitude of "take things one day at a time"

Similarities in centenarians cross-culturally include (15, 30, 40, 71, 102, 103, 133, 137, 139, 166):

1. Moderate diet including fish, fresh fruits and vegetables, and foods with antioxidants, folate, and vitamin B$_6$, limited fat, meat, and dairy products, and food with unsaturated fats.
2. Past and current history of work and exercise, current daily moderate exercise, walking, biking, weight bearing, tai chi, and dance—slow, flowing movements.
3. Consume food in moderation, and no more than 1 to 2 drinks daily of alcoholic beverage, rarely smoke tobacco.
4. Optimistic, happy, relaxed attitude, even-tempered, high self-confidence.
5. Low in time urgency, avoidance of rushing schedules and tension.
6. Healthy stress-resistant lifestyle and personality, manage stress and anxiety through positive attitude and hope, do not dwell on negative.
7. Socialization, staying involved with people, friendly, give and receive support and intellectual stimulation through friendships.
8. Intellectual curiosity, stimulate brain through games, puzzles, reading, painting, and playing musical instruments.
9. Spirituality as the key aspect of life, underlying all activity—including gardening; daily meditation; pray about specific problems.

Supercentenarians, *people who are older than 100*, are becoming more common. The oldest survivor to date is Madame Jeanne Calment, a French woman who lived to be 122 years old (15). In 2000, there were 250 to 300 supercentenarians worldwide and 60 to 70 registered in the U.S. census (70). In a study of 39 elders 110 years or older, the oldest participant was 119 years. Only 2.6% had had a myocardial infarction and only 13% had had a stroke. Seven (22%) were taking medication for hypertension. Eight (25%) had successfully survived cancer. Diabetes mellitus (3%) and Parkinson's disease (3%) were rare. Osteoporosis (44%) and cataract history (88%) were common. The majority (84%) were females. More than 50% had 8 or fewer years of education, as expected since in 1900 the average highest grade attained was eighth grade. (States began advocating for 12 years of education in 1915.) Over 50% were dependent; 41% required minimal assistance or were independent (159).

Assess special needs of the centenarian and foster healthful patterns to enable the person to maintain quality of life. Share what you learn about their healthy lifestyles and attitudes with younger people in this population.

NUTRITIONAL NEEDS

Special problems exist in the nutrition of older people. Educate clients about factors that affect nutrition and their clinical manifestations, which are described in the gastrointestinal section of **Table 16-7** and in **Table 16-8**, Factors That May Affect Nutrition in Later Maturity (41, 44, 45, 67).

Caloric requirements are lower than in earlier life, depending on activity level and physical status (41, 44). The elderly person is likely to consume empty calories from easily eaten carbohydrate foods or desserts. Recommended intake is 25 to 30 cal/kg/day.

Protein requirements are 0.8 g/kg/day minimal. Some experts recommend 1.0 to 1.25 g/kg/day (41, 44). This is probably the greatest dietary problem in meal planning for the elderly person who lives alone, who often wants foods that can be prepared and chewed easily. He or she may seldom eat meat. Milk products may be poorly tolerated, especially in dark-skinned people, because of decreased lactase, the enzyme for digesting lactose. Fermented products such as cheese, yogurt, and buttermilk may be tolerated well and supply needed protein, *calcium* (1,200 mg/day), and *vitamin D* (600 IU) (41, 44). There must be enough vitamin coenzymes to ensure metabolism of these three nutrients and absorption of enough bulk elements to maintain a balance of sodium, potassium, calcium, magnesium, and other trace element cofactors for metabolic needs.

Mineral and vitamin needs generally remain the same for the person over 70 years as for midlife years. Because foods today are subjected to many refinement processes with the loss of some vitamins and essential elements, supplements are often recommended (41, 44).

Teach the elder and family members that the same food groups are the foundation of a balanced diet for the elderly as in any life stage. Plan a diet that follows the recommendations for age and exercise presented in MyPyramid. Refer the person to the MyPyramid. *Emphasize the following points as you teach* (41, 44):

1. Total fat limited to 30% of calories and cholesterol and with the recommended types of fat; no more than 10% of calories from saturated fats
2. Plenty of complex carbohydrates and at least 20 g of fiber
3. Moderate restriction of sodium, as appropriate
4. Adequate calcium (1,200 to 1,500 mg daily), other minerals, vitamins, and protein
5. High nutrient density, especially in the presence of anorexia or feeding difficulties

Emphasize that sufficient water or other fluid intake is essential. Fluid intake is often reduced for several reasons:

1. The aging process reduces the thirst sensation.
2. The senior who has incontinence problems limits fluid intake to reduce output.
3. Fewer meals are eaten; opportunity for fluid intake is less apparent.
4. The senior who takes a diuretic often wrongly assumes fluid intake should be reduced.

Explore ways to overcome or cope with these situations. *At least six or seven glasses (8 ounces) (or 30 ml/kg/day, with a minimum of 1,500 ml/day) of water should be ingested daily to* (a) soften stools, (b) maintain kidney function, (c) aid expectoration, (d) moisturize dry skin, and (e) aid absorption of medications, bulk laxatives, and high-fiber foods.

You can help directly or teach others how to make mealtime pleasant for the elderly person:

1. Encourage the person to prepare menus that are economical and easy to shop for, prepare, and consume.
2. Encourage the person to do meal preparation to the extent possible.

TABLE 16-8

Factors That May Affect Nutrition in Later Maturity

Factor and Process	Effect	Clinical Manifestation
Ingestion		
Loss of teeth; poor dentures; atrophy of jaws	Improper mastication; deletion of important foods from diet	Irritable bowel syndrome; constipation; malnutrition
Dietary habits	Overeating; eccentric diets	Obesity; malnutrition
Psychological losses and changes; changes in social environment; lack of socialization	Poor appetite	Anorexia; weight loss
Reduced income; difficulty with food preparation and ingestion	Excessive ingestion of carbohydrates	Obesity; malnutrition
Decreased fluid intake	Dry feces	Impacted stools
Digestion and Absorption		
Decreased secretion of hydrochloric acid and digestive enzymes	Interference with digestion	Dietary deficiencies
Hepatic and biliary insufficiency	Poor absorption of fats	Fat-soluble vitamin deficiency; flatulence
Atrophy of intestinal mucosa and musculature	Poor absorption; slower movement of food through intestine	Vitamin and mineral deficiencies; constipation
Decreased secretion of intestinal mucus	Decreased lubrication of intestine	Constipation
Metabolism		
Impaired glucose metabolism and use	Diabetic-like response to glucose excesses	Hyperglycemia; hypoglycemia
Decrease in renal function	Inability to excrete excess alkali	Alkalosis
Impaired response to salt restriction	Salt depletion	Low-salt syndrome
Decline in basal metabolic rate	Lower caloric requirements but same amount of food eaten	Obesity
Changes in iron and calcium (phosphorus, magnesium) metabolism	Iron deficiency; increased requirements for calcium	Anemia; demineralization of bone; osteoporosis
Changes in vitamin metabolism	Deficiency in vitamins K and C, especially	Peripheral neuropathy, sensorimotor changes; easy bruising and bleeding tendencies

3. The environment should be a comfortable temperature and well lighted so that food can be seen.

4. Place food, in an institutional setting, where the person can smell, see, and reach it.

5. If needed, either after shopping or in an institution, open cartons and food packets of various sorts and help season the food as necessary.

6. Keep the table or tray attractive, neat, and uncluttered to ensure an appetizing appearance.

7. Select foods that can be easily chewed and digested.

8. Ensure that dentures and eyeglasses are clean and in place on the person at mealtime, instead of in the drawer or on the institutional bedside table.

9. Oral hygiene is important and contributes to greater enjoyment of food. Mouth care also promotes healthy tissues in the mouth, thereby keeping the beginning of the alimentary canal intact and functional.

10. Do not give medications with meals if avoidable, especially if the medication has an unpleasant taste.

11. Encourage the person to eat when hungry rather than only at set meal or snack times. Consult with elderly care agencies to be flexible with providing nutritional needs. Smaller amounts of food served 4 to 6 times during the day and evening are recommended.

12. If necessary, use adaptive feeding devices to help the person feed self.

Adapt your nutrition teaching and keep in mind the altered responses associated with the aging process. Elders are denied many pleasures, and food should not be one of them. Consult with other members of the health team, especially the dietitian and the physician, if there are problems. The family must be included, and can often be of great help when there are cultural, religious, or ethnic reasons for a poor appetite. Often the most important member of the team, the elder, is not consulted enough. He or she should be the first one involved in planning nutritional needs. These same principles can be used as a basis for helping the elder maintain good nutrition in any setting.

Monitor the home situation as necessary when problems of poor nutrition exist. Determine whether the problem stems from lack of funds, physical handicaps, family structure, cultural barriers, or any combination of similar unmet needs. Often you will be the one who helps the client contact community agencies, family, church, and whatever other means may be available.

You may refer elderly persons living alone and unable to shop or to prepare food to obtain assistance of a home health aide—available through some community agencies. You might arrange to have meals sent in from agencies designed to give this type of service. These programs are discussed more fully later in this chapter under the heading Community Planning.

Educate elders, families, and health care providers about nutritional differences for young-old and old-old persons. Eating too much when younger may predispose to disease risk. In old age and for centenarians and beyond, eating too little is a threat to good health. Because of the aging changes previously described, motivating those 100 years or older to maintain adequate nutrients is a challenge. Food sits in the stomach longer, especially if moderate to large servings. Thus more frequent (6 times a day), smaller amounts of easily digested, nutrient-rich servings are essential. Combining meals and socialization or interesting entertainment is effective. The old-old and extremely-old should be given calcium, vitamin D, and vitamin B_{12} supplements. Other supplements may be necessary (41, 44).

In any health care facility that serves food to the elderly, all things connected with *food service* have psychological implications. Food represents life; it nurtures. Mealtime is thought of as a time of fellowship with others and a sharing of pleasure, and this attitude should be retained as much as possible for older people. Making the food more attractive, talking with the person, comforting and touching, and cajoling if need be, may help, especially if food is being refused. Appetizers and special drinks have been successfully used as an aid to therapy.

REST AND SLEEP

Rest is important. Though older adults may not sleep as many hours as they once did, frequent rest periods and sensible pacing of activities provide the added energy for a full and active life. Rest may consist of listening to soft music, reading, thinking of happy experiences, napping, or merely lying with eyes closed. Some older adults have several 15- to 60-minute naps during the daylight hours. Older adults in reasonably good health probably do not require any more sleep than was required during their middle adulthood.

Aging affects the process of sleep in three areas: (a) length of sleep, (b) distribution of sleep during the 24-hour day, and (c) sleep stage patterns. The older adult requires a somewhat longer period to fall asleep, and sleep is lighter, with more frequent awakenings. The total amount of daily sleep declines as the spontaneous interruption of sleep increases. The older adult may actually spend more time in bed but sleep less, waking with the feeling of inadequate sleep. The

time spent in stage IV, the deepest sleep period, and REM sleep decreases (26, 55, 67). This also contributes to feelings of fatigue.

Sleep apnea, described in Chapter 15, occurs in many elderly adults. ∞ Persons with sleep apnea are more sleepy during the day than nonapneic individuals. Apnea during sleep has a detrimental effect on the well-being of elderly adults, even if oxygen desaturation is mild or moderate. Greater levels of depression and cognitive impairment are seen in sleep-apneic elders (26, 45).

Assess for insomnia, a common problem in the older adult (76). *Many factors contribute to insomnia:* (a) the amount and type of daily activity, (b) existence of disturbing environmental conditions, (c) presence of pain, (d) fear or anxiety, (e) lack of exercise, (f) illness, (g) depression, (h) delirium, (i) dementia, (j) metabolic syndrome, and (k) restless legs syndrome.

Review current sleep hygiene measures used. Encourage the person to resist daytime napping and to participate in social activities to improve total sleep time and quality. Suggest stimulus control or reconditioning, soft music, and use of progressive relaxation methods or mental imagery. Use of a dim light can promote better sleep. Recommend that the person try other sleep hygiene measures listed in Chapter 15. ∞ The Epworth Sleepiness Scale can be used to determine daytime sleepiness (26) and design sleep hygiene measures. Cognitive therapy to correct unrealistic expectations about sleep or catastrophic thinking may be useful.

EXERCISE AND ACTIVITY

Physical activity that is sensibly paced and gradually increased will promote and maintain health. Many of the effects of the aging process are controlled by 30 minutes of exercise daily. Weight gain is prevented with 60 minutes daily of moderate to vigorous exercise. Weight loss is promoted with up to 90 minutes a day of physical activity, including gardening, walking, bicycling, and hiking (41, 44, 45). As **Figure 16-4**▢ depicts, the older adult can maintain health by participating in activity with the grandchild.

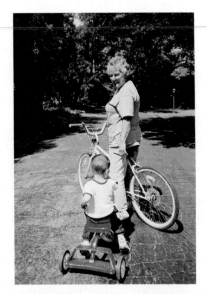

FIGURE ▢ **16-4** The older adult can maintain health by participating in activity with the grandchild.

Exercise has the following benefits for the elder, including the old-old (45, 100, 111, 174):

1. Prolong vitality, balance, and strength; maintain baseline basal metabolic rate (BMR); promote internal heat regulation.
2. Prevent or reduce **sarcopenia**, *muscle weakening, and replacement by fat when muscles atrophy.*
3. Maintain distribution of fat and healthy hip-to-waist ratio. (Divide waist size by hip size; over 0.85 for females and 0.9 for males is a risk factor.)
4. Maintain oxidative capacity and oxygen utilization so muscles can consume more oxygen.
5. Prevent or overcome depression or low self-esteem.
6. Maintain kidney function, excretory function, and fluid balance.
7. Postpone or prevent glucose intolerance, type 2 diabetes mellitus, heart disease, high LDL or cholesterol, arteriovascular disease, hypertension, and osteoporosis—common disabilities with aging.

Most elders will not be as physically active as the 81-year-old man who became the oldest person to scale El Capitan's rock face in Yosemite National Park. This was his second climb; he had also been successful at age 68. He quit skydiving at 78, at the doctor's insistence. Elders, including octogenarians, remain active in other sports, such as competitive swimming. Utilize **Table 16-9** for client education about the physical, psychological, and social benefits of regular exercise (45, 100, 111).

One group of active people is farmers. Farmers age 65 or older generally enjoy better health than city or small-town dwellers of the same age. They generally have fewer medical conditions and excel at performing tasks. Farmers may be healthier because of their lifestyle. If you are looking for a 75-year-old who still works, that person is more likely to farm than do anything else. Most elder farmers say they do not expect to stop working, although they may reduce the amount of strenuous tasks or duration of work periods to enjoy other activities.

Even if the individual has a decreased exercise tolerance, with supervision a plan can be developed to help him or her achieve higher levels of physical fitness, even strength training. It is, however, important that the older adult not start a walking or strength training exercise program without consulting the physician, who would be aware of any needed limitations. See the examples of strength training exercises at the AARP Website, www.aarp.org.

Exercise is increasingly recommended in temperature-regulated swimming pools (no cooler than 83°F). Educate the client, using **Box 16-6**, Positive Effects of Aquatic Exercise (174).

Utilize **Figure 16-5■, Activity Pyramid,** for client education about exercise guidelines. The pyramid stresses the importance of choosing activity each day to achieve maximal health. Twenty nonstop minutes is not essential; all of the activities can log to 20 or 30 minutes for the day. The sedentary person should start at "everyday" activities; most people do not need a physical examination for this level. This baseline level can reduce risk of developing cardiovascular disease. If the person wants to be more active and slow disability, level 2 is recommended. Level 3 is recommended for increasing flexibility and strength. The **Box**, Client

TABLE 16-9

Benefits of Regular Exercise

Physical

1. Helps slow aging process, regardless of age
2. Maintains good health and energy
3. Improves general strength and body agility and balance
4. Improves respiration and circulation
5. Promotes muscle mass, strength, and endurance
6. Protects against ligament injuries
7. Promotes bone mass formation; slows loss of bone tissue
8. Induces better sleep patterns
9. Normalizes blood cholesterol and triglyceride levels
10. Controls blood glucose levels
11. Normalizes blood pressure
12. Improves appetite, digestive processes, and bowel function
13. Promotes weight control (moderate exercise burns 240–420 calories/hour)
14. Reduces risk of heart disease

Psychological

1. Reduces age-related decline in brain's oxidative capacity and improves memory and information processing
2. Promotes faster reaction time
3. Contributes to improved mood and morale
4. Improves cognitive test scores
5. Enhances self-confidence
6. Maintains interest in life and alertness
7. Contributes to sense of control
8. Prevents depression

Social

1. Promotes socialization when exercise is included in group activity
2. Maintains independence

BOX 16-6 — Positive Effects of Aquatic Exercise

Loosens muscles
Increases muscle and joint strength
Improves balance
Prevents osteoporosis
Promotes healing of injured or arthritic joints and sore muscles
Improves cardiovascular function
Makes exercise easy and fun because of buoyancy of water
Provides socialization with others

MediaLink American Association of Retired Persons

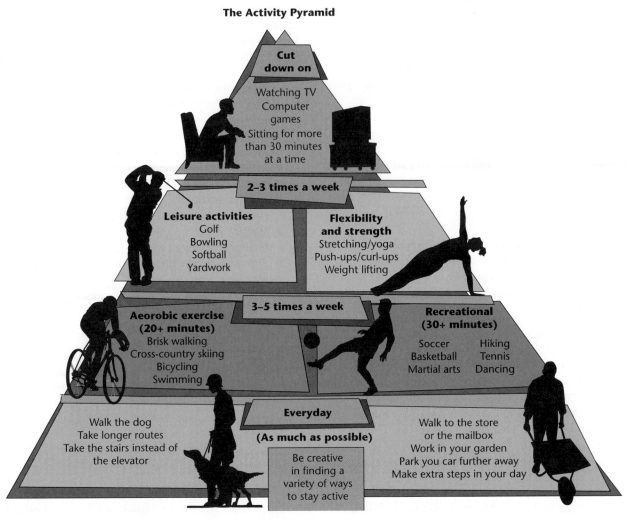

FIGURE ☐ 16-5 Activity Pyramid.

Copyright © 1997 Park Nicollet *Health Source*® Institute for Research and Education. Reprinted by permission.

Client Education

Guidelines for Walking Exercise

1. No single program will work for all elders. Determine first the meaning and perceived value of exercise among sedentary elders before developing the following plan.
2. Begin, if previously sedentary, by walking slightly above a stroll for 15 to 30 minutes.
3. Aim to walk a mile in about 15 to 20 minutes. Then build to 2 miles in 30 minutes.
4. A "training heart rate" is 60% to 90% of your fastest pulse rate per minute.
   - Subtract age from 220.
   - Multiply the result by 0.6 and 0.9 to get the bottom and top of target zone for aerobic training.
5. Walk 3 to 5 times a week, with a heart rate in the target zone for 15 to 60 minutes.
6. Develop a strategy to ensure a commitment to walking.
7. Wear shoes with a firm heel cup for stability, a rocker sole for smooth heel-to-toe motion, and plenty of toe room for push-off. Wear loose, comfortable clothing.
8. Maintain erect posture; lean forward from the ankles, not the waist. Keep head level and chin up.
9. Keep elbows bent at a 90-degree angle and swing arms at the shoulder. The hand should end its forward swing at breastbone height. On the backswing, the upper arm should be parallel to the ground.
10. Stretch before and during the walk and keep a long, smooth stride during the walk.

TABLE 16-10

Consequences of Not Exercising and Being Sedentary

1. Decline in all body systems
2. General weakness
3. Lower energy level
4. Stooped posture
5. Muscle tissue replaced by adipose tissue
6. Atrophy of tissues and functions
7. Higher blood cholesterol and triglyceride levels
8. Greater risk for heart disease
9. Weight gain
10. Lower self-concept, self-esteem
11. Depressive mood

Education: Guidelines for Walking Exercise, provides helpful information (45, 100).

Table 16-10 lists the consequences of insufficient exercise (45, 67, 100, 111, 163). *The elder may be sedentary for various health reasons. However, the person can still engage in exercises* (45, 140):

1. **Arm circles:** Extend arms when sitting on a stool or backless chair. Rotate arms in a circular motion, first forward, then backward. Increase gradually the number of rotations.
2. **Angle stretch:** Lie on bed, legs straight, feet together, arms at side. Move arms and legs outward from body as an eagle spread. Rest. Repeat, increasing the number of spreads.
3. **Stability rock:** Sit erect in chair, feet flat on floor, arms at side. Lean forward and press toes on floor. Lean back and press heels on floor. Continue rocking, taking deep rather than shallow breathes.

Isometric exercises, *tightening and relaxing of muscle groups,* are also effective.

For the individual who is not especially interested in planned exercise programs, suggest bicycling, bowling, golf, swimming, dancing, games such as shuffleboard and horseshoes, and home and garden chores. Jogging should be avoided in late adulthood, perhaps even earlier, because of the potential for joint damage in the hips and lower extremities. Movement therapy programs such as tai chi and other movement patterns contribute to improved morale, self-esteem, and attitudes toward aging. Self-efficacy intervention is useful in promoting physical activity in older adults (5).

MOBILITY ASSISTANCE

When we see persons using canes, walkers, wheelchairs, or electric scooters, we tend to think of them as not being an active part of the community. Actually, various assistive devices, when used correctly, can be a means of promoting mobility and independence, as depicted by the Case Situation. Often, the person who refuses to use a cane or walker develops a shuffling gait, characterized by short steps. Over time, the leg muscles become flaccid, the back may weaken, and posture suffers. The more familiar, older type of walker still has its place in rehabilitation. It can be used as a temporary aid for persons recovering from strokes, fractures, or surgical joint replacements. For long-term use, the new four-wheel walker with adjustable seat is desirable (121).

Electric scooters are another means of providing mobility for some people. They encourage more participation in social activities and aid in the ability to get around in a retirement complex or a nearby store. They can be transported by car to outside events as well: going to the zoo, the shopping mall, or concerts where handicapped access is provided. The theory held by some that an electric cart keeps people from walking is not a valid one. If the client is able to walk at all, he or she should be given an appropriate walking and

Case Situation

Maintaining Independence

Mrs. B., an 85-year-old resident of a life care facility, uses mechanical means to help maintain participation in the life around her, to do volunteer work, to enhance her ability to walk long distances, and to promote a normal posture while walking.

Mrs. B. has had both knees replaced as a result of arthritis. She has osteoarthritis of the spine and rheumatoid arthritis in both hands. She uses a cane for short distances, such as from car to church, shops, or private homes. However, her greatest help is that afforded by a four-wheel walker. It has rack-and-pinion steering, 5-inch wheels, hand brakes, a seat to sit on when tired or waiting in line, and a basket for her purse or packages. Handles are adjustable to allow the person to stand upright, supporting the back in a normal posture. Thus, she

can stride forward without having to lift or turn the walker, because of the ease of steering.

Mrs. B. finds that she uses her walker most of the time, thereby being able to maintain a normal gait and an erect posture, and therefore uses her electric cart less often. She is able to use the shopping carts in supermarkets as she would a walker, and because her walker can be folded, it can go with her on more extensive shopping trips by car or bus. Her electric cart takes her to the swimming pool 6 days a week, where she does water aerobics. Her exercise program, combined with the use of assistive devices, has given Mrs. B. a more enriched life in her elder years.

Contributed by Mildred Boland, MSN, RN.

exercise program by the physician or therapist. Combining the use of cane, walker, and electric scooter or wheelchair with an exercise program is the ideal arrangement.

There are many other assistive devices on the market today to help in the tasks of everyday living. Tools are available to assist in dressing, eating, and various household chores. They can be found in the literature and catalogs that may be obtained through the Arthritis Foundation in most cities.

Health Promotion and Health Protection

There is increasing emphasis on the client and family taking responsibility for personal health promotion, prevention, and management of treatment regimens and general self-care, especially in cases of chronic disease. Each year, over 1 million Americans die from chronic illnesses such as cancer, cardiovascular disease, and diabetes. The problem will increase as the current Baby Boomer population enters old age, especially the old-old stage (87). Because of changes in medical reimbursement and insurance coverage, treatment and care now involves short hospital stays, managed care, and emphasis on care in community settings and the home. *Both risk and protective factors include* (70): (a) severity and trajectory of the condition, including genetic variables; (b) individual age and gender factors; (c) psychosocial characteristics such as depression, self-efficacy, integration of abilities, and diversity factors; (d) family factors such as socioeconomic status and structure; and (e) the environment or community. Independent and self-care lifestyle is also fostered by use of a monitoring company, such as Lifeline, that responds to calls for a need for help or medical assistance—24 hours daily, 365 days a year.

The **Box**, *Healthy People 2010:* Example of Objectives for Health Promotion in Later Maturity, presents health concerns and strategies for this life era, formulated by the U.S. Department of Health and Human Services (185). Refer to the Website www. healthypeople.gov or call 1-800-367-4725.

Health promotion models discussed in Chapter 2 can guide prevention and care for the elderly. ∞ Others are being developed, for example, for late-in-life immigrants (9, 61). A healthy lifestyle based on positive attitudes and behaviors is fundamental to reducing the mortality and morbidity associated with most of the leading causes of death. *Several characteristics or behaviors may contribute to a healthy lifestyle:*

1. Resourcefulness, including learning self-control, self-direction, and self-efficacy.
2. Self-care, being a partner with health care providers in personal health care and help-seeking behaviors when necessary (143).
3. Self-efficacy, expectation and belief that one's actions will make a difference and have a positive outcome (5).
4. Resilience and hardiness, the ability to rebound and adjust to life changes, self-determination, and prosocial behavior in the face of environmental stressors.

Gender differences in longevity result from hormones, genetic makeup, natural immunity, and lifestyle behavior. In the past, lifestyle choices of females gave them an advantage—less drinking of alcoholic beverages, less cigarette smoking, more attention to personal health care, and less exposure to risks at work and play. As females are changing their lifestyles, the gap between the genders in health status and longevity is narrowing. Today's elders, overall, are healthier, better educated, more politically astute, more mobile and youthful in appearance, and more accustomed to changing lifestyles than their counterparts of yesteryear.

Chronic diseases have caused most older deaths throughout the past 50 years. *The most common diseases, which in turn contribute to death, are* (45, 67): (a) cardiac disease, (b) malignant neoplasms, (c) cardiovascular accidents (stroke), (d) chronic lower respiratory diseases, (e) influenza and pneumonia, (f) Alzheimer's disease, (g) nephritis or kidney disease, (h) unintentional injuries, and (i) septicemia or blood poisoning. Rates are similar for both genders, the different aging groups, and racial groups. However, cardiac disease is the leading cause of death for all elders 75 years and older (45, 67). Concerns are being raised about morbidity of the influx of the Baby Boomer population and the chronic illness incidence that will occur because of the epidemic of obesity and their sedentary work and life patterns (87). Arthritis and other neuromuscular diseases, such as Parkinson's disease, decrease functional ability. Decreasing the prevalence would reduce functional limitation.

IMMUNIZATIONS

The elder adult should continue immunizations, as recommended by the Centers for Disease Control and Prevention (CDC). Recommended immunizations and revaccination, including for at-risk elders and elders with uncertain immunization histories or chronic illness, are presented on the CDC Website.

Educate about the importance of maintaining recommended immunizations and keeping a personal record of current immunizations if a historical summary is not available. Explain that tuberculosis, a major killer in their youth, is again increasing in incidence (death rate 1.4 million annually). The elder is at risk and should be tested annually. Since respiratory diseases, especially pneumonia, are a leading cause of death in the elderly, emphasize the importance of influenza and pneumonia immunization. Educate that the immune system response declines in late life. A tetanus-diphtheria (Td) booster is needed every 10 years into old age. Following health-promoting strategies discussed throughout this book and avoiding environmental stresses are beneficial.

SAFETY PROMOTION AND ACCIDENT PREVENTION

Falls are the leading cause of death from injury after age 60. Mortality rates are 33% higher for males than for females, and rates are 10 times higher at age 90 than age 70. The fall may not cause death or even serious injury, but often the person is less able to be as mobile after a fall. Functional decline correlates with being female, being depressed, and falling at home (169). Accidents are directly related to physiologic changes that result from normal aging.

Teach that falls in the elderly may occur for a number of reasons, including:

1. Improper use of or incorrectly fitted assistive devices.
2. Lower-extremity disability.
3. Decrease in functional base of support.

Healthy People 2010

Example of Objectives for Health Promotion in Later Maturity

1. Increase number of women who had mammograms within past 2 years.

2. Increase colorectal cancer screenings.

3. Increase number of people who had cholesterol checked within the past 5 years.

4. Decrease number of people currently smoking.

5. Improve oral health and prevent complete tooth loss.

6. Decrease number of people with no leisure-time physical activity in past month.

7. Decrease prevalence of obesity.

8. Increase number of people who have had flu vaccine in past year.

9. Increase number of people receiving pneumonia vaccine.

10. Decrease number of hip fracture hospitalizations per 100,000 persons.

11. Increase proportion of people eating at least five fruits and vegetables daily.

12. Reduce the proportion of adults who are hospitalized for vertebral fractures associated with osteoporosis.

13. Reduce invasive pneumococcal infections.

14. Reduce the suicide rate.

15. Increase the proportion of primary care providers, pharmacists, and other health care professionals who routinely review with their patients aged 65 years and older and patients with chronic illnesses or disabilities all new prescribed and over-the-counter medicines.

Adapted from reference 185.

---

4. Vision and hearing impairment.
5. Arrhythmias, cardiovascular disease, or strokes.
6. Kinesthetic changes, changes in postural reflexes, or sway.
7. Vertigo and syncopal (fainting) episodes.
8. Peripheral neuropathy.
9. Inadequate swing foot clearance or tripping.
10. Depression or inattention.
11. Excess ingestion of alcohol.
12. Use of certain medications, such as diuretics, sedatives, antibiotics, antidepressants, and antipsychotics.
13. Excess cigarette smoking or osteoporosis, which reduces bone mineral density and can cause fractures resulting from falls.

Educate elders that research indicates that *people who remain active are going to fall less because they* (a) are better able to gauge their position in space and maintain balance, (b) have stronger, better coordinated muscular and more active reflexes for quick response, (c) have greater leg power and grip strength, which reduces risk of falling by 90%, and (d) have a generally better control over the body. Sedentary people who start exercising late in life achieve almost the same extent of benefit as those who have led an active lifestyle (100, 145).

Promote home security and safety. Older adults are particularly vulnerable to fraudulent sales pitches and seemingly honest requests for help by strangers. Educate clients; utilize the **Box**, Client

INTERVENTIONS FOR HEALTH PROMOTION

Teach the following safety measures to be used by the elderly to avoid injury:

1. Use smoke alarms in the home; have a flashlight handy.
2. Place padding on hard edges of wheelchairs and over rough or sharp corners or surfaces of furniture, tables, or countertops.
3. Pad the wooden or metal arms of chairs used by elders.
4. Wear gloves to wash dishes or work in the garden to protect hands.
5. Wear long sleeves to protect arms.
6. Wear long pants and socks to protect the legs and feet.
7. Work and walk more slowly to avoid collisions with objects or falls.
8. Wear flat, rubber-soled, well-fitted shoes; avoid walking in socks, stockings, or loose slippers. Grip handrails (and

place feet on the diagonal if a long foot) when going up and down steps; put nonskid treads on stairs.

9. Use nonslip mats; remove throw rugs; tack rugs to floor if not wall to wall.
10. Use seat and grab bars in bathtub or shower.
11. Maintain exercise to improve gait and mobility; tai chi and yoga also steady movements and improve posture and balance.
12. Keep the house well lit (100-watt bulbs at least), with lights easy to reach. Motion-sensitive lights are useful.
13. Remove or repair unstable furniture or litter/clutter.
14. Have vision and hearing checked annually.
15. Review with physician any medications that could increase risk of falling.

Client Education

Safety in the Home: Do Not Be a Victim of the Con Game

1. **Carpet cleaner:** Ad offers very low price to clean carpeting in one or more rooms of your house. Workers flood room, ruin carpet, and scheme to charge more than quoted to replace damaged material, which may not be replaced.

2. **City inspector:** "Inspector" knocks at the door to check plumbing, furnace, heater, wiring, trees, or whatever. Once inside, he or she may rob you or insist something needs repair and charge excessively for the job.

3. **Home repair:** "Contractor" offers to repair or remodel your home, exterminate pests, or check for radon or offers work with leftover materials from another job in area. The person will find "work" that is unnecessary, resulting in unnecessary expense.

4. **Product demonstration:** Agent offers to describe only (not sell) new product if you will sign paper "for my boss" proving he or she did it. Once inside the house, anything can happen.

5. **Contest winner:** You are told you have won vacation, auto, or other prize but must send $5 for postage or registration or call 800 number for details. Cost for anything will exceed worth.

6. **Lottery:** Person offers to sell you winning lottery ticket he or she cannot cash because "I'm an illegal immigrant," or "I'm behind in my child care payments." Or "law firm" says anonymous donor has bequeathed a winning lottery ticket to you, but first you must send $20 for a computer search to verify your identity.

7. **Land sale:** You are promised cheap land or complete retirement and recreational facilities in a sunny gorgeous site. The land may not exist, even if you paid for it.

8. **Credit or phone card:** Person asks for your credit or phone card number to send you a product, check unauthorized charges, verify insurance, and so on. They can then use your number to charge items.

9. **Governmental service:** Official-sounding firm (e.g., with "Social Security" in name) offers Social Security service that is "required" (e.g., plastic-coated identification cards), "critically needed" (e.g., to help keep agency solvent), or useful (e.g., earnings form). The money sent obtains no service.

10. **Mall-order health care or laboratory tests:** You are promised medical care by mail or laboratory screening for AIDS, cholesterol, cancer, hair loss, and so on. The results are likely to be phony if received at all for the money you sent.

11. **Medical products:** You buy health, beauty care, or "cure" product by mail, or you are sent newspaper clipping extolling magic diet with note scribbled across it. "It works—try it!" signed "J." Avoid such products.

12. **900 number:** Products are offered through special 900 number. Such numbers are common and legitimate but should be avoided.

13. **Obituary:** You are recently widowed; COD box arrives for product "your husband (or wife) ordered." Return unless actually ordered.

14. **Pigeon drop:** Person offers to share "found" money with you if you will put some of your own money with it "to show good faith."

15. **Need help:** Man says his wife is sick, his car has been impounded, he has run out of gas, or some such tale; he needs just $10 or $20, promises to pay it back, and shows extensive identification.

16. **Unknown callers:** Woman with child knocks on door and asks for some favor requiring entrance.

17. **Travel club:** Firm offers bargain airfare or hotel package in glamorous foreign locale. You may never get anything that was promised.

Source: Modified from Marklein, M. (1991). Con Games Proliferate: New Threats Haunt City Folks, *AARP Bulletin, 32*(2), 1, 16–17.

Education: Safety in the Home: Do Not Be a Victim of the Con Game. These strategies help to avoid fraud, scams, or unethical or illegal schemes. Encourage them to report such incidents to the police and family or friends promptly so that safeguards can be instituted in the home (109).

Concerns about older people being *safe drivers* are expressed in the media whenever an elder has an accident. Older drivers generally have fewer accidents per person than the national average, but they have more accidents per mile of driving, especially after 85 years of age. Birthdays are not the cause of accidents—health conditions are (178). *Accidents are frequently due to* (a) medication side effects; (b) eye diseases such as glaucoma or macular degeneration; (c) muscular infirmities, arthritis, or other conditions affecting co-

ordination, strength, and reflex response; (d) confusion about the gas pedal and brake; and (e) cognitive degeneration such as early Alzheimer's disease. However, some people in their 80s drive safely not only the family car but also as part of employment, including driving an ambulance or teaching driver's education.

Educate elders and their families about the importance of safe decisions related to driving, such as during day but not nighttime hours. Explore driver's education for the elder. Explore their ideas about when it would be best for the elder to stop driving. Encourage the elder to voice dismay about losing independence and concern about having transportation needs met. Explore with family or friends how they plan to handle these concerns. Validate that other age groups also have vehicular accidents. Advocate against mandatory specific age restrictions. Periodic testing for the driver's license can foster continued learning of the "rules of the road" and detect either stable or declining abilities as related to driving. Advocate for availability of public transportation and that society has a responsibility to guarantee that elders have a way to get around. Utilize cognitive therapy to foster an attitude of being creative, for example, doing other activities and using money previously spent on car ownership for other plans. Help the elder gain a perspective of challenge and creativity rather than loss.

Refer the elder and family to the following resources:

1. Driver Rehabilitation
   AARP Driver Safety Course (insurance discount upon completion). Phone: 800-424-2410 or www.aarp.org.
2. Self Assessment Tests
   The American Occupational Therapy Association. Self-assessment tests are produced by the AARP and the American Automobile Association. Phone: 301-652-2682 or www.aota.org.

The article by McCullogh (114) on ways to modify the home environment for safety and to promote mobility and independence is an excellent educational source for the elder and family. A number of practical suggestions include installing an entrance/exit ramp, changing door hinges, and using a chair with a seat lift mechanism. These and other modifications listed earlier allow the elder to age in place—at home (114). Walking surfaces outside the home can be covered with kitty litter, kosher salt, or rock salt during icy weather.

Visual Changes Related to Safety Promotion

Changes in visual acuity produce numerous hazards for the older adult. The older adult's problems with color interpretation, light intensity, and depth perception should be considered in the home and institutional environment. Sensitivity to glare, poorer peripheral vision, and a constricted visual field may result in disorientation, especially at night when there is little or no light in the room. The aged person takes longer to recover visual sensitivity when moving from a light to a dark area. **Table 16-4** gives suggestions on how to assist the elder in maintaining vision comfort and safety. Other suggestions follow.

Teach that the environment should be kept free of hazards—no articles on the floor, no furniture with sharp edges, no scatter rugs. Encourage use of a magnifying glass for close vision work, a small flashlight to illuminate dim areas, and properly fitted and cared for eyeglasses. Teach proper care of contact lenses. Teach that nightlights and a safe and familiar arrangement of furniture are essential. Sensory alterations may require modification of the home environment and extra orientation to new surroundings. Furniture and objects should be moved only after discussion with the elder.

Educate administrators of health care agencies and architects or interior designers about special needs of the elder related to aging changes. Environmental factors are important. For example, baseboards, rugs, floors, walls, doorways, and furniture should have contrasting color to avoid confusion and spatial-perceptual problems. The use of contrasting colors in an agency is aesthetic and helps elders locate specific areas, such as the person's room or bathroom. Signs should be prepared with dark backgrounds and light lettering. Blues and greens on signs should be avoided. Numbers on doors, elevators, and telephones should be large enough for the older adult to see.

Teach the elder and family that some signs and symptoms indicate the need for appropriate referral to an ophthalmologist: (a) pain in and around eyes, (b) headaches, especially at night or early morning, (c) mucous discharge from eyes, (d) obvious inflammation or irritation of the eyes and surrounding tissue, (e) avoidance of activities requiring sight, (f) glasses not being worn, missing, or not fitting properly, and (g) change of previous visual habits (requiring different light or reading distance).

When you are caring for a person who is blind, follow the guidelines presented in **Box 16-4.** Teach other health care providers and family members these guidelines also.

Many organizations assist people with low vision, either directly or by helping them find resources in their communities. *Prominent organizations are:*

1. American Foundation for the Blind (AFB)
   11 Penn Plaza, Suite 300, New York, NY 10001
   Phone: 800-232-5463; 212-502-7600
   The Website lists resources in the United States and Canada, www.afb.org.
2. American Health Assistance Foundation
   Lists organizations that sell optical devices and other aids, www.ahaf.org.
3. Lighthouse International
   111 E. 59th Street, New York, NY 10022
   Phone: 800-829-0500; 212-821-9200; 212-821-9713 (TDD), www.lighthouse.org.
4. Lions Club
   300 22nd Street, Oak Brook, IL 60523
   (Check with local branches for assistance.), www.lionsclub.org.
5. National Federation of the Blind (NFB)
   1800 Johnson Street, Baltimore, MD 21230
   Phone: 410-659-9314 or www.nfb.org

Hearing Impairment Related to Safety Promotion

Changes in hearing acuity may predispose the person to accident risks. Many elderly persons have been diagnosed as being mentally ill, whereas in reality they were suffering from a gradual loss of hearing. If one is unable to hear clearly, it is easy to imagine one is being talked about or ignored. This leads to depression, and then behavior often is categorized as irrational, suspicious, or hostile. This produces isolation and further frustrations, and the vicious cycle that ensues may in the end cause real paranoid behavior to develop.

Refer to the suggestions on effective communication with the hearing-impaired person given in **Box 16-5.** Encourage the person to consult with a physician about use of a hearing aid rather than going to a nonqualified practitioner.

Tactile Changes Related to Safety Promotion

Changes in temperature regulation and the inability to feel pain also produce safety problems. Utilize **Table 16-3** for teaching about safety risks and implementing health promotion. The normal body temperature decreases with age.

Pain intensity is difficult to determine even when the person cannot report pain but exhibits what instruments measure as pain behavior (140). Inadequate assessment contributes to poor pain management for the elder (45, 140). Pain perception and reaction may be decreased with age. Use caution when applying heat or cold to prevent burns or frostbite. More accurate assessment of physical signs and symptoms may be necessary to alleviate conditions underlying complaints of pain, such as abdominal discomfort and chest pain.

The elderly usually feel cold more easily and may require more covering when in bed; a room temperature somewhat higher than usual may be desirable. Most hospitals and nursing homes do not have thermometers that register body temperatures below 94°F (35°C). Therefore, statistics are not available on how many elderly persons suffer and die from hypothermia. Mildly cool temperatures of 60°F (15.5°C) to 65°F (18.3°C) can trigger **hypothermia,** *reduction in body temperature to below normal levels.* A nighttime room temperature of 66°F (18.3°C) can be too low for an aged person (45), who may be unaware of extreme loss of body heat, especially when supine and relatively inactive.

Assess for hypothermia risk or presence, as follows (45, 67, 154):

1. Medications to treat anxiety or depression, hypothyroidism, vascular disease, alcoholism, and immobility reduce the body's response to cold.
2. Living alone or anything that increases nighttime accidents can increase risk, as do poverty and poor housing.
3. The elder may insist he or she is comfortable in a cool environment; the person is unaware of the temperature of surroundings.
4. The person is not thinking clearly or acting as usual.
5. Low body temperature, irregular or slow pulse, slurred speech, shallow respirations, hypotension, drowsiness, lack of coordination, and sluggishness may be present, singly or in combination.
6. Coma may occur and is probable when the body temperature is 90°F (32.2°C) or less.

Severe hypothermia can cause complications of kidney, liver, or pancreatic disorders, ventricular fibrillation, and death. Recovery depends on severity and length of exposure, previous health, and the rewarming treatment.

The article by Ruffulo (154) presents detailed information on intrinsic and treatment-related factors that contribute to hypothermia, physiologic effects on a number of body systems, and safe rewarming methods.

Teach the elderly person the following measures to prevent hypothermia in cold weather:

1. Stay indoors as much as possible, especially on windy, wet, and cold days.
2. Wear layered clothing, and cover the head when outdoors.
3. Eat high-energy foods such as some fats and easily digested carbohydrates and protein daily.
4. Keep at least one room warm at 70°F (20°C) or above.
5. Use extra blankets, caps, socks, and layered clothing in bed.

6. Have contact with someone daily.
7. Avoid drinking alcoholic beverages.

Hyperthermia, *abnormal elevation of body temperature unrelated to fever-inducing illness,* may go undetected because the person suffering heat stress may have a temperature of 99°F. This must also be prevented.

Causes of hyperthermia include (a) decreased sweat gland activity and longer response time to heat, (b) less production of perspiration, which leads to less body cooling, (c) loss of subcutaneous tissue, which allows more water loss from deeper tissues through the skin, (d) inability of circulatory system to dissipate heat efficiently due to slower peripheral vasodilation, (e) severe diarrhea and dehydration, (f) elevated body temperature due to illness, (g) sleep deprivation, and (h) taking psychotropic or beta-blocker medications, which interfere with heat regulation (45).

Assess for the three types of heat-related illnesses (45):

1. **Heat cramps.** *Mild disorder that involves large skeletal muscles,* caused by sudden sodium depletion.
2. **Heat exhaustion.** *More serious, not life threatening, but a precursor to heat stroke.* This occurs if the person has inadequate fluid or sodium intake. Signs and symptoms are diaphoresis, thirst, fatigue, headache, elevated body temperature, flushed skin, nausea, vomiting, and possible diarrhea.
3. **Heat stroke. Classic** *occurs during extremely hot weather, during a "heat wave"* when the elder is in a closed apartment with no cooling system or outdoors in the heat. **Exertional** *occurs during strenuous physical exertion (or for the elder with even moderate activity) when temperature and humidity are high.* Increased sweating depletes sodium, but high humidity interferes with ability of the body to lower its core temperature. Several physiologic mechanisms operate to maintain normal body temperature. Thyroid function decreases and aldosterone and antidiuretic hormone (ADH) production increases to conserve body water and sodium. Emphasize that if these mechanisms are overwhelmed, peripheral vasoconstriction conserves central circulatory volume, but the core body temperature rises dramatically.

Signs and symptoms of hyperthermia include (45): (a) fever (103 to 106°F), (b) headache, (c) vertigo, (d) faintness, (e) confusion, (f) hyperpnea, and (g) abdominal distress. At the higher body temperature, skin is hot and dry, respirations are weak, and tachycardia, agitation, delirium, hallucinations, and convulsions may occur.

Complications, especially for heat stroke, include (45): (a) cerebral edema or brain damage, (b) pulmonary edema, (c) liver necrosis, (d) acute renal failure, (e) myocardial necrosis or infarction, and (f) gastrointestinal bleeding or ulceration.

Educate that prompt recognition and treatment of heat-related illness is essential to prevent organ damage or death. *Teach prevention, including* (a) staying in a cool environment, (b) increasing fluid intake, (c) wearing a sunblock outdoors, (d) wearing loose, light clothing, (e) sponging off or taking cooling showers, (f) increasing daily consumption of fluids and carbohydrates, (g) avoiding excessive physical activity, and (h) using a fan or air conditioner.

Treatment includes (a) removing the person to a cool place, (b) applying cool clothes, (c) loosening clothing, and (d) giving fluids. Emergency department care may be necessary to assess for and prevent complications when body temperature continues to rise.

Tactile sensation or *body feeling* is less responsive in a number of areas of the body. The number and sensitivity of sensory receptors decrease with age.

Teach the elder and family about these changes, their implications, and ways to overcome deficits. There may be clumsiness or difficulty in identifying objects by touch. The person may not respond to light touch but needs to be touched. Hair brushing, back rubs, hugs, and touch of shoulder, arms, or hands, if acceptable, stimulate tactile sensation. Because fewer tactile cues are received from the bottom of the feet, the person may get confused about position and location.

Teach health care providers and family that some of the changed behavior discussed under Psychological Concepts is directly related to physical changes in nerve and sensory tissue and influences nursing practice, whether you are giving physical care, establishing a relationship, providing a safe environment, or planning recreational needs. Research indicates that hand, foot, and eye preference becomes more right-sided and ear preference becomes more left-sided with advancing age (45). Adapt nursing care measures to accommodate these changes. *The whole area of client teaching is also affected, because you must understand the altered responses and the changing needs of the elderly before beginning their health education.*

SPECIAL CONSIDERATIONS IN THE PHYSICAL EXAMINATION OF OLDER CLIENTS

The *health history of the elder should include* (54):

1. Current problems.
2. Complete history of past medical problems.
3. Smoking, alcohol, and drug history.
4. Medication list.
5. Psychosocial history and mental status.
6. Nutritional patterns.
7. Review of body systems focusing on functional abilities.
8. Exercise patterns.
9. History of immunizations.
10. Support systems.
11. Caregiver roles, caregiver stress, and possible neglect or abuse.
12. Advance directives.

Physical examination should include (54): (a) vital signs and weight, (b) mobility screening, (c) hypertension and vascular disease screening, (d) cancer screening, (e) hearing and vision screening, (f) breast examination, with mammography for women up to age 75 (and perhaps to age 85), and (g) Papanicolaou smear, if inadequately screened at younger age or if history of abnormalities.

The following are specific ways to *increase comfort during the examination:*

1. Warm the examining room sufficiently (75°F).
2. Use chairs that are high enough to make rising easy.
3. Provide a footstool for getting on and off the table.
4. Place a pillow under the head and perhaps under the knees, as many elders feel a strain on the back when lying supine.
5. Place grab bars near the scale.
6. Minimize positional changes during the examination.

In carrying out any particular physical assessment in the older adult, the nurse may need to modify some procedures to glean the most information. Even helping the patient undress gives the nurse opportunity to observe the patient's ability to perform the task and to note anything unusual, for example, condition of clothing, personal hygiene, or clothing that may be inappropriate for the season or temperature (such as thermal underwear in August). Attention must be given to avoid discomfort, maintain the patient's dignity, and distinguish signs of disease from changes typical of normal aging.

Orthostatic vital signs are valuable in the elderly, as heart rate response to postural change may alter decisions regarding hypertension or hypotension. Another important observation is the palpation of temporal arteries. Checking for tenderness or thickening may raise the possibility of temporal arteritis, especially in a patient with jaw pain, temporal headaches, earache, or unexplained fever.

Other important areas of exploration in the elderly are hearing acuity, condition of dentures, suspicious lesions under the tongue, jugular venous pulse, carotid arteries for bruits, and breast examination, including the skin under pendulous breasts.

Suspected urinary incontinence can be tested by having the patient hold a small pad over the urethral area and coughing three times in a standing position. Cystocele, rectocele, or uterine prolapse should be ruled out. In the male, a digital rectal examination should be done to check the prostate.

Examination of the elder patient's feet is most important. Have the patient sit up and hang the feet down to check the venous flow. Are the patient's shoes appropriate for good balance and prevention of falls? The patient's gait can offer significant clues, for example, the parkinsonian gait shown by short, shuffling steps, short or absent arm swing, and a stooped trunk.

Assess for the **syndrome of frailty,** *weak, physically disabled elders who demonstrate three or more of the following characteristics* (45, 56, 57, 186):

1. Unaccustomed or unintentional weight loss of 10 or more pounds within a year, including **sarcopenia,** *loss of muscle mass.*
2. Exhaustion that prevents normal or enjoyable activities.
3. Weakness, including reduction in grip strength (weakest 20% for age group).
4. Slow walking speed, in the slowest 20% per age group.
5. Low physical activity (males burn less than 380 calories/week, females burn less than 270 calories/week in physical activity).

Up to 25% of people over age 80 are frail. Females are more likely to be frail than males. *Assess for the factors that contribute to frailty:* (a) vitamin and mineral deficiency, (b) other diseases such as anemia or osteoporosis, and (c) low testosterone in males. *Some conditions may be considered triggers for frailty, including* (a) an illness, (b) a heart attack, or (c) a broken hip. Frail people are more likely to fall, be hospitalized, be disabled, or suffer from a variety of diseases and chronic conditions. Inactivity, lack of nutrients, and weakness with loss of muscle mass result in a cycle of decline. Frail people have a higher mortality rate (45, 56, 57, 186).

COMMON HEALTH PROBLEMS: PREVENTION AND TREATMENT

Most Common Disorders

The health problems of the older adult may be associated with the aging process, a disease state, or both. Yet more than 90% of elders need no help with activities of daily living. Consider all of the aspects of aging before deciding on a course of action in treatment, as presentation of illness in older adults is often different from younger persons (6, 54, 64, 123).

CARDIOVASCULAR DISEASE Heart disease is the number-one killer for both genders. *Gender differences occur in the classic warning symptoms. Males* are likely to experience **angina,** *a severe squeezing pain that radiates to the neck, upper abdomen, or left arm and occurs during stress or exertion. Females* are more likely to experience shortness of breath or profound fatigue that occurs in activities they previously found easy to do. Or they may have nausea, heartburn, or indigestion unrelated to anything recently eaten (45, 132).

Stroke (cardiovascular accident) is the third most common cause of death. Excessive adiposity in adults age 65 to 74 seems to influence risk of stroke in conjunction with hypertension, diabetes, and other cardiovascular disease risk factors (45, 100, 111). Therefore, control of weight and fat consumption remains an important concern as people age (41, 44).

Educate the public, including elders, about the *2007 Guidelines for Preventing Cardiovascular Disease in Women, which include the following recommendations* (132):

1. Daily low-dose aspirin therapy, even if at low risk of heart disease and stroke
2. Twice weekly consumption of fatty fish, especially for females
3. Daily saturated fat intake less than 7% of calories, trans fat less than 1% of calories
4. Daily fresh fruits and vegetables, and low-fat dairy products, if consumed
5. Omega-3 supplements for anyone with heart disease or high triglycerides
6. Weight control, increased physical activity
7. Smoking cessation, with counseling and nicotine replacement if needed

Education with the elder and younger family members may also involve constructing a medical genogram for the family, which would include connections to heart disease, as well as to other illnesses of family members. Refer to a local genealogical association or the Website for Your Family History, Your Future, National Society of Genetic Counselors, www.nsgc.org.

OTHER CAUSES OF DEATH Cancer is the second leading cause of death. Pneumonia, influenza, and chronic obstructive lung disease rank next as causes of death. Other prevalent disorders are arthritis, diabetes, hypertension, and osteoporosis (45, 100, 111). El-

derly males are more likely to commit suicide than any other age group in the United States (10), and Caucasians, in contrast to other racial groups, are the most likely to use firearms for suicide (10).

Various other conditions are more frequently observed in the elderly (6), including eating disorders (69), gastrointestinal infections due to *Clostridium difficile (C. diff)*, bacterial skin infection from community-acquired methicillin-resistant *Staphylococcus aureus (CA-MRSA)*, or *extremely drug-resistant tuberculosis* (6).

Diseases That Affect Sexual Function

Health problems associated with the sexual changes of aging are of concern to the older adult. Certain diseases in the elderly female have been linked to estrogen deficiency. There is a rise in atherosclerosis attacking the coronary arteries in aged females (and in younger females who have had ovaries removed). The female hormones apparently are crucial to the enzymatic system in the metabolism of fats and proteins.

Factors that contribute to sexual dysfunction are essentially the same as those that affect performance at any age (10, 45, 100, 111):

1. Disease or mutilating surgery of the genitourinary tract
2. Diverse systemic diseases
3. Emotional responses coupled with societal attitudes
4. Treatment of physical complaints with use of drugs
5. Excessive use of alcohol, marijuana, or other substances that weaken erection, reduce desire, and delay ejaculation
6. Presence of metabolic disorders, overlooked or untreated
7. Presence of anemia, diabetes, malnutrition, and fatigue, which may affect quality of life and cause impotence
8. Obesity, which may impose a hazard for cardiac and vascular integrity and be damaging to a healthy self-image

Many older persons are under the false impression that any sexual activity will increase the danger of chest pain, illness, or even death because of stress on the heart or blood pressure. In truth, oxygen consumption, heart rate, and blood pressure increase only moderately during intercourse and may actually afford a distinct therapeutic and preventive measure (29, 34, 82, 180). In persons with arthritis, for example, the increase in adrenal corticosteroids during sexual activity relieves some of the symptoms. The present-day practice of prescribing exercise for cardiac patients attests that sexual intercourse need not be considered dangerous for anyone able to walk around a room.

Katz (82) presents a useful summary of information that can be shared with cardiac patients in relation to energy requirements, risks, warning signs, sexual difficulties, and resuming sex after a cardiac event.

Radical surgery or dysfunction of the genitourinary tract produces the most devastating effects on sexual capacity and libido. Extensive resectioning due to malignancy may make intercourse difficult if not impossible. Although a decline in desire and capacity for climax may follow hysterectomies, it is by no means inevitable. The loss of childbearing ability and the lack of an ejaculation are for some females and males, respectively, psychologically traumatic. These clients may need some support and guidance.

Human sexuality covers a wide spectrum, and the pattern for each individual is a product of prenatal development and postnatal learning experiences coupled with an inherent sense of personal identity within a gender classification. This basic pattern is not altered simply by age. It continues to mediate one's capacity for involvement in all life activities.

Nursing and health care planning and intervention with the elderly can be effective. Realize the need for sexual expression in some form or other. Be open and nonjudgmental when clients display a desire for warmth, close contact, and companionship. Touch is particularly important to the older person who has been bereft of family ties, perhaps for many years. Some people require more relief from sexual tension than others. If incidents arise that seem unduly unorthodox, such as open masturbation or unusual behavior with the opposite sex, be a support person for counsel. An atmosphere of trust must prevail in which the focus is on the person and not on any specific act.

Explore alternative lifestyles with persons who are single, alone, and old. Teaching that includes information about available therapy when there are emotional or physiologic problems can help the elderly person to choose treatment. Communicate with the families and friends of the older client, as appropriate, and to colleagues the information that will help in dealing with the sexual needs of the aged.

Assess for, educate and counsel about, and intervene related to HIV and AIDS infection. Such infection can occur in this cohort of elders, especially females, considering the male-female ratio. HIV and AIDS infections may be more common in future elderly, considering lifestyle trends, treatment advances, and longevity consequences. In addition to discussion about treatment, counseling may be necessary to resolve past relationship experiences.

Pharmacokinetics and Aging Changes

Changes in brain structure and function in the aging process may potentiate the effects of alcohol and other psychoactive drugs. Total body water content decreases by 10% to 20% from ages 20 to 80, and extracellular fluid volume decreases by 35% to 40%. An increase of 18% to 36% in total body fat occurs in males and an increase of 33% to 45% occurs in females from 20 to 80 years (117). Alcohol, which distributes in body water, has a smaller water distribution volume in the elderly, resulting in higher blood alcohol levels. Medications that are fat soluble have a large distribution volume, lower serum levels for a single dose, longer elimination times, and, thereby, greater cumulative and toxic effects. Serum albumin decreases from a mean of 4.7 mg/dL in the young adult to 3.8 mg/dL in the elderly. Albumin is the major drug-binding protein; a decrease in albumin level may result in higher levels of free medication, less therapeutic effect, and increased drug-drug interactions. Aging affects both the liver and kidneys, reducing the rate of medication elimination and increasing the side effects or toxicity. Blood flow and oxidative enzyme levels decrease with age, which affects disposition of medications and contributes to less therapeutic effects (10, 45, 117).

Educate the elderly about the risk of magnesium toxicity.

Polypharmacy and Adverse Drug Reactions

People in later maturity represent 15% of the population but account for nearly 40% of the prescription drugs consumed in the United States. Over 60% of people over 65 take at least one med-

ication daily. Almost 20% take seven or more prescribed medications daily (10, 45, 112).

Because older persons are more likely to have several chronic illnesses, often complex in nature, they are likely to go to a number of doctors, who each prescribe medication. Thus, a drug side effect, such as confusion, may be mistaken for a new medical condition, such as Alzheimer's disease. The person may get the wrong medication as a result. Often, prescribed doses are too high for elders, related to the lower metabolism and other physiologic changes they are experiencing.

Adverse reactions to medications, a serious health threat, may affect as many as 10 million older Americans each year. Often the symptoms go unrecognized. Yet, excessive medication and medication side effects are responsible for thousands of serious car accidents and hip fractures from falls annually. Many elders have memory loss and cognitive impairment from blood pressure medication, sleeping pills, tranquilizers, and other psychiatric medications. Drug-induced neurologic problems (parkinsonian symptoms and tardive dyskinesia) occur from antipsychotic medications in older adults (10, 45).

Older females are especially vulnerable because they metabolize drugs differently than males, especially antidepressant, antianxiety, and antipsychotic medications. Often recommended doses have been calculated for males. Yet, older females have smaller body size, higher percentage of body fat, hormone fluctuations, and slower gastric-emptying rates. Thus, they may encounter more problems with medication reactions (10, 45, 112).

Teach elders and family members the following:

1. Learn as much as possible about the medication being taken and the disease process.
2. Keep a record of medications, prescribed and over-the-counter, as well as vitamin-mineral supplements and herbs, the doses, times consumed, and any reactions that are unusual.
3. Inform each of the physicians about all of the prescribed and over-the-counter medications that are taken daily.
4. Follow the directions for taking the medications, such as drinking a tall glass of water to reduce side effects.
5. Consult a physician or pharmacist about any questions or symptoms. Report problems promptly.

Substance Abuse

There has been considerable publicity about the recommendation of a small glass of wine daily to lower risk of heart disease. Less has been written about the pitfalls of excessive consumption of alcohol. A safe amount of alcohol is far less than most people think, especially for older adults and females, who are especially vulnerable to intoxication and drug interactions. Whatever the age or gender, *experts do not recommend starting to drink,* because of alcohol's potential for harm and addiction. There are safer ways to protect the heart (10, 18). Further, certain medical conditions require alcohol abstinence: hypertension, cardiac arrhythmias, ulcers, liver disease, and dementia (45, 100, 111). Alcohol also interacts with various drugs, through either potentiation of or interference with medication action. Utilize this information in client teaching, since alcohol and many medications should not be combined.

MediaLink · Magnesium Toxicity

MediaLink · Medical Hazards of Alcoholism

Older adults are especially vulnerable to the effects of alcohol because it is a central nervous system depressant and because of the elder's unique physiology. Aging increases alcohol sensitivity in elders because of slowing metabolism and because their tissues hold less water than that of younger persons (117). Thus, alcohol has greater potential for intoxication, drug interactions (elders typically take two to seven, or more, medications), and side effects (18, 45, 108).

Females are more sensitive to alcohol than males because they produce less of the enzyme that breaks down alcohol. The average female achieves a higher alcohol blood level and becomes more intoxicated after drinking half the amount of alcohol consumed by the average male. Small body size increases alcohol potency because there is less body water to dilute the alcohol, especially in elders, who are more likely to be dehydrated (10, 18, 170).

Alcoholism has a polygenic causation in all ages, but especially in the elderly: a combination of biochemistry and temperament, cultural norms, psychological status, environmental stressors, and inadequate social support systems (10, 18, 156). As many as 10% to 15% are estimated to suffer alcoholism (10, 18). Comparable rates occur in other countries (170). Further, increasing numbers of elders are abusing not only prescription and over-the-counter drugs, but also heroin, LSD, marijuana, and cocaine. Widowers constitute the largest proportion of late-onset elderly alcoholics (10, 170). Stevenson and Masters (170) found that older females who were most at risk for alcohol misuse or abuse scored higher on the T-ACE (revised CAGE instrument), used two or more over-the-counter drugs regularly, consumed large amounts of coffee daily, and used alcohol to fall asleep. Contrary to popular opinion, the elder can be successfully treated.

Your acceptance of, listening to, and assessment of the elderly person in various health care settings can be critical for diagnosis and treatment. You are a liaison between the client and other professionals and can facilitate treatment of the alcoholism and prevention or treatment of various complications. Further, your counseling, education, and support of the family and client can foster their acceptance of the diagnosis and pursuit of treatment.

Failure to Thrive

Annually, a small percentage of frail elders are admitted to hospitals with the diagnosis **failure to thrive,** *a complex presentation of symptoms causing gradual decline in physical and cognitive function that occurs without immediate explanation.* The weight loss, disability, and social withdrawal may be caused by low income, hidden organic illness, polypharmacy, malnutrition, depression, age-related changes, an inadequate support system or living alone, or lack of education. Denial of symptoms, feelings of great loss and grief, helplessness, loneliness, and giving up are experienced. Without adequate care, the person is likely to die prematurely (41, 45, 86, 124).

A holistic focus involving a multidisciplinary team is needed in care and treatment. Explore food choices, which may be less related to preference and more related to income; physical ability to shop, prepare, chew, and swallow food; and food intolerance related to aging, chronic disease, or medication. Individualized intervention will be necessary in these situations. Besides the necessary physical care measures, reminiscence and life review

therapy, and promotion of a relationship and social support system, will be necessary to help the person regain physical and emotional energy and vitality and to survive.

Psychological Concepts

The psychological and socioeconomic concepts about aging are significant for all who work with the aged. You will find older people concerned and needing to talk about the many changes to which they must adjust. Knowledge of the crises in this life stage is necessary if you are to aid clients and families in the attainment of developmental tasks, in meeting the crises, and in the early or appropriate treatment of these crises.

COGNITIVE DEVELOPMENT
Normal Processes

One universal truth that concerns the process of aging is that its onset, rate, and pattern are unique for each person. Within the individual, the various cognitive functions do not change or decline at the same pace. Some will not decrease at all; for example, memorization of facts may be difficult but wisdom will be evident. Psychological and mental changes generally have a later and more gradual onset than physical aging. The brain demonstrates **neuronal plasticity**, *ability to change its structure and function throughout life, governed by an interplay of experience and developmental stages or sensitive periods when neuronal networks are particularly plastic.* The more the neural system is activated, and the more a task is repeated, the stronger the corresponding neural system and its function becomes (45, 67).

Many factors must be considered when assessing the intellectual functioning of older people (6, 15, 16, 32, 33, 45, 67, 117, 133, 140, 148, 162, 166):

1. Overall physical health status, which can affect the level of psychological distress, life satisfaction, and cognitive ability (e.g., anemia, lung disease, sleep apnea, poor circulation, blood pressure or blood sugar changes, hypothyroidism, integrity of the nervous system, pain, and fluid or nutritional imbalance can profoundly affect mental status).
2. Medications (prescribed and over-the-counter) that may slow or interfere with cognitive processes because of toxicity related to slower elimination from the body.
3. Drug overdose or **polypharmacy**, *taking excess and unneeded combinations of drugs that may cause drug interactions, toxicity, confusion, or depression.* Polypharmacy must be avoided with careful monitoring and adjustments.
4. Sensory impairments (vision, hearing) that interfere with integration of sensory input into proper perception, consequent learning, and appropriate behaviors.
5. Sociocultural influences and support systems.
6. Motivation and interest in the task or stimuli.
7. Spiritual beliefs and support systems.
8. Educational level or literacy.
9. Time since school learning.
10. Isolation from others.
11. Deliberate caution.

12. Using more time to do something, which others may interpret as not knowing.
13. Adaptive mechanism of conserving time and emotional energy rather than showing assertion.

The initial level of ability is important: a bright 20-year-old will probably be a bright 70- or 80-year-old. Overall, mental ability increases with age (45, 138). Increasingly, elders are returning for advanced degrees. An example is the 84-year-old graduate who was awarded a Master in Philosophy degree from a large university, fulfilling a vision he began in 1950 but was unable to complete because of numerous life responsibilities and crises. He related well in the classes with late adolescents and young adults and received considerable recognition at pre-commencement and graduation services. The **Engagement Hypothesis** *states that people with high intellectual ability in early life, who have a favorable education and environmental support, engage in a lifestyle with complex demands and thereby promote or retain cognitive, occupational, and social skills* (138, 158). The 84-year-old graduate demonstrated Activity Theory and the Engagement Hypothesis.

The elder demonstrates **crystallized intelligence**, *knowledge and cognitive ability maintained over the lifetime. It is dependent on sociocultural influences, life experiences, and broad education, which involve the ability to perceive relationships, engage in behaviors typical of the Formal Operations stage, and understand the intellectual and cultural heritage.* Crystallized intelligence is measured by facility with numbers, verbal comprehension, general information, and integrative and interpretive ability. It is influenced by the amount the person has learned, the diversity and complexity of the environment, the person's openness to new information, and the extent of formal learning opportunities. Self-directed learning and educational opportunities to gain additional information increase crystallized intelligence after 60 years of age (15, 138, 157, 158). Loss of biological potential is offset by acquired wisdom, experience, and knowledge.

In contrast, **fluid intelligence**, *independent of instruction, social or environmental influences, or acculturation, and dependent on genetic endowment, is less apparent in the elder. It consists of ability to perceive complex relationships, use of short-term or rote memory, creation of concepts, and abstract reasoning.* Fluid intelligence is measured by ability to do tasks of memory span, inductive reasoning, and figural relations. The fluid intelligence may begin to decrease in middle age. There is, however, no uniform pattern of age-related changes for all intellectual abilities, nor is there a consistent decline in all elders (157). In a 7-year longitudinal study of the effects of cognitive training on fluid intelligence, participants in their 70s and 80s performed better than in their late 60s after cognitive training (194).

Intellectual plasticity refers to the fact that the *person's performance or ability can vary a great deal, depending on social, environmental, and physical conditions:* for example, time to do a task, anxiety about evaluation, attention to or motivation for the task, amount of environmental stimulation, or cognitive training or education (15, 138, 156). Use of group discussion, feedback to the speaker, problem solving and memory practice, and leisurely pace of communication also increases cognitive performance (99, 156).

The senior performs certain cognitive tasks more slowly for several reasons (6, 15, 50, 51, 67, 157, 158, 167, 168):

1. Literacy levels at fifth- to eighth-grade level, especially for health-related content, for about half of the elder population
2. Decreased visual and auditory acuity
3. Slower motor response to sensory stimulation
4. Divided attention because of numerous mental associations
5. Greater amount of prior accumulated knowledge and learning that must be scanned and appropriately placed mentally
6. Perceived meaning of task
7. Changed motivation
8. Decreased neurologic and overall physical functioning

He or she may be less interested in competing in timed intellectual tests. Reaction time is also slower when the person suffers significant environmental or social losses, is unable to engage in social contact, and is unable to plan daily routines. The person who is ill often endures environmental and social losses by virtue of being in the client role. Thus, he or she may respond more slowly to your questions or requests (45, 157, 158).

Range of intellectual functioning is quite wide and includes use of multiple intelligences (59) and emotional intelligence (63) similar to past use. There is generally a decline in IQ test scores for people over 60; yet some people over 60 score higher than some of their younger counterparts. Test results are based on speed; they are timed tests. Results of IQ tests may reflect the stress of having to cope with the test more than actual intelligence. Research findings show that there is an age-related decrease in the speed of almost all behavioral processes. Thus, older people carry out the same processes, but at a slower rate, as do younger adults: cue use, encoding, specificity, decision-making speed, design recognition, and spatial memory or awareness of location. Overall, general and verbal intelligence, problem solving, coordination of ideas and facts, judgment, creativity, and other well-practiced cognitive skills and wisdom are maintained even into old age if there is no deterioration caused by extensive physical or neurologic changes. Further, memory can be improved with skills training and motivational incentives (15, 67, 99, 138, 156). Studies indicate that cognitive performances of young and old adults are comparable for assessing content and recall and recognition of factual information when the task is divided or attention has not been interrupted (67, 138). Older females excel over males in verbal ability and speed of reaction.

Older people are able to tolerate extensive degenerative changes in the central nervous system without serious alteration of behavior if their social environments are sufficiently supportive. If their environment was restricted in early life, however, learning is inhibited in later life. *Mental functions, especially vocabulary and other verbal abilities, do not deteriorate appreciably until 6 to 12 months before death, known as* **terminal decline** (138).

Table 16-11 summarizes types of cognitive functions, characteristics of the aging person, and health promotion implications (15, 45, 138, 156, 157, 158, 168). Utilize this information in assessment, client and family education, and your intervention.

Cognition and intellectual development are part of maturity. It is in the last half of life that the person best draws on cumulative experiences to establish social, moral, and ethical standards; render

TABLE 16-11

Cognitive Development in the Aging Person: Health Promotion Implications

Characteristic	Change During Aging	Implication for Health Care
Sensory memory	Large amount of information enters nervous system through the senses; selective attention occurs. Some information is sent to short-term memory for further processing; some is lost because nervous system cannot process. First step of memory process involves recall that lasts a few minutes.	Avoid sensory overload. Assist hearing, visual, and tactile functions. Recognize that person may be inattentive to your teaching or to his or her symptoms or situation. Use variety of teaching methods, include visual aids. Teach importance of health maintenance, as healthy elders maintain general intellectual function.
Short-term memory	Brain holds information for immediate use: conceptualization, rehearsal, memorization, association with long-term memory. Deals with current activities or recent past of minutes to hours. Remains consistent with earlier abilities. Older person can repeat string of digits as well as younger person unless asked to repeat them backward; information about digits fades in about a minute unless person rehearses it. Overall mental status is poorly correlated with short-term memory. Recall is better for logically grouped, chunked, or sequenced information.	Give attention for memory abilities. Teach importance of continuing to use memory, memory retrieval tricks, or cues. Teach person to use variety of associative and memory strategies to enhance recall. Teach relaxation methods to reduce anxiety about memory and enhance attention, rehearsal, motivation, and general function. Teach cognitive tricks or use of lists or ways to organize information to improve memory or remember essential information. Teach person to overcome interferences. Let person set own pace to enhance learning and memory.
Long-term memory	Use of information acquired, transferred for storage, and stored over years. Unlimited, permanent storehouse of memories that may not have to pass through short-term memory. Involves images (mental pictures) and verbalization. Three encoding systems are used: visual-spatial, verbal sequential, and abstraction.	Give attention for memory abilities. Recognize that dysfunctions in short- and long-term memories occur independently. Encourage person to use memories and associations in tasks.
Declarative (episodic)	Conscious memory of specific persons, places, events, or facts that is acquired quickly, but may not be accurately or easily recalled. Requires intact hippocampus. Older person stores long-term memories, but does not retrieve as quickly as younger person unless he or she uses memory tricks.	Give person adequate time for recall. Encourage use of memory tricks and associations.
Recognition	Involves selecting correct response from incoming information rather than recall or retrieval. Ability is retained with age for words, background, familiar objects.	Give support and recognition for ability to recognize and use information.
Implicit (reflexive)	Unconscious learning of information or skill through experience or practice (e.g., playing piano, riding bicycle). Requires intact cerebellum. Ideas, concepts, or ability to perform readily remembered. Does not weaken with age in absence of pathology, as person can demonstrate if not discuss.	Use practice in learning new skills for self-care. Reinforce use of habits. Encourage reminiscence or life review. Use habits and well-practiced skills when possible in teaching or assisting them. Encourage continued practice of implicitly learned tasks or information.

TABLE 16-11

Cognitive Development in the Aging Person: Health Promotion Implications—continued

Characteristic	Change During Aging	Implication for Health Care
Reaction time (RT)	Speed of response slows during life, and is more obvious after age 60 because of central nervous system changes; shorter duration of alpha rhythm in brain wave (RT fastest between ages 20 and 30). RT remains faster in males than females. Reaction time remains accurate even if slower in both sexes in older adult.	If the person is hurried, response quality and quantity will be reduced. Allow person to proceed at own pace in learning, making decisions, or doing tasks. Do not consider slower response the same as confusion or dementia.
Attentional selectivity	Gradual reduced ability in focusing on a specific idea or event, especially as the information-processing demands of the task increase. As capable as younger people in correcting unanticipated errors.	Call attention to specific tasks or ideas that the person must focus on when teaching or counseling. Recognize and reinforce capabilities.
Problem solving	Skills increase steadily into old age; performance unrelated to IQ test scores or formal education. Person adopts simpler judgmental strategies and relies on preexisting knowledge more so than young adult. In low-memory–demand tasks, elder is more efficient than young adult. Is better at complex judgmental strategies than young adult.	Teach importance of continuing cognitive function. Engage person in goal setting and problem solving.
Dialectical thinking	Older people better able to see all sides of a situation and come to conclusion that integrates different viewpoints and contradictory ideas when given time and when experience rather than memory is required. Is better at solving conditional-probability problems than young adult. Is better at telling integrated story than young adult.	Listen to what may appear to be rambling or loose associations, as ideas are likely to be related and pertinent.
Social awareness	Increased knowledge and empathy related to culture, living, value systems, or application of ethical and moral principles. Social responsibility traits remain stable or increase in older adult.	Recognize and reinforce capabilities. Use older people as consultants and teachers of the culture.
Higher mental functions: calculations, abstract reasoning	Involves integrity of several cognitive functions and exercising values and judgment in decision making and problem solving, logical thinking, future planning, comparison and evaluation of alternatives in context of reality and social responsibility, considering consequences of action. These functions are vulnerable to neurologic pathology; loss of abstraction ability may be first sign of disease or dementia.	Encourage person to remain active in situations or roles that require use of cognitive abilities, e.g., volunteer, mentor, teaching aide, organizational committees, political activities.

continued

TABLE 16-11

Cognitive Development in the Aging Person: Health Promotion Implications—continued

Characteristic	Change During Aging	Implication for Health Care
Creativity	Productivity continues into old age. Aesthetic sense and appreciation of beauty continue to develop.	Provide pleasing environment and opportunities for creativity. Teach family and elder that intellectual and creative mastery of the world exists in many forms and manifests itself daily.
General knowledge	Maintains or improves into old age, especially in vocabulary, verbal abilities, and verbal comprehension. General task-specific skills remain equal to those of young adult.	Encourage person to remain active in family and community; participation is a predictor of ability. Reinforce knowledge and wisdom and combat ageism. Teach health promotion, as physical health can affect mental function.
Academic performance	Elderly students in college perform as well as younger students, tend to have fewer problems, and are able to use new technology and equipment.	Encourage elder to participate in classes, continue learning in credit or noncredit courses or in elder hostel.
Spatial discrimination	High-level cortical function related to (1) visual and kinesthetic senses; (2) frontal lobe (motor skill) and parietal lobe (association) functions; (3) ability to produce accurate representations of the way in which objects or parts of objects relate to each other in space; (4) interpretation of directions and top/bottom and visual and spatial cues. Loss of impairment occurs independent of altered sensory function, language dysfunction, or position sense. Older adult tends to need more time and be less accurate in case of maps or finding directions.	Teach spatial cues. Recognize impact on rehabilitation. Test for constructional ability (copy geometric figure or draw face of clock) and general orientation to determine early brain dysfunction. Observe for unilateral neglect of body, inattention to objects or people in left half of sensory field. Assist with and teach family about self-care and safety implications.
Wisdom	Superior knowledge and judgment with extraordinary scope, depth, and balance applicable to specific situations and the general life condition. Increases because of empathy and understanding developed over the years. Depends on cognitive and personality factors as well as virtue (character).	Acknowledge the elder's wisdom, creative ability, and productivity. Encourage family to use elder as confidante and consultant.

BOX 16-7 Effective Memory Strategies

**SELECTIVE ENCODING
(GETTING INFORMATION INTO MEMORY)**

1. Actively and creatively try to find meaning in facts.
2. Underline selectively; outline.
3. Distinguish between important and nonimportant points and facts.
4. Summarize main points.
5. Reconstruct facts; test self.

ELABORATION

1. Use imagery, visualization of content.
2. Use metaphor.
3. Use analogy.
4. Paraphrase in own words.
5. Encode more than one strategy.

ORGANIZATION

1. Understand how information is organized.
2. Choose appropriate and effective retrieval cues.
3. Be aware that related items may cue memory.
4. Reorganize information so new material better relates to previous knowledge.

EXTERNAL REPRESENTATION

1. Take notes; outline.
2. Make charts, diagrams, tables, or graphs.
3. Make a conceptual map.

MONITORING

1. Test self.
2. Check where errors are made; correct errors.

decisions; assist in planning; erect social guideposts; and establish pacific relationships between oncoming generations. The judgmental functions of the mind are most highly developed after midlife (50, 51, 77, 80, 138).

The elder can be taught to remember essential information. **Box 16-7**, Effective Memory Strategies, presents suggestions for client education related to improved cognitive function (15, 45, 99, 126, 138, 156, 158, 167, 177). Teach the young-old, even the late middle-ager, these strategies so that a cognitive-behavioral pattern is developed.

Utilize computer-generated exercises or computer-assisted technology, if the elder is interested, to foster attention, concentration, recall, and learning. Prepare family, friends, and agency staff to assist the elder who is interested in trying new modalities.

Creativity

Creativity is evident in the later years (15, 32, 138, 156, 166):

1. People are not identical to others in creative output at any age. Expected age decrement in creativity varies across disciplines; in some there is scarcely a decline at all.
2. Creative output of the person in his or her 60s or 70s will most often exceed that produced in the 20s as long as the person is healthy.
3. Creative output changes in relation to role changes in career or profession rather than in relation to age.
4. The person with a late start in career or profession usually reaches a later peak and higher output in the last years.
5. Reduced creative output does not mean corresponding loss of intellectual or motivational capabilities.
6. Factors such as health and reduced vigor may interfere with creative output but can be overcome with individual motivation and assistance to the person.
7. Creativity can resurge in life's last years.

The Nun's Study (32, 166) of 678 Roman Catholic nuns over age 70 revealed the continuing cognitive development and creative energy of these females. **Practical creativity,** *solving everyday problems,* has always been evident in elders as they balance maintaining a quality of life with reduced resources and changing physical status. **Fresh connections,** *the sudden burst of imagination or skill or sudden insight,* foster creative ventures, such as in art, music, sculpture, or writing. Sometimes creativity is shown by methodical examination of different possibilities, and a new or different approach, product, or inspiration comes slowly. Many creative outlets need both brain hemispheres and the hippocampus, which specializes in information processing and recall (62, 67).

Various interventions discussed in this and other chapters can be used to foster and acknowledge creativity. Teach family and agency staff not to stifle creative ideas or endeavors, or label them in negative ways. Encourage family and staff to reinforce the elder's creativity as the person implements **activities of daily living** *(ADLs)* and implements **instrumental activities of daily living** *(IADLs). IADLs include* (a) how the elder manages financial affairs, (b) transportation and shopping, (c) meal preparation, (d) use of phone, (e) medication management, and (f) other tasks that require integration of various cognitive abilities.

Reminiscence and Life Review

Two forms of recall serve as therapeutic interventions: reminiscence and life review (15, 45, 49–51, 123, 138, 177). *Reminiscence and life review differ but share some characteristics:* (a) both use memory and recall for enjoyment or to cope with difficulties and look at accomplishments, (b) both can be structured or free-flowing, (c) both are integrative and can involve happy or sad feelings, (d) both serve a therapeutic function, and (e) both are implemented primarily with elders but can be used with middle-agers or young adults, especially in terminal illness.

INTERVENTIONS FOR HEALTH PROMOTION

*Use the following suggestions when you **teach** the elderly:*

1. Always approach the teaching situation in a way that enhances the person's self-concept and self-confidence. Encourage the elder's initiative and self-direction.
2. Accept that elders, like other adults, become ready to learn based on need to function effectively.
3. Keep in mind and assess the elder's experiences, current knowledge, needs, interests, questions, health status and pain, and developmental level as you plan and implement teaching.
4. Minimize distracting noise and distractions; select a comfortable setting.
5. Tell the person that you are planning a teaching session, state the general topic, and emphasize importance. Get the person's attention and increase anticipation.
6. Arrange for the person to be near the teacher, teaching aids, or demonstration.
7. Consider the aged person's difficulty with fine movement and failing vision when you are using visual aids.
8. Provide adequate lighting without glare; do not have the person face outdoor or indirect light.
9. Use sharp or bright colors with a natural background and large print to offset visual difficulties.
10. Explain procedures and directions with the person's possible hearing loss and slowed responses in mind.
11. Use a *low-pitched, clear speaking voice; face the person* so he or she can lip-read if necessary.
12. Teach *slowly* and patiently, with sessions not too long or widely spaced and with *repetition* and *reinforcement*.
13. Mentally "walk through" or imagine a task through verbal explanation before it is to be done to enhance recall. Give examples.
14. Material should be short, concise, and relevant; present material in a logical sequence; summarize often.
15. Break complex tasks or content into smaller and simpler units; focus on a single topic to promote concentration.
16. Match your vocabulary to the learner's ability and define terms clearly and as frequently as needed.
17. Give the aged person time to perceive and respond to stimuli, to learn, to move, and to act.
18. Avoid "yes" and "no" questions. Encourage questions, read the material being discussed, and determine literacy.
19. Help the person make associations between prior and new information and emphasize abilities that remain constant to enhance recall and application.
20. Have the person actively use several sensory modalities to make motions and repeat the content aloud verbally while seeing or hearing it.
21. Plan extra sessions for feedback and return demonstrations and extra time for these sessions.
22. Give emotional support. Express empathy. Often what is being taught to the elder is contrary to current understanding, past learning, personal attitudes, or values. Feelings of loss, related to insistence on accepting new ideas; anger, hostility, and resistance; or denial must be resolved for learning to occur.
23. Whenever possible, include a significant other in the teaching session to ensure further interpretation and support in using the information.

REMINISCENCE The process of **reminiscence** involves *informal sharing of bits and pieces of the past that surface to the consciousness and involves the feeling related to the memories. Thus, this memory process includes affective and cognitive functions.* It is an oral history (15, 45, 123, 177). Reminiscence includes processes, items, and outcomes. *Processes* include talking, listening, and touching to explore the client's historical perspective, education, ethnicity, and the like. The focus is on family, home, community, and life role. *Items* can be crafts, pictures, music, hobbies, and so on. Audio, video, or written records the client may have can be useful.

Goals for use of reminiscence and demonstrated outcomes include to:

1. Provide pleasure and comfort (but sad and angry feelings and memories also come forth).
2. Improve self-confidence, self-esteem, and mood.
3. Improve communication skills and cognitive function; stay oriented.
4. Increase socialization and decrease isolation.
5. Improve alertness and connectedness with others.
6. Increase deeper friendships; put relationships in order.
7. Promote role of confidante.
8. Promote ego integrity and satisfaction with life; find meaning in life cycle.
9. Provide strength to face new life challenges.
10. Facilitate grieving for losses.

Reminiscence may be done with individuals, with family and clients, or with a group of clients. You have a role with all of these.

LIFE REVIEW The process of **life review** *involves deliberately recalling memories about life events; it is the life history or story in a structured, sequential, autobiographical way. It is a guided or directed cognitive process, used with a goal in mind.* It may include reminiscence and affective functions (15, 22, 123, 138, 156).

INTERVENTIONS FOR HEALTH PROMOTION

*During **reminiscence therapy**, your role is to:*

1. Encourage informal, spontaneous discussion.
2. Be supportive and provide a positive atmosphere.
3. Avoid probing or pushing for insight.
4. Allow repetition in the person's discussion.
5. Encourage the person to integrate the happy and sad memories.

6. Allow the person to evaluate implications or prior outcomes as memories are recalled, if desired.
7. Validate and support the meaningful contributions and activities of past life.
8. Use themes or props, if desired, to stimulate discussion, especially in a group. Art and music are useful.
9. Avoid focusing on issues or judgment of memories.

Goals for use of life review include to:

1. Increase self-esteem.
2. Increase life satisfaction or well-being.
3. Increase sense of wisdom; validate wisdom.
4. Increase sense of peace about life.
5. Decrease depression.
6. Integrate painful memories, crises, unmet needs, and unfulfilled aspirations.
7. Promote ego integrity; resolve self-despair.
8. Work through prior crises, events, traumas, and relationships.

Reminiscence and life review, combined as necessary, allow for comprehension and appropriate response and compensate for decline in perception, memory, and slower formation of associations and concepts. Encourage family and friends to listen, engage the elder in oral history conversations, and validate the importance of the life experiences and contributions. Remind family to audio- or videotape conversations and to take pictures and notes for their memories and the genealogical history. Such action raises self-esteem and fosters a sense of continuing generativity and ego integrity in the elder. Further, the time spent together is mutually enjoyable.

Mild Cognitive Impairment

The term **mild cognitive impairment** *(MCI) refers to temporary memory problems or forgetfulness that occur in people the longer they live. These "senior moments"—repeated questions or forgetfulness for recent events or names—present, overall, little difficulty with managing daily affairs* (99, 104, 146). Even in younger persons, the brain processes information more slowly or inaccurately when the person is experiencing anxiety, stress responses, or depression. This phenomenon is magnified as aging progresses. Most elders, even centenarians, maintain cognitive ability. The Senior WISE (Wisdom Is Simply Exploration) study done by McDongal, Becker, and Arheart (115) provides a tool to obtain baseline data about cognitive, affective, and functional ability of elders. It also reports the likely incidence of mild cognitive impairment.

Three types or subgroups of MCI have been identified (104, 146, 195): (a) **single nonmemory domain,** *some impairment in an area that does not rely on memory,* such as an executive ego function or language; (b) **multiple domain,** *mild impairment in several cognitive domains or functions, with or without memory impairment,* which may indicate circulatory problems or eventual progression to vascular dementia; and (c) **amnestic form,** *increasingly severe cognitive impairment that may progress to various dementia illnesses,* such as frontotemporal dementia, dementia with Lewy bodies, or Alzheimer's dementia.

Criteria developed by the Mayo Clinic for MCI are (146):

1. Memory complaint by client is corroborated by an informant.
2. Objective memory impairment is typical for age; person remembers essential information, even if at "last minute."

INTERVENTIONS FOR HEALTH PROMOTION

*During **life review therapy**, your role is to:*

1. Accept the story and accompanying photographs or memorabilia but encourage a life span approach.
2. Convey empathy for experiences and feelings (happy and sad).
3. Validate and support values being expressed.
4. Allow repetition to promote necessary catharsis.
5. Discuss issues that arise so they can be resolved.
6. Reframe events if the person cannot do so.

7. Encourage the person to evaluate prior responses, achievements, or ways of handling a situation.
8. Allow the focus to remain on the person's own self.
9. Validate that which has been meaningful in life to the person.
10. Recognize that the person may not ever really resolve or accept the multiple losses that have occurred (sadness may remain).

3. Largely preserved general cognition is demonstrated.

4. Essentially normal activities of daily living are carried out.

5. No dementia signs or symptoms are demonstrated.

These criteria are present in all ethnic or racial groups.

About 11% to 12% of elders with MCI will develop Alzheimer's dementia if they live long enough. Cognitive decline to dementia is hastened when the elder is admitted to the hospital, by various infections and illnesses, by intense life stressors (intensity is defined by the person's perception), or by transfer from hospital or home to a long-term care facility, especially when there is no choice (10, 146, 195).

Educate the elder and family members on strategies to compensate for age-related forgetfulness (45, 99, 155, 177, 195):

1. Pay closer attention when new information or a new person is being introduced. Repeat aloud the information or name, or write it down. (Keep a small notepad and pen with you.)

2. Avoid conversation, important tasks, or reading with a lot of background noise or distractions, such as loud TV or radio.

3. Do not take on too many mental tasks all at once by yourself. Take breaks in the routine.

4. Eat nutritional meals; get enough sleep and exercise regularly.

5. Engage regularly (daily) in mental games, exercises, and puzzles, ideally with someone who can monitor realistically the ability level.

6. Say "no" to invitations that will add excessively to stress response, even if they are well intentioned or sound interesting initially. High levels of stress and cortisol production damage neurons in the hippocampus and affect memory (67).

7. Interact with other people. Avoid isolating self and excess television.

8. Buy a dated pill organizer to help you remember which medications to take daily.

9. Buy a digital watch with a built-in timer to help remember meetings, events, or errands.

10. Use a calendar (in purse, in plain view in the home, or on the computer) to prompt about future appointments.

11. Avoid polypharmacy. Discuss your medications and treatment plan with your doctor.

12. Limit alcohol, which destroys neurons, and caffeine, which adds to restlessness and confusion.

13. Reduce or stop smoking, which is detrimental to vascular health.

14. Obtain medical care for chronic physical or mental problems.

Listen to the feelings, concerns, and fears expressed by family members. Explore support systems, such as other relatives or friends, the parish nurse and church family, and local agencies that can provide various kinds of assistance. Suggest utilization of the local Alzheimer's Disease Association, which generally provides information on cognitive impairments, caregiver suggestions, and referral to other helpful agencies.

EMOTIONAL DEVELOPMENT

The older person experiences emotions at least as intensely as young adults (50). Emotions, mediated by the nervous system, directly and indirectly influence the immune system. Older adults show greater immunologic impairment associated with depression or negative feelings (67, 85). The physiologic response to emotional stress (for example, increased blood pressure) takes longer to return to baseline in older than younger adults. There is less variability in emotional responses within a day, probably an adaptive response. Further, because the older person's expectations about the ability to control events change with age, the person is less likely to evidence negative affect than would be expected. Emotional responses become less unidimensional with age; for example, love may be less euphoric and become more bittersweet the second or third time around. Positive emotions acquire negative loading over time, and vice versa. Identical events may elicit different emotions over time, and events that elicited emotional response earlier may no longer do so. Multiple roles in old age are linked to greater psychological well-being and flexibility in emotional responses overall (32, 50, 51, 93, 138).

Developmental Crisis: Ego Integrity Versus Self-Despair or Self-Disgust

Erikson (48, 49), describing the eight stages of man, stated the **developmental or psychosexual task of the mature elder person** *is ego integrity versus self-despair or disgust.* A complex set of factors combines to make the attainment of this task difficult for the elderly person.

Ego integrity is the *coming together of all previous phases of the life cycle* (49). *The person accepts life as his or her own and as the only life for the self. He or she would wish for none other and would defend the meaning and the dignity of the lifestyle. Integrity demands tact, patience, contact, and touch—directly and through interaction (these can be difficult in the 80s, 90s, and 100s)* (51). *At the end of life, there is transcendence, a giving to others. The person is what he or she has given* (50, 51). *In order to do that, the person goes beyond the imposed limits and seeks fulfillment* (51). Integrity allows feedback on a long life that can be lived in retrospect, reminiscence, and life review with willpower, a ninth stage of development that is preparatory for death (51). The *person has further refined the characteristics of maturity described for the middle-aged adult, achieving both wisdom and an enriched perspective about life and people.* **Wisdom** *involves not just knowledge, but the capacity to see what is not so evident, to look intently, to listen to the underlying message, and to remember the essence of what is being said* (51). **Box 16-8**, Wisdom: Expert Knowledge (13, 49–54) gives a summary of areas of

---

BOX 16-8	**Wisdom: Expert Knowledge**

1. Knowledge that is both factual and strategic in the fundamental aspects of life

2. Knowledge that considers the context of life and social changes

3. Knowledge that considers relativism of values and life goals

4. Knowledge that considers uncertainties of life

5. Knowledge that reflects good judgment in important but uncertain matters of life

knowledge. Even if earlier development tasks have not been completed, the aged person may overcome these handicaps by associating with younger persons and helping others resolve their own conflicts. Historical situation, family environment, marital status, and individual development all influence the integrity achievement (51).

Use the consultative role to enhance ego integrity. Ask the person's counsel about various situations that relate to him or her personally or to ideas about politics, religion, or activities current in the residence or institution. Although you will not burden the person with your personal problems, the senior will be happy to be consulted about various affairs, even if his or her advice is not always taken. Having the person reminisce and engage in life review also promotes ego integrity. Reintegration and recasting of life events put traumatic events into perspective.

The person who has achieved ego integrity remains creative. Even an octogenarian can expect to produce many notable contributions to any creative activity, as has been witnessed with artists, composers, and statesmen. Creativity in the late years depends on initial creative potential, but creativity may lie dormant during the demanding young adult years. The older adult has many of the necessary qualities for creativity: time, accumulated experience, knowledge, skills, a broader or deeper perspective, and wisdom. Often the changes mandated by retirement and late life trigger new creative levels, including those in ordinary people.

Without a sense of ego integrity, the person feels a sense of **self-despair and self-disgust**. *Life has been too short and futile. The person wants another chance to redo life. Despair reflects the dystonic or dysfunctional aspects of life, regrets about what was done or not done or opportunities missed* (49, 51). *Loss of capacities and disintegration may demand almost all of the person's attention as life space narrows to the small room in an institution or offspring's home, and to concerns about getting daily needs met. Despair in the current life events can be compounded by earlier negative self- or other evaluations* (22, 51). *Many losses and distant relationships add to the sense of despair and hopelessness* (51). If the person has had a sense of trust and fulfilled the other development psychological crisis, the sense of despair can be resolved. Hope, grace, and enlightenment can be felt and extended to others (49–51). Refer to **Box 16-9**, Consequences of Self-Despair or Self-Disgust, for a list of feelings and behaviors that are part of self-despair (49–51). Having no confidant or companion and declining physical health status are both related to the emotional status (48, 49). Suicidal thoughts or attempts may result; this is a growing problem (10). Jung (79, 80) believed the old person could not face death in a healthy manner without some image of the hereafter. He believed the unconscious has an archetype of eternity that wells up from within the person as death nears.

Care for the person in despair involves use of therapeutic communication and counseling principles (presented in Chapter 2), ∞ use of touch and relaxation techniques, and being a confidante so that the person can work through feelings from the past and present ones of sadness and loneliness. The maintenance phase of the nurse-client relationship is important, as the person needs time to resolve old conflicts and learn new patterns of thinking and relating. *The person can move to a sense of ego integrity with the ongoing relating of at least one caring person who* (a) listens; (b) meets physical needs when the person cannot; (c) nurtures and encourages emotionally; (d) brings in spiritual insights; (e) validates the senior's realistic concerns, fears, or points of anguish; and (f) listens to the review of life, patching together life's experiences.

Personality Development

No specific personality changes occur as a result of aging. Values, life orientation, and personality traits remain consistent from at least middle age onward. The older person becomes more of what he or she was. The older person continues to develop emotionally and in personality and adds on characteristics instead of making drastic changes (15, 25, 28, 45, 127, 157). **If he or she was physically active and flexible in personality and participated in social activities in the young years, these characteristics will continue appropriate to physical status and life situation.** If the person was hard to live with when younger, he or she will be harder to live with in old age (**Continuity Theory**). The garrulous, taciturn person becomes more so, and problems of control and dominance are common. Stereotypes describe the older person as rigid, conservative, opinionated, self-centered, and disagreeable. Such characteristics are not likely to be new; rather they are an exaggeration of lifelong traits that cannot be expressed or sublimated in another way (28, 32, 49).

Several characteristics at age 50 are linked to health and happiness at age 75 or 80 (156): (a) history of effective coping skills, (b) not overweight, (c) some exercise, (d) stable marriage, (e) no heavy smoking, and (f) no alcohol abuse. Certain positive persistent trait

BOX 16-9	**Consequences of Self-Despair or Self-Disgust**

1. Discusses unresolved conflicts related to people or life situations
2. Wishes to relive life, redo life course; fears death
3. Is suspicious or hypercritical of others; angry toward others, especially significant others
4. Has a sense of overwhelming guilt, shame, self-doubt, self-disgust, inadequacy
5. Disengages from others; withdraws from people or life's interests

6. Feels worthless, a burden
7. Demonstrates decreasing cognitive competence
8. Discusses lack of accomplishments in life or unfinished endeavors
9. Is lonely, has had few relationships
10. Describes desire for relationships, a confidant, companion
11. Feels hopeless, helpless, sad, depressed
12. Has suicidal thoughts or behavior

patterns contribute in adaptation to aging and may predict health and longevity.

In a longitudinal study that followed four generations for 23 years, self-reported emotions such as restlessness, boredom, unhappiness, and depression decreased with age. Positive emotions, excitement, interest, pride, and a sense of accomplishment tended to remain stable until late life, and then declined only slightly (25). People with neurotic personalities (moody, touchy, anxious) were more likely to report negative emotions, and they tended to become even less positive (25).

The mature elder continues to use multiple intelligences of the past (and may add to the continuum or lose one of the prior skills) (59). Emotional intelligence continues, and even becomes more astute, in the young-old and old-old (63).

Personality Types

Studies of large samples of seniors reaffirm their uniqueness, but researchers have categorized the variety of their behaviors. Most seniors are resourceful and psychologically well.

Four personality types were described by Neugarten (127): integrated, defended, passive dependent, and disintegrated. They are still evident.

The **integrated personality type** is *characteristic of most elderly people who function well and have a complex inner life, intact cognitive abilities, and competent ego. They are flexible, open to new stimuli, and mellow. They adjust to losses and are realistic about the past and present. They have a high sense of life satisfaction.* The integrated group is made up of three subtypes: reorganizers, focused, and disengaged. The **reorganizers** *engage in a wide variety of activities; when they lose old roles and related activities, they substitute new ones. They are as active after retirement as before.* The **focused** are *selective in their activities; they devote energy to a few roles that are important to them rather than being involved in many organizations.* The **disengaged** are *well-integrated persons who have voluntarily moved away from role commitments. Activity level is low. They are self-directed, are interested in the world, and have chosen the rocking-chair approach to life.* Thus, Neugarten defines the disengaged person differently from Cumming and Henry (127).

The **defended personality** is *seen in ambitious, achievement-oriented persons who have always driven themselves hard and who continue to do so. They have a number of defenses against anxiety and a tight control over impulses.* They have a philosophy of, "I'll work until I drop." Some are **constricted**, *preoccupied with their losses and deficits. They have always shut out new experiences and social interactions* (127).

The **passive-dependent personality type** is *divided into two patterns: succorance-seeking and apathetic.* The **succorance-seeking** *have strong dependency needs and seek help and support from others.* The **apathetic** *have an extremely passive personality. They engage in few activities and little social interaction* (127).

The **disintegrated** or **disorganized personality type** *describes a small percentage of elderly who show gross defects in psychological functions and deterioration in thought processes.* They may manage to live in the community because of the forbearance or protection of others around them (127).

The integrated personality type has high life satisfaction. The defended personality type is satisfied with life. These elders follow their normal pattern, although at some point physical, mental, or economic decline may create great stress and crises and adjustment difficulties. They are challenging to caregivers. The passive-dependent personality has medium to low life satisfaction, depending on how caregivers can meet their needs. The disintegrated or disorganized personality is likely to be admitted to a long-term care institution if family resources permit or Medicare benefits can be instituted. Otherwise the family has an increasing sense of burden and will need respite.

Young-Old Personality

The **young-old personality** (ages 65 or 70 to 75, 80, or 85) *is frequently flexible, shows characteristics commonly defined as mature, and is less vulnerable to the harsh reality of aging.* The *person manifests self-respect without conceit; tolerates personal weakness while using strengths to the fullest; and regulates, diverts, or sublimates basic drives and impulses instead of trying to suppress them.* He or she is guided by principles but is not a slave to dogma; maintains a steady purpose without pursuing the impossible goal; respects others, even when not agreeing with their behavior; and directs energies and creativity to master the environment and overcome the vicissitudes of life (49, 50).

Motivations change; the senior wants different things from life than he or she did earlier. Concerns about appearance, standards of living, and family change. Stronger incentives, support, and encouragement are needed to do what used to be eagerly anticipated. He or she avoids risks or new challenges and is increasingly introspective and introverted (80, 83, 128).

The elderly are tough; they often endure against great physical and social odds. Experience has taught the senior to be somewhat suspicious as he or she is likely to be a victim of "borrowings," a fast-sell job for something he or she does not need, thievery, or physical attacks.

Yet generosity is a common trait. The person gives of self fully and shares willingly with people who are loved and who seem genuinely interested in him or her.

The young-old person tries to remain independent and useful as long as possible, to find contentment, and to die without being a burden to others. Increasingly, dependency may undermine self-esteem, especially if the person values independence.

Personality characteristics differ for males and females, especially in relation to assertiveness. The male becomes more dependent, passive, and submissive and more tolerant of his emerging nurturant and affiliative impulses. The female becomes more dominant and assertive and less guilty about aggressive and egocentric impulses. Perhaps the reversal in overt behavior is caused by hormonal changes. Perhaps the male can be more open to his long-unfulfilled emotional needs when he is no longer in the role of chief provider and no longer has to compete in the work world. Perhaps the female reciprocates in an effort to gratify needs for achievement and worth; she expresses more completely the previously hidden conflicts, abilities, or characteristics (128, 130, 131). This personality expression may be dependent on past lifestyle and culture.

Old-Old Personality

The **old-old person** (*age 80 or 85 years and beyond) prefers time for meditation and contemplation, not camaraderie* (45, 138). Camaraderie is for young people who have energy and similarities in background, development, and interest. *Old-old people may be friendly and pleasant, but they are also egocentric. Egocentricity is a physiologic necessity, a protective mechanism for survival, not selfishness. Life space shrinks.* When old-old people get together, certain factors block camaraderie, even if they want to be sociable: varying stages of deafness and blindness, other faulty sense perceptions, and the fact that they may have little in common other than age and past historical era. Old-old people are even more unique in the life pattern than young-old people because they have lived longer. Further, they have less energy to deal with challenging situations, and relating to a group of oldsters can be challenging (45). There is increased interiority in the personality (129).

The person in later maturity, especially in old-old age, may be called childish. Rather, *the person is childlike;* he or she pays attention to quality in others. He or she senses when another is not genuine or honest—as a person or in activities. The old-old person reacts with sometimes exasperating conduct because he or she sees clearly through the facade and lacks the emotional energy to be as polite as earlier. Self-control, willpower, and intellectual response are less effective in advanced age. Many of the negative emotional characteristics ascribed to the elderly may be based on this phenomenon. The use of emotional intelligence described in Chapter 15 is much more common (63). ∞

The old-old have greater need than ever to hold onto others. They are often perceived as clingy, sticky, demanding, loquacious, and repetitious. This often causes the younger person to want to avoid or be rid of the senior, which causes a vicious circle of increased demand and increased rejection.

Preoccupation with the body is a frequent topic of conversation, and other elderly people respond in kind. The behavior is analogous to the collective monologue and parallel play of young children. The talk about the body satisfies narcissistic needs, and it is an attempt magically to relieve anxiety about what is happening. This pattern alienates the young and the young-old, and they tend to avoid or stop conversing with the aged, just when the elder most needs a listener and feedback.

Old-old persons intensely appreciate the richness of the moment, the joys or the sorrows. They realize the transience of life, and they are more likely to start each day with a feeling of expectancy, not neutrality or boredom. Their future is today. As a result, they become more tolerant of others' foibles, more thrilled over minor events, and more aware of their own needs, even if they cannot meet them.

Irritating behavior of the old-old person is frequently related to the frustration of being dependent on others or helpless and the fear that accompanies dependency and helplessness. The tangible issue at hand—coffee too hot or too cold; visitors too early, too late, or not at all; or the fast pace of others—is often not really what is irritating, although the person attaches complaints to something that others can identify. The irritability is with the self, loss of control, lost powers, and present state of being that cannot be changed.

Perhaps the most frequent error in assessing the elderly is the diagnosis of senility or dementia. Conditions labeled as such may actually be the result of physiologic imbalances, depression, inadequacy feelings, or unmet affectional and dependency needs. Psychological problems in the elderly are often manifested in dis-

orientation, poor judgment, perceptual motor inaccuracy, intellectual dysfunction, and incontinence. These problems are frequently not chronic and may respond well to supportive therapy.

Carry out principles of care previously described to meet emotional and personality needs of the elderly. Encourage the uniqueness of the individual. Explain to others that the earlier personality traits are maintained. Help the family and agency staff understand and respond positively to the personality expressed by the elder and to the differences demonstrated by the young-old, the old-old, and increasingly, the centenarian.

ADAPTIVE MECHANISMS

Nursing and all health care professionals need a strong commitment to assist the elderly in maintaining adaptive mechanisms appropriate to this period of life, although each person will accomplish them in his or her unique way, pertinent to life experiences and cultural background. Persons in their older years are capable of changes in behavior but find changing difficult. As new crises develop from social, economic, or family restructuring, new types of ego defenses may be needed.

Developmental Tasks Related to Adaptation

Adaptive mechanisms help the person maintain a sense of self-worth and control over external forces, which in turn promotes a higher level of function.

Peck (142) lists three developmental tasks related to adaptation:

1. **Ego differentiation versus work-role preoccupation** *is involved in the adaptation to retirement, and its success depends on the ability to see self as worthwhile not just because of a job but because of the basic person he or she is.*
2. **Body transcendence versus body preoccupation** *requires that happiness and comfort as concepts be redefined to overcome the changes in body structure and function* and, consequently, in body image and the decline of physical strength.
3. **Ego transcendence versus ego preoccupation** *is the task of accepting inevitable death.* Mechanisms for adapting to the task of facing death are those that protect against loss of inner contentment and help to develop a constructive impact on surrounding persons.

Regression for Adaptation

Certain adaptive or defensive mechanisms are used frequently by the aged. **Regression,** *returning to earlier behavior patterns,* should not be considered negative unless it is massive and the person is capable of self-care. A certain amount of regression is mandatory to survival as the person adapts to decreasing strength, changing body functions and roles, and often increasing frustration. Regression is an adaptive mechanism used by the older adult who is dying, and it is manifested differently than in younger years. The regression is a complex of behaviors not associated solely with a return to former levels of adaptation.

To integrate into self-concept and handle the anxiety created by a complex of losses, changes, and adaptation related to aging and dying, the older person may behave in a way that is confused with dementia or drug reactions. Careful assessment is needed; use a history of the person's normal patterns and history of illness to avoid misdiagnoses.

Other Adaptive Mechanisms

Other commonly used adaptive mechanisms are described in **Table 16-12**. McCrae found in a study that controlled for types of stress that older persons did not consistently differ from younger ones in using 26 of 28 coping mechanisms, including rational action, expression of feelings, and seeking help. Middle-aged and older persons were less likely than younger ones to use immature and ineffective mechanisms of hostile responses and escapist fantasy. Health threats in all ages elicit wishful thinking, faith, and fatalism. Using insight (intellectual understanding) and reminiscence are also adaptive. Resilience is also a part of adaptation (28).

Characteristics of the successfully adjusted older person include (142):

1. **Equanimity:** *balanced perspective of one's life and experiences.*
2. **Perseverance:** *persistence despite adversity or discouragement.*
3. **Self-reliance:** *belief in oneself and one's abilities.*
4. **Meaningfulness:** *realization that life has purpose and the value of one's contribution.*
5. **Existential aloneness:** *realization that each person's path is unique and some experiences must be faced alone.*

The following are *components of an adaptive old age* (45, 49): (a) stable mental status; (b) absence of organic brain damage or disease; (c) high life satisfaction, vitality, interest in and enjoyment of life; (d) active, to extent possible, rather than passive-dependent behavior; (e) adequate income to maintain satisfactory lifestyle, relatively good health; (f) psychosocial stimulation, maintenance of meaningful goals; (g) available family; and (h) acceptance of death and a sense of legacy.

Box 16-10, Characteristics of Successful Aging, summarizes a holistic perspective about successful aging (15, 45, 138, 156). Utilize this information in assessment and health promotion interventions.

TABLE 16-12

Adaptive Mechanisms Used by the Older Adult

Mechanism	Description
Emotional Isolation	*By repressing the emotion associated with a situation or idea while intellectually describing it*, the person can cope with very threatening situations and ideas such as personal and another's disease, aging, and death and can begin to resolve the associated fears. Thus, aged persons can appear relatively calm in the face of crisis.
Compartmentalization	*Narrowing of awareness and focusing on one thing at a time* so that the aged seem rigid, repetitive, and resistive.
Denial	*Blocking a thought or the inability to accept the situation* is used selectively when the person is under great stress and aids in maintaining a higher level of personality integration.
Rationalization	*Giving a logical sounding excuse for a situation* is often used to minimize weakness, symptoms, and various difficulties or to build self-esteem.
Somatization	*Complaints about physical symptoms and preoccupation with the body* may become an outlet for free-floating anxiety. The person can cope with vague insecurities and rapid life changes by having a tangible physical problem to deal with, especially because others seem more interested and concerned about disease symptoms than feelings about self.
Counterphobia	*Excessive behavior in an area of life to counter or negate fears about that area of life* is observed in the person who persists at activities such as calisthenics or youthful grooming or fashion to retain a youthful appearance.
Rigidity	*Resisting change or not being involved in decision making* is a common defense to help the person feel in control of self and life. A stubborn self-assertiveness is compensatory behavior for the person who has been insecure, rigid, and irritable.
Sublimation	*Channeling aggressive impulses into sociably acceptable activity* can be an effective defense to meet old age as a challenge and maintain vigor and creativity. Often the elderly desire to live vicariously through the younger generation, and they become involved with the young through mutual activities and listening or observing their activities.
Displacement	*Expressing frustration or anger onto another person or object that is not the source of the feelings* provides a safe release and disguises the real source of anxiety. The elder may blame another for his or her deficiencies, bang furniture, throw objects, or unjustly criticize family or health care workers.
Projection	*Attributing personal feelings or characteristics, usually negative, to another* allays anxiety, releases unpleasant feelings, or elevates self-esteem and self-concept. Projection is done unconsciously, usually to those closest to the person; a milieu free of counteraggression helps the person feel secure.

BOX 16-10 Characteristics of Successful Aging

HIGH DEGREE OF LIFE SATISFACTION

1. Feels life has been rewarding; has met goals
2. Has few regrets
3. Has positive attitude about past and future
4. Feels life is stimulating, interesting; sets new goals
5. Is able to relax; has good health habits

HARMONIOUS INTEGRATION OF PERSONALITY

1. Has developed ego strength, unity, and maturity over the years
2. Demonstrates self-actualization, satisfaction, individuation, authenticity
3. Makes use of potentials and capabilities throughout life
4. Has an accurate self-concept and body image
5. Has meaningful value system, and spiritual fulfillment

MAINTENANCE OF MEANINGFUL SOCIAL SYSTEM

1. Keeps involved with caring network of family and friends
2. Maintains interest in life through social attachments
3. Feels affection for and from others and sense of belonging

PERSONAL CONTROL OVER LIFE

1. Feels independent and autonomous
2. Makes own decisions, in charge of self to extent possible
3. Maintains sense of dignity, self-worth, positive self-concept

ESTABLISHMENT OF FINANCIAL SECURITY

1. Has made careful and effective financial plans
2. Uses community resources to extent necessary

Your approach during care can either increase or decrease motivation to maintain cognitive and emotional health and adaptive behaviors and, if ill, to participate in treatment or rehabilitation. Acute illness at any age influences aging behavior, affective responses, and cognitive function. These aspects of the person are also affected by chronic illness and pain. Careful assessment is essential. *Helpful approaches toward successful aging and health promotion include* (90, 141):

1. Set a definite goal with the client to embrace the aging process.
2. Reinforce and support the basic drives or character/personality structure of the client. Do not label the preoccupation with achievement or the persistence in practice as obsession or compulsion. Realize that the former "toughness" or "survival traits" of the person are now an asset, not to be diminished by your traditional approach.
3. Convey caring, be kind, and share "power" or control with the client rather than trying to be the boss. In turn, the client will feel, and be, more "cooperative."
4. Encourage or reinforce with attention the person's behavioral attempts as well as achievements.
5. Use humor gently and appropriately to release tension or encourage. Do not use sarcastic humor.
6. Convey a positive attitude that the person can achieve the goal, at least to the extent possible. Avoid negative comments, an attitude that "puts down" the client, or nonverbal behavior that conveys you do not perceive capability.
7. Avoid a power struggle, insistence on the client doing an activity your way, or domination of the client. Let the person go at his or her own pace and in a way that is safe but will still achieve results.

Hoarding: Personal Environmental Adaptation

Hoarding *may be an adaptive behavior, although it is usually regarded as a disagreeable, messy, and unsafe characteristic of the elderly* or a sign of illness or dementia. (It may be maladaptive behavior signaling illness at any age.)

The elderly may hoard and collect various or specific items for various reasons (8, 96, 191):

1. It may be a lifelong habit. In the younger years the person was considered a "pack rat," or someone who always had what was needed in an emergency, or "someone who had everything handy." The behavior, if part of the person's self-concept and previously rewarded, is likely to continue to be valued and practiced.
2. It may be the mark of a creative, intelligent person, an artist, or a former teacher who keeps supplies that can be used in the vocation or hobby.
3. The articles that are saved, potentially useful or likely to be used, represent security, especially if the person (a) lived through the Great Depression and World War II and remembers severe scarcity or poverty, and will not waste; (b) was an immigrant or displaced person from another country; or (c) buys food or supplies in large quantities to save money, even if not used.
4. The articles may be symbolic of a happier past or represent a future.
5. The gathered objects may represent a sense of control.
6. The articles may compensate for loneliness and recent losses or be a way to keep in touch with family or friends now dead or relocated.
7. The collecting, observing, handling, and sorting of objects may be a pleasant diversion, especially for the old who are less socially active.
8. The person may have difficulty categorizing objects or differentiating important from worthless items.
9. Articles may be kept close at hand rather than stored in cabinets or closets to save energy in retrieving them when needed.
10. When cognitive impairment occurs, the person may be unable to discriminate between needed and unneeded objects

TABLE 16-13

Interventions for Hoarding Behavior

1. Discuss the situation with the person. Let the person show you collections and tell the stories; learn the meaning of behavior.
2. Offer to assist with cleanup, filing, or discarding if the person wishes and lacks energy or motivation. Never throw away objects without consent of the person unless dementia is present.
3. Set limits firmly if the hoarding is hazardous; e.g., help the person clean out the refrigerator with spoiled or unedible food, straighten up a room, and make a clear walkway to avoid falls.
4. Do not argue or nag about insignificant articles or out-of-the-way collections.
5. Discuss the need to discard some of the accumulation but tell the person he or she can decide what to discard, store, give to family or friends, and keep.
6. Reward behaviors that reduce hoarding.
7. Arrange for the person to engage in outside activities, groups, and relationships. Keep the person busy with interesting activities.
8. Evaluate the person's need for possible relocation to the home of a family member or to an assisted living retirement center for close supervision and assistance.
9. Refer the person, after consultation with family, guardian, or health care team, to a treatment facility if the behavior is indicative of depression, obsessive-compulsive disorder, paranoia, or dementia.
10. Assist family and friends, if necessary, in determining whether a legal guardian should be appointed.

and thereby keep everything. This difference between benign hoarding and obsessive-compulsive disorder must be determined (8, 10, 96, 191).

Table 16-13 lists interventions that can be used by you, family, or friends if hoarding poses a problem. Educate other health care workers and significant others about strategies for effective intervention.

BODY IMAGE DEVELOPMENT

Physical changes discussed earlier have both private and public components and combine to change the appearance and function of the older individual and thereby influence the self-image. As the person ages, loss of muscle strength and tone is reflected in a decline in the ability to perform tasks requiring strength. The old-old or frail person sees self as weakened and less worthwhile as a producer of work either in actual tasks for survival or in the use of energy for recreational activities.

The loss of skin tone, although not serious in itself, causes the aged in a society devoted to youth and beauty to feel stigmatized. Changing body contours, sagging breasts, bulging abdomen, and the dowager's hump caused by osteoporosis all produce a negative effect. This stigma can also affect the sexual response of the older person because of perceived rejection by a partner.

Loss of sensory acuity causes alienation from the environment. Although eyeglasses and better illumination are of great help in fading vision, the elderly recognize their inability to read fine print and to do handwork requiring good vision for small objects. The danger of injury caused by failure to see obstacles in their paths because of cataracts, glaucoma, or macular degeneration makes the elderly even more insecure about the relationship of body to the environment. Medical help may be sought too late because they do not understand the implications of the diagnosis or the chances for successful correction.

Hearing loss is likely to cause even more negative personality changes in the older person than loss of sight. Behavior such as sus-

piciousness, irritability, impatience, and paranoid tendencies may develop simply because hearing is impaired. Again the person may fear to admit the problem or to seek treatment, through either hearing aids or corrective surgery. Often the elderly view the hearing aid as another threat to body image. Eyeglasses are worn by all age groups and hence are more socially acceptable. A hearing aid is conceived as overt evidence of advanced age. Adjustment to the hearing aid may be difficult for many people, and if motivation is also low, the idea may be rejected.

Hearing needs may not be met as easily as correction of visual problems. Astute observation can change the situation. Consider the elderly woman who returned to her home after colostomy surgery. Although she had been pleasant and cooperative in the hospital, always nodding "yes," she had failed to learn her colostomy irrigation routine. The visiting nurse learned, through being in the home and getting information from the family, that the client was nearly deaf. The client covered her loss by nodding pleasantly. Slow, distinct instructions allowed her to grasp the irrigation techniques, and within several days she was managing well. The nurse also had an opportunity to refer the woman for auditory assessment.

Help the elder keep an intact, positive body image. Encourage talking about feelings related to the changing body appearance, structure, and function. Provide a mirror so that he or she can look at self to integrate the overt changes into his or her mental image. Photographs can also be useful in reintegrating a changing appearance. Help the elder to stay well-groomed and attractively dressed, and compliment efforts in that direction. Touch and tactile sensations are important measures to help the person continue to define body boundaries and integrate structural changes.

MORAL-SPIRITUAL DEVELOPMENT
Moral Development

Moral development, according to Kohlberg, is likely to be in the Postconventional stage by the late 60s or early 70s (91). Perhaps for the first time, the person can stand firm for decisions and actions that embrace ethical and moral principles. Now there is really nothing to lose—certainly job loss is unlikely and family and friends have learned to "go along with the elder to keep peace." Social justice issues, relationships, and generativity to all people are issues to be confronted that middle-agers, even if they agree in spirit, may not have the courage, time, autonomy, or resources to advocate (91).

Kohlberg, shortly before his death in 1987, proposed a seventh stage of moral reasoning (92) that has much in common with the self-transcendence that is discussed by Peck (142), Erikson (48–51), and Eastern religious traditions (91). Now the person questions: "Why be moral?" The answer lies in achieving a deeper, broader, cosmic perspective of the universe and of God, to analyze the whole, to holistically see how all organisms and all of the environment affect each other. Everything is connected. Harm to one unit is harmful to all and rebounds on the doer (92). This view parallels most mature levels of faith, theologically. Most people do not reach this perspective, but elders, as they face their mortality, ponder these concepts.

Spiritual Development

In many societies, the elderly are the spiritual leaders in the community and house of worship (156). Elder African Americans, Asians, Latinos, and Caucasians rate religious faith as significant (15). Most attempt to attend church services, and read religious material, pray, or meditate frequently. Listening to religious programs is a way to express spirituality and religious beliefs. Elder females are more likely than elder males to participate actively in church (156).

Various *factors influence how active the elder will be in church attendance:* (a) physical health problems, (b) transportation, (c) disability accessibility to the building, (d) acoustics in the building, and whether hearing aids are available at the seats if needed, (e) type of music or service schedule, (f) friendliness and helpfulness of other members of the faith community, and (g) activities for volunteerism, leisure, and socialization.

Self-transcendence is related to lower loneliness scores and to mental and spiritual health (149). A strong religious commitment is related to high self-esteem, a sense of well-being, and high life satisfaction in old age (80, 83, 149, 156). Prayer and meditation have been associated with health and longevity (156) perhaps because religious beliefs may reduce behavior that reduces longevity, such as excess smoking, alcohol use, or social isolation (156). Because the elderly person is a good listener, he or she is usually liked and respected by all ages. Although not adopting inappropriate aspects of a younger lifestyle, he or she can contemplate the fresh religious and philosophic views of adolescent thinking, thus trying to understand ideas previously missed or interpreted differently. Such understanding can help to resolve parental-adolescent conflicts about religion. The elderly person feels a sense of worth while giving experienced views. He or she is concerned about moral dilemmas and conflict and offers suggestions on ways to handle them. Basically he or she is satisfied with living personal beliefs, which can serve as a great comfort when temporarily despondent over life changes or changes in the family's life, or when confronting the idea of personal death. The elder is more likely than youth to say that religious belief and practices have a significant influence on health (15, 138).

Spiritual beliefs enable the older person to cope with painful or unexpected events and to be more productive and adaptive in a threatening environment. The spirit can be considered the primary locus of healing, since it is the basic characteristic of humanness. Spiritual health is necessary for physical, emotional, and mental well-being, satisfaction with life, happiness, and a sense of energy. Studies of centenarians reveal the perceived importance of spiritual beliefs and practices to their longevity (32, 40, 102, 103, 133, 139, 144).

Elderly persons who have not matured religiously or philosophically may sense a spiritual impoverishment and despair as the drive for professional and economic success wanes. An immature outlook provides no solace, and, if church members, they may become bitter. They may believe that the church organization to which they gave long and dedicated service has forgotten them as they have less stamina for organizational work. They may feel cast aside in favor of the young who have so many activities planned for them. These persons need help to arrive at an adequate spiritual philosophy and to find some appropriate religious or altruistic activities that will help them gain feelings of acceptance, self-esteem, and worth.

Care of the client's spiritual needs is an essential part of holistic care. This includes talking with the elderly, listening to statements that indicate religious beliefs or spiritual needs, and reading scriptures or praying with the person when indicated or requested. Giving spiritual care to the elderly person may involve providing prompt physical care to prevent angry outbursts and accepting apologies as the person seeks forgiveness for a fiery temper or sharp tongue when feeling neglected. Providing religious music or joining with the person in a religious song may calm inner storms. Acknowledging realistic losses and feeling with those who weep can provide a positive focus and hope. Helping the aged person remain an active participant in church, religious programs, or Bible study in the nursing home can maintain his or her self-esteem and sense of usefulness. Finally, in dying and near death, the religious person may want to practice beloved rituals and say, or have quoted, familiar religious or scriptural verses.

DEVELOPMENTAL TASKS

The following *developmental tasks are to be achieved by the aging couple as a family and by the aging person living alone* (43, 49):

1. Recognize the aging process, define instrumental limitations, and adjust to societal views of aging.
2. Adjust to decreasing physical strength and health changes.
3. Decide where and how to live out the remaining years; redefine physical and social life space.
4. Continue a supportive, close, warm relationship with the spouse or significant other, including a satisfying sexual relationship.
5. Find a satisfactory home or living arrangement and establish a safe, comfortable household routine to fit health and economic status.
6. Adjust living standards to retirement income and reduced purchasing power; supplement retirement income if possible with remunerative activity.
7. Maintain culturally assigned functions and tasks.

8. Maintain maximum level of health; care for self physically and emotionally by getting regular health examinations and needed medical or dental care, eating an adequate diet, and maintaining personal hygiene.
9. Maintain contact with children, grandchildren, and other living relatives, finding emotional satisfaction with them.
10. Establish or maintain friendships with members of own age group.
11. Maintain interest in people outside the family and in social, civic, and political responsibility.
12. Pursue alternative sources of need satisfaction and new interests and maintain former activities to gain status, recognition, and a feeling of being needed.
13. Find meaning in life after retirement and in facing inevitable illness and death of oneself, spouse, and other loved ones.
14. Work out values, life goals, and a significant philosophy of life, finding comfort in a philosophy or religion.
15. Reassess criteria for self-evaluation.
16. Adjust to the death of spouse and other loved ones.

Brown (19) refers to different developmental tasks for young-old and old-old persons because the changing life situations necessitate different attitudes, efforts, and behaviors.

Young-old developmental tasks include to:

1. Prepare for and adjust to retirement from active involvement in the work arena with its subsequent role change.
2. Anticipate and adjust to lower or changed income after retirement.
3. Establish satisfactory physical living arrangements as a result of role changes.
4. Adjust to new relationships with one's adult children and their offspring.
5. Learn or continue to develop leisure time activities to help in realignment of role losses.
6. Anticipate and adjust to slower physical and intellectual responses in the activities of daily living.
7. Deal with the death of parents, spouses, and friends.

Tasks for the old-old or frail-old are to:

1. Learn to combine new dependency needs with the continuing need for independence.
2. Adapt to living alone in continued independence.
3. Learn to accept and adjust to possible institutional living (assisted living, extended continuum of care, or nursing homes).
4. Establish an affiliation with one's age group.
5. Learn to adjust to heightened vulnerability to physical and emotional stress.
6. Adjust to loss of physical strength, illness, and eventual approach of one's death.
7. Adjust to losses of spouse, home, and friends.

Living in the Community: Related Concepts

RETIREMENT

Age, gender, health status, family background, ethnicity, type of job or profession, lifetime work experience, and economic incentives all influence when the person voluntarily or involuntarily ceases the career or job. These variables influence the retirement experience (53, 156). In 2014, there will be 40 million retirees and more grandparents than grandchildren. However, many of the "Baby Boomers" say they will continue to work part-time rather than retire completely (2, 53). As corporations reduce their workforce numbers, the older worker is most likely to be released because of salary and pension costs, despite job discrimination legislation. Yet keeping the older worker may be less costly because of no retraining costs and lower turnover and absenteeism. He or she is knowledgeable, experienced, wise, loyal to the company, flexible about accepting new assignments, and often a better salesperson or manager. Many people are living longer but are working shorter careers; yet the proportion of young to old people is diminishing. In the future it is likely that more older people will be needed in the workplace to relieve the labor shortage (36, 42, 138, 156).

For example, Home Depot and the American Association of Retired Persons (AARP) have formed a partnership. Home Depot will add to its nationwide workforce by recruiting and training older adults as part-time or full-time workers. Home Depot benefits from gaining mature, experienced, skilled, enthusiastic workers. Retirees benefit with the opportunity for job training, sometimes in a new career path, added income, and flexible work schedules. Physical and mental status of the retiree can be stabilized or improved.

Hospitals would benefit by following the plan of Home Depot to stop the exodus of nurses nearing retirement age in order to maintain an adequate number of nursing personnel (42). New roles, flexible scheduling, and financial incentives for nurses who are nearing retirement could induce them to stay or return to professional work. This would help close the gap between dangerous nursing shortages, provide adequate coverage, and relieve the work stress of younger nurses (42). Older nurses bring a wealth of knowledge, wisdom, experience, and skill. They usually cite better staffing levels and more time with patients as incentives to remain in or return to the profession. They would be valuable mentors and benefit personally from the mentorship experience (42).

Retirement affects all the other positions the person has held and the relationships with others. It may mean a reduction in income and benefits (42, 53). Or the person may seek a new job, either part- or full-time, for financial, emotional, and socialization reasons. Inability to keep up with the former activities of an organization or group may result, and a change in status may require a changing social life (138). Utilize **Box 16-11**, Phases of Retirement, for more understanding of the experience and to educate clients in preparation for retirement (42, 45, 53).

Factors linked to well-being in retirement include (156):

1. Length of time retired and resolving loss of job satisfaction.
2. Stable health status and accessible health care services.
3. Adequate income and health care benefits.
4. Active in variety of community or church programs or professional organizations.
5. Higher educational level and ability to pursue new goals or activities.
6. Extended social network of family and friends, including people who were close work colleagues.

BOX 16-11	**Phases of Retirement**

PRERETIREMENT

Remote

Adult works intensely and enjoys fruits of labor, job or professional status, financial security, and competence. Little thought or preparation for retirement.

Near Retirement

Adult begins thinking about and planning time for end of job, structured work, or professional position. Duties and obligations are gradually given up. Active planning for retirement.

RETIREMENT

Adult leaves paid employment, its structure, and its stresses.

POSTRETIREMENT

Honeymoon

Adult is enthusiastic and feels euphoric about change immediately following retirement. Feels enthusiasm and excitement of self-initiated activities. Feels frustrated, angry, and anxious about the future, if forced to retire because of company policy, health, or some other life situation.

Disenchantment

Retiree's plans are beyond financial means, health status interferes, or plans are not as satisfying as anticipated. Feels disappointed, let down, depressed, cynical, or angry.

Reorientation

Retiree comes to grips with reality of retirement, reorients self to the future, and reevaluates goals and strategies for their potential for achievement.

Stability

Retiree determines and implements long-term choices or goals. This stage may occur after the honeymoon; some people do not experience disenchantment and reorientation. Achieves long-term goals with contentment.

Terminal

The person becomes ill, is disabled, or is facing death. Retirement and the associated lifestyle has lost its significance or meaning. Or the person may be dissatisfied with retirement goals, activities, and leisure and reenters employment, usually part-time. Becomes a worker again, sometimes in a field unrelated to earlier career(s).

7. Satisfied with life before retirement.
8. Satisfied with living arrangements, staying in or moving from present home and geographic area.

Major reasons for elders continuing to work in retirement are to (36, 136): (a) maintain financial status, (b) stay physically active, (c) be helpful to others, productive, or useful, (d) do something enjoyable, (e) maintain social ties, (f) learn new information and skills, and (g) pursue a prior goal.

You are often with persons nearing retirement and may be asked directly or through nonverbal cues and disguised statements to help them sort out their feelings as they face retirement. Whatever the elderly person's need, your role is supportive. *Advocate retirement planning* to include financial security, health insurance, legal matters, Social Security benefits, company pension and retirement policies, and health maintenance information. Recommend agencies that may be useful in making plans. One of the most helpful resources is the large supply of government publications available at little or no cost from the Superintendent of Documents of the Government Printing Office in Washington, DC. Current lists of material pertinent to health and social programs may be obtained directly from the National Clearing House on Aging, U.S. Department of Health and Human Services, 330 Independence Avenue, SW, Washington, DC, 20201. You may also *advocate for development of policies, nationally and in the workplace,* that provide opportunities for the older person to remain employed in some capacity, if desired.

Explore the feasibility or desire of the elder to move to a *retirement community*, an apartment complex, a continuous care facility, or some other facility, and the benefits, risks, and obstacles.

Emphasize that they take time to make this major life-changing decision.

Values and life pattern clarifications are essential to establish a secure base in a new life that is often far removed from family, former friends, and familiar patterns of living. Such a move is at least a mild to moderate crisis, even though it has been well planned and executed. Everything is different; the couple or person will undergo an identity change. Utilize crisis intervention principles presented in Chapter 2. ∞

Explore the *spiritual dimension of retirement* with the elder, or refer to someone who can. *The following points can be considered in discussion with the elder about spirituality and this new phase in life* (175):

1. Realize the distance that has been traveled—how far you have come, in every dimension of life.
2. Reflect on the wisdom gained over the years; reminisce and share the insights.
3. Accept both accomplishments and "failures"; discuss frankly to teach others.
4. Write memoirs; preserve a family history for the next generations that includes the spiritual journey as well as other life experiences.
5. Review the panorama of life to better know self and attend to unfinished business; ask for and give forgiveness.
6. Strip away some roles, and take on new roles. Reaffirm and appreciate who you really are and the meaning and purpose of your life.
7. Rework who God has been for you, God's plan for you, and your relationship with God at this phase of your life.

MediaLink Housing

8. Appreciate what you have become. Integrate the past, embrace promises of the future, and refocus energy and goals to realize retirement dreams.

9. Become more comfortable with feelings, with spirituality, and with issues related to retirement.

10. Finish unfinished business; accept mortality of self and others.

11. Enter and relish each moment as personal death is thought about and prepared for as an ongoing process.

12. Appreciate self and others in a new perspective as the reality of eventual death is accepted as a progression of existence, a mystery, another door.

USE OF LEISURE AND THE VOLUNTEER ROLE

The constructive use of free time is often a problem of aging. What a person does when he or she no longer works is related to past lifestyle, continuing activities, accumulated experiences, and the way in which he or she perceives and reacts to the environment. The perception of and activities pursued for leisure by the elder may be similar to or different from the leisure of the young adult, as described in Chapter 14. ∞

Leisure time, *having opportunity to pursue activities of interest without a sense of obligation, demand, or urgency,* is an important aspect of life satisfaction, expression of self, and emotional and social development. Leisure activity is chosen for its own sake and for the meaning it gives to life, but it involves both physical or mental activity and participation. It is a way to cope with change. Elders value most the leisure activity that involves interaction with others or a pet, promotes development, or is expressive and maintains contact with the broader community. Most people have a core of activity that they enjoy. Reading and viewing television are popular pastimes. Considerable leisure time may be spent with grandchildren or great-grandchildren, or children of other family members or friends. **Figure 16-6**☐ depicts the concept of leisure, fellowship, and fun.

The volunteer role is a rewarding use of leisure time. The role is constrained by household income, education, health status, and age. Older Americans participate in many unpaid productive activities at levels commensurate to those reached by young and middle-aged adults. Elders who have been self-reliant and have always worked hard are more likely to incorporate service to others into their leisure and volunteer time (15, 45, 138, 173). Discuss volunteer activities and roles that can be gratifying to the elder.

The AARP is studying the potential impact on people as the United States moves from an industrialized mass society into a more technologically complex but fragmented society. All people will need an education for a life of ceaseless change, for new activities, and for new roles with passing years. Older people can lead the way in creating a better society for all generations. The definition of productivity must be changed from that which involves exchange of money. Family roles are also likely to change, with an older family adopting or nurturing a younger family, giving assistance with child care or other tasks. The elderly will be needed as caregivers across family lines as home care becomes an important aspect of the health care system. The caregiving role can give added meaning to life.

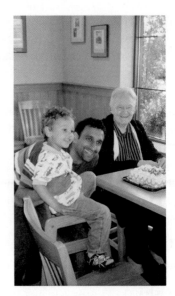

FIGURE ☐ **16-6** Family birthdays provide leisure activity for the great-grandmother.

COMMUNITY PLANNING

Planning and policy and program development must not be bound by ageism and myths about people in later maturity (45). *More and more people who are very old want to remain in their home, are taking care of themselves in their own home, and should be allowed to remain independent to the extent possible* (45, 135). *Elderly African, Asian, and Latino Americans are often nurtured by multi-generational families and churches* in their own homes and communities. Care in the home is related to values, filial responsibility, and economic factors (15).

As people become older and less mobile, a battery of community services is needed, not only to provide social activities and a reason to remain interested in life, but also to enable them to live independently. Most of the federal programs operate at the local level in actual practice, but, in addition, there is much that each community can do to provide needed services. In small communities these services may be limited, but further information is available through any county public health agency.

Be prepared to discuss a new concept with the young-old. A new movement by the Baby Boomer generation now entering the 60s is to build *intentional communities.* This generation grew up in communes in the 1960s and 1970s. They lived through trends of societal fragmentation and alienation. Now they are starting to create new communities and new connections. This kind of collective living, a more sophisticated hippie commune, often includes an extended family—their children and grandchildren. These communities are seen especially in the Southwest and are usually racially and ethnically diverse. A group of couples may own their houses in common and work together to maintain their homes and community, and work at a regular job as well. *Information about this cohousing movement is available from several sources:*

1. Cohousing Association of the United States
   Phone: 314-754-5828, *www.cohousing.org*

2. Federation of Egalitarian Communities
   Phone: 206-324-6822, ext. 2, www.thefec.org
3. Fellowship of Intentional Community
   Phone: 660-883-5545, www.fic.ic.org
4. Global Ecovillage Network
   Phone: 719-256-5003

Discuss values, reasons, risks, and benefits to this type of housing arrangement. Emphasize the need to discuss this concept with the family and friends prior to action.

Community Services

Discuss available and needed services with the elder and family. Refer as appropriate. Advocate for needed services. Educate elders and families about the types of supportive service agencies and the services they render, as described in **Table 16-14**, Community Resources for Older People. These services can be used to promote health, prevent dysfunction, enhance a sense of independence, and aid family caregivers. Educate the public about the need for a variety of services and their accessibility. As a citizen of the community, advocate for initiating and supporting local service agencies and for maintaining high standards of service. Advocate for policy and legislative development and change as needed. Involve the elder population in this process.

You may give direct care to clients, educate or counsel the elders, or serve as a consultant to many of these agencies or services. You may educate agency volunteers or staff about characteristics and needs of the elder and effective services. One type of service is adult day care (see **Figure 16-7**■). Educate the elder and family utilizing information from **Box 16-12**, Criteria for Selecting Elder Day Care.

Extended Care Facility or Campus

The concept of long-term care for the elderly has broadened to be less custodial, more homelike, more holistic, and community focused. The names for the institutions vary: *extended care facility or*

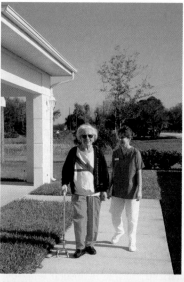

FIGURE ■ **16-7** Adult day care centers offer meals, nutritional counseling, mental health services, exercise classes, physical therapy, and social activites to elders.

campus or senior health care center. The term *nursing home* is used less frequently. The facility must be approved for skilled nursing, although it may have both skilled and intermediate care levels for residents. Criteria are set by Medicare as to what constitutes a person who needs skilled versus intermediate care and what is Medicare-eligible. If the resident or client has little or no financial resources, Medicaid will pay after the elder is approved (45).

Certification of a skilled nursing facility is done by the state agency charged with enforcing the federal Medicare guidelines. The federal government may send out inspectors to check not only the nursing care facilities but also the state inspectors. Licensing of a care facility is done by each state (15, 45).

BOX 16-12 Criteria for Selecting Elder Day Care

1. Is agency certified or licensed? Who sponsors the agency?
2. Is the agency designed in space, furniture, decor and color, equipment, and safety features for the elderly, including frail but ambulatory elderly and the cognitively impaired?
3. What meals are served? Are special diets served? Ask the attendees about food.
4. Are nurses and social workers employed? Physical therapists? Occupational therapists? Are attendants certified? Professionals should be available to the extent that the agency enrolls elders with physical or cognitive problems. The staff/client ratio should be no more than 1:8, with fewer clients if they are impaired.
5. Is transportation provided? Some agencies have van service to pick up and deliver the senior home—within

a certain mile radius and at certain hours—for a nominal fee.
6. How do staff members handle medical or psychiatric emergencies? What is the policy if the elder becomes ill during the day?
7. What is the schedule for the day? Are a variety of activities available? Are trips taken to the community? Are there activities of interest to and for participation by individuals and groups?
8. What is the cost per day? Is financial aid available? Are there extra fees for activities? For clients with special physical or cognitive problems?
9. How do staff members interact with clients and families?
10. How do the clients interact? Do they appear to be satisfied with the care? Talk with them.

TABLE 16-14

Community Resources for Older People

Resource	Service
Adult congregate living facilities (ACLF)	Room, board, and personal services for elderly who would benefit from living in a group setting but do not require medical services; no nursing or medical services available
Adult day care	Provision of comfortable, safe environment for functionally impaired adults, especially frail elderly, moderately handicapped, or slightly confused, who need care during the day, either because they live alone and cannot manage, or because family needs relief from the care to keep the elderly in the home
Adult foster care	Provision for continuous care to a functionally impaired older person in a private home with people who provide all services needed by the elderly individual
Aftercare	Posthospitalization rehabilitation such as cardiac or respiratory rehabilitation or occupational or physical therapy
American Association of Retired Persons (AARP)	Nationwide organization for people over 50 that offers discount drug purchases, health and auto insurance, publications, and other activities
Area Agency on Aging	Federal agency that provides information, referral services, planning and coordination, but not direct or health care services, on a regional or countrywide basis
Congregate nutrition sites	Free or low-cost meals, social activities, and nutrition or health education provided in local churches or senior centers
Congregate living facility	Apartment complex that provides meals and social programs for older people
Elderhostel	An on-campus educational experience, living on campus for duration of the course that includes opportunity for new knowledge, travel to various campuses and national and international geographic areas, new experiences, meeting new people
Foster care	Placement of nonrelated elderly person in private residence for care
Foster Grandparents	Federal program paying people with low income who are over 60 a modest amount for working more than 20 hours a week with children who have mental or physical disabilities
Friendly Visiting	Organized visiting services staffed by volunteers who visit homebound elderly once or twice weekly for companionship purposes if no relatives or friends are available
Gray Panthers	Nationwide politically oriented organization that works to raise awareness about issues affecting older people and to advocate and lobby on these issues in local, state, and national government
Home health services	Agency providing intermittent nursing, social work, and physical, occupational, and speech therapies and other related services to homebound person in the home via qualified health care professional or paraprofessionals
Homemaker/chore services	Agency providing help with light housekeeping, laundry, home chores, meal preparation, shopping for older people meeting income and other eligibility requirements
Hospice	Continuum of care systems for persons with terminal disease and for their family, including home care, pain management, respite care, counseling, family support delivered in the home through outpatient and inpatient care—all within the same licensed program (it is medically directed, nurse coordinated, autonomously administered, and provides care for the physical, emotional, spiritual, and social needs of client and family, using an interdisciplinary team approach)
Long-term care ombudsman committees	Citizen committees appointed by the governor who volunteer their time to investigate and resolve grievances or problems of people in nursing homes and ACLFs
Meals on Wheels	Provision of hot or cold nutritious meals to a homebound elderly person, brought by another person or agency
Medicaid	Governmental coverage of health care and nursing home costs for older people with limited incomes who are eligible
Medicare	National health insurance program for people age 65 and older or disabled, or in some special cases under 65, that is administered by the Social Security Administration (Part A is hospital insurance; Part B covers diagnostic tests, physical fees, outpatient and ambulance costs. Dental, vision, hearing, and preventive services are excluded.)

TABLE 16-14

Community Resources for Older People—continued

Resource	Service
Protective services	Constellation of social services that assists older, noninstitutionalized people who manifest at least some incapacity to manage their money or their daily living or assist those who need protection of life or property
Respite care	Agency providing relief for specified hours, a weekend, or a week, for family caregivers, allowing time for the caregiver to shop, have the time for other reasons, or vacation while care is given to functionally impaired person residing in the home setting
Senior center	Program providing a combination of services; designed to be open 3 or more days a week, with meal, recreational, educational, and counseling services available (sometimes medical services are provided)
Senior Corps of Retired Executives	Agency of retired executives who volunteer their counseling services to small businesses and companies on request
Supplemental Security Income (SSI)	Minimum monthly income to blind, disabled, and aged persons whose income falls below a specified level (personal effects, household goods, and home ownership are not counted as assets, although savings, stocks, jewelry, or car are)
Telephone reassurance	Daily telephone calls to people who live alone, including the aged and disabled, or telephone crisis and information services provided by an agency

The extended care facility may serve as a transitional stop between hospital and home. In some cases, however, the stay is permanent.

Goals of the modern-day facility are to provide (a) supervision by a physician, (b) 24-hour nursing services, (c) hospital affiliation, (d) written client care policies, specialized social services, and (e) specialized services in dietary, physical therapy, occupational therapy, pharmaceutical, and diagnostics. Unfortunately, these are sometimes hollow goals, even though the physical plant is new, licensing is current, and government funds are being used. Often the homes are operated for profit by those outside the nursing or medical profession. The residents are not always physically or mentally able to protest if care is poor, and often families of the residents do not monitor the care. National exposure of blatant neglect in some of the facilities has awakened public and government consciousness; perhaps this exposure will correct the most glaring problems and alert other facilities to their obligation to follow prescribed goals. If standards are met, the extended care facility or nursing home provides an excellent and needed service. Prolonged hospitalization can foster confusion, helplessness, and the hazards of immobility. Further, some elderly cannot care for themselves and have no one to care for them. There are ways to individualize care, give holistic care, and prevent neglect or abuse of residents in long-term care settings (45).

Some facilities go beyond these concepts and provide *independent living options.* They start with offering people meals and clinic access in a congregate (hotel-type) setting. All services and living space are available in one facility. Or the residents may live in a free-standing house or apartment on campus. These independent residents come and go as they please. They choose this living option for the security of the campus and for the assurance that they will get whatever living facility and care that they will need for the rest of their lives.

Refer families who need information about the status of a long-term care facility to "Nursing Home Compare," a tool used by the federal government to compile survey data. Or a long-term ombudsman can be contacted at 202-332-2275.

Educate and reinforce families, and the elder who is alert, to look for the plaque or document shown in **Box 16-13**, Bill of Rights for Residents of Extended Care Facilities. It is meant to remind everyone that the elder resident legally has a right to safe, comfortable, healthy, quality care, given by prepared providers. Every resident should be given a copy on admission to keep and reread.

Assisted Living

Assisted living is a *residential and social model that is an alternative to the medical model of institutionalization for people who are frail or have physical limitations that necessitate help with care beyond the home health care model.* The elder who lives alone, needs help with care, is lonely, and feels isolated may choose this option. Assisted living is staffed with a registered nurse (RN) and other levels of care providers.

The services typically offered in a nursing home are offered in a residential setting, at a lower cost. A comprehensive health, social, functional, and economic assessment is obtained. The RN starts the flow of resources, delegating care to professionals from various disciplines. The resident is to have independence, individuality, choice, privacy, dignity, and greater control over life than would be possible in long-term care. There is not the confinement to one room. There is a choice about activities. Transportation to outside events and shopping is available. This setting, just like the long-term care setting, also requires an ombudsman or consumer protection advocate to ensure the original intent is maintained (14, 45, 120).

Refer the elder and family to information about assisted living standards, licensing, costs, and facilities that can help them make

INTERVENTIONS FOR HEALTH PROMOTION

When you help the family or senior select a long-term care setting, the following questions should be asked:

1. What type of home is it, and what is its licensure status?
2. What are the total costs, and what is included for the money?
3. Is the physical plant adequate, clean, and pleasant? How much space and furniture are allowed for each person?
4. What safety features are evident? Are fire drills held? Are there operable smoke alarms and fire extinguishers?
5. What types of care are offered (both acute and chronic)?
6. What is the staff-to-resident ratio? What are the qualifications of the staff? What staff attitudes are demonstrated toward the elderly?
7. What are the physician services? Is a complete physical examination given periodically?
8. What therapies are available? Are pharmacy services available?
9. Are meals nutritionally sound and the food tasty?
10. Is food refrigerated, prepared, distributed, and served under sanitary conditions? Is eating supervised or assisted?
11. Are visitors welcomed warmly?
12. Are residents aware of their rights? (See **Box 16-13**, Bill of Rights for Residents of Extended Care Facilities.)
13. Do residents appear content and appropriately occupied? (Observe on successive days and at different hours.) Are they treated with dignity and warmth by staff? Is privacy afforded during personal care?
14. Has the local Better Business Bureau received any complaints about this facility?
15. Does the administrator have a current state license?
16. Is the home certified to participate in government or other programs that provide financial assistance when needed?
17. Is an ombudsman available, if not on site, via a phone number or e-mail address, to investigate complaints of residents or family?

BOX 16-13   Bill of Rights for Residents of Extended Care Facilities

1. To be treated with consideration, respect, and recognition of personal dignity and individuality.
2. To receive care, treatment, and services that are adequate and appropriate, and in compliance with relevant federal and state statutes and rules.
3. To receive a regularly updated written statement of services provided by the facility and of related charges. Charges for services not covered under Medicare and Medicaid shall be specified.
4. To have on file physician's orders with proposed schedule of medical treatment.
5. To have all personal and medical records kept confidential.
6. To be free of mental and physical abuse. Except in emergencies, to be free of chemical and physical restraint unless authorized for a specified period of time by a physician according to clear and indicated medical need.
7. To receive from the administration or staff of the facility a reasonable response to all requests.
8. To associate and communicate privately and without restriction with persons and groups of the patients.
9. To manage his or her own financial affairs unless other legal arrangements have been implemented.
10. To have privacy in one's own room and in visits by the patient's spouse, and if both are patients in the same facility, they shall be given the opportunity, where feasible, to share a room.
11. To present grievances and recommend changes in policies and services personally, through other persons, or in combination with others, without fear of reprisal, restraint, interference, coercion, or discrimination.
12. To not be required to perform services for the facility without personal consent and the written approval of the attending physician.
13. To retain, to secure storage for, and to use his or her personal clothing and possessions, where reasonable.
14. To not be transferred or discharged from a facility except for medical, financial, or their own or other patient's welfare, nonpayment for the stay, or when mandated by Medicare or Medicaid.
15. To be notified within 10 days after the facility's license is revoked or made provisional. The responsible party or guardian must be notified as well.

Source: North Carolina Division of Aging and Adult Services. (2007). North Carolina's Adult Care Home Bill of Rights. Retrieved December 1, 2007, from http://www.ncdhhs.gov/aging/rights.htm#r1

BOX 16-14	**Considerations for the Elderly Client in Health Promotion**

1. Personal history
2. Family ties; family history; widow(er)
3. Cultural history
4. Current responsibilities with a spouse or other family members
5. Impact of physiologic changes on functional status and activities of daily living
6. Behaviors or appearance that indicate person is being abused or neglected
7. Implementation of safety measures, immunizations, and health practices
8. Preexisting illness
9. Risk factors, past or current measures used to reduce or prevent them
10. Current illness
11. Behaviors that indicate age-appropriate cognitive status; ability to manage own affairs
12. Behaviors that indicate age-appropriate emotional status, including ego integrity instead of self-despair, and moral-spiritual development
13. Behaviors that indicate that retirement and losses that occur in late life have been grieved and integrated into the self-concept and life patterns
14. Satisfactory living arrangements
15. Involvement in the community to the extent possible
16. Behavioral patterns that indicate adult has achieved development tasks

Review Questions

1. The nurse is assessing a female client in her early 60s. The woman tells the nurse, "I feel like I'm still 25!" Which term associated with aging can the nurse use to describe what the client has verbalized?
   1. Biological age
   2. Social age
   3. Psychological age
   4. Cognitive age

2. An elderly female is brought to the emergency department (ED) by her husband, following a fall down three steps in her home. The nurse notes that this is the second ED visit for an injury for this client in the last 2 months and further notes the client lost 10 pounds since her last admission. When questioned, the client states, "Everything is fine. I just don't feel much like eating." What action by the nurse should be given priority?
   1. Refer the client to a home nursing agency for assessment of the living environment.
   2. Request a consult by a dietitian to address the weight loss issue.
   3. Interview the client privately about her home situation and to assess for indications of abuse.
   4. Suggest that the client enroll in a home meal program.

3. A 60-year-old male client requests a sedative due to his inability to sleep through the night. Which of the following should the nurse include in the assessment of this client? (Select all that apply.)
   1. Evaluate the client's urinary pattern.
   2. Discuss the client's dietary pattern.
   3. Evaluate for food allergies or environmental irritants.
   4. Evaluate for use of prescription and over-the-counter medications.
   5. Evaluate the client's exercise habits.

4. Which of the following should the nurse consider when planning an educational activity for senior citizens?
   1. Visual aids and handouts should be developed in large print.
   2. Materials from textbooks and professional journals can be used without adaptation.
   3. Written and psychomotor testing should be incorporated for evaluation purposes.
   4. One long session is better than several short sessions.

References

1. A new breed of caregivers. (2004). *Mount Sinai School of Medicine Focus on Healthy Aging, 7*(9), 7.

2. Adler, J., Wingert, P., Springer, K., Kent, J., Samuels, A., Raymond, J., & Adams, W. (2005, November, 14). The Boomer files: Hitting 60, *Newsweek,* 51–57.

3. Ahn, T., & Kim, K. (2007). Mutual caring of elderly Korean couples. *Journal of Transcultural Nursing, 18*(1), 28–34.

4. Aldwin, C., & Gilmer, D. (2003). *Health, illness, and optimal aging: Biological and psychosocial perspectives.* Thousands Oaks, CA: Sage.

5. Allison, M., & Keller, C. (2004). Self-efficacy intervention effect on physical activity in older adults. *Western Journal of Nursing Research, 26*(1), 31–46.

6. Amelia, E. (2004). Presentation of illness in older adults. *American Journal of Nursing, 104*(10), 40–51.

7. American Association of Retired Persons. (2001). *In the middle: A report on multicultural Boomers coping with family and aging issues.* Washington, DC: Author.

8. American Psychiatric Association. (1994). *Diagnostic and statistical manual of mental disorders* (4th ed.). Washington, DC: Author.

9. Andrews, M., & Boyle, J. (2003). *Transcultural concepts in nursing care* (4th ed.). Philadelphia: Lippincott William & Wilkins.

10. Antai-Otong, D. (2003). *Psychiatric nursing: Biological and behavioral concepts.* Clifton Park, NY: Thomas/Delmar Learning.

11. Arking, R. (2006). A theory of aging over the life span. In R. Arking, *The biology of aging: Observations and principles* (3rd ed.). New York: Oxford University Press.

12. Arking, R. (2006). Genetic and social aspects of aging in humans. In R. Arking, *The biology of aging: Observations and principles* (3rd ed.). New York: Oxford University Press.

13. Baltes, P., & Standinger, U. (2000). Wisdom. *American Psychologist, 55,* 122–136.

14. Basler, B. (2006, February). Assisted living: 10 great ideas. *AARP Bulletin,* 16–24.

15. Berger, K. (2005). *The developing person through the lifespan* (6th ed.). New York: Worth Publishers.

16. Boland, D., & Sims, S. (1996). Family care giving: Care at home as a solitary journey. *IMAGE: Journal of Nursing Scholarship, 28,* 55–58.

17. Bonnie, R., & Wallace, R. (2003). *Elder mistreatment, abuse, neglect, and exploitation in an aging America, National Research Council of the National Academies.* Washington, DC: National Academies Press.

18. Breslow, R., & Smothers, B. (2004). Drinking patterns of older Americans: National Health Interview Surveys, 1997–2001. *Journal of Studies on Alcohol, 65,* 232–240.

19. Brown, S. (2007, January). Special grandparenting: How to love and help grandchildren with disabilities. *Focus on the Family,* pp. 8–9.

20. Burgess, A., Brown, K., Belt, K., Ledran, L., & Poarch, J. (2005). Sexual abuse of older adults. *American Journal of Nursing, 105*(10), 16–17.

21. Burton, L. (1999). Age norms, the timing of family role transitions, and intergenerational caregiving among aging African-American women. *Gerontologist, 36*(2), 199–208.

22. Butcher, H., & McConigal-Kinney, M. (2005). Depression and dispiritedness in later life. *American Journal of Nursing, 105*(12), 52–61.

23. Butler, R. (2002). *The new love and sex after 60.* New York: Random House.

24. Centers for Disease Control and Prevention and the Merck Company Foundation. (2007). *The stage of aging and health in America 2007.* Whitehouse Station, NJ: The Merck Company Foundation. www.cdc.gov/aging/pdf/saha_2007.pdf

25. Charles, S., Reynolds, C., & Gatz, M. (2001). Age-related differences and change in positive and negative affect over 23 years. *Journal of Personality and Social Psychology, 80,* 136–151.

26. Cole, C., & Richards, K. (2007). Sleep disruptions in older adults. *American Journal of Nursing, 107*(5), 40–49.

27. Cooney, T., & Smith, L. (1996). Young adults' relations with grandparents following recent parental divorce. *Journal of Gerontology: Social Sciences, 51B*(2), S91–S95.

28. Costa, P., & McCrae, R. (1996). Mood and personality in adulthood. In C. Magai & S. McFadden (Eds.), *Handbook of emotion, adult development, and aging* (pp. 369–383). San Diego, CA: Academic Press.

29. Crumlish, B. (2004). Sexual counseling by cardiac nurses for patients following an MI. *British Journal of Nursing, 13*(12), 710–713.

30. Cumming, E., & Henry, W. E. (1961). *Growing old: The process of disengagement.* New York: Guide Books.

31. Curb, J., et al. (1990). Health status and life style in elderly Japanese men with a long life expectancy. *Journal of Gerontology: Social Sciences, 45*(5), S206–S211.

32. Danner, D., Snowden, D., & Friesen, W. (2001). Positive emotions in early life and longevity: Findings from the Nun Study. *Journal of Personality and Social Psychology, 80*(5), 813–814.

33. Deary, I., Leaper, S., Murray, A., Staff, R., & Whalley, L. (2003). Cerebral white matter abnormalities and lifetime cognitive change: A 67-year follow-up of the Scottish Mental Survey of 1932. *Psychology and Aging, 188,* 140–148.

34. DeBusk, R. (2003). Sexual activity in patients with angina. *Journal of the American Medical Association, 290*(23), 3129–3132.

35. Dellasega, C., & Haagen, B. (2004). A different kind of caregiving support group. *Journal of Psychosocial Nursing, 42*(8), 47–55.

36. Deters, C. (2007, January). Boomerang CEOs. *Erickson Tribune,* 1–2.

37. Doka, K., & Merts, M. (1988). The meaning and significance of great-grandparenthood. *Gerontologist, 28*(2), 192–197.

38. Donelan, K., Hill, C., Hoffman, C., Scoles, K., Feldman, P., Levine, C., et al. (2002). Challenged to care: Informal caregivers in a changing health system. *Health Affairs, 21,* 222–231.

39. Douglas, D. (2004). The lived experience of loss: A phenomenological study. *Journal of American Psychiatric Nurses Association, 10*(1), 24–32.

40. Dreifus, C. (2006, March). Why do some people live so long? *AARP Bulletin,* 16, 29.

41. Dudek, S. (2007). *Nutritional essentials for nursing* (5th ed.). Philadelphia: Lippincott Williams & Wilkins.

42. Duffy, J. (2004). Happy un-retirement. *Johns Hopkins Nursing, 11*(11), 16–21.

43. Duvall, E., & Miller, B. (1984). *Marriage and family development* (6th ed.). Philadelphia: J.B. Lippincott.

44. Duyff, R. (2002). *American Dietetic Association complete food and nutrition guide* (2nd ed.). Hoboken, NJ: John Wiley & Sons.

45. Ebersole, P., Hess, P., & Luggen, A. (2004). *Toward healthy aging: Human needs and nursing response* (6th ed.). St. Louis, MO: Mosby.

46. Einstein, G., & McDaniel, M. (2004). *Memory fitness: A guide for successful aging.* Cambridge, MA: Yale University Press.

47. Emami, A., Benner, P., & Ekman, S. (2001). A sociocultural model for late-in-life immigrants. *Journal of Transcultural Nursing, 12*(1), 15–23.

48. Erikson, E. (1963). *Childhood and society* (2nd ed.). New York: W.W. Norton.

49. Erikson, E. (1978). *Adulthood.* New York: W.W. Norton.

50. Erikson, E., Erikson, J., & Kivneck, H. (1986). *Vital involvement in old age.* New York: Norton.

51. Erikson, J. (1997). *The life cycle completed: Erik H. Erikson.* New York: Norton.

52. Erlingsson, C., Carlson, J., & Saveman, B. (2003). Elder abuse risk indicators and screening questions. Results from a theoretical search and a panel of experts from developed and developing countries. *Journal of Elder Abuse & Neglect, 18,* 185–203.

53. Falk, N. (2006). Aging workers in search of employment and health insurance coverage. *Journal of Psychosocial Nursing, 44*(5), 13–16.

54. Fenstermacker, K., & Hudson, B. T. (2004). *Practice guidelines for family practitioners* (3rd ed.). Philadelphia: Saunders.

55. Floyd, J. (2002). Sleep and aging. *Nursing Clinics of North America, 37,* 719–731.

56. Forestalling frailty. (2003). *Harvard Women's Health Watch, 10*(7), 2–3.

57. Fried, L., et al. (2001). Frailty in older adults: Evidence for a phenotype. *Journal of Gerontology Series: Biological Sciences and Medical Sciences, 56,* M146–M157.

58. Fry, P. (2001). The unique contribution of key existential factors to the prediction of psychological well-being of older adults following spousal loss. *Gerontologist, 41,* 69–81.

59. Gardner, J. (1993). *Multiple intelligences: Theory in practice.* New York: Basic Books.

60. Geesamen, B., Benson, E., Brewster, S. et al (2003). Haplotype-based identification of a microsomal transfer protein marker associated with the human lifespan. *Proceedings of the National Academy of Science USA, 100,* 14115–14120.

61. Giger, J., & Davidhizer, R. (2004). *Transcultural nursing: Assessment and intervention* (4th ed.). St. Louis, MO: Mosby.

62. Goldman, C. (2004). *Ageless spirit: Reflections on living life to the fullest in midlife and beyond.* New York: Fairview Press.

63. Goleman, D. (1998). *Working with emotional intelligence.* New York: Bantam.

64. Grey, M., Knaff, K., & McCorkle, R. (2006). A framework for the study of self- and family-management of chronic conditions. *Nursing Outlook, 54*(5), 278–286.

65. Grossman, S., & Lange, J. (2006). Theories of aging as basis for assessment. *Medsurg Nursing, 15*(2), 77–83.

66. Gurung, R., Taylor, S., & Seeman, T. (2003). Accounting for changes in social support among married older adults. Insight from the MacArthur studies of successful aging. *Psychology and Aging, 18,* 487–496.

67. Guyton, A., & Hall, J. (2006). *Textbook of medical physiology* (11th ed.). Philadelphia: Elsevier Saunders.

68. Haber, D. (2003). Introduction. *Health promotion and aging: Practical applications for health professionals* (3rd ed.). New York: Springer Publishing.

69. Harris, M. (2006). Eating disorders across the life span. *Journal of Psychosocial Nursing, 44*(4), 18–26.

70. He, W., Sengupta, M., Velkoff, V. A., & DeBarros, K. A. (2005, December). *65+ in the United States: 2005.* Current Population Reports, Special Studies, U.S. Census Bureau., Washington, DC. Downloaded on May 22, 2005 from www.census.gov/prod/2006/pubs/p23_209.pdf.

71. Health after 100: Secrets of the centenarians. (2001). *Johns Hopkins Medical Letter, 13*(9), 6–7.

72. Herrick, T. (2005). As Baby Boomers age, who will care for them? *Clinical News, 9*(9), 1, 18–19.

73. Hodgson, N., Freedman, V., Granger, D., & Erno, A. (2004). Biobehavioral correlation of relocation in the frail elderly: Salivary cortisol, affect, and cognitive function. *Journal of the American Geriatrics Society, 52,* 1856–1862.

74. Hoonaard, V., & Kistin, D. (2003). Expectations and experiences of widowhood. In J. F. Gubrum & J. A. Holstein (Eds.), *Ways of aging* (pp. 182–199). Malden, MA: Blackwell.

75. Hungerford, T. (2001). The economic consequences of widowhood on elderly women in the United States and Germany. *Gerontologist, 41,* 103–110.

76. Insomnia in late life. (2006). *Harvard Mental Health Letter, 23*(6), 1–5.

77. Jacoby, S. (2005, July–August). Sex in America. *AARP Magazine,* 57–62, 114.

78. Jarvis, C. (2003). *Physical examination and health assessment* (4th ed.). New York: Saunders.

79. Jung, C. (1971). Psychological types. In G. Adler, et al. (Eds.), *Collected works of Carl G. Jung,* Vol. 6. Princeton, NJ: Princeton University Press.

80. Jung, C. (1995). *Modern man in search of a soul.* New York: Harcourt, Brace, & World.

81. Kalins, D., Helms, C., & Chebatoris, J. (2006, March 20). The Boomer files: Art-Design of the times. *Newsweek,* 54–58.

82. Katz, A. (2007). Sexuality and myocardial function. *American Journal of Nursing, 107*(3), 49–52.

83. Kelleber, K. (1992). The afternoon of life: Jung's view of the tasks of the second half of life. *Perspectives in Psychiatric Care, 28*(2), 25–28.

84. Kelley, S. (1993). Caregiver stress in grandparents raising their grandchildren. *IMAGE: Journal of Nursing Scholarship, 25,* 331–338.

85. Kiecolt-Glaser, J., McGuire, I., Rubles, T., & Glaser, R. (2002). Emotions, morbidity, and mortality. New perspectives from psychoimmunology. *Annual Review of Psychology, 53,* 83–107.

86. Kimball, M., & Willams-Burgess, C. (1995). Failure to thrive: The silent epidemic of the elderly. *Archives of Psychiatric Nursing, 9*(2), 99–105.

87. Kirn, T. (2007). Baby Boomers with chronic conditions may overwhelm system. *Clinical Psychiatry News, 33*(6), 2.

88. Kivett, V. (1991). Centrality of the grandfather role among older rural Black and White men. *Journal of Gerontology: Social Sciences, 46*(5), S250–S258.

89. Kivett, V. (1993). Racial comparisons of the grandmother roles: Implications for strengthening the family support system of older Black women. *Family Relations, 42*(2), 165–172.

90. Koehn, M. (2005). Embracing the aging process. *Journal of Christian Nursing, 22*(2), 20–24.

91. Kohlberg, L. (1981). *Essays on moral development.* San Francisco: Harper & Row.

92. Kohlberg, L., & Ryncarz, R. (1990). Beyond justice reasoning: Moral development and consideration of a seventh stage. In C. Alexander & E. Langer (Eds.), *Higher stages of human development* (pp. 191–207). New York: Oxford University Press.

93. Kolanowski, A., & Piven, M. (2006). Geropsychiatric nursing: The state of the science. *Journal of the American Psychiatric Nurses Association, 12*(2), 76–79.

94. Kubler-Ross, E., & Kessler, D. (2000). *Life lessons.* New York: Scritner.

95. Kuhn, M. (2003). Oxygen free radicals & antioxidants. *American Journal of Nursing, 103*(4), 58–62.

96. Lararia, M. (2006). Keep it, repeat it, berate it: Differential diagnosis and treatment of OCD and hoarding. *Journal of American Psychiatric Nurses Association, 18*(1), 10–11.

97. LeDoux, J. (2002). *The synaptic self: How our brains become who we are.* New York: Viking Press.

98. Levinson, D. (1990). A theory of life structure development in adulthood. In K. N. Alexander & E. J. Langer (Eds.), *Higher stages of human development* (pp. 35–54). New York: Oxford University Press.

99. Levy, B., Jennings, P., & Langer, E. (2001). Improving attention in old age. *Journal of Adult Development, 8,* 189–192.

100. Linton, A. D., & Lach, H. (2006). *Matteson & McConnell's gerontological nursing: Concepts and practice* (3rd ed.). New York: Saunders.

101. Litvin, S. (1992). Status transitions and future outlook as determinants of conflict: The caregiver's and care receiver's perspective. *Gerontologist, 32*(1), 68–76.

102. Live to be a healthy 100. (2005). *Mount Sinai School of Medicine Focus on Healthy Aging, 8*(1), 4–5.

103. Living to 100: What's the secret? (2002). *Harvard Health Letter, 27*(3), 1–3.

104. Lopez, O., Becker, J., Jagust, W., et al (2006). Neuropsychological characteristics of mild cognitive impairment subgroups. *Journal of Neurological and Neurosurgical Psychiatry, 77,* 159–165.

105. Maddox, G. L. (1974). Disengagement Theory: A critical evaluation. *Gerontologist, 4,* 80–83.

106. Maddox, G. L. (1994). Lives through the years revisited. *Gerontologist, 34,* 764–767.

107. Mahoney, S. (2006, May). The secret lives of single women. *AARP Magazine,* 70–78, 108.

108. Marklein, M. (1991). Con games proliferate: New threats haunt city folk. *AARP Bulletin, 32*(2), 1, 16–17.

109. Masters, J. (2003). Moderate alcohol consumption and unappreciated risk for alcohol-related harm among ethnically diverse urban-dwelling elders. *Geriatric Nursing, 24,* 155–161.

110. Masters, W., Johnson, V., & Kolodny, R. (1988). *Masters and Johnson on sex and human loving.* Boston: Little, Brown.

111. Mauk, K. L. (2006). *Gerontological nursing: Competencies for care.* Boston: Jones and Bartlett.

112. Mayo Clinic. (2006). *The Mayo Clinic plan for healthy aging.* Rochester, MN: Author.

113. Mayo Clinic. (2006, June). Osteoporosis. Downloaded on May 27, 2007 from www.mayoclinic.com/health/osteoporosis/ds00128/dection-I.

114. McCullogh, M. (2006). Home modification. *American Journal of Nursing, 106*(10), 54–63.

115. McDongall, G., Becker, A., & Arheart, K. (2006). Older adults in the Senior WISE Study at risk for mild cognitive impairment. *Archives of Psychiatric Nursing, 20*(3), 126–134.

116. Mentis, J. (2006). Oral hydration in older adults. *American Journal of Nursing, 106*(6), 40–48.

117. Metheny, N. (2000). *Fluid and electrolyte balance: Nursing considerations* (4th ed.). Philadelphia: Lippincott.

118. Miller, S., & Cavanaugh, J. (1990). The meaning of grandparenthood and its relationship to demographic, relationship, and social participation variables. *Journal of Gerontology: Psychological Sciences, 45*(6), P244–P246.

119. Missouri Coalition Against Domestic & Sexual Violence. (2006). *A framework for understanding the nature and dynamics of domestic violence.* Jefferson City, MO: Author.

120. Mitty, E. (2003). Assisted living & the role of nursing. *American Journal of Nursing, 103*(8), 32–43.

121. Mobility devices can help you remain independent. (2007). *Mount Sinai School of Medicine Focus on Healthy Aging, 10*(4), 3.

122. Moon, A., & Williams, O. (1993). Perceptions of elder abuse and help-seeking patterns among African-American, Caucasian American, and Korean-American elderly women. *Gerontologist, 33*, 386–395.

123. Montbriand, M. (2004). Senior's life histories and perceptions of illness. *Western Journal of Nursing Research, 26*(2), 242–260.

124. Muehlbauer, M., & Crane, P. (2006). Elder abuse and neglect. *Journal of Psychosocial Nursing, 44*(11), 43–48.

125. NANDA International.(2005). *Nursing diagnoses: Definitions & classification 2005–2006.* Philadelphia: Author.

126. Nelson, A., & Gilbert, S. (2005). *The Harvard Medical School guide to achieving optimal memory.* New York: McGraw-Hill.

127. Neugarten, B. (1973). Adult personality: A developmental view. In D. Charles & W. Looft (Eds.), *Readings in psychological development through life* (pp. 356–366). New York: Holt, Rinehart & Winston.

128. Neugarten, B. (1975). The future and the young-old. *Gerontologist, 15*(Part 2), 4–9.

129. Neugarten, B. (1976). Adaptation and the life cycle. *Counseling Psychologist, 6*(1), 16–20.

130. Neugarten, B. (1981). Development perspective of aging. In E. Karl & B. Manard (Eds.), *Aging in America.* Sherman Oaks, CA: Alfred Publishers.

131. Neugarten, B., & Neugarten, D. (1985). Meanings of age in the aging society. In A. Pifer & L. Bronte (Eds.), *Our aging society: Paradox and promise.* New York: Norton.

132. New heart guidelines focus on women's lifetime risk and lifestyle. (2007). *Tufts University Health & Nutrition Letter, 25*(5), 1–2.

133. Nine keys to living to a healthy 85+. (2007). *Tufts University Health & Nutrition Letter,* 1–2.

134. Norris, R. (1989). Commonsense tips for working with blind patients. *American Journal of Nursing, 89*(3), 360–361.

135. Novelli, W. (2006, June). Building livable communities. *AARP Bulletin,* 37.

136. Novelli, W. (2006). Valuing older workers. *AARP Bulletin, 47*(1), 31.

137. Optimistic people live longer. (2003). *Tufts University Health and Nutrition Letter, 20*(1), 4–5.

138. Papalia, D., Olds, S., & Feldman, R. (2004). *Human development* (9th ed.). Boston: McGraw-Hill.

139. Pascucci, M. A., & Loving, G. L. (1997). Ingredients of an old and healthy life: A centenarian perspective. *Journal of Holistic Nursing, 15*, 199–213.

140. Pasero, C., & McCaffery, M. (2005). No self-report means no pain-intensity rating. *American Journal of Nursing, 105*(10), 50–53.

141. Peachey, N. (1992). Helping the elderly person resolve integrity versus despair. *Perspectives in Psychiatric Nursing, 28*(2), 29–31.

142. Peck, R. C. (1968). Psychological development in the second half of life. In B. Neugarten (Ed.), *Middle age and aging.* Chicago: University of Chicago Press.

143. Pender, N., Murdough, C., & Parsons, M. (2001). *Health promotion in nursing practice* (4th ed.). Upper Saddle River, NJ: Prentice Hall.

144. Perls, T. (2006). The different paths to 100+. *American Journal of Clinical Nutrition, 83* (Suppl.), 4845–4875.

145. Perrin, P. (2007). Research helps keep seniors steady on their feet. *Tufts University Health & Nutrition Letter, 25*(3), 4.

146. Peterson, R. (2004). Mild cognitive impairment as a diagnostic entity. *Journal of Internal Medicine, 26*, 183–194.

147. Quinlan, A. (2006, August). Live alone and like it. *Newsweek,* 70.

148. Rancour, P. (2002). Catapulting through life stages. *Journal of Psychosocial Nursing, 40*(2), 33–37.

149. Reed, P. (1991). Self-transcendence and mental health in oldest-old adults. *Nursing Research, 40*(1), 5–11.

150. Reese, C., & Murray, R. (1996). Transcendence: The meaning of great-grandmothering. *Archives of Psychiatric Nursing, 10*(4), 245–251.

151. Reid, J. (1995). Development in late life: Older lesbian and gay life. In A. D'Angeli & C. Paterson (Eds.), *Lesbian, gay, and bisexual identities over the lifespan: Psychological perspectives* (pp. 215–240). New York: Oxford Press.

152. Rosenfeld, D. (1999). Identity work among lesbian and gay elderly. *Journal of Aging Studies, 13*, 121–144.

153. Rubenstein, R., et al. (1991). Key relationships of never married, childless older women: A cultural analysis. *Journal of Gerontology: Social Sciences, 46*(5), S270–S277.

154. Ruffolo, D. (2002). Hypothermia in trauma. *RN, 66*(2), 46–51.

155. Samuels, S. (2003). Forgetfulness: When should you talk to your doctor? *Mount Sinai School of Medicine Focus on Healthy Aging, 6*(7), 4–5.

156. Santrock, J. (2004). *Life-span development* (9th ed.). Boston: McGraw-Hill.

157. Schaie, K., & Willis, S. (1991). Adult personality and psychomotor performance: Cross-sectional and longitudinal analysis. *Journal of Gerontology: Psychological Sciences, 46*(6), P275–P284.

158. Schaie, K., & Willis, S. (1996). Psychometric intelligence and aging. In F. Blanchard-Fields & T. Hess (Eds.), *Perspectives on cognitive change in adulthood and aging* (pp. 293–322). New York: McGraw-Hill.

159. Schoenhofen, E. A., Wyszynski, D. F., Anderson, S., Pennington, J. M., Young, R., Terry, D. F., et al. (2006). Characteristics of 32 supercentenarians. *Journal of the American Geriatrics Society, 54*, 1237–1240.

160. Schultz, R., & Beach, S. (1999). Caregiving as a risk factor for mortality: The Caregiver Health Effects Study. *Journal of the American Medical Association, 282*(23), 2215–2219.

161. Schulz, R., et al. (2001). Involvement in caregiving and adjustment to death of a spouse. *Journal of the American Medical Association, 285*(24), 3123–3129.

162. Sherman, C. (2005). Early sensory input shapes brain's neural structure. *Clinical Psychiatry News, 33*(5), 34.

163. Sheth, P. (2006). What exercise can do for you. *Mount Sinai School of Medicine Focus on Healthy Aging, 9*(10), 1.

164. Sill, J. (1980). Disengagement reconsidered: Awareness of finitude. *Gerontologist, 20*(4), 457–462.

165. Silva, M. (2006). A day in the life of an oldest-old father and his caregiver daughter. *Journal of Psychosocial Nursing, 44*(7), 13–17.

166. Sorrell, J. (2006). Health literacy in older adults. *Journal of Psychosocial Nursing, 44*(3), 17–20.

167. Sorrell, J. (2007). The transparency of aging. *Journal of Psychosocial Nursing, 45*(3), 19–21.

168. Stel, V., Smit, J., Phuijm, S., & Lips, P. (2004). Consequences of falling in older men and women and risk factors for health service use and functional decline. *Age and Aging, 33*, 58–65.

169. Stevenson, J., & Masters, J. (2005). Predictors of alcohol misuse and abuse in older women. *Journal of Nursing Scholarship, 37*(4), 329–335.

170. Stone, K. (2006). The neurobiology of stress and aging. *NeuroPsychiatry Reviews, 7*(12), 18.

171. Stong, C. (2007). Does biology play a role in domestic violence? *NeuroPsychiatry Reviews, 8*(5), 1, 15–16.

172. Streit, M. (2007, April). Do good, feel good—studies show volunteering can improve your health. *Erickson Tribune,* 1, 9.

173. Strength training exercises. (2006, September–October). *AARP Bulletin,* 92–93.

174. Strode, M. (2003). *Creating a spiritual retirement: A guide to the unseen possibilities in our lives.* Woodstock, VT: Skylight Paths Publishing.

175. Strowden, D. A. (1997). Aging and Alzheimer's disease: Lessons from the Nun Study. *Gerontologist, 17*, 150–156.

176. Talerico, K. (2005). Enhancing communication with older adults: Overcoming elderspeak. *Journal of Psychosocial Nursing, 43*(5), 12–16.

177. Ten research-proven tips for better memory. (2005). *Harvard Women's Health Watch, 12*(4), 4–5.

178. The driving decision: Time to give up the keys? (2006). *John Hopkins Medical Letter, 18*(1), 6–7.

179. Thomas, J. (1993). Concerns regarding adult children's assistance: A comparison of young-old, and old-old parents. *Journal of Gerontology: Social Sciences, 48,* S315–S322.

180. Thompson, R., Levis, S., Murphy, M., Hale, J., Blackwell, P., Acton, G., et al. (2004). Are there sex differences in emotional and biological responses in spousal caregivers of patients with Alzheimer's disease? *Biological Research for Nursing, 5,* 319–330.

181. Timiras, M. (2003). The skin. In P. Timiras (Ed.), *Physiological basis of aging and geriatrics* (3rd ed., pp. 397–404). Boca Raton, FL: CRC Press.

182. Timiras, P. (2003). The adrenals and pituitary. In P. Timiras (Ed.), *Physiological basis of aging and geriatrics* (3rd ed., pp. 167–188). Boca Raton, FL: CRC Press.

183. Tompkins, C. (2007). Who will care for the grandparents? *Journal of Psychosocial Nursing, 45*(5), 19–22.

184. United Nations, Department of Economic and Social Affairs, Populations Division. (2005). *World population aging: 1950–2050.*

185. United States Department of Health and Human Services. (2000). *Healthy People 2010: With understanding and improving health and objectives for improving health* (2nd ed.). 2 Vols. Washington, DC: U.S. Government Printing Office.

186. Unraveling the mystery of frailty. (2007). *Johns Hopkins Medical Letter, 19*(2), 4–5.

187. VanEtten, D. (2006). Psychotherapy with older adults. *Journal of Psychosocial Nursing, 44*(11), 29–33.

188. Walker, C., Curry, L., & Hogstel, M. (2007). Relocation stress syndrome in older adults transitioning from home to a long-term facility: Myth or reality? *Journal of Psychosocial Nursing, 45*(1), 39–45.

189. Wallhagen, M., Pettengill, E., & Whiteside, M. (2006). Sensory impairment in older adults: Part I: Hearing loss. *American Journal of Nursing, 106*(10), 40–47.

190. Wallhagen, M., & Yamamota, M. N. (2006). The meaning of family caregiving in Japan and the United States: A qualitative comparative study. *Journal of Transcultural Nursing, 17*(1), 65–73.

191. When keeping stuff gets out of hand. (2006). *Harvard Women's Health Watch, 13*(7), 4–5.

192. White, N., & Cunningham, W. (1998). Is terminal drop pervasive or specific? *Journal of Gerontology, 43*(6), 141–144.

193. Williams-Burgess, C., & Kimball, M. (1992). The neglected elder: A family systems approach. *Journal of Psychosocial Nursing, 30*(10), 21–25.

194. Willis, S., & Nesselroade, C. (1990). Long-term effects of fluid ability training in old age. *Developmental Psychology, 26,* 905–910.

195. Yaffe, K. (2006). Cognitive decline is a major concern in post-menopausal women. *NeuroPsychiatry Reviews, 7*(2), 8–9.

196. You can't teach an old dog new tricks and other myths about the aging process. (2002). *Tufts University Health & Nutrition Letter, 20*(3), 1–3.

197. You, K., & Lee, H. (2006). The physical, mental, and emotional health of older people who are living alone or with relatives. *Archives of Psychiatric Nursing, 26*(4), 193–201.

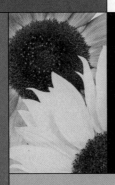

Dying and Death: The Last Developmental Stage

OBJECTIVES

Study of this chapter will enable you to:

1. Explore personal reactions and ethical issues to active and passive euthanasia and the right-to-die movement versus extraordinary measures to prolong life.

2. Contrast the child's, adolescent's, and adult's concept of death.

3. Discuss the stages of awareness and related behavior as the person adapts to the crisis of approaching death.

4. Discuss the sequence of reactions when the person and family are aware of terminal illness.

5. Assess reactions and needs of a dying client and family members with supervision.

6. Plan and give care, with supervision, to a client based on understanding of his or her awareness of eventual death, behavioral and emotional reactions, and physical needs.

7. Intervene appropriately to meet needs of family members of the dying person.

8. Contrast home or hospice care with hospital or nursing home care.

MediaLink

www.prenhall.com/murray

Go to the Companion Website for interactive resources that accompany this chapter.

Glossary	Critical Thinking
Review Questions	Tools
Challenge Your Knowledge	Media Link Applications
Learning Activities	Media Links

Death has been avoided in name and understanding. It is important to prepare emotionally, physically, financially, and socially. Your role is dual—personal preparation and preparation with the client.

Issues Related to Dying and Death

DEFINITIONS OF DEATH

The aged differ from persons in other life areas in that their concept of future is realistically limited. The younger person may not live many years into the future but generally thinks of many years of life ahead. The older person knows that, despite medical and technical advances, life is limited.

Death is the last developmental stage. It is more than simply an end process; it can be viewed as a goal and as fulfillment. If the person has spent his or her years unfettered by fear, has lived richly and productively, and has achieved the developmental task of ego integrity, he or she can accept the realization that the self will cease to be and that dying has an onset long before the actual death. Research on near-death experiences also conveys that death is another stage (74, 78, 85, 88, 94, 97, 103, 126). If death is considered the last developmental phase, it is worth the kind of preparation that goes into any developmental phase, perhaps physically, certainly emotionally, socially, philosophically, or spiritually.

Until this century, death usually occurred in the home. Today most Americans still prefer to die at home, but more than 70% of deaths in U.S. cities occur in institutions, with 23% dying in nursing homes, so death has become remote and impersonal (13, 19).

The Study to Understand Prognoses and Preferences for Outcomes and Risks of Treatments (SUPPORT) identified the shortcomings of American health care in providing compassionate care at the end of life, such as untreated pain and poor communication between providers and patients. In spite of over a decade of attempts to correct these problems, the provision of adequate physical and psychosocial care for the dying remains inadequate (24, 27).

Because of technologic advances, the determination of death is changing from the traditional concept that death occurs when the heart stops beating. The Uniform Determination of Death Act (UDDA), or similar legislation, is recognized in all 50 states. The act defines **death** as *irreversible cessation of circulatory and respiratory functions, or irreversible cessation of all functions of the brain, including the brain stem. Death based on neurologic criteria is true death* (97).

Medically accepted standards for brain death include the following neurologic criteria (97, 120):

1. Underlying cause of condition or brain injury must be known and diagnosed as irreversible.
2. Declaration of death can be made only if patient is not suffering from hypothermia (32.2°C) or receiving central nervous system depressants, either of which may present the appearance of brain death.
3. Person must manifest cerebral unresponsiveness and no reflexes.
4. Apnea testing must not produce spontaneous respiration.

Institutions may also have other criteria for their policies and procedures for pronouncing brain death. Most institutions require an electroencephalogram (EEG) to confirm absence of brain activity. Some require a cerebral radionuclide scan or four-vessel arteriogram to verify absence of blood flow.

Thus, brain death is differentiated from **coma**, *a persistent vegetative state in which the person, not assistive devices, maintains basic vital homeostatic functions and therefore is not dead, even though he or she is not responding verbally or nonverbally.* In **brain death**, *the appearance of life continues when the ventilator is used to deliver enough oxygen to keep the heart beating and skin warm. The ventilation is maintained until there is a decision about tissue or organ donation.* If there is no organ procurement, the ventilator is discontinued (120).

The sophisticated machinery has caused some to ask questions such as, "If we declare someone entirely dead when the brain is 'dead,' even though some of the body continues to function with the help of life supports, then doesn't that body lose its sanctity and become the object of transplant organ harvesting?" The opposition might answer, "Without the present life-support systems, this person would certainly have been dead. Why not take the opportunity to save another person's life with the needed organ or organs?" Some people believe organ donation gives meaning to their own life and death (or that of the family member). Depending on the belief system, the organ donation that allows another to live a long, productive life may be viewed as a kind of immortality. The current issue is not only "When is someone dead?" but "Who decides when to turn off the machines?" Is it the client, medical personnel, a lawyer, the clergy, or the courts?

Ethical considerations in removal of life support from a patient in an end-of-life or vegetative state are (2, 4, 5, 38, 47, 108, 121, 124):

1. Is the existing pathology fatal?
2. If the person lives, can the "goods of life" be maintained: seeking truth, loving others, generating and nurturing future generations, and being part of a community of people?
3. Is death imminent, regardless of therapy?
4. Does resisting the fatal pathology involve effective or ineffective treatment?
5. If therapy is effective, can the "goods of life" be maintained, or will there be an excessive burden to patient or family?
6. What is the intention of the person who removes life support?

Application of the ethical decision-making model is described more fully by Chally and Loriz (23) in relation to the American Nurses Association Code of Ethics. The code emphasizes the respect for human dignity and uniqueness of each person (80, 120).

The family, more than anyone else, must live with the memories of their loved one and the events surrounding death. It is a violation of the family's dignity to rush death. Even though a lesser involved person might say, "Why don't they turn the machines off!" this person should be ignored until all those closely involved with the client can say with acceptance and assurance, "Now is the time." Increasingly, the person is saying that he or she has a right to decide how long machines should maintain personal life or that of a loved one (1).

The moral, ethical, and legal dilemmas of maintaining or withdrawing life support (ventilator, fluids, antibiotics) are debated, especially when the patient can respond verbally or nonverbally, knows his or her name, and says he or she either does or does not want to die. Family, health care providers, the ethical committee, and hospital legal counsel may all be involved in conversations about when to end life. The nurse may advocate for the patient when he or she cannot speak for self (1, 23, 59, 111).

ORGAN AND TISSUE DONATION

As a nurse, you have significant responsibilities regarding declaration of brain death. You help collect, review, and evaluate data that are essential to declaration of death or maintenance on the ventilator. Comfort and support the family as they anticipate death of the loved one. You continue to observe and give thorough care to the person who is being evaluated as if the person was indeed going to live. Identifying a potential donor and referring to an appropriate procurement agency are crucial steps. Until the donor status is confirmed, you continue to administer care and assist in comfort measures and fluid and ventilatory management.

The family must clearly understand the person is dead before they are informed of their legal right to the option of donating, or not donating, tissues or organs. Local organ procurement organizations and tissue and eye banks can supply information and have trained personnel available 24 hours a day to assist families in counseling related to the options. The family needs sensitive communication and a thorough knowledge of the step-by-step process (111).

The procurement coordinator is the best person to talk with the family about donation because he or she is specially trained. A caring, gentle expression of sorrow for the family is necessary. After they have had time to grieve and realize death has occurred, information and support can be given and questions answered. The coordinator can handle cultural or religious considerations. No major religious denomination opposes organ donation; some ethnic or cultural groups may. The family should not be coerced but should be given an opportunity to make an informed decision that is best for them. The family are to be told about the need for organ and tissue donation and how people are helped and that the donation will not disfigure the person, will cost them nothing, and will not delay the funeral (49, 82, 93, 98, 111, 120, 125).

Words are chosen carefully. For example, the coordinator describes the **procurement process** *as receiving, removing, or retrieving organs or tissues*. The unacceptable term "harvesting" is *not* used. The ventilator is not a life-support machine to "keep the patient alive." The patient is referred to as "dead," not as "nearly dead." The patient is referred to by name, not as the donor. If family members disagree, they need time to resolve the conflict.

When the family members agree to donation, you will focus on physical care for the donor, especially eye and skin care, and emotional support for the family. For a grief-stricken family, participating in donation can be a comfort. They will remember your kind and considerate care and be grateful for the opportunity to contribute life to another person, or several persons.

The National Organ Procurement and Transplantation Network, established in 1986, is administered by the United Network for Organ Sharing and, in turn, works with staff from local organ procurement organizations who work with local health care providers. A national waiting list is maintained of people in need of transplantation. The network oversees equitable allocation of organs. Age is no longer a factor for the donor, but donor tissues or organs must be healthy. Thus, patients with extracerebral malignancies or unresolved transmittable infections, such as AIDS and hepatitis B, cannot be donors (93, 95, 98).

The following organs can be transplanted: heart; kidney (can be donated by living donor); liver, lung, and pancreas (segments can be donated by living donor); small bowel; and stomach. A number of tissues can be donated, including cornea, skin, dura, fascia, cartilage, tendons, saphenous veins, heart valves, bone marrow, and bones (rib, femur, tibia, fibula, ilium) (93, 95, 98).

EUTHANASIA

Euthanasia *is legally defined as the act or practice of painlessly putting to death persons suffering from incurable or distressing diseases* (32). Although maintaining life beyond all reason is an ethical dilemma for the nurse, an equally taxing ethical dilemma occurs when the doctor deliberately hastens the client's death by increasing the dose of a narcotic analgesic such as morphine to the point of lethality. Responsible, moral caregivers promote quality of life and the right to die with dignity. If each human life is seen as of infinite value, it will be worth the efforts to ease pain and help the person find meaning in the current situation (5).

Euthanasia is not new. It was practiced in ancient Greece. In the past, African Bushmen and North American Indian tribes abandoned their infirm elderly to die; there was insufficient food for anyone who could not produce his or her own food. Eskimo tribal elders cut a hole in the ice and disappeared when they became burdensome (9). In modern times, some people believe that terminally ill patients have the right to a painless assisted death. This form of euthanasia is accomplished by giving the dying person a prescribed dose of central nervous system depressant sufficient to bring about death.

Euthanasia is illegal throughout the world. In the Netherlands, immunity is granted to the physician who follows specific guidelines (9, 95). Most nurses do not support active euthanasia. Support for it is based on patient autonomy, informed consent, and suffering. Religious beliefs may be the most accurate predictor of the person's stance on euthanasia. Many nurses are opposed to active euthanasia on the basis of sanctity of life and limits to autonomy. They worry about the double effect of giving medication for pain that may also shorten life. They are concerned about their own professional integrity and responsibility. Nurses who support active euthanasia define professional integrity and responsibility as being an advocate for patients who make a decision to end their life (32, 33). To withdraw a patient from life support may allow the patient to die; however, the patient may not die, at least not quickly (101). Those who are disabled, elderly, retarded, or mentally incompetent may not receive the treatment ordinarily given to others.

Most Western countries consider **active euthanasia**, *deliberately hastening death*, as first-degree murder. On the other hand, court decisions have been inconsistent about **passive euthanasia**, *omission of care or inaction to prolong life* (95).

The development of Judeo-Christian law from the beliefs of St. Augustine and St. Thomas Aquinas held that suicide was a sin and against natural law. In the past in American institutions, only physiologic aspects were considered in prolonging life. Today sociologic and economic aspects are also considered. The value or quality of life when the person is kept alive by artificial support systems is considered. Costs to client, family, and society are also considered. Ordinary care is the prevailing standard, not extraordinary means, although what constitutes ordinary care is debated (5, 32, 46, 100, 111, 114).

Euthanasia is based on two fundamental legal premises: (a) the right to privacy and (b) the right to refuse treatment when informed. The competent client may decline treatment based on religious reasons, fear of pain or suffering, exhaustion of finances, and unlikelihood of recovery. The incompetent client is not allowed the right to refuse in similar situations for fear of an irrational choice. Medical practice defers to wishes of the family.

RIGHT-TO-DIE MOVEMENT, THE PATIENT SELF-DETERMINATION ACT, AND ADVANCE DIRECTIVES

Right-to-Die Movement

An increasingly publicized facet with moral and ethical aspects is the right-to-die movement, which was first begun in England, Holland, and the Scandinavian countries and gained momentum in the United States (95). Originally the Right-to-Die Society and the movement insisted that people should have the last word about their own lives, either to maintain or to discontinue treatment when ill or dying. The District of Columbia and many states have adopted **living will laws** *(right-to-die or natural death laws) that permit mentally competent adults to declare, before they are ill, that they do not want life prolonged artificially or by heroic measures.* In states with no formal legislation, living wills have been upheld in courts. Many states have brain death laws that allow withdrawal of respirators when a client no longer shows signs of brain activity. In the case of a lingering, comatose, incompetent person, the relatives, hospital ethics committee, or courts must make decisions about not instituting or withdrawing life-prolonging measures; or the person may have designated someone to have **durable power of attorney**, available in all states, *someone who can make decisions about health care, finances, and property in the event of incapacity* (9, 101).

Patient Self-Determination Act

The **Patient Self-Determination Act** became effective in December 1991. *All health care institutions or agencies receiving Medicare or Medicaid funds are required to give clients written information about these rights in order for the person to make decisions about medical care,* to formulate advance directives, and to refuse treatment.

The institution of health care providers must recognize the *living will* and *durable power of attorney for health care* documents as an advance directive. *Health care agencies must* (a) educate staff about how to talk with patients/clients or families about these issues, (b) maintain written policies and procedures for adhering to these requirements, (c) document the person's status on the medical record, and (d) not neglect or withhold treatment from the person based on the decision. This legislation has forced states to develop mechanisms for instituting the person's durable power of attorney for health care. It has created dilemmas when caring for people who are mentally incompetent (another person then makes the decision as surrogate), in cases of minors needing treatment, when the outcome of an illness is unlikely to be death or in need of heroic measures, or when the person is extremely anxious of facing unexpected death. Will the decision be too hasty? There are concerns. Has the patient fully taken into account the consequences of the treatment decision before completing the written directive? Is sufficient support given to the patient/client, surrogate, and family members? Do patients and families fully understand treatment options? Will a proxy decision maker inappropriately make decisions for a patient with intact decision-making capacities? Are qualified witnesses available? Is the advance directive being followed? Staff also need support as they implement the requirements in unusual or difficult situations (12, 21, 72, 83, 87, 92, 114).

Advance Directives

Various types of treatment directives that a person must consider are (12, 14, 21, 35, 38, 92, 105, 114):

1. The **living will**, *which states what medical treatment a person prefers or chooses to omit or refuse in case he or she cannot make a decision at the time of the illness and which indicates that the person would rather die than be kept alive by artificial or heroic measures if there is no reasonable expectation of recovery.*

2. A **surrogate or durable medical power of attorney for health care**, *which names a trusted person to act as an agent or proxy in making health care decisions in the event of the patient's inability to speak for self.*

3. An **advance medical directive**, *which is a set of documents (living will and durable power of attorney) that explains a person's end-of-life wishes and directs care when the person is no longer able to do so.*

4. A **declaration of desire for a natural death**, *which relates the decisions described above.*

Information about advance directives can be obtained from the following sources

1. MedlinePlus, National Library of Medicine, Advance Directives, www.nlm.nih.gov.
   MedlinePlus is always a good first step for any kind of health information.
2. American Academy of Family Physicians. Advance Directives and Do Not Resuscitate Orders, www.familydoctor.org.
3. Mayo Clinic. Living Wills and Other Tools to Convey Medical Wishes, www.mayoclinic.com.
   Two sites that are very accessible for learning about advance directives. Distinguishes the type of advance directives and the situations they cover.

MediaLink ● Advanced Directives

4. American Bar Association, Commission on Law and Aging, Consumer's Tool Kit for Advance Planning, www.abanet.org. This is more complex than the sites just listed but provides comprehensive information. Sets up legal planning in a structured, sequential manner.

5. Caring Connections, Download Your State's Advance Directives, www.caringinfo.org.

   It is important that these documents conform to state requirements. This Website allows you to download the forms appropriate for your state.

6. Formerly the Electronic Living Will Registry, now called U.S. Living Will Registry, allows an individual's directives to be downloaded from any computer. The registry can be reached at:

   U.S. Living Will Registry
   523 Westfield Ave., P.O. Box 2789
   Westfield, NJ 07091-2789
   Phone: 1-800-LIV-WILL (1-800-548-9455)
   Fax: 1-908-654-1919
   www.uslivingwillregistry.com

Information about advance directives in Canada is available at:

7. Health Law Institute, Dalhousie University, The End of Life Project, Advance Directives in Canada, Frequently Asked Questions.

The consequences of ignoring the living will and the inconsistency that can arise are explained by several authors (21, 28, 123, 124). Having instructions about and planning for the living will document can decrease death anxiety (28, 95). Advance directive decisions may be influenced by the cultural, religious, or racial background of the person (3, 14, 31, 38, 50, 51, 82, 124).

Physicians fear indictment for homicide or aiding suicide, even when following the person's living will, although these laws in all states grant immunity to health care professionals who comply with the declaration. Further, in some states there is a penalty if the physician does not comply. Relatives may sue the physician and/or hospital that refuses to follow the client's wishes reflected in the living will. (Legally, the physician may be charged with battery.)

ASSISTED SUICIDE

Assisted suicide is defined by the American Nurses Association (ANA) as *making a means of suicide available to the patient with the knowledge of the person's intended use of the equipment, medication, object, or weapon. It differs from euthanasia, where the professional directly ends the patient's life.* The ANA has issued a statement against assisted suicide or acting deliberately to terminate a pa-

tient's life. And in most states such action is illegal. The nurse's role is to assist the person, to comfort, and to be present and available as a support (19, 46, 48, 62, 77). Kirk (72) explains how Oregon's Death with Dignity Act, enacted June 5, 1998, affects nursing practice with terminally ill adults. There is potential for neglect of palliative care and the consideration of all options when deliberately promoting the dying process (24, 26, 56, 81, 117, 121, 122).

Certain measures, when covered by a physician's order, fall within ethical principles of double effect, patient autonomy, or not practicing futile interventions (2, 46):

1. Giving a patient who is hypotensive enough morphine to control his or her pain. (Here the principle of double effect applies, in which an action intended to reduce pain and suffering is permissible even if it may have the unintended effect of death.)

2. Giving a dyspneic patient enough morphine to control his or her pain symptoms. (Again, double effect applies.)

3. Sedating a symptomatic or distressed patient at his or her request. (The principle of autonomy applies.)

4. Withholding or withdrawing nutrition or hydration at the request of a patient. (Autonomy applies.)

5. At the patient's and family's request, not treating infections such as pneumonia because recovery will not affect the patient's primary disease process or increase quality of life, and will prolong the patient's suffering. (The principle of not practicing futile intervention applies.)

Benner (7) describes the conflict between heart and conscience when her father, terminally ill with chronic obstructive pulmonary disease and unable to live without a ventilator, made it known he did not want to live that way and wanted the ventilator removed. The family respected his wishes and remained with him. Versed and morphine were given to ease anxiety and pain and to enable him to rest until he died. Death did not come quickly. A new lung infection was not treated. Other medications (heparin, digoxin, and theophylline) were discontinued. A compassionate and competent staff were valued by the family. Both the staff and family continued to talk with the father, although he was in deep sleep, to treat him as a person with dignity and worth. The final pain, twinges of guilt, and self-doubt are poignantly described even though the family had followed the father's wishes. It took him 10 days to die of respiratory failure. Respect for the father as an intelligent man, capable of deciding the difference between living and lingering, respect for his sense of pride and dignity, and respect for him as a person helped to ease the pain for the family (7).

It is possible to buy manuals on how to commit suicide. The demand for these books is increasing as the public realizes it is illegal for doctors to practice euthanasia and that often doctors feel forced to prolong life, in whatever condition. The manuals argue against suicide when the problem is a distortion of judgment or a psychiatric disorder but give a factual guide about the least painful and most effective measures. Violent methods such as shooting, jumping, and hanging are counseled against because they are too traumatic for the survivors.

In contrast, the **Samaritans**, *an international suicide prevention group, professionals who work in hospice care, and the Medical Association of each country* have been sharply critical of such manuals,

---

Practice Point

Nurses and other health care professionals are increasingly having to face questions of conscience, ethics, morals, and legalities in relation to what to say to the client and relatives and whether to assist with initiating heroic measures when it is known that the client does not want them or whether to disconnect life-support machines.

believing that they may pressure terminally ill, depressed, or elderly people to exit early because they believe they are a burden and unwanted. It is as if society fosters rejection instead of seeking solutions to the problem.

According to groups such as the Samaritans, withholding food and water or discontinuing a feeding tube and intravenous fluids to the chronically or terminally ill or those in a persistent vegetative state may become a form of passive euthanasia and assisted suicide if the totality of the situation is not considered. The nurse is taught to be an advocate for the client—a very special charge and a difficult but committed kind of caring related to the client's needs and rights (19, 24, 25, 47, 59, 91, 99, 100, 104, 105, 108, 119, 125). The specifics of each situation must be considered in terms of the medical condition of the patient and the chances for recovery and improved quality of life, the alternatives for palliative care that are possible, the values of the patient and the family, the present wishes of the patient if they can be determined, and the possibilities that technologic means may induce further suffering. Most health care institutions have an ethics committee that can perform consultations and provide a representative to conduct meetings with the patient and family regarding deliberation of such issues and options for further care. However, the timely use of such committees and the presentation of such options to patients and families are severely underutilized.

Several legal cases concerning clients in a persistent vegetative state surviving solely because of the use of respirators and tube feeding have come before the courts, beginning with the Karen Quinlan case in 1977. At least 66% of the court rulings in these cases have allowed the removal of life-support equipment. Many of these people were chronically ill. The cases of Nancy Cruzan and Christine Busalacchi in Missouri involved discontinuance of feeding and hydration. Nancy Cruzan died in 1990, 12 days after a Missouri judge ruled that her feeding tube be discontinued. Three previous co-workers had testified that she had said she "never wanted to live life as a vegetable" (4, 49, 62, 79, 123). In the 1990s, state legislatures began to study bills that would affect an expanded group of physically and chronically ill clients. These bills included the Durable Power of Attorney for Health Care, Health Care Surrogate, and Health Care Consent bills.

The **Hemlock Society** *believes people should be allowed to die. In fact, the society advocates lethal injection as more humane with less suffering.* The international **Anti-Euthanasia Task Force** *believes such action is the forerunner of outright killing of sick, disabled, and vulnerable people,* rather than having a society and professionals committed to caring for these people. The questions to decide concern who will die when and who will decide (4, 5, 95).

Guidelines to help you determine reasons for a patient's desire to die and how to respond without compromising professional principles are presented (2, 46):

1. Talk with the patient about suicidal statements.
2. Assess emotional as well as physical pain and work to reduce both through a variety of pain management methods.
3. Allow the patient to express fears about "losing his (or her) mind" as a result of the disease or aging process and how this can be prevented, prepared for, or coped with in late stages of AIDS, brain cancer, or liver or kidney disease.

4. Assess and treat underlying depression, which is likely to remove the desire to die.
5. Explore losses with the patient and how to cope with or overcome these, and enhance the person's autonomy and control to the extent possible.
6. Discuss the patient's idea of death with him or her. Encourage the person to make plans via advance directives or options of hospice care.
7. Encourage the patient to discuss faith, hope, and meaning of life. Refer to pastoral care.
8. Listen nonjudgmentally, with compassion and concern.
9. Encourage the person to do what he or she can for self and to ask others for help when necessary.
10. When thoughts of suicide persist, the principle of confidentiality does not prevent you from sharing the patient's disclosure with the physician and health care team, or from facilitating discussion between the patient and family.
11. Discuss options for palliative care and hospice with the person (24, 26, 56, 81, 117, 121, 122). Many people do not know about these options and how they can control the distressing symptoms of an illness without resorting to suicide.

As people live longer, they fear there may be a longer period of frailty, disability, depression, and social disconnectedness. Some will choose death rather than survive with pain, isolation, tubes, and machines. There is an increasing movement for the person who is mentally alert but in great pain or disability to make a life termination decision (2, 20, 26, 46, 56, 81, 123, 125).

Nurses must decide the meaning of being a nurse and how that meaning applies to caring for the seriously, chronically, terminally, or vegetatively ill. Further, nurses must:

1. Listen carefully to clients and families about their concerns.
2. Educate society to think and act rationally.
3. Act on values about the sanctity of life and health.
4. Engage in research about the life promotion effects of imagery, faith, prayer, energy work such as Healing Touch, and other complementary methods of healing.
5. Publicize healing events, including the "miracles," so that clients and families can be encouraged and believe in remission and recovery.
6. Let live and let die, discerning when the fight must be for life and when death is inevitable, acceptable, and natural; discerning when to engage in life extension, when to continue life support, and when "to let go" (patient, family, nurses, and physicians).

This issue encompasses the autonomy and individual rights of the patient, the nurse's or physician's role, and society's stake. Each perspective is a complicated issue. We need to establish safeguards so that the true wishes of the patient can be expressed and legally accounted for. Many people know they can write living will directives but do not do so.

The health care professional has seen so much technology for life support that much of the human perspective on dying can be lost. So much emphasis has been placed on scarce resources (e.g., organs), being a gatekeeper, and being an entrepreneur that the concept of aggressive, compassionate, palliative care has been lost,

Case Situation

Mrs. Morton is a 94-year-old widow who has resided in the same farmhouse since her marriage. She has a 45-year history of cardiac disease. She now has a pacemaker and daily takes medication for her heart. She has had a bilateral modified mastectomy but has had no further recurrence of cancer. Several times she has been hospitalized, and during the last two hospitalizations she required resuscitation after suffering cardiac arrest.

Mrs. Morton is a very determined, devout, Christian woman, and each time she has been gravely ill, she has proclaimed her faith and has been discharged to her home. She firmly refused admittance to a senior residence center after the last hospitalization, insisting that if she had a visiting nurse and continued help from her grandson, she could live alone in her farm home. Her grandson, who has shopped for her for the last 10 years, agreed to do more tasks as necessary. Reluctantly, her physician agreed and ordered home health aide and nurse services. Because of her grave condition and inability to walk except for a few steps, the physician also made occasional home visits.

Mrs. Morton is chronically ill. In fact, her cardiovascular condition is so grave that she is considered terminally ill. Within the principles of the euthanasia movement, she could have chosen to die the last time she required resuscitation. However, Mrs. Morton prefers living on in her state of decline.

In the 9 months since her discharge from the hospital, Mrs. Morton has regained her strength and her circulation has improved. She now walks in her home with a walker and cooks meals for herself and her grandson. She does receive help with bathing and vacuuming. Thus she contributes to the employment of several people. Recently her divorced granddaughter, Jean, and two great-grandchildren have come to live with her because Jean is on welfare and cannot pay rent and other expenses.

Mrs. Morton acknowledges that having three more people in her home is stressful but says she believes she must help them. She has loaned, or given, considerable money from her farm income and Social Security checks to all three of her grandchildren and several of her great-grandchildren. Thus she contributes to the economic support of three, and sometimes more, people. She doubts that anyone will ever repay her.

Because Mrs. Morton is very alert, friendly, and indeed very wise, she is a joy to visit. When her many friends come to visit, she shares a piece of cake she has baked and chats about local news. She reminisces some, but not excessively. She seldom complains, even briefly. Although her physical condition is marginal, her mental health is excellent. Possibly because of those healthy components, her physical condition has improved. Mrs. Morton is very much alive and looking forward to her 95th birthday. It is fortunate the emergency team responded by resuscitating Mrs. Morton during her last hospitalization. Indeed, many people would have felt the loss.

Contributed by Ruth Murray, EdD, MSN, N-NAP, FAAN.

except in hospice care. However, palliative care units in hospitals have been established, and there is a new emphasis on this level of care (24–26, 56, 61, 81, 100). Terminal illness and suffering must be seen as a challenge and a responsibility no matter how the health care professional interprets the euthanasia issue. Many references are available, for much has been written about types of euthanasia, moral-ethical issues, and dying and death. This chapter provides only an overview of the subject. The Case Situation describes issues related to extending life and dying.

It is important for you to struggle with the values and issues of death—accidental death, long-term dying, active or passive euthanasia, and right-to-die choices—and consequently the issues and values of life. You will often be asked about your thoughts and beliefs; it is impossible to be value-free, but you can be nonjudgmental and accepting of another's values. How you proceed with nursing care of the chronically ill or dying person will be influenced by your beliefs. Do not force your beliefs and values on another, but often the client will appreciate your open sharing of values and beliefs. Such sharing may even give him or her energy to continue to live, with quality of life, against overwhelming odds. Certainly do what you can so that the person does not face dying and death alone.

Developmental Concepts of Death

As you work with people of all ages, well and ill, you will need to understand how people perceive death. A review is given here of how the child, adolescent, and adult may perceive death. The concept of death is understood differently by persons in the different life eras because of general maturity, experience, ability to form ideas, and understanding of cause and effect. Culture, the religious beliefs, and the historical era also influence the concept of death, how to grieve, and customs for handling the dead person and the mourners.

CHILDREN'S CONCEPTS OF DEATH

Nagy (86) *found three stages in the child's concept of death:* (a) death is reversible, until age 5 years; (b) death is personified, ages 5 to 9; and (c) death is final and inevitable, after age 9 or 10.

The child younger than age 5 sees death as reversible, a temporary departure like sleep or a trip, being less alive or a decrease in life functions, being very still or unable to move. Children think grown people will not die—nothing can happen to them.

There is much curiosity about what happens to the person after death. The child connects death with external events, what is eaten, cemeteries, and absence. He or she thinks dead persons are still capable of growth, that they can breathe and eat and feel, and that they know what is happening on earth. Death is disturbing because it separates people from each other and because life in the grave seems dull and unpleasant. Fear of death in the child of this age may be related to parental expression of anger; presence of intrafamily stress such as arguing and fighting; physical restraints, especially during illness; or punishment for misdeeds. At times the child feels anger toward the parents because of their restrictions and wishes they would go away or be dead. Guilt feelings arising from these thoughts may add to the fear of death. Several authors discuss ways to help the young child cope with loss related to death of an attachment figure or close family member (30, 34, 44, 57, 58, 63, 66, 86, 95, 112, 113). It is important to help a young child deal with death, answer questions, and grieve, and to be loving and supportive.

The child from ages 5 to 9 accepts the existence of death as final and not likelife. Around age 7 (at the Concrete Operations Stage), he or she thinks of death as final, irreversible, and universal. Death is perceived as a person, such as an angel, a frightening clown, or a monster who carries off people, usually bad people, in the night. Personal death can be avoided; the child will not die if he or she runs faster than death, locks the door, or tricks death unless there is bad luck. Dressing in some Halloween costumes (e.g., as a ghost or skeleton) helps the child feel a mastery over the scary, the bad, or death. The biological changes that result in death, are not generally understood. Parental disciplining techniques inadvertently add to fear of death if they threaten that bad things will happen to the child. Traumatic situations also can arouse fear of death (9, 30, 34, 44, 57, 58, 63, 66, 86, 95, 112, 113).

The child, after age 9 or 10, realizes that death is inevitable, is final, happens according to certain laws, and will one day happen to him or her. If he or she is terminally ill, the child may acknowledge approaching death before the parents do (82). Death is the end of life, like the withering of flowers or falling of leaves, and results from internal processes. Death is associated with being enclosed in a coffin without air, being slowly eaten by bugs, and slow rotting unless cremation is taught. The child may express thoughts about an afterlife, depending on ideas expressed by parents and other adults and their religious philosophy (9, 30, 34, 57, 66, 86, 112, 113).

Death is an abstract concept, and Nagy's stages offer a guide. However, not all children's thinking about death fits into those stages. Children may have a concept of death that contains ideas from all three stages. The ability to think abstractly is acquired slowly and to varying degrees by different people. Usually the child is unable to understand death until he or she is preadolescent or in the chum stage, for through a chum he or she learns to care for someone else as much as for self, and loss and grief are better understood.

The child's ideas and anxiety about separation and death and the ability to handle loss are influenced by many factors (30, 34, 44, 66): (a) experiences with rejecting or punitive parents, (b) strong sibling rivalry, (c) domestic or social violence, (d) loss, illness, or death in the family, (e) reaction and teaching of adults to separa-

tion or death, and (f) ability to conceptualize and assimilate the experience. Children who live in a war-torn area have a more complete and different concept of death than do children who grew up in a peaceful environment (57, 95).

The child may think of the parent's death as deliberate abandonment for which he or she is responsible and expect death to get him or her next. The child may fear death is catching and for that reason avoid a friend whose parent has just died. If the child perceives death as sleep, he or she may fear sleep to the point of being unable to go to bed at night or even to nap. He or she may blame the surviving parent for the other parent's death, a feeling that is compounded when the surviving parent is so absorbed in personal grief that little attention is given to the child. The child may use magical thinking, believing that wishing to have the parent return will bring the parent back (9, 30, 34, 44, 57, 95, 112, 113).

The child's fascination with and fear of death may be expressed through the games he or she plays or concern about sick pets or a dead person. Short-lived pets such as fish or gerbils help the child deal with death. Parents should handle these concerns and the related questions in a relaxed, loving manner.

Self-Knowledge of Death

Can the sick child realize his or her own approaching death? Studies by Corr (29, 30) and Waechter (112, 113) showed that despite widespread efforts by adults to shield sick children from awareness of their diagnosis and the inevitability of death, the school-aged children knew of their impending death, although they might not say so directly to their parents. The evasiveness and false cheerfulness of the adults, either parents or staff, did not hide their real feelings from the child.

Often children know more about death than adults may realize, especially chronically or terminally ill children. Children are harmed by what they do not know, by what they are not told, and by their misconceptions. Educate parents about the need to explain honestly and on the child's level of understanding.

Often children acknowledge their lack of future and may say, "I'm not going anywhere." They may request an early celebration of a birthday or holiday. Parents should monitor the child's television viewing carefully, for programs often give an unrealistic impression of death, for example, cartoons and movies that show that death is reversible (or that there is survival or no harmful effects after obviously lethal injuries). A number and variety of secular books are available. The parents' religious denomination can also supply relevant literature.

Children's Attendance at Funerals

There are age-based guidelines for a child's involvement in a funeral. Children from 2 to 3 years can view the body or be given a brief explanation, depending on their level of understanding and relationship to the deceased. But 3- to 6-year-olds benefit from a short private funeral home visit or the service itself. Seven- to 9-year-old children should attend the funeral unless they resist. Eleven- and 12-year-olds can be included in making funeral arrangements and the service itself, if the parents and child desire. In the teen years, friends of the adolescent should be encouraged to share the grief, and all should be treated as adults (see **Box 17-1**, Dos and Don'ts for Discussing Death with Children).

<table>
<tr><td>

BOX 17-1   **Dos and Don'ts for Discussing Death with Children**

DO

1. Ask the child what he or she is feeling. Bring up the subject of death naturally in the context of a dead pet, a book character, television show, movie, or news item.
2. Help the child have a funeral for a dead pet.
3. Help the child realize he or she is not responsible for the death.
4. Tell the child what has happened on his or her level (but not in morbid detail).
5. Explain the funeral service briefly beforehand; attendance depends on the child's age and wishes.
6. Answer questions honestly, with responses geared to the child's age.
7. Remember that expressions of pain, anger, loneliness, or aloneness do not constitute symptoms of an illness but are part of a natural process of grieving.
8. Help the child realize that the adults are also grieving and feeling upset, anger, despair, and guilt.

DO NOT

1. Admonish the child not to cry. It is a universal way to show grief and anxiety.
2. Tell a mystical story about the loss of the person; it could cause confusion and anxiety.
3. Give long, exclusively detailed explanations beyond the level of understanding.
4. Associate death with sleep, which could result in chronic sleep disturbances.
5. Force the child to attend funerals or ignore signs of grieving in the child.

</td></tr>
</table>

ADOLESCENT'S CONCEPTS OF DEATH

Adolescents ponder the meaning of life. They are concerned about their bodies and a personal future. They are relatively realistic in thinking, but because of dependency–independency conflicts with parents and efforts to establish individuality, there is a low tolerance for accepting death. The healthy young person perceives self as invincible and may engage in risky behavior. He or she seldom thinks about death, particularly as something that will happen to the self, although media reports of school violence have focused the thoughts. He or she fears a lingering death and usually views death in religious or philosophic terms. He or she believes death means lack of fulfillment; there is too much to lose with death (9, 29, 30, 66, 86, 89, 90, 95).

Because of inexperience in coping with crisis and the viewpoints of death and wanting to appear in control, the adolescent may not cry at the death of a loved one, peer, or parent. Instead he or she may continue to play games, listen to records, spend more time at the computer, engage in antisocial behavior, withdraw into seclusion or vigorous study, or go about usual activities as if nothing happened. If the young person cannot talk, such activities provide a catharsis. Mastery of feelings sometimes comes through a detailed account of the parent's death to a peer or by displacing grief feelings onto a pet. Also, the adolescent may fantasize the dead parent as perfect or feel much the way a younger child would about loss of a parent. Often the adolescent's behavior hides the fact that he or she is in mourning but carries on an internal dialogue with the dead person for weeks or months. Be attuned to the thoughts and feelings of the adolescent who has faced death of a loved one so that you can be approachable and helpful.

ADULT'S CONCEPTS OF DEATH

The adult's attitudes toward and concept about dying and death are influenced by experiential, cultural, and religious backgrounds. A number of references provide information (3, 9, 13, 33, 43, 45, 60, 71, 73–76, 94, 95, 97, 104, 124). The adult's reactions to death are also influenced by the experience of death of loved ones or of others, and whether the death event is sudden or has been anticipated. Fear of death is often more related to the process of dying than to the fact of death—to mutilation, deformity, isolation, pain, loss of control over body functions and one's life, fear of the unknown, and permanent collapse and disintegration. Premonitions about coming death, sometimes correct, may occur.

Anticipation of Death

There are four responses to viewing death: positivist, negativist, activist, and passivist. Fear or anxiety about death is less in the person who believes that most of the valued goals have been attained. The **positivist** *is a person who is likely to reflect positively on present activities and death as an aspect of the future.* The **negativist** *believes that the time left is short, fears loss of ego integration, wishes that he or she could relive part of life, and fears death.* Refer to Erikson's concept of self-despair rather than ego integrity in Chapter 16. ∞ The **activist** *perceives death as diminishing the opportunity for continued fulfillment of goals. The achieved goals do not offset the fear of death. Death as a foreclosing of ambition is more distasteful than the prospect of loss of life.* Finally, the **passivist** *may not view death with concern or fear but as a respite from disappointments of life because attempts to attain life goals may have been so overshadowed by failure. Death may be accepted as a positive adjustment to life* (9, 45, 95).

Females are more likely to integrate the anticipation and actual experience of widowhood than are males, and greater stability of friendships through the life cycle eases adaptation to loss of spouse. The widow is likely to seek intimacy with same-sex friends, who replace family ties in late life.

The importance of will to live, or lack of it, has been recognized by nurses and others for many years. The person may not be terminally ill yet, but because of loss of a loved one, loss of feelings of self-worth and usefulness, boredom, or disillusionment with life, may lose the will to live and rapidly decline and die. Often there are few or no causes for death apparent on autopsy.

Meaning of Death

To the adult facing death because of illness, particularly the elderly, death may have many meanings. Death may convey some positive meanings: a teacher of transcendental truths uncomprehended during life, an adventure, a friend who brings an end to pain and suffering, or an escape from an unbearable situation into a new life without the present difficulties. Highly creative artists and scientists who believe they have successfully contributed their talents to society and people with a strong belief system may have little fear of death. Death may also convey negative meanings: the great destroyer who is to be fought, punishment and separation, and a means of vengeance to force others to give more affection than they were willing to give in the past (9, 10, 43, 45, 73–76, 80).

The person who is dying may have suicidal thoughts or attempt suicide. Suicide is a rebellion against death, a way to cheat death's control over him or her. The elder may be more likely to commit suicide if the spouse has died or as a way to avoid pain, loneliness, or helplessness.

The time comes in an illness or in later life when both the person and the survivors-to-be believe death would be better than continuing to suffer. The client has the conviction that death is inevitable and desirable and works through feelings until finally he or she has little or no anxiety, depression, or conflicts about dying. The body becomes a burden, and death holds a promise. There is little incentive to live.

Near-Death Experience

A phenomenon that has gained public interest through Moody's publication *Life After Life* (85) is the **near-death experience** *of "coming back to life" after just being declared clinically dead or near dead.* The stories (those told to Moody and those heard before and since) have a sameness, although details and interpretation depend on the personality and beliefs of the person (17, 40, 69, 71, 94, 97, 103, 107, 126).

There is additional publicity about men and women of a wide range of age, education, background, religious and nonreligious belief, and temperament who came close to death and had an **out-of-body experience**, *a feeling that one's consciousness or center of awareness is at a different location than one's body, often reported in relation to being resuscitated* (69, 94, 96, 97, 103, 126). Olson (94) compares these experiences with other states of consciousness, such as dreams, reverie, hypnotic states or hallucinations on falling asleep or awakening, and pathologic states such as hallucinations and depersonalization. When they recall what happened to them after they returned to consciousness, the people describe a sense of comfort, beauty, peace, and bliss. As a result of this experience, the person finds compelling meaning and reason in innumerable small experiences of life. There is a new and deeper spiritual dimension. Nothing is taken for granted. The routine or trivial aspects of life are seen and heard more clearly, and dying and death are viewed from a different perspective than before (39, 69, 71, 97).

Research with people who have been successfully resuscitated or who have been nearly dead and then lived shows that features of the near-death experience include the following (16–18, 39, 69, 71, 85, 97, 103):

1. Feeling of being drawn through a long, dark tunnel or passage at the end of which is a bright light.
2. Looking down from a spiritual body on the resuscitation efforts of the health care team on one's own physical body.
3. Awareness of loud noises or vibrations.

4. Recognizing the presence of and communicating with dead relatives or other deceased loved ones who were there to help make the transition from life to death.
5. Seeing one's own life in review; watching one's own life pass before him or her in color, three dimensions, and third person.
6. Being met or confronted by a brilliant light or many intense colors and the Creator, God, Jesus, a light, or a being of love who asks the person to provide a review of his or her life.
7. Being given acceptance in the presence of the brilliant light, being in the presence of great love, even though the person may feel embarrassment or rejection about the past life.
8. Reaching a threshold but drawing back because of a sense of responsibility for others on earth.

The person may have difficulty describing the feelings, but there has been more researched and written. Individuals are more willing to share what several decades ago was not talked about. People who have experienced a positive near-death experience speak of a spiritual encounter that parallels the writings in the Bible in relation to the afterlife, a paradise, or heaven. They express a stronger spiritual faith and no fear of death. They report a feeling of bliss about a life to come and new meaning in this life. Some people have had a negative, unpleasant, or fear-producing near-death experience; they remain afraid to die unless they turn their life around spiritually.

Health care professionals can cite case studies that verify near-death experiences. Anesthesia, drugs, hallucinations, or wishful fantasies do not account for these experiences. Clinical death has been recorded by absence of electric activity in the brain for 3 to 30 minutes in patients, although at times adequate brain function continued when heart function stopped. Often the person describes exactly what happened when the medical team was working to revive him or her as if the person were looking on from above.

Papowitz (96) describes near-death experiences that have been recounted by various people. She describes guidelines for caring for the person who is being resuscitated in light of the fact that the person may be able to hear and see what is happening. She describes ways to help the person talk about the near-death experience if it is recalled and the importance of listening and taking the necessary time to allow the person to express emotions. Respect that some people view this as a religious experience; some do not. Ask for permission to share the account with family members as a way to enrich their understanding. This trend toward talking about, investigating, and studying death points to a willingness to confront finally an absolute fact: Each of us will die. There is evidence of life after death. Each person must integrate this information and come to terms with it in his or her own life: in memories, memorials, or the mystery of eternity.

Nearing-Death Awareness

Nearing-death awareness differs from near-death experiences. It is an *extraordinary awareness of how death will unfold and what the person will need to die well. This awareness is often communicated symbolically or in obscure messages by people who are dying slowly.* Typically the person describes seeing or being visited by a dead

INTERVENTIONS FOR HEALTH PROMOTION

Use the following principles when caring for the patient who is manifesting a nearing-death awareness and teach these to the family and friends as well (18):

1. *Pay attention to everything the dying person says. All communication has meaning.* Keep a pen and pad at the bedside so notes can be jotted down on any unusual comments or gestures made by the patient.
2. Watch for signs in the patient's behavior that may indicate nearing-death awareness: glassy-eyed look, distractedness, strange gestures (pointing at or waving to someone you cannot see), efforts to get out of bed for no apparent reason.
3. Respond to the patient's statements with gentle, open-ended questions that encourage him or her to explain. When a patient whose mother died long ago says, "My mother's waiting for me," you could say, "I'm so glad she's close to you. Tell me about it."

4. *Accept what the patient says; do not argue.* Do not insist on reality, for example, "Your mother died 10 years ago." When a patient speaks in metaphors, respond in kind. If the patient says, "I've got to catch a train," you might say, "Do you want to get on?" "Do you know anyone on the train?" "Where are you going?"
5. The person may describe something not observed by others, for example, "I keep seeing someone gliding back and forth in front of me" or "Oh, Mary, you are so beautiful" (referring to the Virgin Mary), or "There's been a lot of music and noise around here today." Ask the person to describe as much as possible. Relate what is said to beliefs about "Jesus is coming" or "going to heaven" and talk about approaching death.
6. If you do not understand what the patient is saying, admit it. You might say, "I think you're telling me something important, but I'm not getting it. Don't give up trying—I want to know."

---

loved one or a spiritual figure, and may be heard talking with this visitor. (These are not pathologic hallucinations.) The person may talk of getting in line for a journey (departure from this life) while lying in the hospital bed. (The person is not confused.) The person may call to someone, seeking reconciliation and forgiveness (15, 18, 39, 40, 69, 71, 95). The person may speak of a reunion or a wonderful place; describe heaven, Jesus, or the Virgin Mary; talk about having a dream; or talk about a certain day being sad (and die on that day). For example, a hospitalized elderly farmer, about 12 hours before his death, told a visitor how he had seen "a beautiful man walk back and forth at the foot of the bed all day." "And it's been noisy around here—music and like moving furniture," he added. The visitor confirmed with the hospital staff that he had had no visitors and no furniture was moved. The visitor later felt certain the man had had some heavenly glimpses and had, according to his belief, seen Jesus. This elderly farmer would not have ordinarily called any man "beautiful."

Family members may think the person is losing mental ability when they go through unusual experiences. Reassure them by explaining the nearing-death awareness phenomenon and the need to stay with and talk to the person, and listen and learn. A spiritual care provider should be called to be with the person and family, if desired.

If the patient dies alone, family and staff often express guilt. The patient may have chosen to die alone to spare his or her loved ones. Let the family know this could be considered the dying person's gift to them (18).

The patient may need the family to acknowledge what's happening and give permission to die. If the patient is restless, picking at self or clothing, or struggling, it is often helpful to tell him or her "it's OK to let go," to convey the person will be missed but the

family will be all right (18) and that the person will be lovingly remembered for the life he or she lived.

Keep in mind that dying patients in any setting—intensive care unit, emergency department, home, or hospice—may express nearing-death awareness. Talk to co-workers about this phenomenon, and make sure to chart patients' comments and behavior suggesting it. If we listen with care to our dying patients, we may be able to comprehend their special awareness and help loved ones to share in it—to receive the parting gifts the dying want to give. We, too, may benefit. We have much to learn about dying. Our patients are the best possible teachers.

Behavior and Feelings of the Person Facing Death

When death comes accidentally and swiftly, there is no time to prepare for death. However, death is a normal, expected event to the old, and most older people anticipate death with equanimity and without fear. The crisis is not death but where and how the person will die. The prospect of dying in nonnormal, unexpected circumstances creates the crisis. Widowhood is more expected as the person ages.

AWARENESS OF DYING

When the person approaches death gradually by virtue of many years lived or from a terminal illness, there are several models to describe how he or she will go through a generally predictable sequence of feelings and behavior. Yet, not everyone goes through all of the described behaviors and feelings or exact sequence. However, the models help us understand the person.

Glaser and Strauss (52–54) describe the stages of awareness that the terminally ill or dying person may experience, depending on the behavior of the health team and family, which, in turn, influences interaction with others.

Closed awareness *occurs when the person is dying but has neither been informed nor made the discovery. He or she may not be knowledgeable about the signs of terminal illness, and the health team and family may not want the person to know for fear that "he will go to pieces."* Maintaining closed awareness is less likely to occur if the dying person is at home.

The client and family have no opportunity to review their lives, plan realistically for the family's future, and close life with the proper rituals. Even legal and business transactions of the client may suffer as he or she tries to carry on life as usual, starts unrealistic plans, and works less feverishly on unfinished business than he or she would if the prognosis were known.

Despite the intentions and efforts of the health team and family, however, the client may become increasingly aware. He or she has a lot of time to observe the surroundings, even when very ill. He or she has time to think about the nonverbal cues and indirect comments from the staff, the inconsistent answers, and the new and perplexing symptoms that do not get better despite reassurance that they will improve. At times, others may relax their guard when they think he or she does not understand and say something about the prognosis that is understood.

Suspicious awareness *develops. The person may or may not voice suspicions to others, and they are likely to deny his or her verbal suspicions. The client watches more closely for signs to confirm suspicions.* The changing physical status; the nonverbal and verbal communications of others, with their hidden meanings; the silence; the intensity of or challenges in care; and the briskness of conversation may inadvertently tell or imply what he or she suspects.

Mutual pretense *occurs when staff and family become aware that the client knows he or she is dying, but all continue to pretend otherwise. There is no conversation about impending death unless the client initiates it, although on occasion staff members may purposely drop cues because they believe the client has a right to know.*

There has been a movement toward no pretense, where there is frank discussion between patient and health care providers. The talks may indicate the family members are reluctant to let go or are letting go prematurely. The patient and family are helped to resolve the mutual pretense (16–18).

Open awareness *exists when the person and family are fully aware of the terminal condition, although neither may realize the nearness nor all the complications of the condition and the mode of death.* With the certainty of death established, the person may plan to end life in accord with personal ideas about proper dying, finish important work, and make appropriate plans for and farewells with the family. He or she and the family can talk frankly, make plans, share grief, and support each other. The anguish is not reduced but can be faced together.

The health team in the hospital has ideas, although not always verbalized, about how the person ought to die morally and stylistically. These ideas may conflict with or differ from the ideas of the client and family, and with the cultural backgrounds of the person. The wishes of the client and the family should always have priority, particularly when they ask that no heroic measures be taken to prolong life. Extra privileges, special requests, or the client's discharge to the family can be granted. Most people wish to die without pain, with dignity, in privacy, and with loved ones nearby. Often dying in the hospital precludes both privacy and dignity, and the health team should continuously work to provide these rights.

SEQUENCE OF REACTIONS TO APPROACHING DEATH

When the person becomes aware of the diagnosis and prognosis, whether he or she is told directly or learns by advancing through the stages of awareness discussed previously, he or she and the family may experience a sequence of reactions described by Kübler-Ross (73–76). Although such reactions appear common, any fixed sequence does not appear to be the reality. Grief reactions, whether of the dying person or the significant others, appear and reappear to be worked through as time proceeds (68).

Denial and Isolation

Denial and **isolation** are the *initial and natural reactions when the person learns of terminal illness:* "It can't be true. I don't believe it's me." The person may go through a number of rituals to support this denial, even to the point of finding another doctor. He or she needs time to mobilize resources. Denial serves as a necessary buffer against overwhelming anxiety.

The person is in **denial** *when he or she talks about the future, avoids talking about the illness or the death of self or others, or persistently pursues cheery topics.* Recognize the client's need, respond to this behavior, and let him or her set the pace in conversation. Later the person will gradually consider the possibility of the prognosis. Anxiety will lessen, and the need to deny will diminish (106). Kübler-Ross found that few people maintain denial until the end of life (73–74, 106).

Psychological isolation *occurs when the client talks about the illness, death, or mortality intellectually but without emotion, as if these topics were not relevant. Initially the idea of death is recognized, although the feeling is repressed.* Gradually feelings about death will be less isolating and the client will begin to face death but still maintain hope.

If the client continues to deny for a prolonged time despite advancing symptoms, he or she will need much warmth, compassion, and support as death comes closer. Your contacts with the client may consist of sitting in silence, using touch communication, giving meticulous physical care, conveying acceptance and security, and looking in on him or her frequently. If denial is extensive, he or she cannot grieve or face the inevitable separation.

Practice Point

In your practice, assessment and intervention must be individualized. Do not assume that everyone is experiencing each stage as the research results describe.

Anger

The second reaction, **anger**, *occurs with acknowledgment of the reality of the prognosis. It is necessary for an eventual acceptance of approaching death. As denial and isolation decrease, anger, envy, and resentment of the living are felt.* In the United States, direct expression of anger is unacceptable, so this stage is difficult for the client and others. Anger is displaced onto things or people: "The doctor is no good," "the food is no good," "the hospital is no good," "the nurses are neglectful," and "people don't care." The family also bears the brunt of the anger.

Anger results when the person realizes life will be interrupted before he or she finishes everything planned. Everything reminds the person of life, and he or she feels soon-to-be-forgotten. He or she may make angry demands, frequently ring the bell, manipulate and control others, and generally make the self heard. The person is convincing self and others that he or she is not yet dead and forgotten.

Do not take the anger personally. The dying person whose life will soon end needs empathy. The person who is respected, understood, and given time and attention will soon lower the angry voice and decrease demands. The person will realize he or she is considered a valuable person who will be cared for and yet allowed to function at maximum potential as long as possible. Your calm approach will lower anxiety and defensive anger.

Bargaining

The third reaction, **bargaining**, *occurs when the person tries to enter into some kind of agreement that may postpone death. He or she may try to be on the best behavior. He or she knows the bargaining procedure and hopes to be granted the special wish—an extension of life, preferably without pain. Although the person will initially ask for no more than one deadline or postponement of death, he or she will continue the good behavior and will promise to devote life to some special cause if allowed to live.*

Bargaining may be life promoting. As the person continues to hope for life, to express faith in God's willingness to let him or her live, and to engage actively in positive, health-promoting practices, the body's physical defenses may be enhanced by mental or emotional processes yet unknown. This process may account for those not-so-uncommon cases in which the person has a prolonged, unexpected remission during a malignant disease process. Hope and faith, which are involved in bargaining and which you can support, give each person a chance for more effective treatment and care as new discoveries are made.

Depression

Depression is the fourth and normal reaction and *occurs when the person gets weaker, needs increasing treatment, and worries about mounting medical costs and even necessities. Role reversal and related problems add to the strain.* Depression about past losses and the present condition; feelings of shame about the illness, sometimes interpreted as punishment for past deeds; and hopelessness enshroud the person and extend to the loved ones.

Educate the family and staff about this stage; behaviors are often misunderstood. The family and staff need to encourage the person by giving realistic praise and recognition, letting him or her express feelings of guilt, work through earlier losses, finish mourn-

ing, and build self-esteem. You will need to give more physical and emotional help as the person grows weaker. He or she should stay involved with the family as long as possible.

Preparatory Depression

Preparatory depression *is the next stage and differs from the previous depression. Now the person realizes the inevitability of death and comes to desire the release from suffering that death can bring. He or she wishes to be a burden no more and recognizes that there is no hope of getting well. The person needs a time of preparatory grief to get ready for the final separation of impending loss: not only are loved ones going to lose him or her, but the person is losing all significant objects and relationships.* The person reviews the meaning of life and searches for ways to share insights with the people most significant to him or her, sometimes including the staff. Often the fear that he or she cannot share aspects of life or valued material objects with people of his or her own choosing will cause greater concern than the diagnosis of a terminal illness or the knowledge of certain death. *As the person thinks of what life has meant, he or she begins to get ready to release life, but not without feelings of grief. Often he or she will talk repetitiously to find a meaning in life.*

The family and health team can either inhibit the person during this stage or promote emotional comfort and serene acceptance of death. The first reaction to depressed, grieving behavior and life review is to cheer him or her. This meets your needs but not those of the client. When the person is preparing for the impending loss of all love objects and relationships, behavior should be accepted and not changed. Acceptance of the final separation in life will not be reached unless he or she is allowed to express a life review and sorrow. There may be no need for words if rapport, trust, and a working nurse-client relationship have been previously established. A touch of the hand and a warm accepting silence are therapeutic. Too much interference with words, sensory stimuli, or burdensome visitors hinders rather than helps emotional preparation for death. If the person is ready to release life and die and others expect him or her to want to continue to live and be concerned about things, the person's own depression, grief, and turmoil are increased. He or she wishes quietly and gradually to disengage from life and all that represents life. He or she may request few or no visitors and modifications in the routines of care and repeatedly request no heroic measures to prolong life.

Honor the client's requests but at the same time promote optimum physical and emotional comfort and well-being. Explain the feelings and needs of the client to the family and other members of the health team so that they can better understand his or her behavior. The family should know that this depression is beneficial if the client is to die peacefully and that it is unrelated to their past or present behavior.

Acceptance or Resolution

The final reaction, **acceptance** or a kind of **resolution**, *comes if the person is given enough time, does not have a sudden, unexpected death, and is given some help in working through the previous reactions. He or she will no longer be angry or depressed about the fate and will no longer be envious or resentful of the living. He or she will have mourned the loss of many people and things and will contemplate the* *end with a certain degree of quiet expectation.* Now the *ultimate of ego integrity*, described by Erikson (43), becomes evident. Acceptance is difficult and takes time. It depends in part on the client's awareness of the prognosis of illness so that he or she can plan ahead—religiously, philosophically, financially, socially, and emotionally. *This last stage is almost devoid of feeling.*

Priorities change; family and close friends become more important. Gradually the person is able to plan for the not-too-far future. Money is less important. Negative friends are avoided. The person must adjust to fatigue, changes in body function or structure, effects of chemotherapy or radiation, the continuing treatment appointments, and loss of control.

The healthy aged person will also go through some aspects of the reactions discussed previously, for as the person grows old, he or she contemplates more frequently personal mortality and begins to work through feelings about it.

The Kübler-Ross (73–76) model is helpful. It is built on observations of hundreds of dying persons. Families may parallel the patients in reactions. Do not stereotype responses into these stages. Sometimes the person or family will not go through every one of these stages or behaviors, and the stages will not always follow in this sequence (39, 68). The person or family may remain in a certain stage or revert to earlier stages. Feelings related to several of the stages may exist together.

Do not convey that the client or family should be in a certain stage or reacting a certain way. Avoid social and religious clichés. Rather, be a caring, concerned, available person, willing to do nondramatic, simple, but helpful tasks such as bringing the family member something to drink, watering the flowers sent by a friend, and offering to call a significant person. Equally important is doing physical care procedures in a thorough but efficient manner so that visiting family members can spend as much time with their dying loved one as possible. Listen to feelings when the person wants to talk, but do not probe.

ANNIVERSARY REACTION AND EMOTIONALLY INVESTED DEADLINES

Anniversary reaction *refers to feelings of grief and sadness or a reliving of the mourning process about a year after the death of the loved one. Or the grief and mourning response, including physical symptoms, may be more intense at the person's birth date or at one of several of the major holidays throughout the year.*

PREMONITION OF DEATH AND POSTPONEMENT OF DEATH

The phenomenon of **premonition of death** *is seen in people who, although lacking any signs of illness, emotional conflict, suicidal tendencies, severe depression, or panic, correctly anticipate their own deaths* (11, 20, 22, 64, 110, 115, 117, 118). *The person senses or may be convinced of impending death yet feel no depression or anxiety toward it.* Such clients are resigned to death, as if death is a release from the burden of life or body. Premonition clients may experience less close human relationships and emotional isolation from significant others during their terminal period. Or they may make contact—like a final goodbye to significant others—in person or by telephone, e-mail, or correspondence. For example, one busy woman put aside her tasks one day to visit each nearby neighbor and convey significant messages. That evening she was killed in a car accident on a country road. The neighbors stated "she must have known this was her last day." They felt gratified about the brief exchanges. Her daughter realized later her mother must have tried to telephone that day but the answering machine was not in operation. The daughter felt prolonged grief at realizing there was no last chance to hear her voice, converse, and convey love. The daughter was going to call her mother the next day. Too late!

Death may hold more appeal than life because it promises either a reunion with lost love, resolution of long conflict, or respite from anguish. Death is perceived as a release from continuing in a world in which there are no longer any emotional bonds or reason to remain. Thus there is no fear, anxiety, or depression regarding its approach, but rather a distinctly eager and expectant attitude toward its swift occurrence. Research shows that death comes to the premonition clients about as they have anticipated it would, although medically their condition does not warrant a quick demise or, in some cases, any death at all (15, 20, 22, 118). Premonitions also occur in combat soldiers in the armed forces; sometimes they are not assigned to actual combat at the time of death, but they e-mailed to loved ones about the certainty of death.

A relative or friend may also have a premonition that a loved one is going to die. In fact, such a feeling may cause the person to contact or visit the loved one, and may even prevent death because of intervening actions—either to prevent a suicide or to take the person to emergency care services because of an illness or deterioration in body function. Or the visit may not be accomplished in time, as a grieving daughter and niece each conveyed when they learned of the death of their father/uncle—expected, but not so soon.

Postponement of death *refers to the person making an overt (conscious or spoken) or covert (unconscious) decision about the choice of date or event for time of death. Death seems inevitable but the person holds onto life unexpectedly.* Typically, the choice may be associated with waiting for return of a loved one or an emotionally invested date for the person. Some people die just before entry into a nursing home from their residence or the hospital (15, 20, 29, 39, 41, 95).

Some individuals, despite impending death, maintain hope and endurance and apparently refuse to die and live beyond the time of expected death. A person can program, through unconscious or conscious will or spiritual faith, the onset of illness, recovery from severe illness, or time of death. A strong will to live is often associated with the person's being interested, involved, or active in life or having a loved one, spouse, or dependent whom he or she desires to be with or for whom he or she feels responsible. For some, the death month is related to the birth month in that some people postpone death to witness their birthdays or another important holiday. The person with excessive fear of death may be unable to die until able to express and work through conscious fears or phobias (39, 41, 95).

The choice of the date or event for the time of death seems fitting to the uniqueness of the person. For example, two of the first four U.S. presidents died on July 4, undoubtedly an emotionally invested event for them (95).

LEGAL PLANNING FOR DEATH

While the person is still healthy and capable of making the many decisions in relation to death, he or she can do much to relieve worries and take the burden of those decisions off others. You are in a position to give the following information to others as indicated.

Although not legally binding, the living will is being used by increasing numbers of people. Representatives from some nursing and funeral homes and cemeteries are educating people to keep a folder, revised periodically, of all information that will be used by those making arrangements at the time of death. Such a folder might include names of advisors such as attorney, banker, life insurance broker, and accountant. Personal and vital information should be included, such as birth certificate, marriage license, military discharge papers, and copies of wills, including willing of body parts to various organizations. Financial records (or a copy of those held in a safety deposit box), estimated assets and liabilities, and insurance and Social Security information should be filed and available. Personal requests and wishes, listing who gets what, should be written along with funeral arrangements and cemetery deeds.

Having this information written assumes that the person has made a legal will, has some knowledge of the purposes and functions of probate court, has access to Social Security information, and has decided on a funeral home and burial plot.

Knowledge of how to claim survivor's benefits from Social Security and how to claim the government burial allowance for honorably discharged veterans can ease the loved one's confusion at time of death. These are intellectual preparations. They cannot ease the sense of loss in the living, but they can foster peace of mind, realizing that the deceased's wishes were carried out.

Health Promotion and Nursing Applications

Death is an intensely poignant event, one that causes deep anguish, but one you may frequently encounter in client care.

SELF-ASSESSMENT

Personal assessment, being aware of and coping with your personal feelings about death, is essential to assess accurately or intervene helpfully with the client, family, or other health care providers. How do you protect yourself from anxiety and despair resulting from repeated exposure to personal sufferings? The defenses of isolation, denial, and "professional" behavior are common in an attempt to cope with feelings of helplessness, guilt, frustration, and ambivalence about the client not getting well or the secret wish for the client to die. It takes courage and maturity to undergo the experience of death with clients and families and yet remain an open, compassionate human being. You are a product of the culture, just as the client and the family are, and hence will experience many of the same kinds of reactions. Religious, philosophic, educational, and family experiences and general maturity also affect your ability to cope with feelings related to death.

You may see, consciously or unconsciously, yourself in the dying person. The more believable the identification with the person or family, the more devastating the experience will be as you are forced to recognize personal vulnerability to death. The client may remind you of your grandfather, aunt, or friend, and you may react to the dying client as though he or she were that person.

The dying client may seek an identification and partnership with someone, and often this person is the nurse. You may be unwilling to share the relationship or respond to the dying client. The sense of guilt that results may be as burdensome as the actual involvement.

Dying in the hospital has become so organized and care so fragmented that you are not necessarily vulnerable to personal involvement in the client's death. However, you are more likely to be personally affected by and feel a sense of loss from the client's death if an attachment has been formed to the client and family because of prolonged hospitalization or hospice care, and if the death is unexpected. Also, if you perform nursing measures you believe might have contributed to the client's death, if you have worked hard to save a life, or if the client's social or personal characteristics are similar to your own, you will feel the loss (26, 39, 52–54).

Glaser and Strauss (52) describe how health care workers judge a client's value according to social status and respond accordingly. The client's death is considered less a social loss (and is therefore less mourned by the nursing staff) if he or she is elderly, comatose, confused, of a lower socioeconomic class or a minority group, poorly educated, not famous, unattractive, or considered "responsible" for having the disease. The dying client in these categories is likely to receive less care or only routine care. The client with high social value, whose death is mourned and who receives optimum care by the nursing staff, is young, is alert or likable, has prominent family status, has a high-status occupation or profession, is from the middle or upper socioeconomic class, or is considered talented or pretty.

If the client's death is very painful or disfiguring, you may avoid the client because of feelings of guilt or helplessness. In addition, you may be aware of the callous attitudes of health team members or of the decision of the family and doctor about prolonging life with heroic measures or not prolonging life. These situations can provoke intense negative reactions if you disapprove of the approaches of other members of the health team.

Attempt to deal with the various pitfalls of working with the dying. These include (117): (a) withdrawal from the client, (b) isolation of emotions, (c) failure to perceive own feelings or feelings of client and family, (d) displacing own feelings onto other team members, (e) "burning out" from intense emotional involvement, and (f) fearing illness and death.

SUPPORT FOR NURSES

Sometimes it is essential to say, "I need help in dealing with my feelings about this dying client" just as you would say, "I need help with this procedure." A support system should be available. Specific times should be set aside for staff members to share emotional needs related to a specific dying client or to learn specifics of the dying process. *Often nurses can help each other, but there should also be a specialist with whom to confer:* (a) the master's educated nurse with additional psychiatric consultation liaison skill, (b) a religious leader or nun, or (c) a psychologist or psychiatrist. The specialist should also be available for spontaneous sessions. Yet in many agencies such support is not made available.

INTERVENTIONS FOR HEALTH PROMOTION

Guidelines can assist the nurse who works with dying clients to maintain his or her personal health:

1. Individual staff members should be encouraged to gain personal insight and acknowledge their own limits. Extra support or time off may be necessary when staff members are under a high degree of stress. The needs of clients deserve priority, however. If certain staff members constantly require considerable support, they may be encouraged to seek counseling. A different position in the agency may be helpful.
2. A healthy balance must be maintained between work and an outside life. Although this type of work demands considerable personal involvement, there must be times when staff is totally off call and left to pursue personal affirming activities.

3. The individual must be careful when the "need to be needed" becomes too great and he or she attempts to be everything to everyone. This work is probably best accomplished by a team.
4. The individual must maintain a support system at work and outside the work setting. Hospice units must make provisions for ongoing staff support through the use of visitation, psychiatric consultants for the staff, or weekly staff support meetings.
5. For those working in isolation, it may be wise to consider ongoing sessions with an outside consultant and therapist who can offer guidance and provide support.

Take courses in sociology, philosophy, and religion to gain different perspectives. Join professional organizations in which you can share problems or solutions and gain support. You may need to change departments either temporarily or permanently to feel the accomplishment of working with those who recover. Two nurses can work together in caring for a dying patient so that they can share emotions and support each other.

If you work with cancer clients exclusively, you may also need special assistance. Optimism and logical thinking must be encouraged in the client and maintained in yourself. You may hear many opinions about helpful treatment, both inside and outside the medical establishment. You may see that some of the established treatments have unpleasant side effects. The question arises: Why must the client endure so much?

If you can think of death as the last stage of life and as fulfillment, you can mature and learn from the client as he or she comes to terms with personal illness. The meaning of death can serve as an important organizing principle in determining how the person conducts life, and it is as significant for you as for the client. With time and experience, you will view the role of comforter as being as important as that of promoting care. Then the client who is dying will be less of a personal threat.

ASSESSMENT OF CLIENT AND FAMILY

Assessment of the client and family is done according to the standard methods of assessment. The total person (physical, intellectual, emotional, social, and spiritual needs and status) must be assessed to plan effective care. Learn what the client and family know about the client's condition and what the doctor has told them, to plan for a consistent approach.

Recognize also that people differ in the way they express feelings about dying and death. Mourning may be private or public. Listen to the topics of conversation the person discusses, observe for rituals in behavior, and learn of typical behavior in health from

the client or the family to get clues to what is important. The routines that are important in life may become more important now, and they may assist in preparation for death. Observe family members for pathologic responses—physical or emotional—as grief after loss from death increases the risk of mortality for the survivor, especially for the male spouse or relative who is in late middle age or older.

NURSING DIAGNOSES

The **Box**, Nursing Diagnoses Related to the Dying Person, is a list of diagnoses that may be pertinent to the dying person and are related to assessment and need for holistic care (87).

Stepnick and Perry (104) relate the phases of resolving death according to the Kübler-Ross format to what could be nursing diagnoses. *They list four stages of spiritual development:* (a) chaotic, (b) formal, (c) skeptic, and (d) mystic. They described nursing strategies to assist the client at each stage of spiritual development as the client approaches death.

INTERVENTION WITH THE FAMILY

Supportive Care

The family will be comforted as they see compassionate care being given to their loved one. Your attitude is important, for both family members and clients are very perceptive about your real feelings, whether you are interested and available, giving false reassurance, or just going about a job. Family members often judge your personal relationship with the loved one as more important than your technical skill. Being interested and available takes emotional energy. Without this component in your personality, perhaps you should not be in the profession of nursing regardless of specialty.

Try to help the relatives compensate for their feelings of helplessness, frustration, or guilt. Their assisting the client with feeding or grooming or other time-consuming but nontechnical

Nursing Diagnoses Related to the Dying Person

Death **A**nxiety	Chronic **P**ain
Risk for **A**spiration	**P**owerlessness
Risk for Imbalanced **B**ody Temperature	Readiness for Enhanced **R**eligiosity
Bowel Incontinence	**S**elf-Care Deficit (specify)
Decreased **C**ardiac Output	Impaired **S**kin Integrity
Risk for **C**aregiver Role Strain	Impaired **S**ocial Interaction
Impaired Verbal **C**ommunication	Readiness for Enhanced **S**piritual Well-Being
Ineffective **D**enial	Impaired **S**wallowing
Functional Urinary **I**ncontinence	Ineffective **T**hermoregulation
Impaired Bed **M**obility	
Impaired Oral **M**ucous Membrane	

Source: Reference 87.

aspects of care can be helpful to them, the client, and the nursing staff. The family may be acting toward or caring for the client in a way that seems strange or even nontherapeutic to the nursing staff. Yet these measures or the approach may seem fine to the client because of the family pattern or ritual. It is not for you to judge or interfere unless what the family is doing is unsafe for the client's welfare or is clearly annoying to the client. In turn, recognize when family members are fatigued or anxious and relieve them of responsibility at that point. Encourage the family to take time to rest and to meet needs adequately. A lounge or other place where the family can alternately rest and yet be near the client is helpful.

Show acceptance of grief. By helping the family members express their grief and by giving support to them, you are helping them to support the client. Prepare the family for sudden, worsening changes in the client's condition or appearance to avoid shock and feelings of being overwhelmed. The Abstract for Evidence-Based Practice describes loss and grief reactions.

The crisis of death of the loved one may result in a life crisis for the surviving family members. The problems with changes in daily routines of living, living arrangements, leisure-time activities, role reversal and assuming additional responsibilities, communicating with other family members, or meeting financial obligations can seem overwhelming. The failure of relatives and friends to help or the insistence by relatives and friends on giving help that is not needed is equally problematic. Advice from others may add to rather than decrease the burdens. The fatigue that a long illness causes in a family member may remain for some time after the loved one's death and may interfere with adaptive capacities. You can help by being a listener, exploring with the family ways in which to cope with their problems, and making referrals or encouraging them to seek other persons or agencies for help. Often your willingness to accept and share their feelings of loss and other concerns can be enough to help the family mobilize their strengths and energies to cope with remaining problems.

The most heartbreaking time for the family may be the time when the client is disengaging from life and from them. The family will need help to understand this process and recognize it as normal behavior. The dying person has found peace. His or her circle of interests has narrowed, and he or she wishes to be left alone and not disturbed by any news of the outside world. Behavior with others may be so withdrawn that he or she seems unreachable and uncooperative. He or she prefers short visits and is not likely to be in a talkative mood. The television set remains off. Communication is primarily nonverbal. This behavior can cause the family to feel rejected, unloved, and guilty about not doing enough. They should understand that their loved one can no longer hold onto former relationships as he or she accepts the inevitability of death. The family needs help in realizing that their silent presence can be a very real comfort and shows that he or she is loved and not forgotten. Concurrently, the family can learn that dying is not a horrible thing to be avoided.

This may be the time when the family insists on additional life-sustaining or heroic measures, although they will only prolong suffering. The nurse can listen to their desire to prolong life, explain the needs and what is happening to the patient, act as a mediator when various family members make contradictory statements, calm angry tempers, and start a rational discussion about what's best for the patient. Having a meeting that includes family, nurse, pastoral care, the physician, members of an ethics committee, and other health care workers or significant others is useful. Keeping lines of communication open and maintaining a bond with the family, being nonjudgmental, and encouraging family contact with the patient are essential and challenging, even difficult at times (59, 70, 71, 77, 84, 111, 123, 125).

News of impending or actual death is best communicated to a family unit or group rather than to a lone individual to allow the people involved to give mutual support to each other. This should be done in privacy so they can express grief without the restraints imposed by public observation. Stay and comfort the person facing death, at least until a religious leader or other close friends can come.

Requests by an individual or family to see the dead person should not be denied on the grounds that it would be too upsetting. The person who needs a leave-taking to realize the reality of the situation will ask for it; those for whom it would be overwhelming will not request it.

Sometimes the survivor of an accident may ask about people who were with him or her at the time of the accident. The health

Abstract for Evidence-Based Practice

Lived Experience of Loss

Douglas, D. H. (2004). The lived experience of loss: A phenomenological study. *Journal of the American Psychiatric Nurses Association, 10,* 24–32.

KEYWORDS

bereavement; adaptation, psychological; personal loss; attitude toward death; phenomenological study; thematic analysis.

Purpose ➤ To describe the lived experience of loss and bereavement and their effects upon physical and mental health.

Conceptual Framework ➤ The perspectives of Freud, Lindemann, Kübler-Ross, and the view of the bereaved themselves were incorporated in this study.

Sample/Setting ➤ A convenience sample of 12 individuals, who responded to a newspaper advertisement to join a grief support group in New Orleans, comprised the sample. Inclusion criteria were 18 years of age or over, 3 months past the death of a loved one, and taking no psychiatric medications. The final sample consisted of 8 women and 4 men, ranging in age from 32 to 65 years, all Caucasian.

Methods ➤ Phenomenology attempts to describe an experience as thoroughly as possible from the perspective of the participant. Following written consent, participants were interviewed for approximately one hour using open-ended questions such as: "Tell me about the death of your loved one," or "Tell me how your loss has affected the ways you feel about yourself and others." Verbatim records of the interview were transcribed, and five themes of feeling of loss were derived by the author.

Findings ➤ The five themes that described participants' feelings of loss included (1) profound emotional and physical pain that included anger and suicidal ideation; (2) loss of control to the point that life appeared to have no direction or purpose; (3) irreversible change that required a redefinition of self; (4) new insights into the meaning of life and death, the self, and others; and (5) empathy toward others who are bereaved, and a desire to help others and improve oneself.

Implications ➤ Care offered to the bereaved may be improved by understanding their individual experiences following loss and identifying persistent maladaptive coping responses. Mental health care providers can foster heightened identity, self-understanding, and control through individual therapy and use of role play, assertiveness training, and guided imagery. Group therapy offers the bereaved individual an opportunity to express feelings of loneliness, helplessness, and anger within a supportive context, decreasing feelings of hopelessness and loss of control.

team should confer on when and how to answer these questions. Well-timed honesty is the healthiest approach; otherwise the person cannot adapt to the reality of the accidental death. The person's initial response of shock, denial, and tears or later grief will neither surprise nor upset the medical team who understand the normal steps in resolving crisis and loss. Cutting off the person's questions or keeping him or her sedated may protect the staff, but it does not help the survivor.

The parents who grieve for their dying or fatally injured child must be respected, be given the opportunity to minister to the child when indicated, and be relieved of responsibilities at times. Encourage the parents to share feelings, and work to complement, not compete with, the parents in caring for the child. Also, remember that grandparents, siblings, peers, and sometimes the babysitter will need understanding in their grieving. The timing and type of support given after accidental death of a child are important.

Accident, suicide, and homicide are the leading causes of death before age 40. Thus, survivors often include children and adolescents. The grief and mourning that surround each of these death events differ from an anticipated death. The suddenness of each causes shock, confusion, helplessness, emptiness, and intense sadness. With suicide comes guilt and shame, a sense of being responsible, as well as anger at the person who committed suicide. With homicide comes the feelings of intense anger, rage, and revenge, with the sadness intensified by the imagery related to brutality and what the person suffered in the last moments alive. With each of these types of death, the family longs to undo certain acts and to be able to say good-bye in a loving way. Long-term therapy is often needed.

Intervention with Other Grief Responses

As you care for the family of the dying person, or interact with the family after death, you may perceive that they are not grieving in what is considered the usual or normal way. You may assess their grief and mourning, both in anticipation of and at the time of death, as absent or delayed, complicated, pathologic, neurotic, dysfunctional, or as clinical depression.

Delayed grief response *may be identified when there is no anticipatory grieving or no expression of grief at death. Later, there may be manifestations of not having grieved the loss* (46, 55, 65, 84, 95, 102, 118). *Reactions and behavior include:*

1. Continuing to act as if the person still lives, or looking for the person.
2. Various physical symptoms, such as insomnia, loss of appetite and weight, pain, and actual malfunction of the body.

3. Expressions of frustration or anger that is out of context or excessive, or personality changes.
4. Complaints of excessive stress at work or home.
5. Increased smoking and use of alcohol or other drugs.
6. Difficulty in interpersonal and family relationships.
7. Nightmares, illusions of seeing the person and then realizing the person was someone else, or hallucinations of the person.
8. Statements about "shutting down at the time of death."

Disenfranchised grief *refers to the reaction to a loss that is not socially recognized or sanctioned. The person feels unable to express loss because of the fear of public criticism or even ridicule.* For example, society usually bases legitimate grief on the basis of family relations; thus the death of a dear friend may not elicit the attention given to the death of a sibling, although the two may be identical in terms of closeness. The relationship may also not be publicly recognized or approved, as in the case of the death of a same-gender partner, a partner in an extramarital affair, or someone from a relationship that is ascribed to the past, such as an ex-spouse. Other losses that people may experience as significant but feel are not equally valued by others include miscarriage, perinatal loss, or loss of a pet. At times, the person who is grieving for his or her own situation is not recognized socially. Young children, the very old, the mentally challenged, and the mentally ill are often thought of as beyond grief because of their marginal status in society. The circumstances of a death may also bring about stigma with regard to grief. Situations in which the person appears responsible for the death may elicit judgment. Thus, deaths from AIDS, drug overdoses, suicide, homicide, or abortion may not be seen as legitimate to grieve. Because the grief is hidden, it may be very intense and persist because of the embarrassment over the loss and the reluctance to perform the mourning rituals that would accompany a socially sanctioned loss (8, 36, 37, 68, 116). Refer to Chapter 14 ∞ for the grief responses that may be experienced by the female who has had an abortion.

Complicated grief response *may occur when the person is experiencing unresolved grief associated with the past. It is manifested in several ways* (43, 65, 76, 84, 95, 118):

1. Multiple physical complaints, often with no significant findings on physical examination. (Often the symptoms mimic those of the deceased.)
2. Suicidal ideas or attempts, wanting to join the dead person.
3. Intense grief when speaking of the deceased, inappropriate or angry affect, or the mechanism of emotional isolation (e.g., smiling while talking about the dead person).
4. Withdrawal from others, failure to participate in the usual family or social activities, or radical life changes.
5. Inability to talk about the deceased without intense grief expressions.
6. Intense grief reactions triggered by minor events.
7. Repeated verbalization of themes of loss.
8. Extreme sadness at certain times of the year, such as anniversary dates or special holidays.

Through counseling, the person may remember past losses or rejections and grieve these as well as the current loss.

Dysfunctional grief response *may occur when (a) the person had a very dependent or ambivalent relationship with the deceased;*

(b) the circumstances surrounding death were uncertain, sudden, or overwhelming, such as homicide, or complicated with assault, such as rape or violent attack; or (c) the loss was socially unspeakable or socially negated, such as capital punishment, or death or murder of someone who had been a gang member or molester of children or had a criminal history. If there has been a history of mental illness or suicide, or if the person has minimal support systems, another loss will be more difficult to handle (6, 8, 46, 65, 84, 95).

Pathologic grief response *is an intensification of grief to the point that the person is overwhelmed, demonstrates prolonged maladaptive behavior, manifests excessive symptoms and extensive interruptions in healing, and does not progress to integration of the loss, finding meaning in the loss, and resolution of the mourning process* (46, 65, 84, 95).

Intervention with the grieving person incorporates the communication, relationship, and education principles discussed throughout this and other chapters. Refer the grieving person or family to a grief counselor, as appropriate. Refer them also to their spiritual advisor or other people with whom they can confide. *The following resources may also be helpful:*

1. AARP (American Association of Retired Persons)
   Phone: 800-424-1400, *www.aarp.org*
2. Grief Net, *www.griefnet.org*
3. Grief Share, www.griefshare.org
4. Widow Net, www.fortnet.org

INTERVENTION WITH THE DYING PERSON

As the person moves into the later years of life, life-threatening illness may move the person forward mentally and spiritually faster than anticipated. The person will need to create a gestalt of the life lived, find meaning in accomplishments, and identify the legacy left behind for future generations and the mentoring contributions that were made. This last stage is concerned about completion—the ultimate last stage of dying and death (43). *There are three main tasks* (43, 107):

1. **Recontextualizing:** *Facts of life are reinterpreted from a vantage point of wisdom and understanding. Meaning related to painful events and failures of life is pursued.*
2. **Resurrecting the unlived life:** *Aspects of life sacrificed for another are reclaimed; talents, interests, and passions neglected for some time are envisioned to be pursued in the remaining time.*
3. **Forgiveness:** *Damaged relationships are repaired rather than remaining unresolved.* Asking for or providing forgiveness is a powerful healing tool.

You can be instrumental in fostering **psychospiritual growth**, *the conscious effort to mature, reevaluate, and self-transcend to a greater purpose. Two questions are useful to encourage the client's self-awareness and foster working through disabling chronic disease or approaching death* (43, 91, 105, 108, 119):

1. If your time is indeed shortened, what do you need to get done?
2. Are there people whom you need to contact in order to resolve feelings or unfinished business?

Offer to help patients contact their clergy, relatives, friends, or attorney; such offers can free the person to face the challenge of advance directives or estate planning. *Several questions can help the patient recontextualize the illness expressed* (43, 91, 105, 108, 119):

1. What has surprised you most about yourself through this? About others?
2. If you knew earlier what you know now, would you have made the same choices? If not, what choices would you have made?
3. What do you want to do with whatever time you have left?

Often it is the nurse at the bedside in the middle of the night who is asked questions, who is quietly observed by the patient to determine if it's all right to ask questions. The nurse, through listening and feedback, can help the patient transform despair into a search for personal meaning. The nurse does not have to give answers but rather can wait patiently for the person to arrive at his or her own answers. The nurse can validate that forgiveness is not a feeling, not reconciliation, but a letting go of a hurt. Reconciliation requires both involved parties; it may not be possible to have both involved. Support and acceptance of the patient, whatever the responses, are important.

Home and Hospice Care

The Case Situation describes the death and complexity of feelings experienced by the patient and family that have been previously discussed and the experience of a family member—the son—caring for a dying mother in the home.

Care in an Agency Setting

See the Case Situation, Home Care of the Dying Person, for a holistic practice presentation that incorporates the following discussion of principles and practices. **Much of the following discussion is pertinent to the institutional setting but it is also applicable to home and hospice care.**

Care of the dying client falls primarily on the nurse. You have sustained contact with the client and understand dying and the many needs of the dying person. You know the value of compassionate service of mind and hands. You can protect the vulnerable person and understand some of the distress felt by client and family. You have an opportunity to help the client bring life to a satisfactory close, truly to live until he or she dies, and to promote comfort. The client needs your unqualified interest and response to help decrease loneliness and make the pain and physical care or treatment bearable.

You will encounter frustrations during the care of the dying person for many reasons. There is the challenge of talking with or listening to the client. Will he or she talk about death? Pain may be constant and difficult to relieve, causing you to feel incompetent. He or she may be demanding, nonconforming to the client role, or disfigured and offensive to touch or smell. The family may visit so often and long that they interfere with necessary care of the client. Accusations from the client or family about neglect may occur or be feared. It is no wonder that despite good intentions, religious convictions, and educational programs, you may avoid the dying client and family. They are left to face the crisis of death alone. As you rework personal feelings about crisis, dying, and

death and become more comfortable with personal negative feelings and emotional upset, you will be able to serve more spontaneously and openly in situations previously avoided. You will be able to admit, without guilt feelings, personal limits in providing care, to use other helpers, and yet to do as much as possible for the client and family without showing shock or repugnance about the client's condition.

Physical care of the dying person includes providing for nutrition, hygiene, rest, elimination, and relief of pain or other symptoms; care of the mouth, nose, eyes, skin, and peripheral circulation; positioning; and environmental considerations. Hospital personnel should not focus exclusively on the client's complaints of pain or other physical symptoms or need to avoid the subject of death. Complaints may be a camouflage for anxiety, depression, or other feelings and covertly indicate a desire to talk with someone about the feelings. Analgesics and comfort measures to promote rest can be used along with crisis therapy. Spend sufficient time with the client to establish a relationship that is supportive. Provide continuity of care. Try to exchange information realistically within the whole medical team, including client and family, to reduce uncertainty and feelings of neglect. Clients can withstand much pain and distress as long as they feel wanted or believe their life has meaning (47, 99).

Thorough, meticulous physical care is essential to promote physical well-being but also to help prevent emotional distress. During the prolonged and close contact physical care provides, you can listen, counsel, and teach, using principles of effective communication. But let the client sleep often, without sedation if possible. The many physical measures to promote comfort and optimum well-being can be found in texts describing physical care skills. Nursing care is not less important because the person is dying.

Avoid too strict a routine in care. Let the client make some decisions about what he or she is going to do as long as safe limits are set. Modify care procedures as necessary for comfort. Through consistent, comprehensive care you tell the client you are available and will do everything possible for continued well-being.

During care, conversation should be directed to the client. Explain nursing procedures, even though the client is comatose, as hearing is the last sense lost. Response to questions should be simple, encouraging, but as honest as possible. Offer the person opportunities to talk about self and feelings through open-ended questions. When the client indicates a desire to talk about death, listen. There is no reason to expound your philosophy, beliefs, or opinions. Focus your conversation on the present and the client. Help the client maintain the role that is important to him or her. Convey that what he or she says has meaning for you. You can learn by listening to the wisdom shared by the client, and add to feelings of worth and generativity. Recognize when the client is unable to express feelings verbally, and help him or her reduce tension and depression through other means—physical activity, crying, or sublimative activities.

If the client has an intense desire to live and is denying or fearful of death, be accepting but help him or her maintain a sense of balance. Do not rob the person of hope or force him or her to talk about death. Follow the conversational lead; if the topics are concerned with life, respond accordingly.

Case Situation

Mom's cancer diagnosis shocked us all. She had coped with congestive heart failure for nearly 30 years, and we expected that heart disease would eventually take her life. She dropped weight for months before the cancer diagnosis. The welcome loss of weight was soon accompanied by unpleasant symptoms of nausea and back pain. An MRI revealed the tumor lodged in her pancreas. She grudgingly conceded to the surgery as a diagnostic measure, since no x-ray could determine the extent of the cancer's spread into her lymph glands and other organs.

The surgery provided a makeshift bile duct that was intended to improve her appetite and mitigate the nausea. It also provided a picture of the cancer invading the surrounding lymph glands and liver. The physicians told us of the harsh future: 6 months at best, with mounting pain because the tumor was near the spinal nerves. Mom faced a brief rehabilitation period and a half-year of life with diminishing quality. No one bothered to relate this to my mother in surgical intensive care.

When she first became conscious, Mom asked me, "How long do I have?" As a nurse, I have often been the bearer of grim news and what comfort I could muster. Although I have never been able to withhold the truth from patients, I have learned to mete it out in tolerable doses, for both me and them. Now I had no cards to play; no promises of chemotherapy, medicine, or radiation therapy that could engender a cure or remission. I told her she had 6 months according to the doctors, but she and God would determine the true time allotted to her. She gave me a disgusted look and turned her head to the other side of the room. I had been dismissed.

Family members tried to give Mom the motivation to endure postsurgical recovery. The cliché that "You cannot keep someone alive," rang dissonantly in our ears. Mom refused physical therapy, company, and food, and was rude to the nurses and visiting well-wishers. At one point I summoned the courage to tell her that I was trying to understand how devastated she was by the cancer but felt rejected and angry by her sullen, withdrawn behavior. I was hoping that our remaining time would be different. Mom called me at home for the last time that evening, perfunctorily asked me how my life was going, and then explained what she wanted for the life she had left, even specifying funeral plans. While we had discussed this subject before, I knew her opening this topic meant that she had come to a decision to die. I could argue with her no longer.

I assured her I would support what she wanted. She told me she knew she was beyond cure, that she wanted to be rid of the excruciating pain, and would I please stop irritating her with pep talks to get well.

I called hospice that day; my decision was sealed to bring her home. Ironically, the hospital social worker called me a few

hours later and flatly told me that my mother no longer qualified for the hospital rehabilitation services, or any health services, for that matter. The bottom line, of course, is that her insurance refused to pay for any more care. I made plans to bring Mom home a few days later. I would be her full-time hospice nurse.

The doctors suggested that I reconsider, since Thanksgiving was a few days away and Mom might die on the holiday. My family members were speechless when I told them of my plans. I never knew whether they thought I was crazy or were just shocked that I would entertain such an old-fashioned idea as having a parent die within her home. I was frankly amazed that I would consent to bring Mom home. As a nurse taking care of dying people, I could always leave the floor for the shelter of my home after a shift. Now I would be literally faced with the dreams so many nurses have of not knowing whether they are on or off working time, of finding patients to care for in the rooms of their own homes.

When I told Mom I was taking her home, she just shrugged and refused to discuss my reasoning. I told her that the choice was between her home or a nursing home, but she told me she didn't care. A few days later when she arrived home in the ambulance, she gave me the first smile I had seen in months. The ambulance drivers informed me that she cried throughout the ride home and suggested that I give her pain medication. Mom told me she was crying because she was so happy to be back in the home she never thought she would see again.

Mom's demeanor softened as she settled in the comfortable routines of home. Her irritability, so evident in the hospital, melted into a quiet acceptance of her situation. The mottled skin and pained manner was replaced by a glow and childlike sweetness I had never seen. She was delighted to have visitors and treated them with kindness. However, most came for one visit and did not return. Later, some told me they could not bear to see my mother so sick. Apparently, they could not see the contrast of her racked suffering in the hospital and the acceptance that pervaded her home.

While I had been led to expect that Mom would live a few days at most, she had other plans. *The hospice nurses were sensitive teachers and explained the difference between hospital dying and home dying—which most people don't see anymore.* Patients often return to their accustomed environment and are pumped up with the energy of the familiar, of the color and warmth missing in clinical settings. The depression lifts, pain diminishes, and the course of dying transforms from a steep, staggering one to a gradual ascent into the eternal world.

Mom was truly in a different world at times. She would talk to her mother, my father, and aunts, who had long departed this earth, as if they were at the bedside. She would describe trips she had always meant to take to Paris and other exotic places. She would ask me what I had planned for the day, as if I could put her in the car and take her shopping at her favorite stores. *The hospice nurses explained that these were apt metaphors for the dying process:* (a) contacting those who have gone before, (b) plans for traveling, and (c) wanting to resume formerly pleasurable activities as though the physical body had healed.

A number of times my mother called me because she had "some theological questions" she wanted me to answer. Mostly she repeated the question I first heard in intensive care, "How long do I have?" I honestly told her that I didn't know and that the extent of remaining time was between her and God. At other times, she would ask why we were staying home together and how long would we have to do this. I reminded her how sick she was and told her that I wanted to spend the remaining time with her. She would say, "Oh yes, that's right!" as though she had temporarily forgotten her plight.

My nurse friends were often perplexed at how beautiful my mother looked and her childlike manner. One commented that she was showing that ideal part of us all that is obscured by the hassles of working, paying bills, and managing the thousand compromises that daily life extracts from us. Indeed, Mom had released all such worldly concerns. At times, I would find her staring up at the ceiling with an expression that can only be described as ethereal, a gaze I only saw on the faces of the saints of my childhood holy cards. Mom calmly explained, "I'm just talking to Jesus." *Rather than pathologizing this as delirium, the hospice nurses assured me that this was common in the dying process.*

Mom weathered the Thanksgiving holidays and remained aware clear into Christmas. She would inquire about the date every morning so I taped a large calendar to the bedrails and crossed the days off, and put a large-faced clock at her bedside—those customary nursing interventions to sustain orientation. Although the hospice nurses urged me to celebrate Christmas, I could not bring myself to wrap presents or put up a tree. However, Mom was delighted with the slew of Christmas cards arriving in the mail and asked that I tape them to the wall close to the ceiling so she could admire them as she lay in bed. Family members dropped by throughout the season, and she participated in reminiscences of past holidays.

Mom apparently had planned to live through Christmas. After the holiday passed, she was no longer interested in what day it was and spoke a few bare words to visitors. *The hospice nurses again assured me this was to be expected: that people hang on through the holidays and then let go to resume the dying process.* She frequently forgot who I was, calling me by her father's name at times, but mostly referred to me simply as "nurse."

We did share a few insightful moments, however. Once she asked me what I did in my job as a nurse. I made a sweeping gesture around the room and said, "This is what I do, what we have been doing for the past month." She began to laugh and I followed. We had a brief discussion about the disagreements and grudges we had nurtured and apologized to each other. She was mostly quiet, in that netherworld between waking life and sleep.

Mom's final 2 days had the appearance of death that I saw in the hospital: mottled, cold skin; frequent release of body fluids; mechanical, staccato breathing; and blood-tinged vomit. I had heard about intuitively knowing when loved ones were going to die but was frankly astonished when an inner voice urged me to go to her room. She died within a few minutes as I held her hand and prayed.

I cried mostly from relief. My mother's death relieved me— of vigilance and constant care, from not knowing when and how her end would finally come. *The hospice nurse arrived within the hour; I found a curious comfort in helping her prepare my mother's body for the funeral home, spirits in this kindred profession.* Unlike the hospital, there was no sheet over the face, no body bag. The personality of my Mom was preserved to the end, the funeral directors wheeling her body out the front door, her face and hands uncovered.

Although taking care of my dying mother was the most difficult experience of my life, I would not hesitate to do it again. In a world that denies death and confines it to the technological bounds of hospitals and long-term care facilities, I was allowed the privilege of experiencing dying without the institutional veil. My Mom was able to let go of her life within the context of family, neighbors, and friends and receive care within the familiar rhythms of home rather than on the imposed schedule of a facility. I learned how to rely on others to accomplish this nearly impossible task and to accept nursing care for myself, rather than consistently being on the giving side. And I learned firsthand what the families of dying patients experience and what nursing measures bring the most comfort.

Contributed by Richard Yakimo, PhD, PMH-CNS-BC, N-NAP.

Encourage communication among the doctor, client, and family. Encourage the client to ask questions and state needs and feelings instead of doing it for him or her, but be an advocate if the person cannot speak for self.

Explore with family members the ways they can communicate with and support their loved one. Explain to the family that because the comatose person can probably understand what is being said, they should talk in ways that promote security and should avoid whispering, which can increase the person's fears and suspicions.

Psychological care, regardless of where the dying person is located, includes showing genuine concern, acceptance, and understanding, and promoting a sense of trust, dignity, or realistic body image and self-concept. Being an attentive listener and providing for privacy, optimum sensory stimulation, independence, and participation in self-care and decision making are helpful. You will nonverbally provide a feeling of security and trust by looking in frequently on the client and using touch communication (25, 88).

Spiritual needs of the dying person, regardless of the spiritual beliefs (and regardless of where care is given), can be categorized as follows (48, 67, 105, 119):

1. Search for meaning and purpose in life and in suffering, including to integrate dying with personal goals and values, to make dying and death less fearful, to affirm the value of life, and to cope with the frustration caused by anticipated death.
2. Sense of forgiveness in the face of guilt about unfulfilled expectations for self, accepting nonfulfillment or incompleteness, making the most of remaining life, coming to terms with acts of omission or acts of commission toward others, and resolving human differences.
3. Need for love through others' words and acts of kindness and silent, compassionate presence. If family and friends are not present, the nurse may be the primary source of love.
4. Need for hope, which connotes the possibility of future good. Concrete hope consists of objects of hope within the person's experience such as freedom from pain or other symptoms or ability to perform certain tasks or to travel. Abstract hope or transcendent hope is characterized by distant and abstract goals and incorporates philosophic or religious meanings. Hope may be expressed as belief about afterlife, reunion with deceased loved ones, and union with God, a superior alternative to present existence. If there is no belief in the afterlife, hope may be expressed as belief about transfer of physical energy from the deceased body, belief about contributing to another's life through an organ donation, or belief in leaving a legacy in his or her children or community or organizational contributions.

You may assist with meeting the person's spiritual needs if requested and if you feel comfortable in doing so. Certainly you should know whom to contact if you feel inadequate. The religious advisor is a member of the health team. If the client has no religious affiliation and indicates no desire for one, avoid proselytizing.

Consider the social needs of the client until he or she is comatose or wishes to be left alone. Visitors, family, or friends can contribute significantly to the client's welfare when visiting hours are flexible. If possible, help the client dress appropriately and groom to receive visitors, go out of the room to a lounge, meet and socialize with other clients, or eat in a client's dining room or the unit.

Community-Focused Care

Community health nurses have found two distinct attitudes in families of dying clients. The first attitude is, "If he is going to die soon, let's get him to the hospital!" For these families the thought of watching the actual death is abhorrent. They feel personally unable to handle the situation and feel comforted by the thought of their loved one's dying in a place where qualified professionals can manage all the details. If possible, these families should have their wishes met. Many hospice services have inpatient units that can provide assistance to families needing respite or when the person's physical condition needs to be addressed and stabilized.

The second attitude is, "I want her to die at home. This is the place she loved. I can do everything that the hospital personnel can do." This attitude can be supported by the visiting nurse. The visiting nurse can usually coordinate community resources so that a home health aide, homemaker services, proper drug and nutrition supplies, and necessary equipment can be available in the home. Even the comatose client who requires a hospital bed, tube feedings, catheter change and irrigation, daily bed bath, feces removal, and frequent turning can be cared for in the home if the health team, family, and friends will share efforts. The families who desire this approach and who are helped to carry out their wishes seem to derive great satisfaction from giving this care.

Clients and family members often select the home as the place of care in the terminal stages of disease and as the place to die. Being with family and friends and living in their own home are often high priorities for clients. Home represents their life's work and helps to maintain a sense of dignity, identity, and control over dying. They realize at home they would not have to battle extraordinary measures. The family wants the client at home because it is his or her wish and because they believe they would desire to be at home if they were dying. Clients and families who choose the hospital as the place of death believe clients would receive better care there. Clients do not want to burden their families. Families are concerned about their loved one's comfort.

Perhaps the biggest issue is getting families to explicitly consider the type of care that is wanted for the dying person. This is a difficult issue because although older persons and persons with serious illness want to talk about the dying process, family members are not comfortable discussing this. Health care providers are also not comfortable raising these issues with their clients. The medical system is reluctant to declare that a person is beyond cure and requires more palliative types of care; this is often seen as "giving up" and thus is resisted. Often the referral to palliative care is made long overdue—a short time before death—where little can be done to improve the person's quality of functioning. Another issue is predicting when the end of life will occur. Although this can be done within brief periods, predicting when someone will die over longer periods of time—for example, within a year—is difficult (24, 25, 27, 60, 61, 70, 77, 78).

The Hospice Concept and Care The **hospice** *is an institution and a concept that gives the dying person homelike care either at home with the help of an interdisciplinary team or in an institution with a homelike atmosphere and special attention to the needs of the dying and their families.* The hospice concept is indeed a "care system" that coexists with a "cure system." In the United States, the definition of what constitutes hospice care varies from region to region; the goal, however, is essentially the same. The hospice concept originated in the Middle Ages. St. Christopher's Hospice in England has been the most famous to date. In some hospitals one unit is designated as the hospice area. A modern, free-standing hospice was opened in 1980 in Branford, Connecticut. The first state to regulate the licensing of hospices was Connecticut. In other states licensing depends on the types of facilities and services a hospice provides (60, 77).

Hospice care is designed to (24, 60, 62, 77, 100, 107):

1. Help the client accept and cope with the dying process.
2. Foster communication between client and family.
3. Enhance the client's autonomy and relieve physical pain and other common symptoms.
4. Work with the psychological aspects of late-stage cancer or other disease.

Most hospice care programs enable the family to care for the dying person through a team approach: (a) a visiting nurse does multiple interventions, (b) home health aides do morning household chores, (c) a family physician enables pain control through effective use of medications, (d) a physical therapist helps the person maintain mobility and later teaches the family various transfer techniques, (e) an occupational therapist helps the person maintain functions of daily living, (f) a music therapist brings diversion and suggests exercise to music, and (g) the clergy and church choir visit the home.

At times the client needs to be alone, either at home or in the hospital, as he or she goes through the preparatory depression discussed by Kübler-Ross and is disengaging self from life, loved ones, and all that has been important to him or her. For you to impose yourself at these times might complicate the emotional tasks near the end of life. You should not, however, abandon the client. Give the necessary care but go at his or her pace in conversation and care.

Although most people who are about to die have made peace with themselves, some bargain or fight to the end. Accept this behavior, but do not encourage the client to fight for life when the last days are near with no chance for continuing life. Instead, let him or her know that accepting the inevitable is not cowardly. Remember that fear of death is often found more in the living than in the dying and that this fear is more for the impending separation of intimate relationships than death itself.

After the death of the client, your relationship with the family need not end immediately. Explore with them how they will manage. Some hospice or home care nurses attend a funeral visitation or service; the family typically is very appreciative. Follow-up intervention in the form of a telephone call or home visit by a nurse, minister, social worker, or nursing care coordinator would be a way of more gradually terminating a close relationship and performing further crisis intervention as needed. Use this opportunity to evaluate the effectiveness of care given to the family throughout the client's terminal care period.

EVALUATION

Throughout intervention with the dying client or his or her family you must continually consider and **evaluate** whether your intervention is appropriate and effective, based on their needs rather than yours. Observation alone of their condition or behavior will not provide adequate evaluation. Ask yourself and others how you could be more effective, whether a certain measure was comforting and skillfully administered, and how the client and family perceived your approach and attitude. Assigning a person unknown to the client and family to ask these questions will help obtain an objective evaluation (42). Because of your involvement, you may be told only what people think you want to hear. If you and the client have established open, honest communication that encompasses various aspects of dying and if the client's condition warrants it, perhaps you will be able to interview the dying to get evaluation answers. You might ask if and how each member of the health team has added physically, intellectually, emotionally, practically, and spiritually to the person's care. You may also ask how each member of the health team has hindered in these areas. Through careful and objective evaluation you can learn how to be more skillful at intervention in similar situations in the future (42, 77, 107).

Summary

1. The concept of and reaction to dying and death depend on the person's cultural background and developmental level, the kind of death, the extent of support from significant others, and the quality of care given by nurses and other health care providers.
2. Nurses and other health care workers must work through their own feelings as they face ethical and moral dilemmas related to use of technology and either prolonging or shortening life deliberately.
3. There is much to learn from people who have a nearing-death awareness, a near-death experience, premonitions about death, or other kinds of dying experiences.
4. The dying process and the afterlife are indeed the last stage of development.

Review Questions

1. The parent of a preschool child asks the school nurse how to explain to the child about the impending death of an elderly grandparent. What should the nurse understand about a preschool child's perceptions of death?
   1. Death is perceived as final.
   2. Death is perceived as inevitable.
   3. Death can be avoided by certain behaviors.
   4. Death is perceived as a temporary state.

2. While reviewing documentation in an elderly home care client's chart, the nurse notes that the individual has a terminal condition. The client's children have asked that the client not be told of the diagnosis or its grave prognosis. While planning for a meeting with the client's family, the nurse should be primarily concerned that:
   1. The children's wishes are honored regarding care of the client.
   2. The family will not be able to engage in rituals of life review with the client.
   3. The client will find out the diagnosis by accident.
   4. The nurse has an obligation to the client and should ignore the family's wishes.

3. The nurse is caring for a client with cancer who has a prognosis of 3 months to live. The spouse is concerned because the client recently purchased airline tickets for a vacation that is scheduled 8 months from now. The nurse should explain to the spouse that the client is experiencing which stage of awareness?
   1. Denial
   2. Anger
   3. Psychological isolation
   4. Bargaining

4. The children of a man who is at home and dying tell the nurse they feel helpless because their father does not talk to them, watch television, or read. They are unsure of how to interact with him. How should the nurse respond to the family?
   1. Review the client's medications for any that may be influencing his ability to interact with family.
   2. Request a psychiatric evaluation to rule out depression.
   3. Educate the family about the process of withdrawing at the end of life.
   4. Encourage the children to only visit for short periods of time.

References

1. Andershed, B. (2006). Relatives in end-of-life care—Part I: A systematic review of the literature for the last five years, January 1999–February 2004. *Journal of Clinical Nursing, 15*, 1158–1169.
2. Anderson, P. (2007). Medical fatality: A nurse's viewpoint. *American Nurse Today, 2*(2), 15–17.
3. Andrews, M., & Boyle, J. (2005). *Transcultural concepts in nursing care* (4th ed.). Philadelphia: Lippincott.
4. Aroskar, M. (1990). The aftermath of the Cruzan decision: Dying in a twilight zone. *Nursing Outlook, 38*(6), 256–261.
5. Aroskar, M. (1994). Legal and ethical concerns: Nursing and the euthanasia debate. *Journal of Professional Nursing, 10*(1), 5.
6. Bateman, A., Broderick, D., Gleason, L., Kardon, R., Flaherty, C., & Anderson, S. (1992). Dysfunctional grieving. *Journal of Psychosocial Nursing, 30*(12), 5–9.
7. Benner, K. (1993). Terminal weaning: A loved one's vigil. *American Journal of Nursing, 93*(5), 22–25.
8. Bereavement after homicide for a loved one. (1995). *Menninger Letter, 3*(6), 3.
9. Berger, K. (2005). *The developing person through the life span* (6th ed.). New York: Worth.
10. Bingley, A. F., McDermott, E., Thomas, C., Payne, S., Seymour, J. E., & Clark, D. (2006). Making sense of dying: A review of narratives written since 1950 by people facing death from cancer and other diseases. *Palliative Medicine, 20*, 183–195.
11. Boehnert, C. (1986). Surgical outcome in death-minded patients. *Psychosomatics, 27*, 638–642.
12. Brothers, D. (2005). *Evidence-based advance directives: A study guide for nurses.* Austin, TX: HCPro Inc.
13. Brown Atlas of Dying. Site of death 1989–2001. Retrieved May 29, 2007, www.cher.brown.edu/dying/brownatlas.htm
14. Browning, A. (2006). Exploring advanced directives. *Journal of Christian Nursing, 23*(1), 34–39.
15. Burgess, K. (1976). The influence of will on life and death. *Nursing Forum, 15*(3), 238–258.
16. Callahan, M. (1994). Back from beyond. *American Journal of Nursing, 94*(3), 20–23.
17. Callahan, M. (1994). Breaking the silence. *American Journal of Nursing, 94*(1), 22–23.
18. Callahan, M. (1994). Farewell messages. *American Journal of Nursing, 94*(5), 18–19.
19. Carlson, A. L. (2007). Death in the nursing home: Resident, family, and staff perspectives. *Journal of Gerontological Nursing, 33*, 32–41.
20. Cate, S. (1991). Death by choice. *American Journal of Nursing, 91*(7), 33–34.
21. Cebuhar, J. K. (2006). *Last things first, just in case . . . The practical guide for living wills and durable powers of attorney for health care.* Des Moines, IA: Murphy Publishing.
22. Centerwall, A. (2006). A strange premonition. *Journal of Christian Nursing, 17*, 27–29.
23. Chally, P., & Loriz, L. (1998). Ethics in the trenches: Decision making in practice. *American Journal of Nursing, 98*(6), 17–23.
24. Chochinov, H. M. (2006). Dying, dignity, and new horizons in palliative end-of-life care. *CA: A Cancer Journal for Clinicians, 56*, 84–103.
25. Chochinov, H. M., Hack, T., Hassard, T., Kristjanson, L. J., McClement, S., & Harlos, M. (2004). Dignity and psychotherapeutic considerations in end-of-life care. *Journal of Palliative Care, 20*, 134–142.
26. Clark, W. (2003). Palliative psychiatric nursing care: An emerging role? *Journal of Psychosocial Nursing, 41*(10), 6–7.
27. Collins, L. G., Parks, S. M., & Winter, L. (2006). The state of advance care planning: One decade after SUPPORT. *American Journal of Hospice and Palliative Care, 23*, 378–384.
28. Colmer, R. S., & Thomas, T. M. (2006). *The senior's guide to end-of-life issues: Advance directives, wills, funerals, and cremations.* New York: Eklektika Press.
29. Corr, C. (2005). *Death and dying: Life and living.* New York: Thomson.

30. Corr, C. (2006). *Living with grief: Children, adolescents and loss.* New York: Hospice Foundation of America.

31. Crawley, L. M. (2005). Racial, cultural, and ethnic factors influencing end-of-life care. *Journal of Palliative Medicine, 8*(Suppl. 1), S58–S69.

32. Davis, A., Phillips, L., Drought, T., Sellin, S., Ronsman, K., & Hershberger, A. (1995). Nurses' attitudes toward active euthanasia. *Nursing Outlook, 43*(4), 174–179.

33. Davis, A., & Slater, P. (1989). U.S. and Australian nurses' attitudes and beliefs about the good death. *IMAGE: Journal of Nursing Scholarship, 21*(1), 34–39.

34. De Arteaga, C. (1993). Helping children deal with death. *Journal of Christian Nursing, 10*(1), 28–31.

35. DeAugustine, C. (1998). Advanced directives, considering what is at stake. *Journal of Christian Nursing, 15*(4), 18–25.

36. Doka, K. J. (1989). *Disenfranchised grief: Recognizing hidden sorrow.* Lexington, MA: Lexington Books.

37. Doka, K. J. (Ed.). (2007). *Disenfranchised grief: New directions, challenges, and strategies for practice.* Champaign, IL: Research Press.

38. Doorenbos, A., & Nies, M. (2003). The use of advance directives on a population of Asian Indian Hindus. *Journal of Transcultural Nursing, 14*(1), 17–24.

39. Durham, E., & Weiss, L. (1997). How patients die. *American Journal of Nursing, 97*(12), 41–46.

40. Eadie, B., & Taylor, C. (1992). *Embraced by the light.* Riverside, NJ: McMillan.

41. Eaves, S. (1996). Permission to leave. *American Journal of Nursing, 96*(3), 80.

42. Engelberg, R. A. (2006). Measuring the quality of dying and death: Methodological considerations and recent findings. *Current Opinion in Critical Care, 12*, 381–387.

43. Erikson, J. (1997). *The life cycle completed: Erik H. Erikson.* New York: Norton.

44. Essa, E., & Murray, C. (1994). Young children's understanding and experience with death. *Young Children, 49*, 74–81.

45. Feifel, H. (1959). *The meaning of death.* New York: McGraw-Hill.

46. Ferdinand, R. (1995). I'd rather die than live this way. *American Journal of Nursing, 95*(12), 42–47.

47. Ferris, F. D. (2004). Last hours of living. *Clinics in Geriatric Medicine, 20*, 641–667.

48. Galek, K., Flannelly, K. J., Vane, A., & Galek, R. M. (2005). Assessing a patient's spiritual needs: A comprehensive instrument. *Holistic Nursing Practice, 19*, 62–69.

49. Gavrin, J. R. (2007). Ethical considerations at the end of life in the intensive care unit. *Critical Care Medicine, 35*(2 Suppl.), S85–S94.

50. Geisler, E. (1998). *Pocket guide to cultural assessment* (2nd ed.). St. Louis, MO: Mosby.

51. Giger, J. N., Davidhizar, R. E., & Fordham, P. (2006). Multi-cultural and multi-ethnic considerations and advanced directives: Developing cultural competency. *Journal of Cultural Diversity, 13*, 3–9.

52. Glaser, B., & Strauss, A. (1964). The social loss of dying patients. *American Journal of Nursing, 64*(6), 119ff.

53. Glaser, B., & Strauss, A. (1965). *Awareness of dying.* Chicago: Aldine.

54. Glaser, B., & Strauss, A. (1968). *Time for dying.* Chicago: Aldine.

55. Glass, R. M. (2005). Is grief a disease? Sometimes. *Journal of the American Medical Association, 293*, 2658–2660.

56. Griffie, J., Nelson-Marten, P., & Muchka, S. (2004). Acknowledging the "elephant": Communication in palliative care. *American Journal of Nursing, 104*(1), 48–57.

57. Grollman, E. (1990). *Talking about death: A dialogue between parent and child* (3rd ed.). Boston: Beacon Press.

58. Grollman, E. (1995). Explaining death to young children: Some questions and answers. In E. Grollman (Ed.), *Bereaved children and teens.* Boston: Beacon Press.

59. Haas, B. (1999). Clarification and integration of similar quality of life concepts. *IMAGE: Journal of Nursing Scholarship, 31*(3), 215–230.

60. Hallberg, I. R. (2004). Death and dying from old people's point of view. A literature review. *Aging: Clinical and Experimental Research, 16*, 87–103.

61. Hallberg, I. R. (2006). Palliative care as a framework for older people's long-term care. *International Journal of Palliative Nursing, 12*, 224–229.

62. Hallenbeck, J. (2006). High context illness and dying in a low context medical world. *American Journal of Hospice and Palliative Care, 23*, 113–118.

63. Hames, C. (2003). Helping infants and toddlers when a family member dies. *Journal of Hospice and Palliative Nursing, 5*(2), 103–110.

64. Hearne, K. (1984). A survey of reported premonitions and of those who have them. *Journal of Social Psychiatry Research, 52*, 261–270.

65. Hensley, P. L. (2006). Treatment of bereavement-related depression and traumatic grief. *Journal of Affective Disorders, 92*, 117–124.

66. Hockenberry, M., & Wilson, D. (2007). *Wong's nursing care of infants and children.* St. Louis, MO: Mosby Elsevier.

67. Holloway, M. (2006). Death the great leveler? Towards a transcultural spirituality of dying and bereavement. *Journal of Clinical Nursing, 15*, 833–839.

68. Hooyman, N. R., & Kramer, B. J. (2006). *Living through loss: Interventions across the life span.* New York: Columbia University Press.

69. Kastenbaum, R. (2000). *The psychology of death* (3rd ed.). New York: Springer.

70. Keeley, M. P., & Yingling, J. M. (2007). *Final conversations: Helping the living and dying talk to each other.* Acton, MA: VanderWyk and Burnham.

71. Kennard, M. (1998). A visit from an angel. *American Journal of Nursing, 98*(3), 48–51.

72. Kirk, K. (1998). How Oregon's Death with Dignity Act affects practice. *American Journal of Nursing, 98*(8), 54–55.

73. Kübler-Ross, E. (Ed.). (1969). *On death and dying.* New York: Collier-Macmillan.

74. Kübler-Ross, E. (Ed.). (1975). *Death, the final stage of growth.* Englewood Cliffs, NJ: Prentice-Hall.

75. Kübler-Ross, E. (Ed.). (1981). *Living with dying.* New York: Macmillan.

76. Kübler-Ross, E., & Kessler, D. (2005). *On grief and grieving: Finding the meaning of grief through the five stages of loss.* New York: Scribner.

77. Kuhl, D. (2002). *What dying people want: Practical wisdom for the end of life.* New York: Public Affairs.

78. Lamont, E. B. (2005). A demographic and prognostic approach to defining the end of life. *Journal of Palliative Medicine, 8*(Suppl. 1), S12–S21.

79. Lautrette, A., Ciroldi, M., Ksibi, H., & Azoulay, E. (2006). End of life family conferences: Rooted in the evidence. *Critical Care Medicine, 34*(11 Suppl.), S364–S372.

80. Marco, C. A., & Schears, R. M. (2006). Death, dying, and last wishes. *Emergency Medicine Clinics of North America, 24*, 969–987.

81. Matzo, M. (2004). Palliative care: Prognostication and the chronically ill. *American Journal of Nursing, 104*(9), 40–49.

82. Mazanec, P., & Tyler, M. (2003). Cultural considerations in end-of-life care: How ethnicity, age, and spirituality affect decisions when death is imminent. *American Journal of Nursing, 103*(3), 50–58.

83. Mezey, M., Evans, L., Golub, Z., Murphy, E., & White, G. (1994). The Patient Self-Determination Act: Sources of concern for nurses. *Nursing Outlook, 42*(1), 30–38.

84. Miles, A. (1998). Anger at God after a loved one dies. *American Journal of Nursing, 98*(3), 64–65.

85. Moody, R. A. (1975). *Life after life.* New York: Bantam Books.

86. Nagy, M. (1959). The child's view of death. In H. Fiefel (Ed.), *The meaning of death.* New York: McGraw-Hill.

87. NANDA International. (2005). *Nursing diagnoses: Definitions and classification 2005–2006.* Philadelphia: Author.

88. Noble, A., & Jones, C. (2005). Benefits of narrative therapy: Holistic interventions at the end of life. *British Journal of Nursing, 14*, 330–333.

89. Noppe, I., & Noppe, L. (1997). Evolving meanings of death during early, middle, and later adolescence. *Death Studies, 21*, 253–275.

90. Noppe, L., & Noppe, I. (1996). Ambiguity in adolescent understandings of death. In C. A. Corr & D. E. Balk (Eds.), *Handbook of adolescent death and bereavement.* New York: Springer.

91. O'Brien, M. (2006). Parish nursing. Meeting spiritual needs of elders near the end of life. *Journal of Christian Nursing, 23*(1), 28–33.

92. Oleck, S. (2004). *Taking advance directives seriously: Prospective autonomy and decisions near the end of life.* Washington, DC: Georgetown University Press.

93. Olsen, D. P. (2007). Arranging live organ donation over the Internet. *American Journal of Nursing, 107*(3), 69–72.

94. Olson, M. (1987). The out-of-body experiences and other states of consciousness. *Archives of Psychiatric Nursing, 1*(3), 201–207.

95. Papalia, D., Olds, S., & Feldman, P. (2004). *Human development* (9th ed.). Boston: McGraw-Hill.

96. Papowitz, L. (1986). Life/death/life. *American Journal of Nursing, 86*(4), 416–418.

97. Parnia, S. (2006). *What happens when we die? A groundbreaking study into the nature of life and death.* Carlsbad, CA: Hay House.

98. Peiffer, K. M. (2007). Brain death and organ procurement. *American Journal of Nursing, 107*(3), 58–68.

99. Plonk, W. M., & Arnold, R. M. (2005). Terminal care in the last weeks of life. *Journal of Palliative Medicine, 8,* 1042–1054.

100. Proulx, K., & Jacelon, C. (2004). Dying with dignity: The good patient versus the good death. *American Journal of Hospice and Palliative Medicine, 21,* 116–120.

101. Salladay, S. (2007). Life and death disagreements. *Journal of Christian Nursing, 24*(1), 38–40.

102. Santrock, J. (2004). *Life-span development* (9th ed.). Boston: McGraw-Hill.

103. Schoenbeck, S. (1993). Exploring the mystery of near-death experiences. *American Journal of Nursing, 93*(5), 43–46.

104. Stepnick, A., & Perry, T. (1992). Preventing spiritual distress in the dying client. *Journal of Psychosocial Nursing, 30*(1), 17–24.

105. Sweat, M. (2007). What are the spiritual needs of terminally ill patients? *Journal of Christian Nursing, 24*(1), 22.

106. Telford, K., Kralik, D., & Koch, T. (2006). Acceptance and denial: Implications for people adjusting to chronic illness: Literature review. *Journal of Advanced Nursing, 55,* 457–464.

107. Toombs, S. K. (2004). Living and dying with dignity: Reflections on lived experience. *Journal of Palliative Care, 20,* 193–200.

108. Treloar, L. (1998). Seeking a compassionate death. *Journal of Christian Nursing, 15*(4), 10–17.

109. Vaillant, G. E. (2002). *Aging well.* Boston: Little, Brown.

110. VanDelten, T. (1973). Sudden death...premonition of things to come. *Illinois Medical Journal, 141,* 352.

111. Vergara, M., & Lynn-McHale, D. (1995). Withdrawing life support: Who decides? *American Journal Nursing, 95*(11), 47–52.

112. Waechter, E. (1971). Children's awareness of fatal illness. *American Journal of Nursing, 71*(6), 1168–1172.

113. Waechter, E. (1984). Dying children patterns of coping. In H. Wass & C. A. Corr (Eds.), *Childhood and death.* Washington, DC: Hemisphere.

114. Weber, G. (1993). Tips in implementing the Patient Self-Determination Act. *Nursing and Health Care, 14*(2), 86–90.

115. Weisman, A., & Hackett, T. (1961). Predilection to death. *Psychosomatic Medicine, 23*(3).

116. Werner-Lin, A., & Moro, T. (2004). Unacknowledged and stigmatized losses. In F. Walsh & M. McGoldrick (Eds.), *Living beyond loss: Death in the family* (2nd ed., pp. 248–271). New York: Norton.

117. Wessel, E. M., & Garon, M. (2005). Introducing reflective narratives into palliative care and home care education. *Home Healthcare Nurse, 23,* 516–522.

118. Wiener, L., Alberta, A., Gibbins, M., & Hirschfeld, S. (1996). Visions of those who left too soon. *American Journal of Nursing, 96*(9), 57–59, 61.

119. Williams, A. L. (2006). Perspectives on spirituality at the end of life: A meta-summary. *Palliative and Supportive Care, 4,* 404–417.

120. Williams, L., & Hopper, P. (2007). *Understanding medical-surgical nursing* (3rd ed.). Philadelphia: Davis.

121. Wilson, D. (1992). Ethical concerns in a long-term tube feeding study. *IMAGE: Journal of Nursing Scholarship, 24,* 195–199.

122. Wowchuk, S. M., McClement, S., & Bond, J. (2006). The challenge of providing palliative care in the nursing home: Part I. External factors. *International Review of Palliative Nursing, 12,* 260–267.

123. Zimbelman, J. (1994). Good life, good death, and the right to die: Ethical considerations for decisions at the end of life. *Journal of Professional Nursing, 10*(1), 22–37.

124. Zimmerman, P. (1998). Rest in peace, Rabbi Shapiro. *American Journal of Nursing, 98*(4), 64–65.

125. Zuckerman, C. (1997). Issues concerning end-of-life care. *Journal of Long-Term Home Health Care, 16,* 26–34.

Interview

126. Zentner, R. (1971, March). *Personal story of life after life.*

Appendix A

Nutrition

Nutrient	Major Sources	Major Functions
Protein	Meat, poultry, fish, dried beans and peas, eggs, nuts, cheese, milk. Whole grain cereals are incomplete and must be combined with animal protein. Animal and vegetable protein combined increase use by body of all amino acids.	Builds, maintains, and repairs body cells; is required for amino acids (eight are essential). Constitutes part of the structure of every cell. Supports growth and maintains healthy body cells. Maintains pH balance of blood; acts as buffer system. Regulates osmotic pressure. Constitutes part of enzymes, some hormones, body fluids, antibodies that increase resistance to infection, hemoglobin, plasma proteins. Is source of energy and fuel when inadequate carbohydrate and fat unavailable. Protein degraded and resynthesized continually, daily intake is needed.
Carbohydrate	Bread, potatoes, dried beans, corn, rice, fruit, vegetables, sugar, desserts, candy, jam, syrup, honey.	Supplies energy and forms adenosine triphosphate (ATP) so protein can be used for growth; maintenance of body cells and metabolic processes. Maintains body temperature. Supplies fiber in unrefined products—complex carbohydrates in fruits, vegetables, and whole grains—for regular elimination. Assists in fat utilization.
Fat	Animal fat, shortening, vegetable oil, butter, margarine, salad dressing, mayonnaise, sausages, lunch meats, whole milk and milk products, nuts. No more than 30% of total calories should be from fat. No more than 10% of fat intake should be saturated fat.	Provides concentrated source of energy. Constitutes part of the structure of every cell. Helps control cell permeability. Supplies essential fatty acids. Is necessary for absorption of (carrier for) fat-soluble vitamins (A, D, E, and K). Maintains adipose tissue, which insulates and protects inner organs from trauma. Is component of thromboplastin, used in blood clotting. Adds to food taste, texture, and appearance.
Vitamins Vitamin C (ascorbic acid) (water soluble)	Citrus fruits such as orange, grapefruit, lime, lemon; papaya, mango, kiwi, cantaloupe, pineapple, rose hips, all berries, black currants, melons, cherries, alfalfa sprouts, watercress, parsley, tomatoes, broccoli, sweet peppers, raw potatoes, raw leafy vegetables, cabbage, brussels sprouts, cauliflower, asparagus, bok choy, thyme, horehound root, celery seed, sarsaparilla root, dandelion root.	Antioxidant. Forms cementing substances such as collagen that hold body cells together, thus strengthening blood vessels, hastening healing of wounds and bone fractures, and increasing resistance to infection. Helps develop and maintain healthy bones, teeth, gums, skin, muscles, and blood vessels. Prevents scurvy. Regulates mitochondria and microsomal respiratory cycle. Aids use of iron and folic acid metabolism. Normalizes body cholesterol, decreases risk of heart disease. Aspirin prevents absorption.

continued

Nutrient	Major Sources	Major Functions
Thiamin (B$_1$) (water soluble)	Pork, lean meat, nuts, liver, fish, oysters, crabmeat, dried yeast, milk, whole grains, enriched bread and cereals, pasta, dry beans, peas, lima beans, soybeans, sunflower seeds, brown rice, asparagus, raisins, alfalfa.	Functions as part of coenzyme to promote use of carbohydrate and protein and release of energy. Reduces fatigue and weakness; produces energy. Promotes normal appetite. Contributes to normal functioning of nervous, muscle, and digestive systems. Prevents beriberi.
Riboflavin (B$_2$) (water soluble)	Liver and other organ meats, ham, poultry, milk and milk products, yogurt, cottage cheese, egg yolk, green leafy vegetables, lean meat, whole grains, soybeans, peas, beans, nuts, enriched bread and cereal, brewer's yeast, blackstrap molasses, sunflower seeds, wheat germ, alfalfa.	Is component of flavoprotein involved in biological oxidation. Is essential for building and maintaining body tissues, antibodies, and red blood cells. Functions as part of a coenzyme in the production of energy within body cells. Promotes carbohydrate, fat, and protein metabolism. Maintains nitrogen balance. Is essential for use of oxygen in cells. Promotes healthy skin, eyes, tongue, lips, mucous membranes.
Niacin (B$_3$) (water soluble)	Liver, meat, rabbit, poultry, fish, peanuts, whole grains, brewer's yeast, fortified cereal and bread products, wheat germ, gentian root, licorice root, alfalfa.	Aids use of vitamins B$_1$ and B$_2$. Is essential for tissue respiration. Functions as part of a coenzyme in fat synthesis, protein use, glycolysis and use of carbohydrate, and release of energy. Promotes healthy skin, nerves, digestive tract, blood vessels. Aids digestion and fosters normal appetite. Is required for formation of certain hormones and nerve-regulating substances. Prevents pellagra.
Pyridoxine (B$_6$) (water soluble)	Liver, meat, fish, poultry, whole-grain bread and cereals, wheat germ, brewer's yeast, sunflower seeds, soybeans, nuts, brown rice, bananas, avocado, sweet potatoes, white potatoes, corn, white beans, green leafy vegetables, alfalfa.	Is coenzyme in basic reactions of amino acid, fat metabolism, protein metabolism. Is essential for immune system. Assists antibody, hormone, and red blood cell formation. Is involved with function of neurotransmitters. Helps maintain balance of sodium and phosphorus and metabolism of iron and potassium.
Cobalamin (B$_{12}$) (water soluble)	Organ meats such as liver, kidney, and heart; lean meat, poultry, fish, oysters, clams, sea vegetables (kelp, dulse, kombu), eggs, milk, yogurt, cheese, brewer's yeast, angelica root, alfalfa.	Is essential for all blood cell formation. Is coenzyme for synthesis of materials for nucleus of all cells. Is essential for synthesis of nucleic acids; metabolism of certain amino acids, protein, carbohydrate, fat; and normal cell function. Is especially important for cells of bone marrow, intestinal tract, central nervous system. Strict vegetarians, elders, and persons with malabsorption disorder at risk for deficiency, pernicious anemia.
Folate (folic acid or folacin) (water soluble)	Dark green, leafy vegetables such as collards, mustard greens, turnip greens, kale; organ meats, dried beans, root vegetables, whole grains, brewer's yeast, oysters, salmon, milk, black-eyed peas, lima beans, watermelon, cantaloupe.	Synthesizes nucleic acid and proteins. Acts with B$_{12}$ in making genetic material. Assists metabolism of certain amino acids. Assists in hemoglobin, red blood cell, protein formation. Is necessary for normal cell division. Prevents anemia and birth defects.

Nutrient	Major Sources	Major Functions
Vitamin A (and carotenoids) (fat soluble)	Liver; orange-colored fruits; orange, yellow, and dark green vegetables such as carrots, winter squash, sweet potatoes, broccoli, and greens; eggs, fortified milk, butter, margarine, cheese, horehound root, celery seed, dandelion root, red peppers.	Works as antioxidant in form of carotenoids. Assists formation, maintenance, and repair of normal skin, hair, mucous membranes, increasing resistance to infection. Maintains mitochondrial and liposomal membranes. Functions in visual processes, forms visual purple, thus promoting healthy eye tissue and eye adaptation in dim light or at night. Enhances immune system function. Aids in controlling cell differentiation.
Vitamin D (fat soluble)	Fortified milk, butter, margarine, fish liver oil, salmon, tuna, egg yolk, liver, bone meal, thyme, sunshine.	Regulates calcium and phosphorus metabolism; promotes intestinal absorption of calcium and phosphorus. Regulates blood calcium. Promotes bone mineralization (prevents rickets) and tooth formation.
Vitamin E (fat soluble)	Vegetable oils, liver, wheat germ, whole grain cereals, rice, oats, brewer's yeast, almonds and hazelnuts, peanut butter, foods high in polyunsaturated fatty acids, eggs, molasses, sweet potatoes, leafy vegetables, lettuce, spinach, asparagus, cauliflower, broccoli, angelica root, horehound root.	Is antioxidant at tissue level; maintains tissue. Is essential in cellular respiration. Improves immune system. Prevents abnormal fat breakdown in tissues. Assists in formation of normal red blood cells and muscle. Functions in reproductive system. Prevents buildup of LDL (bad) cholesterol plaque and blood clot formation in blood vessels, thus preventing coronary disease. Protects against exposure to radiation.
Vitamin K (fat soluble)	K_1 is found in lean meat, liver, green plants, green leafy vegetables, tomatoes, cauliflower, peas, carrots, potatoes, cabbage, soybean and safflower oil, egg yolk, blackstrap molasses, wheat germ. K_3 is synthetic therapeutic form. Half of vitamin K in body synthesized by intestinal bacteria as K_2.	Is essential for synthesis of blood-clotting factors; prothrombin (factor I), factors VII, IX, X. Stimulates coagulation proenzymes, II, VII, IX, X. Reduces risk of bone fractures.
Biotin	Egg yolk, organ meats, fish, brewer's yeast, whole grains, legumes, sardines, most fresh vegetables, lima beans, mushrooms, peanuts, bananas, yogurt.	Is necessary for formation of folic acid. Is necessary for carbohydrate, protein, fat metabolism and energy production. Aids in use of other B vitamins.
Pantothenic acid	Organ meats, lobster, oyster, salmon, brewer's yeast, egg yolk, legumes, whole grains, wheat germ, nuts, soy flour, sunflower and sesame seeds, green leafy vegetables, broccoli, cauliflower, potatoes, licorice root.	Aids in formation of some fats, hormones. Aids in metabolism and release of energy from carbohydrates, fats, proteins. Aids in use of some vitamins. Lowers cholesterol. Improves resistance to stress and infection.
Choline	Egg yolk, organ meat, fish, salmon, brewer's yeast, wheat germ, soybeans, legumes.	Aids in normal nerve transmission. Aids metabolism and transport of fats. Aids production of acetylcholine, a neurotransmitter.
Para-aminobenzoic acid (PABA)	Organ meats, wheat germ, yogurt, molasses, green leafy vegetables.	Aids bacteria producing folic acid. Acts as a coenzyme in use of proteins. Aids in formation of red blood cells.

continued

Nutrient	Major Sources	Major Functions
Minerals Calcium	Milk and milk products, chowder, cream soups, puddings made with milk, custards, yogurt; shellfish, salmon, sardines, bone meal; dark green leafy vegetables, egg yolk, whole grains, legumes, nuts, tofu, molasses, broccoli, tomatoes, chamomile flower, cascara sagrada, angelica root, passion flower.	Works with phosphorus, magnesium, vitamin D, other minerals, protein to build bones and teeth. Assists blood clotting. Is necessary for nerve transmission, heart function, muscle contraction and relaxation, cell wall permeability. Intestinal absorption of vitamin D, which decreases with age, necessary for calcium metabolism. Oxalates and phytates in green leafy vegetables and grains interfere with calcium absorption by combining with calcium and creating insoluble compound. Fiber may combine with calcium and limit absorption. Alcohol intake interferes with metabolism. Caffeine and excess salt intake cause calcium excretion.
Phosphorus	Milk and milk products, meat, liver, seafood, whole grains, wheat germ, nuts, egg yolk, legumes, peas, beans, lentils, brown rice, sunflower seeds, brewer's yeast.	Helps formation of nucleic acids. Works with calcium and vitamin D to build and maintain healthy bones, teeth, cell membranes. Aids absorption of glucose and glycerol. Transports fatty acids. Acts as buffer system. Aids energy metabolism.
Magnesium	Whole grains, cereals, nuts, citrus fruits, figs, green leafy vegetables, Swiss chard, dried beans and peas, soybeans, meat, milk, brown rice, wheat germ, chamomile flower, passion flower, senega root.	Promotes healthy nerve and muscle tissue and function. Is component of bones and teeth. Is activator and coenzyme in carbohydrate, fat, protein metabolism. Acts as catalyst in use of calcium and phosphorus. Is essential intracellular fluid cation.
Potassium (electrolyte)	Lean meat, chicken, whole grains, bananas, oranges, apricots, dried fruits, potatoes, broccoli, spinach, raw cabbage, Swiss chard, okra, legumes, lima beans, sunflower seeds, molasses, wheat germ, skim milk, roasted chestnuts, horehound root.	Is major intracellular fluid cation. Controls activity of heart, muscles, nervous system, kidneys. Regulates neuromuscular excitability and muscle contraction. Promotes acid-base balance. Is necessary for glycogen formation and protein synthesis.
Sodium (electrolyte)	Table salt, fish, seafood, kelp, baking powder and baking soda, milk, cheese, meat, eggs, celery, carrots, beets, spinach, cucumber, asparagus, turnips, string beans, coconut, processed foods and cereals, snack foods such as potato chips, pretzels, salted nuts.	Is major extracellular fluid cation. Maintains normal fluid level and osmotic pressure in cells. Maintains health of nervous, muscular, blood, lymph systems. Promotes cell permeability and absorption of glucose. Transmits electrochemical impulse in muscle, resulting in contraction. Promotes acid-base balance; acts with potassium, magnesium chloride; buffers carbon dioxide and ketones.
Chloride (electrolyte)	Table salt, seafood, meats, liver, fish, ripe olives, rye flour, soybeans, egg yolks, peanuts, wheat germ.	Is major extracellular fluid anion. Regulates acid-base balance and chlorine-bicarbonate shift. Maintains osmotic pressure. Stimulates production of hydrochloric acid. Helps maintain joints and tendons.

Nutrient	Major Sources	Major Functions
Trace Minerals Iron	Organ and red meats, fish, poultry, beef, pork, lamb, dried and canned beans and peas, enriched whole-grain breads and cereals, dark green leafy vegetables, mustard and dandelion greens, egg yolk, blackstrap molasses, cherry and prune juice, legumes, nuts, dried fruits (raisins, apricots), chamomile flower, horehound root, senega root, celery seed. Cook in iron skillet.	Is essential for hemoglobin and myoglobin formation. Helps protein metabolism. Is used by cells as component for oxidation of glucose in production of energy. Aids tissue respiration. Promotes growth. Increases resistance to infection. Is more readily used by body when ascorbic acid, copper, folic acid, vitamin B_{12} available. Excess calcium intake interferes with iron absorption.
Zinc	Organ and red meats, sunflower seeds, oysters, herring, seafood, eggs, mushrooms, brewer's yeast, soybeans, wheat germ.	Is component of insulin, serum proteins, reproductive fluid, bone, muscle, eyes, hair, teeth, liver. Aids digestion and metabolism of phosphorus. Is necessary for respiration and digestion. Is important for sensory functioning, normal growth, hair, complexion, sexual function, wound healing. Aids healing and resistance to infection; excess or deficiency interferes with immune function.
Copper	Organ and lean meats, seafood, nuts, legumes, molasses, raisins, bone meal, cocoa, food cooked in copperware.	Absorbs and transports iron and aids in formation of red blood cells. Is component of many enzymes, which, in turn, are necessary for development and maintenance of skeletal, cardiovascular, and central nervous systems. Works with vitamin C to form elastin.
Iodine	Iodized salt, seafood, kelp, green leafy vegetables.	Is necessary for thyroid gland to control cell activities and metabolism. Synthesizes thyroxine, the thyroid hormones, which regulates cell oxidation. Promotes growth. Prevents goiter.
Sulfur	Fish, shrimp, eggs, meat, cabbage, brussels sprouts, asparagus, milk, cheese, nuts, legumes, peas, beans, mustard greens, cauliflower, mashed potatoes.	Is component of amino acids and B vitamins. Is essential for formation of body tissues, collagen, skin, bones, tendons, cartilage. Assists in tissue respiration. Is required for oxidation-reduction reactions. Activates enzymes. Aids in detoxification reactions.
Fluoride	Natural supply in water in some areas of United States, fluoridated water, seafood, bone meal, tea.	Is deposited in teeth and bones. May reduce tooth decay by discouraging growth of acid-forming bacteria. May help to strengthen bones.
Molybdenum	Legumes, whole-grain cereals, milk, liver, dark green vegetables.	Acts in oxidation of fat and aldehydes. Aids in mobilization of iron from liver reserves. Assists in conversion of purine to uric acid.
Manganese	Whole grains, green leafy vegetables, legumes, nuts, pineapple, grapefruit, egg yolk, tea, coffee, cascara sagrada, licorice root.	Is enzyme activator for urea formation, protein and fat metabolism, glucose oxidation, synthesis of fatty acids. Is necessary for normal skeletal formation, brain function. Maintains sex hormone production.

continued

Nutrient	Major Sources	Major Functions
Chromium	Corn oil, clams, whole grain cereals, meat, liver, wheat germ, brewer's yeast, drinking water in some areas of United States.	Stimulates enzymes in metabolism of energy and synthesis of fatty acids, cholesterol, protein. Increases effectiveness of action of insulin in cell, which improves glucose uptake by body tissues.
Selenium	Seafood, tuna, herring, organ and red meat, brewer's yeast, wheat germ, bran, asparagus, mushrooms, broccoli, whole grains, bread, cereals, garlic.	Acts as cofactor in cell oxidation enzyme systems. Is constituent of factor III, which acts with vitamin E to prevent fatty liver. Preserves tissue elasticity. Protects against heart disease.
Water	Water, coffee, tea, milk, soup, fruit juices, flavored gelatin, fruits, vegetables.	Is part of blood, lymph, body secretions. Aids digestion. Dissolves nutrients and enables them to pass through intestinal wall. Regulates body temperature. Transports body wastes for elimination.

Appendix B

Drug Tables

Summary of Legal and Illicit Drugs Related to Nursing Assessment and Intervention

Drug Type/Name	Street Names	Action & Duration	Administration	Desired Effect	Physical & Emotional Effects/Complications
Narcotics Opiates; opium, morphine, heroin, codeine Dilaudid Synthetic nonopiates, Methadone Demerol, Darvon, Percodan, Percoset OxyContin Vicodin	Snow, stuff, H, junk, smack, scag, dreamer, Ska	Central nervous system depressant 3–24 hours Addicting Interaction with alcohol, antihistamine, barbiturates, benzodiazepine, causes respiratory depression.	Oral; smoked; sniffed; injected under skin (skin popping); intramuscular (IM); intravenous (IV); cough medicine containing codeine	Euphoria Prevention of withdrawal discomfort	Drowsiness, sedation, nodding stupor. Eye and nose secretions. Euphoria. Relief of pain. Impaired intellectual functioning and coordination. Constricted pupils that do not respond to light. Excessive itching. Poor appetite. Constipation. Urinary retention. Loss of sexual desire, temporary impotence or sterility Slow pulse and respiration(s); hypotension. Death from overdosage caused by respiratory and cardiovascular depression and collapse. Effects on fetus. Severe infection at injection sites (needle marks and tracks)
Barbiturates Nembutol, Seconal, Amytal, Fiornal, Tuinol, Phenobarbital	Sleepers, downers, goofballs, redbirds, yellow jackets, heavens, red devils, barbs, phennies	Central nervous system (CNS) depressant 1–16 hours Can be lethal with alcohol or other CNS depressants. GABA activity	Oral, or injected IM or IV	Relaxation and euphoria	Relief of anxiety and muscular tension, relaxation, sleep. Respirations slow, shallow. Slowed reactions. Euphoria. Impaired emotional control, judgment, and coordination. Irritability or unusual excitement. Apathy. Confused. Poor hygiene. Slurred, slow speech. Poor memory. Weight loss. Liver, brain, kidney damage from long-term use Death from overdose. Psychosis, possible convulsions, or death from abrupt withdrawal of barbiturates

Tolerance Potential	Physical Dependence	Psychological Dependence	Withdrawal Characteristics	Nursing Care
Yes	High. Controlled substance	High	Abdominal pain. Muscle cramps, tremors, spasms. Nausea, vomiting, diarrhea. Lacrimation, watery eyes. Goose bumps, sweating, chills. Hypertension, tachycardia, increased respirations. Anxiety, irritability, depression. Craving for drugs occurs 48–72 hours after last dose; subsides within a week.	(1) Observe for symptoms of withdrawal and report to physician. (2) Give medications prescribed to suppress withdrawal symptoms. (3) Monitor for vital signs at least qid for first 72 hours following admission. (4) Carry out nursing measures to promote safety, general health, and sense of security. (5) Observe and take precaution for seizure activity. (6) Promote general health and sense of security.
Yes	Moderate. Controlled substance.	Moderate to high.	Nausea, vomiting, diarrhea. Bleeding. Tremors. Diaphoresis. Hypertension or hypotension. Temperature above 99.6°F. Irritability, hostility, restlessness, agitation. Sleep disturbance. Impaired cognitive function. Acute brain syndrome. Seizures.	(1) Observe for withdrawal symptoms and report to physician. (2) Give prescribed medication to suppress symptoms. (3) Provide calm, quiet, safe environment, as free of external stimuli as possible, for acute or severe withdrawal symptoms. (4) Observe for insomnia and nightmares and provide nursing measures to promote sleep.

continued

Summary of Legal and Illicit Drugs Related to Nursing Assessment and Intervention—continued

Drug Type/ Name	Street Names	Action & Duration	Administration	Desired Effect	Physical & Emotional Effects/ Complications
Sedatives Doriden Chloralhydrate, Methaquolone Placidyl		Central nervous system depressant 3–4 hours Can be lethal with alcohol	Oral	Sleep, relaxation	May be same effect as barbiturates but not as severe
Minor tranquilizers Valium Librium Miltown Equanil	Downers, Candy, Tranus	Central nervous system depressant 3–4 hours	Oral, or injected IM or IV	Relaxation, sense of calm	Relieve anxiety. Varied onset and duration of effect according to preparation and administration.
Inhalants (Glue sniffing, aerosols, butane preparations, airplane glue, amyl nitrate, nitrous oxide, any spray, including paint)	Whippits, Poppers, Snappers	Central nervous system depressant Intoxicant lasts a few minutes. Users extend this effect by breathing inhalant repeatedly.	Inhaled through tubes, glue smears on paper or cloth	Intoxication, relaxation, euphoria Rapid high, resembles alcohol intoxication	Excess nasal secretion. Watering of eyes. Tinnitus. Diplopia. Poor muscular control, lack of coordination. Appears dreamy, blank, or drunk. Impaired perception and judgment. Possibility of violent behavior. Sleepy after 35 to 45 minutes or unconscious. Damage to lungs, nervous system, brain, liver, kidney. Death through suffocation, choking, or overdose. Repeated inhalation results in sudden death, especially with abuse of propane or butane.

Tolerance Potential	Physical Dependence	Psychological Dependence	Withdrawal Characteristics	Nursing Care
Yes	Controlled substance	Yes	Anxiety. Insomnia. Tremors. Delirium. Convulsions.	(1) Observe and treat if taken in suicide attempt. (2) Provide environment for safety and sleep. (3) Teach measures to promote sleep and rest.
Yes	Controlled substance	Yes	Anxiety. Irritability. Poor concentration.	(1) Observe for withdrawal symptoms or if a suicide attempt and treat. (2) Provide calm, safe environment. (3) Teach stress management. (4) Promote general health.
Yes	No	Yes	Withdrawal symptoms have not been recorded	(1) Emergency care for respiratory damage or neurological complication. (2) Provide for safety. (3) Implement other nursing measures related to presenting symptoms, especially if this drug has been used in combination with others.

continued

Summary of Legal and Illicit Drugs Related to Nursing Assessment and Intervention—continued

Drug Type/ Name	Street Names	Action & Duration	Administration	Desired Effect	Physical & Emotional Effects/ Complications
Stimulants Amphetamines Dexedrine Methedrine Methamphet-amine ("crystal meth")	Pep pills, uppers, A, speed, heat, crystal, dexies, bennies, lid poppers, black beauties, truck driver crosses	Central nervous system stimulant Varies in duration of action	Oral; or injected under skin or IV. Smoked Snorted	Sense of well-being Alertness, feelings of activity and increased initiative	Giggling, silliness, talk-ativeness. Rapid speech. Dilated pupils. Hyperten-sion, dizzy, tachy-cardia. Loss of appetite, loss of weight. Diarrhea.
Cocaine	Leaf, snow, coke, speedballs Ilake, gold dust, crack, smack, blow Rock Fire Crack C Ice Charlie Toot	2–4 hours Crack, immediate Depression and exhaustion can last several days Dopamine and nor-epinephrine overstimulates CNS	Cocaine sniffed, snorted, IV, or smoking (free-basing)	Excitation Overconfidence	Extreme fatigue. Dry mouth, bad breath. Chills, sweating, increased muscle tension; shakiness, tremors, restless-ness. Irritability. Confused, grandiose thinking. Deep depression. Mood swings. Aggressive behavior. Paranoid ideas which may persist. Feelings of persecution. Delusions. Hallucina-tions. Panic. Toxic psychosis. Possible seizures. Tachycardia may cause heart damage or heart attack. Death from cardiac damage, hypertensive crisis, stroke, paralysis of respiratory center, fatigue or overdose.
Caffeine (Found in tea, coffee, cocoa, cola, and tablet form, including many over-the-counter drugs.)	Kiddie dope (caffeine, ephedrine, phenylo-propanolamine), black beauty, speckled eggs, speckled birds, pink heart, 20–20's, blue and clears, green and clears	Central nervous system stimulant. Cardiac stimulant 2–4 hours High similar to amphetamines	Oral	A "pick-up"; to increase alertness and decrease fatigue. More rapid, clearer flow of thoughts	Restleness. Disturbed sleep or insomnia. Nausea, abdominal distention. Anorexia. Myocardial stimula-tion, palpitation, and tachycardia. Dizzy. Large amounts have led to irrational or hyster-ical behavior and, very large doses, cardiac standstill. Stimulates gastric secretions. Raises BMR by 10%. Diuretic. Reduced fine motor coordination.

Tolerance Potential	Physical Dependence	Psychological Dependence	Withdrawal Characteristics	Nursing Care
Yes	Yes	High	Tremors. Neurological hyperactivity. Paranoia. Assaultive behavior. Irritability. Depression. Possible suicidal behavior or psychotic reaction. Tachycardia, hypertension. Oversensitivity to stimuli. Insomnia. Intense craving	(1) Observe for symptoms of withdrawal and report to physician. (2) Give medication as prescribed to suppress agitated state and prevent exhaustion (3) Take precautions for staff and client safety according to client's paranoia and depression. (4) Monitor vital signs at least qid for first 72 hours following admission. (5) Provide calm, nonthreatening, quiet environment and sense of security. (6) Provide for sleep and nutrition. (7) Cocaine—observe for chronic nose-bleed and perforated nasal septum. (8) Detoxification. (9) Teach stress management, alternate leisure activities.
Yes Develops quickly	Yes	Yes	In moderate heavy users, there may be headache, irritability, nervousness, tremors, lethargy	(1) Introduce substitute decaffeinated beverage (2) Provide for general health needs and teaching (3) Observe for caffeinism; irritability, tremors, tics, insomnia, sensory disturbance, tachypnea, arrhythmias, diuresis, GI distress. (4) Teach cognitive methods and stress management techniques to reduce fatigue, promote alertness.

continued

Summary of Legal and Illicit Drugs Related to Nursing Assessment and Intervention—continued

Drug Type/ Name	Street Names	Action & Duration	Administration	Desired Effect	Physical & Emotional Effects/ Complications
Hallucinogens Synthetic D-lysergic acid (LSD) 4-methyl-2 (STP, DOM) Phencyclidine (PCP) Dimethyltryptamine (DMT) Natural cactus (mescaline, peyote) Mushroom (psilocybin)	Acid, Big D, sugar, trips, cubes Serenity, tranquility, peace Businessman's special	Hallucinogenic, varies: LSD 10–12 hours; STP 6-8 hours Mescaline 12–24 hours	Primarily oral; some are inhaled or injected	Insight. Distortion of senses Exhilaration Increased energy	Severe hallucinations, feelings of persecution and detachment. Amnesia. Incoherent speech Laughing, crying. Exhilaration, depression, or panic alternates with sense of invulnerability. Suicidal or homicidal tendencies. Suspicious. Impaired judgment. Cold, sweaty hands and feet; shivering, chills. Vomiting. Weight loss. Irregular breathing. Exhaustion. Dilated pupils. Hypertension. Brain damage from chronic use. Accidental death. Flashbacks. May intensify psychosis; long-lasting mental illness has resulted. Symptoms may persist for an indefinite period after discontinuation of drug.
Nicotina (Found in cigarettes, cigars, pipe and chewing tobacco, and snuff)		Variable action. Central nervous system toxin. Can act as stimulant or depressant: 15 minutes–2 hours Increases dopamine, acetylcholine.	Smoked, sniffed, chewed	Calmness, sociability Increases alertness.	Can have stimulating and/or calming effect Nausea, Vomiting, Reduces appetite Factor in lung cancer, coronary artery disease, circulatory impairment, peptic ulcer, and emphysema.

IM, intramuscular; IV, intravenous; qid, four times daily.
Adopted from references 13, 42, 79, 96, 104, 119–120, 123–130, 132, 139, 183, 196.
References can be found on pages 485–488.

Tolerance Potential	Physical Dependence	Psychological Dependence	Withdrawal Characteristics	Nursing Care
Yes	Yes	Probable	Severe apprehension, fear, or panic. Perceptual distortions and hallucinations. Hyperactivity. Diaphoresis. Tachycardia.	(1) Have someone who is close to client stay with client at all times to provide support and comfort. (2) Provide nonthreatening environment with subdued, pleasant stimuli. (3) Provide orientation and diversion to pleasant experiences. (4) Avoid use of sedative/ tranquilizers, if possible. (5) Monitor vital signs. (6) Provide for general health needs. (7) Teach stress management and cognitive methods to increase energy, insight, feelings of health, and life satisfaction. (8) Teach alternate leisure activities.
Yes	Yes	Yes	Headache. Anorexia, irritability, nervousness. Decreased ability to concentrate. Craving for cigarette. Energy loss. Fatigue. Dizziness. Sweating. Tremor and palpitations.	(1) Provide support. (2) Explore behavioral changes necessary to quit smoking as well as provide information as to available self-help groups. (3) Provide for general health needs. (4) Teach smoking cessation program.

Summary of Marijuana Drugs Related to Nursing Assessment and Intervention

Drug Type/ Name	Street Names	Action & Duration	Administration	Desired Effect	Physical & Emotional Effects/ Complications
Marijuana (cannabis), *Indian hemp*, which produces varying grades of hallucino-genic material; *hashish*, pure cannabis resin, the most powerful grade from leaves and flowering tops of female plants; *ganja*, less potent preparation of flowering tops and stems of female plant and resin attached to them; *bhang*, least potent preparation of dried mature leaves and flowering tops of male and female plants. *THC* in fat part of cell prevents nutrients from crossing cell membranes: RNA produc-tion and new cell growth reduced; *all* cell functions interfered with	Joints, reefer, pot grass, weed Acapulco Gold The Sticks Hash	Mixed: central nervous system depressant and stimulant. Great variance in duration 2–12 hours THC is fat-soluble, absorbed espe-cially by brain cells and repro-ductive organs. Builds in the brain; 2 ciga-rettes per week for 3 months causes person-ality change. Impairment during non-intoxicated state remains when smoking persists over months.	Smoked or swallowed	Euphoria Relaxation Increased perception Escape	**Nervous system** Stored in fat portion of cells; remains in brain 6 weeks after cessation of smoking Speech comprehen-sion, ability to express ideas, and ability to understand relationships impaired because of damage to the cerebral cortex Memory, decision making, handling complex tasks, ability to concen-trate or focus impaired because of effects on cells in the hypocampus and cerebrum Emotional swings, depression, pessimism, irri-tability, low frustra-tion tolerance, and temper outbursts because of cell damage in limbic system Does not learn adaptive skills or how to cope with stressors Lack of motivation, fatigue, moodiness, depression, inability to cope, loss of interest in vigorous activity or all previ-ously enjoyed activi-ties occurs because of THC effects on various parts of the brain; failure to continue in emotional development

Tolerance Potential	Physical Dependence	Psychological Dependence	Withdrawal Characteristics	Nursing Care
Yes	Yes	Yes	Heavy smokers report irritability, restless-ness, loss of appetite, sleep disturbance, sweating, tremor, nausea, vomiting, and diarrhea, hyperacidity. Ability for memory, thinking, learning, concentration is impaired.	(1) Not usually admitted to acute care settings unless this drug has been used in combination with others, so that a mixed effect occurs. (2) Implement nursing measures listed under *Hallucinogens*. (3) Likely to see increasing number of children and adolescents with physical effects from chronic use or injuries from accidents; appro-priate medical and surgical nursing care should be given. (4) Teach stress management and cognitive methods to relax, cope with stressors, and increase life satisfaction. (5) Explore alternate leisure activities.

continued

Summary of Marijuana Drugs Related to Nursing Assessment and Intervention—continued

Drug Type/ Name	Street Names	Action & Duration	Administration	Desired Effect	Physical & Emotional Effects/ Complications
					Psychosis may occur with one use, delusions of persecution common; each episode increases risk for later schizophrenia
					Insomnia because of damage to cells in the hypothalamus
					Vision blurred and irregular visual perception because of damage to cells in the occipital areas
					Body coordination, maintenance of posture and balance, ability to perform sports or drive a car impaired because of damage to cells in the cerebellum
					Respiratory system
					Upper respiratory infections common because of destruction to mucosal cells from the smoke (more destructive than tobacco smoke)
					Sinusitis, inflammation of the lining of one or more of the sinuses from nasal infection
					Bronchitis, with low-grade fever, chest pain, chronic cough, and yellow-green sputum, common because of inflammation to the bronchial tree caused by smoke inhalation
					Lung cancer more likely because of the numerous chemicals in marijuana (smoking three to five joints a week is equivalent to smoking 16 cigarettes daily for 7 days a week)
					Increased head and neck cancer.
					Emphysema and chronic obstructive pulmonary diseases from long-time smoking and deep inhalation; lung function permanently damaged
					Cardiovascular system
					Cardiac arhythmias and tachycardia related to the dose of THC absorbed (one joint immediately raises heart rate by as much as 50%)
					Hypertension, which may contribute to aneurysm formation or cardio-vascular accident, common

Summary of Marijuana Drugs Related to Nursing Assessment and Intervention—continued

Drug Type/ Name	Street Names	Action & Duration	Administration	Desired Effect	Physical & Emotional Effects/ Complications

					Myocardial infarction possible
					Congested conjunctiva associated
					  with hypertension
					Reproductive system
					Infertility in males from moderate to
					  heavy use because production of
					  testosterone is reduced and low
					  sperm production or production of
					  abnormal sperm occurs
					Impotence, inability to ejaculate
					  sperm
					Gynecomastia, enlarged breast
					  formation in puberty when
					  secondary sex characteristics are
					  being developed (lower testos-
					  terone level causes fat deposits
					  around the breast tissue)
					Hirsutism in females, with increased
					  androgen production resulting in
					  male secondary sex characteristics
					  (increased hair growth on face and
					  arms, deeper voice), irregular
					  menstrual cycles, serious acne, and
					  lack of development of female
					  secondary sexual characteristics
					Infertility in the female because of
					  damage to the ova; menstrual
					  cycle irregularity
					Pregnancy, if present when
					  marijuana is smoked, endangers
					  the embryo and fetus, increasing
					  chance of congenital defects and
					  fetal mortality because THC crosses
					  the placental barrier
					Lactation, if breast-feeding while
					  smoking marijuana, endangers
					  baby's health because THC
					  transfers through breast milk
					Immune system suppressed; prone
					  to infections
					Endocrine system impaired for
					  11- to 16-year-olds
					Marijuana combined with PCP causes
					  psychosis; if taken with other
					  substances, effect of each drug
					  multiplied

Adapted from references 73, 94, 96, 122, 153

Summary of Club Drugs

Drug Type/ Name	Street Names	Action & Duration	Administration	Desired Effect
MDMA (3–4 methyl-enedioxy-methampheta-mine) Synthetic drug chemically similar to metham-phetamine and mescaline	Ecstasy, XTC, X, Hug-drug, Love-drug, ADAM, Beans, Clarity, Lover's speed	Effects occur within 30-60 minutes of taking a single dose. Lasts 3–8 hours. Increases serotonin, dopamine, and nor-epinephrine levels.	Oral-capsule or tablet. Powder may also be snorted for more rapid onset.	Emotional warmth, increased libido, well-being, empathy, physical energy. Enhanced sensory perception. Mental stimulation.
GHB (gamma hydroxy-butyrate)	Liquid Ecstasy, Liquid K, soap, Salty water, Easy lay, vita-G, Georgia Home Boy, Great Hormone Bedtime, Grievous Bodily Harm	CNS depressant. Effective within 10–20 minutes. Lasts up to 4-6 hours. Increases dopamine levels.	Oral—liquid, powder, tablet, capsule—salty, soapy taste. Strong alcoholic drinks can mask taste. Cleared from body within 2 hours and no lab tests to detect it.	Euphoric, intoxicating, sexually stimulating, sedative effects. Counters the stimulating effects of other drugs such as MDMA. Can be used as a "drug-assisted assault "or "date-rape drug."
Rohypnol (flunitrazepam)	Rophies, roofies, roach, rope, roof, forget-me pill, Mexican valium	Potent CNS depressant-benzodiazepine. Not available by prescrip-tion in U.S. Sedation and amnesia occurs within 30 minutes and can last 8–12 hours.	Oral. Can be ground up and snorted. Tasteless and odorless. Dissolves easily in carbonated beverages.	Sedative, anxiety reducing, incapacitating effects. Can be used as "date-rape "drug. Lab detection methods usually fail.

Physical & Emotional Effects/Complications	Physical Dependence	Psychological Dependence	Withdrawal Characteristics	Nursing Care
Animal studies suggest long-lasting damage to serotonin neurons and cardiotoxicity. In high doses, can lead to hyperthermia resulting in liver, kidney, cardiovascular system failure and death. MDMA interferes with its own metabolism—repeated use within short intervals can lead to potentially harmful levels in the body. Adverse effects include nausea, chills, sweating, teeth clenching, muscle cramping, blurred vision, anxiety, restlessness, irritability, sadness, impulsiveness, aggression, sleep disturbances, lack of appetite, dehydration and excessive thirst, reduced sexual interest/pleasure, impaired memory and information-processing.	Yes	Yes	Fatigue, loss of appetite, depression, and difficulty concentrating.	There are no specific treatments for MDMA abuse or any of the club drugs. Education of peer group for prevention since users believe the drugs are safe. Recognition of MDMA abuse based upon history and symptoms of CNS stimulation, which bring the teen to emergency care—agitation, anxiety, tachycardia, and hypertension. Agitation and anxiety can be addressed through provision of a safe environment and therapeutic relationship. To relieve tachycardia and hypertension administer benzodiazepines. Signs of hyperthermia and rhabdomyolosis should be monitored; cooling measures and IV fluids administered.
Coma and seizures may occur with GHB abuse. Combining GHB with other drugs such as alcohol can result in nausea and breathing difficulties. GHB has been involved in poisonings, overdoses, date rapes, and deaths.	Yes	Yes	Insomnia, anxiety, tremors, and sweating. progressing to delirium.	No antidote exists. Collect blood specimen within 4–6 hours; urine specimen 6–12 hours to verify. With supportive care, most patients recover within 7 hours of ingestion. Investigate for intoxication if unexplained or sudden coma. Provide safe, supportive environment in cases of suspected rape.
Can prevent resistance of sexual assault. Can produce anterograde amnesia—inability to remember events experienced while under the drug. May be lethal when mixed with alcohol and other depressants. Adverse effects include decreased blood pressure, drowsiness, visual disturbances, dizziness, confusion, gastrointestinal disturbances, and urinary retention.	Yes	Yes	Headache, tension, anxiety, restlessness, muscle pain, photosensitivity, numbness, tingling of extremities, seizures.	Administer antagonist flumazenil per physician order. Provide safe and supportive environment in case of suspected rape.

continued

Summary of Club Drugs—continued

Drug Type/ Name	Street Names	Action & Duration	Administration	Desired Effect
Ketamine	Special K, K, Vitamin K, Cat valium	Anesthetic—90% legal use is in veterinary settings. Inhibits reuptake of nor-epinephrine, dopamine, and serotonin. Rapid onset with duration of 30–45 minutes.	Liquid form or white powder. Can be injected IM, snorted, or smoked with tobacco or marijuana. Tasteless, odorless, colorless.	Sedative, analgesic effects. Altered perceptions, hallucinations, out-of-body experiences. Can be used as "date-rape drug."
Methamphetamine and LSD are considered "older club drugs." See entries in Table Summary of Legal and Illicit Drugs.				

Adapted from references 13, 72, 101, 109, 120, 121, 130, 162, 164, 195.

Physical & Emotional Effects/Complications	Physical Dependence	Psychological Dependence	Withdrawal Characteristics	Nursing Care
Large doses cause reactions similar to phencyclidine (PCP), such as altered perceptions, hallucinations, and dream-like states. May also result in delirium, amnesia, impaired motor function, high blood pressure, depression, and potentially fatal respiratory problems. Low-dose intoxication results in impaired attention, learning, and memory.	Yes	Yes	Severe addiction and withdrawal syndrome requiring detoxification.	No antidote available. Monitor respiratory and cardiac function. Provide safe environment with minimal stimulation to reduce hallucinations. Provide supportive environment and appropriate emergency care if rape is suspected. Administer midazolam when sedation is necessary.

Appendix C

Answers to Critical Thinking Questions

Chapter 1

Question 1: A student nurse is researching theories on causation of a particular disease process and is reviewing several twin studies. Many of these studies conclude that there is a familial tendency toward this particular disease. These conclusions support which category of theory of human behavior?

Correct answer: Physical-biological

Rationale: Physical-biological theories support that behaviors, characteristics, and illnesses are inherited via the passage of genetic material. There is support that diseases such as alcoholism are linked to DNA. *Ecological-sociocultural* theories would support that a characteristic, behavior, or illness is dependent on environmental or social factors.

    Behavioral theory supports the idea that all behavior is a response to a stimulus, rather than supporting the idea that behavior has a root in familial inheritance. *Moral* theories attribute behavior to adherence with societal norms and values.

Cognitive Level: Analysis

Client Need: Health Promotion and Maintenance

Nursing Process: Assessment

Learning Outcome: Identify major psychological developmental theorists, according to their views about the developing person.

Question 2: A 50-year-old woman is concerned about a persistent "blue" mood and lack of interest in previously enjoyed activities. The nurse may anticipate which measure to evaluate the biochemical cause of this client's condition?

Correct answer: Evaluation of hormone levels

Rationale: Answer 2, *evaluation of hormone levels,* supports the biochemical theories that changes in the hormonal environment, such as occur with menopause, may influence mood and behavior. *A referral to a psychologist* may be appropriate, but does not address the biochemical cause of the mood change. *A social work evaluation* may be appropriate, but does not address the biochemical cause of the mood change. *A recommendation to take a vacation* does not address the client's problem.

Cognitive Level: Application

Client Need: Health Promotion and Maintenance

Nursing Process: Implementation

Learning Outcome: Describe some physiologic theories about aspects of the developing person.

Question 3: The nurse is working with the employees of a community service agency, which due to loss of a major financial grant has been forced to cut several positions. The remaining employees have expressed to the nurse that they are unable to get answers to their questions and concerns about the future of the agency. There is an atmosphere of chaos within the agency. According to General Systems Theory, this can best be described as:

Correct answer: Entropy

Rationale: Entropy is the tendency of a system to go from a state of order to one of disorder.

    A closed system is a system in which information and energy is not exchanged with other systems. *Negentropy* is the tendency of a system to go from a state of disorder to one of order. *Linkage* is the exchange of energy across the boundaries of two systems.

Cognitive Level: Application

Client Need: Health Promotion and Maintenance

Nursing Process: Assessment

Learning Outcome: Discuss Ecological and Systems Theories as they apply to the developing person.

Question 4: The school nurse is working with a parent of a child who has displayed significant behavioral and emotional issues since starting school. The parent is concerned that because the child was adopted as a toddler, the lack of maternal bond in early childhood is the cause of his problems. Which developmental theorist would support the parent's concern?

Correct answer: Sullivan

Rationale: Sullivan's Interpersonal Theory of Psychiatry focuses on relationships, particularly that between mother and child. *Freud's* theory focuses on sexual development rather than the influence of relationships on personality. *Erikson's* theory attributes development of personality to biological, emotional, and sociocultural factors. *Kohlberg's* theory is a moral development theory.

Cognitive Level: Application

Client Need: Health Promotion and Maintenance

Nursing Process: Assessment

Learning Outcome: Identify major psychological developmental theorists, according to their views about the developing person.

Chapter 2

Question 1: A local hospital has offered a reduction in insurance premiums for employees who enroll in an on-site fitness program. This strategy supports the *Healthy People 2010* initiative by:

Correct answer: Encouraging healthy lifestyles

Rationale: Encouraging healthy lifestyles is consistent with the *Healthy People 2010* goals for health promotion and disease prevention. Enrollment in an on-site fitness program does not alter *access to health care* services for employees, but does influence healthy lifestyles. Fitness program enrollment may or may not *enhance screening opportunities* for health problems. *Reducing health care costs* is not a *Healthy People 2010* initiative.

Cognitive Level: Application

Client Need: Health Promotion and Maintenance

Nursing Process: Implementation

Learning Outcome: Relate information about health care issues and national and international initiatives to advance health services.

Question 2: An education session offered at a local middle school for parents of preteen girls regarding the human papilloma virus (HPV) vaccine is an example of what type of activity on the part of the nurse?

Correct answer: Primary prevention

Rationale: Primary prevention includes measures that may decrease occurrence of an illness and include education and immunization. *Tertiary prevention* involves treatment or rehabilitation and follow-up of a diagnosed condition. *Secondary prevention* involves early diagnosis and treatment of an actual health problem. *Screening* is a method of secondary prevention.

Cognitive Level: Application

Client Need: Health Promotion and Maintenance

Nursing Process: Implementation

Learning Outcome: Differentiate primary, secondary, and tertiary levels of prevention, and apply them to health promotion/disease prevention with the client at various developmental stages.

Question 3: Holding frequent hypertension and diabetes screening programs on Native American reservations is an important health promotion initiative for the nurse to engage in because:

Correct answer: These conditions have a high prevalence in the Native American population.

Rationale: Prevalence of diabetes and hypertension in the Native American population is high and is an example of a health disparity that justifies the focus of screening efforts to identify and institute early treatment in members of this population. Diabetes and hypertension, although not curable, are both *treatable* conditions.

Although *dietary issues* are a concern in both conditions, it is the high rates of these conditions that justify screening of the population at risk. Screening this population does not address *lack of access* to care.

Cognitive Level: Analysis

Client Need: Health Promotion and Maintenance

Nursing Process: Planning

Learning Outcome: Relate the focus on improving quality of care to the issue of health care disparities.

Question 4: The nurse is working with a client who expresses a desire to begin taking an herbal preparation for the treatment of depression. In order to effectively teach the client, the nurse should first:

Correct answer: Determine why the client is interested in this particular preparation and what the client knows about its use.

Rationale: Determine why the client is interested in this particular preparation and what the client knows about its use. This is a vital first step to determine if the client's symptoms have changed and for the nurse to evaluate if the client's information is from a credible source. *Tell the client that herbal remedies are generally harmless and there will likely be no ill effects.* This is not necessarily a true statement and the herbal remedy may interact with other pharmacological treatments already in use. *Report this desire to the client's primary care provider for further evaluation.* This approach may be appropriate after the nurse gathers more information from the client. *Tell the client that herbal remedies are never recommended for treatment of depression.* This is not necessarily a true statement. More information is required in order to determine the appropriateness of an herbal remedy.

Cognitive Level: Analysis

Client Need: Health Promotion and Maintenance

Nursing Process: Assessment

Learning Outcome: Contrast complementary and alternative therapies used by various populations to promote health or prevent or treat illness.

Chapter 3

Question 1: A group of college freshmen is discussing marriage and parenthood. When sharing that many of their parents married and started families right out of high school, but do not consider this acceptable for their children, the students are discussing the concept of:

Correct answer: Social time

Rationale: Social time refers to the expectations of behavior for a particular age group in a specific era. *Chronologic age* is the numeric measure of one's lifetime. It is only one factor in determining human development. *Historical time* refers to the political and economic climates that shape a person's life and experiences. *Age-irrelevant societies* refer to groups that have difficulty assigning age designation for periods of adult life, for example, precisely defining adolescence or middle age in America.

Cognitive Level: Application

Client Need: Health Promotion and Maintenance

Nursing Process: Evaluation

Learning Outcome: Describe general beliefs about and principles of development and human behavior.

Question 2: By measuring height, weight, and head circumference during a well-child visit, the nurse is measuring which type of growth?

Correct answer: Incremental

Rationale: Incremental growth is the normal process that results in increases in height and weight. *Development* refers to lifelong changes in thought or behaviors that are a result of maturation. *Psychological growth* results from coping with needs and results in a response to change in self, others, and the environment. *Replacement growth* occurs as a response to the need for repair of tissues and structures that occurs throughout life.

Cognitive Level: Application

Client Need: Health Promotion and Maintenance

Nursing Process: Assessment

Learning Outcome: Define growth, development, and related terms.

Question 3: A woman enrolled in a childbirth preparation class asks the nurse if it is safe to take over-the-counter medications during the last trimester of pregnancy. The nurse should base the response to this inquiry on the fact that:

Correct answer: A critical period of brain development occurs in the third trimester.

Rationale: A critical period of brain development occurs in the third trimester. Rapid neuronal additions occur between 30 and 40 weeks. Some medications may influence this critical period's outcome. *Neurologic development* begins in the first trimester, but other critical periods occur throughout pregnancy. *Some medications are required* during pregnancy and their supervised administration may be required. *Over-the-counter medications* may be safe at certain points in pregnancy and with appropriate supervision.

Cognitive Level: Application

Client Need: Health Promotion and Maintenance

Nursing Process: Implementation

Learning Outcome: Define principles of human growth and development.

Question 4: A parent is concerned that a 3-year-old is not yet toilet trained. The nurse can explain toilet training in this age group by applying the principle of readiness. In using this principle the nurse would explain to the parent that:

Correct answer: This task depends on the nervous system maturity as well as the child's musculoskeletal maturity.

Rationale: The principle of readiness explains that tasks such as toilet training *depend on the nervous system maturity as well as the child's musculoskeletal maturity.*

Development that *occurs from the simplest task to the more complex* is the principle of differentiation. Development that *begins with the head and progresses downward* is descriptive of the cephalocaudal principle. Describing development as *not synchronous and children are not "small adults"* is consistent with the principle of asynchronous growth.

Cognitive Level: Analysis

Client Need: Health Promotion and Maintenance

Nursing Process: Implementation

Learning Outcome: Define principles of human growth and development.

Chapter 4

Question 1: The nurse in a large manufacturing plant is case managing an employee who has developed asthma that is believed to be related to inhaled workplace irritants. The employee, who has worked in the plant for many years, asks why his problem has only recently developed. The nurse's response should be based on the fact that:

Correct answer: The development of the illness may be a result of duration of exposure.

Rationale: The development of the illness may be a result of duration of exposure. Exposure-related illnesses may occur as a result of an extended duration of exposure. *There is no explanation for why illness related to toxic exposure does not occur immediately.* Exposure-related illnesses may occur as a result of extended duration of exposure. *The condition may have existed but the person was asymptomatic.* This statement may be true with some health conditions, but asthma is generally associated with symptoms. *The client likely did not report the condition when symptoms first occurred.* This statement may be true, but there is no information in the scenario to support this.

Cognitive Level: Application

Client Need: Health Promotion and Maintenance

Nursing Process: Implementation

Learning Outcome: Examine the scope of environmental pollution and the interrelationship of various pollutants with each other and their effects on people.

Question 2: The nurse is participating in a community-wide disaster plan. The nurse has been assigned to coordinate the recovery phase of the disaster. Which of the following will be a goal of this phase?

Correct answer: Stress management

Rationale: Stress management is part of the debriefing process that occurs during the recovery phase. *Establishment of communication* is part of the activation phase. *Triage of victims* occurs during the implementation phase. *Secondary assessment* occurs during the implementation phase.

Cognitive Level: Application

Client Need: Safe, Effective Care Environment

Nursing Process: Planning

Learning Outcome: Discuss the importance of disaster planning and management, including bioterrorism.

Question 3: A local hospital has instituted a new security policy requiring all visitors to sign in, produce identification, and have their personal bags searched by a security officer. Instituting these measures addresses which phase of disaster planning?

Correct answer: Mitigation

Rationale: Mitigation is the prevention of a disaster incident from occurring. *Preparedness* is preparation to respond to a disaster situation. *Response* is the immediate action taken by health care workers and emergency management officials in the event of a disaster. *Recovery* is the phase of dealing with the effects of the event and beginning to withdraw emergency aid.

Cognitive Level: Application

Client Need: Safe, Effective Care Environment

Nursing Process: Implementation

Learning Outcome: Discuss the importance of disaster planning and management, including bioterrorism.

Question 4: The nurse in a pediatric office noted that several children from the same household have been treated for repeated otitis media and upper respiratory infections over the last 3 years. During well-child visits, the nurse should question the parents regarding:

Correct answer: Smoking habits of care providers and relatives.

Rationale: Smoking habits of care providers and relatives is important because secondhand smoke can contribute to ear and upper respiratory infections in children exposed. *Proper use of over-the-counter medications* is an important assessment, but does not directly relate to the situation. *Sleeping arrangements of children* is an important assessment issue, but may not be a factor in repeated infections. *Allergy history of the parents* is

helpful information, but may not aid in determining the root cause of the repeated infections.

Cognitive Level: Application

Client Need: Health Promotion and Maintenance

Nursing Process: Assessment

Learning Outcome: Examine your professional responsibility in assessing for and intervening in illness caused by environmental pollutants.

Chapter 5

Question 1: The nurse is visiting a client who is a second-generation American, and who lives in a neighborhood populated by individuals from the same country of origin. Many of the dietary, religious, and lifestyle practices in this neighborhood were brought to the United States by the parents of the neighborhood residents. This group can be defined as a/an:

Correct answer: Subculture.

Rationale: Subculture is a group, such as Italian Americans, within the larger American culture, who maintains an identity, but remains part of the larger cultural group. *Culture* is the total way a group has learned to think, do, and feel over time. *Manifest culture* is what a group is doing or saying in daily lives. *Ideal culture* is what people believe in but may not practice regularly.

Cognitive Level: Application

Client Need: Health Promotion and Maintenance

Nursing Process: Assessment

Learning Outcome: Define culture and subculture and describe various types of cultures and subcultures and their general components.

Question 2: The nurse is concerned that an elderly immigrant client is not eating the food that is served on her meal tray. In order to adequately assess this situation the nurse should:

Correct answer: Ask the client about specific food practices or tastes and determine if those preferences can be accommodated.

Rationale: Ask the client about specific food practices or tastes and determine if those preferences can be accommodated. The cultural component of diet should be addressed on assessment so that food practices and preferences can, if possible, be accommodated. *Help the client to select food choices from the diet menu.* The client may be refusing the food because it does not comply with cultural or religious beliefs about dietary intake. *Request that a dietitian visit the client.* This may be an appropriate intervention; however, it does not address the issue of the cultural component of diet. *Notify the physician that the client has a loss of appetite.* This may be appropriate if it is determined that this loss of appetite is a symptom, rather than a rejection of food that does not meet the cultural requirements.

Cognitive Level: Application

Client Need: Health Promotion and Maintenance

Nursing Process: Assessment

Learning Outcome: Relate ways to give culturally competent care to a person with cultural values and a socioeconomic level different from your own.

Question 3: The nurse in an obstetrics and gynecology clinic is working with a client of Iranian descent who is having difficulty conceiving a child. Which characteristic of this culture should the nurse keep in mind when working with this client?

Correct answer: Childbearing is a source of self-esteem for the women.

Rationale: Childbearing is a source of self-esteem for the women. Islamic cultures view bearing children as the source of a woman's identity. *This group rejects cultural practices regarding childbirth when immigrating to the United States.* Islamic immigrants hold to the birth and childrearing practices of their own culture. *Child rearing is a shared responsibility of husband and wife.* Males are the breadwinners, leaving child and household responsibilities to the wife. *Birth control practices are widely accepted by this culture.* Birth control is not commonly practiced, because motherhood is viewed as the role of the female.

Cognitive Level: Application

Client Need: Health Promotion and Maintenance

Nursing Process: Planning

Learning Outcome: Contrast traditional and current values with values of major diverse racial or ethnic groups in the United States.

Question 4: The home health nurse arrives for a scheduled appointment to be told by a neighbor that the client left to attend a religious service. What is the best action for the nurse to take?

Correct answer: Call the client to reschedule the appointment, then call and confirm immediately prior to arrival.

Rationale: Call the client to reschedule the appointment, then call and confirm immediately prior to arrival. This shows a culturally sensitive response on the part of the nurse and an understanding of this cultural group's response to time. *Send the client a letter about the importance of scheduled appointments.* Some cultures, such as some Middle Eastern groups, have a different view of time from that of Americans. They do not emphasize schedules, but rather what is important to do at the time. A letter may not have an influence on the client keeping appointments in the future. *Call the supervisor and request that the client be informed of agency rules regarding keeping scheduled appointments.* This does not address the cultural difference in response to time and schedules. *Charge the client for the missed appointment and request that the client arrange for another appointment.* This does not address the cultural difference in response to time and schedules.

Cognitive Level: Application

Client Need: Health Promotion and Maintenance

Nursing Process: Implementation

Learning Outcome: Contrast traditional and current values with values of major diverse racial or ethnic groups in the United States.

Chapter 6

Question 1: A student nurse working on a pediatric unit asks the instructor why visitors are allowed to be in the unit with less restriction compared to other units in the hospital. The instructor should base the response to this student on the fact that:

Correct answer: Family presence is important to the development of a child.

Rationale: Family presence is important to the development of a child. Family members are responsible for the child's development. Separation due to hospitalization can disrupt family function and contribute to anxiety in the child. *Children will cooperate when visitors are present.* This may be true in some cases, but maintaining some sense of stability is what is important to the developing child. *Adults require more rest than children.* This is not necessarily true. The purpose of allowing family presence is to support the role of the family in the child's treatment and recovery. *Numerous visitors are less disturbing on a pediatric unit.* This is not necessarily true. The purpose of allowing family presence is to support the role of the family in the child's treatment and recovery.

Cognitive Level: Application

Client Need: Health Promotion and Maintenance

Nursing Process: Implementation

Learning Outcome: Describe the purposes, tasks, roles, functions, and adaptive mechanisms of the family system and their relationship to the development and health of its members.

Question 2: A young woman reports a positive home pregnancy test to the nurse in the student health clinic. The woman tells the nurse that she and her partner intend to marry and raise the baby in a family. Which stage of family development have this couple entered?

Correct answer: Expectant stage

Rationale: Expectant stage. Because this woman is pregnant, the couple will be coping with the developmental crisis of pregnancy. *Stage of leaving home.* This stage is generally defined by young adults leaving home to establish identities through career and intimate relationships. *Establishment stage.* This is the beginning of a committed relationship such as marriage. This couple has not yet married and established a home. *Parenthood stage:* This stage is marked by the birth or adoption of a child.

Cognitive Level: Application

Client Need: Health Promotion and Maintenance

Nursing Process: Analysis

Learning Outcome: Relate the developmental tasks to each stage of family life.

Question 3: A new mother confides in the nurse that she is unhappy with her role as a stay-at-home mother and she is eager to return to work. The client states that she is afraid to tell her husband about her desire to go back to work, because he places great value on his childhood experience with a stay-at-home mother. How should the nurse respond to this client?

Correct answer: "How do you think your husband will respond to your desire to go back to work?"

Rationale: "How do you think your husband will respond to your desire to go back to work?" Asking the client to describe how she anticipates her husband will react opens the conversation to talk about family values and expectations of the role of the mother. *"Do you need to work for financial reasons?"* This question does not address the client's fear about discussing a return to work with her husband.

"It is best to have a parent at home during a child's early years." This places judgment on the mother's desire to work and does not address the concern raised by the client.

"Perhaps joining a group or taking a class will be an alternative to going back to work." This assumes that the client is choosing to work for social reasons and does not address the client's immediate concern.

Cognitive Level: Analysis

Client Need: Health Promotion and Maintenance

Nursing Process: Assessment

Learning Outcome: Analyze variables affecting the relationship between parent and child and general family interaction, including feelings about self and childhood experiences.

Question 4: The school nurse is working with the parents of an adopted child who is entering school. The father feels that the child should be told that he was adopted, but the mother feels that there is no purpose in revealing this information. How should the nurse respond to this couple?

Correct answer: "What are your concerns about telling your child about his adoption?"

Rationale: "What are your concerns about telling your child about his adoption?" This question will give the nurse information regarding the mother's concerns and open the dialogue to discuss potential solutions.

"There may be serious health risks that accompany your decision to withhold this information from your child." This may be true, but will likely make the parent defensive and close conversation. *"Children are very perceptive and on some level, your child may already know that he was adopted."* This statement may not be true and will cause concern for the parents.

"Your child will be very angry if this information is discovered accidentally." This may or may not be true. This statement places judgment on the mother and closes further discussion of the matter.

Cognitive Level: Analysis

Client Need: Health Promotion and Maintenance

Nursing Process: Assessment

Learning Outcome: Analyze variables affecting the relationship between parent and child and general family interaction, including feelings about self and childhood experiences.

Chapter 7

Question 1: While interviewing a client upon admission to the agency, the nurse asks if the client has a religious affiliation. The client responds, "I do not practice a religion, but I am a spiritual person." The nurse understands that:

Correct answer: Spirituality is a quality that goes beyond religious affiliation.

Rationale: Spirituality is a quality that goes beyond religious affiliation. This is an accurate definition of spirituality, which is a dimension that looks for deeper meaning. *Spirituality is a form of religion.* Spirituality is a quality that goes beyond religion to look for meaning. *Those who practice religion do not consider themselves to be spiritual.* Religious people may consider themselves deeply spiritual. *Religion and spirituality have no relationship.* Religion and spirituality, though not synonymous, are related.

Cognitive Level: Application

Client Need: Health Promotion and Maintenance

Nursing Process: Analysis

Learning Outcome: Define the terms *spiritual* and *religious* and the connotations of each.

Question 2: A client tells the nurse about a journal article she read that explained that spirituality and beliefs might be programmed into a person's DNA. The nurse recognizes this as:

Correct answer: A new area of research.

Rationale: A new area of research: Neurotheology is the discipline that studies the biological connection to spirituality. *An ancient belief:* Neurotheology is actually a rather new field that studies the biological connection to spirituality. *Not accepted by Christian faiths:* Neurotheology is the field that studies the biological connection to spirituality. It is not necessarily rejected by Christianity. *A common belief of Middle Eastern faiths:* Neurotheology is the field that studies the biological connection to spirituality. This is a research field and is not descriptive of a Middle Eastern belief system.

Cognitive Level: Application

Client Need: Health Promotion and Maintenance

Nursing Process: Analysis

Learning Outcome: Review research studies and client descriptions related to the spiritual and religious dimension.

Question 3: The nurse is reviewing the medical history of a client who was brought to the emergency room following a motor vehicle accident. The record reveals the client is a Christian Scientist. What effect can the nurse anticipate this religious affiliation will have on the client's care?

Correct answer: The client will likely accept medical care, but not medications.

Rationale: The client will likely accept medical care, but not medications. Those who practice Christian Science do not accept medications. *There will be no conflict of religion and medical care.* Those who practice Christian Science do not accept medications. *The client will reject the spiritual methods of healing.* Christian Scientists turn to the spiritual as a means of healing. *The client will only be treated by a physician of the same faith.* The client may accept treatment from a physician of another faith, but will not consent to medications.

Cognitive Level: Application

Client Need: Health Promotion

Nursing Process: Planning

Learning Outcome: Compare the major tenets of the various branches of Christianity: Roman Catholicism, Eastern Orthodoxy, various Protestant denominations, and other Christian sects.

Question 4: While working with a client at the end of life, the nurse inquires about funeral arrangements and if a clergy member should be notified. The client tells the nurse, "I am agnostic." How should the nurse interpret this statement?

Correct answer: The client feels that one is incapable of knowing if God exists.

Rationale: The client feels that one is incapable of knowing if God exists. This is the meaning of agnostic. *The client is a member of a New Age religious group.* Agnostic means that one is not capable of knowing if God exists. *The client believes that God does not exist.* This defines atheism. *The client is a Christian.* Christians believe in God. Agnostics feel incapable of knowing whether God exists.

Cognitive Level: Application

Client Need: Health Promotion and Maintenance

Nursing Process: Assessment

Learning Outcome: Examine how religious beliefs influence lifestyle and health status in the various religious groups and subgroups.

Chapter 8

Question 1: The nurse is assessing a woman at 15 weeks of pregnancy who has gained 20 pounds. When discussing the weight gain with the client, the nurse should base instructions on the fact that:

Correct answer: Calorie intake at this point should only be about 200 to 300 calories more than the nonpregnant intake.

Rationale: Calorie intake at this point should only be about 200 to 300 calories more than the nonpregnant intake. This is a true statement and can be the basis of diet instruction for the client.

This is an expected weight gain at this point in the pregnancy. A gain of about 10 pounds is expected by the beginning of the second trimester. *High weight gain during pregnancy will result in a healthy baby at birth.* This is not necessarily a true statement. High maternal weight gain may result in an infant large for gestational age and increased risk of childhood obesity. *Higher weight gain is a more favorable situation than not gaining sufficiently.* This is not true. Both high and low weight gain can pose risk for the baby and mother.

Cognitive Level: Application

Client Need: Health Promotion and Maintenance

Nursing Process: Implementation

Learning Outcome: Educate the pregnant woman, and partner if possible, about the normal changes that occur in the developing fetus and in the pregnant female.

Question 2: A recently diagnosed pregnant client tells the nurse that she is a vegetarian and plans to continue this lifestyle during pregnancy. How can the nurse best advise this client?

Correct answer: Many fish and seafoods can pose problems during pregnancy.

Rationale: Many fish and seafoods can pose problems during pregnancy. The mercury content of fish and seafoods can be toxic during pregnancy. Specially farmed fish can be recommended.

Inform the client that a vegetarian diet is contraindicated during pregnancy. A vegetarian lifestyle can be accommodated if appropriate nutrient intake is ensured.

Ensure that the diet includes 100 mcg of folate. Folate should be increased to 600 mcg in order to prevent birth defects. *Avoid dairy products and eggs.* Dairy and eggs are good sources of protein, which is needed by the pregnant female.

Cognitive Level: Application

Client Need: Health Promotion and Maintenance

Nursing Process: Implementation

Learning Outcome: Explore lifestyle variables with the pregnant female, and partner if possible, that are considered to have a negative or teratogenic effect on the embryo/fetus.

Question 3: The nurse is advising a couple who are planning to conceive about the importance of a diet adequate in folate. The couple asks why this nutrient is important to include in the woman's diet even before conception. The nurse should base the response to this couple on the fact that:

Correct answer: Neural tube development begins soon after fertilization and continues into the embryonic stage.

Rationale: Neural tube development begins soon after fertilization and continues into the embryonic stage. Folic acid (folate) has been found to be a vital nutrient in prevention of neural tube defects. Neural tube defects may be prevented by increasing intake of this nutrient before pregnancy.

Good nutrition is vital throughout the life span, not just when planning to conceive. This is a true statement, but it does not address the couple's concern regarding prepregnancy nutrition. *Changing diet before pregnancy will support good nutrition habits throughout life.* This may or may not be true and does not respond to the couple's question. *Folate supplements are not widely available.* This statement is false. This nutrient is found in food sources and can be supplemented via vitamin and mineral supplements.

Cognitive Level: Synthesis

Client Need: Health Promotion and Maintenance

Nursing Process: Implementation

Learning Outcome: Review major physical developmental changes that occur during the 9 months of gestation.

Question 4: A client in the third trimester of pregnancy tells the nurse that she feels bloated and has had some abdominal discomfort. The nurse assesses the client and finds diminished bowel sounds. How should the nurse interpret this finding?

Correct answer: This is a usual change in a pregnant woman's physiologic function associated with the hormonal environment of pregnancy.

Rationale: This is a usual change in physiologic function associated with the hormonal environment of pregnancy. Influence of the hormones estrogen, HCG (human chorionic gonadotropin), and progesterone causes gastric and intestinal motility to decrease, resulting in reduced bowel sounds.

This is an abnormal finding and should be reported to the physician. This is not an abnormal finding, but a common alteration during pregnancy. *This finding is likely a result of poor nutritional intake and requires intravenous fluids.* This finding is likely due to the influence of hormones, not poor intake. *The client likely has a bowel obstruction and should be sent to the emergency department.* This finding is more likely explained by reduced motility and constipation.

Cognitive Level: Analysis

Client Need: Health Promotion and Maintenance

Nursing Process: Assessment

Learning Outcome: Educate the pregnant woman about the normal changes that occur in the developing fetus and in the pregnant female.

Chapter 9

Question 1: The mother of an infant tells the nurse she initially thought that being a parent would be "fun." However, now that the baby has arrived she is very stressed by this new role of a parent. The best response for the nurse to make to this woman is:

Correct answer: "Tell me about what you expected from parenthood."

Rationale: "Tell me about what you expected from parenthood." This response encourages the new mother to talk about her feelings and allows the nurse to gather assessment data.

"New parents have unrealistic ideas." This is a judgmental response that closes communication. *"Didn't your mother tell you how hard being a parent can be?"* This response does not address the new mother's concern. *"It will get easier."* This is a closed comment that does not recognize the client's concern.

Cognitive Level: Application

Client Need: Health Promotion and Maintenance

Nursing Process: Assessment

Learning Outcome: Discuss the crisis of birth for the family, factors that influence parental bonding and attachment, and your role in assisting the family to adapt and meet their developmental tasks.

Question 2: Immediately after birth a healthy infant is handed to the new father. This interaction between the baby and father is best described by which of the following terms?

Correct answer: Engrossment

Rationale: Engrossment is the term used to describe the initial father-baby response. *Attachment* is the term used interchangeably with bonding and is not specific to the father. *Bonding* is not specific to paternal interaction and the term is used interchangeably with attachment. *Parenting* is a term used through the child's development and describes the interaction between the child and caregiver.

Cognitive Level: Application

Client Need: Health Promotion and Maintenance

Nursing Process: Assessment

Learning Outcome: Discuss the crisis of birth for the family, factors that influence parental bonding and attachment, and your role in assisting the family to adapt and meet their developmental tasks.

Question 3: On initial assessment the newborn has a pulse of 110, is crying vigorously with regular respirations, and is moving all of its extremities. The infant's body is pink with cyanosis of the hands and feet. What Apgar score should the nurse assign to this child?

Correct answer: 9

Rationale: A score of 9 is appropriate. One point is deducted for the cyanosis of the hands and feet.

A score of 10 would be assigned if the infant had no cyanosis. *A score of 8* would be assigned if the torso was cyanotic as well as the hands and feet. *A score of 7* is too low as 4 of the 5 areas are able to be scored at 2 out of 2.

Cognitive Level: Application

Client Need: Health Promotion and Maintenance

Nursing Process: Assessment

Learning Outcome: Describe the adaptive physiologic changes in the newborn that occur at birth.

Question 4: A woman who is pregnant with her first child tells the nurse that she would like to have a cesarean section rather than a vaginal delivery so the baby's head will "look normal" after birth. How should the nurse respond to this client's request?

Correct answer: "The infant's head will usually take on a round shape shortly after birth."

Rationale: "*The infant's head will usually take on a round shape shortly after birth.*" This response addresses the client's concern and may stimulate further conversation.

"*The doctor will discuss your options for delivery with you.*" This may be a true statement, but does not address the client's immediate concern. "*Unnecessary surgery may harm the baby.*" This statement may cause alarm if a cesarean birth is required.

"*I will make a note of your request.*" This is a closed response that does not allow the nurse to educate the client on normal changes that occur with the birthing process.

Cognitive Level: Application

Client Need: Health Promotion and Maintenance

Nursing Process: Implementation

Learning Outcome: Describe the adaptive physiologic changes in the newborn that occur at birth.

Chapter 10

Question 1: The nurse is working with the mother of a 2-year-old child who has started to have tantrums when being left at day care. The mother is concerned that she will lose her job as a result of tardiness associated with her child care situation. How should the nurse advise the mother?

Correct answer: "This is normal behavior for a child in this age group. It will likely pass with firm, consistent parenting."

Rationale: "*This is normal behavior for a child in this age group. It will likely pass with firm, consistent parenting.*" This statement reassures the mother that this situation is temporary and will improve with time. It also opens the conversation for further discussion with the parent.

"*Ask your boss if you can come in a little later.*" This is not a realistic option and does not address the issue of the child's behavior. "*The child may need to have a stay-at-home parent.*" This option is not realistic and will enhance feelings of guilt that the parent may already have. "*Leave the child with a relative or neighbor until the behavior is outgrown.*" This statement does not address the mother's concern and offers an unrealistic option.

Cognitive Level: Analysis

Client Need: Health Promotion and Maintenance

Nursing Process: Evaluation

Learning Outcome: Assess a toddler's physical and motor characteristics; general cognitive, language, emotional, and self-concept development; and related needs.

Question 2: The nurse is examining the ears of a 2-year-old child. How should the external ear best be positioned to insert the otoscope?

Correct answer: Pull the ear down and back

Rationale: Pull the ear down and back. This is the optimal position for examination of the ears of a child. *Pull the ear up and back.* This position is best for adult ear exams.

Pull the earlobe straight down. This position will not allow full visualization of the canal. *Do not manipulate the ear.* The external ear should be manipulated to allow visualization of the canal.

Cognitive Level: Application

Client Need: Health Promotion and Maintenance

Nursing Process: Health Promotion and Maintenance

Learning Outcome: Assess a toddler's physical and motor characteristics; general cognitive, language, emotional, and self-concept development; and related needs.

Question 3: Which toy should the nurse suggest that grandparents purchase as a gift for an 18-month-old grandchild?

Correct answer: Tambourine

Rationale: A *tambourine* is an appropriate choice and is consistent with the motor abilities of an 18-month-old.

A *tricycle* is not appropriate in light of the gross motor ability required of an 18-month-old child. A *play kitchen* requires gross and fine motor ability that the child would not yet have. *Garden tools* require fine motor skills that an 18-month-old would not have.

Cognitive Level: Application

Client Need: Health Promotion and Maintenance

Nursing Process: Implementation

Learning Outcome: Assess a toddler's physical and motor characteristics; general cognitive, language, emotional, and self-concept development; and related needs.

Question 4: The nurse recommends to parents the use of bedtime rituals for their toddler because these activities:

Correct answer: Promote a sense of security

Rationale: Rituals *promote a sense of security* because the child can anticipate that certain activities will always occur.

Rituals do not necessarily *promote creativity*. Rituals tend to promote security and trust rather than *encourage dependence*. Rituals are repetitive behaviors and do not necessarily *offer options and choices*.

Cognitive Level: Application

Client Need: Implementation

Nursing Process: Health Promotion and Maintenance

Learning Outcome: Assess a toddler's physical and motor characteristics; general cognitive, language, emotional, and self-concept development; and related needs.

Chapter 11

Question 1: A nurse in the pediatric clinic observes that a 4-year-old female child is being consoled by her father but rejects her mother's attempts to calm her. The nurse concludes that this behavior is:

Correct answer: Normal for a child of this age group.

Rationale: Normal for a child of this age group. Affiliation with the parent of the opposite sex is appropriate behavior for this age group.

    A definitive indication of physical abuse by the mother. This behavior alone would not indicate physical abuse. *A sign of sexual abuse by the father.* Victims of sexual abuse would likely reject affection by their abusers. *Symptomatic of developmental delay.* This behavior is not symptomatic of developmental delay.

Cognitive Level: Analysis

Client Need: Health Promotion and Maintenance

Nursing Process: Assessment

Learning Outcome: Compare and contrast the family relationships between the preschool era and previous developmental eras and the influence of parents, siblings, and nonfamily members on the preschooler.

Question 2: The parent of a 5-year-old is concerned that the child is obese. The child's weight is 22 kg. The nurse should explain to the parent that the child is:

Correct answer: Normal weight for age.

Rationale: Normal weight for age. Children of this age should weigh between 40 and 50 pounds. This child weighs 48.4 pounds.

Cognitive Level: Application

Client Need: Health Promotion and Maintenance

Nursing Process: Assessment

Learning Outcome: Assess and contrast physical, motor, mental, language, play, and emotional characteristics of a 3-, 4-, and 5-year-old.

Question 3: Nutrition education for parents of preschool children should emphasize:

Correct answer: Recognizing that times of not wanting to eat are normal behavior for preschoolers.

Rationale: Recognizing that times of not wanting to eat are normal behavior for preschoolers. Lack of appetite or eating only certain foods is normal in this age group.

    Limiting between-meal snacks. Snacks are necessary in this age group due to the high calorie expenditure of growth and activity. *Providing desserts only as a reward for finishing a meal.* This practice sets the stage for overindulgence in sweets and snack foods as well as the use of food as a reward. *Offering large portions to provide adequate calories.* Children need portions in proportion to their age. Large portions can overwhelm.

Cognitive Level: Application

Client Need: Health Promotion and Maintenance

Nursing Process: Implementation

Learning Outcome: Describe the health needs of the preschooler, including nutrition, exercise, rest, safety, and immunization, and measures to meet these needs.

Question 4: A parent is concerned that a 3-year-old child refuses to play with others, preferring to play alongside other children. The nurse should base the response to the parent's concern with one of the following facts:

Correct answer: Parallel play is a characteristic of this age group.

Rationale: Parallel play is a characteristic of this age group. Playing next to other children while not directly engaging in play with others is typical play behavior.

    Children of this age group usually enjoy games and activities involving groups. This play behavior is characteristic of school-age children. *This play behavior may reflect a developmental delay.* Playing next to other children while not directly engaging in play with others is typical play behavior and not necessarily significant of developmental delay. *The child is too young to play with other children.* Although playing with others usually occurs later, it is more accurate to describe the behavior as parallel play.

Cognitive Level: Application

Client Need: Health Promotion and Maintenance

Nursing Process: Assessment

Learning Outcome: Assess and contrast physical, motor, mental, language, play, and emotional characteristics of a 3-, 4-, and 5-year-old.

Chapter 12

Question 1: The school nurse overhears two 11-year-olds discussing their families. One child states, "My parents are so stupid. They don't know anything!" What is the best action for the nurse to take?

Correct answer: Ignore the comment.

Rationale: Ignore the comment. Without any other related behavior, this is the most appropriate action. Children of this age group commonly question parental authority.

    Notify the parent. Children of this age group commonly question parental authority. Notifying the parents about this comment is not necessary and would not serve a meaningful purpose. *Ask the child about the statement.* Children of this age group commonly question parental authority. Questioning the children may serve only to embarrass them. *Notify the child's counselor.* Children of this age group commonly question parental authority. Notifying the counselor about this comment is not necessary and would not serve a meaningful purpose.

Cognitive Level: Analysis

Client Need: Health Promotion and Maintenance

Nursing Process: Assessment

Learning Outcome: Discuss family relationships of the school-age child and the influence of peers and other adults.

Question 2: A 9-year-old girl complains of breast tenderness. On physical assessment, the nurse notes increased diameter of the areola. The nurse concludes that the child:

Correct answer: Is experiencing changes associated with prepuberty.

Rationale: Is experiencing changes associated with prepuberty. Breast changes are common in girls entering puberty. *Is experiencing precocious puberty.* It is not uncommon for girls in this age group to enter puberty. *Should be scheduled for a mammogram.* Mammography is not indicated as the breast discomfort is an expected developmental change. *Should be counseled regarding birth control.* Breast changes are not indicative of a need for birth control.

Cognitive Level: Application

Client Need: Health Promotion and Maintenance

Nursing Process: Assessment

Learning Outcome: Compare and assess the physical changes and needs, including nutrition, rest, exercise, safety, and health promotion.

Question 3: A 6-year-old child frequently is fatigued during the school day and is not doing well academically. How much sleep should the nurse suggest to the parents is needed by a child in this age group?

Correct answer: 11 hours

Rationale: Eleven hours is the recommended amount of sleep for young school-age children.

Eight hours is the amount of sleep required by most adults and is not enough for a child this age. *Nine hours* is insufficient sleep for children in this age group. *Seventeen hours* is the amount of sleep needed by infants and toddlers.

Cognitive Level: Application

Client Need: Health Promotion and Maintenance

Nursing Process: Implementation

Learning Outcome: Compare and assess the physical changes and needs, including nutrition, rest, exercise, safety, and health promotion.

Question 4: A 12-year-old child responds to the death of a grandparent by playing with younger siblings' toys and displaying behaviors consistent with an earlier age group. The nurse is aware that the child is using the adaptive mechanism of:

Correct answer: Regression

Rationale: Regression is a method of coping with anxiety by returning to an earlier stage of development. *Fantasy* is used to deal with feelings of inadequacy. *Undoing* removes an unacceptable idea by use of ritual. *Projection* is assigning responsibility for an action to another.

Cognitive Level: Analysis

Client Need: Health Promotion and Maintenance

Nursing Process: Assessment

Learning Outcome: Relate the physical and emotional adaptive mechanisms of the schoolchild and how they contribute to healthy development, including to meet the developmental crisis of industry versus inferiority.

Chapter 13

Question 1: A parish nurse is counseling the parents of an adolescent. The parents express concern that the child is refusing to attend church services, which they believe is a crucial part of their family life. The nurse recognizes that by refusing to participate in religious services, the child is probably:

Correct answer: Attempting to establish an identity by rejecting parental values.

Rationale: Attempting to establish an identity by rejecting parental values. Establishment of an identity separate from the parent is the developmental task of adolescence.

Punishing the parents for their rigid limits. Although this may be the child's motivation, the developmental task of the adolescent should be discussed and explored first. *Exhibiting behaviors of substance use by the child.* Changes in behavior can accompany substance abuse; however, attempting to establish an identity is the likely issue if no other symptoms or signs of abuse are present. *Attempting to tell the parents of a desire to join another church.* This may be true, but less likely than the fact that the child is trying to establish an identity independent of the parents.

Cognitive Level: Application

Client Need: Psychosocial Integrity

Nursing Process: Assessment

Learning Outcome: Explore the developmental crisis of identity formation with the adolescent and the parents and the significance of attaining identity formation for ongoing maturity.

Question 2: A client tells the nurse that since her children have left home, she and her husband are finding that they really do not know each other anymore. Which task of family development is this couple struggling with at this time?

Correct answer: Reestablish a mutually satisfying marriage relationship.

Rationale: Reestablish a mutually satisfying marriage relationship. After children grow and become independent, it is the task of the couple to reestablish the relationship of marriage.

Establish a sharing of responsibilities. This is a task of the developing family, but reestablishment of a mutually satisfying marriage relationship is the best response.

Rework relationships with relatives, friends, and associates. This is a task of the developing family; however, the reestablishment of the marriage relationship is the more accurate response in this situation. *Formulate a workable philosophy of life.* This is a task of the developing family; however, the reestablishment of the marriage relationship is the more accurate response in this situation.

Cognitive Level: Application

Client Need: Health Promotion and Maintenance

Nursing Process: Analysis

Learning Outcome: Examine the impact of the crisis of adolescence on family life and the influence of the family on the adolescent.

Question 3: A 12-year-old boy expresses he is upset about not having grown much in the last year. Also, his female classmates are now taller than he is. The nurse should base the response to the child on the fact that:

Correct answer: He will likely continue to grow for several more years.

Rationale: He will likely continue to grow for several more years. This statement is most accurate. Linear growth will continue until the epiphyseal plates at the end of the long bones close. This occurs at the end of adolescence.

Height is genetically determined. This response has some basis in fact; the child will likely continue linear growth until late adolescence. *He has likely reached his full adult height.* Linear growth will continue until the epiphyseal plates at the end of the long bones close. This occurs at the end of adolescence. *Short stature in a male in this age group should be evaluated by a specialist.* This child has most likely not completed linear growth.

Cognitive Level: Analysis

Client Need: Health Promotion and Maintenance

Nursing Process: Analysis

Learning Outcome: Contrast the physiologic changes and needs of early, middle, and late adolescence and compare to changes in preadolescence.

Question 4: When discussing hypertension with a group of adolescents, the nurse should include which of the following relevant facts about this condition? Select all that apply.

Correct answer: Hypertension is not usually a concern in adolescents. High diastolic blood pressure is associated with smoking. Stress is a factor in development of hypertension.

Rationale: Hypertension is not usually a concern in adolescents. However, the incidence of hypertension is rising in this age group. *High diastolic blood pressure is associated with smoking.* Smoking is associated with high diastolic blood pressure. *Stress is a factor in development of hypertension.* Stress does play a role in development of systolic hypertension.

Exercise has no impact on blood pressure. Exercise is helpful in controlling hypertension; lack of exercise is associated with diastolic hypertension. *Caucasian females are most likely to be affected by hypertension.* Although adolescent hypertension is found in all races and both genders, it is more common in Caucasian and African American males.

Cognitive Level: Application

Client Need: Health Promotion and Maintenance

Nursing Process: Implementation

Learning Outcome: Contrast the physiologic changes and needs of early, middle, and late adolescence and compare to changes in preadolescence.

Chapter 14

Question 1: When explaining assessment findings to a young adult female, the nurse should include which of the following points when talking about gender differences in weight?

Correct Response: Females typically have about twice as much body fat as males.

Rationale: Females typically have about twice as much body fat as males. This is a true statement about body fat amounts in the young adult years.

Females typically have about half as much body fat as males. Females typically have about twice as much body fat as males. *Females typically store fat in the abdomen.* Males tend to store fat in the abdomen during this phase of life. *Males typically store fat in the hips.* Females tend to store fat in the breasts and hips during young adulthood.

Cognitive Level: Application

Client Need: Health Promotion and Maintenance

Nursing Process: Implementation

Learning Outcome: Assess the physical characteristics of a young adult.

Question 2: The nurse in the college health office is counseling a female student. The student tells the nurse that her boyfriend is angry because she refuses to have intercourse during her menstrual period. Which of the following research findings can the nurse provide to the student?

Correct answer: Intercourse during menses is not contraindicated, but the student should do what she is comfortable with.

Rationale: Intercourse during menses is not contraindicated, but the student should do what she is comfortable with. There is no physiologic reason to avoid intercourse during menses. However, if the student is not comfortable with this practice she should decide based on her comfort level.

Intercourse during menses can cause tissue damage and is contraindicated. This is a false statement as research indicates no physiologic reason to avoid intercourse during menses. *Intercourse during menses is not contraindicated, but sex drive is diminished.* Sex drive is not usually diminished during menses. *Intercourse during menses may cause increased cramping and discomfort.* There is no physiologic reason to avoid intercourse during menses.

Cognitive Level: Application

Client Need: Health Promotion and Maintenance

Nursing Process: Implementation

Learning Outcome: Assess the physical characteristics of a young adult.

Question 3: A 21-year-old healthy, moderately active male, weighing 170 pounds at 5 feet 10 inches, asks the nurse about the appropriate daily calorie intake to maintain his current weight. Taking into account BMI, physical activity, and digestion and absorption needs, which is the best response for the nurse to offer this student?

Correct answer: 2,880 calories/day

Rationale: The total calories needed for maintenance of the current weight is *2,880 calories/day.*

A value of *1,870 calories/day* represents only the calories needed for the young man's basic energy needs. A value of *2,618 calories/day* represents the calorie needs for the young man's basic energy needs and physical activity, but not those required for digestion and absorption of nutrients. A level of *3,500 calories/day* is higher than required for weight maintenance and will result in weight gain.

Cognitive Level: Application

Client Need: Health Promotion and Maintenance

Nursing Process: Implementation

Learning Outcome: Teach nutritional requirements to the young adult male and female, including the pregnant and lactating female.

Question 4: A young adult who recently started rotating between the day and night shift at his job came to the clinic nurse with symptoms that are consistent with depression. The nurse concluded that the recent onset of depression is likely related to:

Correct answer: Disruption in body rhythms of diurnal cycles.

Rationale: Disruption in body rhythms of diurnal cycles. Shift rotation disrupts the sleep/wake cycle and can contribute to the development of depression.

The client being overwhelmed by new adult responsibilities. This can have an impact on development of depression, but without prior history from this young man it is more likely due to work-associated shift rotation. *Genetic factors that increase risk of depression.* Genetic factors may play a role in the develop-

ment of depression; however, shift rotation is a more obvious cause in this case. *Substance abuse that the client is not admitting.* There is no evidence that the client is abusing substances, but the new shift rotation should be considered as a potential causative factor.

Cognitive Level: Application

Client Need: Health Promotion and Maintenance

Nursing Process: Evaluation

Learning Outcome: Describe factors and health promotion measures that influence biological rhythms and illness, and the desynchronization that may result.

Chapter 15

Question 1: Participants in a local women's group ask the nurse about the benefits and risks of hormone replacement therapy (HRT) to treat menopausal symptoms. Which of the following should the nurse include in the response to the women's questions on this issue? (Select all that apply.)

Correct answer: Increase in heart disease is associated with combination HRT. Use of estrogen-only replacement results in no increased risk of breast cancer. Women taking HRT may have false-positive mammogram results.

Rationale: Increase in heart disease is associated with combination HRT. Studies have shown this to be true in women with existing risk of heart disease. *Use of estrogen-only replacement results in no increased risk of breast cancer.* This is a true statement when compared to use of combination therapy. *Women taking HRT may have false-positive mammogram results.* This is true and is due to increased density of breast tissue.

Women with a history of breast cancer should use combination HRT only. This is false. Women with a history of breast cancer should not use HRT.

HRT is no longer used as a treatment for menopausal symptoms. This is false. Study results have been questioned and HRT is still used to treat menopausal symptoms.

Cognitive Level: Application

Client Need: Health Promotion and Maintenance

Nursing Process: Implementation

Learning Outcome: Describe the hormonal changes of middle age and the resultant changes in appearance and body image, physiologically and emotionally.

Question 2: The nurse is reviewing a daily food journal of a 50-year-old male who is concerned with weight gain in recent years. The nurse evaluates calorie intake with the knowledge that:

Correct answer: BMI decreases with age.

Rationale: BMI decreases with age. BMI declines beginning in the third decade of life and calorie intake should decline as well. *Carbohydrate needs increase during middle age.* Carbohydrate intake should be reduced in the middle years. *BMI increases throughout the life span.* BMI declines beginning in the 20s.

Physical activity is no longer a consideration in the middle years. Calorie intake does need to be adjusted to account for declining physical activity.

Cognitive Level: Application

Client Need: Health Promotion and Maintenance

Nursing Process: Evaluation

Learning Outcome: Analyze the nutritional, rest, leisure, work, and exercise needs of the middle-aged adult, factors that interface with meeting those needs, and your role in helping the person meet these needs.

Question 3: A middle-aged female client is concerned about her risk for heart disease due to the recent death of a sibling to myocardial infarction. The client shows no significant risk factors and indicates she would like to make lifestyle changes to reduce her risk. Which of the following strategies should the nurse suggest to this client?

Correct answer: Increase intake of whole grains and fruits.

Rationale: Increase intake of whole grains and fruits. These foods are good sources of folate and vitamin C, which can reduce the risk of cardiovascular disease. *Maintain a waist-to-hip ratio of 1:2.* Waist-to-hip ratio should be approximately 0.7 or less for females and 0.95 for males.

Take 325 mg of aspirin three times per day. The recommendation is for 81 mg once per day. *Reduce intake of nuts and fatty fish.* The types of fats from these foods are thought to reduce cardiac risk.

Cognitive Level: Analysis

Client Need: Health Promotion and Maintenance

Nursing Process: Implementation.

Learning Outcome: Explore with a middle-aged adult ways to avoid injury and health problems and to promote health.

Question 4: A middle-aged client mentions to the nurse that he would like to return to college but is concerned that it is too late in life to complete a college degree. The nurse can advise this client that:

Correct answer: Success in college has little to do with age.

Rationale: Success in college has little to do with age. Older students are motivated and capable of scholastic success.

IQ test scores decline in middle age, so college performance may be affected. IQ scores in middle age are comparable to those of young adults. *Recall begins to decline in the 20s, so memorization might be difficult.* No major changes are evident in recall ability during middle age. *Ability to learn is reduced by the time one reaches 40.* Learning is a process that occurs at all ages.

Cognitive Level: Application

Client Need: Health Promotion and Maintenance

Nursing Process: Implementation

Learning Outcome: Describe the developmental tasks for this person and your role in helping him or her accomplish these tasks.

Chapter 16

Question 1: The nurse is assessing a female client in her early 60s. The woman tells the nurse, "I feel like I'm still 25." Which term associated with aging can the nurse use to describe what the client has verbalized?

Correct answer: Cognitive age

Rationale: Cognitive age is the individual's own perception of age related to how one looks or feels.

Biological age may be different from the individual's chronologic age and takes into account the functional capacity of the organs. *Social age* is a reflection of the person's dress, use of language, and response to authority. *Psychological age* is a measure of the individual's ability to adapt to change as well as capacity for learning and motivation.

Cognitive Level: Application

Client Need: Psychosocial Integrity

Nursing Process: Assessment

Learning Outcome: Define terms and theories of aging related to understanding of the person in later maturity.

Question 2: An elderly female is brought to the emergency department (ED) by her husband, following a fall down three steps in her home. The nurse notes that this is the second ED visit for an injury for this client in the last 2 months and further notes the client has lost 10 pounds since her last admission. When questioned, the client states, "Everything is fine. I just don't feel much like eating." What action by the nurse should be given priority?

Correct answer: Interview the client privately about her home situation and to assess for indications of abuse.

Rationale: Interview the client privately about her home situation and to assess for indications of abuse. Gathering more information about the cause and frequency of the injuries and to determine if there is any relationship to the weight loss is vital for the nurse to develop an appropriate plan of care.

Refer the client to a home nursing agency for assessment of the living environment. This is an appropriate intervention, but assessment of the home situation and possible abuse is the priority. *Request a consult by a dietitian to address the weight loss issue.* This is an appropriate intervention, but assessment of the home situation and possible abuse is the priority. *Suggest that the client enroll in a home meal program.* This may be an appropriate intervention, but assessment of the home situation and possible abuse is the priority.

Cognitive Level: Analysis

Client Need: Health Promotion and Maintenance

Nursing Process: Assessment

Learning Outcome: Describe signs of and factors contributing to elder abuse and contrast with child and spouse abuse.

Question 3: A 60-year-old male client requests a sedative due to his inability to sleep through the night. Which of the following should the nurse include in the assessment of this client? (Select all that apply.)

Correct answer: Evaluate the client's urinary pattern. Discuss the client's dietary pattern. Evaluate for use of prescription and over-the-counter medications. Evaluate the client's exercise habits.

Rationale: Evaluate the client's urinary pattern. Prostate enlargement common in the older male can be at the root of sleep disturbance due to frequency and nocturia. *Discuss the client's dietary pattern.* Caffeine intake and other diet patterns can contribute to disturbed sleep. *Evaluate for use of prescription and over-the-counter medications.* This is important as medications can disrupt sleep through central nervous system stimulation. *Evaluate the client's exercise habits.* Changes in exercise pattern as well as the time of day that the client engages in physical activity can alter sleep patterns.

Evaluate for food allergies or environmental irritants. Allergies are not generally manifested in sleep disturbance.

Cognitive Level: Analysis

Client Need: Health Promotion and Maintenance

Nursing Process: Assessment

Learning Outcome: Describe physiologic adaptive mechanisms of aging, including in the centenarian, and influences on sexuality, related health problems, and assessment and intervention to promote and maintain health, comfort, and safety.

Question 4: Which of the following should the nurse consider when planning an educational activity for senior citizens?

Correct answer: Visual aids and handouts should be developed in large print.

Rationale: Visual aids and handouts should be developed in large print. Reduction in visual acuity should be considered when developing material for older persons.

Materials from textbooks and professional journals can be used without adaptation. Handouts should be written at a fifth- to eighth-grade reading level for older people. Textbooks are likely at a higher level and often use jargon. *Written and psychomotor testing should be incorporated for evaluation purposes.* Testing may be intimidating for the older adult learner. Motor responses are slower than in younger learners. *One long session is better than several short sessions.* Attention may be enhanced by using shorter sessions and incorporating frequent breaks.

Cognitive Level: Application

Client Need: Health Promotion and Maintenance

Nursing Process: Health Promotion and Maintenance

Learning Outcome: Analyze the cognitive, emotional, body-image, and spiritual development and characteristics of the aged person, their interrelationship, and your role in promoting health and a positive self-concept.

Chapter 17

Question 1: The parent of a preschool child asks the school nurse how to explain to the child about the impending death of an elderly grandparent. What should the nurse understand about a preschool child's perceptions of death?

Correct answer: Death is perceived as a temporary state.

Rationale: Death is perceived as a temporary state. Preschool children often believe that the deceased person is away, asleep, or in other ways temporarily separated and will return.

Death is perceived as final. This realization does not occur until the child is older, age 9 or 10 years. *Death is perceived as inevitable.* This realization does not occur until the child is older, age 9 or 10 years. *Death can be avoided by certain behaviors.* This is typical of the young school-age child in the 5- to 9-year-old age group.

Cognitive Level: Application

Client Need: Health Promotion and Maintenance

Nursing Process: Assessment

Learning Outcome: Contrast the child's, adolescent's, and adult's concept of death.

Question 2: While reviewing documentation in an elderly home care client's chart, the nurse notes that the individual has a terminal condition. The client's children have asked that the client not be told of the diagnosis or its grave prognosis. While planning for a meeting with the client's family, the nurse should be primarily concerned that:

Correct answer: The family will not be able to engage in rituals of life review with the client.

Rationale: The family will not be able to engage in rituals of life review with the client. The lack of planning, life review, and rituals are concerns when in a state of closed awareness.

The children's wishes are honored regarding care of the client. Although this is a concern, the nurse should be aware that closed awareness has implications for all involved. *The client will find out the diagnosis by accident.* The client is more likely to become increasingly aware of the gravity of the situation based on the behaviors and cues of those in his or her environment. *The nurse has an obligation to the client and should ignore the family's wishes.* The nurse should try to bring the family to an increased understanding of the implications of their decision.

Cognitive Level: Analysis

Client Need: Health Promotion and Maintenance

Nursing Process: Evaluation

Learning Outcome: Discuss the stages of awareness and related behavior as the person adapts to the crisis of approaching death.

Question 3: The nurse is caring for a client with cancer who has a prognosis of 3 months to live. The spouse is concerned because the client recently purchased airline tickets for a vacation that is scheduled 8 months from now. The nurse explains to the spouse that the client is probably experiencing which stage of awareness?

Correct answer: Denial.

Rationale: Denial is manifested by planning for the future despite a grave prognosis and imminent death, or may be related to spiritual faith.

Anger is manifested by blaming others or lashing out, as a result of moving toward acceptance of the end of life. *Psychological isolation* occurs when the client talks about the prognosis without expression of emotion. *Bargaining* could be or may be manifested by making deals or vowing to "be a better person" if death is delayed.

Cognitive Level: Analysis

Client Need: Health Promotion and Maintenance

Nursing Process: Assessment

Learning Outcome: Discuss the sequence of reactions when the person and family are aware of terminal illness.

Question 4: The children of a man who is at home and dying tell the nurse they feel helpless because their father does not talk to them, watch television, or read. They are unsure of how to interact with him. How should the nurse respond to the family?

Correct answer: Educate the family about the process of withdrawing at the end of life.

Rationale: Educate the family about the process of withdrawing at the end of life. Although difficult to accept, this is a normal response of a person to impending death. Family members should be assured that their presence is comforting, even if the client is not interactive.

Review the client's medications for any that may be influencing his ability to interact with family. The client near death is naturally withdrawing. Medication side effects generally are not the issue. The family should be encouraged to be silently engaged with the loved one. *Request a psychiatric evaluation to rule out depression.* This is a normal end-of-life response and does not require psychiatric evaluation or intervention. *Encourage the children to only visit for short periods of time.* Family members should be assured that their presence is comforting, even if the client is not interactive.

Cognitive Level: Application

Client Need: Health Promotion and Maintenance

Nursing Process: Assessment

Learning Outcome: Intervene appropriately to meet needs of family members of the dying person.

Glossary of Key Terms

Acceptance Final stage of Kubler-Ross's theory about the stages of dying, in which the person has worked through previous reactions and views death with a degree of quiet contemplation.

Activity Theory The theory that maintenance of physical, mental, and social activity is necessary for successful aging.

Addiction Physical and psychological dependence on a substance for continued function that can involve larger amounts to get the same effect.

Adolescence Period of youth that begins with puberty and continues until the person is physically and psychologically mature, ready to assume adult responsibilities and be self-sufficient.

Adult stem cells Cells that exist in the bone marrow, blood, skin, and other organs. The precursors of new cells in the body.

Affectional functions Functions of the family that meet emotional needs and promote adaptation and adjustment.

Ageism Any attitude, action, or institutional structure that discriminates against individuals on the basis of age, or infers that elderly people are inferior to those who are younger.

Aging A process that begins at conception and ends at death, a process of growing older, regardless of chronologic age.

Agnostic A person who lives by ethical standards, considering him- or herself incapable of knowing whether God exists.

Allostatic Load Model A model that explains the effects of stress on body homeostasis or equilibrium. Integrates the body's response to cortisol secretion and subsequent pathology and integrates other factors that combine to affect the person on a biochemical and cellular level.

Alpha group A group of world religions that includes Christianity, Judaism, and Islam. All adhere to a biblical revelation of a supernatural, monotheistic God.

Alternative medicines/therapies Nontraditional, alternative, or nonmedical approaches that are considered holistic or integrative to promote health, prevent and treat illness, and treat disease.

Anal stage A major developmental accomplishment that relates to the child gaining self-control of basic functions, according to Freud.

Anger A reaction to nearing death, according to Kubler-Ross's theory, that occurs with acknowledgment of its reality. As denial and isolation decrease, feelings of anger, envy, and resentment of the living are felt.

Animistic Endowment of all things with the qualities of life that Westerners reserve for human beings.

Anniversary reaction Feelings of grief and sadness about a year after the death of the loved one, or response at the person's birth date or at one of the major holidays.

Anthropomorphism A mental process in which the child relates God to human beings who are known.

Anxiety Response of tension or dread as the primary motivation for behavior.

Apgar tool Scoring method used to determine the physical status of the newborn, and to measure the newborn's successful transition into extrauterine life.

Assisted living A residential and social care model for people who have physical limitations that necessitate help beyond the home health care model.

Assisted suicide Making a means of suicide available to the patient with the knowledge of the person's intended use of the equipment, medication, object, or weapon.

Atheist A person who lives by ethical standards, believing that God does not exist.

Attachment A close, reciprocal relationship between two people that involves contact with and proximity to one another and that endures over time.

Automatization A process by which thoughts and actions repeated in sequence become automatic or routine, and thereby require less neuron effort.

Autonomy The ability to gain self-control of behavior. Consequence of maturity gained in the toddler era, according to Erikson.

Baby Boomer The largest generation in U.S. history—76 to 80 million middle-agers, who were born between 1945 and 1962. They grew up with unparalleled affluence, opportunity for education, and social mobility—all of which fostered individual path seeking.

Bargaining When the person tries to enter into some kind of agreement that may postpone death and hopes to be granted a special wish or an extension of life, according to Kubler-Ross.

Basal energy expenditure The minimum caloric requirement to sustain life or fuel the involuntary or metabolic life processes in a person in a resting state, after a 12-hour fast.

Basal metabolic rate The body's consumption of oxygen and calories required to fill the involuntary activities of the body at rest after a 12-hour fast.

Basic trust Confidence, optimism, acceptance of and reliance on self and others, belief that others can satisfy needs; sense of hope or belief in the attainability of wishes in spite of problems and without overestimation of results, according to Erikson.

Behavior Overt response to stimuli.

Behavioral Theory A theory that explains behavior by discussing the developing person and behavior using a physical-biological basis and focusing on an identifiable activity, which promotes learning.

Beta group The group of major world religions that includes Buddhism and Hinduism. These religions have their roots in India, their worldview is pantheistic, and they teach that everything is in the being of God.

Bilateral principle The principle that growth that occurs on one side of the body occurs simultaneously on the other side.

Binding-in The active, intermittent, and cumulative process that defines the maternal-child relationship over a period of 12 to 15 months.

Binge drinking Consuming five or more drinks on the same occasion in the past month.

Biological contaminants Bacteria, molds, mildew, viruses, animal dander, cat saliva, house dust, mites, cockroaches, and pollen; all of which may trigger allergic reactions, some types of asthma, and infectious illnesses.

Biological rhythms Self-sustaining, repetitive, rhythmic patterns found in plants, animals, and humans.

Body art Refers to tattoos, piercings, branding, and pocketing, which are increasingly perceived as an aesthetic addition to the self-concept and body image.

Body image The mental image of one's body and its appearance and functions in relation to others.

Body mass index (BMI) A single number representing the ratio of height to weight, without regard for gender or the risk for health problems associated with weight.

Brain death A definition of death that depends on the discontinuation of electroencephalogram (EEG) activity.

Caregiving The prolonged assistance given to meet the physical and emotional needs of a person with functional limitations or incapacity.

Category A agents The Centers for Disease Control and Prevention classification for biological agents that have the greatest potential for adverse impact with mass casualties, and include disease organisms for smallpox, anthrax, plague, botulism, tularemia, Ebola hemorrhagic fever, and Lassa fever.

Category B agents The Centers for Disease Control and Prevention classification for biological agents that have the potential for large-scale dissemination with resultant illness. These have lower mortality potential and include Q fever, brucellosis, ricin toxin, *Salmonella*, and *Shigella dysenteriae*.

Category C agents The Centers for Disease Control and Prevention classification for biological agents that are not believed to present a high bioterrorism risk but could emerge as future threats. Examples are yellow fever and multidrug-resistant tuberculosis.

Centenarian A person who is 100 years of age or older.

Cephalocaudal principle The principle that the upper end of the organism develops earlier and with greater rapidity than the lower end of the organism. Increases in neuromuscular size and maturation of function begin in the head and proceed to hands and feet.

Child abuse A pattern of abnormal interactions and attacks between a parent and child or another person and child over a period that results in nonaccidental injuries to the child physically, emotionally, sexually, or from neglect.

Child maltreatment A broad term including all intentional harm or avoidable endangerment of anyone under 18 years of age. Includes all forms of child abuse and neglect, abandonment, and failure to thrive caused by nonorganic or psychosocial causes.

Chum A special friend of the same sex and age. This is an important relationship because it is the child's first attachment outside the family, when someone else becomes as important as self.

Climacteric The period in life when physiologic changes occur, with the cessation of the female's reproductive ability and the period of lessening sexual activity in the male.

Closed awareness A reaction that occurs when the person is dying but has neither been informed nor made the discovery of approaching death.

Cognitive functions Functions of the family that involve the parent generation educating through internal instruction and by serving as models.

Cognitive style The characteristic way in which information is organized and problems are solved.

Cognitive Theory A theory concerned with how people acquire, interpret, and use information to solve life's problems.

Collaboration Deriving satisfaction from group accomplishment rather than personal success.

Coma A persistent vegetative state in which the person, not assistive devices, maintains basic vital homeostatic functions, even though he or she is not responding verbally or nonverbally.

Complementary medicines/therapies See *Alternative medicines/therapies.*

Complicated grief response Unresolved grief associated with the past. May be manifested in complaints, grief, or withdrawal from others.

Conceptual tempo The manner in which children evaluate and act on a problem. Tempo may be either impulsive, reflective, or analytic.

Concrete Operations Stage Systematic reasoning about tangible or familiar situations with the ability to use logical thought to analyze relationships and structure the environment into meaningful categories.

Continuity Theory The theory that patterns of behavior and personality are the result of a lifetime of experiences and continue into aging. Personality traits remain stable, and early personality function is a guide for the retirement years.

Contraction Stage The life stage for a couple that extends through midlife and the elder years and occurs when children leave home.

Coordination of Secondary Schemata The stage from 8 to 12 months, when the baby's behavior shows clear acts of intelligence and experimentation and the baby uses certain activities to attain basic goals and realizes that someone other than self can cause activity.

Coregulation A relationship in which parents and the child share power. Parents monitor and guide while the child exercises moment-to-moment self-regulation.

Co-sleep An arrangement in which the baby sleeps in the bed with the parents.

Crisis Any temporary situation that threatens the person's self-concept, necessitates reorganization of psychological structure and behavior, causes a sudden alteration in the person's expectation of self, and cannot be handled with the person's usual coping mechanisms.

Critical periods Periods in human development when specific organs and other aspects of a person's physical and psychosocial growth undergo marked rapid change and the capacity to adapt to stressors is underdeveloped. This imbalance increases susceptibility to adverse environmental factors.

Crystallized intelligence Knowledge and cognitive ability maintained over the lifetime; it is dependent on sociocultural influences, life experiences, and broad education, and involves the ability to perceive relationships, engage in formal operations, and understand the intellectual and cultural heritage.

Cult Any group that forms around a person who claims he or she has a special mission or knowledge, which will be shared by those who turn over their decision making to the self-appointed leader.

Cultural competence Behaviors, practices, attitudes, and policies related to embracing cultural differences that health care providers use to function effectively. Adaptations are made that reflect cultural diversity, holistic care, and unique cultural needs.

Cultural relativity Behavior that is appropriate or right in one culture may not be perceived as appropriate in another culture.

Culture The sum total of the learned ways of doing, feeling, and thinking, past and present, of a social group within a given period or place. These ways are transmitted from one generation to the next or to immigrants who become members of the society.

Culture shock Feelings of bewilderment, confusion, disorganization, frustration, stupidity, and the inability to adapt to differences in language and word meaning, activities, time, and customs that are part of the new culture.

Culture-bound illness or syndrome Disorders that are restricted to a particular culture because of certain psychosocial characteristics or because of cultural reactions to the malfunctioning biological or psychological processes.

Cyberdating Dating and establishing relationships over the Internet.

Day care A licensed, structured program that provides daily care for children away from home, throughout the year, for compensation.

Death Irreversible cessation of circulatory and respiratory functions, or irreversible cessation of all functions of the brain, including the brain stem.

Delayed grief response No anticipatory grieving and no expression of grief at death or loss. Later, there may be manifestations of not having grieved the loss.

Denial Failure to recognize an unacceptable impulse, thought, fact, behavior, or situation, or the consequences or implications.

Despair The second stage of separation anxiety in the young child; a quiet stage characterized by hopelessness, moaning, sadness, less activity, and regression to earlier behavior. According to Erikson, consequence of not achieving ego integrity in psychosocial development in old age.

Development Patterned, orderly, lifelong changes in structure, thought, feelings, or behavior that evolve as a result of maturation of physical and mental capacity, experiences, and learning. Results in a new level of maturity and integration.

Developmental processes The physiologic characteristics, environmental forces, culture, and psychological mechanisms that are involved in development.

Developmental task A responsibility that arises at a certain time in the course of development, successful achievement of which leads to satisfaction and success with later tasks. Failure leads to unhappiness, disapproval by society, and difficulty with later developmental tasks and functions.

Developmental Theory A theory that defines the family as a series of complex interacting positions with prescribed roles for each position in each life stage.

Dialectical behavior therapy Counseling therapy that integrates cognitive, behavioral, and psychodynamic or insight-oriented principles.

Dialectical thinking Seeking intellectual stimulation and even crisis, welcoming contradictions and opposing viewpoints, creating a new order, and discovering what is missing.

Dialectical thought Builds on post-formal thought and involves the ability to consider a thesis and its antithesis, and arrive at a synthesis.

Differentiation A developmental principle that emphasizes a progressive separation of feeling, thinking, and acting and an increased polarity between self and others.

Direct food additives Additives to food for a specific purpose, such as salt, herbs, sugar, and spices, which have been added to food for centuries to preserve it and improve flavor.

Discipline Guidance that helps the child learn to understand and care for self and to get along with others.

Disease prevention Behavior motivated by a desire to avoid disease, detect it early, or maintain functioning within the constraints of illness or disability.

Disengagement Stage See *Contraction Stage.*

Diverse society A society in which members of various ethnic, racial, religious, and social groups maintain distinct lifestyles and adhere to certain values within the confines of a larger culture or civilization.

Domestic violence A pattern of assaultive and coercive behaviors that the person uses against current or former intimate partners, those living together, married, or divorced. Abuse is intentional behavior to establish power and control over another through fear and intimidation.

Doubt Feelings of fear, uncertainty, mistrust, lack of self-confidence, and that one is controlled by others rather than being in control of self. Consequence of not establishing autonomy in toddler era, according to Erikson.

Drug dependence A physical need or psychological desire for continuous or repeated use of a drug.

Dysfunctional grief response Reaction that occurs when the person had a very dependent or ambivalent relationship with the deceased, or the circumstances surrounding death were uncertain, sudden, or overwhelming, such as homicide, or the loss was socially unspeakable or socially negated.

Ecological Systems Theory A theory that describes personal development and behavior influenced by a broad range of situations, interactions, and contextual levels.

Ecology A science that studies the community and the total setting in which life and behavior occur.

Educational function See *Cognitive function*.

Ego integrity The culmination of all previous psychosocial phases of the life cycle, according to Erikson. The person accepts life as his or her own, would wish for none other, and would defend the meaning and dignity of the lifestyle.

Egocentric Things and events are seen from a personal and narrow perspective, and are believed to be because of self.

Elderspeak A speech style that infantilizes the elderly and is insensitive to the unique characteristics and competence of the person.

Embryonic stage The stage of in utero development that lasts from the 2nd to 8th weeks, and is the time of rapid growth and differentiation of major body systems and organs.

Embryonic stem cell A cell in the developing microscopic embryo that is capable of becoming any type of cell in the human body.

Emic approach An approach that examines cultures based on the adaptiveness of behavior within the group's own perspective or frame of reference, often by living with the cultural group.

Emotional abuse Excessively aggressive or unreasonable behavior toward a person, deliberate attempts to destroy self-esteem or competence, placing unreasonable demands to perform above the person's capacities, verbally attacking or constantly belittling or teasing, or withdrawing love, support, or guidance.

Emotional intelligence The ability to understand and regulate personal feelings and respond empathically and effectively to the feelings of others.

Emotional regulation Effectively managing arousal responses, such as alertness or activity, to adapt and reach a goal.

Engagement Hypothesis The belief that people with high intellectual ability in early life, who have a favorable education and environmental support, engage in a lifestyle with complex demands and thereby promote or retain cognitive, occupational, and social skills.

Entrainment Models of Timing Models that embody the view that the rate and rhythm of everyday events, such as the sleep-wake cycle, engage people on a moment-to-moment basis through attentional synchrony.

Epigenetic Theory Erikson's theory of development based on the principle of the unfolding embryo; anything that grows has a ground plan and each part has its time of special ascendancy until all parts have arisen to form a functional whole. A result of mastering the developmental tasks of each stage is a virtue, a feeling of competence or direction.

Establishment Stage The initial family stage in which the couple establishes their own identity and home.

Ethnocentrism Behavior based on the belief that one's own group and behavior is superior.

Etic approach An approach that examines cultures from the outside with a cross-cultural or comparative perspective. The researcher is not a member of the group.

Euthanasia The act or practice of painlessly putting to death a person suffering from incurable or distressing disease.

Evil eye A negative condition or disease that is believed to result when a person looks or speaks admiringly at the child of another. Symptoms include headaches, fever, crying, diarrhea, vomiting, weight loss, insomnia, and sunken eyes.

Existentialism A theory that emphasizes the person's uniqueness and existence in a hostile or indifferent world and within the context of history. Emphasizes freedom of choice, responsibility, satisfaction of ideals, the burden of freedom, discovery of inner self, and consequences of action.

Expectant Stage The developmental crisis of pregnancy; many domestic and social adjustments must be made during this stage.

Expressive functions Functions of the family that involve nonverbal and verbal communication patterns, problem-solving roles, control aspects, beliefs, alliances, and coalitions.

Extremely low-birth-weight infant A baby weighing less than 1,000 grams (a little over 2 pounds) at birth.

Failure to thrive Term used to describe infants who are unable to obtain or use calories and other nutrients required for growth. Weight and height are often below the 5th percentile for the child's age.

Family A small social system and primary reference group made up of two or more persons living together who are related by blood, marriage, or adoption or who are living together by agreement.

Family cultural pattern The ways of living and thinking that constitute the intimate aspects of family group life.

Family roles Patterns of behavior assigned to each member, based on status or ability, that fulfill family functions and needs.

Family social system Each person and family that interacts with other systems in the community. Development and function are greatly affected by the interdependence and interrelationships of each component and by all other surrounding systems.

Family structure The legal construction of a family and how its members are genetically and socially connected.

Family Systems Theory A theory of the family as a societal unit composed of interdependent and interacting members. A person is seen as a member of a system and subsystem, but the family is seen as a whole unit, greater than the sum of its parts.

Female health issues Issues of prevention, diagnosis, and management of female health concerns, more prevalent and manifested differently than in males.

Fetal alcohol syndrome The diagnosis when alcohol ingestion by the pregnant female causes deformities in the child.

Fetal Stage The stage that begins at 8 weeks' gestation and continues until birth. Characterized by rapid growth and changes in body form caused by the different rates of growth in different parts of the body.

Fluid intelligence The ability to perceive complex relationships, use short-term or rote memory, create concepts, and reason abstractly. This ability is independent of instruction, social or environmental influences, or acculturation; is dependent on genetic endowment; and is less apparent in the elder.

Folklore Strong cultural beliefs that influence basic aspects of life.

Foodborne illness Disease caused by consuming contaminated foods or beverages.

Formal Operations Stage The most advanced cognitive ability, according to Piaget's theory, characterized by complex cognitive strategies, scientific problem solving, and ability to engage in abstract thinking processes.

Fossil fuels Fuels formed from the fossilized remains of prehistoric plants and animals that drew carbon from the atmosphere.

Functional age A person's ability to function in the physical and social environment, in comparison with others of the same chronologic age.

Gamma group A category of major world religions, including Taoism, Confucianism, and Shintoism, in which people believe either that everything is in the being of God or that there is no personal God.

Gang A group whose membership is earned on the basis of skilled performance of some activity. Its stability is expressed through formal symbols, such as passwords or uniforms.

Gateway drugs Drugs such as alcohol, tobacco, and marijuana, which are easily accessed, popular, and may lead to use of more addictive substances, including cocaine and heroin.

Gender identity The sense of self as male, female, bisexual, homosexual, or ambivalent about sexuality.

Gender roles The behaviors, interests, attitudes, skills, personality traits, and societal roles that are considered appropriate for males or females.

General Adaptation Syndrome According to Selye, describes the physiologic adaptive response to stress, the everyday wear and tear on the person. Includes the alarm, resistance, and general exhaustion stages.

General Systems Theory A theory that presents a comprehensive, holistic, and interdisciplinary study of any aspect of life. Nothing is determined by a single cause or explained by a single factor.

Generation gap The distance between adolescent and adult generations in values, behaviors, and knowledge, marked by a mutual lack of understanding.

Generational stake The tendency to interpret interactions from the view of the respective generation.

Generativity A concern about providing for others that is equal to the concern of providing for the self. A sense of parenthood and creativity; of being involved in establishing and guiding the next generation for the welfare of humankind, typical of middle age, according to Erikson.

Genogram A diagram of family members, their characteristics, and their interrelationships.

Genomics Study of the functions and interactions of all the genes in the genome, including interaction of genes with each other, the environment, and disease.

Germinal Stage The first stage of in utero development, lasting 10 days to 2 weeks after fertilization and characterized by rapid cell division, subsequent increasing complexity of the organism, and implantation in the wall of the uterus.

Gifted child A child with an above average intellectual status (IQ 130 or higher) and a superior talent for or aptitude in a specific area.

Glucocorticoid Cascade Hypothesis The hypothesis that genetic predisposition or exposure to stressful events at a young age disturbs the hypothalamic-pituitary-adrenal (HPA) axis, causing high serum cortisol levels. Eventually the whole body responds to damaged cells in the hippocampus and hypothalamus, which contribute to long-term physical and psychological effects.

Greenhouse gases Gases that contribute to air pollution and illness. Include water vapor, carbon dioxide, methane, nitrous oxide, and ozone, which occur naturally in the atmosphere, and fluorocarbons, which result from human activity.

Growth An increase in body size or change in structure, function, or cell complexity.

Guided participation A form of structured learning that takes place through the intellectual interaction between adults and children, to bridge the gaps between the child's and adult's understanding.

Guilt A sense of defeatism, anger, undue responsibility, and feeling bad, shameful, or deserving of punishment. Consequence of not achieving initiative in the preschool years, according to Erikson.

Hazardous waste Waste that is potentially harmful or dangerous to human health or the environment.

HAZMAT event A situation in which harmful materials are released into the environment.

Health A state of well-being in which the person uses adaptive responses physically, mentally, emotionally, spiritually, and socially, in response to external and internal stimuli or stressors, to maintain relative stability and comfort and to achieve personal objectives.

Health disparities Differences in incidence, prevalence, mortality, and burden of disease and other adverse conditions that exist among specific population groups.

Health promotion Behavior and strategies motivated by the person's desire to increase well-being and health potential.

Helping relationship See *Therapeutic relationship.*

Historical time A series of economic, political, and social events that directly shape the life course of the person.

Hoarding An adaptive behavior of collecting and retaining objects and animals, not for immediate use. Usually regarded as a disagreeable and unsafe characteristic of the elderly or a sign of illness or dementia.

Holistic nursing Nursing practice that examines the relationships among the biological, psychological, sociocultural, and spiritual dimensions of the person and considers the person as an integrated whole interacting with internal and external environments.

Home schooling A form of education in which parents who believe that the public school system is inadequate to teach their children choose to teach at home according to a designated curricular plan.

Hot and Cold Theory of Disease A cultural classification that divides diseases and substances into "hot" or "cold" and attempts to keep the body in balance between the two through use or avoidance of substances or behaviors.

Human sexual response The four phases of excitement, plateau, orgasm, and resolution, which involve the physiologic reactions of vasocongestion and myotonia, as well as psychological components and psychosocial influences.

Humanism A theory that emphasizes self-actualization, satisfaction of needs, the pleasure of freedom, and realization of innate goodness and creativity.

Identity diffusion The outcome that results if the adolescent fails to achieve a sense of identity. The youth feels self-conscious and has doubts and confusion about self as a human being and his or her roles in life, according to Erikson.

Identity formation A stable, unified sense of self that results through synthesis of biopsychosocial characteristics from a number of sources: parents, friends, social class, ethnicity, religion, membership in other groups, and personal experiences, according to Erikson.

Identity moratorium A period of development during which no decisions are made, values and goals are rethought, and the person has begun to examine life's meaning and goals, according to Erikson.

Immigrants People with an international origin who choose to come to a specific location with the intention of taking up permanent residence and citizenship, reunification with family, and employment.

Indirect food additives Agents that become part of food in trace amounts due to packaging, storing, or handling. Used to maintain freshness, prevent spoilage, and improve nutritional value, taste, texture, and appearance.

Indoor air quality The quality of air in an indoor or office environment.

Industry The schoolchild's feeling that he or she can learn and solve problems, the formation of responsible work habits and attitudes, and the mastery of age-appropriate tasks, according to Erikson.

Infant The child during the first 12 months of life.

Inferiority Feelings of inadequacy, defeat, or being unable to learn or do tasks, compete, compromise, or cooperate, regardless of actual competence. A consequence of failure to achieve the task of industry during the school years, according to Erikson.

Initiative Enjoyment of the energy associated with action, assertiveness, learning, increasing dependability, and ability to plan. First seen in the preschool child, according to Erikson.

Instrumental functions Functions of the family that include how routine activities of daily living are handled.

Intellectual plasticity The variance in a person's performance or ability, depending on social, environmental, and physical conditions.

Interactional Theory A theory that defines family members as interacting personalities with little relation to outside influences. Interactions among members have multiple meanings, and study is focused on interacting roles, problem solving, decision making, and teaching effective communication methods.

Interactionist Theory The theory that language develops through interaction between heredity, maturation, encounters with people and environmental stimuli, and life experiences.

Intimacy The young adult reaching out and using the self to form a commitment to an intense, lasting relationship with another person or even a cause, an institution, or creative effort. In an intimate experience there is mutual trust, sharing of feelings, and responsibility to and collaboration with each other, according to Erikson.

Intuitive phase A phase lasting from approximately 4 to 7 years of age, during which the child gains increasing ability to develop concepts, according to Piaget.

Isolation The inability to be intimate, spontaneous, or close with another, thus becoming withdrawn, lonely, conceited, and behaving in a stereotyped manner. A consequence of the adult's inability to achieve intimacy, according to Erikson.

Kangaroo care The practice of holding the neonate so that his or her skin is next to the skin of the mother's chest and abdomen to promote attachment.

Kindergarten A half- or whole-day educational program for the 5-year-old child that may be either an extension of a nursery school or a part of the elementary school system.

Kohlberg's Theory of Moral Development A theory that moral reasoning and behavior develop from childhood through adulthood. Each moral stage is dependent on the reason for the behavior and shows an organized thought system and a focus on universal values.

Kwashiorkor A severe protein or other nutrient deficiency in childhood.

Language acquisition device A hypothesized inborn device that programs children's brains to analyze language and figure out the rules as people speak to them.

Latchkey child A child who lets him- or herself into the home after school because the parents are still at work, and therefore may not see the parents from early morning until late afternoon or evening.

Late childhood A schoolchild from 8 to 12 years of age.

Later maturity The last major segment of the life span. Begins at the age of 65, 70, or 75.

Late-young adulthood A stage of life lasting from the late 30s through the late 40s, or even to 50 years of age.

Learning Theory See *Behavioral Theory.*

Leisure Freedom from obligations and formal duties of work with the opportunity to pursue, at one's own pace, mental nourishment, enlivenment, pleasure, and relief from fatigue of work.

Life-Span Model of Cognitive Development A proposed model in which different abilities are required in different life stages.

Low-birth-weight infant An infant that weighs less than 5.5 pounds or 2,500 g regardless of gestational age at time of birth.

Lower economic level A socioeconomic group of people who are vulnerable, poor, discriminated against, marginalized, or disenfranchised. They experience relatively more illness, premature death, and lower quality of life. Misfortunes are related to lack of resources and increased exposure to risk.

Mal ojo See *Evil eye.*

Male health issues Issues of prevention, diagnosis, and management of health concerns that are unique to males, more prevalent and manifested differently than in females.

Maltreatment Any deliberate pattern of abuse or attack by a parent or an adult on a child's developmental status, sense of self, or social competence.

Man-made disaster A disaster such as war, pollution, nuclear explosions, fires, hazardous materials exposures, explosions, and transportation accidents.

MANopause A 5- to 12-year period during which midlife males go through hormonal fluctuations and physical and psychological changes.

Marasmus A syndrome of protein and calorie deficiency due to physical and emotional deprivation, often seen in failure-to-thrive children.

Marital capital Emotional, social, and financial benefits of marriage.

Maturation An unfolding of the innate growth process, one aspect of development.

Maturational view A view that emphasizes the emergence of patterns of development of organic systems, physical structures, and motor capabilities under the influence of genetic and maturational forces.

Maturity Being holistically developed as a person.

Mendelian Law of Inheritance A law stating that a dominant gene for a trait or characteristic in at least one parent will cause an average of 50% of the children to inherit the trait. If both parents have the dominant gene, 75% of their children will inherit the trait.

Menopause The permanent cessation of menstruation preceded by a gradually decreasing menstrual flow.

Menstrual or reproductive cycle A duration, usually of 28 days, controlled by the intricate feedback system involving the hypothalamus and level of sexual hormones in the bloodstream, which regulates menstruation or onset of pregnancy.

Mentor An adult with experience, wisdom, patience, and understanding who befriends, guides, and counsels a less experienced and younger adult in the workplace or in a social or an educational situation.

Middle age The stage that covers the years of approximately 45 or 50 to 65 and even 70 or 75. Each person also determines the physiologic age, condition of the body, and psychological age—how old he or she acts and feels.

Middle childhood A schoolchild from 6 to 8 years of age.

Middle-middle economic group The socioeconomic group of people who live a comfortable lifestyle and may purchase material comforts considered in the past to be for the upper class. They are well educated and ambitious about the health of themselves and their children.

Midlife crisis A major turning point in one's life, involving changes in commitments to career or spouse and children and accompanied by significant and ongoing emotional turmoil for both the individual and others.

Migrant family A family with children under the age of compulsory school attendance that moves from one geographic region to another for the purpose of working in agricultural production and harvest.

Mild cognitive impairment (MCI) Temporary memory problems or forgetfulness that occurs in people the longer they live. These "senior moments"—repeated questions or forgetfulness for recent events or names—present little difficulty with managing daily affairs.

Mind-body relationship The effect of emotional responses to stress on body functions and the emotional reactions to body conditions.

Mistrust A sense of not feeling satisfied emotionally or physically, an inability to believe in or rely on others or self, due to failure to develop trust in infancy, according to Erikson.

Morality of cooperation The stage at which a child begins to understand the social and moral implications of acts.

Municipal water pollution The contamination of a water source by wastewater from homes and commercial establishments.

Mutual pretense The process that occurs when staff and family become aware that the client knows he or she is dying, but all continue to pretend otherwise. There is no conversation about impending death unless the client initiates.

Myelination The process of encasing the axons with a myelin or fat cell coating of insulation. Begins prenatally and continues after birth and in early childhood. Enables the child to support most movement and increasing physical activity.

Natural childbirth method A method that teaches voluntary or learned physical responses to the sensations of uterine contractions, which reduce fear and pain responses and enhance delivery.

Natural disaster An ecologic disruption or threat that exceeds the adjustment capacity of the affected community or populations, such as earthquakes, volcanoes, hurricanes, floods, and fires.

Near-death experience The phenomenon of "coming back to life" after just being declared clinically dead or near dead.

Nearing-death awareness An extraordinary awareness of how death will unfold and what the person will need to die well. This awareness is often communicated symbolically or in obscure messages by people who are dying slowly.

Neglect The failure to provide a child with basic necessities of life (food, shelter, clothing, hygiene, or medical care), adequate mothering, or emotional, moral, or social care.

Neonate Refers to the first 30 days or 4 weeks of life.

Neo-Paganism A current movement in American spirituality that revives pre-Christian forms of spirituality as an antidote to the perceived rigidity of Christianity and its perceived disregard for the natural environment.

Neuronal plasticity The ability to change neuron structure and function throughout life, governed by an interplay of experience and developmental stages or sensitive periods when neuronal networks are being formed.

Neurotheology A new field of research that examines the biological basis of spirituality.

New Age A current American spirituality movement in which belief is pantheistic and does not dwell on sin or evil. All humans are considered all good, and God is in everything.

Newborn See *Neonate*.

Object permanence The infant's realization that objects and people continue to exist even when out of sight.

Object Relations Theory A theory that the process of separation-individuation takes place during the first 36 months, during which a sense of separateness from the parenting figure is finally established.

Old-old personality Distinct characteristics of a person who is 80 or 85 years of age and older, which reveals adaptability to the demands of life.

Open awareness When the person and family are fully aware of the terminal condition, although neither may realize the nearness, nor all the complications of the condition, nor the mode of death.

Operant conditioning An overt behavioral response that is externally caused and is controlled primarily by its consequences. The environmental stimuli determine how a person alters behavior and responds to people or objects in the environment. Feelings or emotions are not the cause of behavior; they result from the behavior.

Organ reserve The high capacity each organ has for responding to unusually stressful events or conditions that require intense or prolonged effort.

Out-of-body experience A feeling that one's consciousness or center of awareness is at a different location than one's body, often reported in relation to being resuscitated.

Ozone A gas that occurs in the upper atmosphere and at ground level. A thin layer of ozone surrounds the earth and blocks much of the sun's ultraviolet radiation from reaching the earth's surface.

Parasomnias Conditions in which sleep is disrupted by inappropriate activation, either in the brain centers that control body movements or in the autonomic nervous system that governs physiologic and emotional functions.

Parataxic mode The toddler's and preschooler's inability to understand wholeness of experience and cause-and-effect relationships. He or she experiences parts of things in the present; they are not necessarily events connected with past and future.

Parenthood Stage The developmental stage that begins at the birth or adoption of a child. The couple assumes a lifetime status of parents as they become caretakers of a younger generation.

Parish nursing A modern movement in which churches employ nurses in an effort to implement holistic health practices for members of the faith community.

Pathologic grief response An intensification of grief to the point that the person is overwhelmed, demonstrates prolonged maladaptive behavior, manifests excessive symptoms and extensive interruptions in healing, and does not progress to integration of the loss, finding meaning in the loss, or resolution of the mourning process.

Peer aggression Harmful behavior that is deliberately, persistently directed against a victim who is weak, vulnerable, or defenseless.

Peer group dialect A language typical of adolescents that consists of coined terminology and new or extended interpretations attached to traditional terms.

Perceptually bound The inability to reason logically about concepts that are discrepant from visual cues, typical of the young child.

Perimenopausal years A time of gradual diminution of ovarian function and a gradual change in endocrine status from before the menopause through one year after the menopause.

Pesticides Toxic, semivolatile organic compounds used to kill or control pests such as bacteria, fungi, insects, and rodents. Contribute to soil and water pollution.

Physical fitness A combination of strength, endurance, flexibility, balance, speed, agility, and power that reflects ability to work for a sustained period with vigor and pleasure, without undue fatigue, and with energy left for enjoying hobbies and recreational activities.

Physical functions Functions of the family that are met by the parents' providing food, clothing, shelter, protection against danger, provision for body repairs after fatigue or illness, and reproduction.

Physically abusive acts Behavior that is intended to hurt another, such as biting, punching, kicking, beating, burning, shaking, cutting, or physical restraint.

Pica Eating or craving nonfood substances.

Pluralistic society See *Diverse society.*

Polygenic inheritance The combination or interaction of many genes acting together to produce a behavioral characteristic.

Polypharmacy Taking excess and unneeded combinations of drugs that may cause drug interactions, toxicity, confusion, or depression.

Positive self-concept Positive feelings about self, based on positive reactions from others. The person likes self; accepts physical characteristics, abilities, values, and self-ideals; has a positive idea of self in relation to others; and accepts others.

Post-formal thought See *Problem-finding stage.*

Postindustrial society A society in which there are few universal criteria or moral standards to guide or stabilize a culture but also an emphasis on conformity or normalization.

Post-materialistic society A society in which people are generally spiritually oriented but reject mainstream religious beliefs. People are interested in personal development and relationships.

Postmodern society See *Postindustrial society.*

Postponement of death The point at which death seems inevitable but the person holds onto life unexpectedly, by way of overt or covert decisions.

Poverty Having inadequate money to purchase a minimum amount of goods and services. Reflects class and racial stratification and contributes to homelessness and health problems.

Preadolescence Developmental stage that usually begins at 9 or 10 years of age and is marked by a new capacity to be loving, when the satisfaction and security of another person of the same sex (a chum) is as important to the child as personal satisfaction and security.

Precausal thinking Confusing physical and mechanical causation or natural phenomena with psychological, moral, or sequential causes, typical in the young child.

Preconceptual Phase The phase from 2 to 4 years of age, when the child gathers facts as they are encountered but can neither separate reality from fantasy nor classify or define events in a systematic manner.

Premature birth Birth at a gestational age of 37 weeks or earlier, regardless of birth weight.

Premonition of death The phenomenon in which the person, although lacking any signs of illness, emotional conflict, suicidal tendencies, severe depression, or panic, correctly anticipates personal death.

Preoperational Stage Stage of cognitive development from 2 to 7 years old when thought is more symbolic, memory continues to form, and the child internalizes mental pictures of people, the environment, and ideas about rules and relationships, according to Piaget.

Preparatory depression The point at which the person realizes the inevitability of death, needs a time of preparatory grief, and comes to desire the release from suffering that death can bring.

Prepared childbirth method See *Natural childbirth method.*

Preschool years The years from ages 3 to 5, when the child is emerging as a social being, participating more fully as a family member, and spending more time with peers.

Preterm birth See *Premature birth.*

Primary Circular Reaction Cognitive development from 1 to 4 months. The infant's response patterns develop when a stimulus creates a response and gratifying behavior is repeated, according to Piaget.

Primary identification The stage at which the toddler begins to adapt to culture by imitating the parents and responding to their encouragement and discouragement.

Primary prevention Activities that prevent or decrease the probability of occurrence of an injury, physical or mental illness, or health-threatening situation in an individual or family, or an event or illness in the population, by combating harmful forces and by strengthening the capacity of people to withstand these forces.

Principle of asynchronous growth Developmental shifts at successive periods in which parts of the body increase length at different rates.

Principle of differential exposure The principle that the person's inherited characteristics cause differing reactions from people, which in turn affect or shape the personality of the individual.

Principle of differential susceptibility The principle that individual differences in heredity exist that make people susceptible to the influence of certain environments. Given different experiences, a person with certain hereditary potential could develop in different ways.

Principle of differentiation The principle that development in the fetus and child proceeds from simple to complex, from homogeneous to heterogeneous, and from general to specific in structure, function, and behavior.

Principle of discontinuity of growth rate The principle that rate of growth of various structures and organs changes at different periods during the life span. The whole body does not grow as a total unit simultaneously.

Principle of readiness The principle that an ability to perform a task or engage in behavior depends on maturation of neurologic structures and on maturation of the muscular and skeletal systems.

Problem-finding stage A stage beyond problem solving, characterized by creative thought in the form of discovered problems; relativistic thinking; the raising of general questions from ill-defined problems; use of intuition, insight, and hunches; and the development of significant scientific thought.

Prosocial behavior Voluntary activity intended to benefit another.

Protest In the young child, the first stage of separation, which lasts a few hours or days. The need for the mother is conscious, persistent, and grief laden. The child cries continually, tries to find her, is terrified, fears he or she has been deserted, feels helpless and angry that mother left, and clings to her on her return.

Proximodistal principle Principle that growth progresses from the central axis of the body outward to the periphery or extremities.

Psychological abuse Intentional behaviors, activities, or words that intimidate, threaten, humiliate, shame, or degrade the person.

Psychological isolation Occurs when the person talks about the event, illness, death, or mortality intellectually but without emotion as if these topics were not relevant.

Psychological processes The person's perceptions of self, others, and the environment.

Psychologically extended family A family in which people who are not biologically related consider themselves as siblings or "adopted" parent, child, aunt, uncle, or grandparent.

Psychoneuroimmunology A science that focuses on the links between the mind or mental processes, the physiologic brain, and the immune system.

Psychophysiologic See *Psychosomatic*.

Psychosocial development Development that results from the combination of intellectual, emotional, and social components.

Psychosomatic Physical, organic symptoms or diseases that are the result of emotional responses or thoughts.

Puberty The state of physical development between 10 and 14 years for females, and 12 and 16 years for males, when sexual reproduction first becomes possible with the onset of menstruation or spermatogenesis.

Radon An invisible, odorless, radioactive gas produced by the natural decay of uranium in soil and rocks that moves up through the ground and can be harmful at elevated levels.

Reaction range A range of potential expressions of a trait (for example, weight) that are influenced by environmental conditions as opposed to genes.

Reflex An involuntary, unlearned response elicited by certain stimuli.

Reflex Stage First developmental stage, which covers the neonatal period when behavior is entirely reflexive, according to Piaget.

Regional culture A local, regional, or sectional variant of the national culture—for example, rural or urban, or Southern or Midwestern.

Relabeled perspective Shifting the way an adult child strives to be a "good child": not feeling great affection from but showing concern for the well-being of the parent and giving care to the limits of one's ability.

Religion A belief in a supernatural or divine force that has power over the universe and commands worship and obedience. A personal and institutional system of beliefs and a set of practices that are followed. Related to but not synonymous with spirituality.

Religious culture A culture that is shaped by a religion which constitutes a way of believing, living, and behaving, and therefore influences the person.

Reminiscence Informal sharing of past memories and the feelings related to the memories.

Reproductive cycle See *Menstrual or reproductive cycle*.

Resilience The ability to maintain a healthy personality and effective behavioral outcomes in spite of serious threats to adaptation or development.

Resolution See *Acceptance*.

Rites of passage Specific age-related ceremonies or community responsibilities that mark the passage from one life stage to another.

Ritualistic abuse Systematic and repetitive sexual, physical, and psychological abuse of children by adults engaged in group secret activity or cult worship.

Role Theory The theory that each person has ascribed or assumed behavior that contributes to social position, group interaction, and family norms. A person can experience role reciprocity (mutual exchange), role complementarity (differentiation), or role strain (conflict or overload).

Sandwich generation The middle-aged generation that is in the middle in many ways, taking care of parents, children, and grandchildren, and balancing work and caregiving.

Secondary Circular Reaction The stage from 4 to 8 months when a baby learns to initiate and recognize new experiences and repeat pleasurable ones; this leads to intentional behavior.

Secondary identification The preschool child's internalization of attitudes, feelings, values, and actions of the same-gender parent related to sexual, moral, social, and occupational roles and behavior.

Secondary prevention Screening, early diagnosis, and prompt treatment of the existing health problem, disease, or harmful situation, thereby shortening duration and severity of consequences, preventing disability or complications, and enabling the person to return to maximum potential health or normal function as quickly as possible.

Secondhand smoke Inhalation of smoke that people who smoke cigarettes or cigars have exhaled into the air.

Secular growth trend The trend that puberty and physical maturation are occurring at an earlier age.

Self-absorption Regression to younger behavior and focus on self during middle age, passivity, insecurity about life events, and withdrawal from others and responsibilties, according to Erikson.

Self-concept The composite feelings about self and body image, adaptive and defensive mechanisms, reactions from others, and one's own perceptions.

Self-despair The feeling when ego integrity is not achieved that life has been too short and futile. The person wants another chance to redo life, according to Erikson.

Self-disgust See *Self-despair*.

Sensorimotor Period, Internal Representation of Action of the External World The period in which the toddler uses less trial-and-error thinking but uses memory of past experience and imitation to act as if he or she arrived at an answer, according to Piaget.

Sensorimotor Period, Tertiary Circular Reaction The period in which the infant consolidates previous activities involving body actions into experiments to discover new properties of objects and events and to achieve new goals instead of applying habitual behavior, according to Piaget.

Separation anxiety An increased sense of anxiety that occurs when the 7- to 8-month-old baby is separated from the attachment figure.

Set point The body weight that is maintained when no effort is made to gain or lose, the weight that is considered most comfortable by the person.

Set Point Theory of Weight Control The theory that when weight falls below the innate body "ideal," metabolic rate is adjusted downward to conserve fat stores. When caloric intake in-

creases, some people are able to burn the extra calories. Others do not, depending on the compensatory increase in nonexercise energy expenditure.

Sex hormones Biochemical agents that influence the structure and function of the sex organs and appearance of specific sexual characteristics.

Sex steroids Estrogen, progesterone, testosterone, and other androgens released from the gonads.

Sexual abuse Employment, persuasion, inducement, enticement, or coercion of any person to engage in any sexually explicit conduct or stimulation. Rape, statutory rape, molestation, prostitution or other forms of sexual exploitations, or incest are included in the definition.

Sexual harassment Troubling behavior from another toward the self as a sexual object.

Sexual molestation Exploitation of the child for the adult's sexual gratification, including rape, incest, exhibitionism to the child, or fondling of the child's genitals.

Sexual response cycle The four phases of excitement, plateau, orgasm, and resolution, which involve the physiologic reactions of vasocongestion and myotonia, as well as psychological components and psychosocial influences.

Sexuality Sum total of one's feelings as a male or female, the expression of which goes beyond genital response.

Sexuality education Learning about the self as a sexual being.

Sexually transmitted diseases Infections grouped together because they spread by transfer of infectious organisms from person to person during sexual contact, through sexual intercourse, oral sex, or anal sex.

Shame The feeling of being fooled, embarrassed, exposed, small, impotent, dirty, wanting to hide, and rage against self, which develops when autonomy is not achieved, according to Erikson.

Shared sleep See *Co-sleep*.

Sleep deprivation A chronic lack of the required amount of sleep or less than 6 hours of sleep for three or more nights.

Small for gestational age A birth weight of less than the 10th percentile in the intrauterine growth curve, a result of slow intrauterine growth.

Social functions Functions of the modern family that include providing social togetherness, fostering self-esteem and a personal identity tied to family identity, providing opportunities for observing and learning social and sexual roles, accepting responsibility for behavior, and supporting individual creativity and initiative.

Social Learning Theory Bandura's theory that learning occurs without reinforcement, conditioning, or trial-and-error behavior because people can imitate or follow another's behavior, and can think and anticipate consequences of behavior and act accordingly.

Social mobility The process of offspring moving away from the social position, educational level, economic class, occupation, or geographic area of parents, causing offspring overtly to forsake parental teaching and seek new models of behavior.

Social time Social expectations of behavior for each age era.

Socialization The process by which the child is transformed into a member of a particular society and learns the values, standards, habits, skills, and roles appropriate to sex, social class, and ethnic group or subculture to become a responsible, productive member of society.

Socioeconomic level A cultural grouping of persons who have a consciousness of socioeconomic cohesion that affects value formation, attitudes, lifestyle, and health.

Soil pollution Contamination of soil by various substances or agents.

Sound pollution Unwanted or offensive sounds that unreasonably intrude into daily activity. The loudness of sound is measured in units called decibels.

Speech awareness Awareness that is developed in utero, as the fetus hears a melody of language, equivalent to overhearing two people talk through the walls of a motel room. Creates a sensitivity that after birth provides the child with clues about sounds that accompany each other.

Spiritual dimension A quality that goes beyond religious affiliation, that strives for inspiration, reverence, awe, meaning, guidance, and purpose even in those who do not believe in any god. Permeates all of life and integrates values and beliefs.

Spiritual distress The impaired ability to integrate meaning and purpose in life. The person experiences a disturbance in the belief system that is usually a source of strength.

Spiritual functions Functions of the family that involve raising the child to be a moral person with a belief system of some kind.

Spiritual need A lack of any factor necessary to establish or maintain a dynamic, personal relationship with God, or a higher being, as defined by the individual.

Stage of Leaving Home A primary developmental stage of young adulthood which involves independence and separation between children and their parents.

Stepfamily A family that is formed when a divorced, single, or widowed parent with children marries.

Stepgeneration family A family in which grandparents raise their grandchildren or great-grandchildren because the parents are unable or choose not to raise their children.

Stress A physical and emotional state always present in the person, influenced by various environmental, psychological, and social factors, according to Selye. Manifestations of stress are both overt and covert, initially protective, maintaining equilibrium to the extent possible.

Stress overload A feeling of pressure or tension, difficulty in functioning as usual, problems with decision making, feelings of anger and impatience; physical symptoms may occur.

Stress reactions Physiologic and psychological changes, including the alarm, resistance, and exhaustion stages, that may result in illness, unusual or disturbed adaptive behavior patterns, or depression or other negative feelings.

Structural-Functional Theory A theory that defines the family as a system influenced by external forces. Each person is studied in relation to his or her roles within the social system.

Subculture A group of persons within a larger culture who have an identity of their own but are related to the total culture in certain ways.

Superego The part of the psyche that is critical to the self and enforces moral standards, which forms as a result of identification with parents and an introjection of their standards and values.

Suspicious awareness The suspicions of a dying person who is not told of prognosis or approaching death, who may or may not voice suspicions to others, and who is likely to deny verbal suspicions. The person watches more closely for signs to confirm suspicions.

Syncretic speech An early stage of speech in which one word represents an entire sentence.

Syntaxic mode of communication A mode in which the child learns to validate word meanings by talking with the chum and others, typical of preadolesence.

Telegraphic speech A stage of speech in which two- to four-word expressions contain a noun and verb and maintain word order, typical of the toddler stage.

Telehealth practice Electronically transmitted clinician consultation and treatment prescriptions to a client.

Temperament A behavioral style; a characteristic way of thinking, behaving, or reacting in a given situation, first seen in infancy.

Teratogen An agent or substance that causes cell death, malformation, growth retardation, or functional decline in utero or in childhood.

Teratogenesis Development of abnormal structures in uetero. Teratogenesis is time-specific; the stimulus is nonspecific.

Tertiary prevention Restoring the person to optimum function or maintenance of life skills through long-term treatment and rehabilitation and within the constraints of an irreversible problem, thereby preventing progression of sequelae, complications, or deterioration.

Theory of Multiple Intelligences Howard Gardner's theory of factors that reflect the influence of culture and society on intellectual ability. The person may demonstrate more than one of the various cognitive skills or intellectual apptitude.

Therapeutic relationship A purposeful interaction over time between an authority in health care and a person, family, or group, that focuses on client needs, conveys empathy, and utilizes knowledge to achieve healthcare goals.

Toddler stage The stage that begins when the child takes the first steps alone at 12 to 15 months, and continues until approximately 3 years of age.

Transcultural nursing The humanistic and scientific study and comparative analysis of different cultures and subcultures throughout the world in relation to differences and similarities in caring, health, illness, beliefs, values, lifeways, and practices.

Translocation stress syndrome Physical and emotional deterioration as a result of changes or geographic movement.

Transtheoretical Model A model of readiness for change used to help people make lifestyle changes in order to improve health.

Triarchic Theory of Intelligence Sternberg's theory of the three realms of cognition: how thinking occurs, how individuals cope with experiences, and the context of thinking.

Upper-upper economic group The socioeconomic group that comprises the relatively small number of people (about 1%) who has for generations owned a disproportionate share of personal wealth and whose income is largely derived from ownership of investments, business, and property. Their work, profession, or business and family connections provide prestige, status, honor, wealth, and power.

Urban Ecologic Model Person-environment interaction; human behavior and subjective well being are reflected in the social interaction that occurs between the individual and the environment.

Value A learned social principle, goal, or standard held as acceptable or worthy of esteem, which is chosen, affirmed, and demonstrated consistently in various ways.

Vegetarianism Abstinence from consuming animal products.

Voodoo A religious cult practice that dates back to preslavery days in West Africa. A dominant belief is that the person is surrounded by a variety of powerful spirits, good and bad.

Vulnerable children The children closest emotionally to the distressed parent, who are most likely to show signs of distress and later psychiatric disorders.

Vygotsky's Sociocultural Theory The theory that cognitive growth occurs in a sociocultural context and evolves out of the child's social interactions. Knowledge, thought, and language are shaped by the culture, historical time, peers, as well as adults.

Water pollution: point and nonpoint sources The two major origins of man-made water pollution. Point sources discharge pollutants directly into a body of water, such as from an oil spill. Nonpoint sources pollute water indirectly through environmental changes, such as runoff soil from surface-polluted areas or from a fertilized field.

Weapons of mass destruction In the United States, weapons that are categorized as chemical, biological, radiological, nuclear, and explosive (CBRNE) agents.

Widowhood The status change that results from death of the husband or wife, or of a long-term partner. It is a major crisis in any life era, but is more likely to occur first in middle age.

Young-old personality A person of 65 or 70 to 75, 80, or 85 who is flexible, shows characteristics commonly defined as mature, and is less vulnerable to the reality of aging.

Index

Page numbers followed by *f* indicate figures and those followed by *t* indicate tables or boxes.